Color Insert Contents

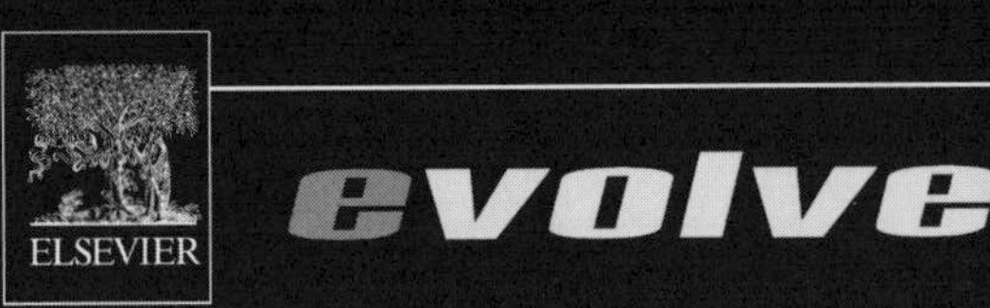

To access your Student Resources, visit the Web address below:

http://evolve.elsevier.com/Lynch/ForensicNursing

Evolve Learning Resources for Lynch: *Forensic Nursing* offers the following features:

- **Key tools and resources for the forensic nurse**
  Important information accessible online for you:
  - Forensic nursing diagnoses
  - Procedures for sexual assault examination in male victims
  - Istanbul Protocol for physical evidence of torture
- **Essential downloadable forms**
  Essential forms for crucial forensic procedures available to you:
  - Body diagrams
  - Evidence collection in sexual assult (adult, child, and suspect)
  - Operative assessment of organ donors
- **Web links**
  A variety of web links organized by book chapter so you can pursue further information and study of key forensic nursing topics

FORENSIC NURSING

FORENSIC NURSING

Virginia A. Lynch, MSN, RN, FAAN, FAAFS
International Consultant in Forensic Nursing Science
Beth-El College of Nursing and Health Sciences
University of Colorado
Colorado Springs, Colorado

with special contributions by
Janet Barber Duval

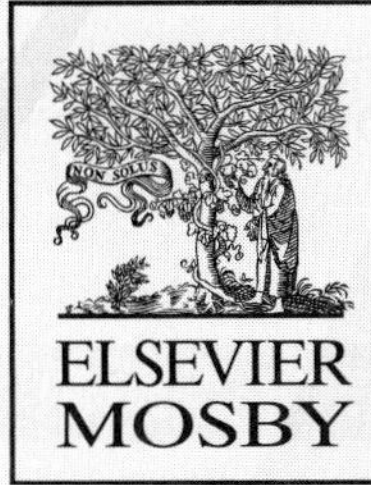
ELSEVIER
MOSBY

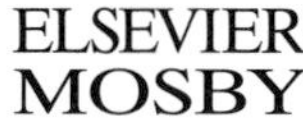

11830 Westline Industrial Drive
St. Louis, MO 63146

FORENSIC NURSING

ISBN-13: 978-0-323-02826-4
ISBN-10: 0-323-02826-8

Executive Publisher: Barbara Nelson Cullen
Senior Developmental Editor: Sophia Oh Gray
Publishing Services Manager: Deborah L. Vogel
Project Manager: Katherine Hinkebein
Senior Designer: Amy Buxton

Printed in the United States of America

Last digit is the print number: 9 8 7 6 5

Dedicated to Janet Barber Duval

Seldom in a lifetime does one have the privilege of sharing an alliance with someone who surpasses the requisite criteria to be a mentor, educator, role model, and friend. Without her extraordinary insight, her exceptional experience, and editorial skills this book would literally not exist.

Contributors

Pamela Assid, MSN, RN, CLNC
General Manager and Founder
IPR Medical Legal Consulting, LLC
Colorado Springs, Colorado
53. *Evidence Collection in the Emergency Department*

Sevil Atasoy, PhD
Director, Professor of Forensic Science
Institute of Forensic Science
Istanbul University
Istanbul
Turkey
56. *Global Perspectives on Forensic Nursing*

John J. Behun
Chief Laboratory Support
Federal Bureau of Investigation Laboratory
Quantico, Virginia
13. *DNA and the CODIS Project*

Patrick E. Besant-Matthews, MD
Forensic Pathology Consultant
Dallas, Texas
19. *Blunt and Sharp Injuries*
20. *Gunshot Injuries*

Ann Wolbert Burgess, DNSc, RN, FAAN
Professor
School of Nursing
Boston College
West Newton, Massachusetts
29. *Stalking Crimes*
30. *Child and Adolescent Sex Rings and Pornography*
36. *Autoerotic Fatalities*

Jacquelyn C. Campbell, PhD, RN, FAAN
Anna D. Wolf Chair
School of Nursing
Johns Hopkins University
Baltimore, Maryland
6. *Violence against Women*

Dora Maria Carbonu, RN, MN, EdD
Hamad Medical Corporation
Emergency Medical Services Department
Doha
Qatar
56. *Global Perspectives on Forensic Nursing*

Victoria Carroll, RN, MSN
Clinical Instructor
University of North Colorado
School of Nursing
Greeley, Colorado
7. *Violence in the Healthcare Workplace*

Cari Caruso, RN, SANE-A
Forensic Nurse Examiner
President and Chief Executive Officer
Forensic Nurse Professionals, Inc.
Pasadena, California
43. *Testifying as a Forensic Nurse*

Susan Chasson, MSN, JD, SANE-A
Lecturer
College of Nursing;
Assistant Lecturer
J. Reuben Clark Law School
Brigham Young University
Provo, Utah
41. *Legal Issues for the Forensic Nurse*

Paul T. Clements, PhD, APRN, BC, DF-IAFN
Assistant Professor
College of Nursing
University of New Mexico
Albuquerque, New Mexico
28. *Bereavement and Sudden Traumatic Death*
31. *Male Victims of Interpersonal Violence*
47. *Suicide Risk Assessment*

Judith W. Coram, RN, MN, FACFE
Forensic Psychiatric Nurse
Spokane, Washington
49. *Psychiatric Forensic Nursing*
50. *Forensic Mental Health Nursing and Critical Incident Stress Management*

Patricia A. Crane, MSN, RNC, NP
Faculty, Graduate Forensic Nursing Program
Duquesne University
Pittsburgh, Pennsylvania
5. *Female Genital Mutilation*

Joseph T. DeRanieri, PhD
Assistant Professor
Thomas Jefferson University
Philadelphia, Pennsylvania
28. *Bereavement and Sudden Traumatic Death*

Theresa G. Di Maio, BSN, RN
Forensic Psychiatric Nurse Consultant
San Antonio, Texas
39. *Sudden Death during Acute Psychotic Episodes*

Pamela J. Dole, EdD, MPH, FNP, ACRN
Nurse Practitioner
Greenwich House
New York, New York
27. *Sequelae of Sexual Violence*
51. *Caring for Offenders: Correctional Nursing*

Janet Barber Duval, MSN, RN, FAAFS
Adjunct Associate Professor
Indiana University School of Nursing
Indianapolis, Indiana;
Clinical Nurse Consultant
Hill Rom Company
Batesville, Indiana
54. *Occupational Health and Safety Issues*

Sheila Early, RN, BScN
Forensic Nurse Consultant, Forensic Nurse Examiner
Surrey Memorial Hospital
Sexual Assault Nurse Examiner Program
Surrey, British Columbia
Canada
56. *Global Perspectives on Forensic Nursing*

Jamie J. Ferrell, BSN, RN, SANE-A, CFN
Forensic Nurse Examiner/Educator
Memorial Hermann Healthcare System
Houston, TX;
Forensic Nursing Consultant
National Forensic Nursing Institute
University of Rochester
Rochester, New York
37. *Postmortem Examination of Sexual Assault Victims*

Lynda Filer, MSc., BSc. (Hons), RGN, PGCEA
Lecturer in Applied Biological Sciences
St. Bartholomew School of Nursing & Midwifery
City University Institute of Health Sciences
London
England
56. *Global Perspectives on Forensic Nursing*

Cris Finn, MS, MA, NP
Affiliate Professor
Regis University
Denver, Colorado;
Principal
Quality Solutions
Monument, Colorado
31. *Male Victims of Interpersonal Violence*

Deborah R. Fulton, RN
Staff Nurse II
Emergency Center
University Hospital
San Antonio, Texas
53. *Evidence Collection in the Emergency Department*

Alice Geissler-Murr, RN, BSN, CRRN, CLNC
Legal Nurse Consultant
Peyton, Colorado
44. *Malpractice and Negligence*
46. *Legal Nurse Consulting*

Mira R. Gökdoğan, PhDFSc, SART/SANE, FNE, RN
Member, Criminal Scene Investigation Unit
Institute of Forensic Science;
Research Assistant, Institute of Forensic Sciences
Istanbul University
Istanbul
Turkey
56. *Global Perspectives on Forensic Nursing*

Bruce A. Goldberger, PhD, DABFT
Director of Toxicology, Clinical Associate Professor
Department of Pathology, Immunology, and Laboratory Medicine
College of Medicine
University of Florida
Gainesville, Florida
14. *Forensic Toxicology*

Gregory S. Golden, DDS, DABFO
Instructor
Loma Linda University
School of Dentistry
Loma Linda, California
16. *Bite Mark Injuries*

Barbara Goll-McGee, MSN, RN
Forensic Nurse Consultant
Canton, Massachusetts
8. *Environmental Terrorism and Mass Disasters*

Gloria C. Henry
Bereavement Specialist
Philadelphia, Pennsylvania
28. *Bereavement and Sudden Traumatic Death*

Belinda Manning Howell, JD, BSN, RN
Registered Nurse
Hospice Austin's Christopher House
Austin, Texas;
Former Nurse Attorney
Mithoff & Jacks, LLP
Austin, Texas
42. *Depositions and Courtroom Testimony*

Kristine M. Karcher, MS-c, RN, D-ABMDI
Adjunct Professor, CSI/Death Investigation,
Southwest Oregon Community College,
Coos Bay, Oregon;
Chief Deputy Medical Examiner,
Coos County Medical Examiner Office,
Coquille, Oregon
48. *Motor Vehicle Collision Reconstruction*

Sarah Kerrigan, BSc, PhD
Independent Forensic Toxicologist Consultant
Houston, Texas
14. *Forensic Toxicology*

Karolina E. Krysinska, PhD
Research Fellow
Australian Institute for Suicide Research and Prevention
Griffith University
Brisbane, Queensland
Australia
47. *Suicide Risk Assessment*

Carll Ladd, PhD
State Police Forensic Science Laboratory
Meriden, Connecticut
12. *Biological Evidence in Criminal Investigations*

Kathleen B. LaSala, PhD, APRN, BC, PNP
Associate Dean and Director of Graduate and Undergraduate Nursing Programs
Beth-El College of Nursing and Health Sciences
University of Colorado
Colorado Springs, Colorado
23. *Child Abuse and Neglect*

Louanne Lawson, PhD, RN, FAAN
Associate Professor
College of Nursing
University of Arkansas
Little Rock, Arkansas
22. *Research with Vulnerable Participants*

Linda E. Ledray, RN, SANE-A, PhD, FAAN
Adjunct Faculty
University of Minnesota;
Director
Sexual Assault Resource Service
Hennepin County Medical Center
Minneapolis, Minnesota
26. *Sexual Assault*

Henry C. Lee, PhD
Chief Emeritus
Connecticut Division of Scientific Services
Meriden, Connecticut;
Professor, Forensic Sciences
University of New Haven
New Haven, Connecticut
12. *Biological Evidence in Criminal Investigations*

Patricia A. Loftus, RN, MSN, MSFS
Former Program Analyst
FBI CODIS Project
Washington, DC
13. *DNA and the CODIS Project*

Virginia A. Lynch, MSN, RN, FAAN
International Consultant in Forensic Nursing Science
Beth-El College of Nursing and Health Sciences
University of Colorado
Colorado Springs, Colorado
1. *The Specialty of Forensic Nursing*
3. *Concepts and Theory of Forensic Nursing*
4. *Human Rights*
6. *Violence against Women*
23. *Child Abuse and Neglect*
33. *The Forensic Investigation of Death*
34. *The Forensic Nurse Examiner in Death Investigation*
37. *Postmortem Examination of Sexual Assault Victims*
55. *Education and Credentialing for Forensic Nurses*
56. *Global Perspectives on Forensic Nursing*
57. *Career Paths for the Forensic Nurse*

Elizabeth McGann, DNSc, RN, CS
Professor and Chair
Department of Nursing
Quinnipiac University
Hamden, Connecticut
25. *Elder Abuse*

John McPhail, PhD, RN
Forensic Nurse Consultant
Pueblo, Colorado
38. *Taphonomy and NecroSearch*

Mary Frances Moorhouse, RN, BSN, CRRN, LNC
Adjunct Faculty
Pikes Peak Community College;
Nurse Consultant
TNT RN Enterprises
Colorado Springs, Colorado
44. *Malpractice and Negligence*
46. *Legal Nurse Consulting*

Barbara A. Moynihan, PhD, APRN, BC
Associate Professor
Master of Science in Nursing Program
Forensic Track Coordinator
Quinnipiac University
Hamden, Connecticut
24. *Domestic Violence*
25. *Elder Abuse*

Steven J. Niezgoda
Forensic Science Systems Unit
Federal Bureau of Investigation
Washington, DC
13. *DNA and the CODIS Project*

Georgia A. Pasqualone, MSFS, MSN, RN, CNS, DABFN
Adjunct Faculty
Fitchburg State College,
Fitchburg, Massachusetts;
Clinical Nurse Specialist/Forensic Nurse Consultant,
Emergency Department Staff Development
Winchester Hospital
Winchester, Massachusetts
18. *Forensic Photography*

Nizam Peerwani, MD
Chief Medical Examiner
Tarrant, Parker, Denton Counties
Fort Worth, Texas
4. *Human Rights*

Robert K. Ressler, BS, MS
Adjunct Assistant Professor
School of Criminal Justice
Michigan State University
East Lansing, Michigan;
Adjunct Assistant Professor of Psychiatry
Department of Psychiatry
Georgetown University Hospital
Washington, DC
35. *Profiling Homicides*

Cynthia Whittig Roach, RN, DNSc
Associate Professor
Beth-El College of Nursing and Health Sciences
University of Colorado
Colorado Springs, Colorado
55. *Education and Credentialing for Forensic Nurses*

Russell R. Rooms, MSN, RN
Assistant Professor of Clinical Nursing
Director, National Forensic Nursing Institute
University of Rochester School of Nursing
Rochester, New York
32. *Approach for Emergency Medical Personnel*

Jane E. Rutty, MSc, BSc (Hons), DPSN, RGN, ILTM
Principal Lecturer
School of Nursing and Midwifery
De Montfort University
Leicester
England
56. *Global Perspectives on Forensic Nursing*

David W. Sadler, MB, ChB, FRCPath, MD
Senior Lecturer
Department of Forensic Medicine
University of Dundee
Dundee
Scotland
55. *Education and Credentialing for Forensic Nurses*

Richard Saferstein, PhD
Instructor
School of Law
Widener University
Wilmington, Delaware
11. *Evidence Collection and Preservation*

Teresa J. Shafer, RN, MSN, CPTC
Executive Vice President and Chief Operating Officer
LifeGift Organ Donation Center
Fort Worth, Texas
21. *Organ Donation*

Paul D. Shapiro, PhD
Assistant Professor of Sociology
Georgia Southwestern State University
Americus, Georgia
32. *Approach for Emergency Medical Personnel*

Laura Slaughter, MD, FACP
Consultant
University of Southern California
Violence Intervention Program
Los Angeles, California;
Consultant
San Luis Obispo County Sexual Assault Response Team (SART)
San Luis Obispo, California
17. *Binocular Microscopy in Sexual Assault Examination*

Catherine C. Smock, RN
Forensic Nurse Consultant
Louisville, Kentucky
15. *Air Bag–Induced Injuries and Deaths*

William S. Smock, MD, FACEP, FAAEM
Director
Clinical Forensic Medicine
Department of Emergency Medicine
University of Louisville
Louisville, Kentucky
2. *Genesis and Development*
15. *Air Bag–Induced Injuries and Deaths*

Z. G. Standing Bear, MSFS, PhD
Associate Professor
Beth-El College of Nursing and Health Sciences
University of Colorado
Colorado Springs, Colorado
10. *Crime Scene Processing*

Deborah Storlie, BSN, RN
Critical Care Nurse
Creighton University Medical Center
Omaha, Nebraska
40. *Mass Graves and Exhumation*

Mary K. Sullivan, MSN, RNC, CARN
Instructor in Forensic Nursing (online program)
University of California
Riverside, California;
Clinical Forensic Nurse Coordinator
Department of Veterans Administration
Phoenix, Arizona
52. *Forensic Nursing in the Hospital Setting*

Cynthia Cupit Swenson, PhD
Associate Professor
Family Services Research Center
Medical University of South Carolina
Charleston, South Carolina
22. *Research with Vulnerable Participants*

Christine Vecchi, MSN, BSc., RN, DABFN
Senior Lecturer in Forensic Nursing
University of Notre Dame, Australia
Fremantle, Western Australia;
Registered Nurse
Emergency Department
Rockingham Kwinana District Hospital;
Nurse Coordinator
Freo StreetDoctor
Fremantle GP Network
Fremantle
Australia
56. *Global Perspectives on Forensic Nursing*

Jane E. Weaver, BSN, RN-FNP, JD
Colonel
US Air Force Reserve
Washington, DC
45. *International Law*

Glenda Wildschut, RN, RPN
Forensic Nurse Consultant
Plumstead
South Africa
56. *Global Perspectives on Forensic Nursing*

M. Fatih Yavuz, MD, PhD
Institute of Legal Medicine and Forensic Science
University of Istanbul
Cerrahpasa
Turkey
56. *Global Perspectives on Forensic Nursing*

Nanako Yoneyama, MSN, RN, PHN
Associate Professor
Akita University
Akita, Akita
Japan
56. *Global Perspectives on Forensic Nursing*

Beatrice Crofts Yorker, RN, MS, JD, FAAN
Director and Professor
School of Nursing
San Francisco State University
San Francisco, California
9. *Nurse-Related Homicides*

Reviewers

Kathleen Brown, RN, NP, PhD
School of Nursing
University of Pennsylvania
Philadelphia, Pennsylvania

Jill Bunnell, RNc, FNE, LNC
The DOVE Program
Summa Health System
Akron, Ohio

John C. Butt, CM, MD, FRCPath, DMJ
Principal
Pathfinder Forum
Vancouver, British Columbia
Canada

Nancy B. Cabelus, MSN, RN, DABRN
Detective
Connecticut State Police, Major Crime Squad
Meriden, Connecticut

Vicki Carroll, RN, MSN
School of Nursing
University of North Colorado
Greeley, Colorado

Mary Pat DeWald, RN, NP, BSN, CCRN, SANE-A
Forensic Nurse Consultant
St. Anthony Central Hospital
Denver, Colorado

Catherine M. Dougherty, MA, RN, FAAFS
Baylor University Medical Center
Waxahachie, Texas

Stacy A. Drake, RN, MSN, FCNS
Harris County Medical Examiner's Office
Houston, Texas

Sonja F. Eddleman, RN, CA/CPSANE, DABRN, SANE-A
Driscoll Children's Hospital
Corpus Christi, Texas

Denise L. Garee, RN, MSN, CEN, CNS, SANE
Henry P. Becton School of Nursing & Allied Health
Farleigh Dickinson University
Teaneck/Hackensack, New Jersey

Amy Grau, RN, MS, SANE-A
Mercy, Unity, United SANE Program
Fridley, Minnesota

Tara Henry, RN, SANE-A
Alaska Regional Hospital
Anchorage, Alaska

Arlene Kent-Wilkinson, RN, MN
Assistant Professor
College of Nursing
University of Saskatchewan
Saskatoon, Saskatchewan
Canada

Thomas W. Kullman Jr.
Chesapeake Police Department
Chesapeake, Virginia

Carl H. Mangum, RN, MSN, PhD(c), CHS
Assistant Professor
Emergency Preparedness Coordinator
School of Nursing
University of Mississippi
Jackson, Mississippi

Jennifer Markowtiz, ND, RNc, WHNP
The DOVE Program, Summa Health System
Akron, Ohio

Linda McCracken, RN
Nurse Clinician
Foothills Medical Centre
Calgary, Alberta
Canada

Stacey Mitchell, MSN, RN, SANE-A, D-ABMDI
Harris County Medical Examiner's Office
Houston, Texas

Melissa M. Prefontaine, RN, MSN, FCNS, SANE
Rivier College
Nashua, New Hampshire

Bonnie B. Price, RN, BSN
Forensic Nurse Examiners
St. Mary's Hospital
Richmond, Virginia

Kelly M. Pyrek
Publisher and Editor-in-Chief
Forensic Nurse Magazine
Phoenix, Arizona

James P. Reed
RockWare Incorporated
Golden, Colorado

Luis A. Sanchez, MD
Chief Medical Examiner
Harris County
Houston, Texas

Valerie Sievers, MSN, RN, CNS, CEN, SANE-A
Colorado Coalition against Sexual Assault
Denver, Colorado;
Memorial Hospital
Colorado Springs, Colorado

Jennifer R. Swinger, BSN, RN, EMT-P, FNE, LNC
Lake Hospital System
West ED
Willoughby, Ohio;
St. Elizabeth Health Center
SANE Program
Youngstown, Ohio

Cindy Teller, RN, BSN, SANE-A
Children's Hospital of the Kings Daughters
Norfolk, Virginia

Lisa B. Valente, RN, BSN
Massachusetts General Hospital Emergency Department
Boston, Massachusetts

Jane E. Weiler, RN, BSN
Forensic Nurse Examiner
Mary Lanning Memorial Hospital
Hastings, Nebraska

Kim Wieczorek, RN, BSN, SANE
Forensic Nurse Examiners
St. Mary's Hospital
Richmond, Virginia

Foreword

The increasing applications of medicine and the forensic sciences to the criminal justice system and civil litigation have made forensic nursing a specialty whose time has come. This first textbook devoted entirely to forensic nursing is as timely as it is necessary.

The role of the healthcare professional in the collection and preservation of evidence from the living and the dead has escalated along with advances in DNA and other forensic sciences. Biological and trace evidence that is properly documented and safeguarded by hospital personnel is vital for the proper functioning of the criminal justice system, so that the guilty are convicted and the innocent are protected.

Today's overburdened and complex healthcare delivery system yields large numbers of iatrogenic injuries caused by the administration of new drugs and other therapies, or by inadequate or misguided medical care. The resultant litigations require review and analysis of medical records by practitioners who can accurately interpret the courses of therapy and the outcomes that may have stemmed from wrongdoings or errors of hospital staff members. When patient injuries or illnesses suggest abuse or neglect, healthcare personnel must be prepared to document findings, conduct evidentiary examinations, and notify law enforcement or appropriate protective agencies. Investigations of claims of sexual abuse, child abuse, elder abuse, police abuse, abuse of prisoners and others in official custody, neglect of vulnerable individuals, and unexpected deaths of hospitalized patients (some who may have been murdered by caregivers, as discussed by Beatrice Crofts Yorker and Mary K. Sullivan in Chapters 9 and 52, respectively) demand the involvement of healthcare personnel who are knowledgeable in the forensic sciences. Forensic nurses are the ideal professionals to interpret and correlate data from clinical records, laboratory results, and autopsy findings. They are able to communicate with stressed physicians and beleaguered police, and are able to challenge the already overwhelmed emergency department and crime laboratory personnel with their findings or suspicions. Nurses can act with passion and compassion, can deal with prosecutors and defense attorneys, and can give comfort and support to the emotionally traumatized victims of crime and their families. In short, the forensic nurse, by training, experience, and interest, is in the ideal position to create liaisons among individuals and diverse groups for the ultimate benefit of the patient and of society.

True to its Latin derivation, the word *forensic* refers to public debate, to the giving of testimony in the public forum. The forensic nurse, like the forensic pathologist, is the advocate for those who have no voice–for the poor, for the disenfranchised, for those who are not receiving adequate medical care, for substance abusers, for the suicidal, and for the victims of interpersonal violence. The forensic nurse must not only speak out for patients and their welfare, but also uphold the principles of objectivity in public inquiry and the application of science and truth, regardless of where they may lead. At times that may require considerable fortitude and personal sacrifice, requiring the "stepping on toes" of hospital or police colleagues, or putting employers or government officials in an uncomfortable limelight.

Virginia Lynch and the 66 contributing authors for this book are among those who have been the pioneers in forensic aspects of healthcare. They represent an awesome international contingent of personnel from medicine, nursing, law enforcement, criminal justice, and other disciplines vital to the success of forensic healthcare. I have been privileged to watch and admire Virginia Lynch for more than 20 years as she has crusaded for forensic nurses to be recognized as able to improve medical care and make unique contributions to the criminal justice system and human rights around the world. I have seen hospitals, medical examiner's offices, and police departments, including Scotland Yard, come forth to embrace this newly defined specialty of forensic nursing.

This forensic nursing textbook will be of great value, not only to nurses, but also to physicians, prosecutors and defense attorneys, judges, emergency department and law enforcement personnel, educators, and all others who endeavor to improve the health and welfare of the victims of violence throughout the world. *Forensic Nursing* is indeed a specialty whose time has come!

–Michael M. Baden, MD

Director, Medicolegal Investigations Unit, New York State Police; former Chief Medical Examiner, New York City; Adjunct Professor (Emeritus), New York Law School; Diplomat and Fellow, The Henry C. Lee Institute of Forensic Sciences, University of New Haven, Connecticut

Preface

Since the advent of forensic nursing, there has been an outcry for a textbook that would serve the growing ranks of experienced and novice nurses who have joined the forensic nursing movement. The long-awaited broad-based and definitive book has arrived. The work represents the thoughts and contributions of 65 leaders within forensic nursing and the forensic sciences that have joined forces to present a truly multidisciplinary view of nursing's most recent discipline.

This combination of talent affords a universal perspective of forensic nursing ranging from basic theory, concepts, and principles to applied practice within a variety of community and clinical environments. This book is more than a basic textbook. It is a series of chapters that carry the reader from novice to expert. It does not stop with "what was and what is"; it looks into the future and considers potential roles and opportunities for the forensic nurse in both healthcare and social justice.

This book is divided into eight units comprising 57 chapters. Each author applies the forensic nursing process to these issues and presents key points, best practices, and case studies, which illuminate core learning about each topic. Unit One, Introduction to Forensic Science in Healthcare, outlines the historical evolution of forensic nursing and presents the foundational concepts and theory.

Unit Two tackles violence as a contemporary social issue that is the *raison d'etre* for the work of the forensic nurse scientist and practitioner. Basic forensic processes and procedures that are essential tools of the forensic nurse investigator or examiner are presented in Unit Three.

Unit Four contains essential content about understanding the mechanics of injury while Unit Five focuses on vitally important, individual issues within forensic nursing. Nursing roles associated with death investigation are highlighted in Unit Six, and Unit Seven helps the forensic nurse appreciate roles and responsibilities within the legal system.

Finally, Unit Eight encompasses various opportunities and challenges in the field of forensic nursing, including global perspectives discussed by a group of international nurse educators and practitioners.

This book also features extensive appendices, a glossary, and a color photo insert. The appendices feature body charts, evidence collection forms, and more. The glossary is a comprehensive alphabetical listing of key terms used within the book and in the field of forensic nursing science. Featured in the color insert is an amazing collection of illustrations provided primarily by Dr. Patrick Besant-Matthews from his archives of forensic medicine and death investigation over 40 years. Other illustrations from Dr. Michael Doberson, Dr. M. G. F. Gilliland, William S. Smock, Kathy Bell, Judith M. Cook, and Teresa M. Roe, as well my own case studies complete an important educational opportunity.

Forensic Nursing offers both a basic text and a living reference. The future of forensic nursing science now lies in the hands of those who read and apply the content of this book, in both clinical forensic practice and death investigation. It is now your responsibility to advance and implement the theory, concepts, skills, and roles that will ensure the victims of crime, the suspects and offenders, the condemned and the executed, as well as the families of each that truth and justice will prevail.

–Virginia A. Lynch

Acknowledgments

The writing and production of this book would have been impossible without the assistance of its 66 contributors who are valued colleagues and friends. With deep regard I acknowledge those who have inspired me and who share my aspirations for the future of forensic nursing. Being a first-time book author can be a tedious process without the expert guidance of someone who has the skills to navigate the world of nursing publishers. For that I thank Alan Sorkowitz, a highly experienced editor who truly realized the potential of forensic nursing in the marketplace.

No single person has contributed more to the success of forensic nursing than Dr. Patrick Besant-Matthews, who mentored me through my first autopsy in 1982 and later opened his teaching files for me when I prepared to give my first lectures. This book would have been incomplete without his illustrations and his exceptional forensic insight.

I wish to pay tribute to Dr. Charles Petty for opening the doors of the Southwestern Institute of Forensic Sciences to me; to Dr. Irving Stone for revealing the mysteries of the crime laboratory; to Dr. M. G. F. Gilliland and her husband, Gary Gilliland, for their sustaining mentorship from the inception of forensic nursing.

To Dr. Nizam Peerwani, my never-ending appreciation for hiring me–the first woman, the first nurse–as a medical investigator in his office. It has been his wisdom, ethics, and dedication to human rights that have challenged me in all I have accomplished.

To Dr. Charles Hirsch, for the 1990 invitation to participate in a homicide investigation fellowship in the New York Office of the Chief Medical Examiner, an opportunity I would have never received in a rural Texas county. Also, for introducing me to Pamela Dole, who mentored me through the Manhattan experience and has remained my close friend.

To the memory of Dr. Samuel Hughes, Graudate Dean, University of Texas at Arlington School of Nursing, who heard my proposal for the first master's degree curricula in forensic nursing science and understood what few could envision at that time. I wish he had lived to see the fulfillment of our mutual vision accepted worldwide. The first among nursing leaders to champion the concept of a forensic nurse examiner was Dr. Ann Wolbert Burgess, who has continued to support and contribute to the progress of forensic nursing. I have also been fortunate to be a protégé of Gwendolyn R. Costello, a long-tenured and dedicated nurse who has devoted much of her career to combating crimes against children.

Dr. William Smock shared my vision of bringing the much-needed and long-overdue field of clinical forensic practice to medicine and nursing in the US. For his conviction and accomplishments, he deserves great accolades.

Dr. George Nichols III foresaw the potential of a forensic specialist in nursing and subsidized the first clinical forensic position in the Office of the Chief Medical Examiner, Commonwealth of Kentucky, for which I am profoundly grateful.

During the early years of forensic nursing, one of my most fortunate acquaintances was Kenneth Pratley, director of forensic medicine at Scotland Yard, who achieved the implementation of the forensic custody nurse through this legendary institution.

Dr. Michael Baden has presented the role of a clinical investigator in the medicolegal management of institutional abuse and death with a zeal that has influenced government healthcare systems and legal agencies of the highest level to implement this position.

Dr. Joseph H. Davis, a forensic legend in his time, embraced my global vision and inspired me to teach in Africa. It has often been his professional influence with others that has given forensic nursing the esteem of a genuine scientific discipline.

Dr. J. F. Els, a true visionary, is recognized as the father of forensic nursing in South Africa. He has stimulated our international movement across developing and war-torn nations. His personal and professional sacrifices are recognized with all my heart.

Dr. C. K. Parikh, a noble name in forensic medicine from Bombay, India, has motivated my desire to take forensic nursing to the subcontinent. He remains one of the most valuable professional associates who have influenced my work both here and in India.

No list of acknowledgments would be complete without Dr. William Maples, who died shortly after his last inspirational presentation at the International Association of Forensic Nurses Annual Scientific Assembly and left an indelible impression on us all.

Another *great* in the annals of forensic nursing whose memory will never be forgotten is Dr. Harry C. McNamara, the first to encourage the inclusion of nurses within the armamentarium of the clinical forensic sciences. I have pursued his mission.

My fellowship among the members of the International Association of Forensic Nurses, the American Academy of Forensic Sciences, and the American Academy of Nursing has provided me with thoughts, opinions, materials, case studies, and motivation. It is the colleagues within these organizations who have helped define what forensic nursing is and what it can be.

No words are adequate to express my gratitude to Dr. Z. G. Standing Bear, my husband and my colleague. He has encouraged me through the years since he heard me present the first scientific paper on forensic nursing at the American Academy of Forensic Sciences meeting in 1986. His first remark was, "Why didn't someone think of this 50 years ago?" He is as much a part of the success of this vision as I.

My family . . . Zac, Kristi, Keri, and Angie, who have given me space and tried to understand when I couldn't be everywhere at once: I hope they realize the significance of what has evolved for the advancement of humanity through nursing.

I cannot sufficiently articulate my appreciation for the assistance of Janet Barber Duval through the trepidations, rejections, and successes of this project. Her skill to manipulate the written word reflects the integrity and ethics of her character. She has critiqued my publications from the beginning of my career and now has helped me bring *Forensic Nursing* to a reality.

–Virginia A. Lynch

Evidentiary Value of Clothing

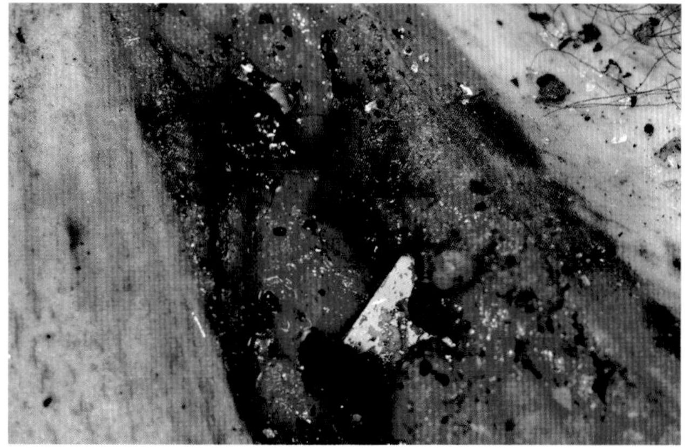

Color Plate 1
Trace evidence related to auto-pedestrian trauma; note blue paint chip.

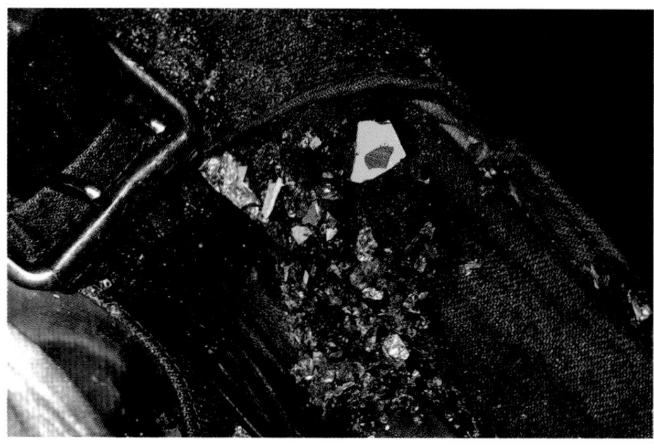

Color Plate 2
Trace evidence in clothing; blue paint chip and broken glass.

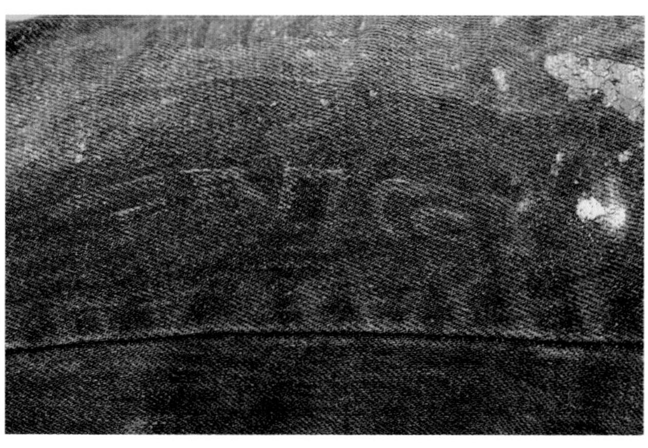

Color Plate 3
Tire imprint on clothing identifying the exact wheel of the vehicle involved.

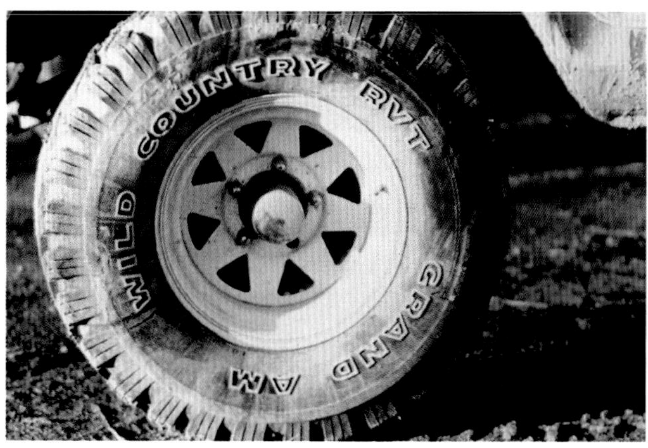

Color Plate 4
Tire matching impact impression on clothing.

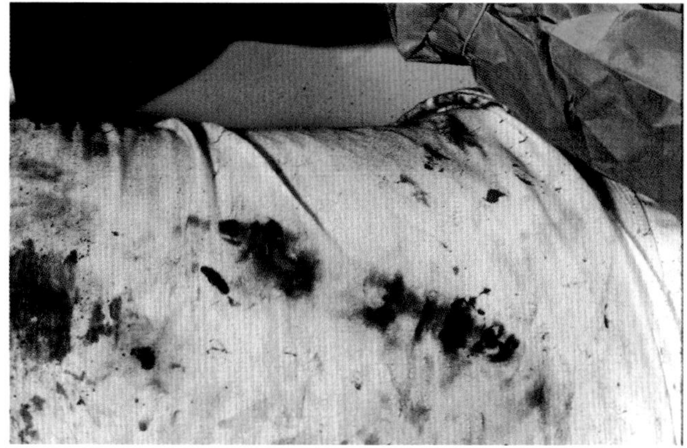

Color Plate 5
Evidence of gun shot residue on clothing reveals grazing gun shot wound.

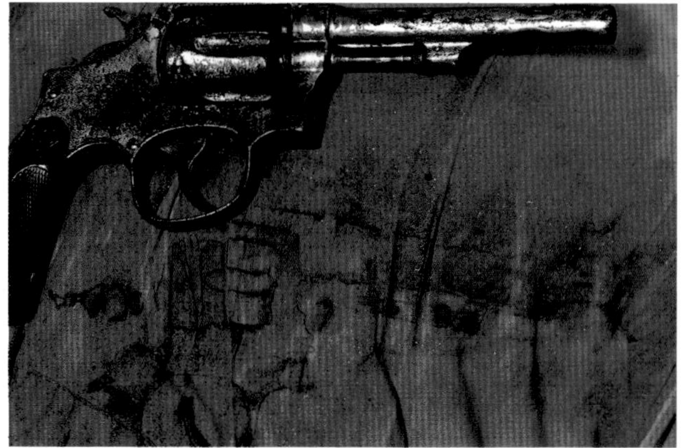

Color Plate 6
Impression of gun revealed on clothing from partially dried blood and rust from weapon.

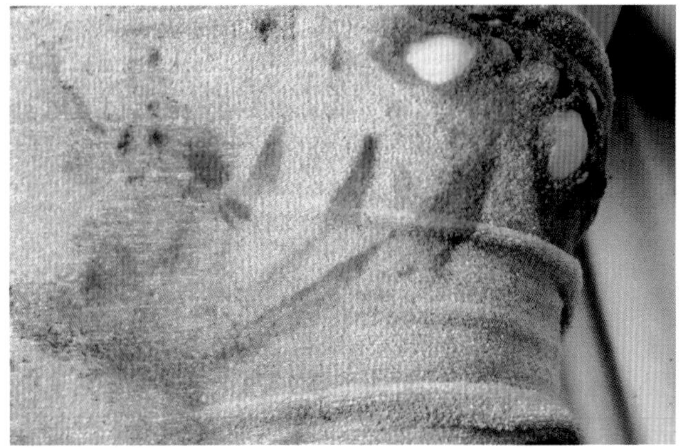

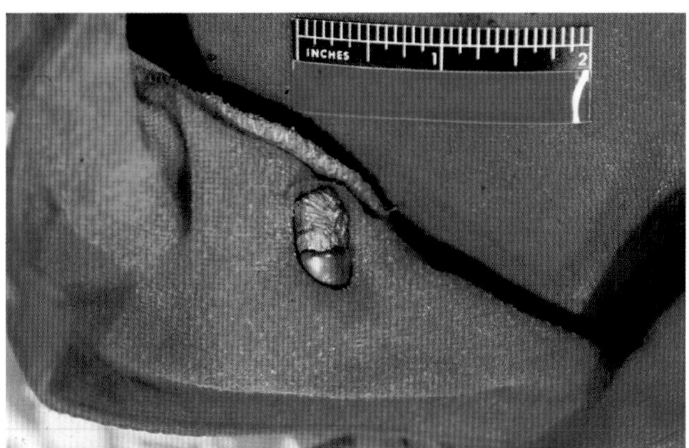

Color Plate 7
Bloody handprint may permit recovery of fingerprints. Note holes in clothing that do not match injury; victim may have been dressed after assault.

Color Plate 8
Bullet found in clothing demonstrates importance of searching clothing for evidence when removing and handling.

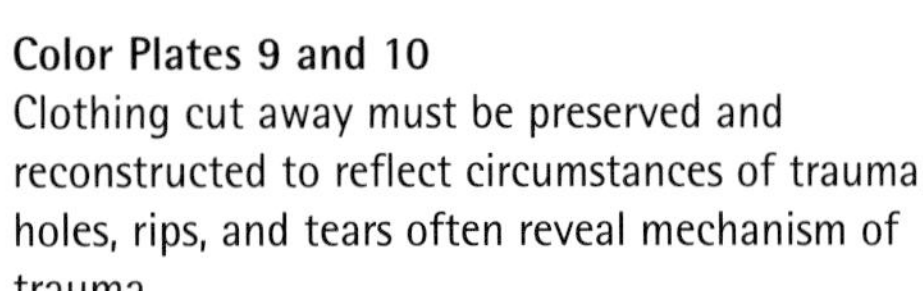

Color Plates 9 and 10
Clothing cut away must be preserved and reconstructed to reflect circumstances of trauma; holes, rips, and tears often reveal mechanism of trauma.

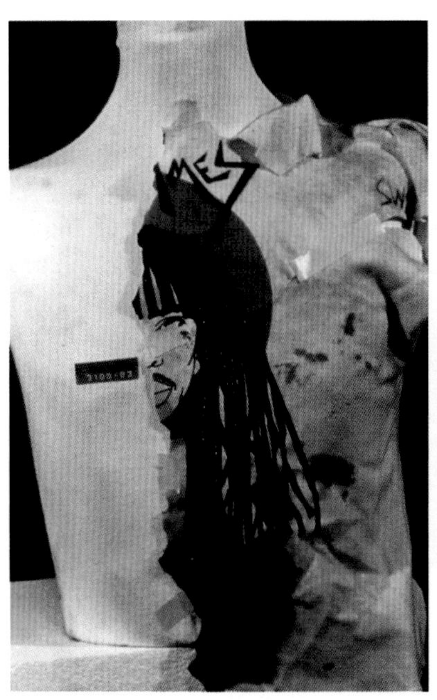

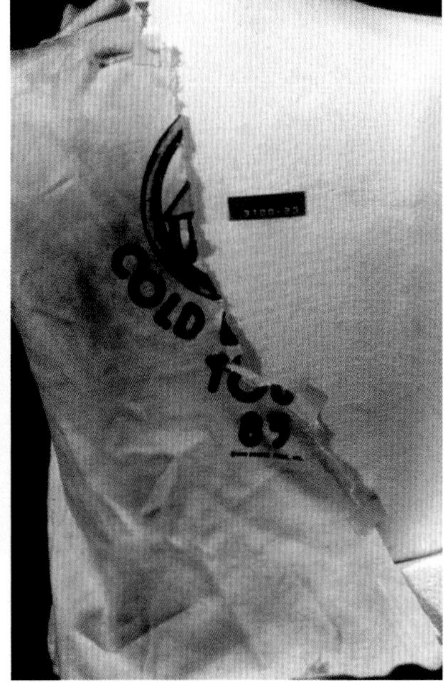

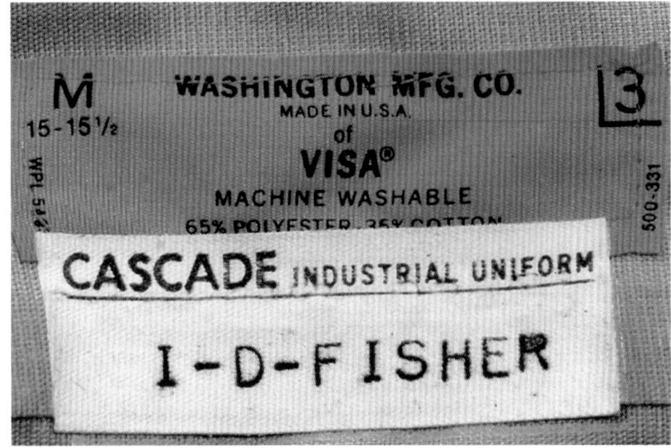

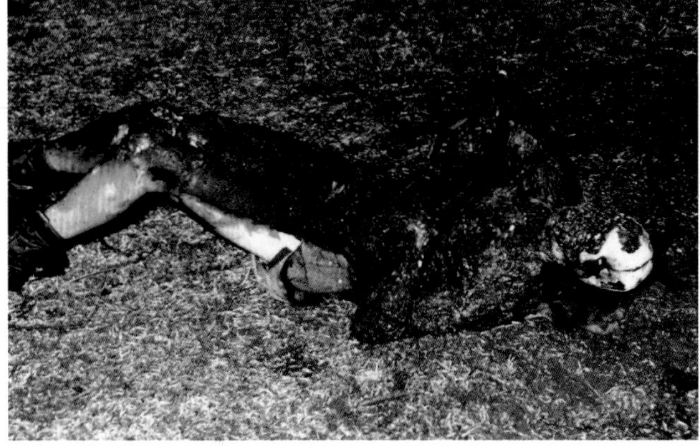

Color Plate 11
Labels of garments may be key to identification of unknown victims.

Color Plate 12
Footwear and clothing are often valuable in identification of badly burned or decomposing bodies.

Blunt and Sharp Injuries

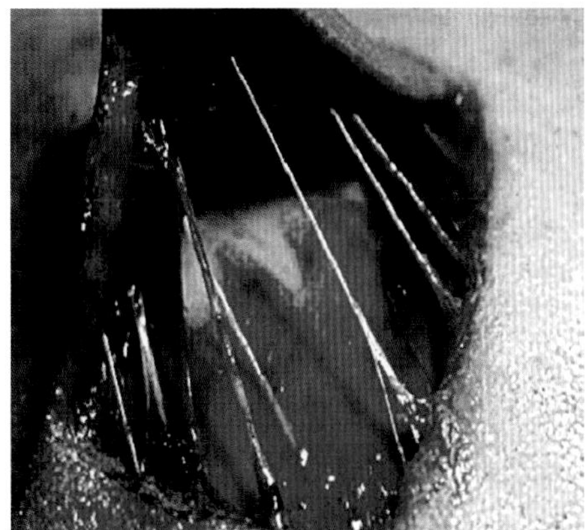

Color Plate 13
Bridging characteristics of blunt force laceration.

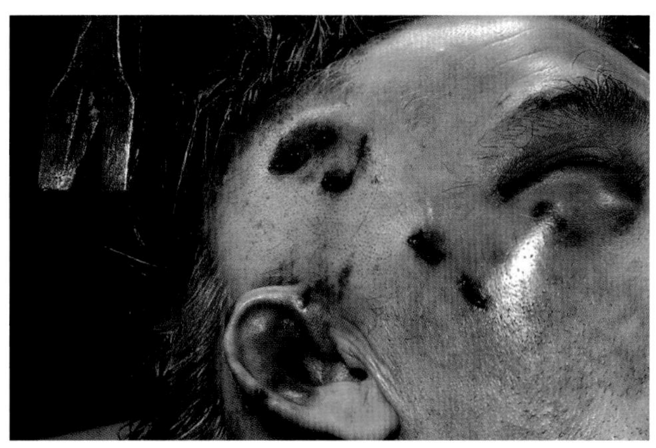

Color Plate 14
Patterned blunt injury from crow bar.

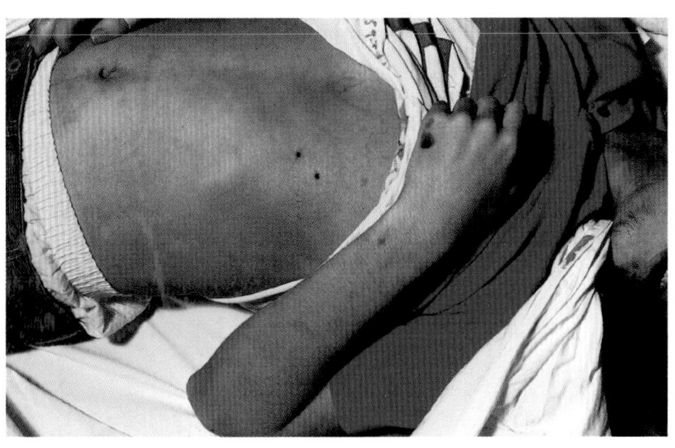

Color Plate 15
Puncture wound to chest; paired injury from carving fork.

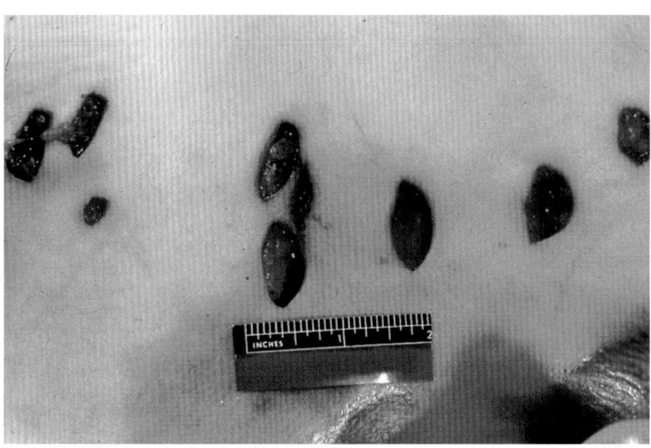

Color Plate 16
Multiple stab wounds to neck with double-edged knife.

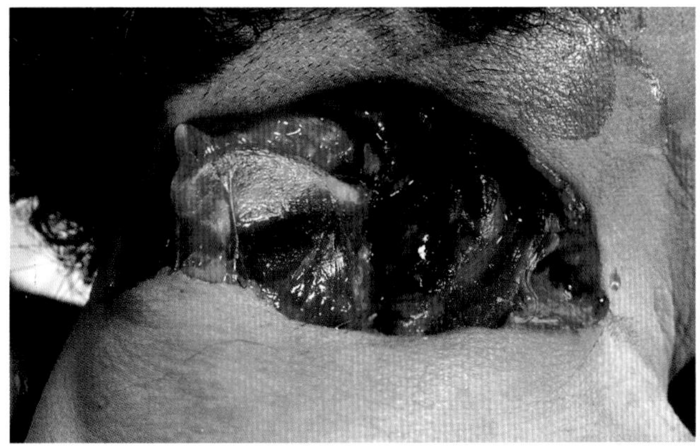

Color Plate 17
Sharp cut wound to posterior neck.

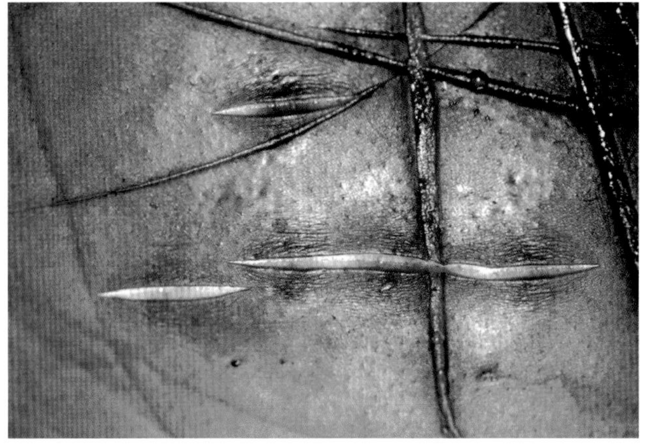

Color Plate 18
Postmortem cut with knife; note lack of bleeding in tissue.

Crime Scene Investigation

Case 1: Suicide on Farm

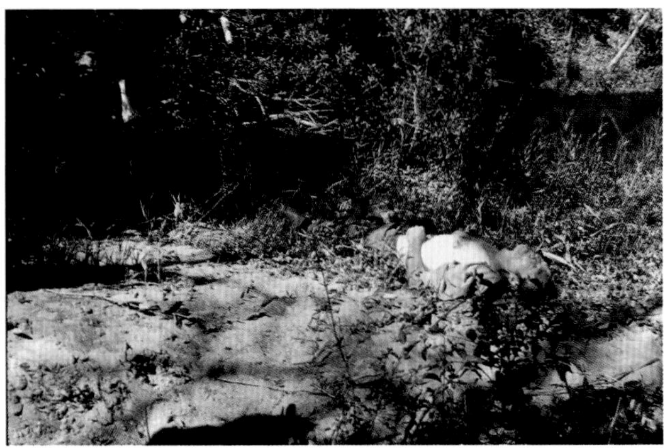

Color Plate 19
Body discovered by creek in rural area, 2 miles from house.

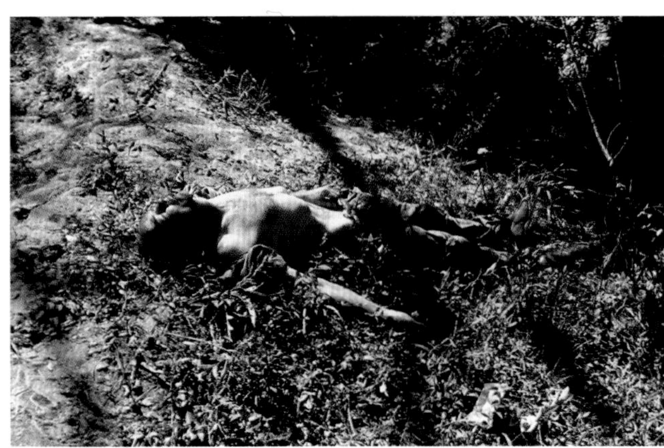

Color Plate 20
Left view of body.

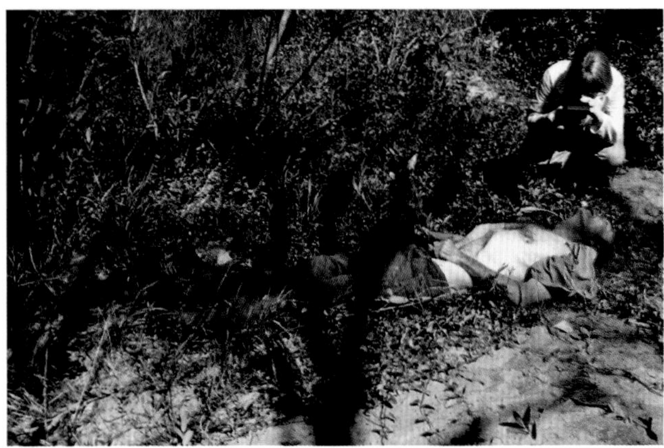

Color Plate 21
Right view of body.

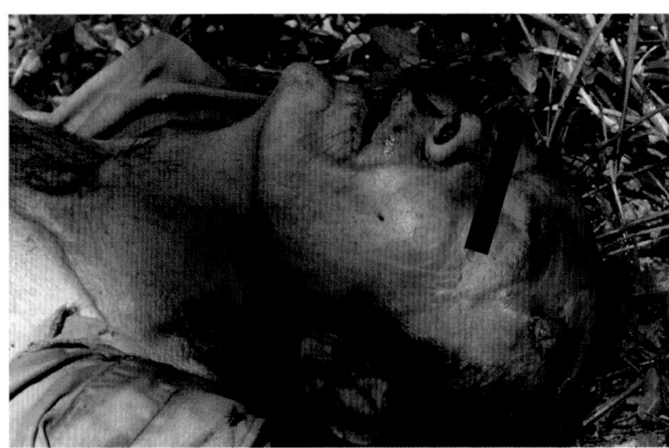

Color Plate 22
Exit wound to left center of head; self-inflicted.

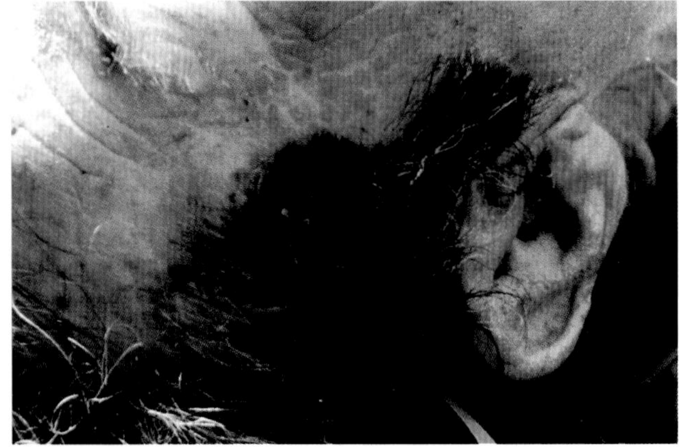

Color Plate 23
Firearm entrance wound to right side of head; note gunshot residue on skin.

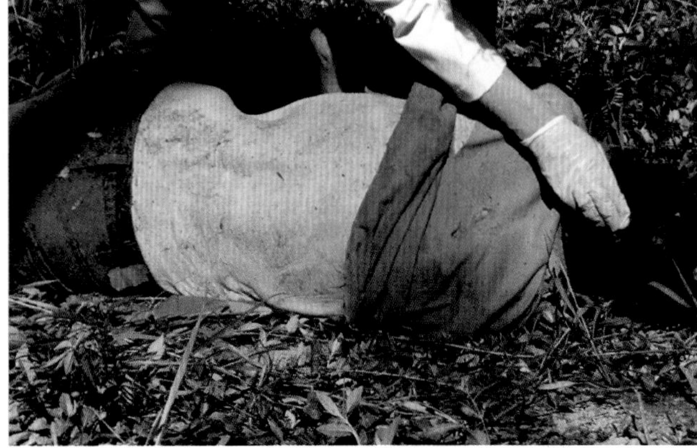

Color Plate 24
Forensic nurse examining back of decedent prior to removing body from scene.

Crime Scene Investigation

Case 2: Skeletal Remains

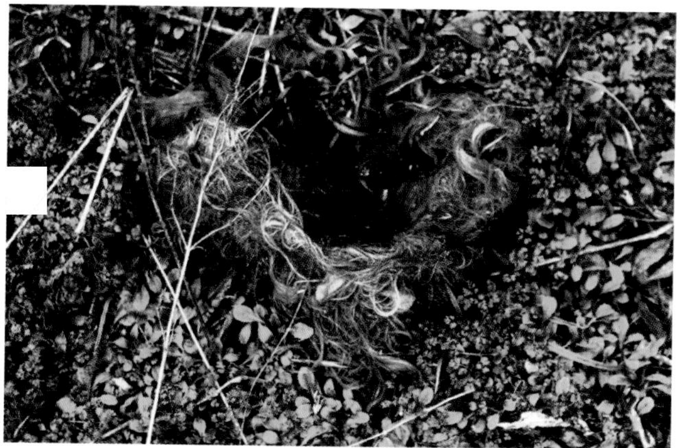

Color Plate 25
Scalp slipped from skull is first evidence of crime scene.

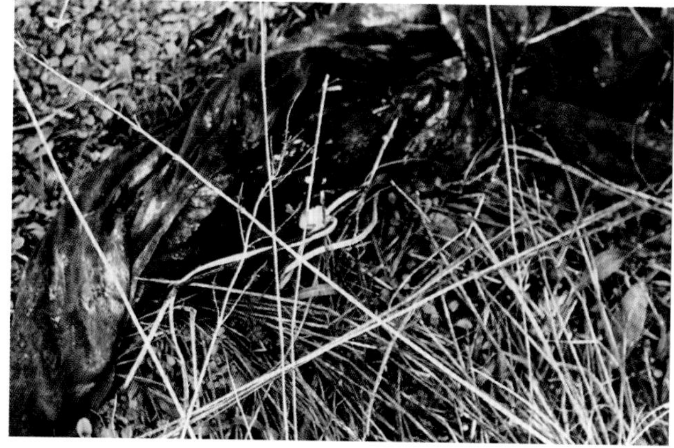

Color Plate 26
View of fabric that had covered the body; note electrical cord used to secure wrapping.

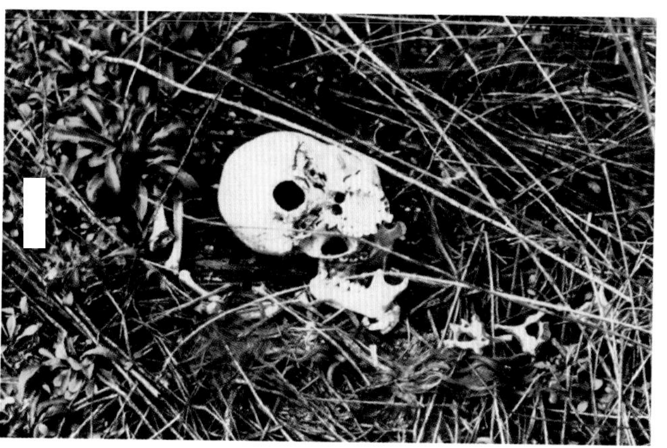

Color Plate 27
Skeletal remains of skull and vertebrae.

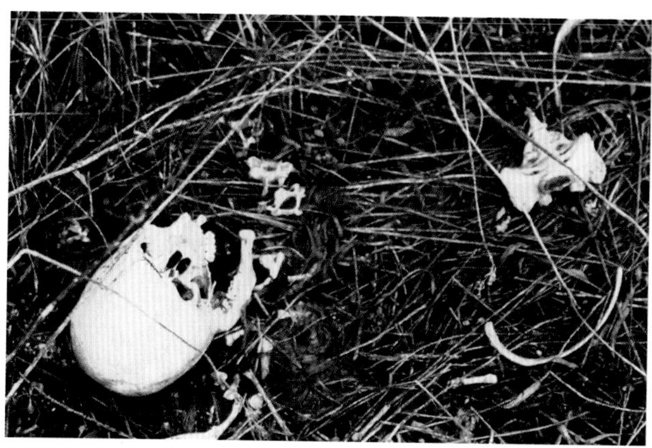

Color Plate 28
Skeletal remains showing coccyx in proximity to skull.

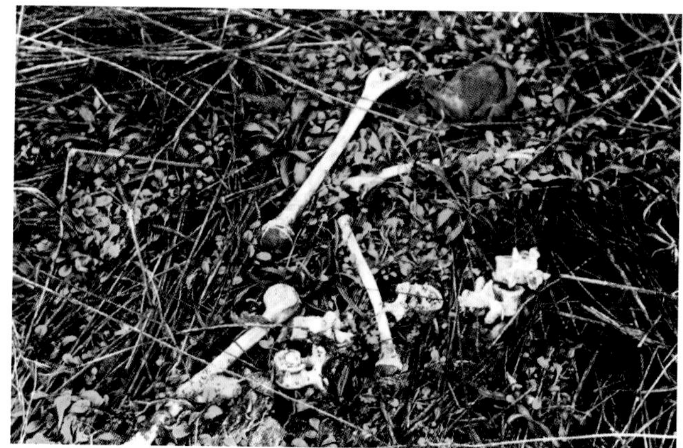

Color Plate 29
Long bones designate central mass of the body; note round brown object near top of long bone, a pair of knotted panty hose assumed to have been used as a ligature.

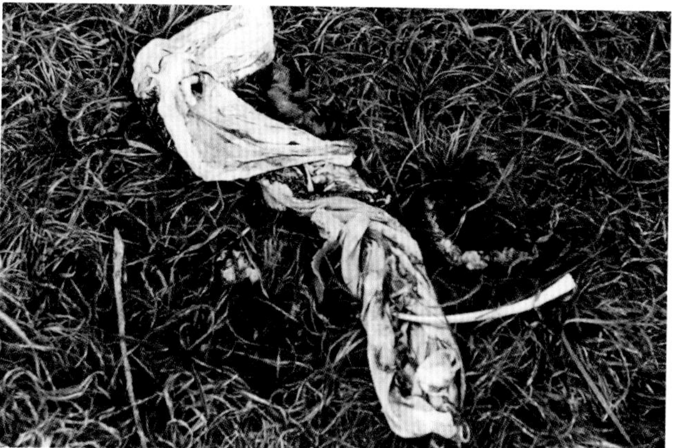

Color Plate 30
Remnant of blouse with adhered rib found 265 yards from the central mass of the body reveals animal activity.

Postmortem Findings and Autopsy

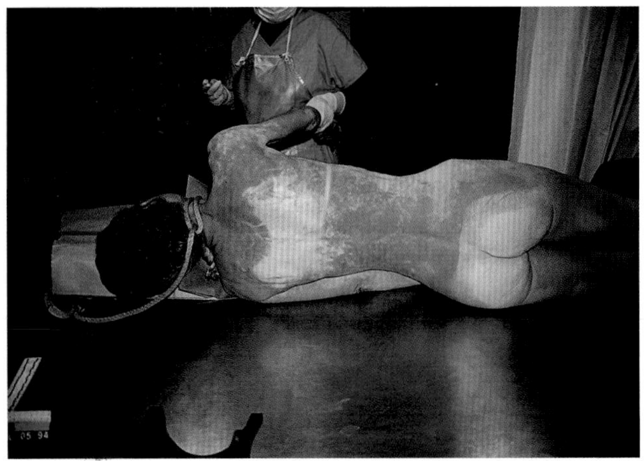

Color Plate 31
Postmortem lividity with pressure pallor.

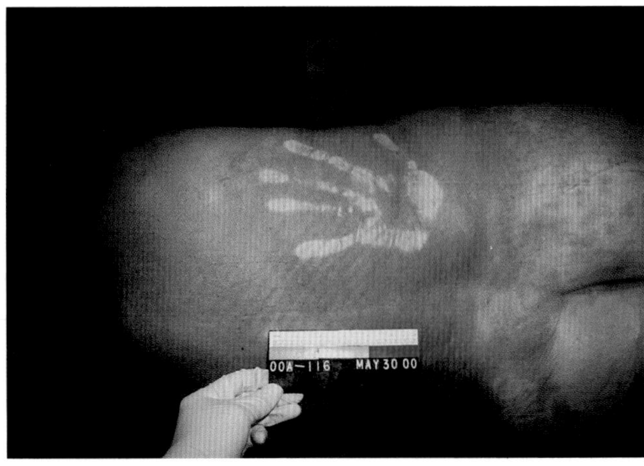

Color Plate 32
Handprint impression indicating nonfixed lividity.

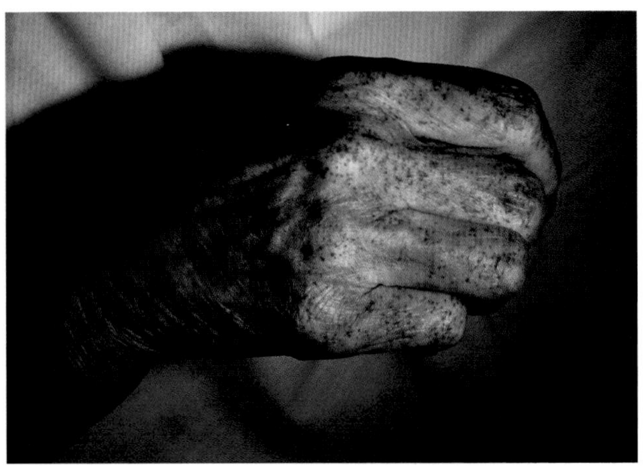

Color Plate 33
Tardieu's spots.

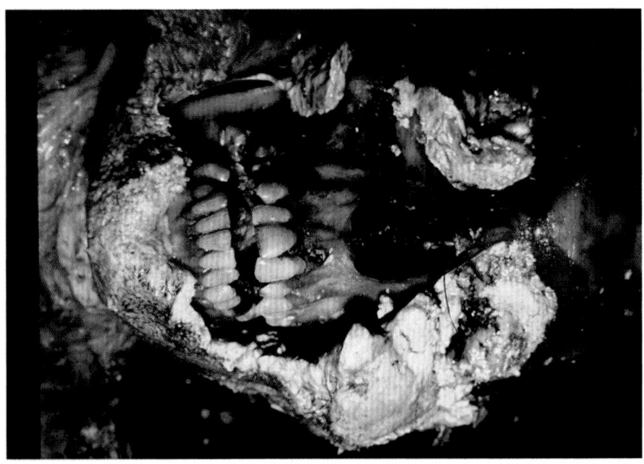

Color Plate 34
Advanced decomposition with adipocere.

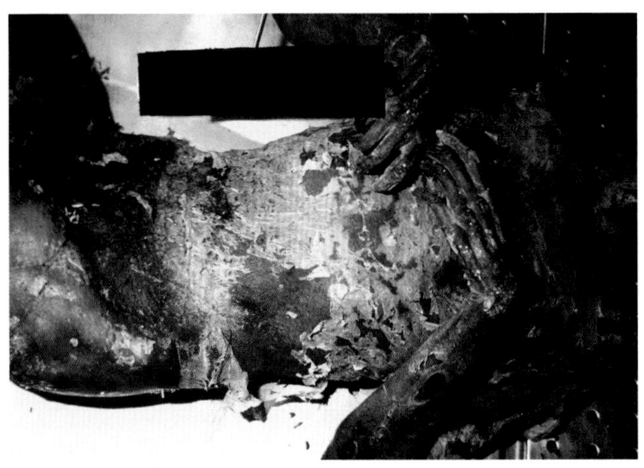

Color Plate 35
Advanced decomposition with sloughing.

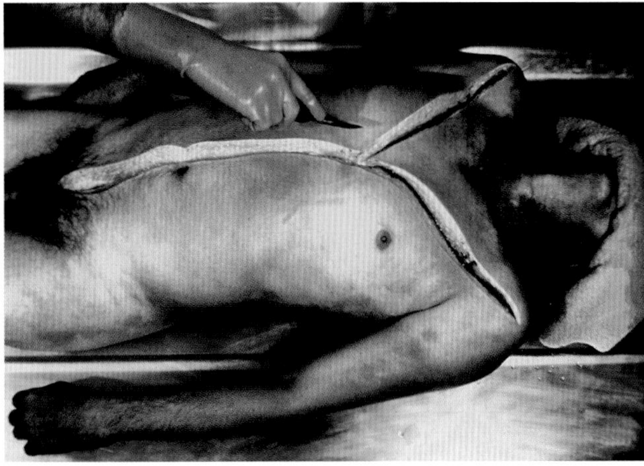

Color Plate 36
Y-shaped autopsy incision.

Childhood Injuries and Neglect

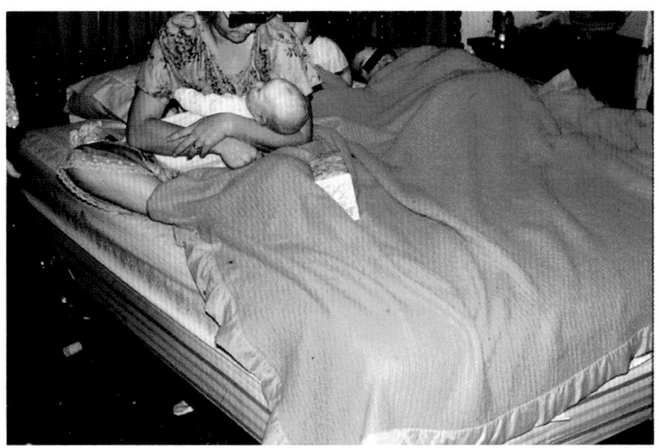

Color Plate 37
Lying-over deaths may be confused with sudden infant death syndrome (SIDS); parent's bed is scene of suffocation death.

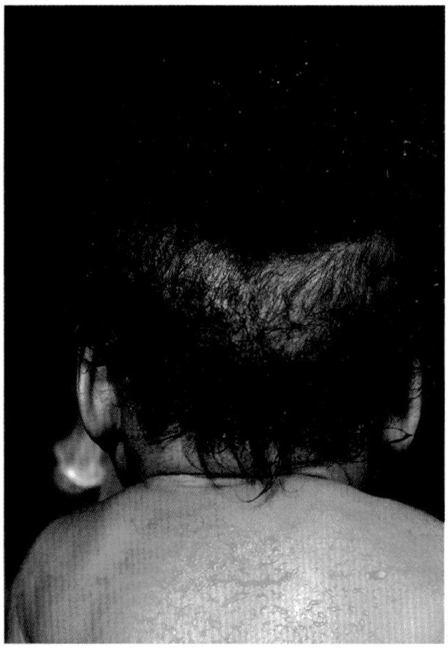

Color Plate 38
Hair loss on posterior head of infant can be normal and must be differentiated from neglect or abuse.

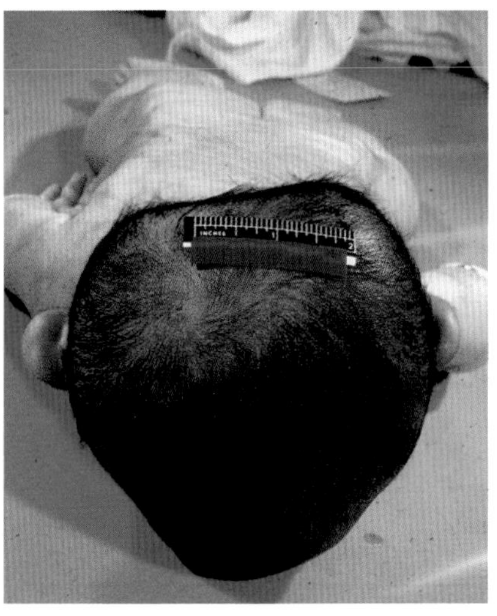

Color Plate 39
Asymmetrical head may indicate abuse.

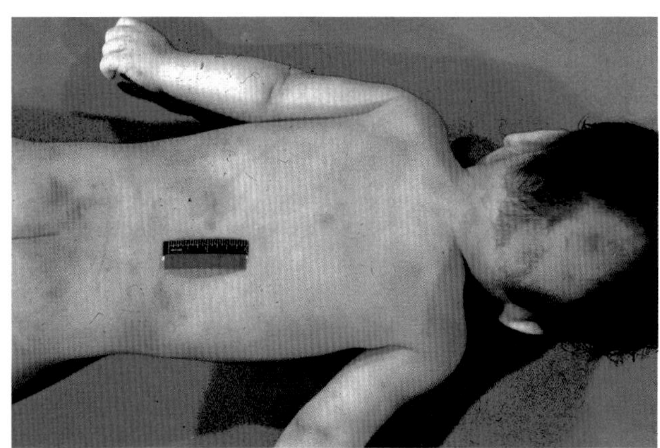

Color Plate 40
Multiple bruises on child's back.

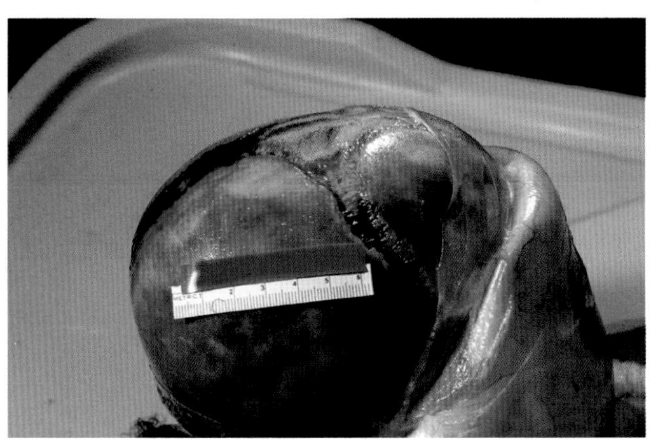

Color Plate 41
Autopsy showing intracranial trauma that is consistent with abuse.

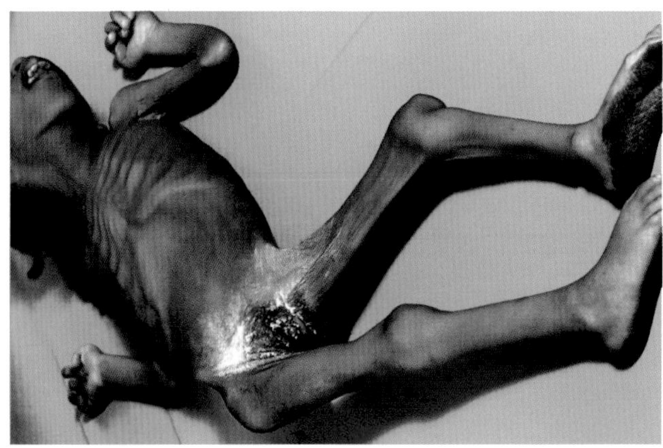

Color Plate 42
Congenital abnormality mimicking starvation.

Sudden Infant Death Syndrome

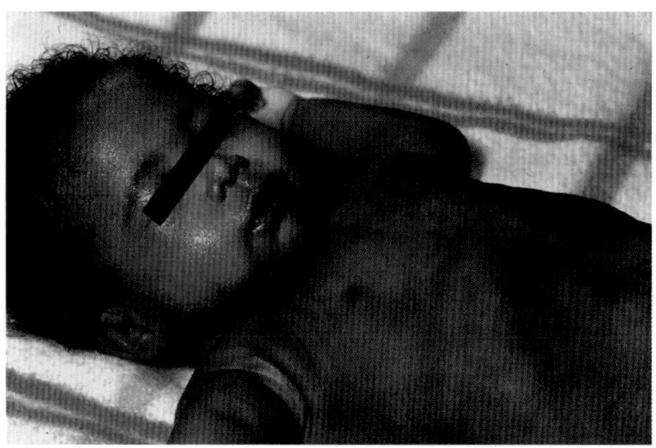

Color Plate 43
Typical appearance of SIDS baby.

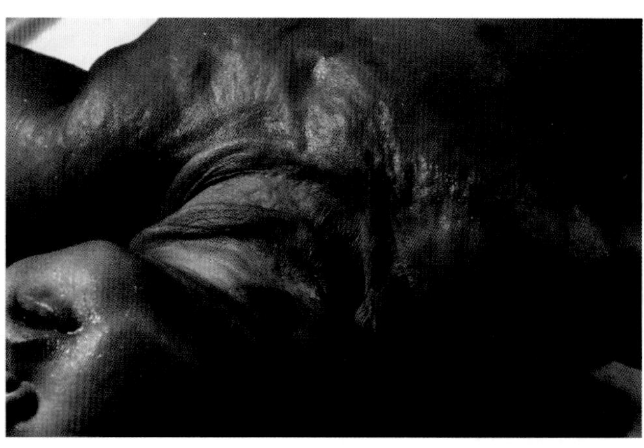

Color Plate 44
Although they may appear to be ligature marks, neck folds of fatty tissue are typical.

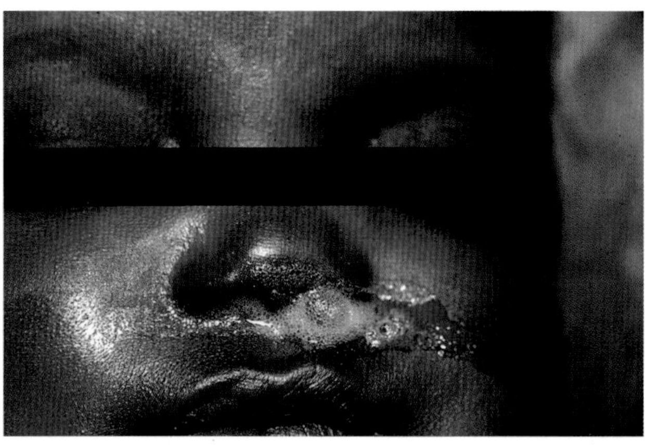

Color Plate 45
Blood-tinged froth at nose is typical with SIDS.

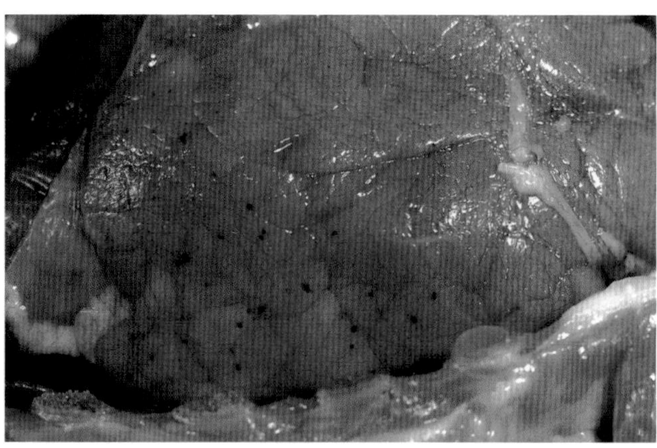

Color Plate 46
Appearance of congested lungs of SIDS baby. Note petechiae.

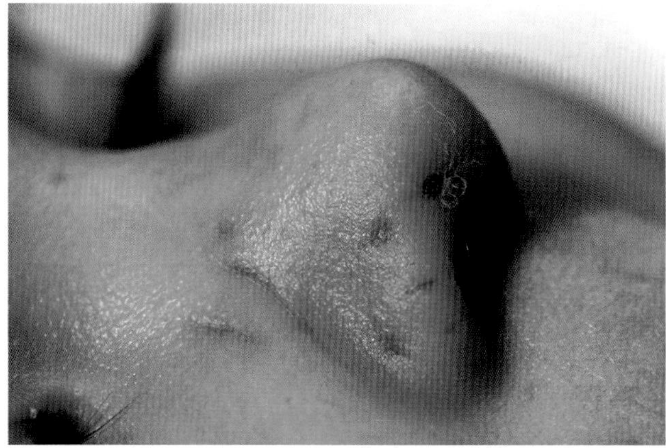

Color Plate 47
Nose injury or scratches are atypical with SIDS and should be studied carefully. Note fibers above right nostril.

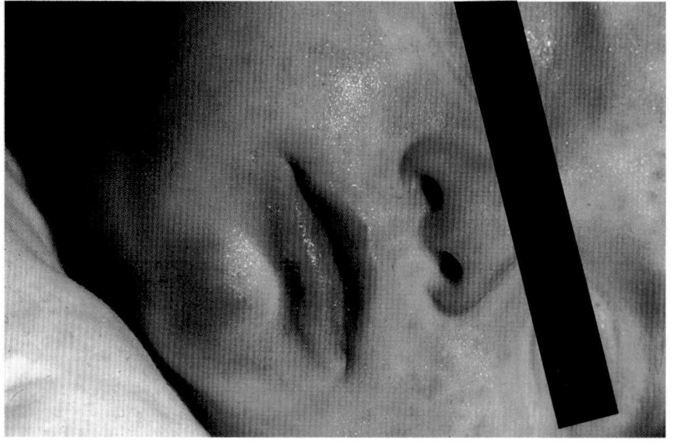

Color Plate 48
Abrasions around nose, mouth, and chin are atypical and may suggest suffocation.

Sexual Abuse and Violent Death

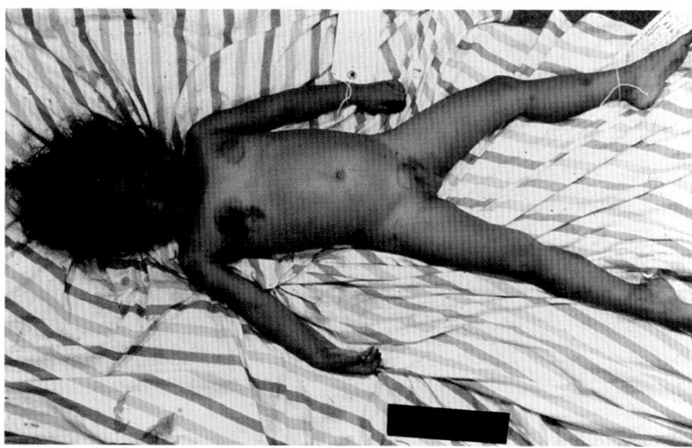

Color Plate 49
Three-year-old victim of sexual homicide.

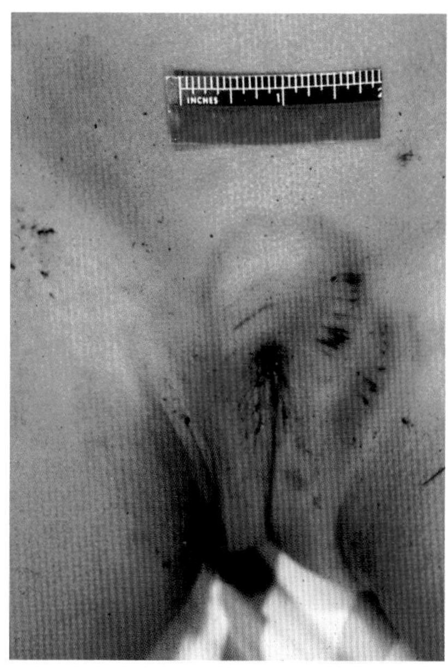

Color Plate 50
Abrasions and contusions associated with sexual abuse.

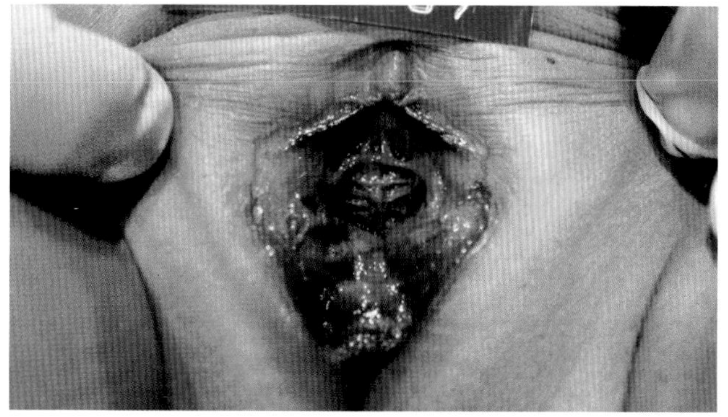

Color Plate 51
Characteristic genital findings of sexual abuse.

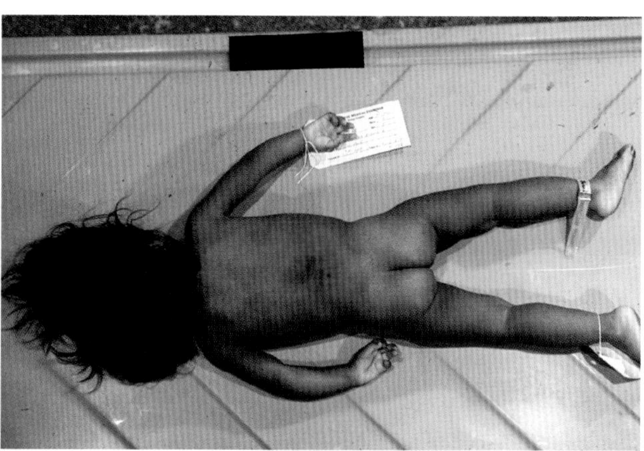

Color Plate 52
Deceased victim of sexual abuse; note patterned injury on back.

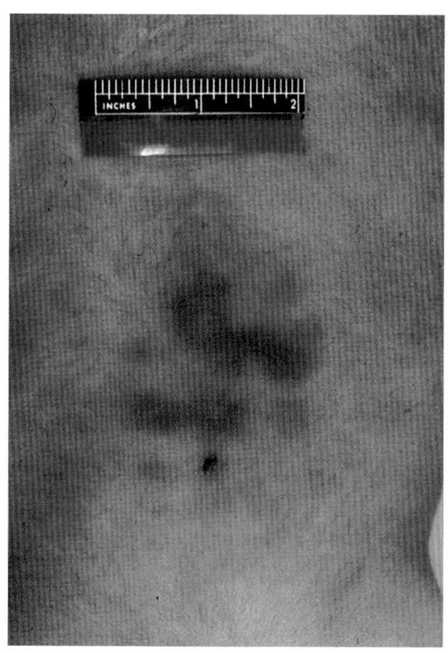

Color Plate 53
Fingertip bruises from restraint during anal penetration.

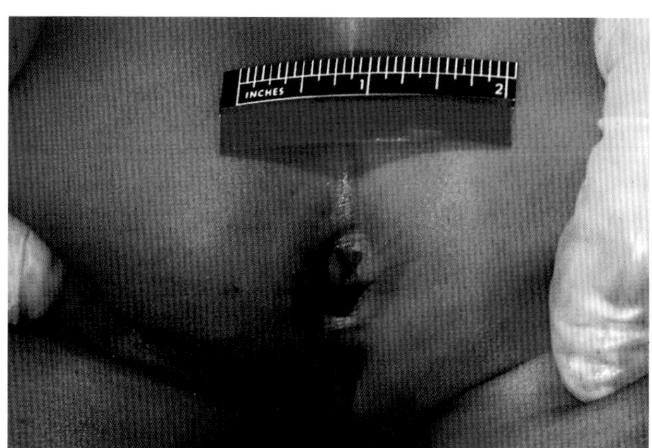

Color Plate 54
Anal injuries characteristic of sexual abuse.

Elder Abuse

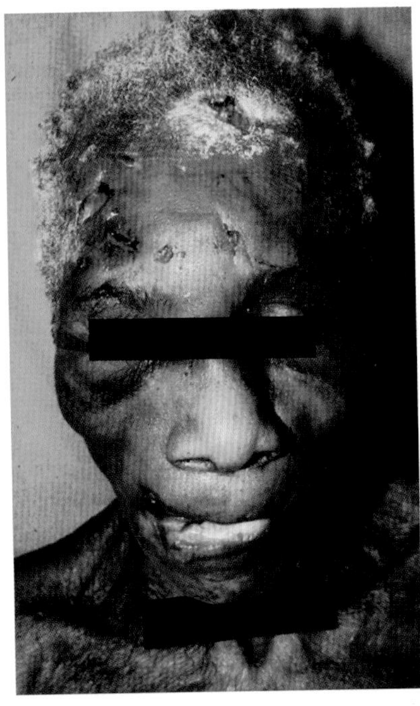

Color Plate 55
Seventy-six-year-old female with injuries to head and eyes.

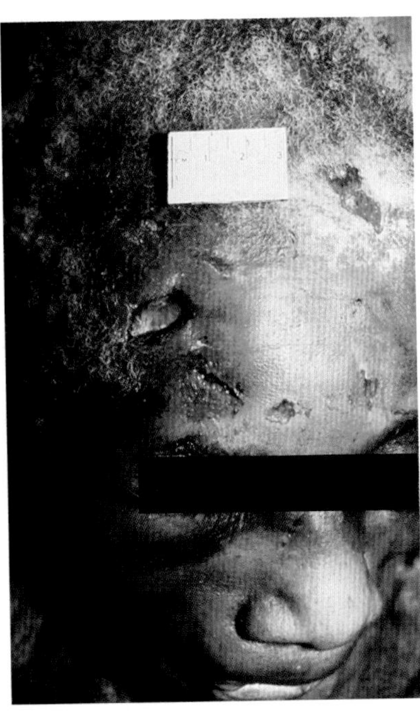

Color Plate 56
Blunt force traumatic injury evidence.

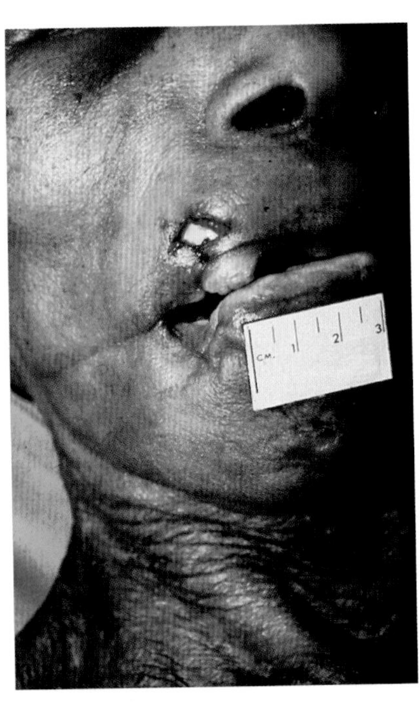

Color Plate 57
Oral trauma with obvious dental injuries.

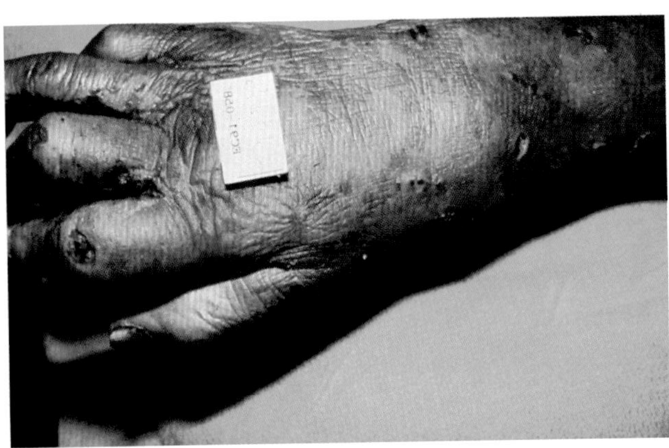

Color Plate 58
Blunt trauma to right hand.

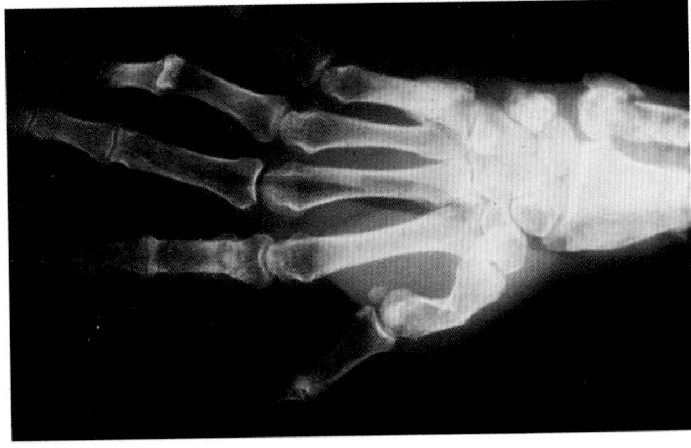

Color Plate 59
X-ray evidence of previous hand trauma; femur, pelvis, and other bones also revealed old and recent fractures.

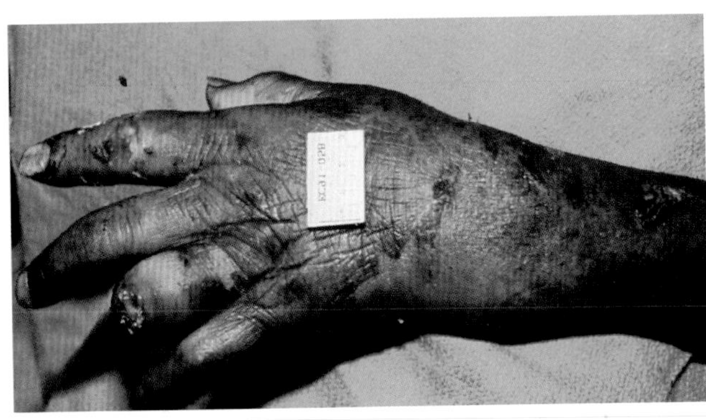

Color Plate 60
Blunt trauma to left hand.

Domestic Abuse and Trauma

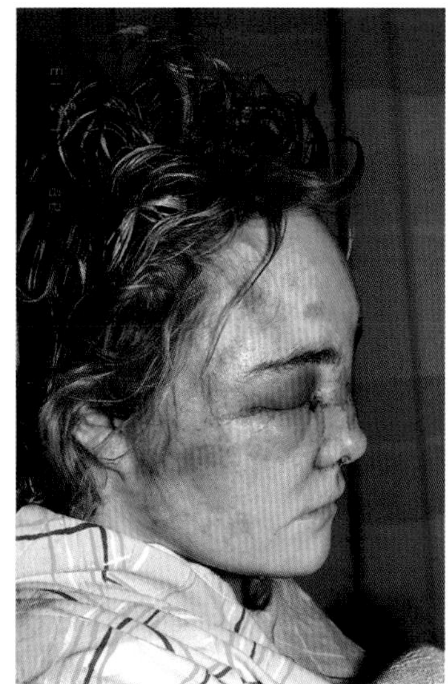

Color Plate 61
Blunt trauma to face from fists of boyfriend.

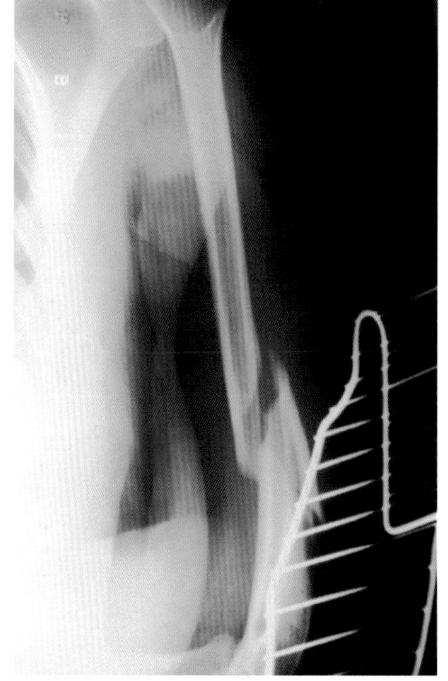

Color Plate 62
Spiral fracture resulting from arm being twisted behind her back.

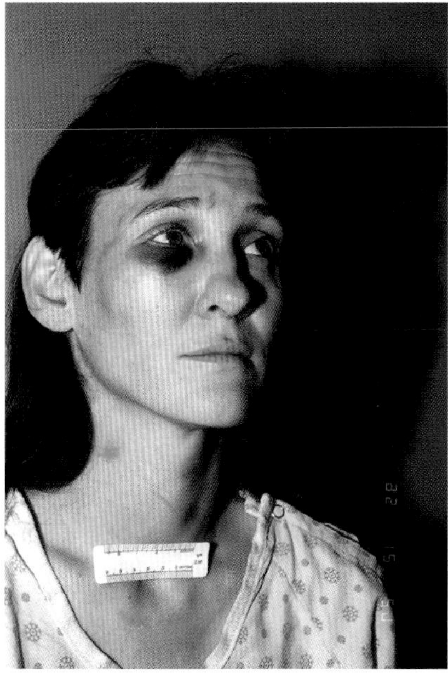

Color Plate 63
Strangulation neck fracture related to spouse abuse.

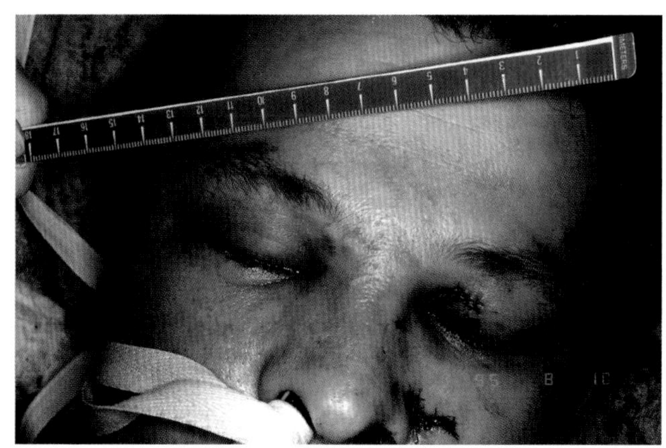

Color Plate 64
Shoe print on face from husband.

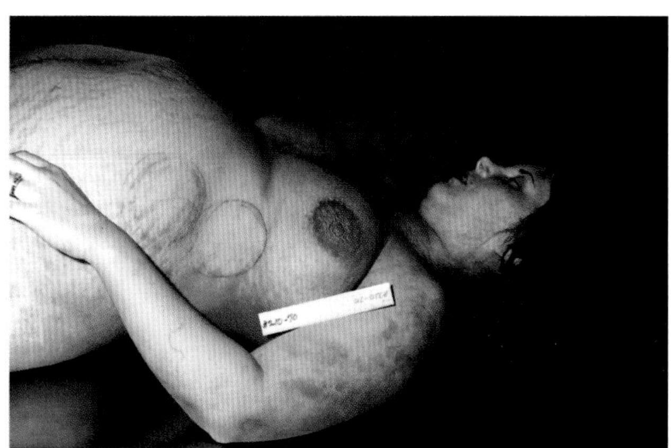

Color Plate 65
Death from late-pregnancy, high-risk sexual activity.

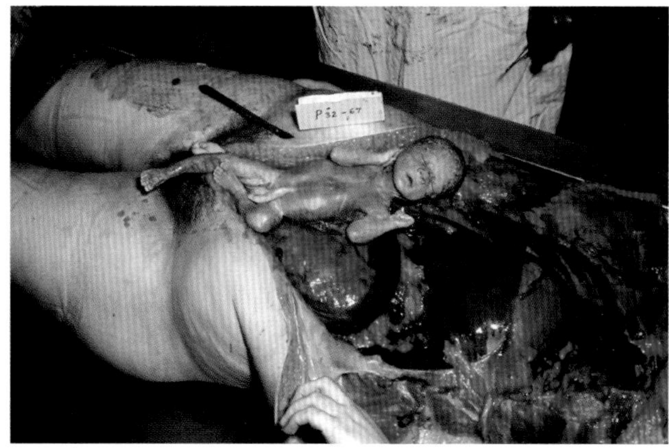

Color Plate 66
Deaths from air embolism induced by sexual activity.

Abuse-Related Trauma

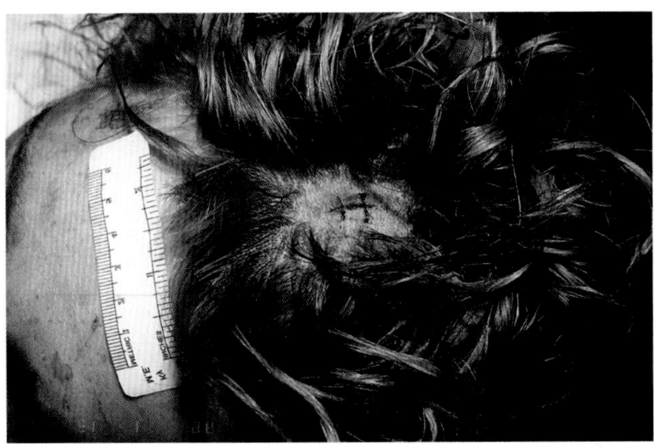

Color Plate 67
Head injury from domestic abuse.

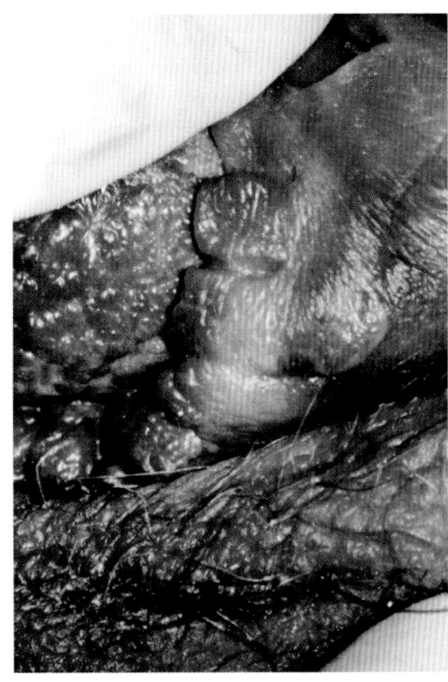

Color Plate 68
Genital bite marks of abusing partner.

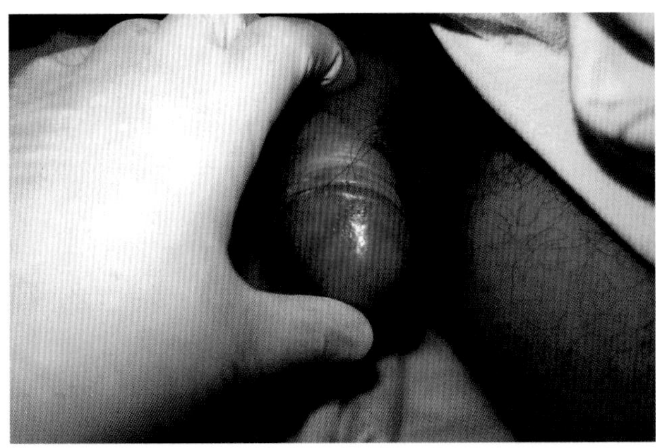

Color Plate 69
Trauma to suspect's penis noted during evidentiary exam.

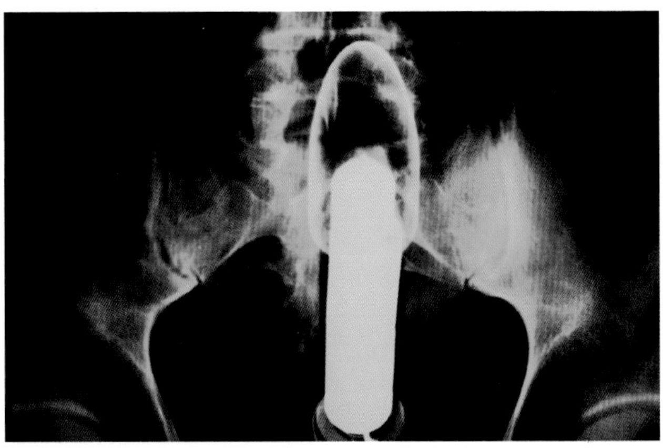

Color Plate 70
X-ray reveals foreign body in orifice inserted by sexual assault assailant.

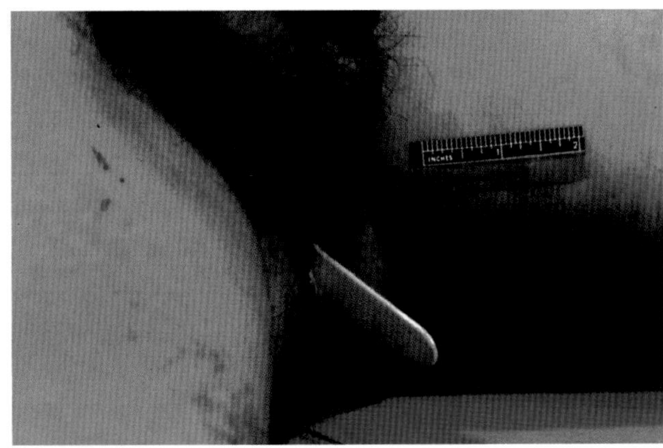

Color Plate 71
When performing premortem examinations, remove all tools or instruments to prevent confusion for death investigators.

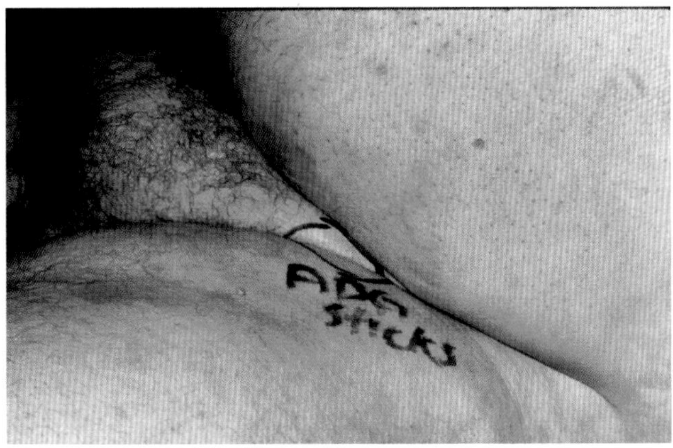

Color Plate 72
Skin markers may be used to differentiate clinical events from abuse or other injuries to soft tissue.

Postmortem Rape-Homicide Examination

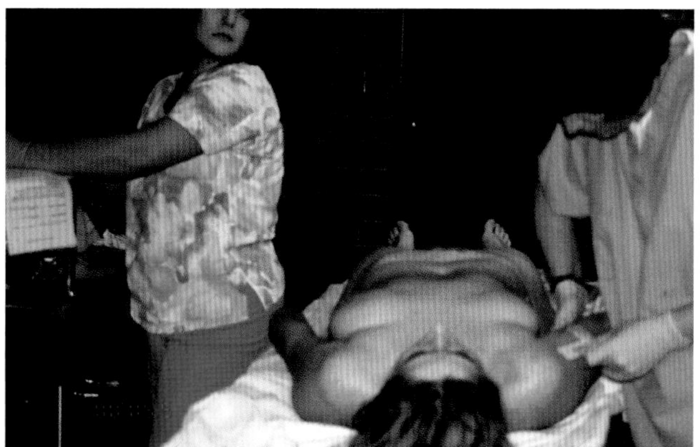

Color Plate 73
Forensic nurses measuring contustions on upper arm and shoulder.

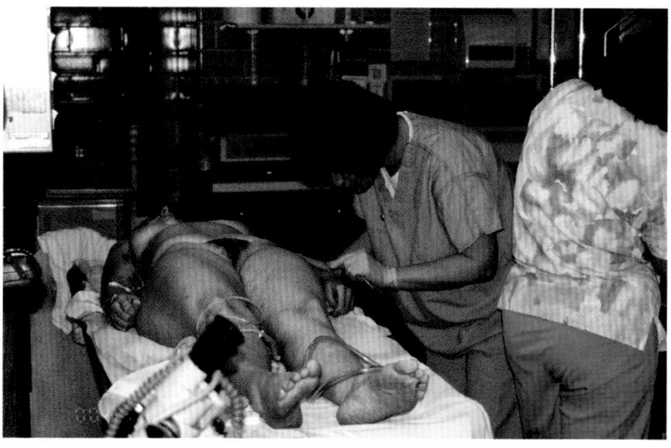

Color Plate 74
Inspecting left arm for injuries prior to obtaining fingernail scrapings.

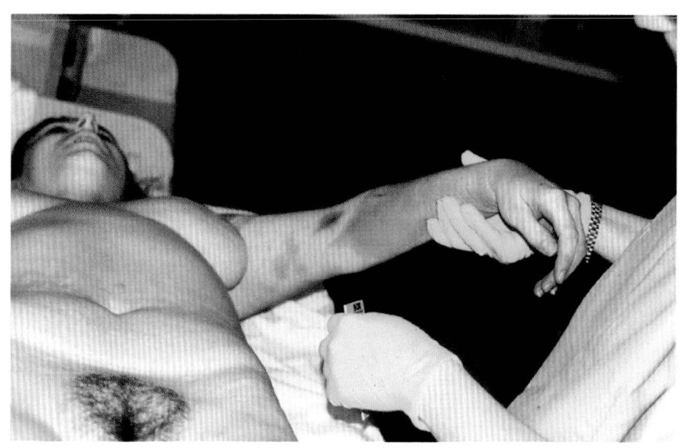

Color Plate 75
Note extensive soft-tissue injuries on upper extremities.

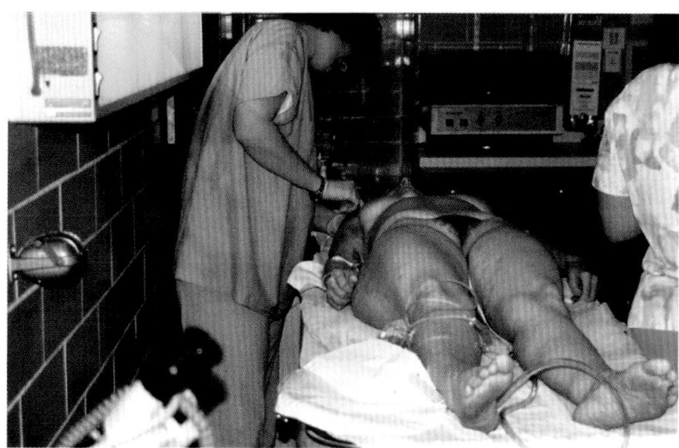

Color Plate 76
Examining right arm for injuries and presence of additional evidence.

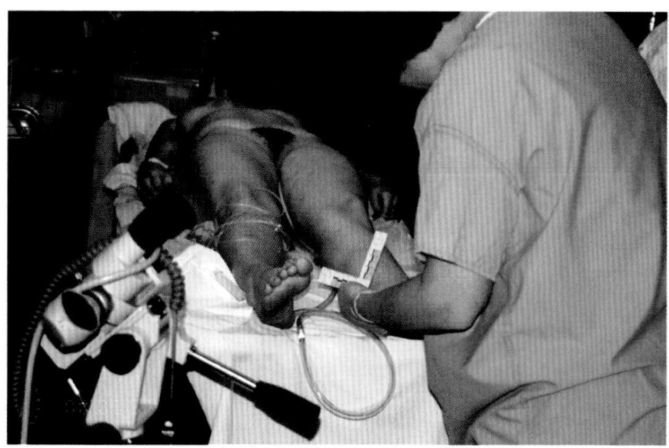

Color Plate 77
Documentation of lower extremity injuries.

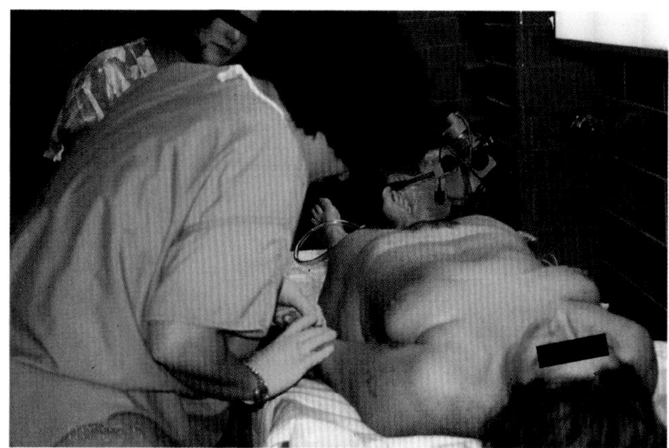

Color Plate 78
Searching extremities for needle marks or other physical evidence.

Death Investigation: Suicide Evidence

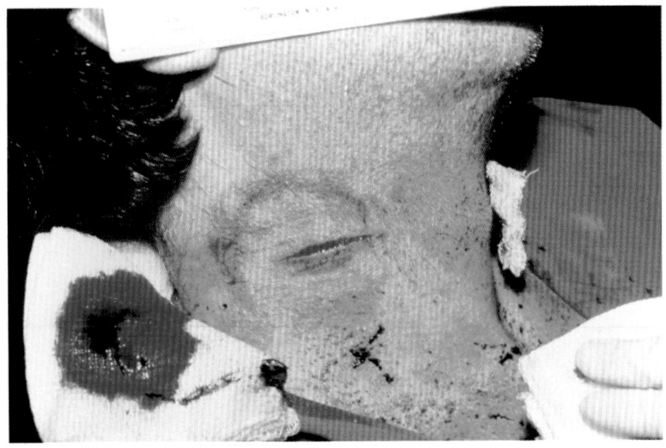

Color Plate 79
Hesitation marks on neck associated with suicide.

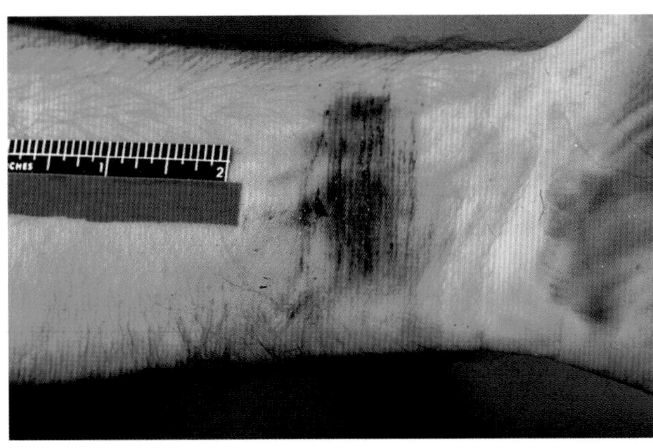

Color Plate 80
Hesitation marks on wrists associated with suicide.

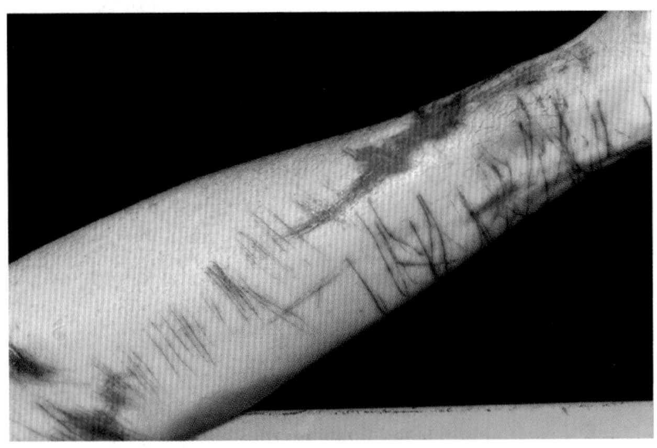

Color Plate 81
Self-multilation and hesitation marks associated with depression and suicide.

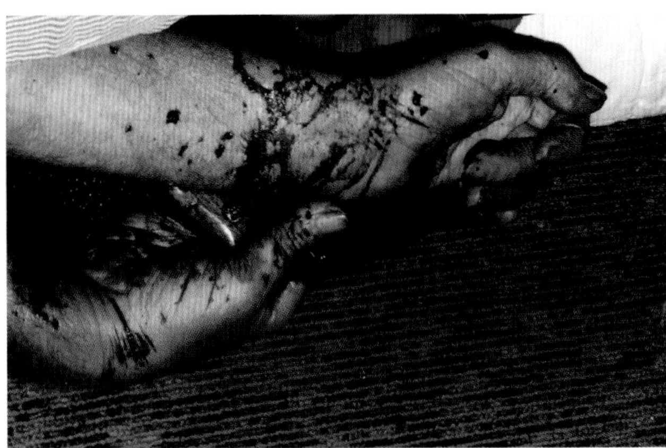

Color Plate 82
Gun and blood blow-back on hands is strong evidence for suicide.

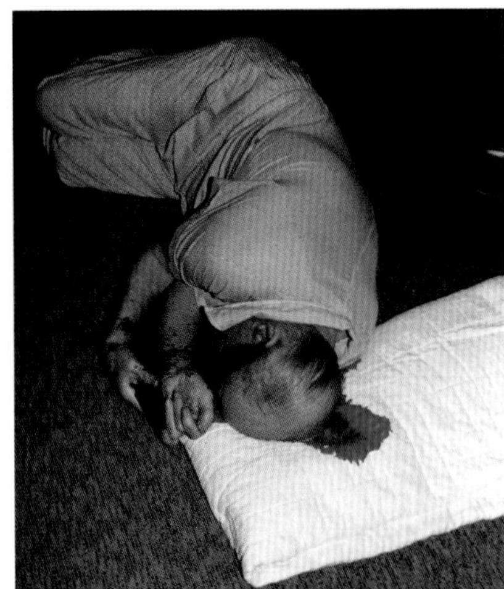

Color Plate 83
Elderly male with self-inflicted gunshot wound; note pillow placement.

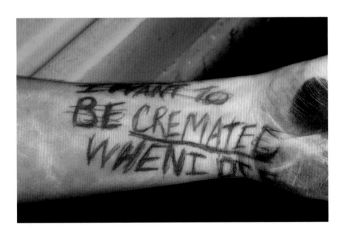

Color Plate 84
Plans for suicide were evident on victim's body.

Death Investigation: Asphyxial Deaths

Hanging and Ligature Strangulation

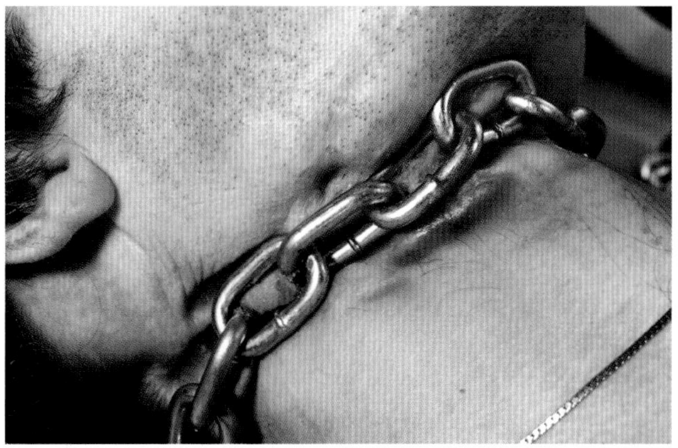

Color Plate 85
Hanging by chain suspension.

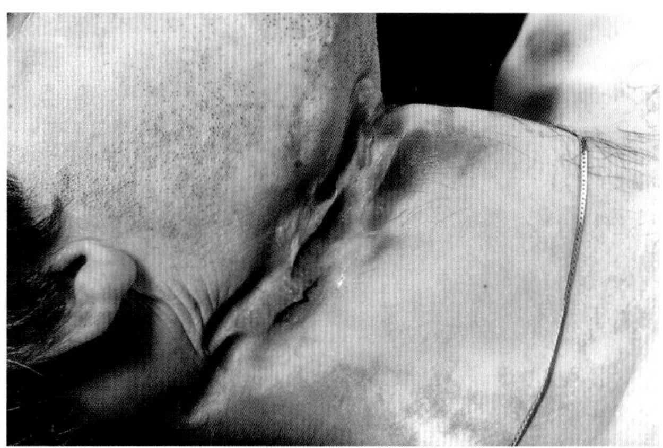

Color Plate 86
Note impression evidence of the chain.

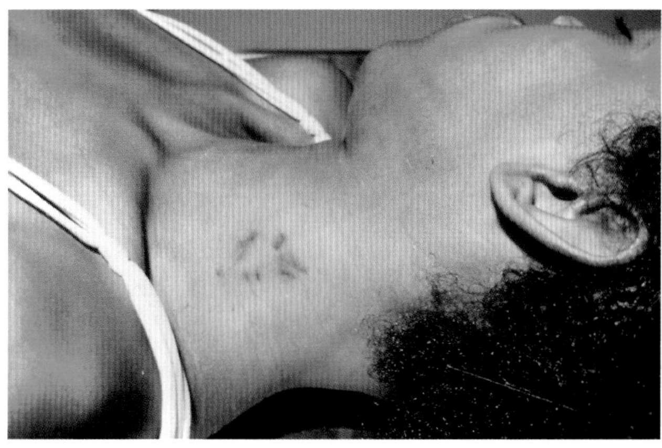

Color Plate 87
Manual strangulation; note fingernail abrasions on neck.

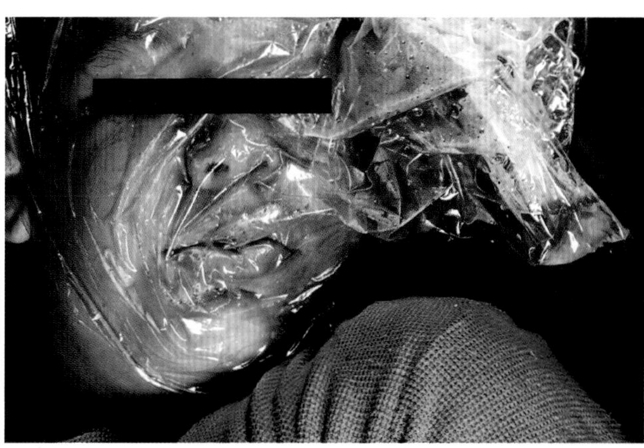

Color Plate 88
Asphyxial death resulting from substance sniffing using plastic bag.

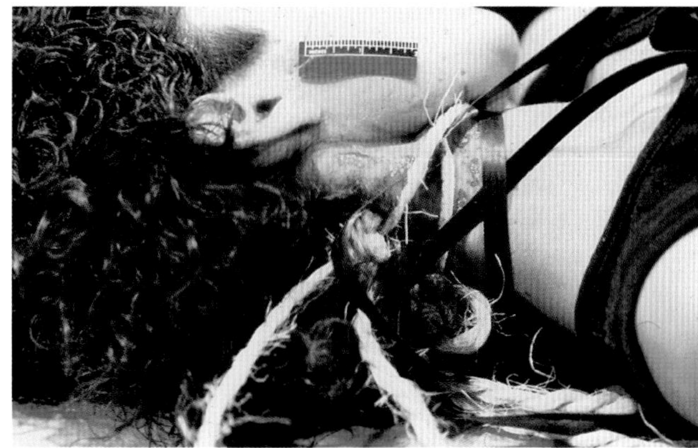

Color Plate 89
Cause of death is asphyxia due to hanging.

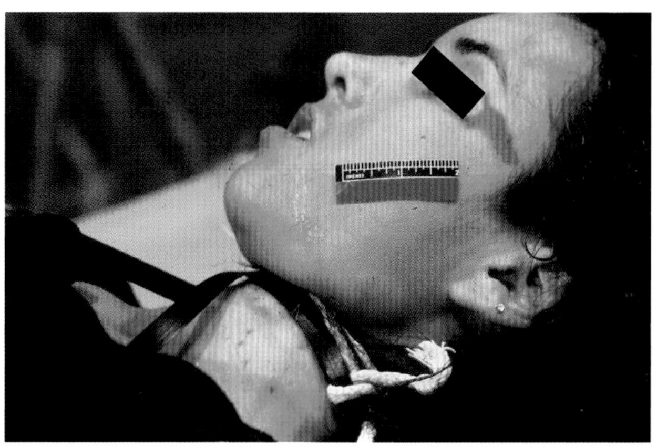

Color Plate 90
Note blunt trauma to left side of face from unknown cause.

Death Investigation: Physical Characteristics

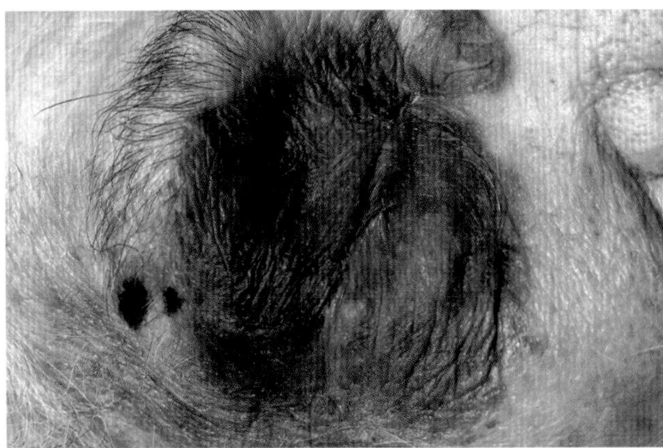

Color Plate 91
Premortem bleeding into soft tissue. Note impressions from nose pad and earpiece of glasses.

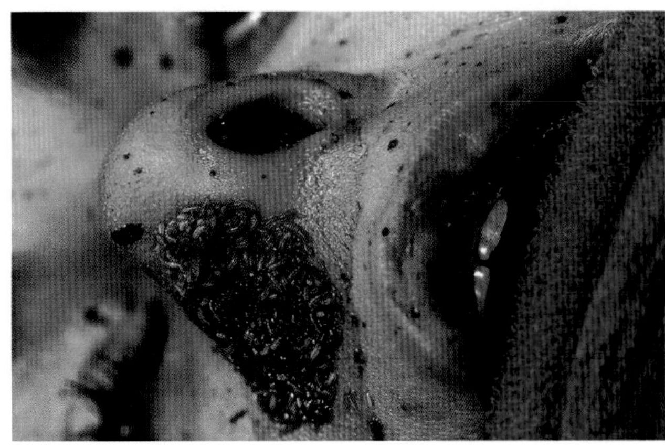

Color Plate 92
Fly larvae in nostril suggesting entomological clue regarding time elapse since death.

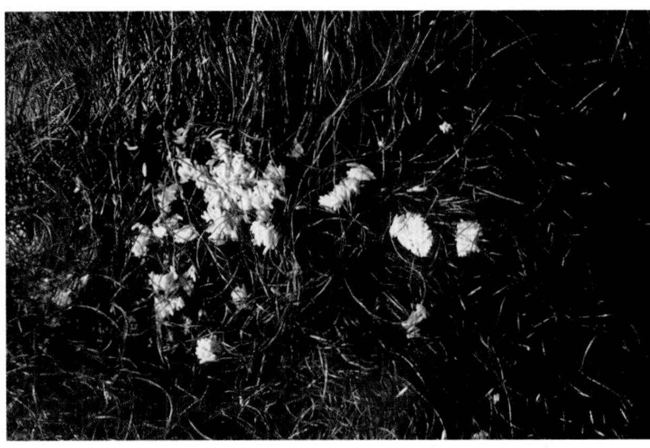

Color Plate 93
Fly larvae in hair suggesting time elapse since death.

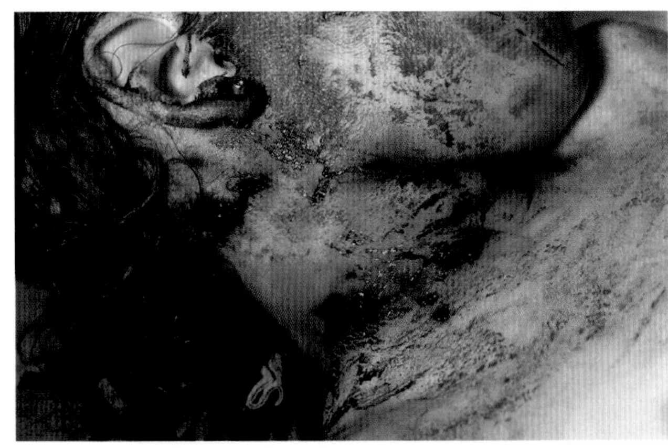

Color Plate 94
Dog bite wound to throat before cleansing.

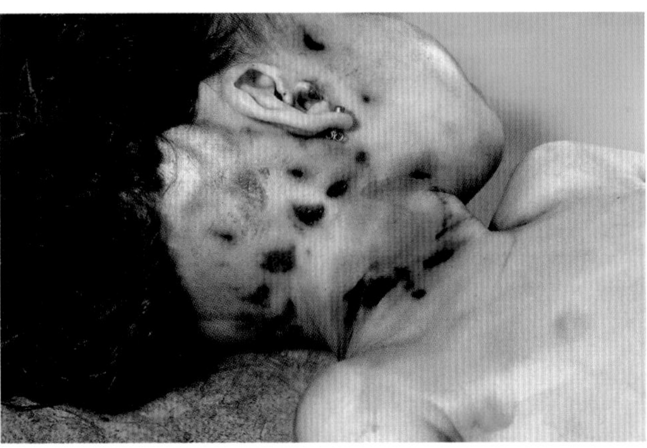

Color Plate 95
Note paired puncture wounds from canine teeth and contusions.

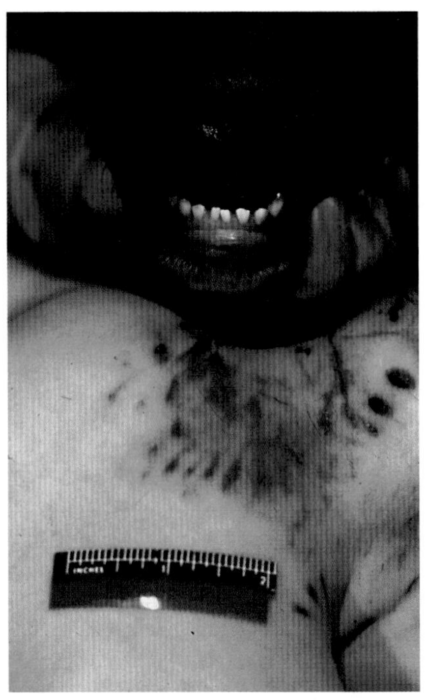

Color Plate 96
Paired injury consistent with protruding canine teeth.

Contents

Unit One
Introduction to Forensic Science in Healthcare

Unit Two

Violence: Contemporary Social Issues and Forensic Science

Unit Five

Special Forensic Issues in Healthcare

21 Organ Donation, 217

Teresa J. Shafer

22 Research with Vulnerable Participants, 235

Louanne Lawson and Cynthia Cupit Swenson

23 Child Abuse and Neglect, 249

Kathleen B. LaSala and Virginia A. Lynch

24 Domestic Violence, 260

Barbara A. Moynihan

Unit One

Introduction to Forensic Science in Healthcare

Chapter 1 The Specialty of Forensic Nursing

Virginia A. Lynch

Forensic nursing is

> *the application of the forensic aspects of healthcare combined with the bio/psycho/social/spiritual education of the registered nurse in the scientific investigation and treatment of trauma and/or death of victims and perpetrators of violence, criminal activity and traumatic accidents. The forensic nurse provides direct services to individual clients, consultation services to nursing, medical and law-related agencies, as well as providing expert court testimony in areas dealing with questioned death investigative processes, adequacy of services delivery and specialized diagnoses of specific conditions as related to nursing. (Lynch, 1991)*

Overview

The application of the principles and standards of the forensic specialist in nursing was recognized as a vital new role in healthcare in the 1990s. Daily, nurses are faced with the extremes of human behavior: child abuse, domestic violence, crimes against the elderly, victims of catastrophic accidents, self-inflicted injuries, blatant neglect, and maltreatment. These cases, based on individual state laws, may be required to be reported to a legal agency and an investigation of this trauma is mandated. Significant concern is also required as nurses interface with patients in legal custody when providing treatment or court-ordered assessments. As trends in crime and violence change, new legislation is implemented as a means of antiviolence strategies; new resources are required in order to meet the needs of society. Nurses have been challenged to share in a mutual responsibility with the legal system to augment resources available to clinical forensic patients and questioned death investigations. This concept represents a new perspective in the holistic approach to forensic nursing (body, mind, spirit, and the law) surrounding patient care in clinical or community-based institutions.

The application of forensic science to contemporary nursing practice reveals a wider role in the clinical investigation of crime and the legal process that contributes to public health and safety (Lynch, 1995). It is not surprising that there is strong support for nursing specialists who possess the combination of knowledge and skills required to go beyond the traditional treatment of patients with liability-related injuries, victims of crime, suspects, or offenders in police custody to fulfill the requirement for forensic expertise in healthcare. This role development is that of a forensic specialist in nursing, not a nursing specialist in forensic science or criminal justice. The major status of the forensic nurse is first and foremost *nursing*.

Forensic versus Forensics

Understanding the definitions of the term *forensic* and the often associated term *forensics* is important to the academic application of language in the development of this new nursing specialty. The majority of healthcare professionals in the US misinterpret the accurate meaning of the term *forensic*. According to *Tabers Cyclopedic Medical Dictionary*, this term is defined simply as "pertaining to the law," specifically related to public debate in courts of law (Latin *forensis*; a forum), implying the debate between the prosecution and defense (Taber's, 2001). It is well to consider that "forensic" is an adjective and should be used in conjunction with a noun, such as in forensic medicine (science, nursing, engineering, etc.). When used as a noun, such as "forensics," it is most correctly implying a college or other scholastic debate team. Although this term is commonly used as a shortened version for forensic science, organizations that promote public speaking may also use "forensic" as the primary term in their title, such as a forensic debate team. For example, in a news article titled "Forensic Honor," a college freshman was named National Forensics League All-American, earning 1647 points and placing fifth among 91,000 student members. It is important to understand the correct application of both terms. Therefore, any subdiscipline of science that practices its specialty within the arena of the law is practicing the principle of forensic science.

Evolution of Forensic Sciences

The Code of Hammurabi created more than 4200 years ago by the King of Babylon established legislation governing the field of medicine and is generally regarded as the oldest known legal code. It was not until the twentieth century, however, that certain specialty disciplines emerged, including forensic science, which eventually gave rise to forensic pathology and clinical forensic medicine (Camp, 1976). As scientific and technological developments escalated in the twentieth century, the basis for forensic science and applications to medicine was firmly established. Sophisticated microscopes and other scientific instruments, advanced techniques in print analysis, radiological procedures, and computers were among the advancements that supported the rapid development and refinement of forensic practice.

At the same time, groups of scientists and medical professionals were creating associations that eventually became the forums for sharing and disseminating advancements within the forensic disciplines. Now there are multiple organizations of specialists dedicated to forensic sciences, enveloping many disciplines and spanning the globe. Among these are the American Academy of Forensic Sciences, International Association of Blood Pattern Analysts, International Association of Forensic Nurses, National Association of Medical Examiners, American Board of Forensic Nursing, American College of Forensic Examiners, International Homicide Investigators Association, American Society of Testing and Materials, Association of Police Surgeons, American Society of Criminology, and the International Association for Human Identification (Lynch & Standing Bear, 2000).

Forensic Science and the Public

Until recently, the American public had little or no knowledge of the disciplines or practices of the forensic sciences. However, actual footage of high-profile cases televised in court has brought recognition of forensic science to the national populous and into university curricula with an impact on career paths as never before. Cases such as the O. J. Simpson trial and the murder investigation of Jon Benét Ramsey raised awareness of the various disciplines and technologies of the forensic sciences, such as DNA analysis, footwear impressions, fingerprinting, geometric interpretation of blood spatter patterns, modus operandi, and preservation of biological evidence.

Dr. R. B. H. Gradwald, a founder of the American Academy of Forensic Sciences (AAFS) in 1948, stated, "There is no fixed border for any forensic science, each has more than necessity to rely on the others. It would thus seem fitting that a central organization be of extreme value in collating and disseminating the fundamentals of all forensic sciences." This includes forensic nursing science (AAFS, 2002).

Based on this principle, the nursing profession has embraced multiple facets of the forensic sciences. The International Association of Forensic Nurses (IAFN) has persistently promoted the global exchange of knowledge and education in the science of forensic nursing. The AAFS has worked to engender the confidence and respect of the nation's courts and to see the ends of justice attained. Together with the AAFS, the IAFN has organized its goals, mission, and organizational structure, opportunities for professional development, education, and research as a forensic specialty in nursing. Based on this ideology, interdisciplinary solidarity will continue to raise the image and profile of forensic nursing and elevate standards in the cause of the forensic sciences (Box 1-1).

Understanding Forensic Terminology

Traditionally in the US, the term *forensic medicine* carries with it the connotation of death, homicide, or murder. This association is due to the fact that previously only one kind of forensic medicine was practiced in North America, forensic pathology, a subspecialty of forensic medicine addressing the scientific investigation of death, as opposed to *clinical* forensic medicine, or "living forensics," involving unrecognized or unidentified trauma and the recovery of evidence in living forensic patients. Whereas clinical forensic medicine has existed for more than 200 years, it has not been recognized as a clinical practice in the US. News media and public communication have also contributed to this misinterpretation of terminology related to forensic science and medicine. However, the newest and perhaps most important advancement in the domain of forensic expertise in the US is the emerging field of clinical forensic practice (or living forensics) as practiced by forensic nurse examiners.

Many remember watching TV serials about medical investigators who searched for the cause of questioned deaths. One popular show featured a forensic pathologist, Dr. Quincy, who was involved in exciting autopsies and sought answers to questions pertaining to homicide, suicide, or accident. Dr. Quincy endeavored to answer the question, "What was the exact time and manner or mechanism of death?" Therefore, in the absence of clinical forensic medicine in the US, it is commonly believed that forensic medicine is entirely related to the deceased patient and is practiced exclusively by pathologists such as Dr. Quincy who gather information during postmortem procedures.

Television programs, such as *CSI: Crime Scene Investigation* and *Cold Case Files*, including forensic pathologists reviewing authentic case histories and videotaped autopsies, far surpass the popularity of *Quincy*. Clinical forensic entertainment has also influenced the well-established and highly praised television series *ER*, which has incorporated the role of the forensic nurse examiner.

Box 1-1 Forensic Science Disciplines within the American Academy of Forensic Sciences

Forensic pathology/biology	Forensic odontology
Forensic anthropology	Forensic documents
Forensic psychiatry/behavioral sciences	Engineering sciences
Medical jurisprudence	Forensic toxicology
Criminalistics	General/multidisciplinary*

*Includes forensic nursing.

From American Academy of Forensic Sciences. (2002). Membership information brochure. Colorado Springs, CO: Author.

Forensic Practice and Public Health

Clinical forensic medicine is derived from the broad field of forensic medicine, a respected discipline in public health over two centuries in many other parts of the world (Lynch, 1995). Therefore, forensic nursing science is considered an integral component of public health. Clinical forensic practice focuses on the civil and criminal investigation of traumatic injury or patient treatment with law-related issues. It encompasses living patients: the victims, the accused, and the condemned.

Forensic pathology, however, addresses the determination of cause, manner, and mechanism of death and incorporates gross anatomical pathology (i.e., autopsies, as well as investigation of the scene of death). Forensic pathology provides insight into why death occurs and makes recommendations for the reduction and prevention of threats to public health and safety. From the beginning of the history of medicine, forensic pathology has established the foundation for all clinical practice. Without consistent determination of the cause of death, preventive practices cannot be initiated. Furthermore, forensic medicine has been the only medical specialty lacking its own skilled nursing associate. The role of the forensic nurse examiner in death investigation (see Chapter 34) provides this long needed and overdue partnership in forensic pathology services as well as in clinical forensic medicine.

Trauma and Public Health

Public health, as opposed to private medical practice, addresses biological and environmental threats to the health and safety of the community population. Public health addresses issues of trauma, communicable disease, and death. All trauma patients are considered forensic cases until suspicion of abuse or questions of liability are confirmed or ruled out. These cases require consideration of intent (an element of crime) necessitating the clinical investigation of injury, illness, or death. Survivors of trauma requiring the investigation of injury are the concern of the clinician, not the pathologist.

The concept of "living forensics" may be attributed to Harry C. McNamara, chief medical examiner for Ulster County, New York. In 1988, McNamara defined clinical forensic medicine as "the

Box 1-2 Categories of Clinical Forensic Cases

All victims of violence	Automobile trauma
Patients in police custody	Workers' compensation
Sexual assault	Medical malpractice
Drug and alcohol abuse	Food and drug tampering
Child maltreatment	Environmental hazards
Domestic violence	Illegal abortion
Elder abuse	Occult-related injury/death
Survivors of attempted suicide	Cults or religion abuses

application of clinical medicine to victims of trauma involving the proper processing of forensic evidence" (McNamara, 1986). See Box 1-2 for categories of clinical forensic cases. Dr. McNamara was one of the first to recognize and encourage the relationship with nursing to this essential field of healthcare. Although wider in its application, this definition stresses the importance of healthcare providers being aware of evidentiary materials and legal issues associated with their patients or clients to preserve national welfare (McNamara, 1986).

Any medical treatment case reported to a legal agency, such as the police department, social services, or child or adult protective services, will require an investigation, may result in charges filed against a suspect, and may ultimately be brought to a civil or criminal trial. The patient may be living or dead and may require testimony involving the healthcare professional who provided forensic intervention and recovery of evidence.

Evidence on Trial

Clinical forensic practice and forensic nursing services represent a new trend in clinical and community healthcare in the US practiced by doctors, nurses, and paramedical services. Forensic nursing science focuses on the areas where medicine, nursing, and human behavior interface with the law and entails both living and deceased patients. Questions related to trauma that may later be of relevance in a court of law may remain unanswered due to ignorance of forensic issues. Frequently cases are won or lost based on the handling of evidence.

Far too often, it is the evidence on trial rather than the accused. US cases have been wrought with criticism regarding the failure to properly recover and secure forensic evidence. These high-profile cases have brought international scrutiny to the validity of methods and technique of our law enforcement agencies and criminal justice systems. With the consistently increasing reliance on DNA evidence in criminal cases, no exception to protocol in recovery of this highly perishable and fragile biological material can be afforded. Examples such as the O. J. Simpson case and the murder of Jon Benét Ramsey have focused on the integrity of the evidence, interview of witnesses, and the destruction of the crime scene. Failure to conduct strict application of policy and procedure when gathering forensic evidence at the scene of crime or in the clinical environs is justice denied.

Violence and Healthcare

An epidemic of violence and its associated trauma is widely recognized as a critical health problem in North America and throughout the world. Among the challenges that face healthcare providers is protection of the patient's legal, civil, and human rights (Lynch, 1995). With a steady increase in reporting of interpersonal violence within our society, nurses are seeing a greater number of victims of criminal acts. These victims, as well as the perpetrators of crime, often come to the hospital for treatment of injuries. As perhaps the first point of contact in the immediate post-trauma period, the nurse is in an ideal position to gather information and physical evidence related to the crime. Forensic nurses must be able to identify injuries from weapons or human abuse and to skillfully interview patients and evaluate the nature and scope of these injuries. Nurses interface with law enforcement and the medical examiner/coroner and provide excellent resources for expert testimony when these cases are tried in a court of law. Forensic nursing demands superb assessment skills, second only to a high degree of suspiciousness. Every injury, illness, or death can have forensic implications. Therefore, a solid forensic education for nurses provides a vital link in the development of clinical acumen required for responding to these forensic circumstances. Forensic nurses are one component of a multidisciplinary team of forensic investigators addressing social injustice. Forensic nurses do not usurp, replace, or supplant any other discipline; rather they fill a void with their unique acumen.

Working Relationships of a Clinical Forensic Team

In a rather comprehensive article, which concentrated on "enhanced involvement in assisting the living," several well-known forensic scientists explored challenges inherent in the role and responsibilities of the emerging clinical forensic medical specialist (Eckert, Bell, & Stein et al., 1986, p. 186). Among these are the following:

- Determination of trauma; physical, sexual, and emotional abuse; assault; rape; and drug abuse.
- Identification of human rights violations, physical and emotional torture, or neglect while in custody of foreign governments, law enforcement agencies, jails, correctional institutions, detoxification centers, juvenile homes, foster and nursing homes, institutions for the retarded, public and private psychiatric institutions, or private homes.
- Determination of unsafe conditions and products, analyses of injuries and illnesses involving electrical burns, fires, toy-related accidents, food and foreign body asphyxiation, ingestion of toxic agents (including lead poisoning), hyperthermia, and hypothermia. Also included within this category would be wider environmental hazards in the workplace and the general environment.

The hospital staff most often comes in contact with police in the emergency department (ED) along with the victims of violence as well as the alleged perpetrators of crime. Every hospital, regardless of size and location, eventually must address problems of conflict with law enforcement agencies regarding patients in legal custody. Policies that increase mutual understanding, define responsibilities, and promote coordination contribute to multidisciplinary, multiagency cooperation. The nurse's role as a clinical investigator provides a vital liaison between the investigative process and courts of law.

If effective forensic protocols for medical-surgical interface are not established, the relationship of these multidisciplinary teams can be damaged if practices are breached. This occurs when police officers and hospital staff are not familiar with procedures that are supposed to be followed by each respective discipline (Lynch, 1995).

Challenges for Clinical Forensic Practitioners

Early recognition of the serious failure to implement clinical forensic standards has led to the development of forensic nursing services. This movement was initiated by forensic pathologists, as well as the Office of the US Surgeon General in attention to violence as a major public health concern.

Forensic pathologists, often the recipient of the consequences of negligent forensic practice in hospital emergency departments, sought to educate nurses and emergency physicians regarding the need to properly document injury and recover evidence prior to alteration of wounds and loss or destruction of forensically significant material. Past US Surgeon General C. Everett Koop challenged healthcare professionals to participate in a close working relationship with law enforcement and the courts involving crimes against persons (National Organization for Victim Assistance [NOVA], 1989).

Interdisciplinary Conflicts

Frequently historical friction has developed between police officers and nurses who fail to recognize their mutual responsibilities in clinical and criminal investigations. This is nothing new.

One early example cited by Friedman concerns a major misunderstanding that occurred in New York City between a nurse and police officers over the care of a handcuffed prisoner (Friedman, 1978). The conflict resulted in the nurse being arrested, handcuffed, and taken to jail. This reflects a common attitude by police that nurses frequently obstruct justice, and the nurses view the police as using unnecessary force or invading the patient's privacy. The Civilian Complaint Review Board, a group of New York City citizens appointed to hear grievances against the police department, upheld the officer's actions on appeal by the nurse.

Historically, far greater complaints by law enforcement officers concerning nurses refer to their constant struggle to save evidence from the well-meaning hands of uninformed clinical practitioners. Oversight in many instances has ruined the prosecution's case against a perpetrator of crime (Turner, 1984). In an effort to reduce the damage to evidence and increase a mutual working relationship between police and ED nurses, Providence Hospital in Oakland, California, devised and implemented a protocol providing information on basic police techniques. Among the most important requests by police was for nurses to preserve clothing removed from injured patients in one piece when possible. For example, cutting through a bullet hole in clothing or tissue may destroy its potential value as evidence.

Another early endeavor to improve coordination and cooperation at Bellevue Hospital in New York City included a "basic ballistic course" for nurses by the New York City Police Department to insure that the ED staff had proper training in the removal, preservation, and identification of projectiles. A most innovative program for improving hospital-police relations occurred in Oakland, California, when nurses were asked to ride along with police officers in patrol vehicles to learn more about police procedures. The program proved to be twofold in its usefulness. Nurses agreed it gave them more insight into the responsibilities of the police, and it also provided police officers with advice on emergency patient care (Friedman, 1978). These informal arrangements strengthen more formal arrangements necessary in times of crisis.

Educational Deficits

In a classic forensic document, Dr. Ivor E. Doney, a forensic medical examiner (FME) in the United Kingdom, emphasized the need for first responders involved in immediate clinical forensic assessment of victims or persons in police custody to establish standards (Doney, 1988). Dr. Doney asserted that the forensic scientist who analyzes the evidence is entitled to know that other members of the multidisciplinary team have provided competent service and that the specimens they are examining are indeed accurate. Doney emphasized that if the first professionals to see the patient are not prepared to give reliable testimony or if vital evidence is overlooked, they are not capable of supplying the experts with the accurate specimens or data required.

Dr. Doney also expressed regret that forensic education has been neglected, resulting in no sufficient guarantee of efficiency from health professionals. If medicolegal standards are not taught, the first responder may compromise clinical judgment when police require medical information. He further emphasized the need for expert witness education and training in the standards and rules of evidence recovery.

Doney cautioned nurses in the ED to recognize and preserve vital fragments of trace evidence before washing it away "in a sea of wound-cleansing liquid" (Doney, 1988). His concern incorporates the physician who would suture a wound with little regard for subsequent examination as to the forensic aspects of the case. He pointed out that it is not possible to have trained personnel everywhere, yet with a call for greater awareness from all health professionals in all countries for standards and protocol, it is hoped that the multidisciplinary forensic team will be able to provide the necessary guidance.

Key Point *1-1*

JCAHO guidelines stress that evidentiary materials must be identified, retained, and safeguarded as part of the screening and assessment processes. (Joint Commission on Accreditation of Healthcare Organizations [JCAHO], 2004)

Advent of Forensic Nursing

Nursing advancements typically parallel those of colleagues in medicine (see Box 1-3). The strong foundations of forensic medicine that were well established on the European mainland were obviously influential in the early development of such nursing roles in those countries. Historical documents reveal that prior to the French Revolution, (nurse) midwives testified regarding sexual assault and pregnancy, undoubtedly an early prototype of the forensic nurse examiner (Camp, 1976). In the United Kingdom, forensic psychiatric nurses have been important members of the clinical forensic team for centuries. As the value of such practitioners was recognized within law enforcement agencies and legal communities, a trend toward the clinical forensic disciplines was ignited in North America as well (Lynch & Standing Bear, 2000).

Framework for Practice

The theoretical model of forensic nursing evolved from the role of the police surgeon or police medical officer of the United Kingdom (Lynch, 1990). This medical officer is contemporarily known as a forensic medical examiner (FME) in order to prevent a

Box 1-3 Comparative Practice Model for Forensic Disciplines

THE FORENSIC ASPECTS OF HEALTHCARE PROFESSIONS

MEDICINE	NURSING
Pathology	Death investigation
Psychiatry	Psychiatric nursing
Clinical forensic physician	Clinical forensic nurse
Sexual assault examiner	Sexual assault examiner
Medical jurisprudence	Nursing jurisprudence
Forensic medical examiner	Forensic nurse examiner
Corrections medical officer	Corrections or custody nurse
Legal medical consultants	Legal nurse consultants

Box 1-4 Chronology of Forensic Nursing

18th and 19th centuries	Development of clinical forensic medical science in Europe, South America, Asia, Russia, etc.
1986	Lynch initiates formal curricula for forensic nursing at University of Texas at Arlington with focus on scientific investigation of death
1988	McNamara introduces concept of clinical forensic practice or *living forensics*
	Lynch develops forensic nursing model
	Lynch expands curricula to include clinical forensic nursing.
1989	Lynch introduces forensic nursing as a scientific discipline
1991	International Association of Forensic Nurses founded
	American Academy of Forensic Sciences formally recognizes forensic nursing
	Clinical Forensic Medical program established at University of Louisville
1995	American Nurses Association's Congress of Nursing Practice grants specialty status to forensic nursing
1997	*Scope and Standards of Forensic Nursing Practice* published jointly by IAFN and the ANA
2000	IAFN celebrates 10th anniversary with membership of more than 2000

misconception of bias associated with the police. This practitioner of clinical forensic medicine is generally hired by the police department, Department of Health, or minister of justice in different countries and is responsible for the crime victim or suspect from the scene of the incident, clinical admission, or court-ordered evaluation throughout the judicial process.

The application of clinical medicine and nursing to trauma patients or those in legal custody involves trauma detection and preservation of forensic evidence. This role emphasizes the importance of thinking critically about the legal issues surrounding patient care. A serious gap in the criminal justice system has been either left open or only partially filled by health and justice practitioners who are essentially without a forensic background (Lynch, 1995). This arena includes not only nurses but also hospital physicians, emergency medical technicians, police officers, and attorneys. These individuals must be able to recognize problems in the existing system and raise the awareness of potential solutions.

In 1991, the American Academy of Forensic Sciences formally recognized forensic nursing as a scientific discipline. In 1992, the International Association of Forensic Nurses (IAFN) was established in Minneapolis, Minnesota, by sexual assault nurses who were meeting to form an organization addressing their special needs (see Box 1-4 for the chronology of forensic nursing). During the discussions, it was agreed that all acts of human violence, not only sexual assault, should be central to the mission of the newly charted nursing organization. In 1993 the IAFN, working in concert with the Center for Professional and Applied Ethics at Valdosta State University and the American Chemical Association, developed its code of ethics (see Appendix A). The IAFN now embraces more than 2500 nurses from a wide variety of subspecialties, including clinical forensic nurses, nurse death investigators, nurse coroners, correctional and forensic psychiatric nurses, sexual assault nurse examiners, nurse attorneys, legal nurse consultants, and several other fields. In 1995, forensic nursing was formally granted nursing specialty status when the American Nurses Association's Congress of Nursing Practice approved the Scope and Standards of Forensic Nursing Practice. These forensic nursing standards are designed to outline the roles and responsibilities of these specialists to assist legislators, law enforcement officers, attorneys, and others to appreciate the framework for forensic nursing practice.

Forensic Nursing Process: a Framework for Accountability

In order to gain full acceptance as a nursing specialty, forensic nursing was required to analyze its practice and define itself in terms of the *nursing process*, a goal-directed, dynamic framework for the roles and responsibilities inherent within the discipline. Although nurses had used a systematic approach to nursing problems for well over a century, it was not until 1973 that the American Nurses Association (ANA) Standards of Practice formalized what is now referred to as the nursing process. The nursing process is a scientific method that nurses use to provide care, beginning with an initial patient assessment and the establishment of a nursing diagnosis. Planning, intervention, and evaluation activities complete the nursing process. The steps of the nursing process, coupled with the knowledge and skills inherent within the discipline, have provided both structure and a common nomenclature to the work of nursing.

The ANA Congress of Nursing Practice requires specific criteria to be recognized as a formal specialty of nursing. The core of forensic nursing has been established to support the nursing process including assessment, analysis, nursing diagnosis, outcome identification, planning, and implementation of interventions and evaluation of responses to its nursing practices. Rules, regulations, and a variety of public policies influence and confirm the validity of forensic nursing as a specialty. The ANA's practice guidelines described in Nursing's Social Policy Statement and Standards of Clinical Nursing Practice are vital elements for both justification and framing of a specialty practice. A fundamental requirement for a nursing specialty is that it influences both the processes and outcomes of nursing care delivery. The Scope and Standards of Forensic Nursing Practice is expected to provide basic direction to educators, researchers, and administrators as well as forensic nurse practitioners.

Process of Specialty Recognition

To receive specialty status, a practice area must be defined distinctly from other areas of nursing in regard to its purpose and functions. In addition, the rationale for the need for the specialty must be well outlined, along with supporting data that there is an existing group of nurses devoting themselves to such a practice arena. These background data are described in a written document submitted to the Congress of Nursing Practice of the ANA for approval. A vital component, of course, is graduate education, evidence of a research-based body of knowledge, and means of dissemination of this research to nurses engaged in the specialty. The presence of the IAFN and its code of ethics, along with a network of publications and scientific meetings, were vital preludes to petitioning the Congress of Nursing Practice for formal recognition (IAFN, 1993).

Nursing's Social Policy Statement requires that a specialty delineate a core of practice including roles, responsibilities, functions, and skills of a unique body of knowledge (ANA, 1995). Dimensions, boundaries, and intersections must be outlined to justify the placement of the specialty practice within the broader collegial and collaborative interfaces with other healthcare and social groups related to the discipline. In the case of forensic nursing, the relevant relationships of law enforcement, public policy, and legal standards were illustrated to explain forensic nursing and describe the environment for its practice. Social consciousness, healthcare delivery trends, emerging technology, and the demands of societal organizations are used to confirm the needs for a practice specialty. The Scope and Standards of Forensic Nursing Practice is designed as a living document, subject to revision, because forensic nursing's structural framework is based on dynamic factors that are reactionary to multiple components of healthcare, social justice, and consumer demands.

The nursing process is likely to be used as a framework for curricula in schools of nursing, and agencies responsible for state licensure and specialty certification use its various components to describe roles and responsibilities of clinicians. The Joint Commission on Accreditation of Healthcare Organizations (JCAHO) has required hospitals and other healthcare facilities seeking accreditation to demonstrate its use of the nursing process. The ANA granted specialty status to forensic nursing based on its demonstrated use of the nursing process.

Forensic nurses care for individuals whose illness, injury, or death stems from acts of violence, maltreatment, abuse, neglect, or exploitation. The forensic nursing process is client centered and establishes a feedback loop that ensures a dynamic mechanism for the reevaluation and revision of care plans. Collaboration is vital to the forensic nursing process. Without strong links to other practitioners within law enforcement and the judicial systems, as well as other healthcare and social support personnel, successful forensic nursing interventions could not occur. Although evaluation is multifaceted and may take place at several points throughout the course of forensic case management, the true evaluation occurs when the victim returns to society and functions at a level consistent with preincident functioning. Perpetrators of abuse and violence are also subjects of the forensic nursing process. Unless there are major efforts to understand and alter the human and social conditions that contribute to abuse, neglect, violence, and exploitation, forensic nursing will fall short of its mission objectives. The major tools and techniques of forensic nursing specialists include forensic assessment and clinical investigative procedures in both the living and the dead. It is obvious that the forensic nursing process is a collaborative one, encompassing a wide array of physical, psychological, social, and legal interventions from both healthcare and jurisprudence domains.

Forensic Assessment and Nursing Diagnosis

The first step of the nursing process is patient assessment, which includes a head-to-toe inspection of the body, history taking, and a review of clinical records or other previous documentation. Because a nurse is typically the first professional to encounter a patient in the healthcare setting, initial observations and information, even selected fragments, significantly impact the steps that follow. The systematic assessment should include both objective physical findings and subjective data based on the patient's perceptions about his or her condition. A perceptive nurse is in a key position to note problems that might otherwise be missed. Skilled assessments are essential to evaluate patients and to ensure that they receive the appropriate treatment and follow-up care. All initial assessments must be supplemented by ongoing evaluations and monitoring to test the working nursing diagnosis and to identify a need for revisions of the care plan. The nurse's abilities to elicit, organize, and convey information from the initial screening process are vital to ensure that significant bits of information are not overlooked or undervalued in later forensic analyses of the incident. All data must be precisely documented, steering clear, however, of making interpretive statements in records. The environment for assessing the forensic patient must ensure that both visual and auditory privacy are assured and that forensic evidence collection is well supported within the space provided.

Key Point *1-2*

All healthcare personnel must be able to use interview skills and physical assessment indicators to detect abuse and neglect.

Nursing Diagnosis: Basis for Nursing Care Plans

Nursing diagnosis is a clinical judgment about individual, family, or community responses to actual and potential health problems/life processes. In 1990 the North American Nursing Diagnosis Association (NANDA) stated that nursing diagnoses provide the basis for selection of nursing interventions to achieve outcomes for which the nurse is accountable.

The nursing diagnosis is a statement that evolves from the interpretation and analysis of data. Each represents a problem, a related phenomenon, and specific manifestations with implications for nursing intervention. Domains of nursing diagnoses relate to physiology (basic and complex), behavior, family, health system, and safety. Functional health status, homeostatic regulation, psychological functioning, lifestyle change, family support, healthcare delivery system use, and safety are all pertinent factors in nursing diagnoses formulation.

For example, in instances of domestic violence or human abuse, pertinent diagnoses might include the following:

- Ineffective coping related to inability to manage situational crisis
- Fear related to perceived ability to control situation
- Sleep pattern disturbances related to anxiety
- Anxiety related to discussion of intimate information, diagnosis and concern for partner

The potential for errors related to the establishment of an appropriate nursing diagnosis may include both shortcomings in data collection and interpretation. A broad, sound knowledge base and pertinent clinical experiences are vital for forensic nurses. Having repeated opportunities to deal with the same or similar problems leads to the development of a keen sense of differentiating normal from abnormal based on pattern analysis. Furthermore, critical thinking skills tend to improve with both time and exposure to common problems.

The value of a well-formulated forensic nursing diagnosis promotes professional accountability and autonomy by defining and describing the independent area of nursing practice. Diagnostic statements also provide an effective way for nurses to communicate among themselves and with other health professionals and are included in the framework for forensic nursing research (see Appendix B).

Planning

Planning to meet the needs of forensic patients encompasses an array of both simple and complex activities and may be directed toward achieving either short-term or long-term objectives. Merely taking steps to provide visual and auditory privacy during a confidential forensic interview and placing a "Do Not Disturb" sign on the room door is a plan, albeit a low level of planning. A more effective option is the Special Exam Suite designated for forensic patients located away from the ED where privacy and accessibility for patients, families, and police officers has become the preferred choice in many hospitals and trauma centers. More typically, when a nursing care plan is outlined, it includes a rather complex series of activities that extend over days, weeks, or even months. It may involve other nurses, other disciplines, and perhaps an array of outside agencies or resources. Optimum nursing plans not only address the patients' priority needs and problems but also enumerate the activities or processes deemed appropriate to minimize or resolve the problems. Planning mandates the formulation of short- and long-term goals. The ideal forensic examination is carefully implemented to decrease emotional trauma while increasing optimal forensic evidence recovery.

Intervention

Nursing interventions are often described as the core of the nursing process. Interventions encompass providing and directing treatment as well as working with a variety of other healthcare workers who also contribute to care provision. In past decades, when nursing interventions were described, they typically represented dependent tasks from the medical plan of care such as giving prescribed medications or doing treatments ordered by the physician. Forensic nurses, however, often function with standing orders, protocols, algorithms, or other directives based on requirements of law enforcement or the judicial processes. As a result, their independence in practice distinguishes them from many other nurses and clearly establishes them in a position of considerable responsibility. Forensic nursing interventions must be continually evaluated and revised based on the response of the patient or specific legal criteria if the patient dies.

Evaluation

The process of evaluation must take into account all data generated in the nurse-patient encounter. For example, the forensic implications of trauma may not be fully recognized until several days, weeks, or even months after the precipitating event. If the patient does not seem to be responding as expected, or if unexpected variables or circumstances arise, the forensic nurse must be ready to respond with alternative strategies to achieve the desired outcomes. Feedback must be derived from the patient and from significant associates and other members of the care team such as advocates, attorneys, therapists, law enforcement officers, and counselors who maintain relationships with the patient and thus have an opportunity to assess responses to interventional strategies. The standard for measuring patient progress and current status is based on established goals and outcomes.

Nursing goals and outcomes are derived from the nursing process and focus on patient responses, *not nursing activities.* Standards are stated in concrete, measurable terms and written to ensure that other members of the healthcare team understand and affirm them. Goals and outcomes represent safe, appropriate nursing care strategies and deemed achievable by the health and justice teams.

Because forensic nurses often encounter patients with the same or similar problems, they may choose to use generic or preformulated care plans. Protocols, policies, and procedures, standing orders, computerized care plans, and algorithms reflect practices designed to achieve care plan standardization. Roles of the forensic nurse examiner often overlap and require specific education and cross-training in other subspecialties of forensic nursing to effectively evaluate a rape victim who is also the focus of a death investigation inquiry. This patient may be both a victim of child abuse, sexual assault, and homicide as well as having survived as a clinical forensic patient for two weeks on artificial ventilation prior to death. This patient may also be a candidate for organ donation requiring further social and legal interventions.

All steps of the nursing process are vital to every patient encounter. Even when the situation or time constraints pose limitations, the forensic nurse must not lose the vision of the systematic and scientific, legal healthcare processes. It should be viewed as a vital problem-solving tool and a way for organizing a logical and responsible course of action.

Key Point *1-3*

The structure of the entire forensic nursing process is predicated on maintaining a certain state of mind—an investigative, interpretive, dogmatic search for the facts and the truth (NANDA, 1990).

As a public service profession, nursing has a responsibility to maintain standards of practice in processing cases involving patients associated with human violence. Due to the vast number of crime victims presenting in the ED from trauma or public health considerations, the need for a forensic specialist has been recognized. A historic lack of interagency cooperation involving law and nursing issues, as well as the absence of forensic education available to nurses, has often threatened the patient's legal rights, resulting in miscarriages of justice. There is growing support among those who understand the significant contribution of the role of the clinical forensic specialist in the advocacy and ministration to this plight. The National Victim's Center has recognized forensic nursing as a movement in *patient advocacy,* whether victim or suspect (NOVA, 1988).

Anyone suspected of a crime that the person did not commit becomes a victim of another kind. The forensic nurse must remain an unbiased, objective clinician throughout the scientific evaluation of injury and documentation of evidence in order to refrain from projecting a preconceived opinion or conclusion prior to adjudication of the defendant.

The problems in society for which this role has been designed to provide solutions are great and multifaceted. These needs require education and expertise that is equally diversified. There are many disciplines that participate in the process of forensic evaluation, working in conjunction with law enforcement agencies in the investigation of injury and death. Among these are forensic pathologists, odontologists, questioned document experts, photographers, entomologists, anthropologists, engineers, attorneys, psychiatrists, and, of course, nurses.

Prevention of Violence

Prevention is a key aspect of traditional nursing care and an imperative one for forensic nursing practice. By educating nurses to think more about the legal issues surrounding patient care and to have a working knowledge of forensic responsibilities, the healthcare system will be able to provide a proactive approach. The identification of crime victims, prevention of further injury or death from recurring cyclical violence, and early detection of potentially abusive situations will help stem society's escalating crime patterns and prove to be cost-effective for governments. Through implementing healthcare policies and practices that address forensic issues in nursing education, critical changes will be effected in the prevention of child abuse and crimes against women and the elderly. These policies will aid law enforcement in meeting the objectives of criminal investigation. Nurse educators must assume the responsibility for establishing formal education programs in this nursing specialty to assist in confronting violence in our society and to alleviate human suffering resulting from this global health problem.

Pilot programs to educate nurses and other healthcare professionals to work in synthesis with law enforcement and the forensic sciences must continue to be developed and implemented. To provide adequate education and scope of practice for the forensic nursing specialist, one first must recognize the combination of knowledge required to go beyond mere treatment of symptoms and injuries and to fill a greater role in medicolegal (forensic) expertise.

It is also important to consider that JCAHO has specific guidance that mandates policies and procedure for handling adult and child victims of alleged or suspected abuse or neglect. A proactive protocol for preventive practice emphasizes the importance of indoctrinating professional staff in the philosophy and practices of clinical forensic science.

Clinical forensic education for ED nurses encompasses forensic photography, jurisprudence, environmental terrorism, wound and bite mark recognition/interpretation, human abuse and neglect, sexual assault, substance abuse, tissue and organ donation, and other essential subjects. This must begin with emergency interventions.

Best Practice 1-1

Every individual who works in a healthcare facility should receive basic forensic education. This is essential to meet JCAHO's standards and limit liability in the event of a failure to recognize indications of injuries associated with sexual assault, child or elder abuse, domestic violence, or other forensic trauma.

Forensic Patient Categories

Research by Pasqualone (1998) distinguishes the *Forensic Categories among Patients Seen in the Emergency Department* and recognizes a general lack of knowledge about forensic issues within emergency healthcare systems:

> *This necessitates a need for the categorization of this unique patient base. A systematic approach to the clarification and delineation of forensic categories is compulsory, should the need arise to provide evidence in a litigious situation. Concise, chronological identification and documentation of these evidentiary groupings is essential as a prerequisite of current and future ED nurses' inevitable direct involvement in judicial proceedings. (Pasqualone, 2003)*

Demographics of the Study

The setting for this study (Table 1-1) was the ED of a small community hospital within 10 miles of a major metropolitan city in eastern Massachusetts. The hospital's ED sees approximately 22,500 patients each year. The categorization system was developed from a retrospective study of ED medical records. The population studied consisted of every person (n = 3436) admitted

Table 1-1 Percentages of Forensic Categories Seen at a Community Hospital Emergency Department

SAMPLE POPULATION BASED ON A 60-DAY SURVEY (N = 3436)
914 PATIENTS (27%) QUALIFIED AS FORENSIC CASES

FORENSIC CATEGORY	FREQUENCY	PERCENTAGE (%)
Occupation-related injuries	289	8.41
Transportation injuries	193	5.62
Substance abuse	160	4.66
Personal injury	125	3.64
Child abuse and neglect	464 per year	2.06*
Forensic psych	49	1.43
Environmental hazards	25	0.73
Assault and battery	22	0.64
Abuse of the disabled	130 per year	0.58*
Human and animal bites	90 per year	0.40*
Questioned death cases	10	0.29
Elder abuse and neglect	56 per year	0.25*
Domestic violence	6	0.17
Clients in police custody	2	0.06
Sexual assault	2	0.06
Sharp force injuries	7 per year	0.03*
Product liability	1	0.03
Transcultural medical practices	1	0.03
Organ and tissue donation	6 per year	0.03*
Burns >5% BSA (body surface area)	3 per year	0.01*
Firearm injuries	7 per 3 years	0.01*
Food and drug tampering	0	
Gang violence	0	
Malpractice and/or negligence	0	

*Data based on a yearly ED population of 22,500.
From Pasqualone, G. (1998). *An examination of forensic categories among patients seen at a community hospital emergency department.* Unpublished master's thesis, Fitchburg State College, Fitchburg, MA.

to the ED during a 60-day period. The chart represents the 24 categories and the percentages of occurrences. The categories of child, elder, and disabled abuse and neglect; human and animal bites; sharp force injuries; organ and tissue donation; burns; and firearm injuries were extrapolated from ED admissions and statistics of mandated reports taken over a 1-year period. Although food and drug tampering, gang violence, and malpractice and/or negligence were not categories identified among the ED population during the study, they are categories having the potential of occurrence at any time in any ED.

Recommendations for Advanced Practice

There is an established need to place advanced practice clinical forensic nurse examiners in hospitals, nursing homes, criminal justice systems, and elsewhere in our communities to act as liaisons between healthcare and the law. Nurses will be prepared to enter into this new career field as medicolegal consultants for attorneys, insurance companies, law enforcement agencies, medical examiner and coroner systems, schools (K-12), university campus sexual assault centers, and healthcare administration and emergency services systems. Questions have been raised regarding the necessity of advanced practice in forensic nursing science. It must be recognized that rationale for advanced education in forensic nursing practice is essential for the same reason nurses have advanced practice in any other specialty of nursing. All nursing care and treatment plans for forensic patients must be designed and managed to ensure that the patient's legal rights are consistently protected as mandated by law or regulatory guidance.

Forensic nurse examiners are responsible for advancing the science of forensic nursing in a broad area of legal issues, such as pronouncement of death, rape examinations, management of prescriptive medication dispensed on discharge, documentation of child maltreatment, expert witness testimony, and research that will define the contributions of forensic nursing to society. Advanced practice does not necessitate all nurses to practice the principles and philosophies of forensic nursing science although this knowledge will enhance all nursing assessments and actions. Three major categories of forensic nursing practice have been recognized: basic forensic nursing, general forensic nursing, and advanced forensic nursing or specialty practice, such as a clinical nurse specialist or nurse practitioner role, which requires a minimum of a master's degree, prescriptive authority, or doctoral education.

One should also consider that in the twenty-first century it is no longer acceptable for any discipline to be identified as a professional practice without a minimal entry-level degree. Consider that forensic nurse examiners will be compared and evaluated by the peers with whom they work and communicate within courts of law. Physicians, forensic scientists, and attorneys are required to have degrees or specialty training beyond basic entry level education, thus becoming the standards by which forensic nurses will be judged.

Role of the Clinical Forensic Nurse

With the ever-increasing medicolegal emphasis in clinical practice, the role of the clinical forensic nurse is emerging. This role is designed to provide one solution to identified medicolegal related problems in clinical or community environs. In addition to medicolegal concerns, sensitivity to victims and families has historically been a responsibility of patient advocates. The policy of advocacy now, however, is to include, to the fullest extent, criminal justice and health service providers (Lynch, 1995). This positive change in policy supports the growing awareness of the need for forensic specialization in the biomedical and social sciences that will incorporate emergency and client advocacy interventions while providing scientific knowledge to combat destructive social, cultural, and political conditions.

The forensic nurse examiner provides a valuable link in interagency cooperation and coordination as well as enhances the care of patients and their significant others. This ever-widening field is being made apparent as more holistic approaches to antiviolence strategies are explored and developed. Roles that promote cooperation contribute to communication and interaction between police officers and the ED staff.

Future Horizons in Clinical Forensic Nursing

The loss of human life and function due to violence constitutes a phenomenon that affects the lives of millions of individuals worldwide. These cases represent a major cost in healthcare as well as an increased burden on the criminal justice systems. Previous resources for victims from law enforcement, social services, and the courts have been identified as inadequate in light of the dimension of the problem (NOVA, 1989). Forensic nursing is one example of an expansion of the role nurses will fill in the healthcare delivery system in the twenty-first century. Forensic nurses have initiated positive change vis-à-vis mutual responsibility with the legal system to protect the patient's legal, civil, and human rights. The role of the forensic nurse as a clinical investigator is one approach to aiding law enforcement and the criminal justice system in combating criminal and interpersonal violence through a multidisciplinary approach.

As a new era of nursing practice approaches, forensic nursing has unlimited potential. With the increasing emphasis on forensic nursing services as one strategic step to interrupt cyclical, interpersonal violence, it is perceived that this paradigm will be considered *as essential as infection control.* Those who understand the need for a forensic specialist in nursing believe it is realistic to expect that JCAHO will one day require every hospital or trauma center to have on staff a forensically skilled nurse to ensure that legal mandates are met with reasonable certainty.

Summary

Prior to the evolution of the clinical forensic specialist in the US, victims or perpetrators of crime who required a forensic evaluation and collection of evidence had to have died from catastrophic circumstances or unknown causes in order to receive a forensic examination. Because only a few physicians are educated in forensic medicine and authorized by law to perform post mortem forensic examinations, collect evidence, and testify in court, individuals who survived were frequently deprived of quality forensic services. The shortage of skilled forensic clinicians has often resulted in a miscarriage of justice, both in the US and in other parts of the world. However, with developing partnerships between healthcare and the law, new paradigms of clinical practice are being realized. The forensic nursing specialist blends nursing's traditional acumen with those of forensic science and criminal justice. This new clinical practitioner has proven to be a valuable asset in the efforts to prevent or reduce interpersonal crimes against vulnerable victims of social crime. Forensic specialization in nursing is emerging in many countries, resulting in a new professional image and exciting global career opportunities.

Resources

Books

American Nurses Association and the International Association of Forensic Nurses. (1998). *Scope and standards of forensic nursing practice.* Washington, DC: Authors.

Joint Commission on Accreditation of Healthcare Organizations (JCAHO). (2004). *Accreditation manual for hospitals, core standards, and guidelines.* Oak Park, IL: Author.

References

American Academy of Forensic Sciences (AAFS). (2002). Membership information brochure. Colorado Springs, CO: Author.

American Nurses Association (ANA). (1995). Nursing's social policy statement. Washington, DC: Author.

Camp, F. (1976). *Gradwold's legal medicine* (3rd ed.). Chicago: Yearbook Medical Publication.

Doney, I. (1988). Who is first on the scene? *Forensic Sci Int, 36*(2), 15-20.

Eckert, W., Bell, J., Stein, R., et al. (1986). Clinical forensic medicine. *Am J Forensic Med Path, 7*(3), 182-185.

Friedman, E. (1978). The men in blue pair up with the people in white. *Hospitals, 52*(22), 153-163.

International Association of Forensic Nurses. (1993). *Codes of ethics for forensic nursing.* Thorofare, NJ: Author.

Joint Commission on Accreditation of Healthcare Organizations (JCAHO). (2004). Accreditation manual for hospitals, core standards, and guidelines. Oak Park, IL: Author.

Lynch, V. (1990). *Clinical forensic nursing: A descriptive study in role development.* Thesis, University of Texas at Arlington.

Lynch, V. (1991). Application for new discipline in forensic nursing. *American Academy of Forensic Sciences.* Archives of the General Section Annual Scientific Meeting.

Lynch, V. (1995) Clinical forensic nursing: A new perspective in the management of crime victims from trauma to trial. *Crit Care Nurs Clin North Am, 7*(3), 489-507.

Lynch, V., & Standing Bear, Z. (2000). A global perspective in forensic nursing: Challenges for the 21st century. In D. Robinson & A. Kettles (Eds.), *Forensic nursing and multidisciplinary care of the mentally disordered offender* (pp. 249-266). Philadelphia: Jessica Kingsley.

McNamara, H. (1986). *Living forensics* (seminar pamphlet). Ulster County, NY: Office of the Medical Examiner.

National Organization for Victim Assistance (NOVA). (1988). *Newsletter, 12*(11).

National Organization for Victim Assistance (NOVA). (1989). President and surgeon general condemn violence against women, call for new attitudes, programs. *Newsletter, 13*(6).

North American Nursing Diagnosis Association (NANDA). (1990). *Taxonomy 1* (rev. ed., pp. 114-117). St. Louis, MO: Author.

Pasqualone, G. (1998). *An examination of forensic categories among patients seen at a community hospital emergency department.* Unpublished master's thesis. Fitchburg, MA: Fitchburg State College.

Pasqualone, G. (2003). Forensic categories among patients seen in the emergency department. *Forensic Nurse Magazine.* Retrieved from www.forensicnursemag.org.

Taber's Electronic Medical Dictionary. (2001). CD ROM v.2.0. Philadelphia: F. A. Davis.

Turner, J. (1984). *Violence in the medical care setting: A survival guide.* Rockville, MD: Aspen.

Chapter 2 Genesis and Development

William S. Smock

Overview

The practice of clinical forensic medicine, the application of forensic medical knowledge and techniques to living patients, has existed in Europe and Great Britain for more than two centuries (McLay, 1990). Professionals in this field go by various titles but most often are referred to as police surgeons, forensic medical officers, or forensic medical examiners. They practice in Asia, Latin America, Russia and Australia as well as Europe and Great Britain.

Until recently, the practices of medicine and nursing in the US have largely ignored the forensic issues of the living patient (Smock, 2002). The coroner, medical examiner, or combined coroner/medical examiner systems in the US, which are responsible for the investigation of unnatural and suspicious deaths, have also not traditionally been assigned the responsibility of dealing with the forensic issues of living patients. This then raises the question of who *is* responsible for addressing the forensic needs of those who by surviving their trauma miss a date for the ultimate forensic medical procedure: the autopsy.

The earliest reference in the American medical literature that directly addresses the practice of forensic medicine on living patients is one by Root and Scott in 1973: "Forensic medicine often is either unrecognized as such or is consciously or subconsciously evaded" by practicing clinical physicians (Root & Scott, 1973). Trained as forensic pathologists, these physicians felt that if vital forensic questions were not answered in the living patient, justice would suffer, criminals would go free, and innocent persons could be convicted of crimes they did not commit.

Forensic Medicine in the Emergency Department

The first article to appear in US emergency medicine literature regarding forensic medicine in the emergency department came a decade later in 1983 (Smialek, 1983). In *Emergency Medicine Clinics of North America,* Smialek stated "medical care of the critically ill in the emergency department has a significant impact on the practice of forensic medicine. Many victims of homicide or accidents receive some degree of medical or surgical treatment prior to expiration." Smialek recognized that evidence, necessary to accurately reconstruct the event, prove guilt, or establish innocence was disappearing in the emergency department. This evidence was being destroyed, either by commission or omission, in the provision of patient care. That same year, Roger Mittleman, MD, a medical examiner for Dade County; Hollace Goldberg, RN, an emergency nurse; and David Waksman, JD, a state attorney for Florida, published "Preserving Evidence in the Emergency Department" in the *American Journal of Nursing* (Mittleman, 1983). This article emphasized the importance of recognizing and preserving evidence on patients presenting to the emergency department.

Key Point 2-1

The failure to incorporate forensic guidelines into the clinical assessment and management of patients may result in far-reaching consequences for the patient, the accused suspect, and, potentially, the hospital and its personnel.

Advent of Forensic Nursing in the US

Due to the identified weaknesses in trauma practices addressed in the literature, combined with professional experiences in death investigation witnessed by Virginia Lynch, her master's thesis advanced the concept of a clinical forensic specialist in nursing. As a graduate student at the University of Texas at Arlington, Lynch finalized her study in 1990, the first published literature titled "Clinical Forensic Nursing: A Descriptive Study in Role Development" (Lynch, 1990). The purpose of this descriptive study was to identify forensic role behaviors and to clarify role expectations of the emergency department nurses working with trauma victims. It further sought to identify and examine the differences between the frequency and perceived importance of selected forensic role behaviors performed by emergency department nurses.

This study promoted the need for a multidisciplinary team approach to the identification of forensic-related trauma and the recovery and preservation of evidence. Research results defined the appropriate application of selected forensic concepts to professional nursing practice and education, as well as to define the potential for a forensic clinical nurse specialist. The overall results of the survey defined 31 forensic role behaviors as appropriate for inclusion in hospital-based emergency department standards for practice. The examination of frequency means revealed a significant lack of performed forensic behaviors of emergency department nurses and physicians.

The perceived importance of the forensic application to trauma nursing indicated that 23 of the 37 role behaviors were identified as "important" to incorporate into practice, indicating that a gap clearly existed between applied practice and level of value. The outcomes of this research demonstrated a consensus among emergency department nurses and provided a strong support and acceptance of forensic nursing practices.

In conclusion, this landmark study set the pace for further examination and the development of a new discipline in the forensic and clinical sciences. Lynch challenged clinical practitioners, nurse educators, and hospital administrators about the responsibilities that nursing must assume in order to meet the needs and demands of our society. Furthermore, nursing education must provide curricula to encompass and support this body of knowledge. Nursing science must not be content to confine its interest to nursing alone, but join with other scientific disciplines and discover new truths within its own domain.

Forensic Science and Living Patients

In 1983, the late William Eckert, the driving force behind bringing clinical forensic medicine to the forefront of contemporary American medical practice, published "Forensic Sciences: The Clinical or Living Aspects" (Eckert, 1990). Eckert's concept of applying forensic techniques to living patients in the US was the basis for a 1986 article by Goldsmith in the *Journal of American Medical Association* (JAMA), "US Forensic Pathologist on a New Case: Examination of Living Patients" (Goldsmith, 1986).

Cyril Wecht, MD, JD, and former president of the American College of Legal Medicine, stated in Goldsmith's 1986 JAMA article that

> *it's a great shame and a source of much puzzlement why a group similar to police surgeons hasn't developed here. Even within our adversarial judicial system and with our guaranteed civil rights–which are much greater than in many of the countries where forensic clinicians are commonly found–I believe that persons with both medical and forensic training could remove much of the guesswork, speculation, and hypotheses from the disposition of accident or assault cases involving living persons.*

Wecht also supported development of forensic training courses for medical students and residents. Eventually Wecht came to lend his support and recognition to the developing specialty of forensic nursing.

Also in 1986, the American Academy of Forensic Sciences published an article by Eckert and several other forensic pathologists (Eckert, 1986). This was the academy's first article addressing the issue of living forensic medicine. Eckert felt very strongly that forensic scientists should expand their roles to "involve the examination of living persons."

With the interest generated by Eckert's writings and presentations, other medical professionals, including emergency nurses and physicians, sought to promote and develop living forensic medicine in the US. The pioneering force behind the development of forensic nursing as a recognized specialty, initially in the US and later internationally, was Virginia Lynch. Lynch also presented an abstract, the first on forensic nursing, at the American Academy of Forensic Sciences (AAFS) in 1986 (Lynch, 1986). By 1991, the academy had become the first to formally recognize forensic nursing as an emerging discipline in the forensic sciences. Based on the discipline description defined by Lynch, the academy extended membership to nurses qualified in clinical forensic practice and in the scientific investigation of death. Since that time, forensic nursing has become the most rapidly growing specialty in the forensic sciences according to the AAFS membership committee.

Forensic Nursing Education Launched

The University of Texas at Arlington established the first formal educational program in forensic nursing (Lynch, 1995). Samuel Hughes, professor and graduate dean of the school of nursing (now deceased), championed this novel addition to nursing education and the program was launched in 1986. The original curricula were designed to prepare the registered nurse as an associate to the forensic pathologist. Death investigation was to be the primary focus. However, with the attention to clinical forensic medicine through the Academy of Forensic Sciences, Lynch determined that the program concept would need to be expanded to include living patients in healthcare environments. When the original program admitted its first students, the curriculum incorporated clinical, bio-psycho-social and necropsy aspects of forensic care. Along with graduate nursing faculty, several elite members of the forensic and legal communities stepped forward to teach and to supervise clinical experiences for students. Nizam Peerwani, MD, chief medical examiner of the Tarrant and Parker County Medical Examiner's District in Fort Worth, Texas, was the first to offer his services as professor of forensic medicine at the University of North Texas to teach necropsy pathology as a core course in forensic nursing. Charles Petty, chief medical examiner of Dallas County, Dallas, Texas, accepted the invitation to teach the principles and philosophies of death investigation, while Irving Stone, chief criminalist at the Southwestern Institute of Forensic Sciences, agreed to incorporate forensic nurses into his courses in criminalistics (crime laboratory and crime scene investigation), as well as a course in expert witness testimony at the Southern Methodist University School of Law. Patrick Besant-Matthews, deputy chief medical examiner of Dallas County, supervised the nurse's clinical experience at the Southwestern Institute of Forensic Sciences.

Peerwani, Petty, Besant-Matthews, and Stone deserve to be commended for their collegiality, endorsement, and encouragement to these initial educational endeavors at the University of Texas at Arlington. Forensic nursing development would surely have been delayed without their support and willingness to volunteer their influence, time, and resources in support of nursing education.

The curriculum for the University of Texas at Arlington program served as a model for other nursing programs in the US and was the first graduate study option in forensic nursing included in the National League for Nursing's listing of specialized programs. Although first in curricular implementation, this program lost its opportunity to remain the premier program worldwide when its academic champion, graduate dean Samuel Hughes, died just prior to the graduation of the first class of students. However, with the publication of Lynch's master's thesis on clinical forensic nursing, the role of forensic science in nursing began to gain momentum.

In the mid-1990s, due to the efforts of Virginia Lynch, Ann Burgess, and other pacesetters, nursing educators began to appreciate the need to include forensic nursing in undergraduate and graduate curricula. Within the US, the University of Virginia at Charlottesville, the University of Massachusetts at Boston, Gonzaga University in Spokane, and Southern Connecticut State University in New Haven were among the first to offer forensic educational components to their nursing students. The Beth El College of Nursing and Health Sciences, University of Colorado in Colorado Springs, and Fitchburg State College School of Nursing in Fitchburg, Massachusetts, offer master's degrees in forensic nursing as others are developing. Other graduate programs, including the clinical nurse specialist master's program at the University of Massachusetts, School of Nursing, have included a 3-hour elective in forensic nursing. Countless schools of nursing have added forensic undergraduate courses, continuing education studies, and online nursing courses. Indiana University, the University of Texas at Austin, the University of New Mexico, and the University of California at Riverside are among these. Several international nurse educators have also introduced forensic nursing into their curricula. The University of Dundee, School of Medicine in Scotland, and the University of Calgary and Mt. Royal College of Nursing in Alberta, Canada, were among the first programs to initiate clinical forensic courses (Lynch, 1995). In 2003, the British Columbia Institute of Technology, an innovative and futuristic institution in Vancouver, implemented a forensic program in nursing and health sciences.

Living Forensic Practice Migrates to Emergency Departments

Harry C. McNamara, the chief medical examiner for Ulster County, New York, proposed in 1987 to provide forensic training to emergency nurses and physicians (McNamara, 1986). McNamara's experience as a medical examiner had demonstrated the existence of a serious gap in the criminal justice system when addressing the forensic needs of living patients. Principally, McNamara recognized that evidence was being destroyed or discarded, wounds were repaired or surgically altered without adequate description or documentation, and forensic opinions were being rendered without a factual basis.

The need, therefore, for forensic training for emergency physicians and nurses could not be overstated. Richard Carmona, MD, a trauma surgeon and US surgeon general, in 1989 reported that a review of 100 charts of trauma patients who presented to a Level 1 trauma center in California revealed poor, improper, or inadequate documentation in 70% of the cases (Carmona, 1989). Additionally, in 38% of cases potential evidence was improperly secured, improperly documented, or inadvertently discarded (Carmona, 1989). The message from the medical and law enforcement communities was clear: A patient's evaluation must be adequately documented narratively, diagrammatically, and photographically, in the patient's chart for possible use in future legal actions. The failure to do so may have far-ranging consequences for the hospital, the patient, the accused, and potentially the treating physician.

Key Point 2-2

The concept of "living forensics" provided the linchpin for the role development and legitimacy of clinical forensic practice in hospital emergency departments and other patient care settings.

Graduate and Post-Graduate Education in the 1990s

In 1990, based on the work and efforts of Eckert, McNamara, and Lynch, many emergency nursing and medicine programs began to see the need to introduce formal clinical forensic education and training (Eckert, 1990). The first clinical forensic medicine conference in the US was a two-day seminar convened in Chicago for emergency physicians in 1990. The program was sponsored by the Illinois chapter of the American College of Emergency Physicians under the direction of Constance Green. This program was suspended after its first year. In July of the same year, Bill Smock, of the Department of Emergency Medicine at the University of Louisville, School of Medicine, and George Nichols II, then the chief medical examiner for the commonwealth of Kentucky, initiated the first formal clinical forensic medicine consultation service in the US (Smock, 1994). A forensic physician, either a forensically trained emergency physician or a forensic pathologist, was made available to respond to the emergency department or other inpatient facility on a 24-hour basis.

In 1990, the primary year of clinical forensic awareness in the US, Lynch studied with police surgeons in London; concurrently, Bill Smock of the University of Louisville was in Scotland, collaborating with the founders of clinical forensic medicine. Unaware of one another's activities, each of these pioneers was gleaning information to form the basis for clinical forensic educational programs that would soon be developed in the US. Since that time, Lynch and Smock have combined forces and continue to advance the skills and practice of clinical forensic nursing and medicine worldwide.

In July 1991, Smock and Nichols II also established the first formal clinical forensic medicine training program for emergency physicians in the US (Smock, 1994). It was designed to introduce forensic topics and techniques into the core curriculum of a residency training program in emergency medicine (Box 2-1). Lectures were given by local, regional, and visiting forensic physicians, prosecuting attorneys, and forensic odontologists as well as by expert criminalists from police agencies and crime laboratories. Later that year, "Clinical Forensic Medicine in the Emergency Department" was presented at the annual scientific assembly of the American College of Emergency Physicians (ACEP) (Smock & Nichols, 1991). This was the first time that forensic medicine had been exhibited at an ACEP forum.

Also in 1991, Lynch published "Forensic Nursing in the Emergency Department: A New Role for the 1990s" (Lynch, 1991). This article clearly charted the course for forensic nursing during the 1990s. Lynch made irrefutable arguments for the inclusion of forensic nurse examiners (FNE) as a functional component of emegency department care. These nursing specialists were expected to expand their knowledge and skills beyond sexual assault examination to include forensic photography, wound identification, evidence collection, and expert testimony.

In 1993, the University of Louisville, School of Medicine, also offered the first fellowship in clinical forensic medicine in the US. This 1-year fellowship is offered to graduates of emergency

Box 2-1 Clinical Forensic Medicine Curricular Topics

Firearms analysis
Blood spatter analysis
Crime scene investigation
Forensic photography
Forensic serology and DNA analysis
Evaluation of the physically assaulted child
Evaluation of the physically assaulted adult
Evaluation and examination of gunshot wounds
Determination of driver versus passenger
Courtroom presentations and expert testimony
Evaluation and examination of sexually assaulted patients
Forensic aspects of pedestrian collisions
Evidence collection and chain of custody
Forensic odontology and the recognition of bite marks
Motor vehicle accident reconstruction
Toxicology and pharmacology
Forensic psychiatry
Forensic analysis of blunt trauma
Forensic anatomy and mechanism of injury

Note: The order and sequence of topics may vary based on actual case presentations in the emergency department and availability of faculty resources.

Table 2-1 Number of Didactic Hours Dedicated to Forensic Topics per Year for Emergency Medicine Residents

TOPIC	HOURS
Forensic evaluation of gunshot wounds	4
Forensic photography	2
Pediatric physical abuse/assault	2
Pediatric sexual abuse/assault	2
Courtroom presentation and expert testimony	2
Forensic evaluation of blunt trauma and domestic violence	2
Firearms and ballistics	2
Forensic odontology and bite marks	1
Adult sexual assault	1
Evidence collection and chain of custody in the emergency department	1
Determination of driver versus passenger	1
Forensic anatomy and injury mechanisms	1
Forensic toxicology and pharmacology	1
Crime scene investigation	1
Forensic serology and DNA	1
Motor vehicle accident reconstruction	1
Investigation of pedestrian collisions	1
Introduction to clinical forensic medicine	1

medicine residency programs and provides advanced forensic training comparable to that received by residents in forensic pathology fellowships. The goal of the 12-month fellowship is to prepare the emergency physician as a forensic expert in the evaluation of nonfatal injuries, just as the forensic pathologist is an expert in the evaluation of fatal ones. In addition, the curriculum provides a well-rounded program for emergency medicine residents in this emerging specialty (Table 2-1).

Nursing Component Adds Value to Louisville Program

In 1996, the University of Louisville's Clinical Forensic Medicine Program hired the first full-time clinical forensic nurse specialists in the US. The program, which began in 1990 with two physicians on 24-hour-a-day call, has grown exponentially. The forensic service the program provides consists of an interdisciplinary team of experts: six forensic pathologists, two clinical forensic emergency physicians, one forensic pediatrician, one forensic odontologist, one forensic pathology fellow, and two full-time clinical forensic nurses. The University of Louisville's Departments of Forensic Pathology and Emergency Medicine's forensic fellows also participate in this collaborative service. Clinical forensic consultations are performed at the request of local, state, and federal law enforcement and child/adult protective services.

Each time a patient presents to the university's emergency department with forensic implications and the case is reported to the police department, the clinical forensic nurse responds along with a police officer. The nurse is in a position to provide an examination to identify injury and collect evidence from the body. If the patient later dies, this evidence is available for the medical examiner at the time of autopsy. Should the patient survive and charges be filed against a suspect, the critical evidence remains within the purview of the commonwealth attorney.

Using state-of-the-art technologies and traditional methodologies, the forensic team assists in the medicolegal evaluation of both victims and alleged perpetrators of crimes and testifies as to its findings in the legal cases that ensue. All examinations are performed with the consent of the victim, the legal caregiver, the protective agency, or a court order.

This clinical forensic interdisciplinary team is called to consult on an average of 300 cases per year. The majority of consultations are performed for the benefit of the pediatric physical abuse victim. The team also performs evaluations on victims of gunshot wounds and domestic assault, as well as suspects in police custody, and determines the roles of occupants in complex motor vehicle collisions.

Members of the team continue to teach and lecture locally, nationally, and internationally to various professional disciplines. Lecture topics have included domestic violence, child abuse, pattern injuries, shaken baby syndrome, elder abuse, gunshot wounds, and clinical forensic medicine and nursing. The original program employing clinical FNEs in conjunction with emergency physicians has been recognized as the ideal in clinical forensic services and has established a precedent for other programs that are developing based on this innovative concept.

The concept of the clinical forensic team is gaining momentum within major trauma centers in the US. One such team in Houston, Texas, has developed a Department of Forensic Nursing Services with a composite of more than 30 nurses. The team was created by forensic clinical nurse specialist Russell Rooms, MSN, RN, EMT-P. Team members are clinical FNEs who provide care for patients with interpersonal violence issues of any type including, but not limited to, adult sexual assault, intimate partner violence, and child physical or sexual abuse. They evaluate patients in all areas of the hospital including the emergency department, intensive care, and medical-surgical units. The surgical operating suite within Memorial Hermann Hospital (Houston) was the first in the nation to use forensic protocols including procurement of gunpowder residue and the use of a forensic drop-box to assure the safeguarding of recovered forensic evidence (Evans & Stagner, 2003). Members of the clinical forensic team also serve as liaisons to the Office of the Chief Medical Examiner and law enforcement agencies in Houston. An established close working relationship with the Office of the Medical Examiner and the city's law enforcement agencies helps in the management of death and near death cases, as well as sexual assault, child abuse, and domestic violence at Houston's Memorial Hermann Hospital. This clinical forensic program has set a precedent for hospitals and trauma centers across the country. In June 2003, its Forensic Nurse Response Team implemented the world's first mobile forensic unit taking forensic nursing services to nine area hospitals. Rooms' Department of Forensic Nursing Services has been visited and studied by R. K. Gorea, head of the Government Medical College in Patiala, Punjab, who has ambitions for establishing a similar program in India.

Best Practice *2-1*

All healthcare personnel, particularly those working in the emergency department, should be educated and trained in the recognition and management of forensic patients, including detection, collection, and preservation of evidence.

Continuing Education Programs and Organizations Emerge

In 1994, the Kentucky Chapter of the American College of Emergency Physicians and the University of Louisville's Department of Emergency Medicine sponsored the first of five annual clinical forensic medicine conferences in Louisville, Kentucky. The keynote speaker at the premier conference in 1994 was George Lundberg, MD, editor of the *Journal of the American Medical Association.* Lundberg, trained as a pathologist, spoke to the need of incorporating forensic medicine into the clinical setting to be applied by nurses and physicians. Other keynote speakers included the internationally recognized forensic scientist Henry Lee; Jason Payne-James, editor of the *Journal of Clinical Forensic Medicine;* Virginia Lynch, founding president of the International Association of Forensic Nursing; Patrick Besant-Matthews, internationally recognized forensic pathologist and photographer; Jamie Ferrell, sexual assault nurse examiner and educator; and John McCann, director of the Child Protection Center at the University of California, Davis, Medical Center. These annual conferences trained more than 1000 prosecuting attorneys, law enforcement officers, nurses, and physicians in the practical applications of clinical forensic medicine and nursing.

The keen interest and support of forensic nursing in the US and around the world prompted forensic nurses to organize the International Association of Forensic Nursing (IAFN) in 1992. Seventy-four nurses, principally sexual assault nurse examiners, founded what was to become the leading organization addressing clinical forensic issues. IAFN's first scientific meeting was held in 1993 in Sacramento, California, with 160 attendees. Within a decade this pioneering organization could boast a membership of nearly 2000. The IAFN members include nurse death investigators, correctional nurse specialists, forensic psychiatric nurses, legal nurse consultants, sexual assault nurse examiners, clinical forensic nurses, forensic pediatric and geriatric specialists, nurse attorneys, physicians, criminologists, and law enforcement officials.

Forensic nursing, as a specialty of nursing, has grown steadily. In 1995, the American Nurses Association officially recognized forensic nursing as a specialty of nursing, further citing it as one of the four major areas for nursing development in the twenty-first century.

Clinical forensic medicine, with the exception of some academic emergency medicine centers and progressive medical examiner programs, has not enjoyed the same success as forensic nursing. In 2000, the ACEP still had no position or statement regarding the role of forensic physicians or police surgeons in emergency departments in the US. The only forensic policy statements for training guidelines related to the collection of evidence in cases of sexual assault and recommending emergency medicine curricula include training in the recognition, assessment, and interventions in child abuse (ACEP, 2000). ACEP has recognized the benefits of sexual assault nurse examiners and strongly supports their utilization in the emergency department for the benefit of patient care (ACEP, 2000).

The development of a new specialty is accompanied by special needs. The University of Rochester's School of Nursing in New York consulted Houston's Russell Rooms, MSN, RN, EMT-P, to assist in developing the National Forensic Nursing Institute (NFNI). The institute's mission is to provide support for forensic nurses including the provision of specially designed evidence collection equipment and forensic program design and implementation. Other mission components include national peer review processes, educational programming, consultation for practicing forensic nurses, and oversight for the post-master's certificate program in forensic nursing at the University of Rochester.

Summary

The fact that clinical forensic medicine has been practiced in most other countries in the world for hundreds of years is a testament to the adage that "nothing is new under the sun." As reports of violence escalate, it is small comfort to think it was ever thus. What is comforting is the increasing awareness of a need to acknowledge this phenomenon and approach its management professionally. The inclusion of forensically skilled nurses to the battery of experts doing just that is an important and critical step toward ensuring the comprehensiveness of the services provided and will improve the quality of life and outcomes in living forensic victims and their cases.

Resources

Books

Anderson, W. R. (1998). *Forensic sciences in clinical medicine: A case study approach.* Philadelphia: Lippincott-Raven.

Olshaker, J. S., Jackson, M. C., &. Smock, W. S. (2001). *Forensic emergency medicine.* Philadelphia: Lippincott, Williams & Wilkins.

Organizations

Association of Police Surgeons

Clarke House, 18 Mount Parade Harrogate, Yorkshire, UK

American Academy of Forensic Sciences

410 North 21st Street, Colorado Springs, CO 80904; Tel: 719-636-1100; www.aafs.org

Journal of Clinical Forensic Medicine

Harcourt Publishers, 32 Jamestown Road, London, England NW1 7BY; Tel: +44 (0) 207-424-4487

References

American College of Emergency Physicians. (2000, January). Child abuse. ACEP Policy Statement, no. 400279.

Carmona, R., & Prince, K. (1989). Trauma and forensic medicine. *J Trauma, 29*(9), 1222.

Eckert, W. (1983). Forensic sciences: The clinical or living aspects. *Inform 16*, 3.

Eckert, W. G. (1990). Forensic sciences and medicine: The clinical or living aspects. *Am J Forensic Med Path, 11*(4), 336-341.

Eckert, W. G., et al. (1986). Clinical forensic medicine. *Am J Forensic Med Pathol 7*(3), 182.

Evans, M. M., & Stagner, P. (2003). Maintaining the chain of custody: Evidence handling in forensic cases. *AORN, 78*(4), 563-569.

Goldsmith, M. F. (1986). US forensic pathologists on a new case: Examination of living patients, *JAMA, 256*(13), 1685.

Lynch, V. (1990). *Clinical forensic nursing: A descriptive study in role development.* Thesis, University of Texas, Arlington.

Lynch V. (1991). Forensic nursing in the emergency department: A new role for the 1990s. *Crit Care Nursing Q, 14*(3), 69-86.

Lynch, V. A. (1986, February). *Forensic nursing: A new field for the profession.* Paper presented to the 38th annual meeting of the American Academy of Forensic Sciences, New Orleans, LA.

Lynch, V. A. (1995). Forensic nursing: What's new? *J Psychosoc Nurs, 33*(9), 1-7.

McLay, W. D. S. (1990). *Clinical forensic medicine*. London: Pinter.

McNamara, H. (1986). *Living forensics* (seminar pamphlet). Ulster County, NY: Office of the Medical Examiner.

Mittleman, R. E., Goldberg, H. S., & Waksman, D. M. (1983). Preserving evidence in the emergency department. *Am J Nurs, 83,* 1654.

Root, I., & Scott, W. (1973, September). The clinician and forensic medicine. *Calif Med, 119,* 68-76.

Smialek, J. E. (1983). Forensic medicine in the emergency department. *Emerg Med Clin North Am 1*(3), 1685.

Smock, W. S. (1994). Development of a clinical forensic medicine curriculum for emergency physicians in the USA. *J Clin Forensic Med, 1*, 27-30.

Smock, W. S. (2002). Forensic emergency medicine. In J. M. Marx (Ed.), *Rosen's emergency medicine: Concepts and clinical practice* (pp. 828-841). St. Louis, MO: Mosby.

Smock, W. S., & Nichols, G. R. (1991, October). *Clinical forensic medicine in the emergency department.* Boston, MA: American College of Emergency Physicians.

Chapter 3 Concepts and Theory of Forensic Nursing

Virginia A. Lynch

Violence-related trauma is central to the role of the forensic specialist in nursing (Lynch, 1990). Whether physical, sexual, or psychological, violence remains the single greatest source of loss of life and function worldwide (Reiss & Roth, 1993). Forensic nursing assumes a mutual responsibility with the forensic medical sciences and the criminal justice systems in concern for the loss of life and function due to human violence and liability-related issues.

The forensic nurse, as a clinical investigator, represents one member of an alliance of healthcare providers, law enforcement agencies, and forensic scientists in a holistic approach to the evaluation and treatment of crime-related trauma. Forensic nurse investigators address relevant areas in the assessment of criminal violence, abuse, and data collection for establishing hypotheses about the interrelationship between healthcare and the law. Forensic nurses do not compete with, replace, or supplant other practitioners–rather they fill voids by accomplishing selected forensic tasks concurrently with other health and justice professionals by providing a uniquely qualified clinician who blends biomedical knowledge with the basic principles of law and human behavior (Lynch, 1991).

Key Point 3-1

When violence is considered within the domain of public health, in addition to criminal justice alone, it mandates that health and justice collaborate on solutions.

In 1979, the US Surgeon General's Report "Healthy People" outlined a strategy for addressing priority areas for improving the health of the nation, which included addressing interpersonal violence, an important contributor to morbidity and premature mortality. One expert noted that public health is in the business of continually redefining the unacceptable, which changes the social norm and eventually changes the problem. Not unlike polio, violence is also a threat to public health (Foege, 1997).

In 1989, US Surgeon General C. Everett Koop challenged healthcare professionals to assume accountability, along with law enforcement, for the problems associated with violence. His workshop on violence and public health addressed domestic violence, child abuse, elder abuse, rape, homicide, murder, and traumatic accidents as pervasive threats to the fundamental public health principle of population exposure. This perspective emphasized that no segment of society can be considered immune from the effects of violence. He remarked that these problems are so pervasive that they can no longer be viewed as acts of individual offenders (Koop, 1989). During the past two decades, the US Department of Health and Human Services has continued to recognize the inevitable outcomes of violence (injury, disability, and death) as the primary benchmarks of public health status.

Theoretical Foundations

As nursing history delineates the principles and philosophies of nursing in general, it has also addressed those of forensic nursing, which parallel traditional nursing care in all specialties within the scope and boundaries of nursing practice. Forensic nursing brings to each nursing specialty specific guidelines that will involve strategies and considerations for meeting the biological, psychological, social, spiritual, and now legal dimensions of patient care in a humanitarian, holistic, and pragmatic orientation. The theoretical perspectives for forensic nursing practice derive their broad construct from several mainstream nursing theories including those presented by Paterson and Zderad (1998), Conway and Hardy (1988), Leininger (1995), Giger and Davidhizar (1991), Chinn and Kramer (1995), and Brenner (1984).

These nursing theories become integrated within the theories of sociology and philosophy, such as the theories of Mead (1934), Plato (427-347 B.C.), and those explored by Farrell and Swigert (1982), to design an integrated practice model for forensic nursing, as philosophers, sociologists, and others have focused on the construction of practice theory in nursing. Forensic nursing integrates their theories into a framework for forensic nursing practice to help describe and explain phenomena specific to forensic nursing science. This common connectedness brings the philosophies of physical science together with the legal dimensions and defines forensic nursing's body of knowledge based on shared theories with other disciplines.

Assumptions Applied and Defined

Assumptions are statements accepted as given truths without proof. Assumptions set the foundation for the application of a particular theory. Central to the forensic nursing theory is the assumption that integrating disciplines of social science, nursing science, and the legal sciences involves the notion that the multiskilled forensic clinician in nursing is mutually beneficial to the patient, healthcare institution, society, law, and human behavior.

Truth

Truth is the mantra of the forensic sciences and central to the field of all scientific investigation. Truth explains the objective methodology of forensic sciences applied across a broad base of disciplines and facilitates the collective search for the truth. Reforms in criminal justice systems have come about through advances in DNA technology that have sustained truth and justice in cases where justice had been denied. The Innocence Project was founded in 1992 to determine the truth as related to the exoneration of incarcerated prisoners through postconviction DNA testing. It cannot be overemphasized that the forensic nurse is not a victim advocate but rather a patient advocate. The patient, however, may be the accused, a convicted felon, the condemned, or the victim.

A forensic nurse is required to remain essentially unbiased and value neutral in all matters–an advocate for truth and justice. Objectivity and neutrality are essential values in the care of forensic patients. The role requires incisive comprehension of fundamental medicolegal issues as well as the ability to prepare and present testimony in a court of law. It is the search for truth.

Truth, as the central implicit assumption to all forensic investigations, brings enlightenment to unknown, unanswered, and questioned issues related to the origin and manifestations of pathological conditions impacting the person, environment, health, and nursing. The philosophy of forensic nursing practice is based on the ancient philosopher's love of truth and of all true being (Plato, 347 B.C.). Without the discovery of truth, diagnosis, treatment, evaluation, rehabilitation, recovery, and prevention would be precluded. Without truth, reconciliation and justice are denied.

Research is an essential element for further developing forensic nursing's concepts, theories, and models of care. Research initiatives and clinical inquiries form the basis of evidence-based practices (Brenner, 1984). Yet it will require appropriate theoretical frameworks for practice, advanced nursing preparation, competency-based training, and experimental work-based academic development to move out of the shadows and forward into the pursuit of truth.

Paradigms, Theories, and Ways of Knowing

Central to all nursing theories is the assumption that human beings are made up of various dimensions and that each dimension is related to health and well-being. Forensic nursing theory incorporates the various human dimensions pertinent to all nursing theories of care, yet it projects beyond the aspects of biopsychosocial-spiritual and cultural beings to introduce and incorporate a dimension of laws. Laws that portend to govern human behavior and social needs represent the direct correlation between the human dimension, health, and well-being. Culture can advance or limit the human dimension. Cultural change can be seen as social learning. Cultural care and cultural interventions are essential components of forensic and clinical investigation of trauma.

Forensic nurse examiners utilize Carper's fundamental patterns of knowing in their practice with a variety of models and theories (Carper, 1978). Patterns of fundamental knowing consist of those described as empirical knowledge, aesthetic knowledge, personal knowledge, and ethical knowing. Other nursing theories and models are symbiotically intertwined and functionally applicable to forensic nursing science.

Components of Theoretical Concepts

The following components are typically addressed in any theoretical concept of nursing practice. They are (1) role clarification, (2) role behavior, and (3) role expectation.

Role clarification identifies shared knowledge and skills. It establishes explicit expectations and boundaries between the role of self and others, and it delineates goals as well as costs and rewards of enacting them. Role clarification also demonstrates the extent to which significant others reinforce or validate role behavior via complementary and counter roles.

Role behavior is the performance or enactment of differentiated behavior relevant to a specific position.

Role expectation is the obligation or demands placed on the individual in a role position. It encompasses the specific norms associated with the attitudes, behaviors, and cognition required and anticipated for a role occupant.

A major component of the integrated model for forensic nursing is *interactionism*. The focus of *interactionism* concerns specific links or associations among persons, environment, concern for persons, social integration, development of meaning and the integration of persons in a social context, as well as processes engaging persons. Not all social systems generate a sense of community, but those that do create a shared culture and social order among their members. Patient advocacy recognizes healthcare as a primary source of physical and emotional stability to the physically or psychologically traumatized patient. Patient advocacy, an aspect of social behavior that protects and provides patients with an emotionally supportive community, serves as one platform for the forensic nurse examiner role. The understanding and explanation of social order as community is the goal of social sciences. This includes the understanding and explanation of criminal behavior and human violence. It focuses on individuals in reciprocal social interaction as they actively construct and create their environment through a somewhat symbiotic interaction. The main focus of this perspective reinforces the need for social order and interdisciplinary coordination in healthcare delivery and the social-justice sciences.

Problematic social situations, such as the escalation of trends in criminal violence, demand new interpretations and new lines of action, which will, in turn, reinforce the need to continually redefine the role of the forensic nurse. This parallels the major focus of forensic nursing as it deals with change, dynamics, and the processes by which individuals creatively adapt to a society in flux. The ongoing problems in society and rapid social change place new demands on public service providers. Their role behaviors, in turn, quickly generate new and valid concepts that contribute to safe, effective patient care.

A dynamic role of the forensic nurse examiner has evolved in clinical and community nursing practice that facilitates specialized and unique behaviors in forensic nursing. This role helps nursing, medical, social, and legal systems to clarify questioned issues in response to the epidemiology and query of murder, suicide, sexual assault, abuse, neglect, intentional trauma, communicable disease, and violent criminal acts that threaten lives daily under existing, destructive social conditions (Centers for Disease Control [CDC], 1995; FBI, 1999, 2001, 2002, 2003). The principle of reciprocal social interaction represents the multifaceted relationships among patient, clinician, and multidisciplinary team members that involve law enforcement agencies, social services, legislative authorities, judicial systems, and healthcare operatives. The reciprocal interaction of interagency coordination and cooperation works to improve the structural and functional management, delivery, and effectiveness of services offered by health and justice institutions.

Assumptions of the Theory

The following assumptions are made concerning this theoretical framework:

- Clinical forensic nursing is a relatively new science, and there is limited awareness of this specialty on behalf of health professionals, law enforcement agencies, and forensic science practitioners, as well as healthcare consumers.
- Evolving healthcare systems ultimately require changes in the role of the professional nurse.
- The conception and perception of the clinical forensic nurse is currently evolving and developing and at times poorly defined.

- The application of clinical forensic science is appropriate for the practice of nursing.
- The registered nurse, qualified by education and experience in a broad range of nursing specialties, is capable of identifying role behaviors of the clinical forensic specialist.
- Human rights are a priority for the majority of society.
- Sensitivity to differences among culturally and ethnically diverse populations are encompassed in forensic nursing care.
- Truth is the central element in the outcome of forensic investigative analysis, which involves patient history, assessment of forensic implications, and correlation with the conditions and circumstances of injury, illness, or death.
- Forensic patients hold equal rights in terms of law and ethics, whether victim, accused, or offender.

Propositions

Propositions are ideas brought forward for consideration, acceptance, or adoption. The basic propositions put forth for consideration of the theory of forensic nursing science include truth, presence, perceptivity, and regeneration. These propositions are explained below:

- Truth as central force in the resolution of questioned issues that involve the physical, psychological, and social health or ills of a human population; includes past and future truths
- Presence, that invisible quality that commands and comforts while directing attention away from one's self and into the being of another, instilling confidence and respect in the self of that being
- Perceptivity as the investigative tool of one who explores human behavior, awareness of the elements of one's environment, sensory phenomena interpreted in light of lived experiences that guide intuitiveness
- Regeneration, a value and a goal of the advanced forensic praxis in patient healing that affects a victim or offender who has experienced the deepest wounds of the soul; becoming once again as before

Application of Propositions

Care that incorporates the nursing process–assessment, planning, intervention, and evaluation, to restore and promote health in the patient throughout the forensic process–is essential. The concepts of truth, presence, perceptivity, and regeneration will guide the forensic practitioner in those ways of knowing, patterns of being, and shared intuition between patient and practitioner.

Best Practice *3-1*

Forensic nurses should augment their usual nursing assessments and objective documentation with preservation and collection of evidence and steps to prevent the psychophysical, psychosocial, and psychosexual health risks associated with trauma and violence.

The objectives of forensic nursing intervention are injury/illness/death assessment, objective documentation, collection and preservation of forensic data and evidence, and the prevention of potential psychophysical/psychosocial/psychosexual health risks. Patient empowerment is also a significant issue, consequential to the criminal trauma, healthcare interventions, and the acceptance or rejection by society regarding the circumstances of the criminal act involved, whether the patient is a victim or an offender.

Theoretical Components of Forensic Nursing

The theoretical support for forensic nursing care involves the dimensions of bio-psycho-social-spiritual-and legal nursing practice. Forensic nursing is holistic in nature, addressing these concepts individually and collectively. The science of forensic nursing has been recognized by the professional bodies of nursing that direct the development of nursing education, research, and practice. Forensic nursing theory identifies interconnectedness with theories of the legal and physical sciences, which are reflected in the Joint Commission on Accreditation of Healthcare Organizations (JCAHO) guidelines and provide regulatory guidance for healthcare practitioners (JCAHO, 2004).

These guidelines regard the identification of crime victims and the recovery and documentation of evidence, as well as the procedures for reporting abuse or suspicious patient behavior to a legal agency, as the foundations of forensic nursing practice. The legal sciences define and delineate the parameters of the law responsible for the behaviors of the nursing professional. Forensic nursing behaviors involve, among others, the identification of crime-related injury, collection of evidence, reporting suspicion of illegal acts to a legal agent, and the abuse or death of patients in custody or that of incarcerated or institutionalized persons. It is, then, the respective dimensions of the health and justice disciplines that integrate a variety of multidimensional theories into nursing practices and define the distinctive conjectures of forensic nursing science.

Key Point *3-2*

Forensic nursing is multidimensional, requiring multitheoretical approaches to explain interactions between healthcare and the law.

Descriptive Theory

In the clinical environs this role is defined as the application of clinical and scientific knowledge to questions of law related to the civil and criminal investigation of survivors of traumatic injury and patient treatment involving court-related issues (Lynch, 1995a). It is further defined as the application of the nursing process to public or legal proceedings; the application of the forensic aspects of healthcare in the scientific investigation of trauma and/or death-related issues involving abuse, violence, criminal activity, liability concerns, and traumatic accidents (Lynch, 1991).

Prescriptive Theory

Nurses have always been expected to care for crime victims, patients in legal custody, and victims of traumatic accidents and other liability-related injuries. However, in the past, there has been no specialty role or explicit education to ensure that these legal responsibilities were reasonably met as a component of nursing care. The complex legal needs of the patient were often in jeopardy due to the ignorance of forensic issues by the emergency medical response team and the nurse or attending physician. Investigating officers generally depended on the nurse or physician to accurately document injury and to recover evidence. Without specialized knowledge, neither objective was fulfilled. Complex recovery of evidence, specificity in documentation, and managing emotionally traumatized patients concurrently with life-saving intervention require separate roles for those who provide emergency intervention and those who provide forensic services.

The introduction of a forensic clinician in nursing has provided healthcare's direct response to violence. This new discipline was intrinsic to the role nurses would fill in the challenge to address the legal issues pertaining to forensic healthcare and to reduce a previously recognized injustice to society. As nurses acknowledged their role in the health and justice movement, they recognized crime-related issues as justifiable elements for healthcare professionals to integrate into their specialty-oriented practice models. They accepted the challenge to reach beyond the immediate treatment environs into the often-shadowed areas of legal issues surrounding patient care. The concept of an integrated practice model in forensic nursing science has initiated an accomplished clinician, cross-trained in the principles and philosophies of nursing science, forensic science, and criminal justice. The recognition and management of medicolegal cases require healthcare professionals to reconceptualize nursing practice and its body of knowledge.

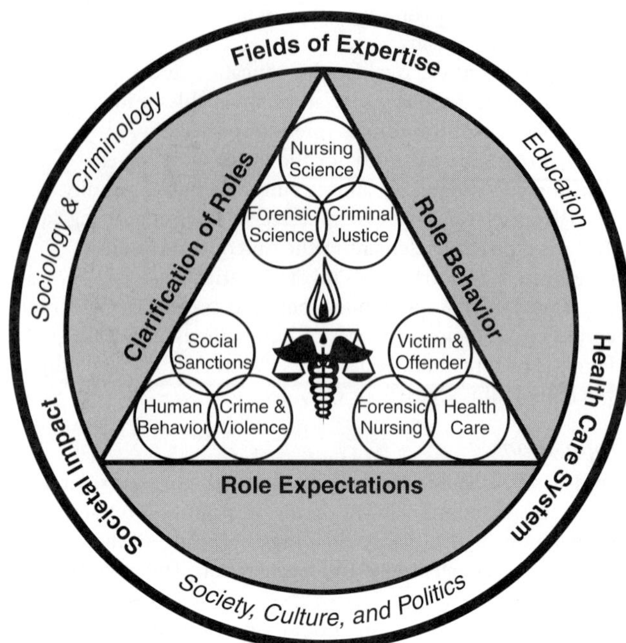

Fig. 3-1 Integrated practice model for forensic nursing science.

Key Point 3-3

Patient care now requires a consideration of legal and human rights as well as an awareness of the greater connection the healthcare delivery system has to other social systems. It is no longer acceptable for the healthcare system to exist in isolation, ignorant of the wider world of interfacing systems.

Practice Theory

An integrated practice model for forensic nursing science incorporates a synthesis of shared theory from a variety of disciplines involving social science, nursing science, and the legal (forensic) sciences. It presents a global perspective on interrelated disciplines and bodies of knowledge that affect forensic nursing practice through social justice. The aspects of a multidimensional theory are activated in the investigation of injury, illness and death, social crime, and liability-related questions. An integrated practice model is especially relevant to the applied health sciences.

An Integrated Practice Model

An illustrative model for the theoretical framework is depicted in Figure 3-1. The pictorial represents the dynamics symbolized in the following conceptual framework.

Forensic nursing science and its humanitarian perspective have the potential to provide new solutions to problems that require a unique multidisciplinary approach. Forensic nursing is a critical component in minimizing the devastating impact of prevalent social and cultural problems in the twenty-first century, which provides a strong theoretical knowledge base for interactional analysis and its prevailing approaches to role development.

Description of the Integrated Practice Model

The model is described as follows: Three principal components embracing the outer triangle constitute the theoretical basis of forensic nursing. The interlocking circles indicate interconnected, interagency coordination, cooperation, and communication essential to public health, safety, and social justice.

- A knowledge base of interrelated disciplines (fields of expertise)–nursing science, forensic science, and the law–use sociological, criminological, and nursing theory to connect role behaviors with the societal consequences of health and human behavior.
- The societal impact components are human behavior (broadly based sociological and psychological notions), social sanctions (legal and institutional sanctions and processes), and crime and violence (both recognized and hidden). Social, cultural, and political factors bring together role expectations within a system of roles.
- A system of roles relates to the victim, the suspected offender or the perpetrator of criminal acts, the significant others of both, forensic nursing science, and the healthcare institution (both individual and institutional roles). Education, both practical (experiential) and theoretical, brings role behavior and role clarification together.

Explanation of the Pictorial Model

At the center of the internal triangle is the symbol of forensic nursing. This symbol, reflecting the legal, forensic medical, physical, psychosocial, and nursing sciences, is composed of the scales of justice, the bundle of public service, the caduceus, and the eternal flame of nursing. The flame illustrates enlightenment of humanity and perpetuates the challenge in nursing to continue to evolve and expand into new roles as societal trends demand. This enlightenment reflects awareness of the greater connectedness that the healthcare system has to other social systems. The caduceus represents medical science, and enmeshed in this symbol is the interdisciplinary collaboration that integrates nursing into the multitude of highly specialized scientific psychocultural arenas. The bundle of public service represents the complexity and weight of public service obligations in which all modern systems in our society are inextricably involved, including the discipline, punishment, and rehabilitation of those who fail society's laws. Finally, the scales of justice emphasize the notion that patient care must require the consideration of legal as well as human rights.

The dynamics of the interlocking circles are omnidirectional. The outer circle, which frames and encompasses these components, is symbolic of the environment and underscores the interaction of society, education, and systems.

The model demonstrates attention to the concepts of *person* (victim, suspect, offender, human behavior), *health* (healthcare institutions, nursing science, individuals, and groups), *nursing* (nursing science, forensic nursing), and *environment* (experience, societal impact, and healthcare systems), as well as to *internal* issues (clarification, expectation, and behavior) and *external* components (sociology and criminology; social, cultural, and political factors; and education).

The model focuses on the necessity for society to respond to problems that develop between the related fields of nursing, forensic science, and the criminal justice system. These systems of roles are not fixed, precisely defined entities. They have flexibility that permits the maintenance of open, evolving systems. This theoretical framework allows for the flexibility needed to achieve a dynamic balance in the role of the forensic nurse examiner. The effectiveness of the forensic nurse is based, in part, on her or his ability to interact with other scientific, legal, medical, and social professionals, victims, suspects, perpetrators, families, and communities. Forensic nursing is not limited to a single context within the definition of a new role. New concepts of forensic nursing will be explored as they continue to emerge within the context of role theory.

This conceptualization embraces an integration of multiple theories derived from other disciplines. As new concepts are integrated into the practice model–such as sociology (sociopolitical impact), criminology (crime, violence, criminal justice, social sanctions, and human rights), clinical and criminal investigation (forensic and nursing science), and education (nursing, medicolegal, staff, patient/clients, and medicolegal specialization)–the cyclic nature of the model speaks to continuance, perpetuation, and balance. Balance is achieved when justice is served–to those who have been victimized, to those accused of crimes not committed, to offenders, and to society as a whole. Justice is served when *truth* is identified, verified, and demonstrated. Thus, the forensic nurse becomes an advocate for justice, an advocate for truth. Truth and justice perpetuate holistic health in the inclusive aspects of biological, psychological, sociological, spiritual, cultural, and legal dimensions of being human.

Explanatory Theory: Interactionism

The properties and components of forensic nursing practice function within society and society's institutions (hospitals, necropsy laboratories, jails and other custodial facilities, courts) that provide the framework within which roles are enacted. The *interactionist* is an individual whose approach is focused on the continual process of interpretation placed on acts and symbols by those interactions with each other (subspecialties within forensic nursing and other forensic specialists) (Conway & Hardy, 1988). From a theoretical perspective, symbolic interactionism can be appropriately applied to the role development of the forensic nurse examiner as these nurses interact with the living and the dead in medicolegal cases. Role theory as it relates to nursing is approached from the perspective of interactionism between healthcare and the law.

The interactionist concept evolves from the belief that flexibility is critical in the development of a role that remains in constant evolution based on the needs and demands of society. The dynamic concepts of role theory, as applied to health professions, identify specific characteristics of the role under development. Thus, the role of the forensic nurse will remain flexible and continue to evolve as trends in crime and criminality mutate and transform into new social and cultural crimes. The following concepts are among the variables that influence the characteristics of the forensic nurse interactionist. A synthesis of role clarification, behavior, and expectation provides the forensic nurse examiner with a framework for culturally sensitive care in which the forensic nurse's role includes such forensic skills as the following:

- Identification of trauma (assessment)
- Investigation (planning)
- Documentation (history) pertaining to the incident (intervention)
- Collection of evidence (specimens)
- Postinvestigation review (evaluation)

The forensic nurse also provides traditional nursing interventions such as crisis care as they interact with traumatized victims, offenders, and their families. These skills may also be extended to various disciplines and colleagues with whom they interact throughout the investigation of trauma and deaths. Those most frequently subjected to pernicious human behavior in forensic cases, such as law enforcement officers, fire fighters, paramedics, often suffer from vicarious or secondary trauma. Conversely, forensic nurse examiners must remain alert to the symptoms of this insidious and debilitating condition, as they may become overwhelmed under such circumstances.

Current literature stresses that our social sciences and legal systems must address the ills of social justice and injustice. The offender of social laws and mores brings a different focus into the practice of forensic nursing. Often, offenders are victims of another kind–and of another crime. Forensic psychiatric nurses and forensic correctional nurses, the primary caretaker of those accused of criminal acts and of the offender patient population, find this to be a group with complex healthcare needs. Caring for offenders is nothing new within the clinical environs. Nurses care for patients in custody in the emergency department, in surgical intensive care, and in the general patient population when physical illness or injuries require medical, surgical, or psychiatric intervention. These patients are often restrained by legal means, generally have armed law enforcement officers in attendance, and are hospitalized in a temporary situation.

Yet caring for the accused, the mentally disordered offender, or the sexual sadist on a long-term basis becomes a formidable task and a challenge to all of a nurse's skills. Although the challenge of caring for this patient population is complex, the duty and responsibility of the forensic nurse remain. Effects of forensic nursing interventions may be hard to assess on an immediate basis, for the psychopathology of the mind is a long-term mystery that requires patience, individualized interventions, reassessment, objective evaluation, and possible changes to more adeptly benefit the client's outcomes or the social system's needs.

One must remember that just as forensic pathology lays the foundation for all clinical medicine (why people die), forensic psychiatrists, behavioral scientists, and criminologists who study and evaluate crimes and criminal behavior (why people commit crimes) lay the foundation for the prevention of crime. It is difficult, if not impossible, to practice prevention without first knowing the underlying causes of human tragedy, death, disease, or crime. Once forensic pathologists can determine the causes of death, clinical physicians can more readily save lives. Once the forensic behavioral scientist can understand why people commit crimes, she or he can begin to reduce and prevent criminal acts. All forensic intervention must begin with a firm scientific foundation, then explore the unknown, unpredictable regions of the human mind. Forensic nursing science has been recognized as one important component to the solution for today's most serious health and justice problem: violence.

Metaparadigms

The dominant constructs of nursing were selected to represent an overriding structure in regard to the role of the forensic nurse. The following constructs are described as metaparadigms applied within the framework of forensic nursing science.

Person (Patient, Victim, Suspect, Perpetrator, Human Behavior)

This primary concept represents the nucleus of the humanistic theory of nursing. In specific relationship to forensic nursing, *person* is defined twofold: the victim of crime and the surviving family members (identified as victims by extension) or the suspect or perpetrator, an individual accused or convicted of a criminal act or socially unacceptable behavior. Human behavior guides human social activity by determining the characteristics that distinguish the role of the victim and the offender of justice. The roles of the accused or suspect and the convicted perpetrator of crime provide a particular relevance that further defines the forensic application of nursing practice. Cultural competence and awareness are essential in the forensic management of patients who have immigrated to the US or seek political refuge. Those who have survived political violence and wars in their countries of origin often experienced crime within the boundaries of the US from discrimination, racism, hatred, and religious persecution–the same crimes they thought they left behind.

Health (Healthcare Institutions, Nursing Science, Individuals or Groups, Physical or Mental)

The implied definition of *health* is influenced by the multiple variables related to the subtheories of forensic nursing within the nursing sciences. The loss of life and function result in disabilities derived from societal crime and violence and are consequentially identified conditions for forensic intervention. However, pain involving the violation of the spirit is a phenomenon that challenges health service practitioners' potential to the greatest extent. If life prevails, yet the distress of the human spirit remains impaired, health remains dysfunctional. Sensitivity to victims and families is a fundamental concept that distinguishes forensic nursing care to the emotionally and spiritually compromised patients. Health is not merely a person's physical well-being; but helping that person "become more as humanly possible in a particular life situation" (Paterson & Zderad, 1998, p. 279) describes one core component of forensic nursing praxis. The concern of forensic healthcare provides for needs beyond survival and functioning, assumes responsibilities beyond the immediate treatment environment, and now includes the legal care that may dictate the patient's future well-being.

Nursing (Nursing Science, Forensic Nursing Science, and Practice)

For the purpose of this description, the forensic nursing role is based on the concept of a continuously evolving scientific base that challenges health professionals to enhance, reinterpret, and redefine their roles. These roles were designed to face the issues of societies in transition by moving into a social condition that requires nurses to incorporate new knowledge, to reach out to other scientific-based disciplines. There is no stereotype for nurses. Nurses create their own image–based on their responses to others and their compassionate and nonjudgmental intervention to decrease racism, religious or ideological animosity, or economic superiority–without fears or prejudice.

Nurses must affirm a support for community services outside the clinical setting. It is necessary to react to injustices. To gain a new understanding of the phenomenon known as empathy is crucial. The nurse's ability to look directly at the negative human behavior that engenders fear and prejudice in society and implement empathic nurse-patient interactions of coping and accommodation is as essential to recovery as physical intervention when facing degradation of the human spirit.

The forensic nurse is viewed as an integral member of the multidisciplinary investigative team consisting of healthcare professionals, law enforcement agencies, social science advocates, and forensic scientists. The effectiveness of the forensic nurse is based in part on the nurse's ability to interact with other professionals and to view the victim or offender in the humanitarian nursing perspective, a unique kind of nursing. As health is viewed on a continuum, it is essential to provide clients with interventions and resources that will help them to reestablish a sense of balance. The forensic nurse examiner strives to facilitate optimum functioning, which begins with objectively assessing the problem, applying the nursing process to achieve mutually established goals, and providing a humane, caring interaction.

Environment (Human Experience, Societal Impact, Healthcare Systems, Correctional Facilities, Courts)

The complex milieu of forensic nursing practice incorporates interactions between the healthcare systems and the external social context. This social climate (societal behaviors, laws) dictates role expectations unique to the forensic application of nursing. A more abstract forensic interpretation of the environment may focus on social stress or stressors by viewing the environment as hostile and the human-environment interaction negatively (crime, human abuse, death). Thus, the environment develops characteristics relevant to guide role behaviors appropriate to the treatment and prevention of physical and emotional trauma, psychopathology, unacceptable social behavior, and contamination and violation of the physical world, as well as spiritual degradation of human existence. A more positive symbolic relationship views the environment as one of a contextual space and conditions where forensic nursing intervention is applied and outcomes evaluated on interactions with the life-and-death process.

Best Practice *3-2*

The forensic nurse must protect the constitutional and human rights of the living, the severely compromised (near-death) individuals, the deceased, and their families during that interval between life and possible death.

The environment of the forensic nurse may reflect ambiguity and conflict. The medicolegal management scenarios vary widely and challenges abound in this new practice area, where the focus is on preventing further injury or death and repairing the lives of those who have suffered indignity. The major components of this environment are sources of stimuli emotionally charged with human conditions, at once nurturing and protective, yet constantly challenged with scientific and legal issues that have the potential to impact standards of nursing practice. This includes improving the quality of life and advancement of humanity.

Relevance and Roles

As healthcare reforms create complex systems for healthcare delivery, the professional nurse must be aware of ethical and legal considerations within those systems. A pattern of accountability revolves around four areas: the public, the patient, the profession, and the law. The forensic practitioner must know the boundaries and circumstances of both autonomy and accountability in order to provide forensically competent care. Issues of autonomy and accountability are subject to either criminal or civil law. The primary care practitioner must adhere to these principles.

Forensic intervention draws on all nursing skills and knowledge to fully address the bio-psycho-socio-spiritual-cultural and legal dimensions of the patient whose health and justice needs require the application of forensic nursing scope and standards of practice (International Association of Forensic Nurses [IAFN], 1997). This client population is divided equally in the social context of victims and offenders; for each victim there is a perpetrator of criminal acts.

The role and relevance of forensic nursing practice incorporates the nursing care of individuals of all ages with perceived physical or emotional alterations, which may be diagnosed or undiagnosed and may require immediate or long-term intervention with implicit legal implications. Forensic nursing care is scheduled or unscheduled pertaining to the specific environment in a specific care setting–that is, special forensic exam unit, emergency department, mobile unit, child advocacy facility, suicide prevention center, forensic mental health institution, remand center, correctional setting (jail, prison), or institute of legal medicine. Thus, forensic nursing practice is episodic (domestic violence, drug abuse) and acute (gunshot wounds, sexual assault), as well as primary, secondary, and tertiary in nature.

Relevance

Central to all programs of health delivery and promotion (physical, mental, cultural, and social well-being) is the concept of prevention, which includes forensic healthcare and involves three levels:

- Primary prevention is "pure" prevention, or preventing the health problem from occurring at all, such as determining the cause, manner, and mechanism of death in order to prevent future deaths of a similar nature; providing recommendations for public health and safety (avoidance of tobacco smoking, preventing polio through vaccination); or recommending the elimination of unsafe products or health hazards in the workplace. Clearly, this is the ideal and most cost-effective approach. Primary prevention is often referred to as health promotion, the process of enabling people to increase control over and to improve health through forensic assessment and interventions.
- Secondary prevention involves prompt detection and successful management or treatment of the health condition so as to avoid actual damage to the person's health. For example, the early detection and treatment of communicable diseases can prevent epidemics that result from uncontrolled infections; likewise, diagnosing early indicators of domestic violence or child or elder abuse can lead to medicolegal intervention (reporting, etc.), counseling, and shelter placement, which may prevent further injury and death.
- Tertiary prevention seeks to limit the impairment, increase the quality of life, and prolong life. Examples would include forensic interventions in cases that involve serious bodily harm or violent deaths with attention to evidentiary data and removing the offender from the home or the community, thus preventing further threat or death; or rehabilitative services and documentation of evidence for torture victims to help secure political asylum and prevent deportation to country of origin, resulting in summary execution.

Roles

In introducing practicing nurses to the importance of forensic protocol and tailoring forensic education designed to protect the legal rights of trauma victims in the clinical arena, one must first clarify the roles of a forensic nurse. This constructive action will reduce the actual threat associated with uniformed personnel and help toward the resolution of legal action by and for victims. Role definitions include the following:

- *Clinical forensic nurse.* Provides care for the survivors of crime-related injury and deaths. This specialist has a duty to defend the patient's legal rights through the proper collection and documentation of evidence that represents access to social justice.
- *Forensic nurse investigator.* Employed in a medical examiner or coroner's jurisdiction; represents the decedent's right to social justice through a scientific investigation of the scene and circumstances of death. This role may also include the investigation of criminal behavior in cases of long-term care, institutionalized care, insurance fraud and abuse, or other aspects of investigative exigency.
- *Forensic nurse examiner.* Provides an incisive analysis of physical and psychological trauma, questioned deaths, or psychopathology evaluations related to forensic cases that involve interpersonal violence (i.e., child abuse, domestic violence, elder abuse, sexual assault, or injury resulting from lethal weapons, torture, police brutality, etc.).
- *Sexual assault nurse examiner.* A registered nurse specially trained to provide the forensic/medical examination and evaluation of sexual trauma while maximizing the collection of biological, trace, and physical evidence and minimizing the patient's emotional trauma.
- *Forensic psychiatric nurse.* Specializes in the assessment and intervention of criminal defendants, patients in legal custody who have been accused of a crime or have been court mandated for psychiatric evaluation.
- *Forensic correctional, institutional, or custody nurse.* Specializes in the care, treatment, and rehabilitation of persons who have been sentenced to prisons or jails for violation of criminal statutes and require medical assessment and intervention.
- *Legal nurse consultant.* Provides consultation and education to judicial, criminal justice, and healthcare professionals in areas such as personal injury, product liability, and malpractice, among other legal issues related to civil and criminal cases; investigates questioned documents such as medical records, health histories, or medication instructions pertaining to

abuse, neglect, maltreatment, or death; recovers evidence from the context of such documents rather than from the scene of the crime or the body.
- *Nurse attorney.* A registered nurse with a jurist doctorate degree who practices as an attorney at law, generally specializing in civil or criminal cases involving healthcare-related issues.
- *Nurse coroner.* A registered nurse who serves as an elected officiator of death, duly authorized by state and jurisdictional statutes to provide the investigation and certification of questioned deaths; to determine the cause and manner of death; and to determine the circumstances pertaining to the decedent's identification and notification of next of kin.

Each of these primary roles and other subspecialties of the forensic nurse examiner is investigative in nature, requiring specific knowledge of the law and the skill of expert witness testimony. The prevalence of criminal and negligence-based trauma indicates a growing need for healthcare providers to intercede on behalf of social justice; to require the recognition and reporting of crime-related injury; to ensure accurate documentation and security of evidence; and to evaluate, assess, and treat social offenders.

Prevention and Risk Reduction

The prevention of violence requires a direct response from healthcare professionals. Most perpetrators of crime repeat their criminal acts. To identify risk reduction and preventive measures, one must first identify victims of crime. Preventive measures are provided through forensic interventions, such as identification of crime-related injuries and documentation of evidence that will in turn link the victim to the perpetrator or to the crime scene, which assist in identifying criminals and interrupting the cycle of violence. Within the clinical or community environs, forensic nurse examiners apply sound methods of legal and ethical care by providing a crucial role in the clinical investigation of trauma and may determine the outcome of legal decisions or survivor benefits.

Best Practice *3-3*

It is the obligation of forensic nurses as well as other healthcare workers to suspect that violence has occurred, to inspect the patient for physical signs of abuse or neglect, to protect and respect the patient and family members, and to recover evidence in an objective manner.

If the healthcare professional providing immediate treatment to victims of criminal or liability-related trauma fails to incorporate forensic guidelines, the misinterpretation, omission, or loss of evidence may result in a miscarriage of justice. Moreover, inappropriate evidence recovery in healthcare facilities involving complex situations such as criminal cases may obscure the most important forensic evidence and complicate subsequent investigations. Medical care of the critically ill in the emergency department remains a responsibility that cannot be compromised. Trauma practitioners can best serve the needs of society when they can simultaneously recognize and safeguard evidence.

The application of forensic science to clinical nursing reveals a wider role in the legal process that facilitates the medicolegal management of forensic patients from trauma to trial. The forensic psychiatric nursing specialist has been recognized as an asset in the evaluation of criminal suspects through remand evaluations and examination that will impact the adjudication process and patient outcome. As the Scope and Standards of Forensic Nursing Practice (IAFN, 1997) identifies a significant contemporary phase of healthcare progress, the growing interest among medical and nursing professionals implies a need to further define these roles in terms of forensic specialization and role evolution. Uniquely skilled nurses educated in forensic techniques enhance clinical investigative capabilities and forensic science functions.

Nurses specializing in the care and treatment of victims of pernicious human behavior offer, in addition to traditional nursing care, a composite of skills in the identification of covert and latent patterned injuries, recognition and collection of human bite mark evidence, photo-documentation, recovery and preservation of genetic evidence, and crucial intervention in emotional trauma. The forensic nurse is equally obligated to protect the constitutional rights of those who have been accused of criminal acts through accurate forensic cognitive assessment as well as the clinical documentation of evidence pertaining to the innocence or guilt of the client.

Predictive Theory

Forensic nursing science has progressed greatly since it was first introduced in 1986 as a formal specialty in nursing at the University of Texas at Arlington, and it continues to do so. Forensic nursing is not only a reflection of society's needs, but it is also a plan for prevention in the future. After centuries of barbarian punishment in an attempt to deter crime without success, these methods were abandoned and society began to approach crime from an *intelligent* perspective. It was not until the 1830s that society began to fight crime in a positive manner, *thinking* of solutions to the problem of crime rather than reacting to it. As intellectual foundations of fighting crime with science rather than with brutality were being considered, new concepts were explored. In 1835, the publication of *On Man* by Lambert Que'telet, a criminologist who stated, "society contains within itself the germs of all future crimes," projected a concept that takes one into another dimension of human behavior, one in which the prediction of dangerousness becomes a self-fulfilling prophecy. Crime and criminals will exist. Victims will exist (Que'telet, 1835).

What is the function of forensic nursing science, and what is its future? Futurists who study forensic science predict that in the next century the focus will be on the prevention of crime rather than the detection of crime. With the current innovations in science and technology, the research that led to the development of DNA, lasers, infrared photo-documentation, and other exciting scientific developments will continue. Throughout the twentieth century, the emphasis was on trying to analyze the psychopathology of the criminal mind through various means of scientific and nonscientific methods. Thus far, the criminal mind remains elusive. The one conclusion is that crime is a mental activity; the criminal makes choices, which is not to say that it is a controlled or uncontrolled decision. From the early literature, Dostoyevsky's *Crime and Punishment* became a study not only of the criminal mind but of criminology. In a vivid and impressionistic portrayal of the criminal mind–decisions, retribution, and pride–Dostoyevsky challenged us with a dramatic combination of the mental, physical, and metaphysical description of the mechanics of criminality (Dostoyevsky, 1866).

The mechanics of the criminal mind have not changed, crime has not increased; only trends in crime change with the trends of the time. According to criminologists, those who study the rise and fall of crime statistics, as well as the diseases of the mind that result from the germs of societal crime, it is the types of crimes that change, as opposed to the steady increase of crime itself. Therefore, if crime is the outcome of the germs of society resulting in a disease that takes control of the mind and renders it an anomaly, toxic, deviant, or malignant, then forensic nurse professionals must recognize their responsibilities in the identification of the problem: assessment, planning, intervention, and the evaluation of cause, manner, and mechanism of crime-related injury and death.

The roots of crime have been identified. Poverty, aggression, alienation, negativity, hate, lack of structure, lack of identity, revenge, rage, resentment, feelings of inadequacy, greed, power, and other organic and inorganic diseases of the mind: the germs of society. Aggression has been defined as a manifestation of disorganized purpose. Aggression results in extreme forms of behavior. The extremes of human behavior face nurses daily: child abuse, domestic homicide, suicide, sexual criminality, and emotional devastation (Campbell, Pliska, & Taylor et al., 1994; CDC, 1995, 1999; Crane, 2002; Ellis, 1999; Ledray & Arndt, 1994). There is no simple answer for such complex concerns for a better world. Forensic nurse examiners, however, have been identified as one step in the reduction and prevention of crime.

Awareness, perception, and insight pertaining to the roles and behaviors expected of each respective specialist must become synthesized into one voice: for victims, for the accused, for the offender, and for the health and security of society. Forensic nurses cannot assume the burden of treatment, rehabilitation, and cure for society's ills alone. These are multifaceted problems for which the cause and the cure will require commitment of each interrelated discipline. If crime is a mechanism of the mind, it stands to reason that the forensic and nursing sciences must focus intellect and energy on the mentally disordered offender, to consider the social and behavioral sciences in addition to the physical and medical sciences as a requirement of forensic nursing education. The need to incorporate the Scope and Standards of Forensic Nursing Practice as essential knowledge in traditional nursing preparation must be addressed in order for nursing students to face the reality of the patients they will care for.

The scene of the crime is in the mind. The mind comprises the body of the crime in as much as the corpus delicti is the essence of the crime. Crime scene investigators, forensic nurse examiners, and forensic medical scientists look to the body of the victim as a primary tool of the investigation of trauma, of crime, and of the criminal. Detectives look for psychological clues as well as the physical evidence at the crime scene. The sexual impulse is primarily a mental process; like murder, it begins inside the mind. The sexual assault nurse examiner looks for psychological clues as well as physical evidence. The nurse death investigator or coroner evaluates the trauma to determine whether or not the killer was a sexual pervert or a sexual sadist. The mind, then, must be the central organism that bonds each of these disciplines together in health and justice, in the living and the dead. No one role is more or less important than the other. As in the final analysis of the crime, the autopsy of the physical body, the psychological autopsy is equally important in understanding the corpus delicti.

Often, nurses, nursing students, and nurse educators express abhorrence when discussing the role of the forensic nurse examiner who works with offenders–the mentally disordered offender or offenders who remain in control of their minds. Equally, an innate resentment exists for attorneys who defend the criminal at trial. The role of the sexual assault nurse examiner and the nurse death investigator or coroner is often considered with aversion. Society must approach these concerns from a more positive perspective, viewing forensic nurse examiners as those who do not shy away from the reality of crimes involving the degradation of society, who choose not to remain wedged in the archaic philosophy of isolationism and limited capacity but rather move toward more holistic solutions. Serious attempts to eliminate crime must begin with an understanding of the criminal mind and the rehabilitation of the criminal. Most criminals repeat their criminal acts. Statistics indicate that the recidivism rate of the average offender is great. Punishment is a useless expedient; expectation to reform society must be addressed by example and humanness. Forensic nursing science has a role to fill in this attempt to create positive change. The medicolegal management of both victims and offenders in healthcare systems will have a crucial impact on the outcomes of court-related cases.

Deterrent to Crime

Execution has been studied from earliest history; each era has attempted to resolve crime with heinous methods of execution. Generations who have practiced execution as a form of punishment have documented their own opinion and that of statesmen, human rights activists, and criminals themselves that capital punishment is no deterrent to crime. Nor is the swiftness of capital punishment seen as a solution, as pickpockets have been observed working a crowd of spectators as another pickpocket was being hanged, drawn, and quartered (which included disemboweling and placing hot coals in the abdominal cavity). History documents the impact of executions on society (when 10-year-old children and pregnant women were hanged), as well as their impact on the executioners, a number of which went mad or committed suicide. Considering the vast number of those executed in the name of justice, crime should not exist today. Yet crime continues to exist. Only when society is able to understand the mentality of social aggression will true prevention be practiced. To expect society to set the appropriate example, radical changes must emerge.

A learned society recognizes that the most critical aspect in need of change is the parenting and socialization of its children. Studies of the phenomena of serial killers have indicated that the majority of these criminals are physically and psychologically damaged from childhood. It also notes that this human radical wears a "mask of sanity to hide his perverse desires from the world" (Norris, 1991). If hope exists to change the world, to reduce and prevent human violence, it will begin with the protection of the world's children. Diversity in human violence requires diversity in nursing knowledge. To keep pace with the physical and psychological sequelae of the germs of society, a process of multidisciplinary exchange of purpose and shared responsibility must exist. In such a milieu, forensic nurses will contribute, not only to the recovery of the victim or the apprehension of the criminal but also to a new insight into the healing of society.

Summary

Millions are sufficiently injured each year to seek medical assistance in hospitals and clinics for injuries sustained due to human violence. An enlightened healthcare system must be oriented toward change: to replace traditional concepts with new philosophies and new specialists to carry out these changes. As a change agent, the forensic nurse is often the crucial link between the untoward events of the real world and the more remote scientific undertaking of the legal sciences. According to criminologists, the lack of forensic knowledge can and will wreak havoc on an otherwise well-functioning system. Historically, these two worlds have not meshed philosophically or practically, which puts the forensic nurse in a unique position that can be both potentially difficult and influential (Standing Bear, 1995).

Forensic science is at the threshold of an explosion of technical advancement. In combating increasingly sophisticated crime, new and improved methods of identification and apprehension of the criminal will revolutionize the ability to bring those who commit violent crime, particularly the serial rapist and murderer, to justice. It is imperative that clinical professionals support law enforcement agencies in this quest to transmit developing knowledge through services that include forensic nursing interventions. Nursing education must engage in inquiry that is not immediately applicable to current clinical practice. It must be continually reevaluated in terms of societal needs and scientific discoveries. This requires nurse researchers to incorporate a variety of approaches to nursing's perspectives. The scope of the forensic nurse goes beyond that required for current clinical praxis.

Nurses are beginning to realize their potential for discovering particular knowledge that is relevant to other disciplines and essential to nursing (Newman, 1979, 1983). There is often a lag between the discovery of knowledge and its implementation in practice (Marsden-Scott, 1988). Forensic nursing, in its effort to decrease the lag between learning and applying forensic skills and services, has not only a responsibility but also an opportunity to chart new directions. It is important that the knowledge presented here become a part of the role preparation for the basic, generalist, and specialist practicing the forensic aspects of nursing. The answer lies within a combination of the emerging roles encompassing forensic nursing and quality public services.

This chapter has presented an overview of the evolution of forensic nursing science and forensic nursing services as they have developed and continue to advance. This framework is not intended to remain static but to evolve as new concepts and new knowledge are presented to the body of nurses who practice their skills within the arena of the law. This framework must also reflect the need for *holistic forensic nursing care* that encompasses the law designed for protection of legal and human rights.

Each individual has inherent dignity, worth, and responsibility to society. The universal mission of the forensic nurse examiner is to recognize the unique and complex human needs that are communicated through a variety of ways in the processes of living and dying. As the spectrum of forensic nursing expands, subspecialties of forensic nursing will continue to evolve where nursing and patient care interface with the law.

Resources

Organizations

American Academy of Forensic Sciences

410 North 21st Street, Colorado Springs, CO 80904; Tel: 719-636-1100; www.aafs.org

American Academy of Nursing

611 East Wells Street, Suite 1100, Milwaukee, WI 53202; Tel: 414-287-0289; www.aannet.org

Web Sites

Nurse Scribe, a lifelong learning resource for nursing students and nurses

www.enursescribe.com/nurse_theorists.htm

University of San Diego, Hahn School of Nursing and Health Science, nursing theory

www.sandiego.edu/nursing/theory

Valdosta State University, College of Nursing, nursing theory

www.valdosta.edu/nursing/history_theory/theory.html

References

Brenner, P. (1984). *From novice to expert: Excellence and power in clinical nursing practice.* Menlo Park, CA: Addison-Wesley.

Campbell, J. C., Pliska, M. J., & Taylor, W., et al. (1994). Battered women's experiences in the emergency department. *J Emerg Nurs, 20*(4), 280-288.

Carper, B. A. (1978). Fundamental patterns of knowing in nursing. *ANS Adv Nurs Sci, 4*(1), 253-259.

Centers for Disease Control (CDC). (1999). Nonfatal and fatal firearm-related injuries–United States, 1993-1997. *Morb Mortal Wkly Rep, 48*(45), 1029-1034.

Chinn, P., & Kramer, M. (1995). *Theory and nursing: A systematic approach* (4th ed.). St. Louis, MO: Mosby–Year Book.

Conway, D., & Hardy, L. (1988). *The use of knowledge.* Norwalk, CT: Appleton & Lange.

Crane, P. (2002, Spring). An historical timeline of rape. *On the Edge. 8*, 1

Dostoyevsky, F. (1866, 1980). *Crime and punishment: The Russian messenger.* 1866. Norwalk, CT: Easton Press.

Ellis, J. M. (1999). Barriers to effective screening for domestic violence by registered nurses in the emergency department. *Crit Care Nurs Q, 22*(1), 27-41.

Farrell, R., & Swigert, V. (1982). *Deviance and social control.* New York: Random House.

Federal Bureau of Investigation (FBI). (1999). *Uniform crime reports: Crime in the United States 1998.* Washington, DC: US Department of Justice.

Federal Bureau of Investigations (FBI). (2002). *Crime in the United States 2001.* Washington, DC: US Government Printing Office.

Federal Bureau of Investigation (FBI). (2002). *Uniform crime reports: Crime in the United States 2001.* Washington, DC: US Department of Justice.

Federal Bureau of Investigations (FBI). (2003, June). *Preliminary Uniform Crime Report, 2002.* Retrieved June 28, 2003, from www.fbi.gov/ucr/cius_02/02prelimannual.pdf.

Foege, W. (1997, November). Cited in L. B. Winett, Constructing violence as a public health problem. *Public Health Reports* (vol. 113, issue 6, pp. 498-499) Washington, DC: US Department of Health and Human Services.

Giger, J., & Davidhizar, R. (1991). *Transcultural nursing: Assessment and intervention* (2nd ed.). St. Louis, MO: Mosby.

International Association of Forensic Nurses (IAFN). (1997). *Scope and standards of forensic nursing practice.* Washington, DC: American Nurses Publishing.

Joint Commission on Accreditation of Healthcare Organizations (JCAHO). (2004). *Accreditation manual for hospitals.* Oakbrook Terrace, IL.

Koop, C. E. (1989). President and surgeon general condemn violence against women, call for new attitudes, programs. *National Organization for Victim Assistance Newsletter,* vol. 13.

Ledray, L., & Arndt, S. (1994). Sexual assault victim: A new model for nursing care. *J Psychosoc Nurs Ment Health Serv, 32*(2), 7-12.

Leininger, M. (1995). Cited in J. George, *Nursing theories: The base for professional nursing practice* (chap. 20). Norwalk, CT: Appleton & Lange.

Lynch, V. (1990). *Clinical forensic nursing: A descriptive study in role development.* Thesis, University of Texas, Arlington.

Lynch, V. (1991, February 12). *Proposal for a new scientific discipline: Forensic nursing.* Presentation to the general section at the annual meeting of the American Academy of Forensic Sciences, Anaheim, CA.

Lynch, V. (1995a). Clinical forensic nursing: A new perspective in the management of crime victims from trauma to trial. *Crit Care Nurs Clin North Am, 7*(3), 489-507.

Lynch, V. (1995b). Forensic nursing: What's new? *J Psychosoc Nurs* 33(9), 1-7.

Marsden-Scott, S. M. (1988). The discovery and practice of knowledge. In D. Conway & L. Hardy, *The use of knowledge.* Norwalk, CT: Appleton & Lange.

Mead, G. H. (1934). *Mind, self, and society.* Chicago: University of Chicago Press.

Newman, M. (1979). *Theory development in nursing.* Philadelphia: F. A. Davis.

Newman, M. (1983). The continuing revolution: A history of nursing science. In N. Chaska (Ed.), *The nursing profession: A time to speak* (pp. 385-393). New York: McGraw-Hill.

Norris, J. (1991). Cited in B. Marriner, *On death's bloody trail: Murder and the art of forensic science* (chapter titled "Facets of Murder–The Way Ahead," pp. 40, 165). New York: St. Martin's Press.

Paterson, J., & Zderad, L. (1998) Nursing theories: The base for professional nursing practice. In J. E. Patterson & L. T. Zderad, *Humanistic nursing* (pp. 287-299). New York: National League for Nursing Press.

Plato. (427-347 B.C.). *The Republic* (pp. 309). Translated from Greek to English by B. Jowett. Norwalk, CT: Easton Press.

Que'telet, L. (1835). *On man.* In B. Marriner (1991), *On death's bloody trail: Murder and the art of forensic science* (chapter titled "Crime and Punishment," pp. 40, 165). New York: St. Martin's Press.

Reiss, A. J., & Roth, J. A. (Eds.). (1993). *Understanding and preventing violence.* Washington, DC: National Academy Press.

Standing Bear, Z. G. (1995). Forensic nursing and death investigation: Will the vision be co-opted? *J Psychosoc Nurs Ment Health Serv, 33*(9), 59-64.

Unit Two

Violence

Contemporary Social Issues and Forensic Science

Chapter 4 Human Rights

Nizam Peerwani and Virginia A. Lynch

Universal Declaration of Human Rights Preamble

Whereas recognition of the inherent dignity and of the equal and inalienable rights of all members of the human family is the foundation of freedom, justice, and peace in the world.
—United Nations, 1948

Overview

As the world celebrated the fiftieth anniversary of the Universal Declaration of Human Rights in 1998, violence was beginning to be viewed as a health problem rather than merely a legal one. Human violence is the major cause of trauma worldwide. Contemporary healthcare professionals have been challenged to contribute to health and human services due to the caustic consequences of intentional violence inflicted by governments, as well as the atrocities of violence that stem from social and political degradation. Just as some forms of world currency have been devalued, human life has also been devalued and tragedies such as apartheid, ethnic cleansing, and genocide have occurred as a result. Public health and human rights organizations have recognized a covenant with the rule of law that will address and advance human well-being. A mutual responsibility with health and human rights is essential to create a positive and profound change in the world's moral code of ethics (Mann, Gruskin, & Grodin et al., 1999).

Human Rights: The Role of Forensic Examiners

In 1973, Amnesty International (AI) sponsored a major conference in Paris to focus on the issue of torture. As a result of this effort, the first AI medical group was formed in Copenhagen in 1974. Since then, physicians and nurses from many countries have assisted AI and similar organizations, such as Physicians for Human Rights (a nongovernmental organization [NGO] based in Boston, Massachusetts) and the American Academy of Nursing (a professional organization based in Washington, DC), in opposing torture. These groups are taking action on behalf of detained physicians, nurses, and prisoners of conscience, and they are promoting and protecting human rights and ethical standards within the medical and nursing profession.

The role played by forensic experts is vital for ensuring a scientific investigation. In addition to examining victims of torture and fatal injuries in custody, forensic experts are now involved in a variety of activities including performing clinical forensic evaluation to document crimes against humanity and genocide as well as helping to identify human remains. Forensic examiners draw from many specialties including forensic pathology, nursing, anthropology, dentistry, toxicology, and various criminalistics disciplines including ballistics, serology, and DNA.

Mann's Health and Human Rights Triad

Historically, health and human rights have always been linked. In describing this linkage and providing a framework, Jonathan M. Mann et al. (1999) focused on three relationships. The first concerns the potential impact of health policies, programs, and practices on human rights. The second expresses the idea that violations or lack of fulfillment of any and all human rights have negative effects on physical, mental, and social well-being, both in peacetime and particularly so in times of conflict and extreme political repression. The third expresses the notion that health and human rights act in synergy. Hence, promoting and protecting health requires explicit and concrete efforts to promote and protect human rights and dignity, and, likewise, fulfillment of human rights necessitates attention to health and its social determinants.

Modern concepts of health have developed from three related, although quite different disciplines: medicine, nursing, and public health. Medicine generally focuses on curative services for the individual in the context of physical and, to a lesser extent, mental illness and disability. Nursing approaches health from a holistic perspective, including physical, psychosocial, and spiritual concepts of individuals, families, and communities. In contrast, public health focuses on the health of populations and the conditions in which people can avoid illness (Mann, Gruskin, & Grodin et al., 1999). More recently, public health has included a distinct health-promoting emphasis, focusing on the prevention of disease, disability, and premature death.

Global Health and Human Services

In 1946, the World Health Organization (WHO) developed the most widely used modern definition of health. It stated that "Health is a state of complete physical, mental and social well-being and not merely absence of disease or infirmity." With this declaration, WHO has helped to broaden the scope of "health" beyond a limited, biomedical, pathology-based perspective, beyond individual diseases or viruses, to the all-encompassing perspective of "well-being" incorporating psychosocial dimensions. These broader societal perspectives were illustrated in the Declaration of Alma-Ata (1978), which stated that health is a "social goal whose realization requires the action of many other social and economic sectors in addition to the health sector" (WHO, 1986, pp. 50-76).

Healthcare around the world is provided through many diverse public and private mechanisms. However, the primary responsibilities of public health are carried out in large measure through laws, policies, and programs promulgated, implemented, and enforced by or with support of the state. In many situations, this is the Department of Health and Human Services or Ministry of Health. Central to all programs of health delivery and promotion (physical, mental, and social well-being) is the concept of prevention, which involves three levels (Declaration of Alma-Ata, 1978). In a similar framework, the forensic nursing model addresses interfaces of body, mind, spirit, and the law (see Chapter 3).

- *Primary prevention is "pure" prevention, or preventing the health problem from occurring at all* (e.g., preventing cancer through avoidance of tobacco smoking or preventing polio by vaccinating children with a polio vaccine). Clearly, this is the ideal and most cost-effective approach. Primary prevention is often referred to as *health promotion*, the process of enabling people to increase control over and to improve health (International Federation of Red Cross et al., 1999).
- *Secondary prevention involves prompt detection and successful management or treatment of the health condition so as to avoid actual damage to the person's health* (e.g., early detection and treatment of high blood pressure can prevent the strokes or kidney damage that result from uncontrolled hypertension).
- *Tertiary prevention seeks to limit the impairment, increase the quality of life, and prolong life* (e.g., providing emergency care for victims of automobile crashes or rehabilitative services to help maximize activity and independence after a stroke or heart attack).

Promotion of prevention in the public health setting necessitates assessing health needs and problems, developing policies designed to address priority health issues, and assuring programs to implement strategic health goals (Ottawa Charter, 1986). Assessment is the first and primordial step, without which adequate policy development and assurance of service are greatly handicapped. Assessment means collecting and analyzing data in order to identify and understand the major health problems facing a community.

Prediction and Prevention

The main tool of assessment is the science of epidemiology, which studies the distribution and determinants of health-related states and events in populations, with the primary goal of providing critical information for control of health problems. It is in this arena that the forensic scientist plays a critical role in public health. Through the establishment of sound forensic programs, reliable and accurate mortality data (which includes the cause, manner, and mechanism of death) can be gathered. This is not limited to trauma but also includes deaths due to diseases.

Best Practice *4-1*

Nurses should assess all traumatic injuries and deaths in terms of the potential for preventing the same injury or death under similar circumstances and should initiate an active nursing plan involving primary, secondary, and tertiary prevention strategies.

Forensic Health Science and the Law

Definitely, the role played by forensic health science goes beyond the domain of public health. No other scientific specialty plays a more important and vital role in the domain of human rights. This is because of the critical need for a legitimate authority, which is best summarized by Thomsen (International Federation of Red Cross et al., 1999):

> *There is a need for forensic expertise in the detection of human rights violations. The concept of legitimate authority is central to the practice, indeed to the principle, of forensic medicine that is the application of medicine to the resolution of issues in a legal context. Without legitimate authority applying the law in accordance with international norms, the very concept of forensic medicine is undermined (p. 29).The evolution and acceptance of what constitutes violation of human rights or of International Humanitarian Law has been slow and painful. Following the 1945 Nuremberg Tribunal, which judged the accused war criminals and medical personnel of Nazi Germany, the international community pledged that never again would it allow monstrous crimes against humanity or genocide to take place. In 1948, the United Nations (UN) general assembly adopted the Convention on the Prevention and Punishment of the Crime of Genocide. In 1949, a Diplomatic Conference for the Establishment of International Conventions for the Protection of Victims of War, held in Geneva, adopted four new Geneva Conventions (the first was adopted in 1864), which codified the humanitarian action of soldiers in times of war. The four Geneva Conventions more specifically outlined the humane treatment of wounded, sick, or surrendering combatants, prisoners, and civilians and banned the willful taking and killing of hostages. In 1997, two additional protocols were added to the Geneva Conventions and together with customary law regarding just war, these form the body of International Humanitarian Law.*

In somewhat of a parallel track, the framework of what constituted human rights law was developed and gradually adopted. A little more than 50 years ago, a UN committee chaired by the former First Lady Eleanor Roosevelt proposed, and the UN General Assembly adopted, the Universal Declaration of Human Rights (UDHR). Although this document is nonbinding in international law, it sets the ideal to guarantee all people security, dignity, and well-being in every place in the world (Thomsen et al., 1984). In Articles 1 and 2, the UDHR states that all human beings are born free and equal in dignity and rights and they are endowed with reason and conscience and should act toward one another in a spirit of brotherhood. Furthermore, everyone is entitled to all rights and freedoms without distinction of any kind, such as race, color, sex, language, religion, political or other opinion, national or social origin, property, birth, or other status. This declaration was drafted as a response to the horrors of World War II and was to be taught around the world, in every institution of learning and at every level of education. Every year the UN publishes small pocket-sized handbills in all its official languages for worldwide distribution.

Conflicts and Warring Factions

Yet, 50 years later, horrendous crimes against humanity, genocide, and ethnic cleansing are still witnessed. Indeed, as the world marched into a new millennium, every continent witnessed unfolding horrors and humanitarian crises (e.g., Democratic Republic of Congo, Afghanistan, Palestine, Kashmir, Chechnya, Angola, Colombia, Mozambique, Sri Lanka, Burundi, Somalia, and Kosovo). There is no doubt that some of the most serious threats to international peace and security are armed conflicts that arise not among nations but among warring factions within a state. Although initially they are situations of internal or regional conflict, they often spill over borders, endangering the security of other states and other peoples and resulting in complex humanitarian emergencies. The human rights abuses prevalent in internal conflicts are now among the most atrocious in the world.

In 1996 so-called high-intensity conflicts cumulatively led to between 6.5 million and 8.5 million deaths. In the same year, there were also 40 "low-intensity conflicts," each causing between 100 and 1000 deaths. Another 2 million deaths can be added to these figures if one includes situations of internal violence that had deescalated in 1996. Incredibly, the number of conflict-related deaths is only a small indication of the tremendous amount of suffering, displacement, and devastation caused by conflicts. Assaults on the fundamental right to life are widespread and include massacres, indiscriminate attacks on civilians, execution of prisoners, and starvation of entire populations (Thomsen et al., 1984).

Torture is common in internal conflicts, as are measures restricting people's freedom of movement including forcible relocation, mass expulsions, and denial of the right to seek asylum or the right to return to one's home. Women and girls are raped by soldiers and forced into prostitution, and children are abducted to serve as soldiers. Regrettably, tens of thousands of people detained in connection with conflicts "disappear" each year, usually killed and buried in secret, leaving their families with the torment of not knowing their fate. Thousands of others are arbitrarily imprisoned and never brought to trial or, if they are, are subject to grossly unfair proceedings. Homes, schools, and hospitals are deliberately destroyed. Relief convoys, which try to assist civilians by providing humanitarian aid, are attacked. Just as human rights are a key element in peacekeeping and peacebuilding efforts, the protection of human rights during humanitarian operations is now recognized as a priority.

Reconciliation and Justice

To break the cycle of violence, past abuses against civilian populations must be addressed. Accountability and justice are important elements in the reconciliation and prevention of further atrocities.

Although International Humanitarian Law has been established for some time, venues for its application have been tenuous. Despite the success of the UN's direction of the International Law Commission in drafting a statute for an International Criminal Court, disagreement among member states on the jurisdiction of such a court has hindered its actual implementation. Key nations, including the US, continue to oppose key requirements for effective functioning of such a tribunal.

Genocide

Genocide is a value-laden word and does not include killings in the setting of a traditional war or border skirmish. Genocide is distinguishable from all other crimes by the motivation behind it. Toward the end of the Second World War, when the full horror of the extermination and concentration camps became public knowledge, Winston Churchill stated that the world was being brought face to face with "a crime that has no name." History was of little use in finding a recognized word to fit the nature of the crimes in Nazi Germany. Raphael Lemkin, the Polish-born adviser to the US War Ministry, saw that the world was being confronted with a totally unprecedented phenomenon and that "new conceptions require new terminology." In his book, *Axis Rule in Occupied Europe*, published in 1944, he coined the word *genocide*, constructed it from the Greek *genos* (race or tribe) and the Latin suffix *cide* (to kill). According to Lemkin's work, genocide refers to the destruction of a nation or of an ethnic group and implies the existence of a coordinated plan, aimed at total extermination, to be put into effect against individuals chosen as victims purely, simply, and exclusively because they are members of the target group. In today's news stories, genocide is often referred to as "ethnic cleansing."

In Rwanda, civil strife and internal violence led to genocide on a vast scale. From April to July 1994, a systematically planned genocide by extremist Hutu militia claimed the lives of between 500,000 and 1 million persons (Destexhe, 1995). The main victims of this carnage were members of the Tutsi minority and moderate Hutus. The civil war forced hundreds of thousands of Rwandans to flee to neighboring countries. By mid-July, more than 2 million Rwandan refugees were living in camps in Burundi, Tanzania, and Zaire. Many thousands more had been displaced internally within Rwanda. In November 1994, the UN Security Council created the International Criminal Tribunal for the Prosecution of Persons Responsible for Genocide and Other Serious Violations of International Humanitarian Law Committed in the Territory of Rwanda. The gathering of forensic evidence to establish and prosecute the perpetrators of genocide was undertaken by Physicians for Human Rights under the auspices of the UN Security Council. According to Article 2 of the Convention on the Prevention and Punishment of the Crime of Genocide, genocide is any act committed with intent to destroy, in whole or in part, a national, ethnic, racial, or religious group (Box 4-1).

Thus, using the definitions of both Lemkin and the convention there have been four genuine examples of genocide during the course of the twentieth century: the Armenians by the Young Turks in 1915, the Jews and Gypsies by the Nazis during World War II, the Bosnian Muslims by Serbs in former Yugoslavia from 1993 to 1995, and in 1994, that of the Hutus and Tutsis in Rwanda.

There are several objectives in performing forensic evaluation of genocide. These include the following:

- Documenting and collecting forensic evidence to assist in criminal prosecution
- Identifying human remains in order to repatriate the remains and thereby bring closure
- Recording scientific facts to abort revisionist history

Considering the paucity of forensic clinicians throughout the world, and the insufficient education of many, it stands to reason that the opportunity for the emerging role of the forensic nurse examiner will provide forensic expertise, historically absent in most of the world.

Box 4-1 Acts of Genocide

- Killing members of the group
- Causing serious bodily or mental harm to members of the group
- Deliberately inflicting on the group conditions of life calculated to bring about its physical destruction in whole or in part
- Imposing measures intended to prevent birth within the group including forced pregnancies by men outside the group
- Forcibly transferring children of one group to another group

The Role of the Forensic Nurse Examiner

The forensic nursing examiner has a vital role in the identification of victims of human rights abuse as well as in the investigation of violations of international humanitarian law in conflict situations. Forensic nursing as a clinical subspecialty provides an important resource to clinical forensic medicine, justice systems, and the human rights community. As an emerging discipline, forensic nursing assumes a mutual responsibility with forensic scientists as well as the criminal justice and national security systems in concern for the loss of human life and function due to the intimidation, domination, or control of political, religious, cultural groups, or other forms of interpersonal oppression. The unique skills of nurses educated in forensic technique enhance investigative and rehabilitative capabilities, as well as preventative public health functions (Lynch, 1995).

Nurses specializing in the care and treatment of victims of pernicious human behavior offer, in addition to traditional professional nursing care, the complex skills of assessment of covert and latent patterned injuries, recognition and collection of human bite mark evidence, photo-documentation, and recovery and preservation of genetic evidence, as well as provide crucial intervention in emotional trauma associated with human rights violations.

A forensic specialist in nursing is ideally qualified to design and implement forensic guidelines regarding accurate assessment and documentation, as well as to address the educational needs of staff to ensure compliance with forensic protocols. These distinct responsibilities include the role of assessor, educator, and therapist for individuals, families, and communities, both survivors and potential or actual perpetrators of cruel and inhuman treatment. The forensic nurse examiner may also assist institutional staff members with critical incident stress debriefing, survivor follow-up, and conducting research about this nursing specialty.

Sexual assault is a violent act resulting in serious physical and emotional sequelae, often repeatedly, inflicted upon victims of social and political torture. The forensic nurse as a sexual assault examiner provides advanced physical assessment and stabilization of the victim's emotional equilibrium, collection of forensic evidence, and courtroom testimony for all cases, regardless of whether medical treatment is required. Forensic nurse examiners specializing in the scientific investigation of death collaborate with forensic pathologists in questioned death cases. Participation in this area includes investigation at the crime scene, postmortem examinations in the autopsy laboratory, exhumation of clandestine gravesites, and disaster site recovery. Others forensic nurses apply their skills as nurse attorneys or legal nurse consultants, in the clinical setting of forensic mental health in the community as hostage negotiators, and in academe conducting research or developing new roles on the frontier of violence.

The academic and professional development of the forensic clinical nurse specialist (FCNE) provides an incisive exploration of the principles and philosophies of the forensic sciences that include the following:

- Forensic psychopathology
- Signs and legal aspects of death
- Certification of death
- Forensic odontology
- Bioethics and health law
- Victimology and traumatology
- Sexual and domestic violence
- Forensic pathology
- Organ/tissue recovery
- Biochemical and mass disasters
- Medicolegal documentation
- Forensic photography and criminalistics
- Structure and function of institutions of legal medicine
- Interpersonal violence, abuse and neglect
- Accident scene and occupational health
- Rules of evidence and expert testimony
- Human rights

Forensic education prepares nurse clinicians with enhanced and focused observation, assessment, clinical communication skills, legal documentation, and maintenance of evidence skills, as well as in prevention and rehabilitation issues essential to caring for individuals who have sustained intentional trauma, including those violated by government institutions and terrorists.

Nursing's theory base and scope of practice support forensic interventions for survivors of torture and human rights violations. Nurses can bring empathy, compassion, and respect for human rights victims combined with advanced expertise in forensic fields. Forensic specialization in the biomedical and social sciences incorporates emergency advocacy for individual victims while simultaneously providing scientific knowledge to systematically combat destructive social and political conditions in the tradition of population-based public health interventions (United Nations, 1964).

Further, forensic nursing, due to its holistic orientation, helps provide a humanistic approach to the application and protection of internationally recognized human rights standards. This new *Health and Justice* specialist provides uniquely qualified clinical professionals, blending biomedical knowledge with the basic principles of international law and of human behavior in caring for survivors of torture (Rocky Mountain Survivors Center, 2000).

Forensic Nursing Responsibilities

The skills of physicians, nurses, and other healthcare workers along with those of biomedical and forensic scientists are uniquely valuable in the investigation and documentation of human rights violations. Many relevant investigative tasks, ranging from physical examination to exhumation of mass graves, often produce more credible evidence of abuse, which is less vulnerable to challenge than traditional methods of case reporting. Contemporary roles in forensic nursing join with health and human rights specialists in the investigation of genocide, documentation of torture, mass grave exhumations, and collection of evidence that supports or refutes allegations of government-sanctioned torture, rape, and extrajudicial executions (Lynch, 1995).

International standards outlaw arbitrary deprivation of life. The Universal Declaration of Human Rights states, "Everyone has the right to life, liberty, and security of person." In the past 10 years, the UN has made many recommendations on the standards for incarceration, the investigation and prevention of torture, arbitrary or summary executions, and the investigation of deaths among detainees. Yet forensic services are a neglected aspect of medical and judicial systems as well as human rights programs. If forensic services are funded at all, they are generally low on the agenda of most government officials who fail to prioritize the moral duty of governments to use their power and influence to prevent assault and cruelty in prisons and refugee and detention camps (Watson, 1995).

Further protection is accorded in Article 5, which states specifically, "no one shall be subjected to torture or to cruel, inhuman, or degrading treatment or punishment. In particular no one shall be subjected without his free consent to medical or scientific experimentation." The UN General Assembly defined additional obligations when it adopted the Convention against Torture in December 1984. The convention is legally binding on member states that no issue, irrespective of its merits, can serve as a justification for torture. Presently, 123 member states have signed the convention, including the US.

Despite having signed the UN Convention against Torture and Other Cruel, Inhuman or Degrading Treatment or Punishment (1987) and the Covenant on Civil and Political Rights (1966, 1992 for US), now considered universal international standards, many official governments do not meet these standards.

International Humanitarian Law

International Humanitarian Law (IHL) dictates that healthcare professionals restricted to humanitarian roles in times of war are entitled to special protections as noncombatants. Medical and nursing personnel are generally accorded this special consideration during armed conflict if they abstain from any roles as combatants or from working in warehouses or aircraft being used to support combat. Further, healthcare providers eligible for the legal Geneva Convention protections usually must carry a special identification card and display the emblem of the International Red Cross, Crescent, or Star of David. These protective privileges or rights are enumerated in detail in the Geneva Conventions of 1949 (ratified by the US in 1955). As globalization increases in importance for healthcare professionals, the need for a curriculum that covers issues related to both human rights and international humanitarian law must be considered. The professional responsibilities nurses have in nonmilitary clinical and community settings (besides the traditional roles of alleviating the suffering among victims of human rights violations) must be better defined. Nursing professionals are tasked to take action relating to armed conflict as never before (Hoffman, 1995). The sequela of war demands a need for health services across a broad continuum including acute emergency services as well as rehabilitation and reintegration of civilian casualties into the public domain. With each subsequent armed conflict or peacekeeping mission, a greater number of forensic nurse examiners will be needed to provide forensic services. Forensic expertise in war and armed conflict is an essential ingredient documenting criminal acts or war crimes. It includes identifying human remains, preserving evidence related to violations of international humanitarian law, addressing issues of torture, and assisting in the establishment of a sustainable post-conflict rehabilitation and justice scheme.

International Human Rights Law

The body of international law protecting human life and dignity in peacetime is commonly referred to as human rights law. As IHL designates the framework for nursing professionals during armed conflict, human rights law is broader and further sets forth the conceptual legal framework identifying all person's rights and duties during peacetime, including laws relating to nursing in prisons.

The International Council of Nurses (ICN) has passed a resolution providing that nurses "having knowledge of physical or mental ill-treatment of detainees and prisoners take appropriate action including reporting these matters to appropriate national and or international bodies." Fulfillment of this responsibility is essential to advancing global human rights advocacy. Nurses should be the first to understand that even single, seemingly minor human rights violations can have significant health consequences including the following:

- Physical manifestations, emotional distress, disruption of physiological functioning, loss of self-esteem and confidence
- Psychological and sexual torture
- Loss of faith in healthcare providers
- Loss of motivation to participate in civil society
- Loss of interest in parenting and other forms of social withdrawal
- Epidemic infectious diseases spread by overcrowding, lack of sanitation facilities for refugees
- Lack of access to healthcare resulting in untreated chronic disease
- Starvation

Violations of human rights standards include the following:

- Breaches of medical neutrality
- Forced deportations
- Use of indiscriminate weapons
- Mass executions
- Other violent actions affecting entire populations
- Purposeful destruction of health facilities
- Forced pregnancy or spread of infectious disease from nonconsensual sex
- Slavery
- Forcing children to become soldiers

Nurses and Global Torture: A Health and Justice Dilemma

Torture is one of the most severe problems in the world–a plague in modern times. The scale of torture in the world is broader than is generally perceived. The UN indicates that government-sanctioned torture occurs in more than 78 countries, approximately a third of the members of the United Nations (Glittenberg, 2004)

Inge Genefke, MD, honorary director and founder of the International Rehabilitation Center for Torture Victims, stresses that torture is designed to destroy a person as a human being. When survivors of torture are helped to regain health and strength, the torturer's weapon has been essentially destroyed (Glittenberg, 2004).

Torture did not just emerge in the twenty-first century but has existed throughout the millennia of human existence. Archaeological evidence indicates that torture has been practiced since at least 1500 B.C., as skeletal remains from Mesopotamia reflect forensic evidence of involuntary, violent death. Throughout countless millennia torture, like slavery, has been accepted as the right of a ruling society to control its citizens, yet the extreme burden of torture increases when whole groups of subjects are prosecuted and society fails to mount any opposition. As the world became more populated and less enamored of recognizing human rulers as gods, global wars and their aftermath, as well as massive human rights violations, triggered more concern for human victims and a desire to set forth minimal standards of universal human rights. The concept of protecting human life and freedoms has thus gained wider acceptance (see Box 4-2) (Glittenberg, 2004).

Box 4-2 Torture Defined

Any act by which severe pain or suffering, whether physical or mental, is intentionally inflicted on a person for such purposes as obtaining from them or a third person information or a confession, punishing him/her for an act he/she or a third person has committed or is suspected of having committed, or intimidating or coercing him or a third person, or for any reason based on discrimination of any kind, when such pain or suffering is inflicted by or at the instigation of or with the consent or acquiescence of a public official or other person acting in an official capacity. It does not include pain or suffering arising only from, inherent in or incidental to lawful sanctions.

—UN Convention Against Torture and Other Cruel, Inhuman or Degrading Treatment or Punishment of December 10, 1964, which entered into force in June, 1987.

Two countries with the largest populations on earth, China and India (particularly in Kashmir), are still known for human rights abuses. The Middle East, including Turkey, Iran, and Iraq, are also part of the particularly severe state-sponsored torture zone where institutionalized torture is organized and not merely local or accidental. As torturers are selected and trained, new methods of torture spread rapidly inside the torture profession affecting long-term medical consequences and psychological damage long after the torture has stopped.

Export of Terrorism

In the past, some manufacturers of military and police supplies in the US have exported stun guns, mace, laser devices, and other instruments. Although far from their perceived intended use, they sometimes fell into the wrong hands and many of these items eventually were used for acts of torture within the international community. In 1989, the Antiterrorism and Arms Export Amendments Acts was passed. The aim of this legislation was to halt exportation of such devices to countries that sponsor international terrorism (US Senate Proceedings, 1989).

This legislation was designed to combat international terrorism and further the national security and foreign policy interests of the US. It imposed a ban on the export of arms from the US to countries that sponsor international terrorism and also imposed tighter controls on nonmilitary exports to such countries. The bill's purpose was to reaffirm, strengthen, and clarify this nation's prohibition on exports of military weapons and equipment to countries that have been designated by the secretary of state as supporters of international terrorism. Further, it imposed new criminal and civil penalties on violators. Unfortunately, however, there is no single standard in law for the following:

- Determining whether a country supports international terrorism
- Identifying which US official should make such a determination
- Identifying which arms are subject to restrictions
- Identifying the criteria that empower the president to waive statutory restrictions
- Informing Congress of arms exports, including covert exports

The inconsistent provisions of existing law have blunted the effectiveness of US antiterrorism policy, both in terms of government actions and the activities of private American citizens who look to the law for guidance.

Addressing Torture in Nursing

The international health community has organized against torture by bringing together a collective group of experts to address this complex social crime against humanity. Although initially health professionals were recognized mainly as trauma care providers, and their early focus was primarily on healing those who had survived torture, their skills in communication and behavior modification have risen to the fore in searching for conflict-prevention strategies. Forensic nurses have a key role in breaking the cycle of violence tied to heredity, poverty, cultural oppression of women and children, and the all-too-common complicity of military police and judicial systems. To begin with, more than 200 centers throughout the world specialize in the rehabilitation of torture survivors (Glittenberg, 2004).

Rehabilitation of Torture Survivors

The concept of rehabilitating torture survivors began through Amnesty International (AI) when it appealed to the medical profession around the world for help to combat torture. In 1973, a conference was convened in Paris titled, "Conference on Abolition of Torture," and as a result the first medical group was organized in Denmark in 1974. This group of physicians began to examine claims of torture by people in Chile and Greece. In 1975, a group of Danish nurses also organized to work toward greater understanding of torture. In 1978, AI organized an international seminar in Athens, Greece, involving medicine and nursing and focused specifically on rehabilitation of survivors. Denmark became the first center of rehabilitation and the first survivors, found to have special needs to reduce their fears, came to Copenhagen in 1982. This endeavor has become recognized the world over as the International Rehabilitation Center for Torture Victims (Glittenberg, 2004). Two centers are located in the US, one in Denver, Colorado, and another in Minneapolis, Minnesota.

Nursing has had a role in establishing these global rehabilitation centers. This declaration is specific to the care of people in prisons where torture took place. The ICN Statement on Nurses and Torture specifically requires that the nurse provide professional nursing care to victims of torture without fear of reprisal from authorities. Nurses are also prohibited from engaging or participating in any activities that were conceived of as torturous, such as depriving anyone of nursing treatments. The ICN document clearly describes risk situations in which a nurse might be engaged and how the nurse has protection to seek advice and counsel from the profession in these difficult situations (Jacobsen & Smidt-Nielson, 1997). In 1975, the ICN adopted the Declaration of Singapore on the *Role of the Nurse in the Care of Detainees and Prisoners* (The Declaration of Singapore, 1975).

Key Point *4-1*

Nurses should be aware of their responsibility in safeguarding human rights as defined by the International Council of Nurses and other professional nursing associations' codes of ethics. Nurses should be familiar with their responsibilities when caring for prisoners and detainees and must understand that it is an unethical practice to participate in acts of torture or execution in any setting.

Box 4-3 Mission Statement of the Rocky Mountain Survivors Program

To promote compassionate refuge by engaging survivors of human rights abuse through the provision of specialized human services within the community; thereby contributing to the elimination of torture and other violations of human rights.

From Rocky Mountain Survivors Center for the Assistance of Survivors of Torture and War (2000). Educational brochure. Denver, CO: Author

Advancing Forensic Nursing in Human Rights

Sadly, torture is a growth industry, still practiced by nearly two thirds of the world's countries. Amnesty International estimates that between 30% and 50% of refugees and asylum seekers have suffered human rights abuses, including torture from countries with the most deplorable human rights records. One endeavor to raise awareness of the role of forensic nurse examiners in the documentation of torture, evaluation of injury related to torture, and classification of other human rights violations has been addressed through the Rocky Mountain Survivors Center (RMSC) for victims of torture in Denver, Colorado.

This organization represents one of the few centers specifically created to provide information, counseling, and support services for survivors of torture and their families (Box 4-3). The RMSC also provides training and education to personnel from other organizations that directly assist survivors and immigrants. The RMSC is profoundly impressed by the dignity and courage of survivors of torture. The determination of survivors to transcend the victim identification and reacquire strength in their lives demonstrates that ordinary people who suffer extraordinary trauma can make extraordinary recoveries (Rocky Mountain Survivors Center, 2000).

Since 1996, the RMSC has successfully provided direct services to the survivors of torture in the Rocky Mountain region regardless of their immigration status. Clients include refugees, asylum seekers, and newly arrived immigrants in search of permanent status–basically all people who cannot return to their home countries without endangering their lives and the lives of their families. And as people previously stigmatized by torture, subsequently having been disfigured or disabled, are willing to trust again, they are able to seek services from culturally competent and understanding healthcare providers. The need for the services provided at the RMSC continues to grow as the US continues to offer refuge to displaced people of the world.

A grant awarded to the RMSC specifically addressed the need for refugees seeking assistance and political asylum through the US Court of Immigration to "receive a forensic evaluation by a nurse." This funding recognizes the forensic expertise of nurses who have been educated in forensic science and nursing, including the mechanics and specifics of physical and emotional trauma secondary to interpersonal violence, sexual assault, traumatic witnessing of catastrophic death or near-death incidents, surviving a hostage or kidnapping event, as well as the dynamics of torture rehabilitation.

In light of the global shortage of forensic examiners, the advent of the forensic nurse provides a new, reliable resource in addressing the ever-increasing needs of forensic services previously unavailable to this population of clients. In light of the dimension of needs for these services, the health and justice communities are recruiting and training nurses in developing and industrialized countries worldwide.

Working with Torture Victims

Torture victims frequently demonstrate the symptoms associated with post-traumatic stress disorder (PTSD). RMSC provides psychological evaluations and counseling through both individual and group therapy programs with particular expertise in cross-cultural counseling and body-centered psychotherapy designed for torture and trauma recovery. *Secondary trauma* experienced by the staff is often a consequence associated with the emotional distress resulting from exposure to the primary trauma of the clients who have been exposed to unthinkable brutality.

Unique trauma training programs address secondary trauma for the interpreters and therapists who may be affected by their continued interface with human rights atrocities. Such acts include kidnapping, disappearances, rape, ethnic cleansing, and massive raids perpetrated by political regimes aimed not at discovering information but at destroying the personalities or will to live of the potential opponents of the torturing regime. Too often, initial torture is compounded when after discovery torturers are not prosecuted. New powers may wish to keep a facade of harmony. Impunity often occurs in spite of verbal opposition because victims are either unorganized or lack the means to bring perpetrators to justice. Unfortunately, the freedom of the press is not mentioned specifically in the UN Convention on Torture, but citizens need to know, and vital information is too often withheld. Torture is hard to prove, as the practice is done in secret and often the tortured, if they survive, leave the region out of fear of further torture and become part of the 100 million displaced persons (refugees and asylum seekers) worldwide.

Description of Torture

To develop treatment and advocacy plans, acts of torture need to be studied. Torture is unlike random acts of violence, commonly investigated in forensic nursing, for the goal of torture is to strike fear in the community (Glittenberg, 2004). Torture exists to mentally destroy. The more extreme the pain and torment, the more horrifying the message will be for the not yet captive or still dissenting population (Chester, 1988). Extreme acts of cruelty are used to break the will of the tortured and unrelenting fear is instilled to shatter the will of the populace. Torture via extreme forms of trauma deliberately and strategically attacks the body, psyche, and spirit of the individual in order to destroy all levels of meaning (Chester & Jaranson, 1994).

Methods of Torture

Physical torture methods include beating, dental torture, suspension, and painful positions of the body, suffocation, electric torture, mutilation, pharmacological torture, and burning. Psychological torture methods include deprivation (e.g., sleep, isolation, food). Vicarious torture of others is often a strategy via projection of fellow prisoners' screams, being forced to watch the torture of others (public amputations and executions in soccer stadiums under the Taliban), or being given grave preparation duties. Threats of sham executions and waiting in anticipation constitute psychological torture. Another form of torture is exile–being forced to leave home and belongings, loss of familiar language, friends, and family, loss of social status, complete denial of identifying papers–which comprises a less physically invasive yet demeaning threat to self.

The nature and extent of prolonged and repeated trauma in groups under repression has an impact of destroying important relationships and, in some cases, multigenerational ties and health. Untold trauma occurs when the entire social context is interrupted and transformed. Those in power target the most vulnerable and strategically destroy communities and families (Ramsay, Grost-Unsworth, & Turner, 1993). Many in the US attribute the increased incidence of hypertension among African Americans to the hardships for generations of forced exile, slavery, and mistreatment.

Sexual Torture and Rape

Sadistic sexual homicide evokes fear and powerlessness in the minds of the public. Sexual torture evokes the same emotions of those in captivity. Mass rape of women during wartime has historically been considered a spoil of war. Women, impregnated by their enemies as a cruel form of ethnic cleansing, leaves a generation of human beings unwanted and often despised. Sexual torture is demeaning, and its purpose is to evoke shame in the family and community. The despair of helplessness that shadows the conquered is beyond words

The gruesome motive of sexual torture is to humiliate the victim (Jacobsen & Smidt-Nielson, 1997). Universally, victims are restrained to increase the helplessness they endure while mutilation and electric shock assault sexual organs; clothes are torn away while victims are placed and tied in embarrassing positions; and victims are forced to masturbate and take part in the rape of other prisoners. Specially trained dogs assault both men and women; instruments, such as broken bottles, are forced into the anus or vagina. Electric probes are forced into the male urethra. It is believed that one third to two thirds of women and girls seeking treatment for sequelae of torture have been raped or sexually violated (Chester, 1992).

Healing the Tortured

As for other acts of criminal cruelty, forensic nursing adds to the cadre of skilled, compassionate health providers in the rehabilitation of torture survivors. When political forces become fearful and oppressive, torture raises its ugly head (Glittenberg, 2004). Being alert to threats against democracy is one means of preventing torture. As nurses are involved globally, such alertness is part of nursing care. As a part of the international community engaged in eliminating torture, nurses oppose the oppressive behaviors of humankind. As citizens of the world, nurses need to acknowledge their responsibility in mobilizing forces against torture and in maintaining moral standards to ensure a civil society.

Psychologist Barbara Chester who directed the first US center for rehabilitation of torture victims in Minneapolis, Minnesota, in 1997 wrote: "torture is an act that defies the boundaries of language. We reserve the thought to express anguish deeper than pain. Ultimately, however, working with torture survivors has taught me that the fact of pain beyond pain leaves only the hope of uncovering a calm, healthy, and entire soul within a distressed and devastated body, that if there is pain beyond pain, there is also tranquility beyond reason" (Robin, 2000). Chester (1992) believes:

> *You have to grieve for your lost fantasy of the world as a just, fair place where people are kind to you. The world's been turned upside down. The experience leaves a mark on your mind, if not your soul. You need to be able to acknowledge the evil you've lived through but also see there can be meaning in life now, even if you can't undo the scars. (p. 209)*

Nursing, as do all health professions, must begin the rehabilitation of torture victims through a commitment of the heart. As stated by Mahatma Gandhi, "Love is the sole medicine to treat hatred and flourishes only inside the hearts of people without fear." Nurses are such caregivers without fear. Rehabilitation in torture parallels the goals of forensic nursing: *to provide a continuum of care from trauma to trial* (Lynch & Burgess, 1998). Yet far too often, there is no trial for the survivors of torture. The event of torture needs to be rebuilt through remaking the survivor's world, always dealing with the whole person (Chester, 1992).

Those who work with torture survivors find it challenging and in need of research. The *DSM-IV-R* of PTSD is useful in guiding psychotherapy for survivors in trying to deal with the nightmares, insomnia, depression, and anxiety. Therapists are researching the process to develop a subtype of PTSD specific for torture victims. An example of the subtype is what Chester describes above.

In medical nomenclature torture has been described as a "disorder of despair," a "disorder of hope," and a "loosening of the world." The nurse therapist helps lift the veil that separates the "unmade world of the tortured" and a "remade world" of new meaning (Bosoglu, 1993; Westermeyer, 1985). There is a way to integrate these lost fantasies and cruel tortures, but it demands a great deal of therapy and begins when the survivor seeks help (Sumnier, Vesti, & Kastrup et al., 1993). How many survivors walk about, still feeling half naked, humiliated, and guilty? As nursing becomes more aware of the symptoms of torture, nursing can respond in a manner unique to nursing to undo the scars. Forensic nursing will be an advocate for this humanistic approach to nursing practice.

Global Forensic Nursing

From the founding of the International Association of Forensic Nurses (IAFN), a concern has focused on maintaining the international aspects of this organization. An international perspective was expressed at the initial organizational meeting in 1992, as the charter members voted to ensure the association would have a global scope and focus. In 1996, the executive board of the IAFN signed the petition to support the US ratification for the Convention on the Rights of the Child. Issues regarding human rights have been addressed within the board's strategic plan and were discussed in open forum at the 1997 IAFN conference in Irvine, California. IAFN members promptly agreed to support and endorse the global perspective of its mission to "develop, promote, and disseminate information about the science of forensic nursing nationally and internationally" (IAFN, 1994).

In 1999, the executive board voted unequivocally and without reservation to endorse the human rights movement by the inclusion of "Advancing Humanity" within its mission statement. It is believed that this message will best convey the character of the organization and the philosophy of members that the world can change. To fail to appreciate the intention of this statement is to fail to realize the global potential of forensic nursing as an international movement and the International Association of Forensic Nurses potential in a leadership role in response to human violence.

IAFN program objectives reflect this vision, and its members hope to inspire others to join in establishing nursing initiatives that advance universal human rights and dignity. The IAFN's international mission has now been affirmed: the fundamental principles embrace humanity and are committed to protect and promote the triad between health, justice, and human rights. The IAFN will continue to address global health challenges related to human rights in collaboration with forensic physicians, human rights advocates, and kindred organizations. The relationship between forensic nursing and the central core issues of human rights demands no less.

It has been suggested that there are ways that forensic nurses could complement the scarce resources of the International Criminal Court to assist in the investigation of human rights atrocities. Many human rights authorities share the belief that forensic nursing is appropriately poised to significantly contribute to the implementation of the International Convention on the Elimination of All Forms of Discrimination Against Women, the Convention on the Rights of the Child, the Convention on Torture and other Cruel, Inhuman or Degrading Treatment, Female Genital Mutilation and Reproductive Rights, as well as local, national, and regional human rights movements to eliminate racial discrimination; intolerance based on religion or belief; and lack of access to food, basic health services, and education.

The IAFN is properly aligned with the larger nursing profession, which worldwide has joined with international advocates and bodies promoting gender equality, such as the UN, Physicians for Human Rights, Amnesty International, and the Human Rights Watch, among others. The International Council of Nurses, the American Nurses Association, and the American Academy of Nursing reflect this commitment to promote and protect public health, individual rights and human dignity in the position statements adopted by their more than 5 million members.

Changing the world depends on the direction and nature of societal change, which reflects the personal and professional philosophies of the individual leveraged by the collective actions of the organizations the individual joins. Only communally embraced value systems will prevail and thrive. If nurses believe deeply in changing the world, of creating an environment of peace for the next generation of the world's children, then they will join in the spirit of forensic nursing and seize the vision of advancing humanity (Box 4-4).

Box 4-4 American Academy of Nursing

Role in Advocacy, Education, and Research

As a voice of the US profession of nursing, the American Academy of Nursing's Expert Panel on Violence presented policy recommendations to address *Nurses Caring for Victims of Torture*. This historic event builds from over a decade of work by the expert panel on various levels of violence in the US and the world, including *Violence: Nursing Debates the Issues*, presented in 1994.

The recommendations are based on the following beliefs:

- Nursing must acknowledge the United Nations Universal Declaration of Human Rights (1948) and Article 5, the prohibition of torture under international law and the UN Convention against Torture (1964), which need to be upheld in all parts of the world.
- Nursing as a caring profession with international linkages needs to speak forcefully and compassionately in appropriate venues by insisting that torture must cease and respect for human dignity and the rights of all must prevail.
- Nursing needs to support the ongoing work in the established treatment centers of survivors of torture and, when appropriate, create additional centers.

The following policy recommendations were made:

- Advocate for funding and administering educational training and support for nurses who will develop nursing care plans to assist victims of torture in finding hope and healing.
- Develop linkages with centers of treatment to add nursing expertise.
- Support a conference or institute on the topic of torture and survivors of torture.
- Augment nursing educational training to add expertise in the treatment of victims of torture.
- Consider a Wingspan conference to develop a white paper on torture.
- Extend the academy's support of recommendation to the ANA and ICN to honor nursing's covenant to bring healing to survivors of torture (AAN, 2001).

Summary

Human rights violations remain the major cause of trauma worldwide, despite the attention they have been given since the late twentieth century. Although myriad health and human services continue to monitor and report the consequences of intentional violence, human rights violations persist and even flourish in some regions of the world. Ethnic cleansing and genocide have remained a constant in civil and national wars. To achieve a positive and profound change in the world's moral code of ethics and to address the atrocities of violence, a strong partnership of human rights advocates, healthcare organizations, and forensic scientists is imperative.

Resources

Organizations

Amnesty International, USA

322 Eighth Avenue, New York, NY 10001-4808; www.amnestyusa.org

Department of Health and Human Services

200 Independence Avenue SW, Washington, DC 20201; www.dhhs.gov

Doctors Without Borders US Headquarters

333 7th Avenue, 2nd Floor, New York, NY 10001; www.doctorswithoutborders.org

Human Rights US Resource Center

229 19th Avenue S, Suite N-120, University of Minnesota Law School, Minneapolis, MN 55455; www.hrusa.org

International Association of Forensic Nurses

East Holly Avenue, Box 56, Pitman, NJ 08071-0056; www.forensicnurse.org

International Rehabilitation Council for Torture Victims

Borgergade 13, PO Box 9049, DK-1022, Copenhagen, Denmark; www.irct.org

Physicians for Human Rights

2 Arrow Street, Suite 301, Cambridge, MA 02138; www.phrusa.org

Rocky Mountain Survivors Center

1547 Gaylord Street, Denver, CO 80206; www.rmscdenver.org

United Nations

UN Headquarters, First Avenue at 46th Street, New York, NY 10017; www.un.org

Convention on the Prevention and Punishment of the Crime of Genocide

Universal Declaration of Human Rights

Covenant on Civil and Political Rights

Convention against Torture and other Cruel, Inhuman or Degrading Treatment or Punishment

Convention Relating to the Status of Refugees

Convention against Genocide

International Conventions for the Protection of Victims of War (Geneva Conventions)

Convention on the Rights of the Child

Convention on Elimination of Discrimination against Women

World Health Organization

WHO Headquarters, Avenue Appia 20, 1211 Geneva 27, Switzerland; www.who.int

References

American Association of Nursing. (2001). Position statement 2001. Washington, DC: Author.

Basoglu, M. (1993). The prevention of torture and care of survivors: An integrated approach. *JAMA, 270*(5), 606–611.

Chester, B. (1988, December 19). For ultimate survivors, a place to heal. *US News & World Report.*

Chester, B. (1992). Women and political torture: Work with refugee survivors in exile. *Women Ther, 13*(3), 209–220.

Chester, B., & Holtan, N. (1992). Working with refugee survivors of torture. *West J Med, 157*(3), 301–304.

Chester, B., & Jaranson, J. M. (1994). The context of survival and destruction: Conducting psychotherapy with survivors of torture. *Clinical Quarterly, 4*(1), 17–20.

Declaration of Alma-Ata, Health for All. (1978, September 12). Series No. 1. Geneva: World Health Organization.

Destexhe, Alain. (1995). *Rwanda and genocide in the twentieth century.* New York: New York University Press and Pluto Press.

Glittenberg, J. (2004). A transdisciplinary, transcultural model for healthcare. *J Transcult Nurs 15*(1), 6–10.

Hoffman, M. (1995). *International humanitarian law and the nursing profession: The current framework and challenges ahead.* Presentation at the American Academy of Nursing, Washington, DC.

Institute of Medicine. (1988). *Future of health.* Washington, DC: National Academy Press.

International Association of Forensic Nurses. (1994). Mission statement. Tyson's Corner, VA: Author.

International Council of Nurses. (1975). Declaration of Singapore on the role of the nurse in the care of detainees and prisoners.

International Federation of Red Cross and Red Crescent Societies and François-Xavier Bagnoud Center for Health and Human Rights. (1999). Public health: An introduction. In *Health and human rights: A reader* (pp. 29–35). New York: Routledge.

Jacobsen, L., & Smidt-Nielsen, K. (1997). *Torture survivor: Trauma and rehabilitation.* Copenhagen, Denmark: International Rehabilitation Council for Torture Victims.

Lempkin, R. (1944). *Axis rule in occupied Europe.* Washington, DC: Carnegie Endowment for International Peace.

Lynch, V. (1995, November 15–17). *Forensic nursing: Defending human rights.* Presented at the seventh international congress for heathcare professionals on caring for victims of torture, Cape Town, South Africa.

Lynch, V., & Burgess, A. (1998). Forensic nursing. In A. Burgess (Ed.), *Advanced practice psychiatric nursing* (pp. 474–490). Stamford, CT: Appleton & Lange.

Mann, J. M., Gruskin, S., Grodin, M. A., et al. (1999). International Federation of Red Cross and Red Crescent Societies and François-Xavier Bagnoud Center for Health and Human Rights. Public Health: An introduction. In *Health and human rights: A reader* (pp. 1–20). New York: Routledge.

Ottowa Charter for Health Promotion, Ottowa , Canada, held 17-21 November 1986.

Ramsay, R., Grost-Unsworth, C., & Turner, S. (1993). Psychiatric morbidity in survivors of organized state violence including torture: A retrospective series. *Br J Psychiatry, 162*(1), 55–59.

Robin, R. W. (2000, August). *Commemoration of the life of Barbara Chester.* Hopi Foundation award ceremony for clinicians who work with torture victims in Tucson, AZ. Hotevilla, AZ: Hopi Foundation.

Rocky Mountain Survivors Center for the Assistance of Survivors of Torture and War. (2000). Educational brochure. Denver, CO: Author.

Sumnier, F., Vesti, P., Kastrup, M., et al. (1993). Psychosocial consequences of torture: Current knowledge and evidence. In M. Basoglu (Ed.), *Torture and its consequences: Current treatment approaches* (pp. 56–71). Cambridge: Cambridge University Press.

Thomsen, J. L., et al. (1984). Amnesty International and the forensic sciences. *Am J Forensic Med. Pathol., 5,* 4.

United Nations. (1948). *Declaration of human rights.*

United Nations. (1948). *Convention on the prevention and punishment of the crime of genocide.* Document A/810 at 71.

United Nations. (1964, December 10). *Convention against torture and other cruel, inhuman or degrading treatment or punishment.* Speech from United Nations Declaration on Human Rights.

US Senate. (1989, November 21). Proceedings, p. S16578.

Watson, W. (1995, November 15–17). *International standards in the investigating and prevention of arbitrary and summary executions and torture.* Presentation at the seventh international congress for healthcare professionals on caring for victims of torture, Cape Town, South Africa.

Westermeyer, J. (1985). Psychiatric diagnosis across culture boundaries. *Am J Psychiatry, 142,* 798–805.

World Health Organization. (1986). *Constitution in basic documents* (36th ed.). Geneva: Author.

Chapter 5 Female Genital Mutilation

Patricia A. Crane

Denouncing the practice of female genital mutilation (FGM) can make some countries feel superior and self-righteous, but it certainly does not solve the problem. Our purpose should not be to criticize and condemn. Nor can we remain passive, in the name of some bland version of multiculturalism. We know that the practice of genital mutilation is painful and can have dire consequences on the health of the baby girl and, later on, of the woman. But we must always work from the assumption that human behaviors and cultural values, however senseless or destructive they may appear to us from our particular personal and cultural standpoints, have meaning and fulfill a function for those who practice them. People will change their behavior only when they themselves perceive the new practices proposed as meaningful and functional as the old ones. Therefore, what we must aim for is to convince people, including women, that they can give up a specific practice without giving up meaningful aspects of their own cultures.

—Statement of the director general to the World Health Organization's Global Commission on Women's Health (WHO, 1996)

The clinical forensic role is found applicable in many professional positions where the nurse faces intersecting ethical challenges, cultural issues, and legal matters affecting the provision of healthcare. One of the newest crimes of interpersonal violence to confront nursing, female genital mutilation or female circumcision (FGM/FC), is achieving great international notoriety in political, human rights, and women's reproductive health arenas in the US and Canada. In the face of unfamiliar and often inhumane acts that may be confronted on a daily basis, the forensic responsibility must be integrated into the nursing process. Integral to professional practice is the ability to honor individual human rights and to maintain professional and legal objectivity, as well as cultural sensitivity and respect for patients.

Key Point 5-1

Integral to professional practice is the ability to honor individual human rights and to maintain professional and legal objectivity, as well as cultural sensitivity and respect for patients.

An overview of the history of FGM/FC, its psychological and physical health consequences, and the possible legal ramifications will provide a background for the development of appropriate assessment, diagnosis, and intervention. Reviewing case studies supports the need for cultural competence and patient education, while accessible resources are available throughout the nursing process for follow-up and referral of patients and families for evaluation. With the combination of cultural competence and forensic knowledge to the application of the nursing process, enhanced patient outcomes are assured.

Significance of the Issue

Worldwide, more than 130 million women and ultimately their families are affected by the practice of FGM/FC. The World Health Organization (WHO, 2000) admittedly underestimates that nearly 2 million more are subjected to the ritual daily. The age at which a young woman undergoes FGM/FC varies greatly but may be from sometime in the first year of life up to 18 years old. In villages and communities with limited access, the person performing the ritual procedure may travel through the area every four to five years, so girls in a wide age range are expected and often forced to undergo the procedure by peers and parents. According to the Program for Appropriate Technology in Health (PATH, 1997), the rural population is not as likely to support FGM as are the employed and educated women. In larger cities, a ritual practitioner may be available for hire on a daily basis. For others, a celebration and feast takes place after a season of superfluous crops and is associated with fertility. The village elder decides which group of marriageable girls will participate in an associated FGM ritual (Hosken, 1981), and it has been reported that the younger the girls are, the better, because small girls are easier to restrain when cut and are less likely to remember the pain and terror. There is more education regarding the practice and a greater awareness as girls grow older, hence more verbal and physical rebellion (PATH, 1999).

Large university surveys of students in Khartoum, Sudan, report that more than half are mutilated. It seems promising for the future generations that 88% of the women and 78% of the men want the practice to be abolished (Herieka & Dhar, 2003).

Early estimates stated that more than 168,000 people from countries where FGM is practiced had entered the US by 1997, either as immigrants or as refugees. Within this group, those who may be at risk for FGM/FC are under the age of 18 and number more than 60,000 (E. T. Ortiz, personal communication, January 30. 1997). Bringing the tradition with them, indigenes are leaving their countries of origin for new opportunities in various countries throughout Europe, Canada, and South America. In the US, large pockets of FGM/FC-practicing populations are settling together in communities in major metropolitan areas such as Los Angeles, Washington, DC, Dallas, Denver, New York, and Boston. Hence, health personnel and educators who face the issue on a daily basis may have little or no knowledge of how to initiate conversation regarding the problem or how to control their reaction when it comes up in a medical interview or examination.

Girls are subjected to the inhumane tradition of FGM/FC across all continents. Although the practice is not mandatory or supported by Islam, Christian, or Judaic law, it is found to be performed and encouraged at various times in history by members of all religions. Hosken's (1981) extensive investigation on worldwide genital cutting resulted in reports, with few actual medical studies, of such ancient practices being found in South America, Mexico, Europe, Australia, Asia, India, and primarily in Africa. Genital mutilation is not unknown in the US. In the 1950s, such procedures were documented as a treatment for control of women

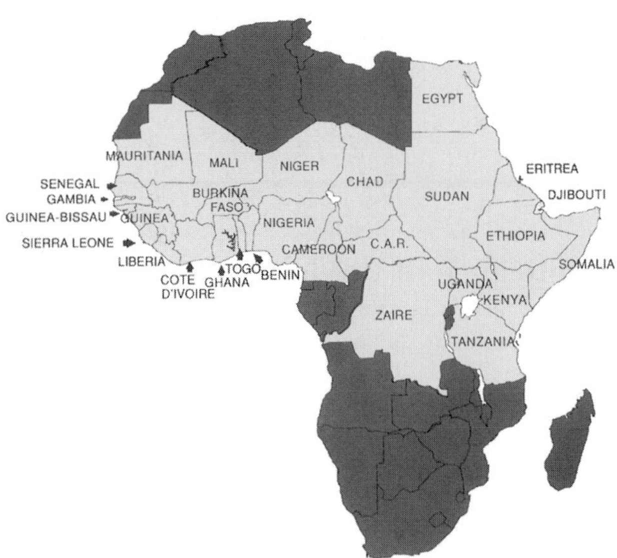

Fig. 5-1 Countries in Africa where FGM is practiced.

with hysteria and sexual problems. Medical reports and statistics indicate that FGM/FC is utilized, with varying degrees of severity, primarily across the central belt of Africa in more than 28 countries (Fig. 5-1) and a few isolated groups in Asia and the Middle East (WHO, 2000). They follow local indigenous religious customs and Islamic law. However, Muslim leaders are adamantly opposed to references to FGM/FC as a religious practice. In fact, they are sought out and used in the movement to eradicate FGM/FC in Africa and in the US because of their highly influential roles as teacher and authority.

Criminalization of FGM/FC

All states in the US have developed laws criminalizing the practice of FGM, or they consider child abuse law adequate to guarantee protection of individual human rights. Congress amended the US Code as part of the Illegal Immigration and Reform and Immigrant Responsibility Act of 1996, by adding "whoever knowingly circumcises, excises, or infibulates the whole or any part of the labia majora or labia minora or clitoris of another person who has not attained the age of 18 years shall be fined under this title or imprisoned not more than 5 years, or both." The Center for Reproductive Law & Policy (1997) claims that no criminal court cases based on the statutes have been reported.

Key Point 5-2

The criminalization of FGM in the US requires that forensic nurses be prepared to deal with its associated issues with immigration groups and experts in immigration law, as well as the courts in order to protect the human rights of the patients who have been victimized by the practice.

Criminalizing the offense in the US can have drastic effects on noncitizens depending on the judge, the skill of the attorney, and the extent of their knowledge of immigration law (Brady & Tooby, 1997). For many authorities, little is known about the practice of FGM and its health implications, despite its emergence in the US. Adverse consequences, such as deportation even without a conviction, is possible, with no consideration for the person's length of residency. Persons participating in the perpetration of the crime in the US can be faced with fines and jail sentences but must also consider their personal value of keeping the family together and the survival outcomes for the family members who may be left behind should deportation or incarceration occur. Brady and Tooby also strongly advise contacting an immigration organization and experts in immigration law to best meet the needs of clients who are not citizens.

Hundreds of young women, after being educated and given the choice, seek to escape their country of origin and inhumane rituals, often seeking asylum in Europe, Canada, or the US. The asylum standard in the US requires three elements: (1) persecution, (2) a well-founded fear, and (3) an act of persecution that was based on the grounds of race, religion, nationality, or membership in a particular social group. Despite the need for education, ultimately a decision on the matter would rest with the asylum officer or immigration judge. Asylum law is in need of reform and may not offer much in the way of protection for a woman (Stern, 1997). There may be detrimental effects on a woman's physical and psychological health, and yet being granted asylum may be impossible or take years. However, case summaries of gender asylum clearly show that increasing numbers of immigrant women from many different countries are succeeding in being granted asylum.

On a global perspective, the international health community has addressed the practice through many forums for at least half a century. The Universal Declaration of Human Rights in 1948, the United Nations (UN) Convention on the Rights of the Child in 1959, the African Charter on the Rights and Welfare of the Child in 1990, the UN Declaration on Violence Against Women in 1993, the UN High Commission on Refugees Statement Against Gender-Based Violence in 1996, to name a few, express opposition to the practice and strongly encourage enforcement of the law in countries where it is forbidden. The International Council of Nurses' position statement (1992) advises that nurses pay particular attention to protecting children from all forms of abuse so they can grow up in health and dignity. Human rights are essential to quality of life, regardless of ethnicity or sex. Many feel that outlawing FGM/FC in other countries was a move to please the advocates in the Western world whose voice and money have influence. Family or community decisions to cease a ritual practice that is deeply rooted and of incalculable value are not likely to be made based on foreign policy alone, although this may carry weight in the long run. Laws in the European Community and Canada have resulted in arrests that have gained international notoriety but resulted in little change in FGM-practicing countries.

In the US, as with other crimes of violence, many feel that making the act illegal could drive it underground where it will flourish, shrouded in secrecy. There are reports from immigrant groups in California that circumcision is being surreptitiously performed on immigrant girls. In personal conversations with young African immigrant working mothers, they relay fears that family members or babysitters, perceiving that the practice is still of social value and a necessary cultural tradition, may locate an individual with little medical training to perform circumcisions. Returning from work to find the baby mutilated is a constant fear. As documented in the University of California Hastings gender asylum case summaries (2000), the fear that young daughters will be taken and circumcised is prevalent in mothers who try to leave this ritual behind. On the other hand, wealthy families may send their daughters on "holiday" to be circumcised (Reichert, 1998).

Historical Basis for FGM/FC

Ritual ceremonies that involve the cutting of women's genitalia are rooted in tradition thousands of years old. As with many cultural practices, the original rationale is recondite. Documented history is lacking with much of women's health behavior, such as birthing and circumcision rituals. However, the reasons most often given for FGM/FC were of a psychosexual, sociologic, or hygienic nature (Gibeau, 1998). Passed down through generations of oral history, there is no foundation for rationalizing such practices today.

Some say eliminating a woman's sexual desire reduces any undue sexual demands of her husband, who may have several wives to enhance his progeny and wealth. In addition, destruction of the clitoral nerve endings would prevent her from seeking sexual pleasure with other men. The clitoris was also seen as masculinizing and the rumor was that it would grow very large and turn a woman into a man unless it was removed when she was young. To others the clitoris is thought to be poisonous to the man or to the newborn, and those who were to touch it would die.

Hygienic reasons required that the clitoris and labia be removed to make the woman clean and beautiful. Closing the vagina ensures virginity and a high bride price, critical issues in an area where families may depend on the price of daughters and cattle to keep the family subsistent. Not only can the surgery keep her virginal before marriage, if the man is away for long periods of time hunting, trading, and protecting herds of grazing animals, a woman may have the vagina resutured, reinfibulation, to assure her virtue in his absence and prevent rape.

If originally instituted for any or all of these stated reasons, the most often quoted reason for FGM/FC in recent times is that it is simply the tradition. No man would think of marrying a woman who had not been cut (Hosken, 1993).

Female relatives consider that it is something they must do to maintain their daughters' marriageability, family status, and honor. It is not felt to be mutilation.

Naming the Ritual

What to call the procedure varies from international conferences to meetings of policy makers. Unequivocally, in healthcare and policy settings, the Program for Appropriate Technology in Health (PATH, 1999) claims that the WHO terminology female genital mutilation is accepted. Admittedly, the reason the surgery takes place is not to mutilate one's daughter. To insinuate the idea is insulting to the ancestors and sets up an impenetrable barrier in communication between patient and provider. However, mutilation is often the end result. In the country of origin, those who practice the procedure may refer to it as being made clean, being cut, or excision. Others refer to it as circumcision, and it is linked with premarital celebrations and coming-of-age rituals at the time of adolescence. In reality, there is little resemblance to the circumcision of males, which refers to the foreskin of the penis being removed. An Arabic word, sunna, meaning tradition, is the only word known for FGM/FC in some countries. In personal communication, a physician said that if she used any other word the women would not know what she was saying. The WHO has developed descriptions of four categories of FGM/FC: Type I, Type II, Type III, and Type IV (WHO, 2000).

Type I

Type I may include removal of the prepuce or hood of the clitoris and partial or total removal of the clitoris. This is typically the procedure known as sunna.

Type II

Type II may be known as excision and includes removal of clitoris and labia minora. The vagina is typically not covered, but copious scar tissue and adhesions may obliterate the vaginal introitus over time.

Type III

Type III, also known as infibulation or pharaonic circumcision, includes removal of the clitoris, labia minora, and part of the labia majora. The two sides of the remaining vulvar tissue are closed over the vagina in a crude fashion often with suture or acacia thorns. A small hollow reed from a local plant may be left in place while the injury is healing. This allows for a small opening to be left for the passage of urine and menstrual flow. The girls' legs may be bound together for several weeks. It is not uncommon for the incision to require opening at the time of marriage or childbirth. Many women request that they be resutured afterward, as local practice and the woman's family may dictate.

Type IV

Type IV is an unclassified grouping of all other mutilations of the female genital area such as pricking, piercing, cutting, and scraping of vaginal tissue, incisions to the clitoris and vagina, and burning, scarring, or cauterizing of tissue. (See Figures 5-2, 5-3, and 5-4.)

Physical Consequences

Despite often noted horrific outcomes, many variables influence the severity of scarring and damage to the genital area after cutting, backed by little scientific evidence (Morison, Scherf, & Ekpo et al., 2001). In areas where the trend is toward medicalization, the educated, trained professionals perform procedures with proper surgical technique using up-to-date sterile equipment so there is less risk involved. Where practiced, medicalization is not the norm, however. As the severity of cutting increases, so do the gynecologic and obstetrical problems (Jones, Diop, & Askew et al., 1999).

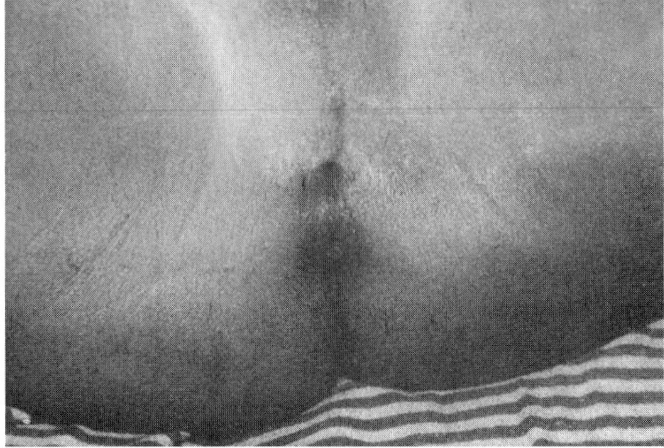

Fig. 5-2 Seven-year-old victim of FGM.

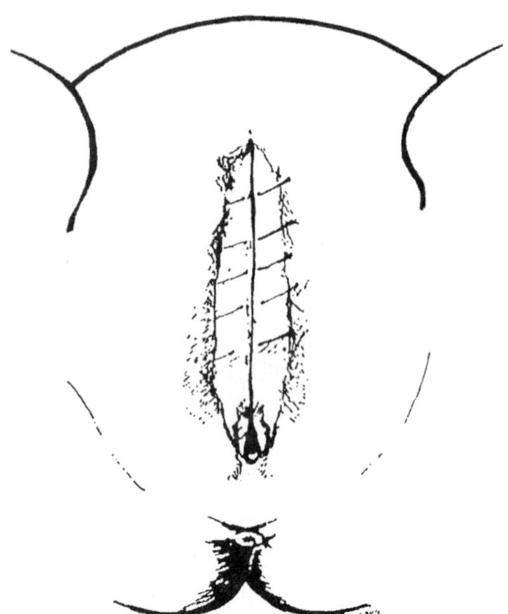

Fig. 5-3 Illustration of thorns used for infibulation.

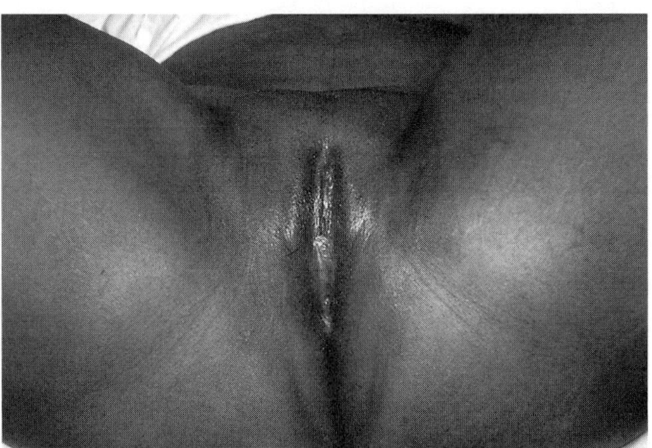

Fig. 5-4 Adult FGM victim deinfibulation. Note extensive scarring and disfigurement.

Often the village midwife, traditional birth attendant (TBA), local barber, or a male or female circumciser performs the procedure. Routinely, these are not highly educated people, and they have little or no knowledge of anatomy, asepsis, disinfectant, or medications and rarely use anesthesia. They may have a reputation throughout the region and have learned to earn a living in this manner through several generations of women. Local educators often provide circumcisers with less primitive equipment as well as education on asepsis in an attempt to curb some of the problems.

Despite the use of applications of local herbs, animal products, and primitive closure of the vagina with thorns, hemostasis may not be accomplished, resulting in hemorrhage as well as an irreversible state of anemia. Immediate physical problems include shock, not only from hemorrhage but also from severe pain due to the tragic degree of sensory nerve damage, an irreversible condition. If the circumciser is using items such as a rusty razor, sharp stone, shell, piece of glass, machete, or scissors, it is not difficult to comprehend frequent and widespread infections. Tetanus is fatal in as many as 50% of the cases (PATH, 1999). The risks of exposure to human immunodeficiency virus (HIV), various forms of hepatitis, and other pathogens are greater when instruments are used on a group of girls, which is often the case. Damage to surrounding organs and lack of knowledge of nerves and arteries in the genital area end in tragic results, including gangrene. Urinary retention can occur with the blockage of the urinary opening with eventual irreversible kidney damage. Urinary tract infections can be immediate or occur more frequently the rest of a woman's life. Over the long term, damage to the urethra from the cutting, frequent infections, and growth of scar tissue undoubtedly cause chronic pain, urinary hesitancy, and incontinence. Women and girls often report that it takes 10 to 15 minutes to complete urination. The bartholin gland openings near the vaginal introitus may be covered with scar tissue, a blockage that can lead to cysts, abscesses, and tumors in the vulvar area up to 10 cm in diameter.

Childbirth itself is a risk because scar tissue reduces the elasticity of the birth canal and limits the local tissue response to hormones designed to make this natural process occur with minimal discomfort. Hence, the women undergo more pain and tissue damage. Laceration and fistula formations between the vagina and rectum or vagina and urethra are not uncommon. An obstructed birth canal can prolong second stage labor and increase the likelihood of stillbirth or irreversible brain damage to the newborn (Morgan, 1997). Hosken (1993) stated that infant and maternal morbidity and mortality rates are highest in communities where FGM/FC is the norm.

In the US, healthcare providers are often called on to manage the devastating effects of these primitive surgeries. Additional incisions anterior and posterior to the vaginal opening may be necessary at the time of childbirth (Lightfoot-Klein & Shaw, 1991). Healthcare providers may be asked to resuture the women postpartum in a manner that leaves the vaginal opening as small as it was before delivery. An inspection by the husband, an older woman, or a midwife is not unusual to confirm that the vagina was sutured enough. Women report that marital problems arise if resuturing the vagina after childbirth is not done properly (Hosken, 1993).

Menstrual problems are quite common following FGM/FC. The sutured and scarred tissue may block menstrual flow, leading to the inappropriate drainage of blood backward into the peritoneal cavity. With the retention of menstrual blood, there is abdominal distention and pain as it is resorbed, as well as the increased risk of infection and scarring of internal reproductive organs. Social problems abound when there is no evidence of monthly menstrual flow, which leads others to misinterpret symptoms and assume a young unmarried woman is pregnant. This brings dishonor on the family and leads to negative repercussions and ostracism. Extreme pain with menses is common following genital tract infections. Abscesses, keloids, and hypertrophic scarring add to the physical agony and contribute to infertility. In a culture where children increase a family's wealth, infertility is a cause of disrespect, diminishing a woman's worth, and is likely to lead to her rejection by the family or community. Ironically, FGM is thought by many who practice it to increase a woman's fertility.

Psychosexual Problems

Damage to vulval nerve endings, neuromas, and scarring are not only causes for lifelong intractable pain; they also limit the blood flow to the rich body of sensitive tissue responsible for the initiation and completion of the human sexual response cycle.

Depending on the damage and scarring, orgasmic pleasure may be delayed or unattainable. Lack of scientific studies, lack of open discussion regarding women's sexual experiences, and the cultural overlay make information in the area limited. However, from Hosken's surveys (1993), the act of intercourse is considered a duty and provides no pleasure to most women who have been subjected to acts of genital mutilation.

Equally as tragic aftereffects are the psychological responses to FGM. Women may harbor deep psychological fears, losing trust and confidence in women and caregivers in general. Chronic depression and anxiety are commonly confounded by psychotic episodes. Deep-seated behavioral problems and marital conflict result (WHO, 2000). Oddly, healthcare providers are confronted with the disconcerting challenges associated with individuals who are choosing not to carry on the practice as well as those who have endured it in their past. Eliminating a practice thousands of years old is causing upheaval in highly regarded family values. With little support, women and their families may suffer physically and mentally if they maintain the practice illegally and in secret or if they seek to put an end to it.

Medicalization

In many countries, there are movements to medicalize the procedure in order to maintain asepsis and curb the mortality rate. Physicians claim to have been taught the "right" way to do it (sterile with less severe cutting), while in medical school and in many areas this continues. Healthcare providers have also promoted the use of Type I, supposedly to incur less tissue damage, in their local communities in an attempt to help mitigate the serious health risks associated with the routinely practiced infibulation. To satisfy the family and community demand for the ritual, it was felt that progress was made if the practice could be reduced to a simple clitoridectomy.

However, the WHO (2000) claims that the inequitable position of women is seen as a threat to their health and development as well as social and economic development as a whole. Hence, the movement to eradicate the dangerous and life-threatening practices in any form must be the priority. Negative repercussions are advised for those who perform FGM in any of its forms or profit from it in any way. The human rights approach for children and women is suggested as the best approach. In the US, with the recognition of the practice being perpetuated in secret and requested of physicians, the consensus is that adamant refusal of any form of sexual mutilation of females must be maintained.

Some see the cessation of FGM/FC as the main priority for survival of women affected by it, while the women themselves may not see it that way (WHO, 2000). Those outside the ethnic or cultural group must realize that they may never understand such practices. Even within a single country, the tribal, sexual, and genetic differences vary greatly. In the Gambia, for instance, FGM is nearly universal in one ethnic group, the Mandinkas, but it is rare in the Wollofs (Morison, Scherf, & Ekpo et al., 2001). In three Nigerian tribes, the Igbo, Yoruba, and Hausa women's meanings, beliefs, and practices varied also, according to religion, education, and occupation in the US and in Nigeria. Researchers caution that importing foreign values will promote resistance and drive the practice further underground (Anuforo, Oyedele, & Pacquiao, 2004).

Families who move to the US in general seek to improve their lives and health and that of their children by letting go of old ways that are harmful while appreciating the new opportunities available to them. Indeed, across African countries as well, PATH data (1999) denotes that generation to generation there is a reduction in the number of girls circumcised from 4% to 10% in countries that staunchly defended the tradition in the past. Reproductive Health Outlook (2004) quotes development experts as recommending numerous small steps rather than grand solutions.

The need to adhere to the value-laden societal norm keeps populations self-enforcing a tradition that has long lost its origins. Mackie (1996) compared FGM/FC to the outdated practice of foot binding in China. Methods of eliminating an outdated practice initially involve educating the population at risk about the physiological facts regarding the practice. This has been going on for close to a century in Africa, with health workers in the communities and civic leaders providing supportive education to the young and old alike, particularly in refugee camps. Information regarding the laws in other countries is explained to emigrants with special focus on matters such as FGM being a crime that could result in jail and deportation. The second point Mackie made is that an international attitude regarding the issue must be conveyed. This is evident in the international denunciation of FGM by the health councils, organizations concerned with world health, and laws passed in European and North American countries making FGM illegal. Finally, all those concerned, from international organizations to the individual healthcare workers, must exhibit tact and respect for the enduring and motivating fact that families love and value their children and want what is best for them. Critical to the elimination of dangerous practices is that individuals at all levels in the at-risk group must commit to change.

The Nurse's Role

Congress passed legislation in 1996 delineating the responsibility of the healthcare community through the Department of Health and Human Services (DHHS), which was then to compile data on numbers of women who may be affected by FGM/FC, specifically those under the age of 18. The DHHS also was required to identify communities that practice the ritual and develop and implement outreach activities in collaboration with the ethnic groups. Third, the DHHS was to develop and distribute information on FGM/FC and its complications to educators and students in medical training. These steps can be viewed as the assessment of the range of need, the development of a care plan, and patient education when viewing the community as client in the nursing process (Lundy & Barton, 1995). Traditional nursing courses and nursing textbooks do not teach these issues as a role responsibility of the general nurse, however. The subject of FGM, the US federal laws regarding FGM, and the responsibilities of the healthcare provider are not adequately addressed, with the exception of courses in forensic or transcultural nursing, or human rights issues.

Lynch (1993) clarified that "the application of forensic principles and standards represents a new perspective in the holistic approach to the treatment of victims and perpetrators of criminal acts." Furthermore, Lynch added that "forensic science is relevant to contemporary curricula and will ensure that clinicians are prepared to identify and report" all manner of abuse and suspicious trauma. The discipline of healthcare unites with law enforcement and forensic science in their common concern for human acts of violence. Goals articulating the full spectrum of knowledge are necessary to address the safety and public health issue of FGM/FC.

Despite the fact that opinion and policy oppose FGM/FC, being politically correct is not always culturally sensitive. The more culturally competent the provider, the more likely he or she is to stimulate changes in healthcare behaviors and attitudes, whether one is choosing patient care, advocacy, or the activist role outside the clinical arena. It is imperative that the clinician confront her or his own prejudice just as those affected by the practice will need to confront the issue for themselves. Overt prejudice exhibited by the provider may be experienced as another violation of patient's rights, the right to sensitive and respectful healthcare despite ethnic and cultural differences (Black & Matassarin-Jacobs, 1997).

Incorporating cultural competency, the nursing process enhances the logical, holistic approach to problem solving. Preliminary to the initial assessment, nurses must examine their own prejudices and convey respect for the values, beliefs, and customs of the patient. Sensitivity to their culture must be perceived, and focusing on finding similarities will produce familiarity while reducing prejudice. Nursing care focused on differences is threatening. Attention must be given to the unique positive features of each culture. The Foundation for Women's Health, Research, and Development (FORWARD) produced a guide for health professionals listing such positive attributes as strong family support, improved parenting strategies such as breastfeeding and close contact of mothers and babies, and community involvement in child rearing (Adamson, no date available).

Initial assessment with acceptable communication style will build rapport. Information offered about the health effects of a practice one wishes to discourage will be more likely accepted and viable replacement alternatives considered. Alternative ceremonies instituted in 1996 by Maendeleo Ya Wanawake Organization (MYWO) included a weeklong rite-of-passage ceremony with the ritual singing, flowers, and gifts for girls, leaving out the mutilation of the genitals. The women were given accurate health information along with the expectations inherent in the role of wife and mother. Individual families are also being encouraged to have their own parties in the girls' honor (PATH, 1999). Utilizing successful approaches, such as these new rituals, are promoted also in the US as part of the education campaign that includes videotapes of the celebrations.

Best Practice *5-1*

Nurses who do physical assessments or who perform procedures on female patients should be alert to the anatomical, physiological, and psychological changes that may accompany female circumcision or associated ritualistic procedures of certain cultures. They must anticipate changes in medical or surgical procedures involving female genital anatomy.

Intervention and management plans for patients may be multifaceted, taking into account the medical concerns for which the woman has sought care as well as the possible need for a referral for mental health counseling (Box 5-1). When initial contact with a woman who has been subjected to FGM in the past is in the labor and delivery suite or emergent care setting, marshaling all resources as quickly as possible may be necessary. Medical risks of childbirth, language spoken, the sex of the healthcare provider, and the fact that the provider may never have seen a patient who has undergone FGM add to the challenge of assessment and management in these situations (Reichert, 1998). Stories abound concerning the gasps of shock and amazement when, unknowingly, a nurse or physician unfamiliar with FGM first views the infibulated vagina. Prevention of such a response can be best managed by educating healthcare providers about FGM and being aware of local resources.

Box 5-1 Selected Nursing Diagnoses for FGM/FC Patients

- Low self-esteem due to abuse from family or coworker
- Pain related to tissue, nerve, or vessel disruption from penetrating trauma
- Risk for infection due to loss of skin integrity
- Sexual dysfunction related to injury
- Fear related to perceived inability to control situation

Healthcare professionals must have accessible educational material, colleagues sensitive to the issue, awareness of the prevalence of FGM in a given community, and knowledge of their forensic responsibility.

Best Practice *5-2*

According to JCAHO, accredited hospitals must develop and use criteria to identify possible victims of physical assault, rape or other sexual molestation, domestic abuse, and abuse or neglect of older adults and children, and they must educate and train all personnel to use interview and physical assessment skills to detect abuse and to initiate appropriate referrals to other healthcare providers or agencies for follow-up care.

Documentation of the initial assessment is critical as well as the patient's expectations after delivery. A proactive stance is to provide patient education on the fact that reinfibulation is not legal, nor is the perpetuation of FGM on female infants. Because of its value in some ethnic groups, significant family members and influential elders should be involved in any such educational process.

Opportunities for counseling on psychosocial and physical problems associated with FGM must be in place for use with patients in the ambulatory and inpatient settings. Options for surgical intervention or deinfibulation that are not associated with childbirth should be included. It is standard practice in discussion of a procedure that the patients provide informed consent. Barstow (1999) explained that consent must be voluntary. Second, the patients must have the mental capacity to make a decision. Third, patients must receive information on the pros and cons of the procedure in a language they understand. Last, patients must not be coerced physically or emotionally. Most healthcare providers are familiar with informed consent as a universal process in patient education. Barstow has claimed that women who have undergone FGM procedures and request them for themselves or their daughters are not able to give informed consent. Since FGM is a relatively new forensic issue in the US, there remain many questions to be answered and much to be learned about how to handle families that desire to have the ritual performed on the minor child or themselves. In addition to assessment of risk and education, involving law enforcement may be considered a choice, as with other forensic or medical legal challenges such as domestic violence, sexual assault, and other forms of child abuse. Having a protocol in place for such situations, with counselor and adjunct support staff on hand, is critical.

Participants in a focus group in California working on interventions for possible recurring FGM discussed corrective surgeries that had been done at no charge to the women requesting it. The possibility of reconstructing vulvar and urethral tissue to some semblance of normalcy, providing nerve blocks for intractable pain, removal of scar tissue that entraps nerve bundles, and fistula repair are invasive, specialized, and expensive management for the results of FGM. What is the likelihood of surgery being available through local gynecologists, private, or federally funded health insurance plans? Coding the diagnosis and potential surgical treatments remain unresolved issues. There are clinics and physicians who specialize in treating patients suffering from the long-term health effects of FGM and offer surgical solutions. However, they are not the norm and are seen in few communities such as Boston and Washington, DC, where the political and legal climate helps to generate financial support of the agencies. In the UK, where FGM has long been illegal, specialists routinely perform reconstructive surgery at specific clinics and can be contacted for consultation if the need arises.

Law and justice professionals and educators are in need of education and support, as well as are healthcare providers. Few are sensitized to the issue, and most have little knowledge of what to do if it is reported. Kmietowicz (2000) surveyed 16 international health and welfare agencies and found that fewer than half were aware of the legal position on FGM. To test the responses of local authorities, several practitioners in California made anonymous phone calls to child protection agencies and law enforcement regarding cases of FGM in the local area. The reports were rebuffed with claims of ignorance regarding California law, knowledge of FGM, and what they needed to do.

Evaluation of the success of nursing interventions must be ongoing. This may include phone calls and follow-up visits in conjunction with all health professionals involved in the initial treatment plan. As yet, there are limited protocols for evaluation. Results of mental and physical health treatments must be documented, including a review of the law and its repercussions, particularly if there are plans to subject the children to FGM. Advocacy and support agencies with counselors of the same ethnicity may be the most effective support for the practitioner, and a concerted effort must be made for ongoing communication between the agencies involved.

Health workers in the front lines will most likely be the initial contact for patients at risk. It is essential that information be presented to professionals and the public in general about the denouncement of inhumane acts and the progress being made in the human rights arena with laws and community movements. Hosken (1993) has strongly encouraged those in opposition to support in any way they can the grassroots organizations that have implemented eradication movements in Africa. She explains that no matter what is done in Western countries, the real changes must take place with the millions of people in Africa carrying on the tradition. However, with the legislation criminalizing FGM/FC and its initial discovery likely to occur in the healthcare setting, it is incumbent on all healthcare providers in the US to play a more active role.

Key Point *5-3*

A culturally valued tradition of an extremely personal nature that is illegal in the US and laden with controversy demands a sensitive approach. From a holistic forensic healthcare perspective, it is imperative that all involved understand it to be a violation of human rights.

Gender Asylum Case Summaries

It is inaccurate and illegal to justify the continuance of FGM on the grounds of necessity. More appropriately, it involves child abuse and violence against women (Morison, Scherf, & Ekpo et al., 2001). Respect for the lives at risk must take precedence over a cultural tradition antithetical to professional ethics and the law. Legal mandates, resources, and knowledge of its health implications allow nurses to confront FGM with the forensic responsibility inherent to their role. These gender asylum cases amplify the problems associated with immigration laws and practice.

Case Study 5-1 Nigerian Applicant

A Nigerian woman with two young daughters, both born in the US and therefore citizens, applied for asylum. She is Catholic and strongly opposed to FGM/FC.

At the time of her marriage, the fact that she had not been subjected to FGM was not disclosed to the husband's family. The husband's mother is a village elder who performs FGM on the village girls and put pressure on the woman to have the daughters cut. The applicant hid the girls 24 hours a day in fear of the relatives taking them.

Because of her refusal to submit, her husband began to beat her. She was locked in the home, raped, and psychologically abused. Often she was beaten into unconsciousness, and once she was hospitalized. Her family members reported the situation to the police, who interviewed the husband but refused to intervene because it was a marital matter. Once, after threatening the woman with a loaded gun, the husband managed to bribe the police, succeeding in getting them to drop the matter.

The government was unwilling to take action to prevent enforcement of the traditions supporting abusive treatment of women and girls, doing less than other African countries to protect her.

The woman fled to the US and continues to receive threatening letters for her refusal to allow the daughters to undergo FGM. The husband blames her for the death of another child she left in Africa and for his poor health. If deported, the daughters will be forced to undergo FGM, and the mother will suffer violence at the hands of her husband.

In 1999, the immigration judge granted her asylum.

Case Study 5-2 Malian Applicant

The applicant is a Malian woman with a young daughter and son who were both born in the US. The father of the children, her husband, is a Malian citizen living in the US.

The woman suffered the persecution of FGM herself as a child and strongly opposes the practice for her daughter. She fears that the husband's family will subject her daughter to FGM if they are forced to return to Mali, and she can do nothing to prevent this mutilation. She will endure violence and be ostracized by both of their families.

She is violating a deep-rooted family and cultural tradition. Over 95% of the women are subjected to FGM in her hometown, and no laws in Mali prohibit it.

Although the application for asylum was made in 1996, the immigration judge did not grant asylum until May of 1999.

Case Study 5-3 Ethiopian Applicant

The applicant is of the Harari ethnic group in Ethiopia, of which close to 100% of the women are subjected to FGM in early childhood. Her daughter is a US citizen, and the applicant fears her daughter will be tortured in the same manner if returned to Ethiopia.

Although Ethiopian officials are aware of the prevalence of FGM, they have passed no law specifically outlawing it. The woman feels sure that her family will force the daughter to be mutilated and anything else necessary to bring her in line with the traditions of the group. As an unmarried mother with a child of mixed heritage, she will face extreme scrutiny and be ostracized.

The immigration judge denied asylum, but withholding removal was granted.

Case Study 5-4 Guinean Applicant

The applicant was considered to be a person with no one to protect her rights when her monogamous father died in Guinea. Her mother became the fourth wife of an uncle. She was forced to undergo the torture of FGM at age 5 and was mistreated in the household.

Later the applicant fell in love and had a child by a man whom the uncle refused to let her marry. The uncle beat her often, causing her lose a subsequent pregnancy. Eventually he had the father of her children imprisoned and beaten, then forced her to marry a 60-year-old man with three other wives.

She was beaten, abused, raped, drugged, and threatened with death. Escape attempts were followed by beatings. Eventually she managed to enter the US with a friend's help and a false passport.

She fears that her daughter will be forced to endure FGM as the family has threatened. She will be an outcast if she is returned, or she will be killed.

The immigration judge granted her asylum in February 1998.

Resources

Organizations

Equality Now USA

PO Box 20646, Columbus Circle Station, New York, NY 10023; www.equalitynow.org

FORWARD International (Foundation for Women's Health, Research, and Development)

Unit K, 765-767 Harrow Road, London, England NW10 5NY; www.forwarduk.org.uk

Immigrant Legal Resource Center

1663 Mission Street, Suite 602, San Francisco, CA 94103; www.ilrc.org

National Immigrant Law Center

3435 Wilshire Boulevard, Suite 2850, Los Angeles, CA 90010; www.nilc.org

PATH (Program for Appropriate Technology in Health)

1455 NW Leary Way, Seattle, WA 98017; www.path.org

Rainbo (Research Action Information Network for Bodily Integrity of Women)

Suite 5A, Queens Studio, 121 Salusbury Road, London, England NW6 6RG; www.rainbo.org

WIN News (Women's International Networks News)

187 Grant Street, Lexington, MA 02420; www.feminist.com/win.htm

References

Adamson, F. (no date). *Female genital mutilation: A counseling guide for professionals*. London: FORWARD.

Anuforo, P. O., Oyedele, L. & Pacquiao, D. F. (2004). Comparative study of meanings, beliefs, and practices of female circumcision among three Nigerian tribes in the United States and Nigeria, *Journal of Transcultural Nursing, 15*(2), 103-113.

Barstow, D. G. (1999). Female genital mutilation: The penultimate gender abuse. *Child Abuse Negl, 23*(5), 501-510.

Black, J. M., & Matassarin-Jacobs, E. (1997). *Medical-surgical nursing: Clinical management for continuity of care* (5th ed.). Chicago: Saunders.

Brady, K., & Tooby, N. (1997). Protecting defendants from immigration consequences. *Crime Crim Justice, 24*(3), 54.

Center for Reproductive Law and Policy. (1997). *Legislation on female genital mutilation in the United States*. New York: Author.

Gibeau, A. M. (1998). Female genital mutilation: When a cultural practice generates clinical and ethical dilemmas. *JOGN Nurs, 27*(1), 85-91.

Herieka, E., & Dhar, J. (2003). Female genital mutilation in the Sudan: Survey of the attitude of Khartoum university students towards this practice. *Sex Transm Infect, 79*(3), 220-223

Hosken, F. P. (1981). Female genital mutilation in the world today: A global review. *Int J Health Sci, 11*(3), 415-430.

Hosken, F. P. (1993). *The Hosken report* (4th ed.). Lexington, KY: Women's International Network News.

International Council of Nurses. (1992). *Resolution: Elimination of female genital mutilation*. Geneva, Switzerland: Author.

Jones, H., Diop, N., Askew, I., et al. (1999). Female genital cutting practices in Burkino Faso and Mali and their negative health outcomes. *Stud Fam Plann, 30*, 219-230.

Kmietowicz, Z. (2000). MPs recommend tightening the law on female circumcision. *Br Med J, 321*(7273), 1365.

Lightfoot-Klein, H., & Shaw, E. (1991). Special needs of ritually circumcised women patients. *JOGN Nurs, 20*(2), 102-107.

Lundy, K. P., & Barton, J. A. (1995). Assessment: Data collection of the community as client. In P. J. Christensen & J. W. Kenney (Eds.). *Nursing process: Application of conceptual models* (4th ed., pp. 102-119). St. Louis, MO: Mosby.

Lynch, V. (1993). Forensic aspects of health care: New roles, new responsibilities. *J Psychosoc Nurs Ment Health Serv, 31*(11), 5-6.

Mackie, G. (1996). Ending footbinding and infibulation: A convention account. *Am Sociol Rev, 61*(6), 999-1017.

Morgan, M. A. (1997). Female genital mutilation: An issue on the doorstep of the American medical community. *J Leg Med, 18*, 93-115.

Morison, L., Scherf, C., Ekpo, G., et al. (2001). The long-term reproductive health consequences of female genital cutting in rural Gambia: A community-based survey. *Trop Med Int Health*, 6(8), 643-653.

Program for Appropriate Technology in Health (PATH). (1997). *Female circumcision/female genital mutilation: The facts*. Washington, DC: Author.

Program for Appropriate Technology in Health (PATH). (1999). *Female genital mutilation–The facts*. Retrieved from www.path.org/resources/fgm_the_facts.htm.

Reichert, G. A. (1998). Female circumcision: What you need to know about genital mutilation. *AWHONN Lifelines, 2*(3), 29-34.

Reproductive Health Outlook. (2004). Harmful traditional health practices. Retrieved from www.rho.org/html/hthps_overview.htm.

Stern, A. (1997). Female genital mutilation: United States asylum laws are in need of reform. *J Gender Law,* 6, 89-109.

University of California Hastings. (2000). Gender asylum case summaries. Retrieved from
http://sierra.uchastings.edu/cgrs/summaries/summary74.html
http://sierra.uchastings.edu/cgrs/summaries/summary76.html
http://sierra.uchastings.edu/cgrs/summaries/summary58.html
http://sierra.uchastings.edu/cgrs/summaries/summary172.html

World Health Organization. (2000). *Female genital mutilation information pack*. Retrieved from www.who.int/frh-whd/FGM/infopack/English/fgm_infopack.htm.

World Health Organization. (1996). H.R. Doc. 104-863, 104th Cong., 2nd Sess.

Chapter 6 Violence against Women

Jacquelyn C. Campbell and Virginia A. Lynch

Traditionally, violence against women within societies has been viewed as a cultural practice. From an emic (from within the culture) or cultural relativism view, cultural norms and practices are considered to be outside the purview of international law or sanction. To impose cultural norms on another culture or society (usually less industrialized or less economically powerful) is considered by some to be cultural imperialism. However, since the advent of the League of Nations and the United Nations (UN), practices that are destructive to human beings, even if they are sanctioned within the cultural norms of a given society, have been increasingly acknowledged as violations of human rights. They are therefore subject to international sanction through universal declarations and courts. Examples of such violations are genocide, slavery, and torture. However, violence against women (VAW), including rape, wife-beating, and female genital mutilation (FGM) (or the more culturally acceptable term *female genital cutting* [FGC]), were not declared to be violations of human rights by the UN until 1993. The atrocities against women in Afghanistan are reminders that serious problems still exist. This chapter will highlight selected international examples of violence against women and explore the cultural norms that support and facilitate such practices. The need for a global response and involvement of forensic nursing will be emphasized.

Information presented in Western social sciences and popular literature has isolated much of the world from the truths about VAW (Crowell & Burgess, 1996). However, the more recent publications in the 1990s began to elucidate the problems (Campbell, 1997; Dobash & Dobash, 1998; Gaffney, Choi, & Kwanghyoung et al., 1997; Richie, 1996; Wessel & Campbell, 1997). In much early anthropological work, wife beating, rape, FGC, and other forms of violence against women were reported and examined as cultural practices, but primarily by male anthropologists using male informants (Campbell, 1985), with the notable exception of Beatrice Whiting's 1965 work (Whiting, 1965). Feminist scholarship began to identify the commonalities of forms of violence against women worldwide in the late 1970s (Daly, 1979). In the late 1980s and early 1990s, anthropologists began to examine violence against women within the context of other scholarship on the topic (Counts, 1990; Counts, Brown, & Campbell, 1999). Finally, by the late 1990s, disciplines that address VAW in Western literature (e.g., anthropology, criminal justice, medicine, nursing, psychology, public health, sociology, social work) have begun to present the problems of various cultures and countries throughout the world.

The Declaration on the Elimination of Violence against Women was passed in 1993 by the UN General Assembly, and the first UN Special Rappateur on VAW was appointed in 1994 to investigate abuses of human rights among women. The 1995 UN World Conference on Women held in Beijing strengthened the language of needed action based on powerful testimony from women around the world about harm from these practices. The first official recognition of VAW as a health problem in the world governing bodies was acknowledgment of its relationship to population control at the 1994 Cairo Conference and the 1995 Pan American Health Organization (PAHO) Initiative on VAW. Finally, the World Health Organization (WHO) officially recognized VAW as a public health priority in 1996. In spite of these signs of progress, healthcare professionals, including nurses, have been slow to respond to the far-reaching effects and overall impact of a global epidemic of VAW. The WHO "Safe Motherhood" campaign still does not include VAW, notably abuse during pregnancy, as threats to maternal/infant morbidity and mortality. This continued resistance to both the criminalization and medicalization of violent practices toward women is illustrated by attempts to classify practices such as marital rape as a "private matter" as recently as the 2000 UN Conference. WHO launched a multicountry research project to study the adverse health-associated effects of VAW. Brazil, Japan, Jordan, Namibia, Sweden, and Thailand are among the initial countries where data are being collected. It is quite apparent that there are many exciting opportunities for nursing practice, nursing research, and policy development addressing issues associated with VAW around the world.

Concepts and Definitions

Violence against women can be conceptualized as encompassing the entire range of violent and aggressive acts (intentional behaviors causing harm to another) committed against women of all ages. In Western society, certain acts of VAW are well understood. There is a wide range of acts constituting physical and sexual assault, emotional deprivation, and verbal abuse perpetrated by intimates and others. In addition to these types of VAW familiar in Western society, acts such as dowry deaths (also known as bride burnings), violence against domestic workers or wives by mothers-in-laws, FGC, abortions of female fetuses, and intentional food deprivation of female infants are experienced in other parts of the world. Because of the breadth of these acts and their relationship to women's status and cultural norms, some scholars use the terminology *gender-based violence* or *violence against women and girls* (Heise, Ellsberg, & Gottemoeller, 1999).

A concept particularly relevant to an international context is the distinction between *wife beating* and *wife battering* developed by Counts (1990) and then Counts, Brown, and Campbell (1999). The differentiation was important to clearly reflect the views and languages of the international community when addressing violence against women by intimate partners. *Wife beating* was defined as at least an ambivalently condoned, most often occasional (although sometimes frequent), and most often not seriously or permanently injurious act of physical aggression against at least some of the female partners in a culture. As such, this practice is close to universal in terms of occurrence by group (not individual), estimated by Levinson (1989) to occur in 85% of small-scale societies and found in all of the industrialized countries in the world (Heise, Ellsbergy, & Gottemoeller, 1999). In contrast, *wife battering* was defined as repeated physical or sexual assault within a context of coercive control. This kind of domestic violence tends to increase in severity and frequency over time, is relatively rare, and is not generally sanctioned in most societies. Some theorists in the Western social sciences have also used this conceptual division. For instance, Johnson (1995) differentiated between "common couple violence" and "patriarchal terrorism" in the US on similar lines.

Best Practice *6-1*

Use quotation marks to document verbatim wording in the subjective assessment. This is especially essential when naming a suspect. The objective data or assessment, in addition to photographs, then provides the succinct descriptions or depiction of noted injuries.

Individual psychological factors within a context of cultural tolerance (not necessarily acceptance) (Greenblat, 1985) may be most predictive for acts of wife beating (a particular man hitting a woman occasionally and not seriously throughout the course of a relationship). On the other hand, societal, cultural, political, and economic factors tend to control or facilitate that individual's acts of violence toward his spouse becoming more frequent and severe. This pattern of escalation is the most usual case according to evidence from the Straus and Gelles (1990) American national sample and other data (Jacobson, Gottman, & Gortner et al., 1996). It is a pattern also found in other countries and cultures (Johnson, 1995; Levinson, 1989).

In some cultures, including North America, women also commit acts of violence against male partners. American survey data can be interpreted as demonstrating close to equal numbers of acts of violence toward male partners as that directed toward females (Straus & Gelles, 1990). Self-defense is not separated out in that approach. Most US data suggest that serious violence (battering) is primarily directed toward female partners (Bachman & Saltzman, 1995; Dobash, Dobash, & Wilson et al., 1992; Tjaden & Thoennes, 1998). This is supported by Levinson's (1989) sample of small-scale societies worldwide, where husband beating happens in a majority of households in only 6.7% of cultures (compared to wife beating in all or a majority of households in 48.7% of the sample) and even occurs in 26.9% of societies (versus 84.5% for wife beating). Husband beating never occurred in a culture where wife beating did not. These patterns were also found in a sample of international societies, used by Counts, Brown, and Campbell (1999).

Using both Levinson's (1989) and other cross-cultural data (Counts, Brown, & Campbell, 1999; Heise, Ellsberg, & Gottemoeller (1999) Wessel & Campbell, 1997) as well as studies from Westernized cultures (Campbell & Humphreys, 1993; Dobash, Dobash, & Wilson et al., 1992), battering, in contrast to partner beating and mutual violence, is concluded to be a phenomenon almost exclusively directed toward women. This includes other kinds of coercive control as well as ongoing and severe acts of violence not seen as usual by others in the society (Campbell & Humphreys, 1993). Although there is definitely a correlation between wife beating and wife battering in any culture, battering is often less ubiquitous and less frequent than wife beating even when cultural norms display acceptance of wife beating (Counts, Brown, & Campbell, 1999). Both beating and battering can cause physical and mental health problems, and neither is condoned, but it is battering that is most amenable to societal level interventions directed at changing cultural norms, and battering is most likely to come into the purview of forensic nursing.

Best Practice *6-2*

The social, cultural, ethnic, and religious characteristics of the patient and family must be considered when assessing and managing incidents of physical or emotional abuse. However, these factors should not deter the nurse from intervening, from making appropriate referrals for care and protection, or for reporting indications of abuse to law enforcement personnel.

Best Practice *6-3*

The nurse should make inquiries regarding injuries and safety in an objective, nonjudgmental, nonassuming, and culturally conscious manner respecting privacy and patient wishes (e.g., in some cultures, male nurses cannot attend a female patient unless the husband is in the room).

Prevalence of Violence against Women

Studies from developing and industrialized countries have uniformly reported high rates of domestic violence. A review of 35 studies from developing countries found that one quarter to as high as one half of women who were queried reported physical abuse by a current or former male partner (Heise, Pitanguy, & Germain, 1994). Examples of surveys from a variety of countries follow. In a 1995 demographic and health survey in Colombia, 21% of interviewed women reported lifetime physical abuse; over 5% of women reported having been raped. Almost one half of these rapes had been committed by the husband or partner (Profamilia, 1995). A demographic and health survey in Egypt found that one third of women sampled reported having been beaten since marriage, with 45% of these women reporting beatings to have taken place in the year prior to the survey (El-Zanaty, Hussein, & Shawky et al., 1995). In a study in Sierra Leone, two thirds of women surveyed reported having been beaten by their spouse or partner, and half reported having been forced to have sexual intercourse against their will (Coker & Richter, 1998). A study in Bangkok, Thailand, found that 20% of husbands interviewed reported having subjected their wives to physical abuse (Hoffman, Demo, & Edwards, 1994). Finally, a study of domestic violence in Korea found that 38% of women reported having been battered by their spouse within the last year; 12% of women experienced serious battering (Kim & Cho, 1992). These cultural issues reach beyond these borders, involving US women, specifically in the Native American and Hispanic populations.

In spite of the increasing number of studies, it is difficult to make exact comparisons of prevalence between countries because studies used widely differing definitions of domestic violence, sampling frames, settings and interview methods, and time frames (lifetime prevalence, versus current relationship prevalence, versus past year prevalence). Even so, it is possible to ascertain variations across nations and between communities and cultural groups within nations, even when general economic conditions, legal proscriptions, and ethnic backgrounds are similar (Dobash & Dobash, 1998; Miller, 1992).

A review of 49 studies from 36 different countries (26 developing countries) provided more comparable data from population-based studies demonstrating a variation of past year prevalence from 1.3% (the lowest of the US population based studies; the others ranging from 8.3% to 13.6%) to 52% with the highest (greater than 20%) prevalence found amongst Arabs and Palestinians in Israel and in Nicaragua, Korea, and New Zealand. Other relatively high prevalence areas included Antigua, Barbados, Egypt, Ethiopia, Bangladesh, India, Kenya, Nigeria, Papua New Guinea, Uganda, Turkey, and the UK. In comparison, the US, Canada, the Philippines, Switzerland, and South Africa lifetime prevalence ranged between 20% and 30%, whereas Cambodia, Norway, Paraguay, Puerto Rico, South Africa, and Zimbabwe were between 10% and 20%. Although exact comparisons are still not possible, it is noteworthy that developed and industrialized countries from every region of the world and of each major racial group are represented in each of the categories.

Cultural Norms Regarding Women

The relationships between cultural norms and VAW are complex. Although there is definitely a relationship between women's status and wife battering around the world, it may be a curvilinear rather than directly linear. Wife battering appears to be relatively low in societies where women's status is the lowest, as there are other norms that effectively control women (Campbell, 1985). Women's status and power are complex variables with many manifestations (Rosaldo, Zinubalist, & Lamphere, 1974; Whiting, 1965). Where women's status is changing and in contention is where battering is expected to be highest and where there is the most equality, rates are expected to be low. In fact, Gartner and colleagues (Gartner, Baker, & Pampel, 1990) found that perceived challenges to male dominance place women at especially high risk for homicide from their spouses. In addition, such development agencies as United States Assistance Independent Democracies (USAID) and the World Bank are finding that increasing women's economic viability in a culture of low female status sometimes increases the prevalence of wife beating in communities and may increase the severity of wife beating within individual couples (Carrilo, 1992; Davies, 1994; Schuler, Hashmi, & Riley et al., 1996).

Studies of the relationship between women's status or power and wife assault have been confounded by various measures of both variables. For instance, Levinson (1989) found women's family status variables (economic, decision-making, and divorce restrictions) more predictive of wife beating than societal level variables (control of premarital sexual behavior, place of residence, property inheritance). An important exception was female economic work groups, which was predictive of absence of wife beating (not differentiated from wife battering). Similarly, a study in Bangladesh by Schuler et al. (1996) reported that membership in group-based savings and credit programs was associated with significantly lower rates of domestic violence, ranging from one-half to two-thirds lower relative to nonmembers. Another study in India reported that higher age at wife's marriage and her greater control over resources were both associated with significantly lower risks of domestic violence (Jejeebhoy & Cook, 1997). The same is true in the US, where economic dependence of women and male decision-making norms within couples are associated with wife battering (Kalmuss & Straus, 1990; Straus & Gelles, 1990), yet individual male attitudes toward women and sex role stereotypes do not consistently differentiate abusive men from others (Dutton & McGregor, 1992; Stark, 1990; Tolman, Richard, & Bennett, 1990).

Male sexual jealousy can be viewed as an expression of a socialized view of women as *property* of men and is accompanied by other aspects of male controlling behavior (e.g., economic coercion, social isolation). In small-scale or kinship societies, there is a general pattern of strong male sexual jealousy and other expressions of male ownership of women (e.g., female chastity before marriage as critical to the value of a woman, dowry payments, forced sex in marriage, and physical punishment by other male kin). In societies with serious wife battering and very little jealousy and ownership symbols among peoples, there is almost no wife battering and far less beating of wives (Counts, Brown, & Campbell, 1999). For instance, two studies from India indicated that disputes over dowry payments–cash and gifts provided by the family of the bride to the groom's family at the time of marriage–played a significant role in precipitating domestic violence (Jejeebhoy & Cook, 1997; Rao, 1997). However, some societies present exceptions to the pattern. For instance, Equadorian Indians hold female chastity and other aspects of male control as the ideal, but there is actually considerable female autonomy (Counts, Brown, & Campbell, 1999). The economic power of women, coupled with female decision making authority in the home, seems to protect the women from the degree of battering that the otherwise machismo ethics and beating norms would seem to dictate. Yet the ideal for women is passivity, and women and men are perceived to have very different natures, with men destined to be dominant in marriage. A simplistic feminist model does not hold up well with these people, who exhibit much of quintessential patriarchy yet relatively little battering. Obviously, there are other aspects of the status of women and relative presence of patriarchal norms that affect physical violence.

Even so, women having some sort of significant power in the culture outside of the home, economic or otherwise (e.g., magical), provides at least some protection against wife battering in many cultures. There are caveats to this generalization in places such as Taiwan and Indo-Fijian communities where societal development has afforded economic possibilities for wives but battering continues, albeit somewhat lessened (Counts, Brown, & Campbell, 1999). However, it can be argued that the strong continuing ethic of females as property, coupled with the societal norms supporting the beating of wives in those cultures, is now creating a contentious female status in society resulting from the development of autonomy in women. Iran also offers an interesting case of the opposite trajectory of women's status where the temporary Westernizing of the society apparently decreased (although did not eliminate) wife battering for that time period. Later when there was a return to a strictly interpreted patriarchal Muslim structure, the abuse increased again (Counts, Brown, & Campbell, 1999). Thus, societal sanctions were apparently stronger than other forces, and the increased relative power of women, even though temporary, decreased violence against them.

Religion

As with woman's status, the complexities of religious premises and their relationship to VAW argue against simple generalizations.

Islam as a religion is generally thought of as strictly patriarchal with strong beliefs in women as property and sanctions for the beating of wives for correction. However, the Qur'an itself does not prescribe wife beating, and it is only in some of the wide range of cultural, state, and local religious interpretations of the Islam religion that practices such as wife beating and FGC are given an Islamic justification. Two very different Islamic cultures illustrate the extensive variations of cultural practices related to VAW (Counts, Brown, & Campbell, 1999). The islanders of Mayotte (off the southeastern coast of Africa) strongly proscribe premarital sexual activity, but women otherwise wield a comparatively substantial amount of political power and personal autonomy, even post-marital sexual autonomy. Yet husbands perform a ritual defloration of their wives, who are usually young girls, a practice often considered another instance of violence against women (Heise, Ellsberg, & Gottemoeller, 1999). However, the act is not experienced negatively on Mayotte and is often monitored by grandmothers, which could be interpreted as an act of female solidarity protection. In contrast, Iranian brides respond to a similar act (in outcome yet very different in quality) conducted in private, with great shame and negativity. This illustrates the fallacy of equating acts of "violence" toward women across cultures without careful consideration of context. To continue the contrast, wife beating on Mayotte is extremely infrequent and battering unknown, while in Iran, under the fundamentalist Muslim regime, battering is horrifyingly frequent and severe. Divorce is easy for women amongst the Mayotte, and their kin will actively intervene if the violence appears to be getting out of hand. Violence against wives is negatively sanctioned among the people of Mayotte, whereas it is quietly condoned in Iran. Although the basic religious premises are the same, the practices of VAW may be entirely different.

Sanctions and Sanctuary

Counts, Brown, and Campbell (1999) found evidence in their sample of 15 societies from all over the world that it is a combination of community level sanctions against wife battering and sanctuary for abused women that is the most powerful influence against wife beating becoming battering. This may explain wide variations of wife beating and battering within national boundaries among different cultures such as in Papua, New Guinea (Counts, Brown, & Campbell, 1999), and among different communities in Bangladesh (Koenig, Hossain, & Ahmed et al., 1999; Schuler, Hashmi, & Riley et al., 1996). In addition, sanctions and sanctuary look different in different cultures. The four societies in that sample without any battering (three with a low level of wife beating) had significant sanctions against battering if the wife beating started to become severe, and these societies offered sanctuary for the woman if she was beaten. For the Nagovisi, a small-scale society in the Solomon Islands of Papua New Guinea, the sanctuary takes the form of the man leaving to his family and village of origin in cases of conjugal dispute. Female groups in the Wape, also of New Guinea, provide the active community intervention against potential beating, presenting a compelling image of women surrounding a home where there is marital conflict until the wife comes outside to join them. Similarly, there is female solidarity of the Garifuna (of Belize in Central America) around violence against women, taking the form of the community women shaming the man. When taken in conjunction with Levinson's (1989) data, this evidence suggests that female solidarity groups around any issue may be protective against wife battering, in addition to the negative sanction specifically against battering provided in these examples. This can be contrasted with the divisions among women in the Taiwanese, Bun, and Indo-Fijians societies of high levels of battering.

To add complexity, the majority of the cultures in the Counts, Brown, and Campbell (1999) sample demonstrated differential sanctions between beating and battering (the former always more acceptable). For instance, on Mayotte and even more striking among the Garifuna, there is some acceptance for wife beating although none for battering. There is also kin intervention to prevent battering (not beating) based on ideas of male kin ownership of women in Mayotte and the Kailai (also of New Guinea), thus combining a female ownership premise with a sanction against battering. Community intervention in the Kaliai and the Kung (of Botswana, Africa) is evoked when there is battering, not beating. Also confounding of simple premises is the contrast between the aboriginal use of violence toward wives as an expression of anger not dominance, as opposed to the clear dominance purpose of Ecuadorian Indians males, yet approximately equal levels of both battering and beating in the two groups. In addition, the cultures with strong conventions of female passivity (Taiwanese, Indo-Fijian, Ecuador-Indian, Iranian, and Indian) have different degrees of wife battering, and many Kaliai and Bun (New Guinea) women, hardly passive, are being rather severely battered. An absence of female passivity as the ideal is more associated with an absence of mutual violence than battering.

In China, the historical preference for male children has resulted in significant wife abuse around issues of infertility and a female child being born first (Xu, Campbell, & Zhu, 2001). Studies from Bangladesh and India (Rao, 1997; Schuler, Hashmi, & Riley et al., 1996) have also found that living male children conferred significant protection to women against the risk of violence. The study by Rao (1997) in South India also found that the wife having been sterilized significantly increased the likelihood of reported violence, which the author attributed to heightened fears concerning the wife's fidelity, combining the issues of jealousy and fertility.

These studies suggest that individual couple data are meaningless without the societal and historical context. Everyone can find examples of women who beat their male partners or women who have substantial power in a society where other women are beaten. This does not disprove the feminist explications for wife battering. In fact, the evidence in the Counts, Brown, and Campbell (1999) and Levinson (1989) studies supported feminist theory more than any of the theories purporting to explain VAW, but it illustrated the need for nuanced, contextual, culturally specific formulations and operationalizations (Dobash & Dobash, 1998; Heise, Ellsberg, & Gottemoeller, 1998). There was only limited support for the cultural/subcultural, resource, and social learning theories as now articulated, while the sanctions against battering evidence was supportive of exchange theory but the wide variety of isolation across degrees of battering nonsupportive. The evidence suggests that systems theory needs to either separate wife abuse (almost universal across societies) from child abuse (relatively rare in kinship societies) or differentiate between child beating and child battering to work across cultures. And although feminist theory had considerable support, mutually violent couples and the use of violence by women needs to be acknowledged and explained by those theorists.

Health Effects of Violence against Women

There have also been increasing studies of the effects of violence on women's health throughout the world. Echoing the strong research evidence of abuse during pregnancy as a significant maternal child health issue in the US (Gazmararian, Lazorick, & Spitz et al., 1996; McFarlane, Parker, & Soeken, 1996) and Europe (Ellsberg, Pena, Herrera, Liljestand & Winkvist 1999; Hedin, 2000; Schei, 1990), research has demonstrated that abuse during pregnancy in Nicaragua is a significant risk factor for adverse maternal and infant outcomes. Studies in India and Bangladesh have implicated violence as a cause of maternal morbidity by homicide and suicide (Counts, Brown, & Campbell, 1999).

The intersections of HIV and VAW are increasingly being documented in developing countries and the US, with VAW increasing the risk of women for HIV through forced sex and the inability to negotiate safe sex, and HIV positive disclosure by women leading to beatings (Gielen, O'Campo, & Fadin et al., 1997; Levinson, 1989; Maman, Campbell, & Sweat et al., 2000). Other gynecological problems associated with both intimate partner violence and childhood sexual assault in the US and around the world include chronic pelvic pain, sexually transmitted infection, urinary tract infections, and sexual dysfunction (Campbell & Lewandowski, 1997; Levinson, 1989).

Other physical health problems range from chronic pain and chronic irritable bowel syndrome to injury and death from both homicide and suicide, again in both industrialized and developing countries (Campbell & Lewandowski, 1997; Counts, 1990; Gartner, Baker, & Pampel, 1990; Levinson, 1989). A study in Mexico has shown intimate partner violence to be associated with functional neurological problems (Diaz-Olavarrieta, Campbell, & Garcia de la Cadena et al., 1999). Abuse accounts for significant morbidity in terms of effects on women's mental health, especially depression and post-traumatic stress disorder. Although most of the evidence on the effects of VAW on mental health has been accumulated in the US (Campbell & Lewandowski, 1997; Golding, 1997), there is a beginning recognition of the role of VAW in explaining the two-to-one female-to-male gender ratio of depression around the world (Astbury, 2000; Levinson, 1989). Controlled studies in Nicaragua (Ellsburg, Pena, & Herrera et al., 1999) and Pakistan (Fikree & Bhatti, 1999) have demonstrated that VAW accounts for a large proportion of self-reported emotional distress and depression in these two developing countries. Furthermore, when children witness acts of violence, the effects are astounding. It has a significant impact of their emotional development and sometimes their psychological and even physical development.

Implications for Forensic Nursing Practice and Policy Development

Wife beating or battering is contemporarily referred to as intimate partner violence and has existed for centuries. Yet only since the late twentieth century have healthcare providers recognized it as a public health epidemic and assumed it as a healthcare responsibility. It extends into families regardless of ethnicity or race, age, socioeconomic status, educational background, religious belief, or sexual orientation. With the advances in modern medical and scientific technology that have expanded the life span significantly, partner violence may continue far into the later ages of women's lives.

General Guidelines for the Forensic Nurse

The forensic nurse should understand what constitutes human abuse and be prepared to accurately describe specific acts in proper terms. Intimate partner abuse can be characterized by physical, sexual, and emotional abuse. It is rare that physical injuries occur without precedents of emotional abuse, neglect, and exploitation. Note that these definitions are broad and may be applied to children, women, the elderly, and other vulnerable subjects.

- Human abuse is the willful infliction of injury, unreasonable confinement, or cruel punishment of another individual. Acts that cause mental or emotional injuries or that negatively impact growth, development, or psychological functioning are also acts of human abuse.
- Neglect is the failure on the part of a caregiver to provide the goods or services that are necessary to avoid physical harm, mental anguish, or mental illness for someone under his or her care, or to leave that person in a situation where he or she could be exposed to serious harm.
- Exploitation is the illegal or improper act or process of using the resources of an adult, child, elderly dependent, or disabled person for monetary or personal benefit.

It is not uncommon for nurses to become emotionally involved with patients who have been abused and want to assume a protective role in their behalf. However, guard against trying to rescue the victim while reassuring the person that there is help. As a concerned ally, do not judge or preach to the victim. Admonishment or patronizing behaviors are counter-productive. Remaining objective, providing appropriate nursing and safety interventions, and displaying a professional caring demeanor will help to build trust between the nurse and the victim.

Primarily, be aware of the signs and symptoms of abuse. Take action. Say something like, "I see you have a lot of bruises. You can talk to me about how they happened." Listen carefully and always express concern for the abused victim's safety and welfare. Explore whether or not children are in the household too, since they may also be victims. Provide telephone numbers of local resources, (e.g., hot lines, shelters, etc.) even though the individual may be reluctant to take them. A discreet card that can be hidden in a wallet is appropriate.

Sometimes nurses feel that intimate violence between adults "is their own concern." The principles and philosophies of forensic nursing compel them to take an active role in domestic violence by careful interviews and assessments and by generating the required report forms. The philosophies of a caring nursing practice will guide the interaction and the relationship that is being established.

Assessment of VAW

There is not an emergency/casualty department in any hospital in any country that does not come into contact with domestic violence victims. Many women seeking to escape from interpersonal violence turn to healthcare professionals for help. In the US, victims of intimate partner violence visit their doctors eight times more often than women who are not abused; yet only approximately 10% of these women are identified as abused ("Stalking 101," 2001). This can be attributed to the healthcare professional's lack of information, education, and the reluctance to ask the right questions. Healthcare workers are often hesitant to get involved in intimate partner violence.

The Emergency Nurses Association and the Joint Commission on Accreditation of Healthcare Organizations (JCAHO) have set forth recommendations for instituting protocols in facilities to manage victims of domestic violence. In the US, the Healthy People 2010 objectives include such goals as reducing the rate of physical assault by former or current intimate partners, reducing the annual rape or attempted rape rates, and reducing physical assaults. Forensic nursing can have a direct effect in achieving these goals.

Detailed screenings, interviews, referrals, and treatment of injuries may be tedious and time consuming, especially considering the intense workload in the emergency/casualty department. Some survivors of intimate violence have reported they felt twice victimized, once by the abuser and again by the healthcare workers who failed to recognize violence against women and instead treated the injuries and ignored the cause. Screening for intimate-partner violence and providing help for victims through referral processes are ways to interrupt the cycle of violence, thus reducing further injury or even death for thousands of victims. Important concepts for forensic nurses when dealing with this victim are confidentiality, safety, objectivity, and caring.

Universal Screening

Terminology varies whether asking about abuse is called screening, routine inquiry, or assessment, but the need is for early identification and intervention. Statistics based on international data have shown that there is a universal need to screen for intimate partner violence all females presenting to the clinical environs regardless of the chief complaint. Increasing nurses' awareness and education about intimate violence and how to ask about it can ensure an increase in early recognition.

Although several countries mandate universal screening and reporting of abuse or neglect, there are no requirements in many developing countries. Universal assessment can provide appropriate nursing interventions to the victims and possibly keep them from becoming another statistic in the annals of forensic pathology.

Identification of Victims

Researchers have identified characteristics common to victims of domestic violence that include low self-esteem, anxiety, depression, suicidal ideation, and psychosomatic illness. The suspiciousness factor should indicate awareness when injuries seem inconsistent with the patient's explanation of them, the injuries are concealed by clothing, there was a delay between injury and the seeking of medical treatment, and there is evidence of untreated or old injuries. Patients may also have repeated emergency department visits or a history of many accidents documented in their medical records, a previous history of suicide attempts, or drug and alcohol abuse. VAW must be viewed as life threatening. Healthcare personnel cannot afford to miss patterns of abuse or clues of injuries associated with violence that might have been recorded in the medical record during previous healthcare contacts. Of course, even though time consuming, all body surfaces should be routinely inspected for subtle or obvious injuries of abuse during routine clinic visits as well as during all emergency/casualty department encounters.

Best Practice *6-4*

During encounters with potential victims of abuse:

1. Always obtain the medical records from previous admissions.
2. Undress the patient completely for the head-to-toe examination.

A skilled nurse interviewing a patient that may have abuse-related injuries will see that the assessment is accomplished in a safe, private area. The nurse should make every effort to interview the patient alone. Asking in the presence of the abuser or anyone else can be dangerous for the patient and rarely elicits accurate information. In the clinical setting, getting the patient alone may not be easy, but confidentiality and safety should be assured. Questioning should be direct and nonthreatening for screening procedures to be effective. The ability to achieve and maintain trust with the patient will facilitate disclosure of abuse incidents. The nurse prefaces her or his assessment with the statement, "I always ask these questions when I'm dealing with an injured female patient. I see lots of women with injuries like yours who are hurt by their partners. Is this happening to you right now?"

These introductory remarks permit the patient to feel more at ease in revealing what has happened within her home. She will know immediately that she is not alone in what she may be experiencing and that someone is willing to talk about this weighty topic without hesitation. During the interview, the nurse should be attuned to statements from the woman that might reveal characteristics of her partner that are known to be associated with abuse. These include the following:

- Has an explosive temper
- Repeatedly "puts down" partner
- Wants to control the partner
- Manipulates the healthcare system
- Makes all family decisions
- Is overprotective, jealous, suspicious
- Abuses alcohol or drugs

The nurse can begin with a statement such as, "Intimate partner violence is so common in women's lives that we have a policy that everyone is questioned about it." The following are recommended queries:

- Have you ever been emotionally or physically abused?
- Have you been hit, slapped, pushed, shoved, punched, kicked, strangled, or otherwise physically hurt by someone close to you in the past year? If so, who did it to you?
- Within the past year, has anyone forced you to have sexual activities against your will? If so, who did it to you?
- Have you ever been hit, slapped, kicked, or otherwise physically hurt by someone during a pregnancy? If so, who did it to you?
- Are you afraid of anyone close to you?

Asking these questions may be uncomfortable for the nurse at first, but early identification is the first step in appropriate treatment for the domestic violence victim and has a tremendous impact on the outcome of the situation. If done regularly, screening will become as comfortable as any routine nursing assessment and will give patients the message that nurses care about the safety, as well as the health, of their patients.

After healthcare workers gather the healthcare history in an objective format for the purposes of diagnosis and treatment, other personnel conduct investigative interviews. Nurses perform a thorough head-to-toe examination, taking steps to document injuries. Photographs and body diagrams are useful in documenting the location and extent of visible trauma. Special care should be taken when the patient is pregnant, as blunt abdominal trauma is not uncommon. Obstetrical consultation is recommended promptly because both maternal and fetal injury potential is high. Consequences of abdominal injury in the pregnant patient include abruptio placenta, preterm or premature labor, uterine rupture, disseminated intravascular coagulopathy, and fetal death. If sexual assault is reported, the nonpregnant patient should be offered contraceptive options and treatment for sexually transmitted infection, even if the perpetrator is the spouse. Forensic evidence should be collected using the usual procedures (see Chapter 26).

Physical Assessment

When inspecting a body for physical findings, a head-to-toe approach should be used. Injuries are common on central zones of the body (e.g., chest and breasts, abdomen, and genitals). Examiners should not overlook the areas that might provide clues to a strangulation injury. These include front and back of the neck, mastoid region behind the ears, eyelids, jaw, and upper chin. Other indicators of strangulation include a sore throat, scratch marks, raspy or hoarse voice, difficulty swallowing, coughing, petechiae under the eyes, on the cheeks or neck, and neurological changes. It is important to note that most strangulation victims (85%) have no visible injuries.

Key Point *6-1*

Be sure to avoid the word *choking. Strangulation* is an intentional attempt to asphyxiate the victim by applying manual pressure to the throat; *choking* implies an unintentional obstruction of the airway.

The nurse should document the type of injuries, identifying specific wound characteristics, and note whether or not there is a pattern associated with the time of injury. The history of how the injury occurred is vital in determining the potential for abuse. If the injury is incompatible with the history, if there are multiple injuries in various stages of healing, or if there are patterned injuries (i.e., the injury reflects the implement used in the abuse process, such as a belt buckle, rope, or hands), this suggests abuse. Be especially aware of confinement injuries caused by being tied or restrained.

Pay special attention to clustered bruises or other injuries on the torso, upper arms, buttocks, thighs, or neck. These areas are usually spared during accidental falls or collisions with objects and may represent injuries of abuse.

Assessment for physical injuries should also include noting fractures or dislocations, lacerations, cuts or burns, head injuries with unknown mechanisms of injury, missing patches of hair, contusions on the body in various stages of healing, poor hygiene, unexplained dehydration, and weight loss. Genital complaints and sexually transmitted infections also deserve investigation. Nurses should also note the patient's psychological state, noting depression, withdrawal, or thoughts of suicide.

If the patient is fearful of the partner who offers a differing history of injury causation, or if there is unusual concern about the patient relating to the medical staff in private, it should be a red flag for the nurse. Other factors that should be of interest are that the caregiver is overly concerned with the cost of care or is overtly hostile or intimidating to the patient. In addition to careful annotation in the medical record, photos and voice recorders and granted patient consent may augment documentation of physical findings.

Stalking as VAW

Among the common crimes against women, stalking remains relatively unidentified in legal statutes internationally. Stalking is the willful, malicious, and repeated following and harassing of another person, affecting approximately 1.4 million Americans. Although unknown by the term *stalking* in other countries, it is well recognized worldwide, specifically by women, by the actions involved. Stalking crimes are motivated by interpersonal aggression rather than by material gain or sex. The purpose of stalking resides in the mind of stalkers who are compulsive individuals with a misperceived fixation (Wright, Burgess, & Burgess et al., 1995).

The stalker is looking for attention and seeking positive reaction from the victim. These individuals are afflicted with an emotional conflict, driven by an unseen force that impels them to follow, harass, and communicate with a person with whom they perceive to have an affectionate or intimate relationship, yet no relationship exists except in the delusional fantasy of the stalker.

The target of a stalker, the victim, finds himself or herself the object of an unsolicited focus of unwanted attention. When the target fails to respond positively, the stalker will accept negative attention because it will still be misinterpreted as being a part of the victim's life. Although most stalking does not escalate to violence, the threat of violence is a serious potential. Before any action can be taken in a stalking case, it is imperative that law enforcement agents validate a threat analysis. Conflict comes when the stalker begins to accept the fact that he or she is not part of the victim's life and that he or she is being rejected, perhaps for the last time. Because of the threat of violence, victims of stalkers endure fear and anxiety on a daily basis.

Laws related to stalking are continually evolving. Most stalkers harass their targets for long periods of time without ever breaking the law, preventing law enforcement intervention. Many state laws require that a threat of violence be made to the victim for the activity to be legally considered stalking. In 1994, the Model Anti-stalking Code was introduced, and law enforcement realized that a threat does not necessarily require words ("Stalking & Harassment," 2001). Insinuated threats may include implied threats with the intent to harass, annoy, or alarm another person; strikes, shoves, kicks, or following a person in public; and the spoken or written word. Greater numbers of workplaces and schools are getting involved with stalking issues due to the restraining orders or orders of protection that could potentially include these locations to protect the victim or the children of the victim. Because local, national, and international laws vary, anyone who finds himself or herself the target of a stalker should research the specific laws concerning this issue.

Stalking is a crime of extreme emotional abuse, causing fear and anxiety to the victim, and it may escalate to threats or actual physical violence. Stalking psychodynamics range from delusional, where no actual relationship exists, to nondelusional in nature, where an historical relationship has existed with close interpersonal association, such as marriage or common-law relationships. Although stalkers fall into various classifications, the two primary categories are the nondomestic (with no domestic partnership) and the domestic stalker (with a domestic partnership, generally past). Of these, the most dangerous offender is the domestic stalker. This offender attempts to control a relationship in the stages of termination or to reestablish a previous but failed partnership. This generally occurs during a divorce or breakup of a relationship involving a former lover or husband, including nondomestic long-term relationships.

Although the offender is generally male and the victim is female, it can involove a female who has become obsessed with a male in the same circumstances. Women in domestic relationships have much to be concerned with if they believe they are the target of a stalker. Too often, triggered by rejection, the man's attempt to control the situation escalates into a violent event, and kidnapping, murder, or suicide may be a result of the final rejection. Generally the victim has had a history of prior abuse or conflict with the stalker, and the victim describes the past relationship in terms of control issues, smothering, or domination. Others in the victim's life can also become potential victims of the stalker when they try to protect the victim or children, to conceal the victim's new residence or safe house, or to provide a safe working environment.

Victims of stalking must be aware of the danger and notify law enforcement agents of this type of abuse. Forensic psychiatric nurses or forensic psychiatrists who study and treat victims should be aware of the psychological impact as well as the life-threatening danger. Forensic nurses should provide a nursing diagnosis and safety plan that addresses the following issues:

- Denial
- Bargaining with the stalker
- Exhaustion, emotional and mental
- Depression
- Self-blame

Whatever the reason, being the target of a stalker is real and terrifying. Forensic nurse examiners in clinical and community settings are valuable resources to clients who may be experiencing symptoms that are not recognized as emotional sequelae related to stalking. The forensic clinical investigation of these clients also provides a valuable resource to law enforcement agents. Anywhere VAW is prevalent, stalking is a potential crime that must be recognized, assessed, and evaluated.

Although some countries recognize stalking as a criminal act, few have antistalking laws that may be effective in reducing potentially violence events. The most dangerous and most often fatal category of stalking identified as domestic stalking is most commonly associated with VAW in any geographical location or any culture where intimate partner relationships are disintegrating and the woman is attempting to leave the existing exploitative relationship.

However, as stated earlier, in countries where antistalking laws do exist, women may not know of this act by the term *stalking* or know that it is against the law. In Zimbabwe, Africa, women were not familiar with the term *stalking* but were well aware of the act of stalking and expressed their past experiences under these circumstances. However, they did not know that this behavior was called *stalking* or that it was considered a crime or abuse. They also expressed surprise that antistalking laws existed in the US to protect victims from this type of crime (Lynch, personal communication). Police departments in larger cities and metropolitan areas of the US often have "threat assessment" units to investigate stalking cases and consider stalking a serious crime against women.

Violence in Zimbabwe

In spite of the political violence and social unrest in Zimbabwe, nurses have demonstrated their concern and commitment to reducing and preventing intimate violence through the establishment of a forensic nurse examiner program. Emelia Hlatywayo, founder of the Zimbabwe chapter of the International Association of Forensic Nurses, recognized this futuristic insight into prevention of VAW and human rights violations through forensic nursing services.

In a personal conversation with Virginia Lynch, Hlatywayo emphasized her vision for forensic nursing in her country, stating, "Forensic nursing is a new concept in Zimbabwe and it is a considerable challenge to encourage more nurses to train with in the field so we can improve the community response to human abuse and interpersonal violence." As a forensic nurse examiner, Hlatywayo has brought a new focus on caring for survivors of torture and human violence in a country faced daily with the ruling government's issues of power and control. Forensic nursing has assumed a strong responsibility in this area, and nurses work directly with forensic physicians to identify and document these crimes against humanity, thereby helping to protect lives and promote cost-effective, holistic healthcare.

In Zimbabwe, trauma is among the top 10 reasons for outpatient's attendance and constitutes 10% to 15% of all registered deaths. There is also an increase in reported violent injuries such as torture, homicide, rape, and domestic violence, as well as hundreds of deaths associated with existing political conflicts. In 2004, Zimbabwe had one forensic pathologist in a country of roughly 13 million people where nurses staff all rural clinics. Therefore, nurses trained in clinical forensic issues can fill a significant gap, ultimately improving the healthcare delivery system and the healthcare provider's responsibility to the law and legal agencies (Benak, 2000). In June 2001, the first forensic nursing practice was established in Harare and is now influencing healthcare policies throughout Zimbabwe.

Pitfalls in Documentation

The forensic nurse should take great care to precisely document the following:

- The name and relation of the abuser
- How many time the abuse has occurred
- The worst episode of abuse that the victim can recall
- What was used to hurt the victim

If any children were at home during the abuse it is imperative to determine whether the children might have been injured during the violent episode.

When recording or describing the presenting problem or complaint, the nurse should avoid using the term *alleged* because it has a negative connotation, suggesting disbelief. In a court of law, the term can be prejudicial, predisposing the magistrate or the jury to determining that the complaint lacks merit or cannot be well substantiated. The nurse should also preface the documented statements with the words, "Patient states" in order to avoid being held liable or having information excluded as hearsay evidence. Under US federal rule of evidence, statements made to healthcare practitioners for purposes of diagnoses and treatment can be admissible in court through the hearsay exception. It is therefore crucial that the nurse accurately document what the patient is sharing in the history.

All injuries should be annotated on a body map. Photography, with consent of the victim, should also be a part of the routine documentation of trauma. Photographs continue to reveal the injuries long after the patient has healed. All consultations and referrals for follow-up care should be carefully recorded. In some settings, the nurse is also responsible for collecting, safeguarding, and transmitting forensic evidence that may link the victim to the abuser.

Key Point *6-2*

Remember, proper collection of evidence could help to assure a conviction, whereas improper collection could result in an acquittal. Evidence procedures must be flawless.

Patients should be aware of the danger signs of escalating violence. They include the following:

- Threat of weapons
- Extension of violence to children and pets
- Isolation of the victim from others
- Accusations of infidelity
- Forced sexual encounters
- No remorse exhibited by perpetrator

Because further abuse is likely if the patient returns to her home, a lethality checklist should be completed.

Interventions for VAW

If the patient screens positively for indicators of abuse, it is important to remain supportive, caring, accepting, and nonjudgmental. The nurse should stress to the patient that she is not to blame; no one deserves to be beaten. Inform her that resources are available, and make the appropriate referrals. Next, the patient's safety must be assessed and protected. The nurse may consider making a safety plan if the patient decides to return to the abuser. This should include emergency numbers for the police, the emergency department, and shelters; reserved money; house and car keys; important documents such as birth certificates, proof of insurance, and driver's license; an escape plan; and counseling referrals. If the patient screens negatively, the patient should still be educated about the cycle of violence and should be encouraged to share the information with others. Depending on the laws, nurses may also be responsible for notifying appropriate agencies in regard to child protection (i.e., if the children have been hurt, if evidence of trauma on the children accompanying the woman is observed, or if the victim relays past abuse toward the children by the abuser).

The forensic nurse examiner may be expected to assume several roles, including that of a patient advocate and educator, providing reassurance and information that assist the patient in making her own decisions. The nurse must remember to let the patient make her own choices even if the nurse disagrees or does not understand the patient's decisions or actions.

Partner Violence during Pregnancy and Postpartum

Violence among intimates frequently begins or escalates during pregnancy and the postpartum period. Several studies have revealed an escalating incidence of intimate violence during pregnancy. It is believed that 8% to 10% of pregnant women may be victims. Because most perpetrators are in their twenties to thirties, the victim is also likely to be young. Physical abuse during pregnancy may lead to miscarriage or fetal injury or death, low-birth-weight infants, drug and alcohol toxicity in infants, and homicide of the abusing partner.

Healthcare workers in settings such as obstetrical offices, outpatient testing facilities, obstetrical units, operating rooms, and emergency should be especially sensitive to this VAW issue because women battered *during* pregnancy are more likely to seek healthcare for injuries than women battered *before* pregnancy. Occupational health nurses employed by companies or workplaces may see a victim for complaints during or after a pregnancy and should be aware of the signs of abuse. Furthermore, as these women are seen for prenatal care, the nurses and physician have an opportunity to note injuries characteristic of abuse. Examples of abuse during pregnancy include bite marks, sexual battery, slapping, threats, confinement, intimidation, and strangulation.

During postpartum visits, the nursing staff should be attuned to observe for problems that may suggest continuing abuse. These include infant feeding problems, extended depression, poor communication between parents, and reports of sexual coercion or sexual assault. Emotional and behavior clues include a change in the appointment pattern, depression, anxiety, sleep disturbances, alcohol and drug abuse, low self-esteem, and self-blaming. A change in the behavior or school performance of siblings may also be observed.

When pregnant patients are seen in any setting, nurses should obtain and review all medical records. The patient should be completely undressed for screening examinations. It is recommended that a domestic violence screening form be used during prenatal and postpartum visits.

Key Point *6-3*

All intrauterine trauma and stillbirths are forensic cases, because maternal trauma from an intimate partner has been shown to be a precursor for such adverse outcomes.

Case Study 6-1 Violence during Pregnancy

A 29-year-old pregnant wife of a graduate student from Saudi Arabia was brought by ambulance to a city-county emergency department in Texas. A neighbor had called the ambulance after the panicked young woman in her second trimester of pregnancy experienced considerable vaginal bleeding. Although she had tried to contact her husband at the school, she could not reach him since he was in the midst of graduate preliminary examinations.

The frightened woman, who barely spoke any English, would not talk to doctors or nurses in the emergency department who were trying to manage the bleeding and to help her understand what was happening with her care and treatment. When the husband was finally reached and he arrived at the emergency department, he was outraged that the wife had been examined by both male paramedics and the emergency department physician in his absence. Although she continued to bleed and was horrified at the thought of losing her first pregnancy, the woman received no comforting attention from her husband who continued to exhibit anger and resentment toward the doctors, the nurses, and his wife.

The woman was admitted against her husband's wishes and a social services representative was called for assistance. A cultural interpreter, a Middle Eastern nurse, was summoned to the facility to assist with the crisis. She helped the staff to understand that female patients who are admitted to a hospital without their husbands being present during examinations and treatment are viewed as dishonoring their spouse. In such instances, these women may be subjected to beatings and other abuse when they return to the home. They may even be killed in order to preserve the honor and dignity of the male. These "honor killings" stem from Arabic and Asian tradition that has been practiced for centuries; thus these deaths are not viewed as homicides by the social or judicial systems in those societies. Although the nurse seemed successful at partially defusing the husband's volatile behavior and the fears of his wife, social services arranged for counseling and follow-up with the family in an attempt to resolve the crises between the couple. An in-service program was also planned for the emergency department staff and the local emergency medical personnel to assist them in understanding the cultural beliefs and traditions of other countries.

Public Health and Safety

There is a considerable challenge in healthcare facilities to convince personnel that the potential for abuse is high during the maternity cycle. However, the facts must be continually stressed. Perinatal nurses are in an ideal position to recognize and interrupt the cycle of violence and must remain familiar with updates in the law related to these issues.

Public Health Service Act, Section 330H, 42 USC 254C-8, addresses the legislative authority to develop or enhance systems that identify pregnant, preconceptional, or postpartum women experiencing family violence and provide appropriate information and linkages to interventions within a clearly defined system of care. Barriers to access should be significantly reduced so that women are actively supported in their desire to utilize services within a coordinated, confidential network of medical and psychosocial providers, women's shelters, legal and law enforcement agencies, and other support services. A community-based consortia of individuals and organizations that provide significant sources of healthcare services should consider incorporating forensic nurse examiners as viable resources for achieving quality patient assessment and early identification of women at risk.

A Model for Suspected Abuse or Neglect Reporting Procedures

Many countries do not require reporting of abuse and neglect to the police. However, in the US, anyone reporting or assisting with the investigation of suspected abuse or neglect is immune from any civil or criminal liability unless one is surreptitiously reporting one's own conduct or is making the report in bad faith or maliciousness. In most states, the failure to report abuse or neglect constitutes a misdemeanor. There is a mandate to report any injury suspected of being caused by neglect or being willfully inflicted by the caretaker, regardless of the victim's age. In the US, reporting child abuse is mandatory. Any professional person reporting suspected child abuse is exempted from liability. Every nurse should become familiar with the specific laws of the country, at the state, province, and federal levels, regarding reporting, as well as the hospital's policy for management of the suspected child-abuse case.

The US requires that in all states a report must be initiated in cases of suspected abuse or neglect, even if death or apparent injury is not obvious. Some states also require the reporting of runaways, because their circumstances often placed them in harm's way for acts of violence and poor living conditions, which are consistent with neglect. Reports may be generated for local or state law enforcement agencies, the Department of Human Services, or any other agency that has some responsibility for the welfare of the individual. Reports must contain the name and address of the victim and any known persons who are responsible for the individual's welfare, as well as any other information that would assist in investigating the suspected base or neglect case. Reports must be made promptly when there is reason to believe that abuse or neglect has occurred. Usually the initial report is accomplished in oral form by telephone or in person. Within an established time period, usually one to three days, the oral report must be followed by a written report.

First Line of Defense

Healthcare personnel, teachers, police officers, and others may be specifically mentioned as those who must assume the responsibility for reporting suspected cases. Within law enforcement agencies, there are specially trained agents who investigate these cases and report them to the proper authorities. Within healthcare facilities, the forensic nurse examiner as a specially trained clinician has responsibilities that include identifying crime victims and alerting law enforcement investigators as well as documenting evidence prior to emergency trauma care. The medical record is vital evidence in all cases. Documentation constitutes criminal evidence and may be subpoenaed for courtroom trials.

The forensic nurse examiner employed by the police department's Child Protective Unit, prosecutor's office, or the forensic pathologist has responsibilities that reach beyond the clinical environment into the community setting. These investigations may involve interviewing teachers, baby-sitters, neighbors, or others who have firsthand knowledge of the child's home or family life. In Atlanta, Georgia, a forensic nurse examiner responds to domestic violence calls with police investigators, interviewing the female partner from a health perspective while police interview the male partner. Police have stated that the presence of a forensic nurse tends to have a calming effect on both parties, providing greater safety in a potentially volatile environment. Domestic violence research indicates that it is one of the most dangerous types of investigations for law enforcement officers as well as for the woman. Her life is in greater danger at the moment she tries to break away from an abusive relationship than a police officer's is in the line of duty. The forensic nurse also provides an immediate and on-the-spot universal assessment, collects data for research, and assists police with sensitive questioning.

Violent physical abuse in intimate partnerships occurs worldwide and is not limited to any particular culture, socioeconomic class, geographic area, or historical period. Where cultural factors affect the context of violent conflict in domestic circumstances, it represents an expression of dominance and control in intimate relationships. Culturally specific nursing interventions should be directed toward the reduction and prevention of violence against women and children. These interventions should begin with evaluating the hospital policies and community resources that include the following:

- Establishing or reviewing institutional policies on domestic violence
- Providing education to clinicians about domestic violence and healthcare including physical and emotional signs and symptoms
- Seeking out community resources and making those available to clinicians/victims
- Reporting abuse and violence to appropriate agencies
- Identifying women and families at risk before injuries occur
- Educating women and families about life span developmental tasks so that behavioral expectations are realistic
- Teaching conflict-resolution skills as one method for problem solving in the home
- Monitoring and supporting media that depict violence and its consequences responsibly and realistically
- Advocating programs and social policies that prevent (or reduce) violence
- Putting the philosophy of caring into practice

Adult Protective Services

In countries where adult protective services is a new concept, whether it involves VAW, elder abuse, or psychological impairment, women again constitute the majority of victims who require protection among the most vulnerable subjects. An important premise in adult protective services is that the patient *is mentally competent* to act in his or her own behalf. Therefore the abused or neglected adult should be involved in decisions about her or his care and custody. Nurses should avoid the paternalistic, rescue attitudes. The patient often knows best and should be an active partner in deciding what course of action would be best; it is the healthcare professional's responsibility to provide the victim with alternatives, education, and plans, and to offer support during the decision-making process. In addition, healthcare workers accept the patient's right to refuse help as long as the patient is competent to understand the consequences of his or her decisions. Because the patient should be permitted maximum freedom in resolving the problem, extreme actions such as the appointment of a guardian or institutional placement should be last resorts. If legal issues such as these arise, the adult has a right to an attorney who will represent his or her interests in problem resolution.

Adult protective services ordinarily are charged with investigating complaints of abuse within 24 hours. They also are required to assess the individual's capacity to understand the imminent danger of remaining within an abusive or neglectful environment. When deemed necessary, they make arrangements for protective services, although they remain mindful of the patient's rights to self-determination. When court orders are indicated, they seek them. Many states charge adult protective services agencies with the review and monitoring of abuse investigations conducted by other agencies. They also are responsible for preparing official reports for the legislature and other branches of government, as well as advocacy groups.

Domestic violence is being reported with increased frequency as women worldwide are recognizing their human value and the laws that protect them. The nurse needs to be aware of this growing awareness and must complete universal screening on all female patients that show indicators of abuse. By incorporating abuse screening into health history, case findings will improve, which provides an opportunity to interrupt the cycle of abuse. The patient should be interviewed alone and may require the assistance of security officers when the male partner refuses to comply. The nurse should maintain a caring, nonjudgmental attitude and attempt to treat the patient in a safe and confidential environment.

A resource for guidelines in any country should involve the accreditation agency for hospitals and clinics, as well as for healthcare providers in jails or prisons. Amnesty International has acknowledged the prevalence of VAW in correctional facilities, where it may involve interpersonal violence, sexual assault, forced prostitution, intimidation, humiliation, and lack of proper healthcare. It is suggested that problems of this nature may be improved through the forensic education of the correctional nurse and adoption of international laws specific to health-related issues and VAW in departments of corrections worldwide.

In the US, the Joint Commission for the Accreditation of Healthcare Organizations has established guidelines for the identification and management of victims of abuse in private and public institutions (Box 6-1) (JCAHO, 2004).

Box 6-1 Victim Identity Guidelines

- Possible victims of abuse are identified using criteria developed by the hospital.
- Staff are trained in the use of these criteria; criteria must focus on observable evidence and not on allegations alone.
- Staff members are able to make appropriate referrals for victims of abuse and neglect.
- Patient care assessment standards include the recognition of forensic patients and mandates that evidence is collected and preserved.

Summary

The emerging role of the forensic nurse challenges antiquated or absent healthcare policies and helps to erode barriers between healthcare and the law. In societies where the triad of abuse against women involves culture, tradition, and religion, forensic nurses are in an ideal position to address issues of victim empowerment. Through a global alliance with forensic science operatives, healthcare systems, and criminal justice agencies, nurses can subtly influence a more positive status for women within society.

The emergency/casualty department in any country is most often the first source of help for women and children seeking intervention and refuge in cases of domestic violence. The forensic nurse is a vital link in the early detection of these patients and has the potential to empower women to interrupt the cycle of abuse, providing options for safe termination of toxic relationships.

Resources

Organizations

Ending Violence against Women

Population Report, Population Information Program, Johns Hopkins School of Public Health, 111 Market Place, Suite 310, Baltimore, MD 21202-4012; Tel: 410-659-6300; www.jhuccp.org/pr/l11edsum.stml

Gay Men's Domestic Violence Project

PMB 131, 955 Mass Avenue, Cambridge, MA 02139; Tel: 617-354-6056; Crisis Line: 800-832-1901; www.gmdvp.org

Information and resources for gay men in violent relationships.

Institute on Domestic Violence in the African-American Community

University of Minnesota School of Social Work, 290 Peters Hall, 1404 Gortner Avenue, St. Paul, MN 55108; Tel: 877-643-8222; www.dvinstitute.org

National Domestic Violence Hotline

800-799-SAFE (800-799-7233), TDD 800-787-3224; www.ndvh.org

Network for Battered Lesbians & Bisexual Women

P.O. Box 6011, Boston, MA 02114; Tel: 617-695-0877; Hotline: 617-423-SAFE; www.thenetworklared.org

Office on Violence against Women

810 Seventh Street, NW, Washington, DC 20531; Tel: 202-307-6026; TTY: 202-307-2277; www.ojp.usdoj.gov/vawo

Web Sites

Defense Task Force on Domestic Violence

www.dtic.mil/domesticviolence

Focus is on systemic changes required to strengthen the Department of Defense's comprehensive domestic violence in the military program.

Intimate Partner Violence During Pregnancy: A Guide for Clinicians

www.cdc.gov/nccdphp/drh/violence/ipvdp.htm

Screening for Abuse in Spanish-Speaking Women

www.vachss.com/help_text/archive/abuse_spanish.html

References

Astbury, J. (2000). *Promoting women's mental health.* Geneva: WHO.

Bachman, R., & Saltzman, L. (1995). *Violence against women: Estimates from the redesigned survey.* US Department of Justice (abstract).

Benak, L. (2000, Winter). Zimbabwe's forensic nurse crusader. *On the Edge* (vol. 6:5). Pitman, NJ: International Association of Forensic Nurses.

Burgess, A. W. (1995). Investigating stalking crimes. *J Psychosoc Nurs Ment Health Serv, 33*(9).

Campbell, J. C. (1985). The beating of wives: A cross-cultural perspective. *Victimology, 10,* 174–185.

Campbell, J. C., & Humphreys, J. (1993). *Nursing care of victims of family violence.* St. Louis, MO: Mosby.

Campbell, J. C., & Lewandowski, L. A. (1997). Mental and physical health effects of intimate partner violence on women and children. *Psychiatr Clin North Am, 20,* 353–374.

Carrillo, R. (1992). *Battered dreams: Violence against women as an obstacle to development.* New York: United Nationals Development Fund for Women.

Coker, A. L., & Richter, D. L. (1998). Violence against women in Sierra Leone: Frequency and correlates of intimate partner violence and forced sexual intercourse. *Afr J Reprod Health, 2*(1), 61–72.

Counts, D. A. (1990). *Domestic violence in Oceania.* Honolulu, HI: University of Hawaii Press.

Counts, D. A., Brown, J. K., & Campbell, J. C. (Eds). (1999). *To have and to kill: Cultural perspectives on wife-beating,* (2nd ed). Chicago: University of Illinois Press.

Crowell, N., & Burgess, A. W. (1996). *Understanding violence against women.* Washington, DC: National Academy Press.

Daly, M. (1979). *Gyn/Ecology: The metaethics of radical feminism.* Boston: Beacon Press.

Davies, M. (1994). *Women and violence.* London: Zed Books.

Diaz-Olavarrieta, C., Campbell, J., Garcia de la Cadena, C., et al. (1999). Domestic violence against patients with chronic neurologic disorders. *Arch Neurol, 56,* 681–685.

Dobash, R. E., & Dobash, R. P. *Rethinking violence against women.* Thousand Oaks, CA: Sage, 1998.

Dobash, R. E., Dobash, R. P., Wilson, M., et al. (1992). The myth of sexual symmetry in marital violence. *Soc Probl, 38,* 71–91.

Dutton, D. G., & McGregor, B. M. S. (1992). Psychological and legal dimensions of family violence. In D. K. Kagehiro & W. S. Laufer (Eds.), *Handbook of psychology and law.* New York: Springer-Verlag. Pp. 318–334

Ellsberg, M. C., Pena, R., Herrera, A., et al. (1999). Wife abuse among women of childbearing age in Nicaraugua, *AJ Public Health,* (89), 214–244.

El-Zanaty, F., Hussein, E. M., Shawky, G., et al. (1995). *Egypt demographic and health survey.* Calverton, MD: National Population Council and Macro International.

Fikree, F. F., & Bhatti, L. (1999). Domestic violence and health of Pakistani women. *Int J Gynecol Obstet, 65*(2), 195–201.

Gaffney, K. F., Choi, E., Kwanghyoung, Y., et al. (1997). Stressful events among pregnant Salvadoran women: A cross-cultural comparison. *JOGN Nurs, 26*(3), 303–310.

Gartner, R., Baker, K., & Pampel, F. C. (1990). Gender stratification and the gender gap in homicide victimization. *Soc Probl, 37,* 593–612

Gazmararian, J. A., Lazorick, S., Spitz, A. M., et al. (1996). Prevalence of violence against pregnant women: A review of the literature. *JAMA, 275,* 1915–1920.

Gielen, A. C., O'Campo, P., Fadin, R., et al. (1997). Women's disclosure of HIV status: Experiences of mistreatment and violence in an urban setting. *Women's Health, 25*(3): 19–31.

Golding, J. M. (1997). Intimate partner violence as a risk factor for mental disorders: A meta-analysis. *J Fam Violence, 14,* 99–132.

Greenblat, C. (1985). Don't hit your wife . . . unless . . . : Preliminary findings on normative support for the use of physical force by husbands. *Victimology, 10,* 221–241.

Hedin, L. W. (2000). Postpartum, also a risk period for domestic violence. *Eur J Obstet Gynecol Reprod B, 89,* 41–45.

Heise, L., Ellsberg, M., & Gottemoeller, M. (1999). *Ending violence among women.* Population Reports. Series L, No. 11. Baltimore: Population Information Program, Johns Hopkins University School of Public Health.

Heise, L., Pitanguy, J., & Germain, A. (1994). Violence against women: The hidden health burden. Discussion paper 255. Washington, DC: World Bank.

Hoffman, K., Demo, D. H., & Edwards, J. N. (1994). Physical wife abuse in a non-Western society: an integrated theoretical approach. *J Marriage Fam, 56,* 131–146.

Jacobson, N. S., Gottman, J. M., Gortner, E., et al. (1996). Psychological factors in the longitudinal course of battering: When do the couples split up? When does the abuse decrease? *Violence Vict, 11*(4), 371–392.

Jejeebhoy, S. J., & Cook, R. J. (1997, March). State accountability for wife-beating: The Indian challenge. *Lancet, 349,* SI10–SI12.

Johnson, M. P. (1995). Patriarchal terrorism and common couple violence: Two forms of violence against women. *J Marriage Fam, 57,* 283–294.

Joint Commission for Accreditation of Healthcare Organizations Manual for Accreditation (JCAHO). (2004). Oak Park, IL: Author.

Kalmuss, D. S., & Straus, M. A. (1990). Wife's marital dependency and wife abuse. In M. Straus & R. Gelles (Eds.), *Physical violence in American families* (pp. 369–382). New Brunswick: Transaction Press.

Kim, K., & Cho, Y. (1992). Epidemiological survey of spousal abuse in Korea. In E. C. Viano (Ed.), *Intimate violence: Interdisciplinary perspectives.* Washington, DC: Hemisphere Corporation.

Koenig, M. A., Hossain, M. B., Ahmed, S., et al. (1999, May). Individual and community-level determinants of domestic violence in rural Bangladesh. Johns Hopkins Population Center Working Paper No. 99-04.

Levinson, D. (1989). *Family Violence in Cross-Cultural Perspectives.* Newbury Park, CA: Sage.

Maman, S., Campbell, J. C., Sweat, M., et al. (2000). The intersection of HIV and violence: Directions for future research and interventions. *Soc Sci Med.*

McFarlane, J., Parker, B., & Soeken, K. (1996). Abuse during pregnancy: Associations with maternal health and infant birth weight. *Nurs Res, 45,* 37–42.

Miller, B. D. (1992). Wife-beating in India: Variations on a theme. In D. A. Ayers, J. K. Brown, & J. C. Campbell (Eds.), *Sanctions and sanctuary: Cultural perspectives on the beating of wives.* Boulder, CO: Westview Press.

National Population Council and Macro International, Inc., Calverton, MD.

Profamilia. (1995). *Demographic and health survey for Columbia.* Calverton, MD: Macro International.

Rao, V. (1997). Wife-beating in rural South India: A qualitative and econometric analysis. *Soc Sci Med, 44*(8),1169–1180.

Rosaldo, M. Z., & Lamphere, L. (1974). Women in politics. In *Women, culture and society* (pp. 89–96). Stanford, CA: Stanford University Press.

Schei, B. (1990). Psycho-social factors in pelvic pain: A controlled study of women living in physically abusive relationships. *Acta Obstetrical Gynecological Scandinavia, 69,* 67–71

Schuler, S., Hashmi, S. M., Riley, A. P., et al. (1996). Credit programs, patriarchy and men's violence against women in rural Bangladesh. *Soc Sci Med, 43*(12), 1729–1742.

Soeken, K., Parker, B., McFarlane, J, et al. (1998). The abuse assessment screen: A clinical instrument to measure frequency, severity, and perpetrator of abuse against women. In J. C. Campbell (ed.), *Empowering survivors of abuse: Health care for battered women and their children.*, Newbury Park: Sage, p. 195–203.

Stalking 101. (2001, April 29). Retrieved from www.stalkingvictims.com/stalk.htm.

Stalking and harassment, 2001. (2001, April 29). Retrieved from www.stalkingvictims.com/stalk.htm.

Stark, E. (1990). Rethinking homicide: Violence, race and the politics of gender. *Int J Health Serv, 20,* 3–26.

Straus, M., & Gelles, R. (1990). *Physical violence in American families.* New Brunswick: Transaction Press.

Tjaden, P., & Thoennes, N. (1998). *Prevalence, incidence, and consequences of violence against women: Findings from the national violence against women survey* (Rep. No. 718-A-03). Washington, DC: National Institute of Justice.

Tolman, R., & Bennett, L. (1990). A review of quantitative research on men who batter. *J Interpers Violence, 5,* 87–118.

Wessel, L., & Campbell, J. C. (1997). Providing sanctuary for battered women: Nicaragua's Casas de la Mujer. *Issues Ment Health Nurs, 18,* 455–476.

Whiting, B. (1965). Sex identity conflict and physical violence: A comparative study. *Am Anthropol, 67,* 123–140.

Wright, J. A., Burgess, A. B., Burgess, A. W., et al. (1995). Investigating stalking crimes. *J Psychosoci Nurs Ment Health,* 33(9), 38–43.

Xu, X., Campbell, J., & Zhu, F-C. (2001). Intimate partner violence against Chinese women: The past, present, and future. *Trauma Violence Abuse, 2*(4), 296–315.

Yllo, K., & Straus, M. A. (1990). Patriarchy and violence against wives: The impact of structural and normative factors. In M. A. Straus and R. J. Gelles (Eds.), *Physical violence in american families,* New Brunswick: Transaction Press, p. 383–399.

Chapter 7 Violence in the Healthcare Workplace

Victoria Carroll

The increasing violence on our streets and in our communities in America has invaded hospitals and other healthcare facilities, threatening the safety and well-being of those caring for the sick and injured. The forensic nurse is well prepared to serve as an advocate for the prevention of workplace violence in healthcare situations. Forensic nursing has been described as focusing on the areas in which medicine, nursing, and human behavior interface with the law (Lynch, 1995).

Prevention is key in addressing workplace violence. The proactive, multidisciplinary perspective of the forensic nurse examiner (FNE) will be effective in the development of a workplace violence reduction plan. Through effective planning and problem solving, nurses can collaborate with other nurses, disciplines, and administration to enhance the future of healthcare and develop safer workplaces. Just as one advocates for safe and quality healthcare for our clients, one must be a champion for creating a safer work environment for everyone.

The Problem

In 1997, the Colorado Nurses Association (CNA) established a Task Force on Workplace Violence that surveyed nurses in seven states: Colorado, Delaware, Kansas, Missouri, Illinois, Alabama, and Hawaii. The first question on the survey asked what the term *workplace violence* meant to them. The responses from 586 nurses indicated that more than 90% felt workplace violence included verbal abuse, sexual assault, and physical assault with or without a weapon. Seventy-eight percent included sexual harassment in the definition of workplace violence (Carroll & Morin, 1998). Incidences of violence occurring in healthcare facilities include assault and battery, hostage situations, homicide, kidnapping, armed robbery, arson, theft, vandalism, and bomb threats.

One of the biggest problems in addressing workplace violence is the phenomenon of denial: it won't happen here. No hospital or healthcare agency is immune. According to the Bureau of Labor Statistics in 1994, 38% of nonfatal workplace assaults occurred in healthcare settings. Studies by the California Division of Occupational Safety and Health (CAL-OSHA) (1999) and the New York Committee for Occupational Safety and Health (1995) have found that the rate of nonfatal assaults is considerably higher for nurses than for law enforcement personnel. Homicide is now the leading cause of workplace death for women. The latest National Traumatic Occupational Fatalities database indicates that there were 106 homicides of healthcare workers from 1980 to 1990 (Goodman, Jenkins, & Mercy, 1994).

Key Point 7-1

Healthcare environments are not immune from violence among employees. More than one third of nonfatal workplace assaults occur in healthcare settings.

More than 30% of the nurses participating in the CNA survey reported having been the victims of workplace violence in the previous year. Because only 5% of the nurses who responded are emergency department (ED) nurses, it is possible that the number of nurses assaulted on the job is actually much higher. Some studies have shown that ED nurses are at the highest risk for being assaulted at work (Mahoney, 1991; Stultz, 1993). Most of the nurses in the Colorado survey had been assaulted by patients. Many clients treated in hospitals, and in home health, and long-term care situations, have a high risk for violence. Problems associated with violence include hypoglycemia; electrolyte imbalances; anemia; hypoxia; alcohol intoxication; pain; the use of cocaine, PCP, LSD, and other drugs; and dementia.

Violence exists on a continuum from verbal abuse to physical assault to homicide. The escalation from verbal abuse to physical assault can occur quickly. A man who was angry about his father's death in surgery was verbally threatening to the hospital staff at a hospital in California. Later the same day, he returned to the hospital's ED and opened fire with a gun, killing a nurse and an emergency medical technician student and wounding a physician.

The wave of deinstitutionalized mental health patients has increased the numbers of disturbed and potentially dangerous patients appearing in community emergency departments. The victims and perpetrators of gang violence are treated in hospitals, as are the victims of domestic violence. Long-term care facilities are facing the challenges of caring for those responsible for violent crimes. Home health nurses often work alone and in high-crime neighborhoods. As staffing levels and lengths of stay have decreased, the frustration levels of patients and families have increased. Security departments are often understaffed, lacking adequate training and resources. Training for employees in recognizing potential violence, defusing violence, and dealing with the aftermath of violence is sorely needed in many hospitals and healthcare agencies. In the Colorado study, 71% of the 586 participants indicated this training was needed where they worked.

In addition, healthcare settings are not immune to other causes of workplace violence, such as poor and overly authoritative management practices and the actions of disgruntled current or former employees.

Prevention

Prevention is key in addressing workplace violence, and the success of any violence-reduction plan is strongly correlated to the degree of management commitment and staff participation. A safety team should be selected, and the responsibilities of the team should include the oversight of threat assessment, training and prevention, and trauma response (Baron, 1996). The team should include members from human resources, security, and public relations departments; personnel from high-risk areas; the FNE; and an employee assistance program professional. Information from consultants in workplace violence, legal experts, and law enforcement personnel may be required during the planning stages and at times of crisis (Carroll, 1997).

Assessment

The US Department of Labor/Occupational Safety and Health Administration (OSHA) recommend a worksite analysis. This worksite analysis provides the hospital or facility with a diagnosis that facilitates planning that is tailored to the environment. A multidisciplinary, participative assessment enhances consensus. Staff should be surveyed to identify their concerns and suggestions for a safer workplace. Areas of concern are most often identified by those who work in those areas. The administration's commitment to an effective prevention plan should include listening to staff.

Key Point 7-2

In addition to a comprehensive program of education about workplace violence, a facility must ensure that it has a well-designed and well-rehearsed crisis action plan that can be launched promptly by employees in any setting.

Retrospective data about violent incidence should be collected, as well as prospective data using the easiest reporting system for the specific unit to provide a comprehensive picture of assaults. Policies, such as those regarding patient restraint, hostage situations, and sexual harassment, should be reviewed. In-services should be presented on these and other security policies on a regular basis, and staff should know where to locate these policies. A policy that places employee safety and health on the same level of importance as patient and client safety should be in place (CAL-OSHA Guidelines, 1993). The assessment should also include reviews of state and local laws, staff training, security presence and training, crisis management plans, and counseling available for assaulted staff (Carroll, 1997).

An assessment of the environment would include questions such as the following:

- Is the lighting in the parking areas adequate?
- Are the parking areas patrolled frequently?
- Is crime increasing in the geographical area?
- Are metal detection systems in place at emergency and outpatient entrances?
- Are there curved mirrors at hallway intersections?
- Are waiting areas comfortable and designed to minimize stress?
- Are alarm systems installed in appropriate areas?
- Are seclusion rooms designed with patient and staff safety in mind?
- Do the pharmacy, newborn nursery, and other highly sensitive areas have strictly enforced limited access systems?

The assessment should be more than one question deep. For example:

- Does the facility have closed-circuit television sets?
- If so, are they operational?
- Who monitors them?
- Are the images on the television sets recorded, and if so, how long are the videotapes saved?

Work practice reviews would include questions such as the following:

- Are patients, visitors, and employees aware that violence is not permitted or tolerated?
- Are employees required to wear photo identification tags?
- Do employees ever work alone?
- Is inadequate staffing a common problem?
- Are employees required to fill out an incident report after a violent incident?
- Are employees assisted in filing charges if assaulted?
- Do employees wear keys or other potential weapons around their neck?
- Are patients asked to undress and wear a patient gown, so that weapons can be revealed and removed?

Policies and Procedures

The safety team would be responsible for the development and implementation of policies and procedures designed to make the workplace more secure. Examples of policies that provide for a safer workplace include the following:

- Sexual harassment
- Prevention of infant abduction
- Visitor restriction
- Weapon possession prohibition
- Drug testing of employees
- Hostage situation plans

Sexual harassment is against the law, and most hospitals and healthcare facilities have a strong written policy prohibiting it. To prevent infant abduction, it is recommended that all healthcare personnel wear conspicuous color photo ID badges plus another form of unique identification. The policy should ensure that babies are never carried and are always pushed in a bassinette (Carroll & Conejo, 1999/2000). A weapon policy prohibiting the carrying or use of any weapon on the premises is needed. Usually this policy has an exemption for sworn public law enforcement officers, except in psychiatric treatment areas. When M. Powell, RN, BS, published the hostage situation policy for Martha Jefferson Hospital, it drew high praise from law enforcement (Powell, 1991). The policy designates that an overhead code be called when a serious incident has occurred, indicating that all personnel should avoid entering that area until further notice. The policy also provides basic guidelines for surviving a hostage situation. The FNE specializing in forensic psychiatric nursing and trained in hostage negotiation by the FBI has also served as a skilled negotiator in hostage situations by local law enforcement agencies. Such a forensic nursing specialists can serve as a consultant to risk management, police, and hospital management (Coram, 1993). Giving specialized training in this area to an FNE on staff provides several benefits, including policy development, staff education, the ability to monitor sensitive situations as they develop rather than reacting to a crisis, and increased communication with legal agencies should a crisis develop.

Education

Education is essential in preventing workplace violence. All employees, including security and physicians, must be trained to recognize and manage aggressive behavior. It is not appropriate to be arguing about various approaches during a violent or threatening incident.

The training should cover topics such as the following:

- Early recognition of escalating behavior
- Ways of preventing or diffusing volatile situations or aggressive behavior
- Progressive behavior control methods and safe methods of restraint application
- Procedures for obtaining medical care, counseling, workers' compensation, or legal assistance after a violent episode or injury (OSHA, 3148, 1996)

Perhaps the most important lesson to be learned is to take threats seriously. When a post-operative patient in a Colorado hospital threatened to kill the next person who came to get him out of bed, the night nurse did not pass that information on. The next morning, two physical therapists were stabbed with forks.

Best Practice *7-1*

All threats of violence will be taken seriously and communicated to others who might be in danger. Initial steps for a crisis action plan will be instituted at once, including official notifications to supervisors and hospital security forces.

Since the early 1990s, in-service education and training programs on how to assess and manage assaultive behavior have become common in most American psychiatric facilities. Research has shown that a decrease in the rate of assault can be achieved. Staff concerns and liability issues are diminished as a result of these training programs. In these training programs, verbal deescalation techniques are taught, such as the use of a slow, calm voice, as well as therapeutic communication techniques, such as acknowledgment of what the person is feeling. People should be treated with dignity using the least amount of physical force as possible. People should, however, be held responsible for their behavior.

One such technique, known as verbal judo, was originally developed as a tactical course enabling police officers to communicate more effectively when interacting with difficult people. It has proven extremely effective in hospital environments when dealing with intoxicated, angry, and mentally ill individuals. Verbal judo teaches the skill of remaining centered and focused while redirecting behavior and generating voluntary compliance. These techniques provide a safer environment for staff, patients, and the public.

Dr. George J. Thompson based the principles of verbal judo on physical judo. Often the goal in a mental health or hospital setting is to calm individuals who have become confrontational. This type of behavior is understandable, for when an individual is in distress and in need of assistance, it generally is not without anxiety, fear, or anger. The healthcare professional is trained in many areas, but by and large, the least amount of education lies in the sphere of spoken communication. Verbal judo addresses this deficiency by providing practical, easy-to-use strategies for use in verbal encounters of all types.

Hiring and Firing

Violence can happen between peers, and between supervisors and staff. Policies must be quickly and fairly implemented. Michael Mantell (Mantell & Albrecht, 1994), a consultant on workplace violence issues, has suggested that the best deterrent to nonstranger or coworker violence is not to hire violence-prone individuals in the first place. Effective preemployment screening is very important. Firing should be handled with concern for the individual as well as for the safety of those still employed (Duncan, 1995). Employee assistance programs (EAP) in some hospitals are asking for the help of all employees in identifying the potential disgruntled worker or "avenger" by printing early warning signs in a hospital newsletter and asking that threats be taken seriously and reported immediately.

Reviews

An annual review should be conducted of implemented plans. Any incidents should be reviewed to determine if additional security measures are needed. Trends should be analyzed and addressed.

Case Study 7-1 Revenge

Mr. X was terminated from his job in a hospital microbiology laboratory after multiple attempts of the supervisors to salvage his job through counseling and work improvement initiatives. Mr. X had worked in the lab for many years, but he was a loner who seldom joined others for breaks or lunches. Others often remarked that "he was negative about everything." He even complained when the hospital announced a program to honor the Employee of the Month by giving the winner three days off and free parking in a prime spot in the administrative lot for a year. He professed that the whole program was for "the boss's pets" and that it was a waste of time and money to give employees' days off with pay when the hospital was already financially challenged. Mr. X met every change in departmental procedures with resistance and failure to comply. Many thought that from time to time he may have even falsified documentation of specimens and results, but no one was ever able to confirm the suspicion. Eventually, his waning performance and his negative attitude resulted in termination. Although he did not discuss his job loss with coworkers, it was generally known that he was extremely angry and had threatened to "get even with the place" someday.

A few weeks after he was fired, Mr. X returned to the hospital front desk with neatly wrapped cream-filled pastries and asked that the pastries be delivered to the lab for its regular staff meeting to be held that morning. During the evening, night, and next day, everyone who had eaten the pastry began to feel ill, to vomit, and to experience diarrhea. Eventually it was determined that the pastries had been inoculated with a salmonella serotype identical to a specimen that was found to be missing from the lab inventory. When Mr. X was questioned, he readily admitted to the act and stated, "It serves them right. I guess I got the last laugh, didn't I?"

Crisis Response

What if a violent incident does occur? The hope is that there is a quick response by security, the crisis response team, or the police. The crisis response team must be able to be activated quickly at any time of the day or night. The members of this team must have the training needed to respond safely to an incident. The incident should be documented and reported.

A crisis management plan should be in place that has established levels of authority and defined roles, with only one person

Box 7-1 Selected Nursing Diagnoses for Victims of Workplace Violence

- Fear related to perceived inability to control situation
- Ineffective coping related to inability to manage situational crisis
- Low self-esteem due to abuse from patient, family, or coworker

in charge. Crisis management is the process of identifying, acquiring resources, rehearsing, and applying resources requisite to resolving a crisis. A crisis might be loss of power to the facility, a natural disaster, a loss of computer access, an employee strike, or public disclosure of improper or unethical practices.

EAP counseling and debriefing sessions should be provided, and healthcare workers should utilize these services if assaulted. Marilyn Lanza (1992) studies nurses who have been assaulted, and the reactions include headaches, sleep disturbances, depression, self-blame, and decisions to leave nursing. Potential nursing diagnoses for the victim, which can be addressed by the nursing staff, are discussed in Box 7-1. It is important to discuss the incident, learn from it, and share that information with other healthcare workers.

Nursing's Role

The nurse is in a position to promote a vision that everyone can be safer at work. The nurse can do the following:

- Serve on the safety committee
- Participate in the development of policies and procedures
- Document incidents where patients or healthcare workers are threatened with or actually receive abuse
- Take threats seriously and report them to security, the supervisor, and others on a need-to-know basis
- Promote increased and continuing education on workplace safety on a personal, unit, institutional, state, and national level
- Encourage a risk-management approach to the problem of workplace violence

The forensic nurse will have the background to serve as a link between healthcare and law enforcement. The nurse managers need to take an active role in addressing workplace violence in their facilities.

Employer responsibilities would include the following:

- Maintain a safe work environment
- Assess the workplace for the potential for violence
- Provide in-service programs on security hazards
- Provide training in the management of assaultive behavior
- Encourage employees to report incidents and suggest ways to reduce risks
- Develop and implement a violence-reduction plan
- Provide counseling for the assaulted employee

Staff members have responsibilities as well. Employee responsibilities would include the following:

- Report hazards, incidents, and suspicious individuals
- Participate in the violence assessment
- Attend security in-service programs
- Use communication skills learned in training programs
- Work to develop policies and procedures, if none are in place
- Utilize counseling if assaulted

Participation in a violence-assessment project and in the development of a violence-reduction plan empowers healthcare workers, increases awareness, enhances communication between administrators and staff members, and improves the safety of the workplace.

Best Practice *7-2*

Nurses should be consistently vigilant in observing the behaviors of coworkers and should not hesitate to report threats, intimidation, or escalating signs of hostility toward the employer, supervisor, patients, or workplace.

Summary

Prevention is the primary key in addressing workplace violence. The proactive, multidisciplinary perspective of forensic nurse examiners can be effectively utilized in planning and implementing a violence reduction plan within the workplace. One vital aspect of such a program is for all staff members to understand the characteristic profile of offenders.

Individuals who engage in workplace violence typically devalue others and challenge authority. They are often argumentative, with the anticipation of escalating a confrontation. Violating policies and procedures, bypassing the chain of command, stealing from the organization, and framing coworkers are other characteristics. Blame for problems is invariably placed on others, and they overtly undermine authority by refusing to follow changes in policies and procedures, conveying that they do not value their job or the jobs of others who might be affected by their behavior. Individuals with high stress levels and a history of violence are especially prone to committing aggressive acts that endanger their own safety or the safety of others within the workplace.

The innate abilities of nurses to be astute observers of human behavior place them in an ideal position to identify potential violent employees or the escalating work environmental stress that contributes to violence. Nurses are also skilled in collaborative actions and problem solving with other nurses, disciplines, and administration, all imperative factors for successful implementation of an effective program to curb workplace violence.

The heightened awareness of forensic skills and intensified training brings a new perspective of the suspiciousness factor to the forefront of nursing challenges in a collaborative network of observation and awareness. Having a cadre of forensic nurse examiners on duty throughout large trauma centers or a single FNE in small community hospitals can provide personnel essential to identifying and combating dubious circumstances before they escalate into a life-threatening situation.

Resources

Publications

Workplace violence: Can you close the door on it?

American Nurses Association, Tel: 800-274-4ANA

Guidelines for Preventing Workplace Violence for Healthcare and Social Service Workers

US Department of Labor, OSHA, 3148-1996; www. osha-slc.gov80/Newinit/Workplaceviolence/index.html

References

Baron, S. A.(1996). Organizational factors in workplace violence: Developing effective programs to reduce workplace violence. *Occup Med, 11,* 335–351.

CAL-OSH. (1999). *Guidelines Health and Safety Code 1257.7 and 1257.8.* San Francisco: State of California, Division of Occupational Safety and Health.

Carroll, V. (1997). Workplace violence: Shared responsibilities. *Surgical Serv Manage, 3*(7), 17–19.

Carroll, V., & Conejo, P. (1999, December–2000, January). Infant abduction: Lowering the risk. *AWHONN Lifelines,* 25–27.

Carroll, V., & Morin, K. H. (1998). Workplace violence affects one-third of nurses. *Am Nurse, 30*(5): 15

Coram, J. (1993) *J of Psychosoc Nurs Mental Health.*

Duncan, T. S. (1995). Workplace homicides. *FBI Law Enforcement Bull, 64,* 20–25.

Goodman, R., Jenkins, L., & Mercy, J. (1994). Workplace-related homicide among healthcare workers in the US. *JAMA, 272,* 1686–1688.

Lanza, M. L. (1992). Nurses as patient assault victims: An update synthesis and recommendations. *Arch Psychiatr Nurs, 6,* 163–171.

Lynch, V. A. (1995) Clinical forensic nursing: A new perspective in the management of crime victims from trauma to trial. *Crit Care Nurs Clin North Am,* 7(3), 489–507.

Mahoney, B. S. (1991). The extent, nature, and response to victimization of emergency nurses in Pennsylvania. *J Emerg Nurs, 17,* 282–294.

Mantell, M., & Albrecht, S. (1994). *Ticking bombs: Defusing violence in the workplace.* Burr Ridge, IL: Irwin.

New York Commission OSH (1995) Violence in the workplace: The NY state experience, Author.

Powell, M. K. (1991). Hostage-situation policy statement for the emergency department. *J Emerg Nurs, 17,* 313–314.

Stultz, M. S. (1993). Crime in hospitals, 1986-1991: The latest IAHSS surveys. *J Healthc Prot Manage,* 2, 1–25.

Thompson, G. J. (1982). Rhetoric: An important tool for police officers. *FBI Bulletin.* April, 1–7.

Thompson, G. J. (1983). *Verbal Judo: Words as a Force Option.* Springfield, IL: Charles C. Thomas.

Thompson, G. J. (1993). *Verbal Judo: The Gentle Art of Persuasion.* New York: Quill/Morrow.

Thompson, G. J. (1994). *Verbal Judo: Redirecting Behavior with Words.* Jacksonville, FL: IPTM.

US Department of Labor, OSHA. (1996). Guidelines for preventing workplace violence for healthcare and social service workers, US Department of Labor, OSHA 3148-1996. Retrieved from www. osha-slc.gov 80/Newinit/Workplaceviolence/index.html.

Chapter 8 Environmental Terrorism and Mass Disasters

Barbara Goll-McGee

In times of global terrorism, the future seems to hold escalating threats to society and episodes of tragedy that will consume lives and economic security. Air travel plans may be marred by terror alerts, and children are sent to school on the defense, in fear of some act of violence. The threats of terrorism are everywhere, it seems, impacting the sense of safety we associate with travel, our attendance at public events, and even our everyday necessities such as food sources, air, and water. Unfortunately, these grim views are not merely pessimistic; they reflect reality. It is not surprising, therefore, that each successive threat or real act of terrorism brings fear into the lives of millions of people and undermines their sense of security.

Due to instant and sophisticated communications technology and media coverage, a disaster that affects multiple to thousands of lives can be exposed within minutes to an expectant and apprehensive population. It is no longer a question of if another catastrophic event will happen; it is a matter of when and what type. Where will the next mass homicide or suicide, terrorist bombing, building collapse, plane crash, or tornado take place? How many people will be injured and killed, and how will it be managed as a medicolegal event? Because acts of terror are becoming almost regular occurrences, they tend to receive significant media attention only when they create mass casualties or cause widespread damage. When a violent act causes more casualties than did previous attacks, terrorists are given widespread publicity for and reaction to their cause (Simon, 2000).

The Need for Forensic Nurses

To keep from living in fear and helplessness, elements of society must prepare and respond to terrorist threats in a proactive manner. Nurses are among the professions that are ideally suited for disaster responses, and those who specialize in forensic nursing have a role mandated by the theoretical framework and social sanctions that guide professional role behavior in response to crime and violence.

Historically, nurses have been involved on the front line due to the attention they give to casualties of war and the palliative care they administer to victims of natural catastrophe. As early as the days of Florence Nightingale, nurses have been a vital clinical and humanitarian resource in times of emergent need. A review of the literature finds nurses working within military response and other organized response efforts. The Red Cross, established in 1863, is cited as "the most significant large scale and long standing organized disaster relief effort in contemporary society" (Komnenich & Feller, 1991, p. 124). With the development of the Department of Defense and the Federal Emergency Management Agency, church groups and private voluntary organizations such as the National Committee of Voluntary Organizations increased documented knowledge about human responses to mass emergencies by victims and caregivers (Komnenich & Feller, 1991).

The Disaster Relief Act defines a disaster as "any major man-made or natural event of such severity and magnitude to warrant disaster systems" (US Congress Office of Technology Assessment, 1993). Military nursing in wartime is among the first documented disaster nursing response to a human-caused event; however, the disaster nursing response has been developing quickly, adapting and responding to threats of environmental terrorism and other criminal incidents. This adaptation continues as research is initiated and personal accounts of nurses' experiences are shared in an effort to provide substantial information from which further role function in disaster nursing can be customized and evolve.

It may be premature to determine the role clarification of disaster nursing as it relates to the to the events of September 11, 2001, when American commercial aircrafts were used as suicide missions killing thousands of innocent people and leaving countless victims by extension with financial, psychological, and environmental damage too profound to be assessed. The horrific assault on New York City's World Trade Center left a world in shock and disbelief. Premeditated acts, especially against civilians, are impossible to accept and difficult to endure. The aftermath of such events, teeming with human and physical devastation, is the operating climate for the forensic nurse examiner responding to a mass disaster.

It is beyond the scope of this chapter to specifically discuss every element of environmental terrorism and natural catastrophe. However, describing and understanding past disasters can be the first stage to preventing or ameliorating the effects of future disasters (Illing, 2000). Through analyses of a well-known act of terrorism and a study of potential events, one can more easily understand the central elements in disaster response and appreciate the role of the forensic nurse examiner responding to disasters. (See Figures 8-1 and 8-2.)

An example of emerging disaster nursing response is found in a discussion of chemical warfare or chemical terrorist attacks. Chemical agents are poisons that incapacitate, injure, or kill through their toxic effects on the skin, eyes, lungs, blood, nerves, and other organs (US Congress Office of Technology Assessment, 1993). Initially, acts of chemical warfare were considered to be completely devastating and only a threat to unprepared and unprotected groups of people. The Chemical Casualty Care Office reported that the ignorance was particularly striking in view of the seven-decade-long history of modern chemical warfare and the well-publicized use of mustard and nerve agents during the Iran-Iraq War in the 1980s. Through education and experience, medical professionals involved in Operation Desert Shield/Desert Storm learned that medical defenses were possible and effective, that chemical casualties could be saved and returned to duty, and that mortality could be minimized (Chemical Casualty Care Office, 1995).

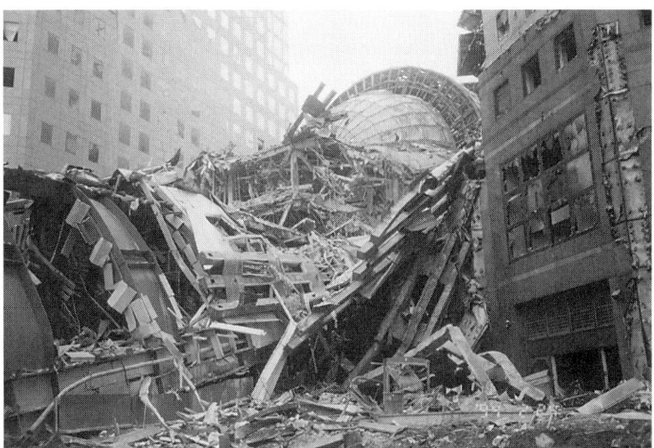

Fig. 8-1 The World Trade Center collapse on September 11, 2001, was a wake-up call for all citizens regarding the threat of terrorism and disaster.

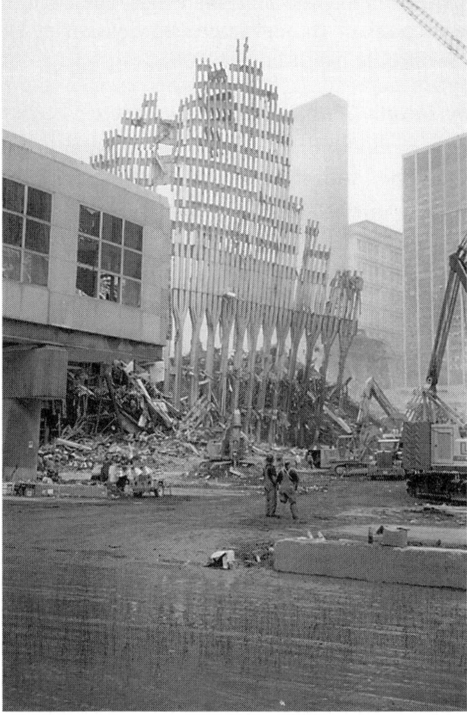

Fig. 8-2 Experienced disaster workers stand in awe of the mass destruction of the World Trade Center several days after the event.

A plan prepared in defense of chemical warfare and chemical terrorist attack (nerve gas poisoning in particular) includes training medical personnel to recognize and treat symptoms, wearing protective gear to minimize exposure, stockpiling antidote, and immediately accessing military expertise regarding specific agents and their dissemination. One of the most chilling terrorist acts of 1995 was the gas attack on the Tokyo subway on March 20 by the Aum Shinrikyo cult. This attack indicated that terrorism involving chemicals was no longer confined to combat operations but that civilians could also be targeted. After an investigation, the Japanese police also charged the cult for the sarin gas attack in June 1994 in Matsumoto that killed 7 and injured about 500 (Center for National Security Studies, 1995).

Chemical agents, specifically riot control agents like Mace (CN) or its synthetic derivative (CS) are most likely to be encountered during a small-scale event. Nerve agents, vesicants, cyanide, and lung-damaging agents may be seen at small- or large-scale scenarios (Chemical Casualty Care Office, 1995). The secondary effects of chemical agents can account for devastating injuries such as the jet fuel showers from aircraft hitting the New York City World Trade Center and Pentagon causing large body surface area burns to those bystanders below and around the area of impact. Chemical agents may also be used in product contamination. The level of scientific expertise needed to develop chemical or biologic weapons for terrorists is not high, nor is it cost prohibitive (Simon, 2000).

Biological Agents

Biological warfare agents involve a deliberate use of disease or natural poisons to incapacitate or kill people. Microorganisms such as bacteria, rickettsia, fungi, and viruses that cause infection or liberate incapacitating amounts of lethal toxins are used (US Congress Office of Technology Assessment, 1993). Biotechnology and genetic engineering have led to the creation of more potent and environmentally stable biological agents (Simon, 2000). The detection of these biological agents is particularly difficult because symptoms may not be seen for hours or even days. It was not until more than a year after the Salmonellosis community outbreak, which affected 751 people, that the event was found to be caused by the intentional contamination of restaurant salad bars by members of a religious commune (Torok, Tauxe, & Wise et al., 1997). Forensic nurses may assist in detecting such occurrences by careful epidemiological study of the incident, including case-finding, surveillance strategies, and documentation of forensic evidence.

Bacillus anthracis and *Clostridium botulinum* are some of the agents likely to be used by terrorists (Simon, 2000). These organisms cause anthrax and botulism, respectively. Anthrax (rarely seen in modern hospitals) and botulism are reportable to the Centers for Disease Control and Prevention. Ricin, a plant by-product used in the past for assassination attempts, has been delivered by an "umbrella-type weapon in the form of a pellet" (Simon, 2000, p. 1727). Since October 1, 2001, media attention has focused on anthrax due to the increased numbers of anthrax exposure through the US mail (Pittman, 2001). An active bioterrorist threat drives the demand for information and discussion of other potential biological agents including smallpox, plague, and tularemia. Thousands of concerned citizens are worried about anthrax exposure, eliciting new responses from healthcare personnel, including forensic nurses. Readiness, or disaster preparedness, is the primary action that keeps this societal dilemma and pervasive fear from becoming a clinical disaster. It is also the action that will most likely offer the most efficient control for different types of future incidents.

Ionizing Radiation

Any radiation, as either particles or electromagnetic energy, that has sufficient energy to produce ions in matter is referred to as ionizing radiation (Voeltz, 1999). The efficiency of radiation for producing mass destruction and the death of thousands was confirmed as a result of the atomic explosions at Hiroshima and Nagasaki (Warren, 1977). A report on radiation accidents reveals heavy morbidity and mortality around the Chernobyl reactor incident in Russia in 1986. At least 2897 people were exposed to significant radiation doses, and 28 deaths were reported. There were 8 deaths due to exposure to a high-level sealed source in Morocco in 1984 (Voeltz, 1999). The detonation of an atomic bomb or accidents involving a nuclear reactor are examples of how ionizing radiation can pose particular nuclear threats to society. Other potential dangers have been threats of "dirty bombs" or explosives that contain particulate radioactive material. These weapons are cheaper alternatives to an atomic bomb and require less sophisticated methods for manufacture and deployment. Their potential has not yet been fully realized, however.

The Disaster Response System

Disaster Preparedness

Preparation for the potential use of nuclear, biological, and chemical (NBC) agents receives attention at every level. Locally, emergency nurses are trained for heightened awareness, casualty management, decontamination, and NBC defense equipment. Forensic nurses who practice and prepare for NBC disaster response are obvious resources to hospitals and communities planning for this type of scenario. The forensic nurse examiner responding to disasters may be integral in the attempts of industry, individual governments, and international organizations to develop and implement procedures for preventing or minimizing the effects of potential or actual disasters (Illing, 2000). The management of patients suspected of use or exposure to these agents includes a detailed analysis of the mechanisms of injury, as well as the how and why of their occurrence. This type of assessment, particularly involving living victims, is within the operational domain of the forensic nurse examiner (Goll-McGee, 1999).

The forensic nature of human-caused disasters exists because the event itself is a criminal act. Forensic science can serve as a deterrent by increasing the likelihood that the terrorists will be apprehended before fully launching a successful attack (Franz, 1999). The medicolegal aspects of terrorist attacks extend into natural disasters too, as our litigious society will surely look to determine fault and gain monetary restitution when there are adverse secondary effects.

When a disaster occurs, local first responders and the mayor or county executive perform a joint preliminary damage and needs assessment. The local emergency operations center (EOC) is activated. Depending upon the magnitude of the event and the local availability of resources, the local EOC may then, in turn, request aid from the state governor. The state EOC may declare a state of emergency and informs the regional director of the Federal Emergency Management Agency (FEMA). The FEMA director, in cooperation with the Catastrophic Disaster Response Group (CDRG), emergency support team (EST), and other federal agencies, contacts the president of the US in tandem with a request from the state EOC for a presidential declaration of a federal emergency or major disaster. Federal and state coordinating officers are appointed to set up and support a disaster field office and emergency response team, which provide emergency support functions, recovery, and mitigation programs. Disaster field operations occur on a local, state, and federal level and respond with any one, a combination, or all needs. These may include transportation, communications, public works and engineering, firefighting, information and planning, mass care, resource support, health and medical services, urban search and rescue, hazardous materials management, food, and energy (FEMA, 1999).

Emergency Mobilization Preparedness Board

In the early 1980s, the US government recognized the need to improve emergency preparedness by establishing the Emergency Mobilization Preparedness Board (EMPB). Its response to the presidential mandate for health program development resulted in the creation of a single system charged with the responsibility to care for large numbers of casualties from either a domestic natural or human-caused disaster or conventional overseas war. Services are expanded to include health and medical assessment, surveillance, equipment and supplies, evacuation, definitive care and food, drug and device safety. Considerations are also given to veterinary services, worker health and safety, inherent NBC hazards, mental health services, public information, vector control, potable water sources, solid waste disposal, and mortuary services. The National Disaster Medical System (NDMS) was a cooperative asset-sharing partnership of four federal departments and agencies, including the Department of Health and Human Services (DHHS), Department of Defense (DoD), Department of Veterans Affairs (VA), and FEMA, which has been redefined under the auspices of the newly created division of Homeland Security (Twomey & Goll-McGee, 1999).

Specialty Teams

Further customization of the healthcare disaster response has been accomplished with the formation of specialty teams in disaster medical assistance (DMAT) and disaster mortuary operational response (DMORT). These teams may be fully equipped and self-sufficient enabling their immediate response to an austere environment or to augment the response of previously deployed teams and even to support overwhelmed local or state resources as necessary. The dynamic response is dictated by need and is situationally dependent. Specific pediatric, burn, trauma, critical care and international specialty teams augment the efforts of a responding DMAT as worldwide catastrophic events dictate, just as specific death investigation, mental health, and forensic specialties enhance the efforts of a responding DMORT. Teams may be predeployed for consequence management of potential weapons of mass destruction scenarios, adding special decontamination teams to the system (Twomey & Goll-McGee, 1999). A focus on those affected by disaster directs the content expertise of a particular response team. In light of the medicolegal aspects and potential of human-caused and natural disasters, forensic nurses who serve on both DMAT and DMORT squadrons bring the ideal cross training, versatility, and expertise on which the teams rely for the specificity and success of their responses.

Readiness for Deployment

Members must have personal gear and federal identification to leave within the optimal 12-hour period after notification. The specialty of forensic nursing encompasses a broad acumen, allowing its members to assume several diverse roles within the same disaster scenario. These may include functioning in the capacity of a clinical forensic nurse or serving as an antemortem data interviewer or a processing technician for a disaster management support agent. Deployed nurses may be assigned to work in a hospital intensive care unit as staff augmenters for the facility or to function in the austere environment of a DMAT mobile medical tent (Figs. 8-3 and 8-4). Forensic nurses are not restricted in

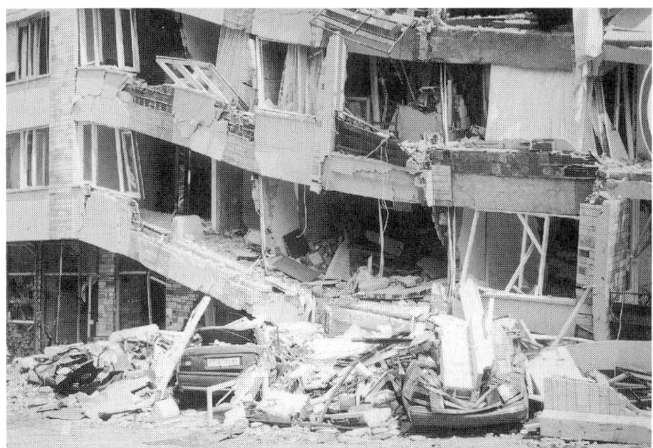

Fig. 8-3 Earthquake devastation demands clinical response, family assistance, and forensic processing.

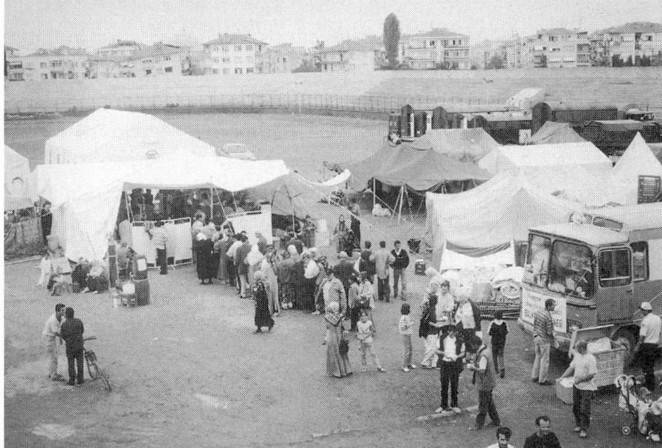

Fig. 8-4 This temporary field hospital was used for Turkish earthquake victims.

their potential roles in disaster, providing they have the education and experience required for each and practice within the broad scope and standards of forensic nursing.

The Forensic Nurse's Role in Disasters

The scope and standards of forensic nursing practice define the victim as a client, the family, the perpetrator, and the public in general (International Association of Forensic Nurses [IAFN], 1997). Disaster responses satisfy advocacy to all these areas. The clients and the families affected directly by the catastrophic event will benefit from the initial work of the forensic nurse; the general public will be served secondarily in several ways ranging from education and emotional support to environmental safety and security. In human-caused disasters, the event itself must be treated as a medicolegal incident or a crime scene. Evidence collection and appropriate documentation are crucial responsibilities of nurses on the scene.

It is important to also note that natural disasters are seldom void of forensic issues. During and after disasters such as tornados or hurricanes, there may be injuries and deaths that result from looting or violent competition for shared survival resources including food, water, and shelter. Other facets of natural catastrophes may constitute culpability or directly contribute to deaths and injuries. For example, faulty construction of a building may lead to excessive deaths and injuries during an earthquake, or failure to have properly marked and accessible building exits may prevent egress of victims when a fire or explosion occurs. Therefore, the forensic nurse must be ever mindful of careful assessment and documentation of factors that may be important later in judicial proceedings (see Figures 8-3 and 8-4).

In a disaster response, the forensic nursing role is divided into three parts: clinical response, family assistance, and forensic processing.

Key Point *8-1*

The forensic nurse specialist serving disasters provides direct care services that are quantitatively and qualitatively different from those provided by other responders. Clinical experience in emergency or critical care settings is the basis for the development of expertise in clinical forensic nursing disaster management. The forensic nurse specialist prepares for this expanded role by becoming involved in community disaster planning, state emergency management, and hospital disaster protocols. The extent of involvement in disaster medical assistance depends on the active membership of the team and the specialties, which the clinical forensic nurse specialist fosters.

Clinical Response

In a customized DMAT response, increased clinical specialties may increase the likelihood and opportunity for deployment. Forensic nursing in and of itself is a specialty, but within the realm of forensic nursing there is a professional commitment to subspecialties such as clinical forensic nursing; critical incident stress management; and disaster nursing such as the medical disaster-response model (Schultz, Koenig, & Noji, 1996), the Incident Command System, or knowledge of NBC agents and previous humanitarian crises. This versatility and preparedness is what also opens up opportunities to respond with other various medical relief organizations and efforts. Forensic nurses need to develop a dynamic personal philosophy in this role and throughout their careers; this will keep them at their highest level of effectiveness and their lowest level of risk. The notion of being involved in the disaster management system *before* a critical incident occurs is paramount for the forensic nurse specialist interested in being a part of a disaster response team.

Mass Casualty Incident (MCI)

This response comprises four basic elements: search and rescue, triage and initial stabilization, definitive medical care, and evacuation (Briggs & Leong, 1990). The version of triage–that is, to do the greatest good for the greatest number of people–functions as an analytical sorting process in classic MCIs of limited scope (Briggs & Leong, 1990). The clinical forensic nurse examiner provides expert care as a registered nurse for victims in various stressful, fast-paced, and often demanding clinical situations assessing vital signs, managing pain and wounds, and maintaining the homeostasis and hemodynamic stability of the patient. "The medicolegal patient population, however, require that these same goals *plus* forensic concerns be addressed" (Goll-McGee, 1999, p. 9). Expert clinical care is vital as disaster nursing and other healthcare roles are often expanded to meet the acute demands of the situation. A unique dimension of nursing assessment of disaster patients involves an index of suspicion to discern the mechanisms of injury or illness that placed them within the scope of a specific disaster team.

Documentation

The forensic aspects of clinical disaster response will be discussed later; however, the single most important aspect must be documentation of injuries, conditions, and deaths for future data collection and research. This is accomplished to satisfy the medicolegal management of disaster victims and the continued education of healthcare professionals and the public in general regarding a critical incident or disaster.

Learning and Adaptation

What is learned from one disaster must be shared in order to avoid pitfalls and to design a more effective response for future events. The knowledge acquired in one event may lead to early detection of problems in future events and will ultimately lead to improved medical management of victims and less morbidity and mortality.

Case Study 8-1 Working Together

The shifts caring for the burn victims of the World Trade Center were busy and long, but after work, concerns of medical personnel rapidly moved to management issues and plans for replacement, as physicians knew the long-term nature of caring for burn trauma patients. It became evident that burn intensive care unit (ICU) nurses who could take the place of the disaster nurses already deployed over the next six to eight weeks were needed. At the time, only 30 burn ICU nurses were registered within the NDMS, 7 of which were already there. An urgent call went out through the American Burn Association and to ICU nurses. Rapid applications were processed as nurses from around the country continued to respond to this demand. This is a real-life occurrence in which interagency cooperation and the disaster nurse's advance practice disaster management skills directly affected the mortality and morbidity of living forensic patients and resulted in an improved and enlarged pool of disaster nursing resources for use in future events. Substantial efforts in training, monitoring, and reviewing actions in the field now take place in all agencies set up for disaster response (Birggs & Leong, 1990).

Family Assistance

The Aviation Disaster Family Assistance Act of 1996 requires the National Transportation Safety Board (NTSB), air carriers, and the American Red Cross (ARC) to provide an integrated family assistance center (FAC), which offers support to family survivors of mass casualties (Wright, Peters, & Flannery, 1999). The purpose of FAC is to provide the relatives of victims with information and access to the services they may need in the days following the incident; to protect families from the media and curiosity seekers; and to allow investigators, the medical examiner (ME), and coroner access to families so they can get information more easily (Emergency Management Institute, 1996). This response to a federal mandate challenges forensic nurses to develop forensic nursing care practices that are consistent with the FAC guidelines.

Forensic nursing activity provides care for bereaved families of those involved or thought to be involved in a catastrophic event and addresses the needs of bereaved families through participation in interagency organization and cooperation (American Red Cross, 1997). The American Red Cross has specific policies and services for the FAC. The American Red Cross works with local governments in the assessment of response capability and the coordination of services for emergency care, mental health support, and victim identification (Wright, Peters, & Flannery, 1999). The forensic nurse who possesses knowledge of family assistance strategies and techniques can assume an important role in planning and implementation with the American Red Cross or with the local ME's or coroner's office that assumes the responsibility of victim identification and family support (Wright, Peters, & Flannery, 1999).

Within the FAC, the forensic nurse interfaces with family members and assesses the informant's state of being and needs for referral services defined within educational, emotional, psychological, or medical categories. A "panic button" is available for emergency security if these indicators establish a threat of danger or violence against the forensic nurse interviewer. Assessment in this phase of interface also relates to the collection of antemortem data, consisting of personal and medical data essential for timely, efficient, and accurate victim identification.

Antemortem Interview

The outcome for these assessments results in each informant, whether a family member, friend, loved one, coworker, neighbor, or the individual involved in the disaster, having an antemortem interview completed. An evaluation is made so that those potential informants are not children under the age of 12 and are not individuals who are totally distraught or under the influence of drugs and alcohol at the time the interview is to take place. The result is a safe exchange that elicits information that is as complete as possible by cueing and guiding objective data collection from possibly multiple informants.

The forensic nurse interviewer obtains a valid description of the individual involved in the critical incident determining if the information/informants are credible. The forensic nurse interviewer must realize the importance of interviewing not only next of kin or family members but also boyfriends, girlfriends, or others who may know personal attributes, surgeries, behavioral habits, and other privileged information that might assist in identification. Consider the mother who is unaware of her daughter's tattoo or breast implants or a husband who is not aware that his wife has an implanted birth control device. This information may be vital to the identification efforts for this individual. For various reasons, it is not all that uncommon for this type of information to be withheld. The forensic nurse interviewer is aware of such factors and uses unique skills to determine if individuals to be interviewed are likely to disclose information about someone who may have been involved with the incident in question. The forensic nurse interviewer discerns this and eliminates those individuals who want to give information about pets, possessions, or people unlikely to be involved. These concerns are referred to and addressed elsewhere within the FAC.

The forensic nurse interviewer records personal information and transmits it for entry into software programs. This typically initiates the systematic identification efforts. The interviewer identifies areas of missing information and directs informants in procedures for obtaining pictures, dental records and dentist's names and locations, hospital records, and other data sources. All informants are identified within the FAC database, and each will be provided with a personalized plan for obtaining information sources that will guide decisions about medical care, mental health and spiritual support, communications, accommodations, and even funeral arrangements. The bits of information gleaned from many and varied sources will help to eventually construct a template for the disaster team.

Referrals and Counseling

Mental health referrals address grief counseling, emotional defusing of witnesses and others close to the disaster scene, and subsequent critical incident stress debriefing. Healthcare providers may treat some individuals with medication or may transport them to a healthcare facility if local resources are not already overwhelmed. Medical assistance provides basic checkups or first aid to those within the FAC, for example, victims of falls, accidents, or assaults. They may also provide DNA blood sampling from next of kin or provide medication for those who do not have personal medication supplies at hand. Medical safety may also be considered if those responding to the FAC are suspect of contamination or contagion. Spiritual guidance, which is diverse or nondenominational, is provided for those interested in seeking it. Communications should be provided for telephone or computer links for notifications, inquiries to obtain missing information, and to facilitate conversations with distant friends and relatives. Accommodations should generally be provided within the FAC if it has been established at a hotel; if not, nearby accommodations are desirable that are located away from, but nearby, the disaster site. Funeral arrangements are made with assistance from volunteer staff, death notification officers, or forensic nurse examiners within the center. Informants of living victims and deceased victims should be separated whenever possible, and body processing specifics and formalities must be addressed if the options for body disposal are limited or restricted due to exposure, contamination, or dissemination. Resources for possessions and pets must be available using appropriate airline, security, or officiating personnel.

Individual outcomes will depend on the effectiveness and preparedness of the FAC and, of course, will hinge on the nature of the incident. Flexibility is necessary for optimal outcomes in every effort to meet people's needs. Forensic nurses and others working within the FAC must realize their personal limitations and the limitations of available resources. Using the forensic nursing process will assist in the determination of priorities of care and help to ensure collaboration within the FAC.

Death Notification

When the forensic nurse works with local medical examiner's (ME) or coroner's systems to prepare for the FAC, forensic nurses may be positioned to direct activities and to staff the antemortem interviewers, thus assuming a role in death notification. Nurses must communicate with the ancillary personnel of the FAC, which includes, but is not limited to, medical assistance teams, mental health workers, spiritual leaders, American Red Cross volunteers, police and security, hotel and airline representatives, or participating agency and communications personnel. This role is possible only with an underlying knowledge of the FAC, advance planning, participation, and implementation by the forensic nurse with the American Red Cross and the ME's or coroner's office. In transportation disasters, the National Transportation Safety Board oversees this function. Otherwise, it will be managed at the level of the American Red Cross.

Forensic nurses can use a rapid needs assessment in order to obtain relevant information quickly for planning and implementing responses (Payne & Baumgartner, 1996). The medical incident management system under an incident command structure is suggested as the most efficient method in disaster type scenarios (Irwin, 1989). Assessment, diagnosis, outcome identification, planning, and implementation do not always designate a restricted order of activity but act as an integrated approach between standards, an ever-changing dynamic approach used by the forensic nurse specialist to meet the demands of the FAC.

Best Practice *8-1*

The forensic nurse shall function collaboratively within a multidisciplinary team, combining healthcare with criminal justice and law enforcement agencies and other resources to implement a prescribed regime within the scope of professional nursing practice (IAFN, 1997).

The outstanding goal of the FAC is to serve families and those affected by a disaster by providing positive identification in a timely manner through a working association with the ME's or coroner's office and healthcare institutions and with the return and receipt of victims, their property, and their dignity. The forensic nurse specialist, in order to maintain and determine the effectiveness of the FAC, utilizes ongoing assessment and research. Follow-up with those involved with the FAC should be queried near the anniversary date for victim's informants and within a few months of the incident for those working within the FAC. This questionnaire for quality improvement helps to identify methods and areas for improvement and focus.

Challenges, successes, and strategies are documented and procedures reviewed. Originally a response for aviation disasters, the notion of the FAC and the role of the forensic nurse within it can be utilized for response to various other disaster scenarios. Forensic nurses can also be a resource for the ME/coroner's office being upscaled or downsized to meet the demands of every unique catastrophe whether it is a train crash with hundreds of victims or a car crash involving six to eight victims. The World Trade Center event led to the use of the FAC in an extended role for the incorporation of a missing persons database and, in the absence of human remains, the early distribution of death certificates authorized by city officials.

Forensic Processing

In the event of a mass fatality incident, human remains should be recovered onsite and prepared at the forensic processing center (Wright, Peters, & Flannery, 1999). A forensic processing center (FPC) acts as a collection area, organized in a methodical, efficient, and scientific manner to process large numbers of bodies and body parts, thereby expediting victim identification. This makeshift morgue facility is utilized when the regular morgue is insufficient to accommodate the large volume of victims of an incident or whose location is not conducive to immediate transport of remains to the facility. Requirements for a temporary morgue or FPC include convenience to the scene but far enough away to be out of harm; adequate capacity; complete security; easy access by vehicles; adequate ventilation; hot and cold water; drainage; and electrical capacity for necessary equipment, communication, office space, rest and debriefing area, and restrooms (Emergency Management Institute, 1996). An FPC may be located in an airplane hangar or a field tent. In the absence of adequate facilities for an FPC, the National Foundation for Mortuary Care, in support of the National Disaster Medical System's DMORT teams, maintains a mobile mortuary container depot, an aggregation of equipment and supplies for deployment to a disaster site at any time. The depot contains a complete morgue with designated workstations for each of the necessary processing elements, prepackaged equipment to maintain the workstations, along with expendable supplies (National Disaster Medical System, 1999).

The flow of operations within an FPC is flexible but will include reception, radiology, dental, autopsy, fingerprinting, and embalming areas. Depending on the situation, forensic processing may not include the autopsy, for example, which could be carried out at the regular morgue site. "When a catastrophe occurs, the large numbers of bodies and mutilations make identification difficult and require the involvement of multidisciplinary teams" (Martin-de las Heras, Valenzuela, & Villanueva et al., 1999, p. 428). The FPC and morgue may utilize DMORT team members also depending on the magnitude of the incident and the resources of the local response. Under the incident command structure, no power is given to or taken away from specific individuals or agencies that respond to assist. When activated, DMORT teams provide local authorities with technical assistance and personnel to recover, identify, and process deceased victims (National Disaster Medical System, 1999). Teams include medical examiners, coroners, pathologists, anthropologists, medical records, fingerprint experts, forensic odontologists, mental health debriefers (for the team only), forensic nurses, police, supply specialists, and computer experts dispatched in whole or in part depending on scope of the disaster (National Disaster Medical System, 1999).

The role of the forensic nurse examiner functioning within the FPC is varied and diverse. Again, forensic nurses are challenged to develop strategies to promote new professional standards in accordance with existing forensic nursing standards while organizing or working within the FPC.

The FPC reception area is a secure entrance where transported remains from the disaster site are first logged. The time and date of arrival and name(s) of delivery personnel are documented here. The remains, already bagged and tagged by recovery teams, are validated by number and issued a corresponding case file containing worksheets for all of the forensic processing stations. The remains are accompanied by an FPC staff member (possibly a forensic nurse) who records contents as the bag is opened, its contents photographed, and personal items such as clothing and jewelry are removed and logged. The remains are now ready to continue through the processing workstations.

Fingerprints

Obtaining fingerprints is mainly a matter for law enforcement. However, forensic nurses trained in fingerprinting technique may be an instrumental resource in obtaining fingerprints by injecting tissue builder into dried digits to plump up the surface area of fingertips or "even to the extent of removing peeled skin or finger tips where a body is putrefied" (Knight, 1997, p. 33). Local police will conduct postmortem fingerprinting using various methods, including the use of image enhancement techniques (Moler, Ballarin, & Pessana et al., 1998). The FBI fingerprinting team usually is called to mass fatalities incidents to provide assistance (Emergency Management Institute, 1996). Fingerprints are then compared to others available on file for identification. Because many individuals will not have had antemortem fingerprints taken, investigators will sometimes be forced to examine personal items from the victim's home or automobile to obtain fingerprints for comparison.

Radiographs

Remains are radiographed to sort out debris and for comparison with antemortem medical records of osteopathic injuries, implanted surgical devices, projectiles, and other anomalies. The comparison of antemortem and postmortem radiographs is accepted as a fundamental method in forensic dental identification (MacLean, Kogon, & Stitt, 1994). The prime situation here is the mass disaster, such as an air crash where the passenger list can be used to obtain dental records for positive identification (Moler, Ballarin, & Pessana et al., 1998). The importance of dental evidence in the identification of burn victims has been emphasized in a number of case reports and in papers dealing with mass disasters (Martin-de las Heras, Valenzuela, & Villanueva et al., 1999). The teeth are the most resistant tissue in the body and may sometimes be the only things that defy total decomposition and even severe fire (Knight, 1997). Upon examination by an expert, the teeth can give general information regarding the age and gender of an individual and the bones give information regarding age, gender, race, height, and weight or stature.

Role of ME and Coroner

The ME or coroner acquires legal custody of the body until it is released from jurisdiction and is required by jurisdiction statutes to perform autopsies on certain classifications of deceased individuals (Hoyt & Spangler, 1996). The forensic autopsy functions to discover some or all of the following facts:

- The identity of the body
- The cause of death
- The nature and number of injuries
- The time of death
- The presence of poisons
- The expectation of duration of life for insurance purposes
- The presence of natural disease and its contribution to death (especially where there is also trauma and the interpretation of the injuries, either criminal, suicidal, or accidental)
- The interpretation of any other unnatural conditions, including those associated with surgical or medical procedures (Knight, 1997)

The body is examined, photographed, and trace evidence is collected. Appearances and interventions are meticulously recorded. Various bloods, body fluid, and tissues samples are taken for blood grouping, toxicology, and DNA testing. Cytological smears have been reported to be a possible source of DNA reference samples, which can be compared to DNA recovered from found human remains (Sweet, Hildebrand, & Phillips, 1999). Forensic nurses trained in death investigation can assist in the autopsies performed on the victims of catastrophic events.

Releasing the Body

The ME or coroner may also waive the autopsy after initial investigation of the death and release the body to the next of kin (Hoyt & Spangler, 1996). The number and extent of autopsies depend on the situation and type of mass fatality. Due to the medicolegal nature of aviation disasters, for example, the National Transportation Safety Board requires the autopsy of crewmembers. The ME or coroner also has the right to order embalming for sanitation and preservation. At this station, the best process for embalming of the remains is chosen and the body wrapped in absorbent material and placed in a heavy-duty opaque pouch with a name (if available) and number (Emergency Management Institute, 1996). The casket is also labeled and transported by professional hearse to the point of shipment or receiving funeral home. Common tissue or human tissue that is not identified because of commingling or sheer amount is buried at a common grave.

Identification of Human Remains

This function is dependent on the availability of sufficient antemortem information obtained from records and relatives and the existence of sufficient postmortem material for the recording of identification data (Matin-de las Heras, Valenzuela, & Villanueva et al., 1999). When the processing is completed, the manner and cause of death are determined and the remains are then released to the family (Wright, Peters, & Flannery, 1999). The identification of victims of a mass disaster is essential for humanitarian, religious, as well as for judicial reasons (Martin-de las Heras, Valenzuela, & Villanueva et al., 1999). The timely and efficient identification of disaster victims satisfies the natural inclination and emotional strain of loved ones to give remains a proper burial and allows for the coordination and fulfillment of certificates, wills, and other matters.

Key Point 8-2

Within each domain of disaster response (clinical, family assistance, and forensic processing), the forensic nurse examiner practices standard care activities, which include evidence collection, documentation, and crisis intervention. Disaster-type scenarios may emphasize and complicate these forensic aspects of care. For example, the forensic nurse's ability to discover, identify, and collect physical and nonphysical evidence may play an important role in the investigation of a disaster. It is imperative that the forensic nurse discerns what may be evidence and how and if it should be collected.

Evidence Collection in Disasters

In clinical disaster response, the forensic nurse examiner may be the person most familiar with physical and testimonial evidence collection and may be required to instruct the healthcare team as to why it should be collected and to provide instructions about collection procedures. Chain of custody must also be considered, taught, and maintained.

Physical Evidence

Wound debris, projectiles, and clothing are among the most commonly found physical evidence on individuals; however, additional evidence may be collected accordingly. For example, from a building explosion or package bomb, bomb residue swabbing may be collected. A sputum sample may be evidence in the confined noxious gas inhalation of a terrorist attack. Life-threatening conditions may compromise the possibility of physical evidence collection in the clinical environment as decontamination efforts destroy physical evidence. In disasters of sudden onset, whether natural disasters or terrorist bombings, the absence of warning and the potential for large numbers of injuries or deaths can at best evoke only a reactive medical response, not only among the first responders but also among the professionals who are first at the scene (Briggs & Leong, 1990). Physical evidence collection is most likely to occur with assistance from the forensic nurse examiner at the autopsy in the FPC. Many situations are possible and require the advanced thought, preparation, and skill of the forensic nurse serving disaster populations. In a disaster situation, forensic nurses are protected from liability.

Testimonial Evidence Collection

Testimonial evidence collection is emphasized in clinical and family assistance disaster response domains and includes assessment of psychosocial history, predisposition toward violence, abuse, self-mutilation including suicide attempts, or trauma recidivism. Nonphysical evidence collection involves separating the injuries from the story. A comprehensive history from a patient or informant includes medical background, development, family, household, support systems, and physical appearance, as function and circumstances of presentation are observed and objectively documented. Any experience before a disaster should be carefully paid attention to as it may disclose the precursor to a tragic episode, the location of other survivors, or insight into the series of events. Victims of the World Trade Center attack divulged stories of building lobby fireballs and flaming elevator back drafts. Forensic nurses should be prepared to document these utterances and share them quickly with other members of the multidisciplinary response team.

Documentation

Record keeping occurs in all three of the disaster response domains and poses a challenge to the forensic nurse functioning in a fast-paced, high-stress, and demanding environment. Goll McGee wrote, "Meticulous documentation provides evidence that something is done or not done, exists or does not exist" (Goll-McGee, 1999, p. 5). Scrupulous documentation provides evidence for a victim and testimony for the court. Proper documentation technique that will stand up to scrutiny and will supply education around disaster response is best achieved with timely and efficient methods such as photography, diagrams, and recordings.

Crisis Intervention

This may be the most challenging experience for nurses to endure and practice because it relates to issues that require a personal, professional, and frequently an emotional commitment (Goll-McGee, 1999). Goll-McGee's account to the response at the World Trade Center illustrates the impact of this commitment:

> *We scrambled for extra supplies we might need, but were otherwise unprepared. All of us needed hardhats, facemasks, and goggles. Some got work boots, gloves, and rain gear from the donation area.*

A few of us procured additional nebulizer masks and ophthalmic supplies from a now vacant, make-shift, trauma-receiving area for the hundreds of injured who were expected to be found, but never came. We were off. The eight block trip took almost two hours as security was tight at several checkpoints along the way. The threat of serious weather eliminated most of the surrounding lights. An ominous cloud of smoking debris which continued to emanate from the grave of the World Trade Center collided with giant gray thunder clouds.

Suddenly I didn't want to see any more. I wished this horrible event had never happened, especially as a police officer began to recount his experience of the disaster. He thought he had died because the sky went black in the middle of the day and he couldn't hear or see anything. So many of his friends were gone–from his home, a city that itself was grieving. It actually hurt him to look at the place where the towering landmarks once stood.

I thought about all the hurt and psychological terror that these people had endured and with which, were still being assaulted [Fig. 8-5]. Perhaps the hardest part was touching and caring for the direct victims of the disaster and knowing their families and their prognosis. The acute nature of burn trauma in patients with large body surface area burns accompanied by an inhalation injury component carries with it a high incidence of mortality or a long, tough, disfiguring road to recovery. For the first time I began hearing personal stories of the victims from nurses' reports or by descriptions of family members. Burns from fireballs passing through the tower lobbies, back drafts from elevator shafts and jet fuel showers, and desperate attempts to survive were no longer just stories. The victims of such horrors were living patients under our care.

Every morning or evening as we left our work environment we could see the hundreds of missing faces taped to the nurse's station, the elevators, the exit and entrances, and on the streets. The walk to where we lived just across the street seemed like a long passageway of grief and disbelief. How terribly sad to be able to see the flickering of candles at a candlelight vigil from the computer where I documented my patients' vital signs. Two nights in a row we came to work and two nights in a row we coded and lost a person. For the first time I was feeling actual rage and anger towards the terrorist responsible for the attack. It became personal.

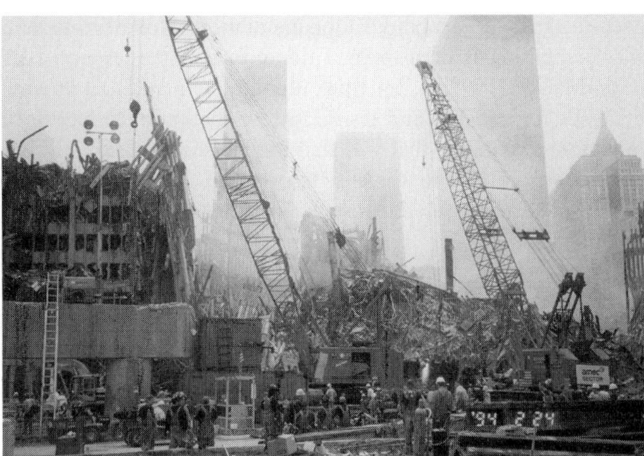

Fig. 8-5 The aftermath of the disaster on September 11, 2001, evoked devastating psychological responses for citizens worldwide. Smoldering ruins complicated recovery processes for several months after the event and were a constant reminder of the horrors associated with the World Trade Center bombing.

Best Practice *8-2*

The forensic nurse must use caution in treating patients as victims when indeed they may be perpetrators, in interviewing informants as they may be infiltrating media, or processing remains when they may be contaminated. The nurse must be acutely aware of surroundings, attitudes, and emotions while maintaining an index of suspicion.

Scene Security

Scene security issues are satisfied with daily changing identification badges for whatever disaster response domain one is working. Media responses are given only by a designated individual, and the forensic nurse is not to disclose any information without proper authority. Confidentiality in disaster response is crucial to protect the dignity of the responders, the hope of the families, and the safety of the victims. Crisis intervention also may involve use of the forensic nurse in death notification or as a resource for the family viewing deceased disaster victims. Forensic nurse examiners intervening in such crises will require critical incident stress management skills and are sometimes assigned to this duty exclusively.

Disaster-Related Conditions

The forensic nurse responding to disasters will see, think, and do things differently beyond ordinary assessment and treatment of traumatic, medical, and psychologic disaster-related conditions. It is important for the forensic nurse to recognize this and teach other healthcare professionals in disaster response the methods and dimension of thought that support medicolegal management of the disaster population. A disaster is not always outside the scope of a responding Level I Trauma Center, for example. Clinical forensic nursing practice on a daily basis can only enhance the efficiency and likelihood of the response in matters of larger-scale disasters. Some of the following conditions may be encountered in a clinical environment, and becoming familiar with these conditions can enhance the forensic nurse's response by increasing her or his ability to recognize, intervene, and document their clinical presence.

Pressure Wave Injuries

When an explosion occurs, the exploding material is converted into a large volume of gas with release of a tremendous amount of energy (Marshall, 1977). A person in the vicinity can experience an isolated blast injury, dismemberment, or complete annihilation and dissemination. The person can also be injured by pressure or shock waves, which spread concentrically from the blast center (Marshal, 1977). The organs most likely to be affected are the tympanic membranes of the ears, lungs, bowel, cardiovascular, and central nervous system. The resulting blast injury may help to ascertain proximity to the explosive device. In the outer injury zone, there is ordinarily no immediate mortality from primary injuries, and secondary or tertiary blast injuries accompanying them (Mellor, 1992).

The secondary blast injury may also contain evidentiary material such as fragments of burned safety fuse, torn and twisted pieces of clock mechanism, batteries parts, bits of wire, parts of switches, electrical tape, and container pieces (Marshall, 1977). At the scene, wounds may be wrapped or left unwrapped. If the wound is dressed, the forensic nurse will examine the bandage and the wound for particulate evidence, which may be removed and then irrigate the wound. A basin can be placed under the blast injury during irrigation. The irrigant may be saved and later strained further for collection of any debris that may be useful in determining the type of incendiary device used. When in doubt as to whether something is evidence, it should be collected. Obvious rules for evidence collection and handling apply, and under no circumstances should the condition of the patient be compromised in order to collect evidence. Of particular importance is what the patient may have heard or seen before an explosion. This is carefully documented and shared with investigative personnel. The perpetrator may have been injured when handling the device.

Burns

Burn injuries often accompany miscellaneous blast injuries and may be of varying depths. The most common type of burn during an explosion includes the flash burn, an often superficial burn that may be patterned to illustrate position during the explosion. A photograph of this type of burn injury and other patterned burns is the best documentation of any injury that may later reveal proximity and location of a patient involved in a blast. Burns may be present in varying degrees. The location of a burned patient may be more important in explosions of smaller scale such as a pipe or letter bomb in a closed environment. The presence of an accelerant may also give insight into the origin of a burn. Also, chemicals and radiation passing through tissue may cause burns.

Blunt Force Injury

This type of injury is sustained by absorbing energy and is divided into four categories: abrasions, contusions, lacerations, and fractures (DiMaio & DiMaio, 1993). Tertiary blast injury is blunt force trauma due to the victim being thrown against an object (DiMaio & DiMaio, 1993). The forensic nurse examining blunt force injury will use techniques of forensic wound identification described in Chapters 19 and 20 and will photograph and collect evidence from the wound site. Documentations about injuries during a disaster are of particular importance for later data comparison to similar events. For instance, during the 1992 Hurricane Andrew in Florida, blunt trauma was the foremost cause of accidental death in that 8 of the 15 reported deaths were a direct result of the hurricane's physical forces on land and water (Lew & Witli, 1996). Blunt forces from flying debris and crush injuries also are commonly seen together in tornadoes, earthquakes where buildings collapse, and other natural and human-caused disaster scenarios. Documentation of injuries during a disaster gives healthcare responders an idea of what they might potentially face during future emergencies of a similar type. Records may also be used to provide testimony in a court of law when victims subsequently seek justice and restitution.

Radiation

The management of radioactive contaminants includes early recognition of the problem, avoidance of a secondary spread of contamination within a hospital, and skin decontamination by washing or showering (Voeltz, 1999). Under no circumstances is loose radioactive material collected for evidentiary value. Because of the delayed effect of radiation exposure, a forensic nurse may be suspicious of populations that present with cataracts, acute radiation syndrome, chromosomal aberrations, genetic mutations, or cancer (Voeltz, 1999). Disaster-related medical conditions may involve toxic inhalation, poisoning, or bacterial or viral infection. The pulmonary route of entry generally involves a volatile substance, gas, dust, smoke, or aerosol (Winek, 1977). At the World Trade Center, a firefighter developed situational asthma as a result of inhaling soot, gypsum dust, and asbestos.

Inhalation Injuries

Poisoning and bacterial or viral infections are generally inhaled, aspirated, or ingested. Anthrax can be contracted through cutaneous exposure. Inhalational anthrax starts with flulike symptoms of fever, sweats/chills, severe fatigue, cough, nausea/vomiting, shortness of breath, and abdominal pain and is the more fatal form of the disease (Pittman, 2001). Smallpox symptoms begin with fever, headache, backache, and sore muscles, followed quickly by a maculopapular rash that first appears on the face (Pittman, 2001). Evidence collection may include sputum samples and bronchial washings, or specimens of blood, urine, and stomach contents (Smialek & Schwartz, 1999).

Forensic nurses should be alert to potential therapeutic misadventures that sometimes occur as a result of excessive concentrations of antidote (Winek, 1977). They must also be aware of the requirements for reporting specific infections or toxic inhalations to the Centers for Disease Control. The presence of bacterial and viral infections should remind caregivers to avoid contagion and contamination and engage in scrupulous and frequent hand washing and wear personal protective clothing, masks, and gloves as prescribed in Standard Precautions (see Chapter 54). Again, complete and precise documentation of the circumstances is vital to the management and follow-up of this disaster population.

Psychological Effects

Disaster-related psychological effects are profound, not only to the physical victims of a disaster but to those secondary victims who experience the loss of a loved one or possessions. They too may perceive a real sense of violation and concerns for their personal safety. Critical incident stress management (CISM) offers services ranging from precrisis preparedness to acute care services to post-intervention procedures. These services address the psychological aftermath of critical incidents and prevent or mitigate the potential onset of post-traumatic stress disorder (PTSD) (Everly & Mitchell, 1993).

Skilled forensic nurses should be aware of the acute and delayed sequelae experienced by survivors. If they are not trained to provide CISM, they should know how to elicit the resources required to provide CISM debriefing sessions within the first 24 to 72 hours following a critical incident (Martin, 1993). A majority of victims experience acute stress disorder with disruptions in reasonable mastery, caring attachments, and meaningful purpose in life, the three domains associated with good physical and mental health (Flannery, 2000). The forensic nurse trained in CISM should recognize the three stages: ambiguity, depression, and PTSD (Flannery, 2000). Finally, nurses who work with disaster scenarios must understand their own role conflict during a disaster situation and appreciate the emotional reactions that they may experience in the aftermath in order to recover a sense of control in life (Stanley, 1990).

Summary

Human-caused and natural disasters present unique and sometimes insurmountable challenges to forensic nurses preparing to meet their demands. There is nothing in the forensic nursing standards and scope of practice that could encompass an adequate response to these types of societal catastrophic events. By exploring the existing resources, the forensic aspects of disaster response, and disaster-related conditions, preparation has begun for a role in disaster responses at clinical, family assistance, and forensic processing levels.

A goal of the forensic nurse who participates in disaster responses should be to return to routine living and working conditions in a healthy physical and emotional state, postdisaster. To ensure this outcome, forensic nurses must possess a sound clinical and experience acumen for their roles, and they must amass the skills, techniques, and human resources that will ensure their emotional well-being during and after disaster response participation.

Resources

Government Reports

Chemical and Biological Terrorism: Research and Development to Improve Civilian Medical Response. (1999). Washington, DC: National Academy Press.

Health Aspects of Biological and Chemical Weapons, Second Edition, World Health Organization.

Organizations

Association for Professionals in Infection Control and Epidemiology (APIC)

1275 K Street NW, Suite 1000, Washington, DC 20005-4006, Tel: 202-789-1890; www.apic.org

APIC Scientific and Policy/Procedure Resources include:
Anthrax as a Biological Weapon
Biological and Chemical Terrorism: Strategic Plan
Bioterrorism Agent Sheets
Bioterrorism Agent Wall Chart
Bioterrorism Readiness Plan
Botulinum Toxin as a Biological Weapon
Epidemiology of Bioterrorism
Mass Casualty Disaster Plan Checklist
Medical Management of Biological Casualties Handbook
NATO Handbook on the Medical Aspects of NBC Defensive Operations
Plague as a Biological Weapon
Potential Biological Weapons Threats
Smallpox as a Biological Weapon

American Hospital Association

One North Franklin Avenue, Chicago, IL 60606-3421; Tel: 312-422-3000; www.aha.org

Hospital Resources for Disaster Readiness (report)
Hospital Preparedness for Mass Casualties (report)
A Review of Federal Bioterrorism Preparedness Programs from a Public Health Perspective (testimony)
The Silent War: Are Federal, State, and Local Governments Prepared for Biological and Chemical Attacks? (testimony)

Web Sites

American College of Emergency Physicians

www.acep.org

American Medical Association

www.ama-assn.org

American Nurses Association

www.ana.org

Emergency Nurses Association

www.ena.org

Joint Commission on Accreditation of Healthcare Organizations

www.jcaho.org

References

American Red Cross. (1997). *Plan for implementation of the Federal Family Assistance Act for Aviation Disasters.* Washington, DC: Author.

Briggs, S., & Leong, M. (1990). Classic concepts in disaster medical response. In J. Leaning (Ed.), *Humanitarian crises: The medical and public health response.* Boston, MA: Harvard Publishing.

Center for National Security Studies. (1995). Recent trends in domestic and international terrorism. Washington, DC: US Government Printing Office.

Chemical Casualty Care Office, US Army Medical Research Institute of Chemical Defense. (1995). *Medical management of chemical casualties handbook* (2nd ed.). Washington, DC: US Government Printing Office.

DiMaio, D., & DiMaio, V. (1996). *Forensic pathology.* Boca Raton, FL: CRC Press.

Emergency Management Institute, National Emergency Training Center. (1996). *Mass fatalities incident response course manual SM-386.* Washington, DC: US Government Printing Office.

Everly, G. S., & Mitchell, J. T. (1999). Critical incident stress management (CISM): A review of the literature. *Aggress Violent Behav,* (5) 23–40

Federal Emergency Management Agency (FEMA). (1999). Federal Emergency Management Agency (FEMA). Washington, DC: US Government Printing Office.

Flannery, R. B.(1999). Treating family survivors of mass casualties: A CISM crisis intervention approach. *Int J Emerg Ment Health, 1*(4): 243–250

Franz, D. (1999). Biologic and chemical terrorism. In R. Bowler & J. Cone (Eds.), *Occupational medicine secrets.* Philadelphia: Hanley & Belfus.

Goll-McGee, B. (1999). The role of the clinical forensic nurse in critical care. *Crit Care Nurs Q, 22*(1), 8–18.

Hoyt, C., & Spangler, K. (1996). Forensic nursing implications and the forensic autopsy. *J Psychosoc Nurs Ment Health Serv, 34*(10), 24–31.

Illing, P. (2000). Toxicology and disasters. In B. Ballantyne, T. Marrs, & T. Syversen (Eds.), *General and applied toxicology* (2nd ed.). London: Macmillan Reference.

International Association of Forensic Nurses (IAFN), American Nurses Association. (1997). *Scope and standards of forensic nursing practice.* Washington, DC: American Nurses Publishing.

Irwin, R. (1989). The Incident Command System (ICS). In E. Auf der Heide (Ed.), *Disaster response: Principles of preparation and coordination.* St. Louis, MO: CV Mosby.

Knight, B. (1997). *Simpson's forensic medicine* (11th ed.). New York: Oxford University Press.

Komnenich, P., & Feller, C. (1991). Disaster nursing. In J. Fitzpatrick, R. Taunton, & A. Jacox (Eds.), *Annual review of nursing research 9.* New York: Springer.

Lew, E., & Wetli, C. (1996). Mortality from hurricane Andrew. *J Forensic Sci, 41*(3), 449–452.

MacLean, D., Kogon, S., & Stitt, L. (1994).Validation of dental radiographs for human identification. *J Forensic Sci, 39*(5), 1195–1200.

Marshall, T. (1997). Explosion injuries. In C. Tedeschi, W. Eckert, & L. Tedeschi (Eds.), *Forensic medicine: A study in trauma and environmental hazards.* Philadelphia: W. B. Saunders.

Martin, K. (1993, May). Critical incidents: Pulling together to cope with the stress. *Nursing,* 39–43.

Martin-de las Heras, S., Valenzuela, A., Villanueva, E., et al. (1999). Methods for identification of 28 burn victims following a 1996 bus accident in Spain. *J Forensic Sci, 44*(2), 428–431.

Mellor, S. (1992). The relationship of blast loading to death and injury from explosion. *World Surg, 16,* 893–898.

Moler, E., Ballarin, V., Pessana, F., et al. (1998). Fingerprint identification using image enhancement techniques. *J Forensic Sci, 43*(3), 689–692.

National Disaster Medical System. (1999). *D-MORT teams: Disaster mortuary teams.* Washington, DC: US Government Printing Office.

Payne, J., & Baumgartner, R. (1996). CNS role evolution. *Clin Nurse Spec, 10*(1), 46–48.

Pittman, T. (2001, December 6). PFLC educates public about chemical and biological warfare: Anthrax and other potential bioterrorist threats. *Caring Headlines, 7.*

Schultz, C., Koenig, K., & Noji, E. (1996). A medical response to reduce immediate mortality after an earthquake. *N Engl J Med, 334*(7), 438–445.

Simon, J. (2000). The emerging threat of chemical and biological terrorism. In B. Ballantyne, T. Marrs, & T. Syversen (Eds.), *General and applied toxicology* (2nd ed.). London: Macmillan Reference.

Smialek, J., & Schwartz, G. (1999). Forensic emergency medicine. In G. Schwartz (Ed.), *Principles and practice of emergency medicine* (4th ed.). Philadelphia: Williams & Wilkins.

Stanley, S. (1990). When the disaster is over: Helping the healers to mend. *J Psychosoc Nurs Ment Health Serv, 28*(5), 12–16.

Sweet, D., Hildebrand, D., & Phillips, D. (1999). Identification of a skeleton using DNA from teeth and a PAP smear. *J Forensic Sci, 44*(3), 630–633.

Torok, T., Tauxe, R., Wise, R., et al. (1997). A large community outbreak of Salmonellosis caused by intentional contamination of restaurant salad bars. *JAMA, 278*(5), 389–395.

Twomey, J., & Goll-McGee, B. (1999). Answering the call when disaster strikes. *Nurs Spectr, 3*(13), 5.

US Congress, Office of Technology Assessment. (1993). *Proliferation of weapons of mass destruction: Assessing the risks* (OTA-ISC-559). Washington, DC: US Government Printing Office.

Voeltz, M. (1999). Radiation. In G. Schwartz (Ed.), *Principles and practice of emergency medicine* (4th ed.). Philadelphia: Williams & Wilkins.

Warren, S. (1977). Effects of occupational and environmental exposure to ionizing radiation. In C. Tedeschi, W. Eckert, & L. Tedeschi (Eds.), *Forensic medicine: A study in trauma and environmental hazards.* Philadelphia: W. B. Saunders.

Winek, C. (1977). Injury by chemical agents. In C. Tedeschi, W. Eckert, & L. Tedeschi (Eds.), *Forensic medicine: A study in trauma and environmental hazards.* Philadelphia: W. B. Saunders.

Wright, R., Peters, C., & Flannery, R. (1999). Victim identification and family support in mass casualties: The Massachusetts model. *Int J Emerg Ment Health, 1*(4), 237–242.

Chapter 9 Nurse-Related Homicides

Beatrice Crofts Yorker

Five previously published epidemiologic studies have linked nurses to clusters of mysterious cardiopulmonary arrests. This chapter presents three case studies to illustrate the connection between factitious disorder and these caregiver-associated epidemics. A review of the literature on factitious disorder by proxy (often called Munchausen syndrome by proxy) and factitious disorders in occupational settings provides a background for these three cases in which nurses who exhibited signs of a factitious disorder were ultimately convicted of murder. It seems factitious disorder by proxy is not isolated to familial victims but also occurs between healthcare providers and dependents in their care.

On May 17, 1993, a jury convicted a British pediatric nurse of four murders, three attempted murders, and six assaults of patients in her care. This is not the first such case. Since 1975, there have been at least 14 other criminal trials of healthcare providers associated with epidemics of adverse patient outcomes. Each case has seriously shaken the community in which it occurred, and the medical setting has been scrutinized for its role in detecting and handling the situation.

Five previous articles, three in the *New England Journal of Medicine* (Buehler, Smith, & Wallace et al., 1985; Isrtre, Gustafson, & Baron et al., 1985; Stross, Shasby, & Harlan, 1976), one in the *Journal of the American Medical Association* (Sacks, Stroup, & Will et al., 1988), and one in the *American Journal of Public Health* (Sacks, Herndon, & Leib et al., 1988), have been devoted to the epidemiologic studies performed following epidemics of mysterious cardiopulmonary arrests. The Centers for Disease Control contributed to these studies in hospitals in Michigan (Stross, Shasby, & Harlan, 1976), Texas (Isrtre, Gustafson, & Baron et al., 1985), Toronto (Isrtre, Gustafson, & Baron., 1985), Maryland (Sacks, Stroup, & Will et al., 1988), and Florida (Sacks, Herndon, & Leib et al., 1988). The studies concluded that the presence of a specific healthcare provider was associated with increased numbers of deaths and cardiopulmonary arrests. Additionally, toxicology studies performed following resuscitative efforts revealed the presence of lethal levels of medication commonly found on hospital units.

There are several recommended preventive measures, including heightened surveillance of time, place, and person; control of the suspect agent; and prompt toxicologic studies. These recommendations were found effective in a subsequent investigation of increased patient deaths in a 1985 Georgia case (*Rachals v. State*, 1988). However, other cases have not been handled as effectively. Factors that contribute to prolonged epidemics with no criminal convictions include the difficulty in establishing clusters of adverse outcomes in a timely fashion, the prevalence of temporary agency staff, the lack of sophisticated forensic toxicology input, a general reluctance on the part of healthcare professionals to suspect a provider as the cause of an epidemic, and the need to obtain evidence before making accusations (Forrest, 1992).

Rothman (1985) wrote an editorial titled "Sleuthing in Hospitals" after two of the epidemiologic studies that were published in the *New England Journal of Medicine* associated the presence of a particular healthcare provider with mysterious clusters of cardiopulmonary arrests. He challenged the authors of the studies and the readership of the *Journal* to go beyond the published exercises in applied epidemiology and to provide "some more searching causal conjectures; for instance, what are the relevant aspects of the psyches and backgrounds of Nurse A and Nurse 32?" (Rothman, 1985). Summarizing three cases will illustrate a theoretical linkage to factitious disorders, specifically Munchausen syndrome by proxy.

Factitious Disorders or Munchausen Syndrome

Munchausen Syndrome

The *DSM-IV* lists 300.19 Factitious Disorder with Predominantly Physical Signs and Symptoms as a disorder characterized by the intentional production of physical symptoms (American Psychiatric Association [APA], 1994). The best studied form of factitious disorder with physical symptoms is known as Munchausen syndrome named after the legendary Baron von Munchausen who traveled widely and told fanciful tales. In 1951, Asher (1951) described individuals who presented at hospitals with self-inflicted or fabricated illnesses. These patients typically engage in uncontrollable and pathologic lying about their history or symptoms. The types of illnesses induced include hypoglycemia, hemoptysis, rashes, abscesses, fevers, hematuria, seizures–even AIDS and cystic fibrosis (Orenstein & Wasserman, 1986) have been cleverly mimicked. The *DSM-IV* concludes: "All organ systems are potential targets, and the symptoms presented are limited only by the person's medical knowledge, sophistication, and imagination" (APA, 1994).

There has been no evidence of psychosis or decreased mental competence in persons diagnosed with Munchausen syndrome. Although Goodwin discusses the relationship between dissociative disorders and Munchausen syndrome (Goodwin, 1988), the area of possible overlap remains unclear. Factitious disorders are conceptualized in the literature as predominantly consciously motivated, carefully and intelligently crafted, and quite believable until diagnostic technology shows inconsistencies that could not occur unless deliberate interference took place. The *DSM-IV* considers true physical disorders with extensive hospitalizations during childhood, employment in a medicine-related field, and a significant, if not traumatic, prior relationship with a physician as predisposing factors (APA, 1994).

Factitious Disorder in the Occupational Setting

Although the concept of factitious disorders within an occupational context is a relatively new one, emerging literature discusses suspicious critical incidents that occur in the line of duty as manifestations of factitious disorder. DiVasto and Saxton (1992) published an article in the *FBI Law Enforcement Bulletin* on Munchausen's syndrome in law enforcement. Police officers sometimes appear to be creating emergencies that include self-inflicted gunshot wounds, bruises, or lacerations and then claim the injury occurred as a result of a dramatic incident with alleged perpetrators.

The authors described the two dynamics involved:

1. Officers who are experiencing a significant amount of interpersonal stress, or threat of loss, and are unable to cope. Creating an incident allows the officer to receive support and sympathy without giving up control. The officer is at once a victim and a hero.
2. Affiliation. In order to be accepted as a peer in the informal hierarchy among police organizations, officers must experience certain highly intense and life-threatening situations. There is a tremendous pressure to achieve parity in a law enforcement environment. The authors conclude: "An officer who feels the need to fabricate a critical incident may be manifesting perceived ego deficits or may simply be reacting to that pressure, often combined with boredom" (DiVasto & Saxton, 1992).

Although this particular description is limited to law enforcement, there are similar examples of people creating emergencies in their line of work for attention or other psychological reasons. There have been firefighters who have been associated with actually starting fires. For example, two volunteer firefighters were arrested in connection with the Malibu, California, fires. The primary motives appear to be excitement of the event and appearing competent in a crisis (Murphy, 1991).

Key Point *9-1*

Nurses are usually the first hospital staff members to identify cases of unexpected and adverse patient events that may be precipitated by the hands of a caregiver. They are also typically the first to request an investigation of suspicious events.

Factitious Disorder by Proxy

The term *factitious disorder by proxy* is defined by the *DSM-IV* as the intentional production or feigning of symptoms in another person who is under the individual's care. Munchausen syndrome by proxy (MSBP), a highly documented variant of factitious disorder in which a parent fabricates or induces illness in a dependent, was first coined by Money and Werlwas (1992) and Meadow (1977) in the latter 1970s. In a study of 117 cases of MSBP, Rosenberg found that 98% of the perpetrators were biological mothers and the most common methods of assault included suffocation, poisonings with ipecac or laxatives, and induced seizures (Rosenberg, 1987). Schrier distinguished the mothers who actively induce symptoms (compared to those who simply fabricate symptoms) as having the following key clinical features (Shrier, 1992):

- Pathological lying
- Causing repeated serious harm to the infant
- Manifesting a compulsive need to repeat the behavior
- Taking unnecessary risks
- Displaying a kind of gleeful excitement just at the moment when the infant's life hangs in the balance

Professional Factitious Disorder by Proxy

In September 1992, a California foster mother who had received national acclaim for her care of medically fragile foster children was charged with child abuse and alleged Munchausen syndrome by proxy. Physicians in the local hospital began an investigation after they discovered one of the children's intravenous tubes was cut and punctured with traces of fecal bacteria on the plastic. Another child who died in her care was found to have excessive amounts of sodium and potassium in his body. The mother denied any wrongdoing, although the medical condition of the remaining children improved significantly after removal from her care (Gunnison, 1996).

Meadow (1977) listed having a previous history of feigning or inducing one's own illness as a risk factor in individuals who later develop MSBP. Of the unusual clusters of adverse patient outcomes associated with the presence of a nurse, at least five of the nurses convicted of murder have a history that suggests they showed signs of having a factitious disorder (Yorker, 1994). Although the term Munchausen syndrome by proxy has traditionally been reserved for family caretakers, there is now sufficient anecdotal evidence to suggest using a child or a helpless dependent as a "proxy" for fabricated or induced illness is not isolated to familial caregivers and can occur in professional settings.

Legal Case Studies

A dissertation that studied a total of 37 caregiver-associated serial killings (CASK) supports the presence of a history of factitious disorders or Munchausen syndrome in several of the perpetrators (Forrest, 1992). These perpetrators' situations also resemble the dynamics found in law enforcement Munchausen syndrome (e.g., the need to appear competent or gain attention). The following three cases of nurses convicted of murder illustrate the most salient features related to factitious disorder.

Case Study **9-1 England, 1991-1993**

During a 60-day period of employment for a newly qualified nurse, the 15-bed pediatric ward of a small acute-care hospital experienced an unprecedented 24 adverse patient incidents including cardiac arrests, respiratory failures, and heart attacks. In the past, the average was two per year. Four children died, another three suffered permanent brain damage, and six others survived following sometimes multiple resuscitative efforts. It was doctors in the pediatric intensive care unit at the hospital where five of the children had been transferred who finally insisted on an investigation.

Police installed video surveillance and began examining ward records. At the same time, toxicologic studies on some of the children who suffered mysterious attacks began to be analyzed with heightened scrutiny. They were considering the possibility of a virus that attacked heart muscles or Legionnaire's disease. Then a vial of blood on a child who had died registered 500 milliunits of insulin per liter of blood. This information suggested that a person might be at the source of the adverse incidents. Officers began interviewing all of the staff on the unit to ask about visiting nurses from temporary agencies and other persons seen on the ward. They made a graph of staff assignments with critical incidents. The occurrences clustered on the evening/night shift, and the only person present during all 26 incidents was a 22-year-old newly graduated nurse who had been turned down for a job in a children's hospital because she needed more experience with very sick children.

The nurse was taken into custody for questioning, and her home was searched. Officers found the ward allocation book and a syringe. The nurse was relieved from work but released on bail. A second blood analysis came back with 43,167 milliunits of insulin per liter of blood. However, it still took several more months to accumulate enough evidence to charge the nurse with murder. X-rays examined later showed one child had presence of an air embolus in the axilla and another child had fractured ribs. Potassium levels in other blood samples were high (Davies, 1993).

In the month that followed, the press and law enforcement personnel compiled a history of the nurse's life. She was born the second of four children to a father who worked in a tractor factory and a mother who had industrial sewing and cleaning jobs and who worked in a school cafeteria in a small village. Friends remembered little exceptional about the family, but when the nurse was 13 or 14 she began having problems with her health. She had a reputation for being very helpful, an excellent babysitter, and seemed to have little trouble other than incredible accident-proneness. Her friends secretly wondered if she might be exaggerating her need for bandages and reports of headaches and backaches.

Evidence of problems was clear from examining her nursing school records. As a student nurse, she had made 24 visits to the emergency unit for complaints such as urinary retention, multiple injuries to her wrists and hands, a false pregnancy, headaches, and other complaints. She reported sick for a total of 160 days of her training, 94 days during 1990 alone, and had missed so much school that she had to make up clinical experiences on the ward that ultimately hired her as a new graduate. At one point a physiotherapist told police that it was obvious the woman's injuries and her explanations of how they occurred were inonsistent. They were self-inflicted.

Once the nurse was arrested, her medical problems flared up again. She precipitously lost half her body weight and was reported to be suffering from anorexia nervosa. News reports revealed her forceful vomiting was from ingestion of feces. She was also in the infirmary for breast tenderness that nurses concluded was from injecting herself with water. She developed fevers during the night, and as the verdicts were read at the conclusion of her trial, she was so ill that she could not attend court. Fed through a nasogastric tube, she sent a written consent for her lawyers to represent her in her absence (Davies, 1993).

At the conclusion of the trial, Dr. Roy Meadow, the famous British physician who is considered the leading expert on Munchausen syndrome by proxy, testified how this nurse showed the key features. His testimony was kept from the jury members until after their deliberations so that it would not influence them either to lessen any findings of guilt due to psychiatric incompetence or to enhance her guilt in their eyes based on presence of a syndrome.

Parents of the children who suffered cardiac or respiratory arrests were initially grateful to the nurse for "saving" their children. One couple made her the godmother of their surviving twin daughter because she had so completely won their admiration. Ultimately, the nurse was convicted of four murders, three attempted murders, and infliction of grievous bodily harm to six other children.

Case Study 9-2 New York, 1987-1989

Administrators of a hospital in Long Island, New York, became suspicious when 25 patients died following breathing failures in a six-week period. Nurses on the nightshift noticed that their competent charge nurse was always on duty when codes happened, and that he was invariably the first to initiate resuscitations. They were reluctant to think the charge nurse could be in some way contributing to the patient arrests, as he was well respected for his clinical acumen and professionalism. After one successful resuscitation, the frightened patient told another nurse that the charge nurse had come into his room during the early morning hours and said he was going to give the patient something to make him feel better. The accused nurse injected the intravenous tubing with something from a syringe, which immediately caused frightening changes in the patient's body and made him unable to breathe. The nurse who heard this confronted her colleague, who indignantly denied the accusations. The nurse who had listened to the allegations remained unconvinced, however, and told her supervisors the next day. The administrators asked that she keep her suspicions private until they could investigate further. They felt that they would need concrete evidence to take action against the accused nurse because of his good reputation and impeccable credentials (Linedecker & Burt, 1991).

The investigators analyzed blood and urine samples of the verbal patient who survived. Both specimens and the intravenous tubing were found to have traces of Pavulon (a nondepolarizing neuromuscular-blocking agent) in them. The accused nurse was suspended while an exhaustive investigation was launched, which included exhuming patients, reviewing charts of 37 patients who died or experienced life-threatening events while in the nurse's care, and searching the nurse's locker and home. Vials of Pavulon, Anectine, and potassium chloride were found in his possession. Once arrested, the nurse provided a lengthy confession. He elaborated on the vials of Pavulon at his home, saying he had conducted experiments using it on field mice. He had been a highly respected volunteer fireman, and he told police detectives that he was like the people who set fires so they can rush in and be a hero or perform a noble service. He said he felt inadequate and that he had to prove himself to the staff (Holzberg, 1989).

Former neighbors of the nurse said he was a quiet, gentle boy who must have been crying out for attention. His parents were schoolteachers and his family was described as nice and middle class. He had been an altar boy in his Catholic church and an Eagle Scout. Although the defense tried to convince the jury that the nurse had a mental illness and could not be legally responsible for his actions, the prosecution pointed out the calculated, deliberate way in which he induced breathing failures in helpless patients. He was convicted of the second-degree murder of two patients, second-degree manslaughter of another patient, and criminally negligent homicide of a fourth patient. First-degree convictions require intent to commit murder; thus, the defense argument that the nurse had not intended to kill his patients carried weight with the jury (Linedecker & Burt, 1991). Additionally, he was found guilty of assault for injecting the patient who survived to testify against him.

Case Study 9-3 Florida, 1984-1988

A Florida medical examiner requested an epidemiologic and criminal investigation following 12 patient deaths in a two-week period. The expected number of deaths was 2.5 for the whole month. A review of employee schedules revealed a consistent and strong association between the duty times of two nurses and the onsets of the terminal episode and the times of the patient deaths (Sacks, Stroup, & Will et al., 1988). The criminal investigation intensified following a suspicious incident in which one of the nurses identified by the epidemiologic investigation was found lying on the floor of a patient's room with a bleeding wound to the stomach. She was also linked to an arson incident at the nursing home. The nurse said she had been attacked by a prowler. A background check revealed that this nurse had been fired from a previous job in another state for stabbing herself in the vaginal area with a pair of scissors. In fact, her license was suspended in that state because of her self-inflicted injuries and mental instability (Linedecker & Burt, 1991).

After her arrest, the nurse's ex-husband talked to the press about other troubling incidents. After their then seven-year-old son was repeatedly admitted to the hospital, drug studies showed he was being overdosed by medication prescribed for his mother. She was charged with repeatedly poisoning her son; the court threatened foster placement and then gave the father custody. Since 1970, her medical records showed multiple hospitalizations for a broken arm, gallbladder surgery, ulcers, a hysterectomy, a colostomy, and five surgeries to remove tumors or treat other stomach problems. The nurse was hospitalized during the investigation and psychiatrists determined she indeed had Munchausen syndrome. Ultimately, the nurse and her attorneys worked out a plea bargain, reducing the first-degree murder charges to second-degree murder and keeping the attempted murder charge. She was sentenced to 65 years imprisonment.

Analysis of Cases

Each of these three cases shares features with the factitious disorders. The two female nurses have documented histories of their own Munchausen syndrome. The male nurse likened himself to volunteer firefighters who set fires themselves. These nurses fit the professional Munchausen syndrome described in law enforcement (DiVasto & Saxton, 1992); however, the nurses injured others, making it "by proxy."

Rosenberg's exhaustive review of the Munchausen syndrome by proxy literature describes characteristics of perpetrators in more than a hundred cases. She noted "an overwhelming number of mothers were described as having an affable and friendly demeanor and being socially adept" (Rosenberg, 1987). Twenty-four of the perpetrators had features of their own Munchausen syndrome; however, many histories were not available. Although 40% of the maternal perpetrators' occupations were unknown, a striking 27% had nursing training, 3% were medical office workers, 2% were social workers, and one was an orderly. The perpetrators' admissions or denials were unknown in 60% of the cases, with 15% completely admitting their participation in the deception, 7% partially admitting, and 18% completely denying their actions (Rosenberg, 1987). Rosenberg's study suggests, unfortunately, that people who use the healthcare system with factitious disorders or for attention-seeking purposes have an affinity for the nursing and healthcare professions. It should not be surprising, then, that the factitious disorder by proxy dynamics are not restricted to familial victims but can also occur in professional caretaker-dependent relationships (Box 9-1).

Cautionary Notes and Backlash

This extremely limited information is not intended for drawing general conclusions about caregiver-associated serial killings. It simply provides a partial answer to Rothman's question about the backgrounds of nurses associated with epidemics of adverse patient outcomes. The link to factitious disorders can be made in these three cases, but others are less clear.

Box 9-1 Reducing Risk of Caregiver-Associated Epidemics

Ensure that employment and hiring practices comply with the Americans with Disabilities Act and other civil rights:

- Verify credentials and qualifications from originating source.
- Routinely obtain some demographic information that can be verified purely for the purpose of assessing truthfulness (e.g., educational background, siblings, occupation, location of parents).
- Call and verify employment for three prior positions.

In addition, take routine preventative steps:

- Conduct routine toxicology screens immediately following cardiac arrest for all patients, regardless of the presumed cause or manner of the event.
- Obtain monthly code and death statistics by unit, shift, and total hospital. Compare units to each other and to themselves; monitor any trend changes.
- Use strict pharmacy/unit-level accounting for all doses of medication.

Key Point *9-2*

Compulsive fabrication of incidents for secondary gain, regardless of social or personal danger, is consistent with the dynamics of factitious disorder.

Effects on the Nursing Profession

One of the key aspects in each of the 14 cases of nurse-associated epidemics is the victimization that occurs to all nurses during the investigations and as a result of media coverage. In three criminal trials, the nurses' due process was violated on multiple occasions. All of the nurses who worked on the units involved, or even in the institution, felt harassed during parts of the investigation. The media tend to highlight the nursing occupation of the suspect, far more than in other murder trials (Yorker, 1994). Often overlooked is the fact that frequently other nurses were the first to notice the unusual adverse occurrences and to request investigations.

Psychiatric Diagnoses

Another legal and ethical issue involves labeling when psychiatric diagnoses are applied to clusters of behaviors. They can be used to enhance guilt (e.g., these behaviors fit a profile; therefore, the person must have committed the crime) or to mitigate guilt through the insanity defense (e.g., this person has a syndrome; therefore, the person is mentally incompetent to commit the crime). Caution should be exercised when using syndrome evidence in criminal proceedings. There are many instances when a landmark treatise that describes common features of a group such as known perpetrators (e.g., sex offenders) or known victims of crime (e.g., battered women) have been misused or taken out of context to influence criminal proceedings (Myers, 1993).

Brian Morgan (1993) wrote a thought-provoking letter to the editor following the conviction of a nurse in England. He pointed out that the Munchausen syndrome diagnosis keeps being applied to new groups. Originally, Asher (1951) used it to describe "hospital hobos," people who induced illness and traveled from hospital to hospital. Then Money and Werlwas (1992) used the *by proxy* term to describe parents who produced psychosocial dwarfs. Meadow (1977) then wrote the classic description of mothers who fabricated illness in their children to gain medical attention. Subsequent accounts of MSBP include fathers and nonrelated caretakers as perpetrators, and now it is being applied to serial murderers. Morgan has interviewed a dozen mothers who have been labeled MSBP who believe they were given the diagnosis because clinicians were unable to find the cause of their child's symptoms. Some are being vindicated by the courts or with more expert diagnosis. One mother in a group called Parents against Injustice warns that MSBP "could become a dustbin diagnosis for lazy clinicians," and Morgan asks whether it could do the same for criminality (Morgan, 1993) (Fig. 9-1).

Best Practice *9-1*

When hiring new personnel, ensure that credentials, work experiences, and job qualifications are verified by reliable sources including the immediate three employers.

Hospitals Working with Nursing Administrators and Staff

In several cases, nurses were the first to alert hospital authorities about suspicious activity. In an Indiana case, the head nurse who blew the whistle was treated in a hostile manner by administrators, fired, then reinstated. By that time she had such severe stress-related symptoms that she had to take workers' compensation for a period of disability. She will never work as a nurse again. In Florida, the stress of the investigation turned the new nursing home administrator away for a career in healthcare. On the other hand, the head nurse in the Georgia case collaborated so well with law enforcement that she continues to present risk management protocol to other hospitals.

In many of the cases, however, members of the nursing staff reported feeling mistreated during the investigation. In Michigan, procedural violations resulted in an overturned conviction. There was also a nursing organization backlash, arguing that there were racist and sexist elements to the investigation.

In Canada, the public outcry over the treatment of all the staff nurses during the investigation, including the arrest of an innocent nurse after she refused to answer questions without her lawyer present, precluded prosecution of the statistically correlated nurse (Boxes 9-2 and 9-3).

Box 9-2 Nonsurveillance Methods of Detecting Caregiver-Associated Incidents

- Nursing or other personnel report their suspicions
- A member of the patient's family complains that she or he was given a drug that made that person feel sick, stop breathing, tingle, or have an otherwise serious adverse reaction.
- Autopsy results are suspicious (e.g., air embolus, fluid in lungs, toxic levels of drugs).
- A caregiver exhibits Munchausen syndrome or falsifies his or her own health status and suspicious patient events occur.

Box 9-3 Hospitals Working with Law Enforcement

In many cases, prosecutors found hospital administrators and physicians to be uncooperative. In some cases, they were simply stonewalling; in other cases, they actually obstructed the investigation. Some reasons for their uncooperative behavior include the following:

- Fear of negative publicity
- Fear of civil suits for negligence
- Fear of civil suits by nurses being investigated
- Poor record keeping

Note: In a Georgia case, the hospital worked so effectively with state authorities that the epidemic only lasted three months, a surveillance protocol deterred any further suspicious adverse patient incidents, and smoking-gun evidence was collected once the statistically likely nurse was identified and the protocol was lifted. This was accomplished without alerting the nursing staff to the presence of a criminal investigation and without any concerns about a witch-hunt or civil rights violations.

Summary

A study of several cases of nurse homicides reveals the shocking truth that nurses can and do murder patients who are under their care. The three cases of nurse-associated epidemics of clinical murders induced by therapeutic agents in the environment provide insight into the underlying dynamics of these crimes and why coworkers did not intervene promptly when they suspected foul play. The forensic nurse examiner as a clinical investigator is an ideal resource for epidemiological surveillance and systematic study of such incidents that may later prove to be serial in nature if not handled swiftly.

Resources

Journals

Journal of Clinical Forensic Medicine

Official Journal of the Association of Police Surgeons, Journal Subscription Department, Harcourt Publishers, Foots Cray High Street, Sidcup, Kent DA14 5HP, UK

Journal of Forensic Sciences

Official Journal of the American Academy of Forensic Sciences, Michael A. Peat, PhD, Editor, 7151 West 135th Street, PMB 410, Overland Park, KS 66223

Organizations

American Academy of Forensic Sciences

410 North 21st Street, Colorado Springs, CO 80904, Tel: 719-636-1100; www.aafs.org

American College of Forensic Examiners

2750 East Sunshine, Springfield, MO 65804; Tel: 800-423-9737; www.acfei.com

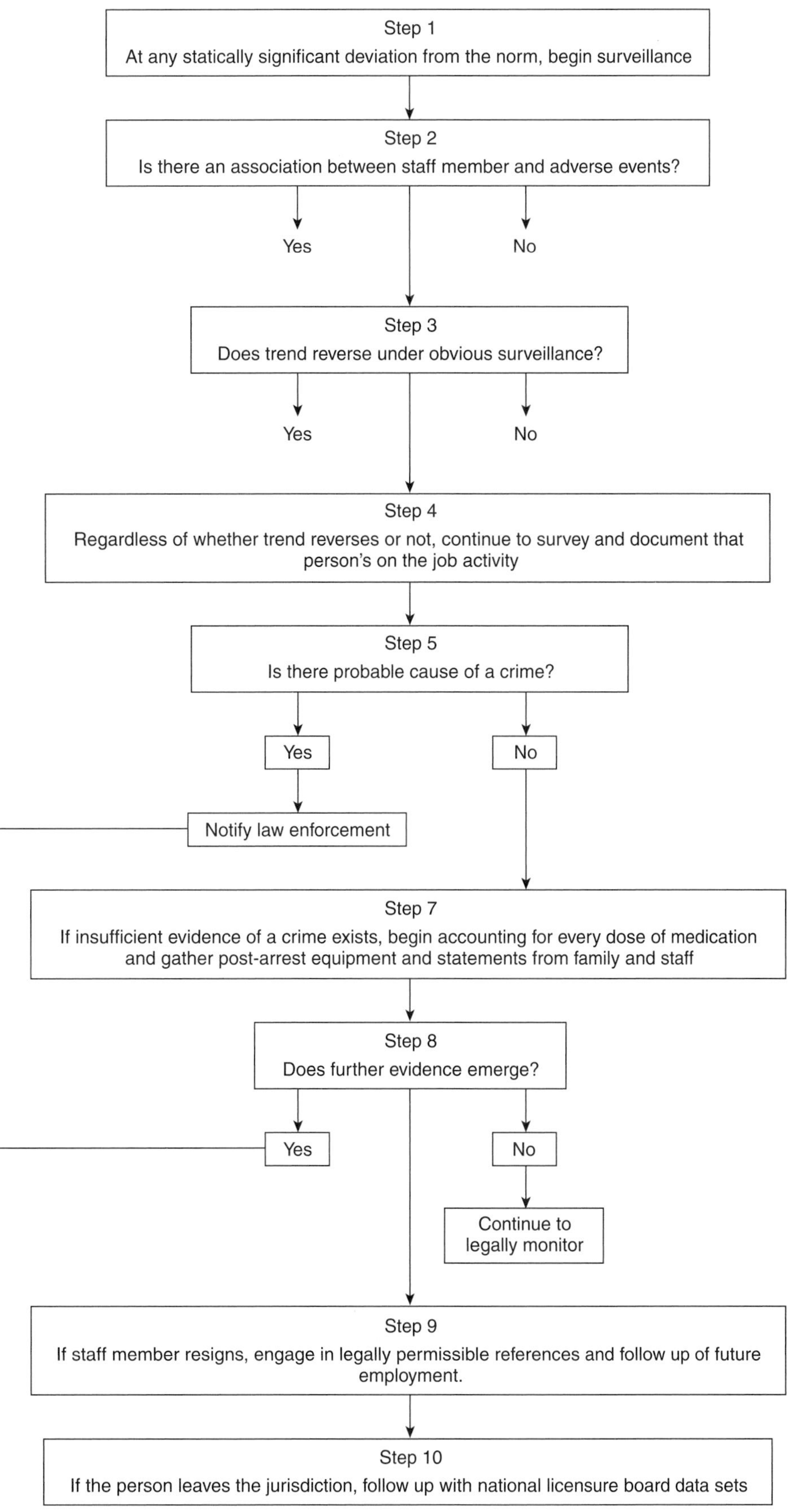

Fig. 9-1 Algorithm: Mitigating morbidity and mortality of caregiver-associated epidemics.

International Association of Forensic Nurses

East Holly Avenue, Box 56, Pittman, NJ 08071-0056, www.forensicnurse.org

References

American Psychiatric Association (APA). (1994). *Diagnostic and statistical manual of mental disorders* (4th ed.). Washington, DC: Author.

Asher. R. (1951). Munchausen's syndrome. *Lancet, 1*, 339–341.

Buehler, J. W., Smith, L. F., Wallace, E. M., et al. (1985). Unexplained deaths in a children's hospital: An epidemiologic assessment. *N Eng J Med, 313*, 211–216.

Davies, N. (1993). *Murder on ward four*. London: Chatto & Windus.

DiVasto, P., & Saxton, G. (1992). Munchausen's syndrome in law enforcement. *FBI Law Enforce Bull, 61*(4), 311–314.

Forrest, A. R. W. (1992). *The investigation and prosecution of health care workers who systematically harm their patients*. Unpublished dissertation, Florida State University, Tallahassee.

Goodwin, J. (1988). Munchausen's syndrome as a dissociative disorder. *Dissociation 1*, 54–60.

Gunnison, R. B. (1996, October 23). Woman accused in deaths of 3: Investigators say mental disorder made her kill foster children. *San Francisco Chronicle*.

Holzberg, B. (1989, November 20). A nurse who said he just wanted to be a hero. *Natl Law J*.

Istre, G. R., Gustafson, T. L., Baron, R. C., et al. (1985). A mysterious cluster of deaths and cardiopulmonary arrests in a pediatric intensive care unit. *N Eng J Med, 313*, 205–211.

Meadow, R. (1977). Munchausen syndrome by proxy: The hinterland of child abuse. *Lancet, 2*, 343–345.

Money, J., & Werlwas, J. (1992). Folie a deux in the parents of psychosocial dwarfs: Two cases. *Bull Am Acad Psych & Law, 4*, 351–362.

Morgan, B. (1993, May 24). Letters to the editor. *The Independent*.

Murphy, D. E. (1991, December 17). When the firebug happens to be a firefighter. *L.A. Times*, A1 ff.

Myers, J. E. B. (1993). Expert testimony describing psychological syndromes. *Pac Law J, 24*, 1449–1465.

Orenstein, D. M., & Wasserman, A. L. (1986). Munchausen syndrome by proxy simulating cystic fibrosis. *Pediatrics, 78*(4), 621–624.

Rachals v. State (1988). 364 SE 2d 867 (Georgia).

Rosenberg, D. A. (1987). Web of deceit: A literature review of Munchausen syndrome by proxy. *Ch Abuse Negl, 11*, 547–563.

Rothman, K. J. (1985). Sleuthing in hospitals. *N Eng J Med, 313*, 258–259.

Sacks, J. J., Herndon, J. L., Leib, S. H., et al. (1988). A cluster of unexplained deaths in a nursing home in Florida. *Am J Pub Health, 78*, 806–808.

Sacks, J. J., Stroup, D. F., Will, M. L., et al. (1988). *JAMA, 259*(5), 689–695.

Shrier, H. A. (1992). The perversion of mothering: Munchausen syndrome by proxy. *Bull Menninger Clinic, 56*(4), 421–437.

Stross, J. K., Shasby, D. M., & Harlan, W. R. (1976). An epidemic of mysterious cardiopulmonary arrests. *N Eng J Med, 295*, 1107–1110.

Yorker, B. C. (1994). An analysis of murder charges against nurses. *J of Nursing Law, 1*(3), 35–46.

Unit Three

Principles and Techniques of Forensic Science

Chapter 10 Crime Scene Processing

Z. G. Standing Bear

This chapter addresses the proper processing of crime scenes where interpersonal violence, either physical or emotional, is involved, as may be seen in the crimes of murder, manslaughter, negligent homicide, rape and other sexual assaults, maiming, aggravated assault, robbery, and torture. Not detailed in this chapter is the examination of scenes of catastrophic events (such as acts of terrorism in which many persons are killed or disasters such as commercial aircraft crashes), where scene search procedures and protocols are far more extensive and multifaceted than reported here and involve the deployment of specialized teams of investigators. Disaster scene investigation procedures have been meticulously developed by such organizations as the United States National Transportation Safety Board (1999).

The violent crime scene brings together healthcare, emergency service, criminal justice, and forensic science personnel who may have a wide variety of backgrounds, such as police officers, emergency medical technicians and paramedics, forensic nurses, police investigators, fire fighters and fire investigators, and possibly highly specialized individuals (such as forensic engineers, forensic entomologists, or forensic anthropologists). Proper care of a victim of violent crime and the professional, careful, and complete processing of the crime scene require that certain tasks be carried out *in a specified order*. Many adequate publications prescribe and describe proper techniques of searching a crime scene and for collecting, preserving, and identifying physical evidence. Currently, however, only one source, an earlier version of this chapter (Standing Bear, 1999) has spelled out, in succinct fashion, the exact steps to be taken in the thorough examination of a crime scene involving violence. This chapter details an updated protocol for procedures to be followed in responding to a complaint of a crime of violence. It is important that properly skilled personnel, trained in violent crime scene search techniques and the collection/preservation of evidence, be employed in the scene investigation of these offenses. When forensically unskilled officials are first to respond to the incident scene, they should perform steps in this protocol only up to the point at which the scene is secured; then they should arrange for scene security until skilled personnel arrive.

It is important to gauge the experience and expertise of the uniformed law enforcement and investigative personnel one will be working with at crime scenes. If expertise in crime scene processing is lacking, as is often the case, the time to get training is *before* the scene is examined. Joint training sessions will prepare personnel to work together as a team. Lack of training on the part of any member of a crime scene processing unit invariably leads to interagency disputes and diminished effectiveness.

This chapter details a sequential format to be followed. Performing the scene investigation out of sequence may alter or destroy important evidence. One need review only a few of the recent "celebrity cases," such as the O. J. Simpson investigation or the Jon Benet Ramsey case, to get the picture that all is *not* well in the conduct of crime scene examinations.

Virtually anyone can discover a crime scene. It is understandable that well-meaning but unskilled citizens may alter a scene to the detriment of case solution. However, there is no reason why professionals who deal with emergencies and major crimes on a frequent basis, such as emergency medical technicians and paramedical personnel; emergency, flight, or forensic nurses; and police officers and investigators, should not be able to secure and process a crime scene in an effective manner. Although some of the following sequential steps may seem simplistic, they are of utmost importance in the proper processing of a major crime scene. Certain responders, such as emergency medical technicians and paramedical personnel, may have a limited role in the actual processing of a crime scene. Nonetheless, it is important for them to realize the steps that must be followed in order to facilitate the effective processing of the scene, because even their limited role may jeopardize effective evidence collection. The serial killer or rapist who is permitted to remain at large owing to poor evidence collection or crime scene processing will return again to revictimize and tax the resources and emotions of the entire community. Accordingly, good crime scene examination is not solely within the province of the police but is the responsibility of every member of the emergency response team.

Key Point *10-1*

Although some of the steps in the sequential crime scene search seem simplistic and intuitive, often crime scenes are irreparably damaged by failure to observe these procedures.

The scene investigation in a major incident must be undertaken in a systematic, sequential manner by trained and skilled investigators in order to ensure that all valuable evidence is identified, accurately documented, and effectively recovered, preserved, and secured, so as to permit optimal laboratory or other expert examination. At the same time, the chain of custody must be maintained so that the evidence is admissible. The scene investigation in a major crime is among the most important initial activities in a chain of events that may significantly affect the outcome (successful suspect identification and prosecution, consideration of the victim, public safety and security) of a serious criminal offense.

Preparation

Investigation of the scene of a violent criminal offense cannot be carried out effectively without adequate preparation prior to the initial report of the incident. Because timeliness of response to such scenes is of paramount importance in the discovery, security, recovery, and preservation of evidence, the prior possession and maintenance of adequate supplies and equipment are essential.

Crime Scene Search Equipment

Scene Security Supplies and Equipment

Adequate scene security supplies and equipment must be maintained. That includes physical barriers, such as sawhorses and crime scene barrier tape, as well as rain protection devices, such as large plastic containers (in the event footprints or tire tracks must be protected from inclement weather) and waterproof tarpaulins.

Scene Documentation Supplies and Equipment

Prior to notification of a violent incident, scene documentation supplies and equipment must be immediately available to scene investigators, including clipboards, paper, pencils and pens, measuring devices (small inch/centimeter rulers for photographic documentation and 100-foot tape measures for scene measurement), flags and other markers for outdoor scene identification, photographic equipment (35-mm camera, photoflash capability, and film), and adequate portable lighting. Contingency plans should be formulated for the rapid replenishment of supplies and equipment should a scene examination require extraordinary resources, such as additional photographic supplies or intensified lighting (available through many large fire departments). Examples of such scenes are a basement during a power outage and a forest at night.

Evidence Recovery Supplies and Equipment

Evidence recovery kits for the investigation should contain sufficient quantities of suitable containers (test tubes, bottles, plastic and paper bags, boxes, rubber gloves, rubber bands, tweezers, print and impression recovery materials, and syringes) to recover a variety of substances. A method must be in place to replenish stock once depleted. In one death case, the host of a party was found dead the next morning in his home and it was suspected that he had been poisoned. At the scene were 87 drinking glasses containing various levels of liquids and residue, each of which had to be examined.

> **Key Point *10-2***
>
> Gathering of supplies to process a variety of crime scenes requires imagination, and premanufactured crime scene search "kits" usually fall short of what is needed. Stock test tubes for collecting liquids by the gross, not the half-dozen.

Maintenance of Equipment and Vehicles

All equipment and the vehicles used to transport the investigators and equipment to the scene must be properly maintained and ready to respond to a crime scene 24 hours a day. Equipment and supplies must be adequately stocked on a continuous basis. Written inventory control and replenishment procedures for equipment and supplies should be in place and a specific individual designated as responsible for maintenance and replenishment.

Attire at the Scene

Although suitable field uniforms are commercially available for scene search work, any comfortable and durable clothing that may become soiled or damaged without concerning the wearer and is suitable to the scene temperature may be adequate in all but the following specialized cases:

- Scenes that contain biohazards, toxic materials, or vapors may require specialized protective clothing for scene investigators.
- Large crime scenes or scenes where several investigating agencies may be working and investigators are not familiar with each other (such as a killing involving drug traffickers or a suspected serial killer) may require special identifying uniform clothing (or other controls such as badges or photo identification) in the interests of operational control.

Portable Lighting and Other Specialized Equipment

Adequate battery- or generator-powered portable lighting should be available to investigators at all times in the event of outside scenes that must be searched during hours of darkness or indoor scenes that must be searched where electrical lighting is not available, either because of location (cellars, closets, attics) or a power outage. Responsibility for maintaining portable lighting and batteries should be contained in written operating procedures. Also, the appropriation of other specialized equipment and equipment operators (e.g., metal detectors, scaffolding erectors, heavy equipment such as cranes or recovery vehicles, fumigators) should also be written into procedures. Often, memorandums of understanding can be promulgated with fire departments and other specialized organizations for the provision of portable lighting and other specialized equipment when necessary, as such departments usually maintain lighting and other equipment as a matter of standard practice.

Notification and Response

In investigating violent crimes, procedures must be in place for an organized and orderly response well in advance of notification of the occurrence of such a crime. Procedures must be in writing and shared among all the agencies that potentially may become involved in an incident. It is as important for each participant to understand what the function and role is of each member responding in an interagency sense as it is to understand the function and role within a particular agency (intra-agency responsibilities).

> **Key Point *10-3***
>
> Know in advance what the special capabilities are of each member of the crime scene search team and capitalize on those capabilities. In the words of General George S. Patton, Jr.: "Know what you know and know what you do not know!" (Williamson, 1988).

These advance understandings will do much to ensure a smooth and effective scene processing and should eliminate much of the on-scene confusion and squabbling too often encountered.

Organization for Response

In violent crimes, several investigators should be mobilized if possible. For example, sexual assault investigations generally require a minimum of three responding investigators: at least one to process the crime scene, one to interview the victim and assist the victim through the remainder of the investigative process, and one to locate, apprehend, interview, and process the suspect. Until all initial phases of the investigation (scene searches, interviews, and medical examinations) have been completed, the suspect(s) and victim(s) should be kept separate from one another and should never be transported in the same vehicles or occupy the same treatment, waiting, or interview rooms so at to avoid cross-contamination of trace evidence, allegations of possible cross-contamination, collusion (such as a possible attempt by the perpetrator to have the victim drop the complaint), and confrontations. Although cross-contamination of evidence is nearly impossible (e.g., from both the victim and the suspect walking across the same hospital parking lot at different times), the perception of the possibility may become very real in court.

Contemporary agencies are implementing a conjoint team approach involving both law enforcement investigators and forensic nurse examiners, specifically in sexual assault, homicide, child abuse, elder abuse, and domestic violence cases. For example, in San Diego, California, police investigators request sexual assault nurse examiners (SANEs) at the scene and at the examination facility to assist in identifying crucial biomedical evidence often unrecognized by investigators without a medical background. Increasingly, investigative agencies are preferring that sexual assault examinations be performed by a credentialed SANE nurse following standards set by the International Association of Forensic Nurses (IAFN). SANE Council Standards of Practice (International Association of Forensic Nurses, 1996) and those sexual assault investigation standards are presently developed by the American Society for Testing and Materials (ASTM), Committee E-30 (1998).

Proceeding to the Scene

Transport to the crime scene should be done in a safe and lawful manner, with team organization (such as the fixing of responsibility for scene security, scene search, witness interviews, and area check) decided in advance so that the typical confusion present at violent crime scenes will not be exacerbated by an arriving group of disorganized investigators.

Initial Actions at the Scene

Upon arrival at the scene of any violent crime, certain actions must be accomplished quickly and competently so as to gain control of the circumstances and the scene.

Note Time, Date, and Weather Conditions

The time, date, and weather conditions at the scene should be noted by the investigator(s) immediately upon arrival. This seemingly small detail may become important weeks or months later when alibis of potential suspects are checked and when testifying in court as to the sequence of events at the initiation of the investigation. Attorneys who call into question an investigator's competence by exclaiming, "You mean you do not even remember what day it was?" have embarrassed investigators on the witness stand. Also, weather conditions may contribute to the cause or effect of the incident, and these possibilities may not be realized until some time after the results of the incident have been discovered.

Make Initial Observations of the Scene

Several assessments of a scene must be made simultaneously by arriving investigators so as to evaluate relative danger, scene scope, control of individuals at the scene, and the coordination of responsibilities.

Nature of Scene (Immediate Danger)

A rapid assessment of the condition of the scene should be made in order to rule out potential danger to the investigator(s) or others. Such dangers may include the presence of dangerous person(s), weather problems, toxic or otherwise dangerous gases or substances, seismic activity, electrical hazards, fire danger, potentially dangerous plants or animals, and possible avalanche, mudslide, or rock slide, or dangerous structures.

Suspects, Victims, and Witnesses

The identification of suspect(s), victim(s), and witnesses at the scene, if any, should immediately be made and decisions reached as to the treatment of each. As a minimum, suspect(s) and victim(s) should be separated and, when possible, witnesses should be separated from each other and interviewed separately so that one does not color another's perception of an incident. As soon as a suspect meets the legal requirements for apprehension, that individual should be placed in police custody. Even though an individual at the scene does not appear, at the moment, to be a suspect, victim, or witness, complete identification (including address and telephone number) is still needed in the event there is a need to recontact that person in the future.

Police

All police officials present at the scene should be identified. If more than one law enforcement agency is present, it should be determined which has primary jurisdiction. The senior official present of the agency or office with primary jurisdiction will take charge of the scene. Often, a crime scene may share primary jurisdiction with several agencies, as when a sexually assaulted dead body is found and the body itself is the responsibility of the medical examiner's investigator while the remainder of the scene is the responsibility of police investigators. In certain cases, specialized agencies may also share jurisdiction, such as the Drug Enforcement Administration (an assault in a drug trafficking case) or the state Department of Wildlife (an assault in a wild animal poaching case). In these circumstances it is imperative that both senior officials work in an organized and coordinated way to ensure optimal identification, collection, and preservation of evidence. The senior individual representing the agency with primary jurisdiction at the scene must insist upon inspecting the credentials (badges, photo identification, etc.) of other officially authorized persons seeking admission to the investigation or the scene. This inspection is especially important if the senior official does not personally know the individuals. Accordingly, the senior official must be familiar with the authorized credentials issued by other agencies.

Other Agencies

Often, individuals from agencies other than the police with an interest in the crime scene may be represented. Officially authorized agencies, such as coroner or medical examiner's offices, public agency or contracted forensic nurses, emergency medical services, or public safety agencies (fire departments, environmental protection agencies, etc.) may have specific authority and jurisdiction for certain functions at the scene and must be coordinated and cooperated with to the benefit of all concerned. Agencies without official authorization but with an interest in the scene, such the news media, insurance companies, management or labor representatives, various activist/advocacy groups, and property owners, must be controlled and not permitted access to the scene. Such interest groups should be referred to the police public information officer or the chief of police for information and guidance. Often personnel from unauthorized agencies may use subterfuge or intimidation to gain access to a scene; such practices must be guarded against.

Assure Medical Aid

Any seriously injured or ill persons (at risk of loss of life or limb) at the scene must be provided immediate medical aid, regardless of the necessity to locate, recover, and preserve evidence. Minor illnesses or injuries may be treated at the expense of the loss of identification and recovery of evidence at the discretion of the senior law enforcement official with primary jurisdiction in coordination and consultation with healthcare professionals at the scene.

Although paramedical personnel are primarily concerned with lifesaving interventions, caution to preserve forensically significant evidence should be an important concern as well. Paramedical personnel should be trained in advance in the ability to render emergency treatment swiftly while preserving evidence, such as the rapid removal of clothing when necessary without altering defects or contaminating the clothing at trauma sites.

Locate Senior Police Official or Most Significant Witness

Responding healthcare personnel and investigators should coordinate with the individual possessing the most knowledge about the scene and the incident to prevent interference in the securing and investigation of the crime scene and to establish the physical parameters of the scene. For example, normally in a situation where a sexual assault occurred within a single-family residence, the secured area of the scene would include the house and the adjoining property. However, if a witness saw an individual run from the house in a certain direction, leap a fence, and run through three adjoining vacant lots before getting into a car parked on the next block, the size of the scene to be secured may be greatly expanded.

One important consideration cited by police for the conjoint team approach with forensic nurses concerns the ability of the nurse to elicit often sensitive information from victims and grieving families who may be in shock or may be intimidated by a uniformed officer. This technique may be commonly lacking with officers who may not be skilled in psychosocial intervention.

Key Point *10-4*

A crime scene cannot be adequately secured until one is sure about what that scene entails. Careful preparation in advance, although often tedious, pays off in the end.

General Scene Security

The scene should be secured using physical barriers (crime scene/police line tape installed waist high where practical, guarded by uniformed official security personnel) until the scene has been examined and cleared for release to the appropriate owner or tenant.

Environment Security

Nonhuman environmental elements, such weather, animals, and nonnatural elements, may act to damage or obliterate a crime scene and should be stabilized to the maximum extent possible, not only to preserve evidence but also to provide for the safety of those examining the scene.

Weather Security

The scene should be protected from weather elements when necessary. Fragile evidence, such as tire tracks and footprints, should be covered and guarded until the weather clears and recovery efforts can begin.

Animal Security

A crime scene may be destroyed, damaged, or significantly altered by any number of animals in a variety of settings. Scene security procedures should include protection of the scene from not only birds, insects, and other wild animals, but domestic animals as well. Also, although some animals may not be particularly dangerous to evidence at the scene itself, they may be quite dangerous to investigators searching the scene. Accordingly, investigators should use extreme caution when working in the unknown habitats of such animals as poisonous snakes, spiders, scorpions, and exotic animals kept as pets.

Security in Emergencies

In some situations emergency response personnel, such as firefighters, hazardous materials specialists, and engineers, must make rapid decisions to protect life and property from further danger and destruction. Often, this action requires the employment of water, chemicals, explosives, or other interventions. Although evidence discovery and preservation may have to occupy a secondary place in the face of emergency action, continuous coordination and cooperation should be maintained with emergency response personnel to minimize evidence destruction.

Scene Security and the Human Element

Scenes of violent crimes are generally more prone to alteration from human beings than from environmental factors. Although one tends to think of suspects tampering with scene evidence as being the main danger from human involvement with crime scenes, far more evidence is rendered useless or of limited use from the inadvertent contamination or destruction by unknowing witnesses and official investigative personnel.

Security Concerning Suspects

Once the scene is secured, a quick check should be made to determine the presence of any suspects or others who are potentially a danger to the scene or the individuals processing it. Places in which a human could escape detection, such as closets, attics, basements, under beds, and outbuildings, should be carefully checked. Occasionally, a suspect is trapped in a scene that has been discovered and is forced to go into hiding. It is rather disconcerting for an investigator, carefully searching the minute details of a crime scene, to come face to face with an armed suspect upon opening the door of a closet. Persons found at the scene who could be considered suspects should be placed in custody.

Security Concerning Witnesses and Victims

Witnesses, victims, and others ("bystanders") should be identified (correct names, addresses, and telephone numbers noted) and removed from the scene. Even if a person present at the scene may originally appear unconnected with the incident, further investigation may reveal that the individual possesses significant incident-related knowledge. This individual may need to be contacted at a later date. Victims should be initially interviewed to determine what parts of the crime scene should receive particular attention. Beyond the initial interview, victims should be transported to the appropriate healthcare facility for examination and continued investigation.

In cases involving all forms of assault, the victim's body is, in and of itself, a crime scene. Thus, victims transported to a treatment or examination facility should be kept separate from others, be they suspects, witnesses, or other victims. In addition, an official member of the investigative team should remain with the victim at all times. Victims should not be permitted to bathe in any way (including washing of the hands) or change clothes until examined.

It is often difficult to ensure that certain scenes be cleared of victims and witnesses, especially if that scene is located at the home of a victim or witness. For example, prudent investigative procedure would have dictated that the wealthy parents of a small girl reportedly kidnapped (whose body was later found in the basement of their home) be immediately required to exit their home and be lodged in a hotel while the scene is examined. There are numerous skillful and diplomatic ways in which such situations may be approached, but prior training in these techniques is required.

Key Point *10-5*

Proper crime scene procedures, including the treatment of potential witnesses, should be followed in a uniform manner, regardless of the socioeconomic status of the individuals involved.

Security Concerning Officials

Often, high-ranking officials may wish to visit the scene for a variety of purposes. Ideally, anyone not directly involved in the search of the scene for evidence should be excluded. However, reality dictates that investigators searching a crime scene are occasionally interrupted by officials demanding to inspect the scene. When this occurs, investigators should suspend their search, accompany the inspecting officials, and ensure that officials do not disturb or alter the scene in any way.

Security Concerning Investigators

Occasionally, a crime scene may be inadvertently altered or contaminated by an investigator who does not recognize the presence or the importance of physical evidence. This evidence then may become obscured, destroyed, or damaged. This precaution is especially germane to sexual assault investigations, in which trace evidence is common and difficult to detect. Because of this, investigators must move through crime scenes with utmost caution until the search is complete. It is equally important for investigators to avoid bringing items into the scene and setting them down for convenience, such as clothing items (jackets, etc.) and crime scene equipment containers (evidence collection kits, camera bags, etc.). The scene should be kept "clean" and individual items of equipment and supplies should be brought into the scene only as needed.

Although sometimes irresistibly convenient, investigators must never use any telephone, appliance, or other convenience (such as lights, sink, or toilet) at the scene unless absolutely necessary to process the scene. Even the necessity of turning on or off lights or turning off gas or a motor should be done so that evidence such as fingerprints are not disturbed.

Security Concerning Admission

Once the scene is secured, it must stay secured. Only one entrance/exit to the scene must be permitted, and that point must be guarded and controlled by a competent official, preferably an experienced police officer. It must be made clear exactly who is to be permitted into the scene and that all others are to be excluded unless the senior official in charge of the scene grants an exception. A detailed log must be maintained of the times, dates, and complete identities of all persons entering and exiting the scene. This log becomes a permanent part of the investigative case file.

When the Treatment Room Is a Crime Scene

Death or serious injury may occur in the clinical environs: the trauma room, operating room, emergency department, delivery room, etc. Consideration must be given to protecting and securing these areas in the same manner as other violent crime scenes. Particular attention should be paid to access, inventory of supplies and medications, and records, including computerized records. It is especially important in these cases that an individual on the investigative team possess medicolegal forensic skills and education in order to minimize conflicts of interest between the institution and the investigation (Lynch, 1991).

Searching the Scene

One may think that once the prior discussed needs have been met, one may begin searching immediately. Such is not the case, however. Up until this point, the scene has been prepared for search, but further details must be explored before the physical search can begin.

Preparation for Search

Before a scene is physically approached with a view toward the search, certain immediate preparatory steps must be undertaken to ensure a complete and orderly search and to document the prior condition of the scene before the physical search began.

Conduct Preliminary Interviews

As previously stated, preliminary interviews of persons with knowledge of the scene and incident should be conducted. Armed with such information, investigators can begin searching the scene with some frames of reference that will permit specific attention to various areas of the scene.

Take Overall Scene Photographs

Overall photographs of the scene should be taken prior to beginning the search in order to preserve an image of the scene before the evidence search and recovery process disturbs it. These photographs also help to resolve any future questions concerning the original condition of the scene or if scene reconstruction becomes necessary. It may be appropriate to have aerial photographs taken of the scene, especially if the scene is outdoors and contains many items of physical evidence.

Determine the Method of Search

The search should be conducted using a pattern that accommodates the physical nature of the scene. At least six crime search patterns are generally offered by the criminal investigation literature. Table 10-1 lists the different search patterns.

Line or Strip Search. The line or strip search method is used to cover large, open areas and involves personnel who typically form a long line, maintaining an arm's distance between each individual. As the line moves forward as a unit, it essentially creates parallel lanes to search; each member concentrates on one

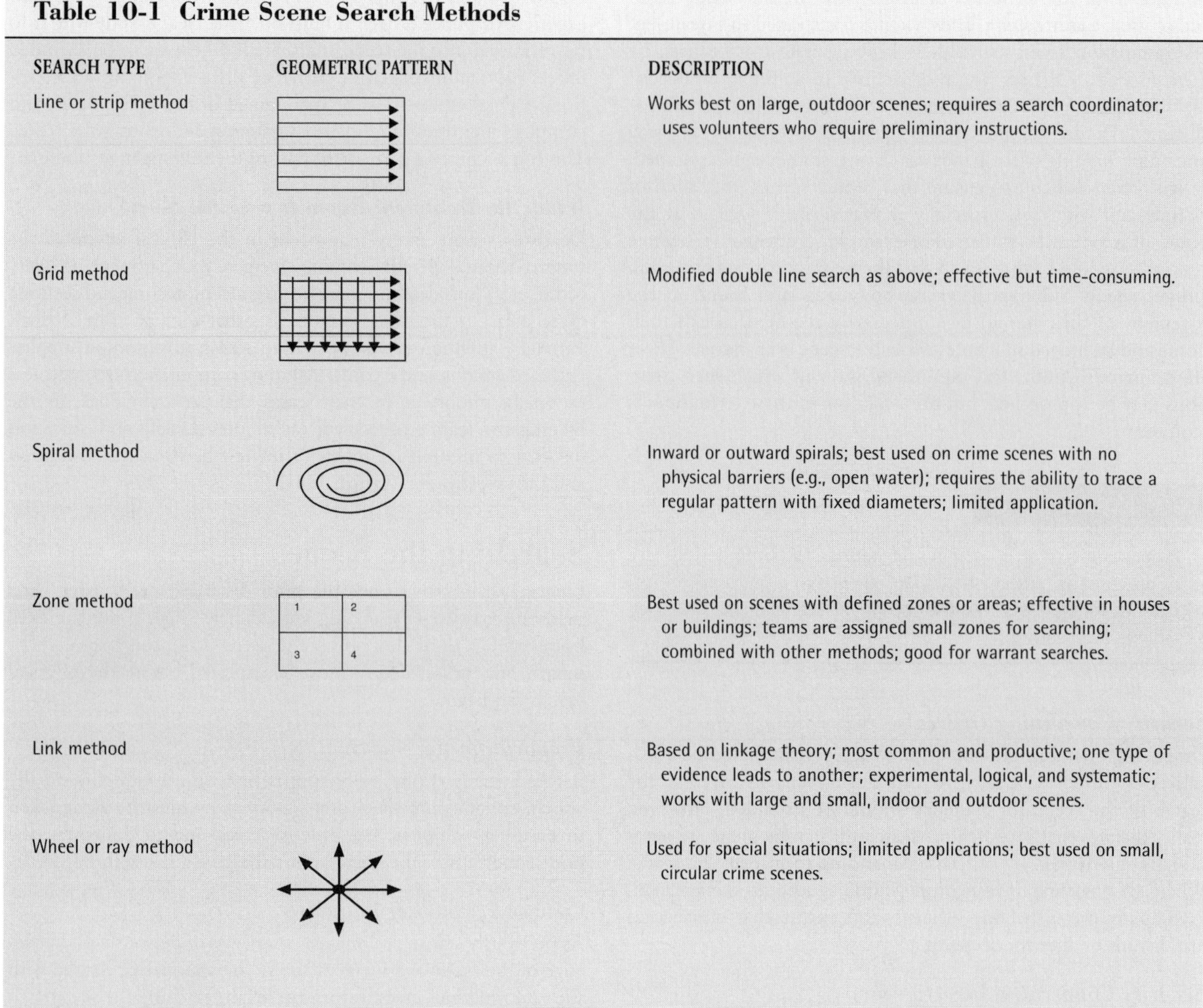

Table 10-1 Crime Scene Search Methods

SEARCH TYPE	GEOMETRIC PATTERN	DESCRIPTION
Line or strip method		Works best on large, outdoor scenes; requires a search coordinator; uses volunteers who require preliminary instructions.
Grid method		Modified double line search as above; effective but time-consuming.
Spiral method		Inward or outward spirals; best used on crime scenes with no physical barriers (e.g., open water); requires the ability to trace a regular pattern with fixed diameters; limited application.
Zone method	1 2 3 4	Best used on scenes with defined zones or areas; effective in houses or buildings; teams are assigned small zones for searching; combined with other methods; good for warrant searches.
Link method		Based on linkage theory; most common and productive; one type of evidence leads to another; experimental, logical, and systematic; works with large and small, indoor and outdoor scenes.
Wheel or ray method		Used for special situations; limited applications; best used on small, circular crime scenes.

From James S. H., & Nordby, J. J. (2003). *Forensic science: An introduction to scientific and investigative techniques.* Boca Raton, FL: CRC Press.

lane. This technique is useful when the scene is long and narrow, such as a roadside area.

Grid Search. The grid search involves covering the same area twice, using linear lane patterns (described under line search). In a grid pattern, the group searches along both a horizontal and a vertical axis. This method is suited to small outdoor crime scenes that do not involve obstructions (such as underbrush) that may pose physical or visual obstructions.

Double Grid Search. The double grid search is a linear search that involves doubling back upon the original search pattern at 90-degree angles to provide multiple coverage of the same area from different points of view. This search pattern is useful in outdoor scenes where vegetation may obscure vision.

Spiral Search. Spiral searches are useful in large outdoor crime scenes. The search usually begins from the "center" of the crime scene (where the principal item of evidence is, such as a dead body, where an assault reportedly took place, or where the majority of the physical evidence is located); however, it may also originate on the periphery (outside limits) and move inward toward principal evidence.

Zone Search. Indoor crime scenes are generally approached using the zone search. Specific zones are identified within a crime scene and then individually searched. Close coordination between investigators is needed to ensure that all zones are accounted for and searched.

Link Method. In the link method, one piece of evidence leads to another. For example, an empty wallet leads to a knife, a trail of blood-spattered leaves, a body face-down with stab wounds. This method is not favored among experienced investigators due to its lack of a systematic approach to the scene.

Wheel Search. The wheel search, usually advanced as a supplementary search in outdoor areas, is not particularly effective because of the ever-increasing space between search lanes as the searchers move out farther away from the center of the scene.

Scene Search and Sketch

Once the search method has been decided, the scene should be thoroughly searched and sketched simultaneously. At this time, evidence is merely located; it is not further processed unless immediate action is necessary to prevent damaging or destroying the evidence.

Searching

The crime scene should be thoroughly searched, using one of the first five scene search patterns. Particular attention must be paid to the possible existence of trace evidence, such as hairs, fibers, and stains, in very small quantities. This attention to detail requires the use of enhanced lighting, alternative light sources, and magnification devices.

Sketching

A (not-to-scale) sketch of the scene should be prepared simultaneously with the search. The main point at this stage of the search is to locate and document the location of the evidence at the scene, rather than to recover the evidence. Recovery is accomplished *after* the search is complete and all the evidence is identified. The progress of a crime scene search to locate evidence should be interrupted only in the event of two situations: First, if fragile evidence in danger of immediate destruction or deterioration is located and must be photographed, measured, recovered, and preserved immediately, this should be done at the time of discovery. Second, if intruders such as high-ranking officials invade the scene, they should be dealt with and escorted in such a way that they are not permitted to contaminate the scene.

Spotting the Evidence

As evidence is identified, some mechanism must be in place to mark the location so that the evidence can be recovered. Such a mechanism must also serve as a warning to others working in the scene that this specific location contains evidence. This marking is especially valuable in outdoor scenes where plant growth or other obstacles may obscure the location of the evidentiary material. Small colored flags attached to stiff wires are often useful in achieving this task in outdoor scenes.

Best Practice *10-1*

Unless discovered evidence is so fragile or so perishable that immediate processing and collection are required, it is best to complete the scene search uninterrupted before evidence is further processed.

Evidence in Natural and Artificial Light

In addition to searching the scene in natural light, using battery-powered, portable artificial lighting in daylight may help to reveal evidence because small objects may reflect light at certain angles. The use of battery-powered artificial light at crime scenes with insufficient natural light (such as at night or in places with inadequate lighting) may be necessary as well, and therefore, such equipment must be available for immediate use.

Locating Evidence with Alternative Light Sources

Often, especially in sexual assault cases, portable ultraviolet lighting is useful in detecting articles and stains that may fluoresce under ultraviolet light while remaining invisible in other light sources. For example, semen stains readily fluoresce in ultraviolet light but are often difficult to detect otherwise. The Omnichrome 1000, used on deceased bodies, is now used on living victims of sexual assault (Arndt, 1999). Infrared videography may assist the investigator in the detection of bruises not visible in conventional lighting and is especially useful in the investigation of crimes involving child abuse and battered victims.

Scene Processing

Measurement and Photography

Once all the evidence is located at the scene, each item of evidence should be photographed in place (before it is moved) both in its natural state and with a measuring device in the photograph. It is also useful for the measuring device to be fitted with a gray scale card (usually preferred by laboratory examiners) or a color card, thus enabling photographic laboratory personnel to ensure that the colors in the evidence photographs are accurate. Color accuracy is especially important when the determination of color is important to the investigation of the case, such as in incidents involving paint chips or dyed fibers. Pasqualone (1996) provides an excellent guide to photographic documentation in the emergency department (see Chapter 18).

Best Practice *10-2*

All evidence should be documented in regard to its distance from a fixed point in the crime scene to aid in later scene reconstruction.

Fix Locations of Evidence and Measure to Fixed Objects

In the event that the scene may need to be reconstructed, measurements must be taken fixing the location of each piece of physical evidence to stationary objects so that the exact location may be again determined at a later date. Usually this process consists of measurements from three fixed objects (such as the base corner of a building, or the base corner of a room or door, or large nails driven into the base of trees or telephone poles) to three definable points on each piece of evidence. Measurement points should be indicated on the scene sketch, and measurements between points should be recorded in a logbook.

Rephotograph Entire Scene with Evidence Spotted

Photographs of the entire scene should show where evidence has been spotted so as to provide an impression of the relationship of each piece of evidence to the other. Again, outdoor scenes and especially large scenes with many items of evidence may benefit greatly from aerial photography.

Marking the Evidence

Prior to recovery, where possible, the evidence should be properly marked for future identification and to assist in the integrity of the chain of custody. Evidence marking is often difficult, and caution must be exercised so that the process of marking does not obliterate or damage any of its evidentiary features.

Nature of Identifying Mark

Generally it is sufficient to mark evidence with the time and date of recovery, along with the initials of the investigator recovering the evidence. The marks should be applied so that they are difficult to remove, but they must not obscure any potential evidentiary features.

Best Practice 10-3

Identifying marks should be placed on an object as far away as possible from surfaces of the object that are going to be examined. When small objects are involved, only the container in which the evidence is placed should be marked.

Location of Identifying Marks

Identifying marks should be placed on an object as far away as possible from surfaces of the object that are going to be examined. In many situations, and especially when small objects are involved, only the container in which the evidence is placed should be marked. Because of the various capabilities of firearms and tool mark examiners in examining cartridges and projectiles under magnification, persons recovering such items at a scene should never mark upon these items. If in doubt, such as in the case of clothing that may harbor latent stains or invisible laundry marks, it is best to avoid marking the individual piece of evidence at all and to simply mark the container into which the evidence is placed. This method should not be problematic if the integrity of the chain of custody is maintained.

Evidence Recovery

There is extensive literature pertaining to the recovery of physical evidence at crime scenes. Such procedures fill volumes (Saferstein, 2003; Fisher, 1993; Hazelwood & Burgess, 1987; Geberth, 1997). Although specific directions concerning the recovery of the various types of physical evidence one may find at a crime scene is beyond the scope of this chapter, a few general precautionary notes are germane.

Evidence Preservation and Integrity as Primary Concern

The key focus in evidence recovery is to ensure preservation of the evidence in order to maximize the capabilities of the forensic laboratory. Achievement of this goal requires not only close attention to the recovery and preservation protocols, but close coordination with laboratory personnel to ascertain the latest preferred methods of recovering and preserving evidence. Such collaboration will provide maximum utilization of the instrumentation in the forensic laboratory. An important part of maintaining the integrity of physical evidence is to ensure that the chain of custody is not broken and that the evidence is adequately identifiable from the time of recovery until the disposition of the case. Marking evidence for identification that is fragile or small presents difficult challenges. Improper marking may taint or obliterate important evidentiary materials. Accordingly, it is generally safest to recover the evidence in an uncontaminated state when possible, marking the container in which the evidence is placed with the time, date, and initials of the recovering investigator. For example, a firearm projectile or cartridge casing should be placed in a hard-sided clear plastic container and anchored with cotton so that the item is visible from the outside, and the container is then sealed and marked. Marked in this way, the only person needing to unpack the item will be the laboratory firearm examiner. Others who wish to see the evidence, such as the prosecutor or defense attorney, may view it from the outside of the container. Again, not placing marks directly on the evidence should not pose a problem if the chain of custody is intact.

Recovery of Possible Print Evidence

Evidence that may possibly have fingerprint or other print evidence should be marked as such. Precautions must be taken to prevent abrasions on the surface of an item that may obliterate or obscure print evidence.

Recovery of Trace Evidence

Trace evidence should be recovered as intact as possible. In recovering stains, hairs, or fibers, for example, the material on which the item is found should be recovered along with the item, if practical. For example, in the recovery of a hair adhering to a stain on a garment or a large cardboard box, it would be advisable to recover the entire garment or a portion of the cardboard box.

Recovery of Perishable Biological Evidence

Particular attention should be paid to the recovery of perishable biological evidence to prevent further deterioration. Generally, if wet evidence can be quickly transported to a laboratory, this should be quickly arranged. However, if time or distance precludes immediate transmittal to the laboratory, biological stains (blood, semen, etc.) should be air-dried without heat in as dust-free an atmosphere as possible. Plastic packaging should be avoided due to the possibility of condensation, which might cause evidence deterioration. Commercial evidence packaging materials firms have made great strides recently and should be contacted for advice on new packaging advances.

In many medical facilities, standard operating procedures require that contaminated materials, such as clothing, be placed in biohazard plastic bags. In such a situation, the contaminated garments should first be placed in a paper bag that is then sealed and suitably marked. The paper bag should then be placed in the plastic biohazard bag, leaving the biohazard bag open for air circulation (Lynch, 1991).

Scene Closure

After the rigors of systematically searching a crime scene, often the competent closure of the scene is neglected, frequently resulting in problematic results, such as forgotten materials, security breaches, and lawsuits.

Evidence Removal

All evidence identified and recovered at the scene should be inventoried, logged, and removed, maintaining preservation and security of the evidence. The inventory and log becomes a permanent part of the case file.

Equipment Removal

The scene should be resurveyed to ensure that all materials brought into or near the scene have been recovered, such as crime scene search equipment, cameras, and other materials. Although this step sounds simplistic, in over two decades of practice, some rather incredible lapses of judgment have been observed, such as investigators leaving behind cameras, their badges and credentials, their own clothing, and even individual items of evidence.

Arrangement for Continuing Security

A completed crime scene cannot simply be abandoned. Significant property loss or vandalism can occur if arrangements are not made for continuing security. At the time a crime scene is

Case Study **10-1 Abandoned Vehicle**

Responding to an abandoned vehicle notice, Wyoming State Patrol officer Vernon Caldwell checked on an old pickup truck that was unoccupied by the side of a dirt road that emptied onto the west side of a paved two-lane north-south US highway in southern Wyoming. The truck was parked facing the paved highway on the right side of the dirt road about 40 feet from the intersection with the paved road just forward of a cattle guard on the dirt road. The location was on US Highway 285 connecting Laramie, WY, and Ft. Collins, CO, about 4 miles north of Tie Siding, WY. The truck was unlocked with the key in the ignition and was registered to Melodie Foxx of Casper, WY. Seeing nothing in the immediate vicinity on the rangeland, the trooper noticed some bird activity over a range fence about 80 yards off the east side of the highway. The trooper climbed over the fence and discovered the body of a male clad in typical rancher clothing. There was some decomposition and evidence of bird scavenging activity, but no signs of trauma were seen on the body. Close by, an empty wooden box lay open in the brush. The box was sturdy, appeared to be hand-made, and was about 14 inches square and 8 inches deep with solid sides, top, and bottom. It looked as if the box had been thrown or dropped and had sprung open because the metal latch was broken. On the dead body, the trooper found a wallet with $23 in bills and miscellaneous identification, including a Wyoming driver's license issued to Mitchell Grinsby, age 46, with an address in Casper, WY. The body seemed to match the age and weight of the individual described on the license. The trooper also found a key ring on the body containing four keys. Two of the keys were to the pickup truck on the side of the road. There was nothing else remarkable about the truck except that there were six empty chicken cages in the rear bed of the truck. Although the cages were old and fairly dirty, they did not contain the minute feathers and fecal matter usually associated with chickens.

searched, it is under the supervision and authority of a public agency. When that agency relinquishes jurisdiction, continuing security must be assured. In some cases, usually major crimes, the scene is sealed for possible later reinvestigation. In these cases, the scene remains in control of a public agency. In other cases, the scene is relinquished to the legal occupier of the property. In these latter cases, assistance and advice should be provided as to how the property owner may resecure the property if, for example, a forced entry had occurred.

Scene Departure

The final step, scene departure, marks a formal exit from the scene by investigators, with the intent not to return. If, for any reason, there is doubt as to the finality of this move, the scene should not be released and should stay the subject of continued security until such time as it is considered suitable for release.

Summary

As important as the proper discovery, recovery, and preservation of physical evidence at a crime scene is the necessity to approach and process the scene in a sequential manner. Without invoking the sequential steps described, valuable evidence may be lost or damaged beyond usefulness. Strict adherence to forensic protocol, in the order presented, should help avoid many mistakes made in the past.

Although it may not be the direct responsibility of the healthcare or paramedical personnel, forensic nurses, flight nurses, nurse coroners, and others who may be first on the scene to ensure scene security and integrity, it is a professional responsibility to anticipate the needs of subsequent investigators (police, prosecutors, defenders) and systems (law enforcement, courts) that must invariably be involved in crimes of violence. The better all persons and agencies involved in a major crime coordinate and cooperate with one another, the better the quality of life will become in our communities. The effective examination of major crime scenes brings perpetrators swiftly to justice (and out of circulation) and seeks to free the wrongly suspected or accused. This high level of performance is accomplished only through a coordinated team effort.

Resources

Organizations

American Academy of Forensic Sciences

410 North 21st Street, Colorado Springs, CO 80904; Tel: 719-636-1100; www.aafs.org

American College of Forensic Examiners

2750 East Sunshine, Springfield, MO 65804; Tel: 800-423-9737; www.acfei.com

Federal Bureau of Investigation

935 Pennsylvania Avenue NW, Room 7350, Washington, DC 20535; Tel: 202-324-3000; www.fbi.gov

Journals

Journal of Forensic Sciences

Journal of the American Academy of Forensic Sciences, Michael A. Peat, PhD, Editor, 7151 West 135th Street, PMB 410, Overland Park, KS 66223

Journal of Clinical Forensic Medicine

Journal of the Association of Police Surgeons, Journal Subscription Department, Harcourt Publishers, Foots Cray High Street, Sidcup, Kent DA14 5HP, UK

References

American Society for Testing and Materials. (1998). Standard guide for sexual assault investigation, examination, and evidence collection. *Annual book of ASTM standards*, Vol. 14.02, Standard E 1843-96. Philadelphia: Author.

Arndt, S. (1999, February 15). *Specialized technology in sexual assault investigation.* Workshop in Forensic and Nursing Science: Role of the Forensic Nurse Examiner in Sexual Assault Examination. Annual Meeting of the American Academy of Forensic Sciences, Orlando, FL.

Fisher, B. A. J. (1993). *Techniques of crime scene investigation*, 5th ed. Boca Raton, FL: CRC Press.

Geberth, V. J. (1997). *Practical homicide investigation checklist and field guide.* Boca Raton, FL: CRC Press.

Hazelwood, R. R., & Burgess, A. W. (Eds.). (1987). *Practical aspects of rape investigation: A multidisciplinary approach.* New York: Elsevier.

International Association of Forensic Nurses. (1996). *Sexual assault nurse examiner standards of practice.* Thorofare, NJ: Slack.

Lynch, V. A. (1991). Forensic nursing in the emergency department: A new role for the 1990s. *Crit Care Nurs Q, 14*(3), 69-86.

Pasqualone, G. A. (1996). Forensic RNs as photographers: Documentation in the ED. *J Psychosoc Nurs Mental Health Serv 34*, 10.

Saferstein, R. (2003). *Criminalistics: An introduction to forensic science* (8th ed.). New Jersey: Prentice-Hall.

Standing Bear, Z. G. (1999). Crime scene responders: The imperative sequential steps. *Crit Care Nurs Q, 22*(1), 75-89.

United States National Transportation Safety Board. (1999). The investigative process. Washington, DC: US Government Printing Office. Retrieved from www.ntsb.gov/Abt_NTSB/invest.htm.

Williamson, P. B.(1988). *General Patton's principles for life and leadership*. Tucson, AZ: Management and Systems Consultants.

Chapter 11 Evidence Collection and Preservation

Richard Saferstein

Forensic science begins at the crime scene. If evidence cannot be recognized, retrieved, and preserved at the scene, little can be done at the forensic laboratory to remedy the problem. The healthcare professional is in a unique position to facilitate evidence collection. In some situations, the healthcare professional will be in the presence of police personnel at critical moments during the collection and preservation of physical evidence. At other times, the clinical investigator may be the sole determiner of what evidence to collect. The permutations of crime are so varied that one cannot reduce to simple sentences or paragraphs scenarios depicting when the healthcare professional will need to step forward to make critical decisions on evidence preservation. Well-written chapters in this volume already amply depict the basics of crime-scene investigation and the role of DNA profiling in criminal investigation (see Chapters 10 and 13). What follows is a short primer on the collection and preservation of key items of physical evidence.

Key Point 11-1

Forensic science begins at the crime scene. If evidence cannot be recognized, retrieved, and preserved at the scene, little can be done at the forensic laboratory to salvage the situation.

Evidence Sources and the Environment

The conditions under which forensic evidence is gathered are not always ideal and it may be that the first opportunity to collect evidence will take place in a hospital environment. For this reason, it's imperative that physicians and nurses present in emergency department situations be knowledgeable in recognizing and preserving relevant forensic evidence. This discussion is written with the objective of sensitizing the healthcare professional to physical evidence and to teach an appreciation of how to optimize the role science plays in criminal investigation.

Best Practice 11-1

The patient's body, hospital supplies and equipment, medical documentation, and the healthcare environment itself can be important sources of evidence in a criminal investigation. Nurses should be prepared to identify, protect, collect, preserve, and transmit certain items of evidentiary value.

Locard's Principle

Locard's principle states that when a person or object comes in contact with another person or object, there exists a possibility that an exchange of materials will take place. This exchange can prove very useful when investigating the circumstances surrounding a crime or accident. The presence or absence of physical evidence can corroborate or disprove a person's recollection of events. Physical evidence can implicate a person to the commission of a crime, or it can exonerate those wrongly suspected or accused. Physical evidence is an invaluable tool that law enforcement authorities use for the reconstruction of the circumstances surrounding the incident. However, evidence is of value in an investigation or in a court of law only if its integrity is upheld through careful handling, proper collection, and a documented chain of custody.

Chain of Custody

Chain of custody documents link each person who handles a piece of evidence. Transferring evidence from one person or one location to another must be accompanied with written documentation. The end result is a paper trail that records where the evidence was, on what date, and who held responsibility for it from the time it was collected until the time it is presented in court. It's best to use chain of custody forms designated by the organization one works for. This form should provide a clear and concise presentation for any exchanges of the physical evidence. Once an evidence container is selected for the evidence, whether it is a box, bag, vial, or can, it also must be marked for identification. A minimum record would show the collector's initials, location of the evidence, and date of collection. If the evidence is turned over to another individual for care or delivery to the laboratory, this transfer must be recorded in notes and other appropriate forms. In fact, every individual who has occasion to possess the evidence must maintain a written record of its acquisition and disposition. Frequently, all the individuals involved in the collection and transportation of the evidence may be requested to testify in court. Thus, to avoid confusion and to retain complete control of the evidence at all times, the chain of custody should be kept to a minimum. In the clinical setting, a locked evidence cabinet with one key should be used to maintain security of clinical evidence. The key should be kept by the evidence custodian, preferably the FNE on duty, and should never be turned over to another person without that person signing the chain of custody, in the same manner a narcotics key is managed.

Documentation of Evidence

The first step of proper evidence collection is thorough documentation. Descriptive notes and observations should be recorded as soon as possible. Make note of the condition in which the patient arrived, as well as how and when the patient came into the emergency department. If possible, encourage appropriate personnel to photograph the patient and each specific injured area prior to medical treatment. However, above all else, the foremost concern is the patent's health and well-being. No forensic protocol should inhibit a patent's care. Nevertheless, sensitivity on the part of attending medical personnel to potential forensic investigations may prevent the unnecessary destruction of vital evidence. If photography is a reasonable undertaking, one should avoid cleaning the wound area prior to photography. A patient's consent should be obtained before the photographs are taken so that legal complications regarding inadmissibility of evidence can be avoided. When a patient is unable to consent, try to obtain consent from a relative. It is important to document who gave the consent and their relationship to the patient. Current forensic protocol is to include permission to document injury with photography within the same line as permission to treat, thus having one form needing a signature.

Best Practice *11-2*

A consent form must be obtained prior to taking evidentiary photographs. Patient's parents, guardians, or other representative may provide consent if the patient is unable to do so.

Photodocumentation

Photographs of the patient should include the face, along with the injured areas. A photo log should be kept and should include pertinent information such as a patient's name, date, time, photographer's name, type and speed of film, and the specific exposure numbers. When an injured area is photographed, include an object of measurement for delineating the size of the injury. For example, placing a quarter next to a bullet hole will allow an investigator to easily interpret the size of the hole when viewing the photographs later. More ideally, an ABFO (American Board of Forensic Odontologists) ruler should be employed (see Chapter 16 and Appendix H). As the condition of the injured area changes, subsequent photographs should be taken to reflect such changes. Remember that the film and photographs will become part of the chain of custody. Therefore, they should be handled and documented in the appropriate manner. Along with photographs, handwritten notes describing injuries should also be taken.

Anatomical Charts and Diagrams

An anatomical chart is a handy tool to record all the marks on the body (Fig. 11-1). The description of each mark must include size, shape, color, location, and the characteristics of the edges around the wound. Also, the presence of any foreign material in or around the wound should be noted. Emergency department personnel are often one of the first human contacts a patient will encounter. Verbal statements made by the patient should be recorded using quotation marks. The value of thorough documentation will prove significant later during the investigation into what occurred. An inventory list that includes what items were collected, the time and location of collection, the name of the person who performed the collection, and the name and badge number of the officer who received the evidence should be maintained.

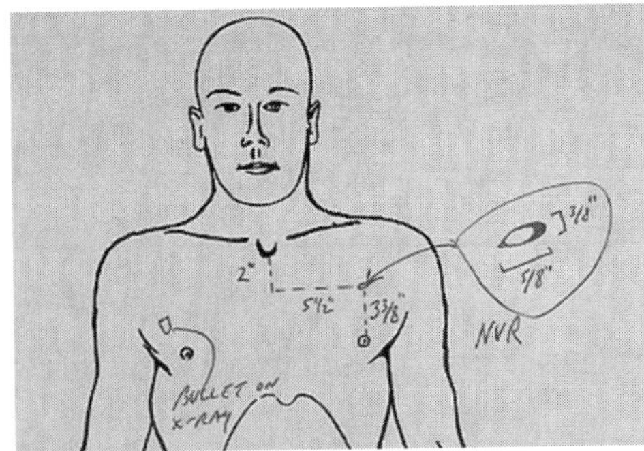

Fig. 11-1 Body map used to document location of gunshot wounds. Note that specific defects are annotated in relation to easily referenced anatomical landmarks.

Best Practice *11-3*

Hospital personnel must ensure an accurate inventory of all evidentiary items and observe strict chain of custody procedures.

Evidence Kits

Commercial evidence collections kits are a convenient and useful means for assuring the availability of appropriate evidence containers. Commercial evidence containers will also have appropriate chain of custody information printed on the outside of the container. The kit normally includes a variety of small metal cans for the collection of debris, paint chips, glass particles, or metal fragments. Paper envelopes of different sizes are present to package bullets, cartridge cases, or hairs and fibers. Ziploc bags provide packaging for soil samples, drugs, or dried plant materials, excluding clothing or biological material, which should be packaged in paper. Evidence seals are an important component of the kit. They seal the various containers within the kit so that evidence tampering is not possible. Any attempt to gain access to the container will require the obvious breaking and disruption of the seal (Fig. 11-2).

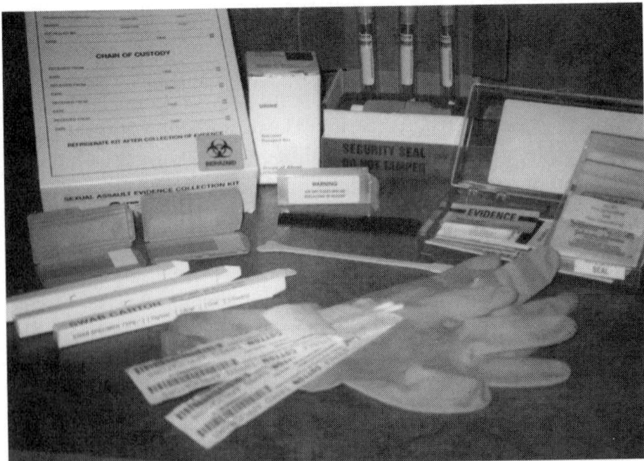

Fig. 11-2 Commercial forensic evidence kit with several types of containers for biological, physical, and trace evidence. The kit also contains tamper-proof tape, labels, and gloves.

Evidence on Clothing

The recognition of physical evidence is not always an easy task. Often, materials that are transferred from one object to another will exist in only trace amounts. However, by learning to recognize where and how such exchanges take place, emergency department personnel can aid in the collection and preservation of potential forensic evidence. In a hospital environment there probably is no more important an item of physical evidence than the patient's clothing. For example, a shooting victim's clothes may contain a multitude of information. When a bullet penetrates a piece of clothing, characteristic material is usually deposited on the garment. Partially burned and unburned gunpowder particles can be scattered around the bullet hole. The shape and distribution of these particles will reveal information about the distance between the firearm and the victim. For example, a shooting victim may claim to have been intentionally attacked. However, the assailant may claim the shooting was in self-defense and ensued during a struggle. Careful examination of the clothing surrounding the bullet hole may give some important clues. A minute amount of gunpowder residue given off by a firearm may refute the self-defense theory and suggest the weapon was fired at a significant distance between the shooter and the target. Even when no gunpowder residue is deposited on the garment, important information can be obtained from a dark ring, known as bullet wipe, surrounding the bullet hole. Bullet wipe is composed of material transferred from the surface of the bullet onto the target as the bullet passes through the fabric (Fig. 11-3).

Another piece of significant evidence that can be retrieved from bullet holes in clothing are the rip patterns caused by a penetrating bullet. When a firearm discharges within direct or very close contact with material a star-shaped rip pattern may characterize the bullet hole. Often, fibers surrounding the hole made by a contact or near-contact shot will be scorched or melted as a result of the heat from the discharge. Cuts in clothing arising from sharp objects such as a knife blade contain important forensic information. Careful laboratory examination may reveal the type of knife blade used or whether the assailant hesitated while inflicting the knife wound.

The removal of clothing from a patient must be performed in a careful and conscientious manner. Cutting along seams and away from the injured area will help reduce any interference with physical evidence. Whenever possible, cuts should not be made through bullet holes, stab wounds, or any rip or tear caused by a foreign object. In the case of a patient who is either dead on arrival or dying while in the emergency department, all clothing, including the shoes and any linen in contact with the patient, is kept with the body when it is turned over to the medical examiner. Whenever possible, leave any evidence in its original condition on the body. However, if transportation may lead to loss of evidence, properly collect and package those materials.

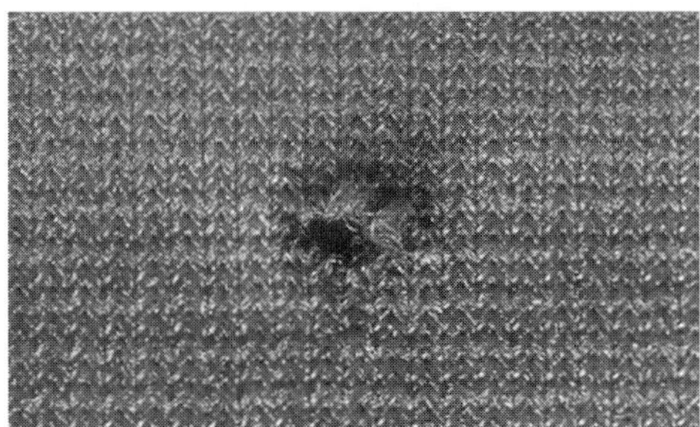

Fig. 11-3 Bullet wipe consisting of soot, carbon, and other soiling materials is noted on the bloody clothing of a shooting victim.

Best Practice *11-4*

Clothing should be cut away along seam lines and away from the injured area in order to protect the integrity of physical evidence. All clothing and clothing fragments must be retained as evidence.

Preservation of Clothing-Related Evidence

Crimes involving the contact of a victim with another person or object are particularly fertile for the retrieval of physical evidence. In keeping with Locard's principle that every contact leaves a trace, the clothing of a hit-and-run victim becomes a focus of attention. The blunt force placed upon the body by a vehicle will often leave an impression of the material on the car's surface. Therefore, the clothing will be helpful if a suspect vehicle is apprehended. Paint chips and debris could also dislodge during this type of accident. When removing the clothing, be aware of the possible presence of such debris. Anything that is found should be documented in detail as to where it was located (i.e., left pant leg), properly packaged, and labeled. After the clothing is removed, it should be placed in a paper bag. As has already been noted, paint chips are most likely to be found on or near persons or objects involved in hit-and-run incidents. The recovery of loose paint chips from a garment must be done with the utmost care to keep the paint chip intact. Paint chips may be picked up with a tweezers or scooped up with a piece of paper. Paper druggist folds and glass or plastic vials make excellent containers for paint. If the paint is smeared or embedded in garments or objects, the investigator should not attempt to remove it; instead, it is best to package the whole item carefully and send it on to the laboratory for examination (Fig. 11-4).

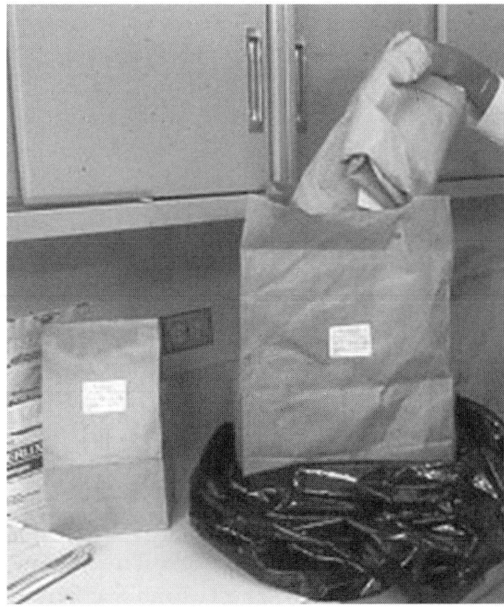

Fig. 11-4 This forensic nurse is ensuring that each evidentiary item is handled carefully and individually packaged in a paper bag.

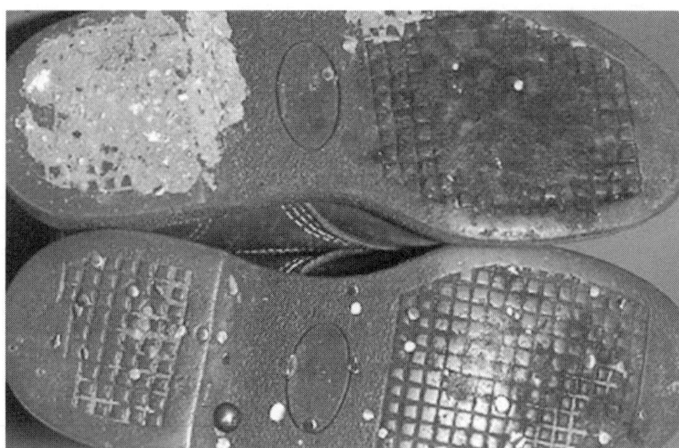

Fig. 11-5 These shoes must be handled with great care to ensure that important evidence is not altered or lost.

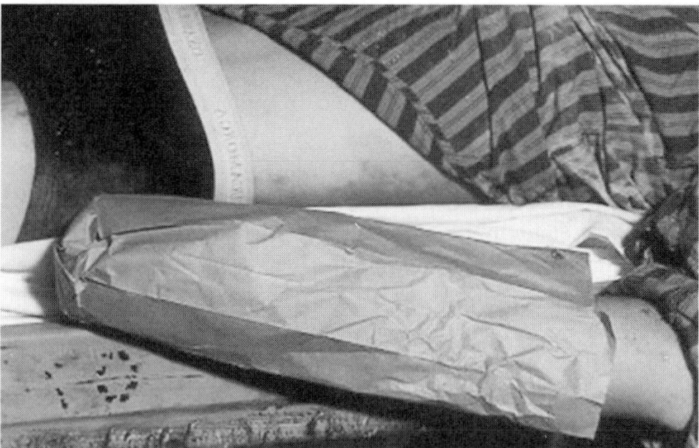

Fig. 11-6 Victims of firearm injuries should be protected by covering the hands with a paper bag to prevent the accidental loss of vital evidence.

Best Practice *11-5*

Each item of evidence must be packaged separately. The forensic scientist treats all objects placed in the same container as one evidentiary item. Each item of clothing or any physical evidence must be placed in its own separate container to maintain its forensic integrity.

If any article is wet or damp, air-dry it in a secured area. Never place clothing in plastic bags. A plastic container can cause moisture to accumulate that may destroy possible evidentiary materials. If possible, try not to fold the clothing. Paper should be placed between any materials that must be folded against each other. Each bag containing a piece of clothing should be labeled with pertinent information including a detailed description of its contents, patient's name, and the name of the person who collected the evidence, as well as the date and time the evidence was collected.

Package each item of clothing separately. It's important to remember that all objects placed in the same container are treated as one as far as the forensic scientist is concerned. Each item of clothing or any item of physical evidence must be placed in its own separate container in order to maintain its forensic identity (Fig. 11-5).

Best Practice *11-6*

All evidentiary items that have become wet or damp must be thoroughly air-dried before placement into a paper evidence bag or other suitable container.

In addition to collecting the clothing of a patient, precautions should be taken to preserve other types of evidence. Washing the hands or rubbing the hands against a foreign object will cause the removal of gunshot residues from the hand's surface. If circumstances permit, persons involved with a shooting, regardless if they are the alleged victim or assailant, should have their hands placed in paper bags that are sealed with tape to the wrist. This procedure prevents the loss of primer residue that may be present on the hands until an appropriate investigator can sample the hands (Fig. 11-6).

Preservation of Firearm Evidence

Bullets, cartridge casings, and other types of debris such as glass or metal fragments are sometimes found near or within a patient admitted into an emergency department. All such evidence is fragile, and necessary precautions need to be taken to ensure that all original conditions remain intact as much as possible. When bullets and other types of debris are collected, rubber-tipped forceps or gloved hands should be utilized. Do not wash bullets; rather, air dry them thoroughly before packaging. Recommended packaging for this type of evidence includes individual manila-clasp envelopes or Ziploc bags for each piece collected.

Case Study 11-1 Proper Handling of Evidence

A middle-aged man was admitted to a city trauma center with full- and partial-thickness burns over 25% of his body. The burns involved his chest, upper abdomen, and both arms. He said that he was preparing to light the grill for cooking when the fire flared and his clothing caught fire. He admittedly had been drinking prior to the incident. The emergency department forensic nurse (FN) on duty saved the burned shorts, T-shirt, and sneakers that the man was wearing. The FN placed each item of clothing into a separate paper bag and labeled them and ensured that photographs were taken and body diagrams marked to document the extent of the burn prior to debridement. While taking the close-up photos, the FN noted a small round hole in the man's left midthigh adjacent to, but not contained within, the burned tissue. The hole was surrounded by slight ecchymosis but minimal bleeding. It appeared to be an entrance point for a bullet, perhaps, but no associated wound was noted. An x-ray confirmed the presence of a bullet just anterior to the femur. A small plastic container and rubber-tipped forceps were taken to the operating room for the surgeon's use in extracting and collecting the bullet. Local law enforcement was called to further investigate the incident.

Other Physical and Trace Evidence

Glass Fragments

The gathering of glass evidence must be thorough if the examiner is to have any chance to individualize the fragments to a common source. If even the remotest possibility exists that fragments may be pieced together, every effort must be made to collect all the glass found. For example, collection of evidence at hit-and-run scenes must include all the broken parts of the headlight and reflector lenses. This evidence may ultimately prove to be an invaluable means of placing a suspect vehicle at the accident scene by actually matching the fragments with glass remaining in the headlight or reflector. If the person's shoes and clothing are to be examined for the presence of glass fragments, they should be individually wrapped in paper and transported to the laboratory. It is best that the field investigator avoid removing such evidence from garments unless it is thought absolutely necessary for its preservation.

Soil

Soil found on a victim or suspect must be carefully preserved for analysis. If it is found adhering to an object, as in the case of soil on a shoe, the evidence collector must not remove it. Instead, each object should be individually wrapped in paper bag, with the soil intact, and transmitted to the laboratory. Similarly, no effort should be made to remove loose soil adhering to garments; these items should be carefully wrapped individually in paper bags and sent to the laboratory for analysis. Care must be taken that all particles that may accidentally fall off the garment during transportation will remain within the paper bag. When a lump of soil is found, it should be collected and preserved intact. For example, an automobile tends to collect and build up layers of soil under fenders, body, and so on. In some situations, the impact of an automobile with another object may jar some of this soil loose. Soil found in this form imparts greater variation, and hence greater evidential value, than that which is normally associated with loose soil.

Hair

When questioned hairs are submitted to a forensic laboratory for examination, they must always be accompanied by an adequate number of control samples from the victim of the crime and from individuals suspected of having deposited hair at the crime scene. Hair from different parts of the body varies significantly in its physical characteristics. Likewise, hair from any one area of the body also can have a wide range of characteristics. For this reason, it is imperative that the questioned and control hairs come from the same area of the body; for instance, one cannot compare head hair to pubic hair. It is also important that the collection of control hair be carried out in a way to ensure a representative sampling of hair from any one area of the body.

As a general rule, forensic hair comparisons involve either head hair or pubic hair. The collection of 50 full-length hairs from all areas of the scalp will normally ensure a representative sampling of head hair. Likewise, a minimum collection of two dozen full-length pubic hairs should cover the range of characteristics present in this portion of the body. In rape cases, care must first be taken to comb the pubic area with a clean comb to remove all loose foreign hair present before the victim is sampled for control hair. The comb is to be packaged in a separate envelope. Typically, the evidence collector will have an evidence collection kit assembled or approved by the local forensic laboratory. This kit will contain combs and packaging envelopes necessary to facilitate the collection of evidence at a hospital site. Because a hair may show variation in color and other morphological features over its entire length, the entire hair length is collected. When examining a victim of a sexual assault, this requirement is best accomplished by clipping the hairs at the skin line. This approach is more desirable than pulling hairs out of the skin because it avoids additional discomfort for the victim. Current laboratory protocols for conducting hair comparisons do not necessitate that hair roots be associated with hair control exemplars.

Fiber

Fiber evidence can be associated with virtually any type of crime. It's the kind of evidence that will not usually be seen with the naked eye and thus can be easily missed by someone not specifically looking for it. In order to optimize the laboratory's chances for locating minute strands of fibers, the task becomes one of identifying and preserving potential "carriers" of fiber evidence. Relevant articles of clothing, including shoes, should be packaged carefully in paper bags. Each article must be placed in a separate bag to avoid the possibility of cross-contamination of evidence (Fig. 11-7). Scrupulous care must be taken to prevent articles of clothing from different people or from different locations from coming into contact with one another. Such articles must not even be placed on the same surface prior to their packaging. If a body is thought to have been wrapped at one time in a blanket or carpet, adhesive tape lifts of exposed body areas may reveal fiber strands upon examination in the laboratory.

Best Practice *11-7*

Items of clothing from different individuals should not be permitted to come into contact or to be placed on the same surface to prevent accidental transfer of hair, fibers, blood, or other vital evidence.

Occasionally, it may be necessary to remove a fiber from an object, particularly if the possibility exists that loosely adhering fibrous material will be lost in transit to the laboratory. These fibers must be removed with a clean forceps and placed in a small

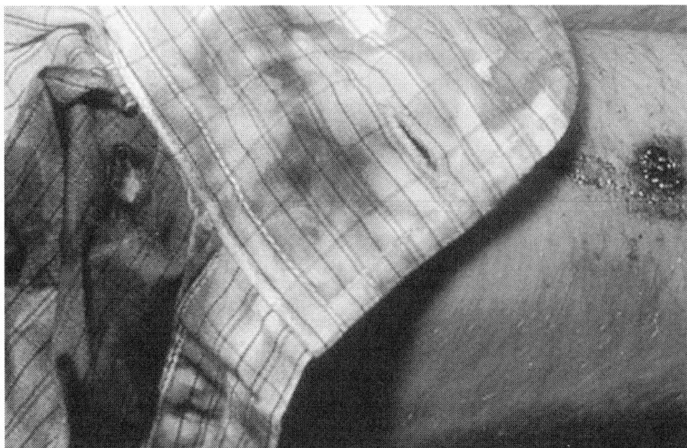

Fig. 11-7 Note the bullet hole and fire soot on this victim's shirt. After photographing the site, the bloody clothing item should be air-dried and packaged in a paper bag to prevent deterioration of evidence.

sheet of paper, which, after folding and labeling, can be placed inside another container. Again, scrupulous care must be taken to prevent fibers collected from different objects or from different locations from coming into contact with each other.

Arson Evidence

On occasion, hospital personnel may have to deal with an injured person who is suspected of being involved in the commission of the crime of arson. One important piece of evidence that is not to be overlooked by arson investigators is the clothing of the suspect perpetrator. If this individual is arrested within a few hours of initiating the fire, residual quantities of the accelerant may still be present in the clothing. The forensic laboratory can detect extremely small quantities of accelerate materials, making the examination of a suspect's clothing a feasible investigative approach. Each item of clothing should be placed in a separate airtight container, preferably a new, clean paint can. Paint cans are very convenient containers for this type of evidence as they are airtight, unbreakable, and unreactive with volatile hydrocarbons.

Best Practice *11-8*

Clothing suspected of containing hydrocarbon residues should never be placed in plastic bags, as the plastic will react with the vapors and ultimately consume trace quantities of petroleum residues that may be present on the garment.

Sexual Assault Evidence

The finding of seminal constituents in a rape victim is important evidence for substantiating the fact that sexual intercourse has taken place, but their absence does not necessarily mean that a rape did not occur. Physical injuries such as bruises or bleeding tend to confirm the fact that a violent assault did take place. Furthermore, there is a distinct possibility that the forceful physical contact between victim and assailant will result in a transfer of physical evidence–that is, blood, semen, hairs, and fibers. The presence of such physical evidence will help forge a vital link in the chain of circumstances surrounding a sexual crime.

To protect this kind of evidence, all the outer- and undergarments from the involved parties should be carefully removed and packaged separately in paper (not plastic) bags. The packaging of biological evidence in plastic or airtight containers must always be avoided, because the accumulation of residual moisture could contribute to the growth of DNA-destroying bacteria and fungi. Each potentially stained article should be packaged separately in a paper bag or in a well-ventilated box. If the rape victim can stand to disrobe, a number of precautions should be implemented. Place a clean bed sheet on the floor and lay a clean paper sheet over it. The victim must remove her shoes before standing on the paper. Have the person disrobe while standing on the paper in order to collect any loose foreign material falling from the clothing. Collect each piece of clothing as it is removed and place it in separate paper bags in order to avoid cross-contamination of physical evidence. Carefully fold the paper sheet so that all foreign materials will be contained inside.

Items suspected of containing seminal stains must be handled carefully. Folding an article through the stain may cause it to flake off, as will rubbing the stained area against the surface of the packaging material. If, under unusual circumstances, it is not possible to transport the stained article to the laboratory, the stained area should be cut out and submitted with an unstained piece as a substrate control.

In the laboratory, efforts will be made to link seminal material to a donor(s) by utilizing DNA typing. The fact that individuals may transfer his or her DNA types to a stain through the medium of perspiration requires that investigators handle stained articles with care, minimizing direct personal contact.

The evidence collector must handle all body fluids and biologically stained materials with a minimal amount of personal contact. All body fluids must be assumed to be infectious; hence, wearing disposable gloves while handling the evidence is required. Gloves will also significantly reduce the possibility that the evidence collector will contaminate the evidence.

The rape victim must undergo a medical examination as soon as possible after the assault. At this time, trained personnel collect the appropriate items of physical evidence. It is to be expected that evidence collectors will have an evidence collection kit that has been disseminated by the local crime laboratory (see Fig. 11-2). Box 11-1 highlights items of physical evidence to collect from the rape victim.

When collecting pubic hair combings, the examiner should place a paper towel under the buttocks and comb the pubic area for loose or foreign hairs. The pubic hair control samples must be clipped close to the skin line. Two dozen full-length hairs from the pubic area are recommended for a suitable exemplar sample. The genital area and the inner thighs should be swabbed with two lightly moistened applicators. After the collection is made, the swabs must be air-dried for approximately 5 to 10 minutes before placement in a swab box that has holes to permit air circulation. The swab box can then be placed in a paper or manila container for transmission to the crime laboratory. The vaginal area should be swabbed with two applicators. These swabs should also be air-dried before packaging. Using two additional swabs, repeat the swabbing procedure and smear the swabs onto separate microscope slides, allowing them to air-dry before packaging in a swab box. Collected swabs must never be packaged while moist. If the history warrants rectal swabs or smears, the perianal area should be swabbed with two lightly moistened applicators in order to prevent contamination of the rectal swabs from vaginal fluid drainage that may be present on the anus. Two swabs should be done simultaneously; swab the rectal canal, smearing one of the swabs onto a microscope slide. Allow both swabs to air-dry before

Box 11-1 Evidence to Collect from a Rape Victim

- Pubic combings
- Pubic hair controls
- Genital and thigh swabs
- Vaginal swabs and smear
- Rectal swabs and smear
- Oral swabs and smear
- Head hair
- Blood sample
- Fingernail scrapings
- Urine specimen
- All clothing worn at the time of the attack

packaging in a swab box. If oral-genital contact has occurred, two swabs should be used simultaneously to swab the buccal area and gum line. Using both swabs, prepare one smear slide. Allow both swabs and the one smear to air-dry before packaging in a swab box. Head hair exemplars should be clipped at the skin line. A minimum of five full-length hairs should be obtained from each of the following scalp locations: center, front, back, left side, and right side. It is recommended that a total of at least 50 hairs be clipped and submitted to the laboratory. Blood samples are collected in sterile vacuum tubes containing the preservative EDTA (ethylenediamine tetraacetic acid). EDTA inhibits the activity of enzymes that act to degrade DNA. The blood samples can be used for DNA typing, as well as for toxicological analysis if it is required. Prior to delivery to the laboratory, the tubes must be kept refrigerated (do not freeze) while awaiting transportation to the laboratory. Besides blood, there are other options for obtaining control DNA specimens. The least intrusive DNA control specimen that can readily be used by nonmedical personnel is the buccal swab. Here, cotton swabs are placed in the subject's mouth and the inside of the cheek is vigorously swabbed, resulting in the transfer of buccal cells onto the swab (Fig. 11-8).

Fingernail scrapings are obtained by scraping the undersurface of the nails with a dull object over a piece of clean paper to collect debris. A separate paper should be used for each hand. Thirty milliliters or more of urine should be collected from the victim for the purpose of conducting a drug toxicological analysis for Rohypnol, GHB (gamma hydroxybutyrate), and other substances associated with drug-facilitated sexual assaults. Finally, all clothing should be carefully packaged as described earlier.

Often during the investigation of a sexual assault, the victim will report that a perpetrator engaged in biting, sucking, or licking areas of the victim's body. The high sensitivity associated with DNA technology offers investigators the opportunity to identify a perpetuator's DNA types from saliva residues collected off the skin. The most efficient way to recover saliva residues from the skin is to first swab the suspect area with a rotating motion using a cotton swab moistened with distilled water. A second swab, which is dry, is then rotated over the skin to recover the moist remains on the skin's surface from the wet swab. The swabs are air-dried and packaged together as a single sample.

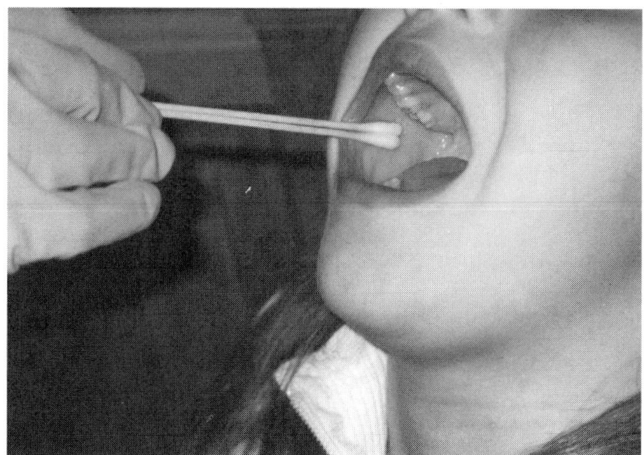

Fig. 11-8 DNA evidence can be obtained by a buccal swab. Two swabs are used to collect cells from inside the cheek and along the gum line. (Photo courtesy of Eileen Allen, MSN, RN, FN-CSA, SANE-A.)

If a suspect is apprehended, the following items are routinely collected:

- All clothing items believed to have been worn at the time of assault
- Pubic hair combings
- Pulled head and pubic hair controls
- A blood or buccal swab sample
- Penile swab (taken within 24 hours of assault when appropriate)

The persistence of seminal constituents in the vagina may become a factor when trying to ascertain the time of an alleged sexual attack. Although the presence of spermatozoa in the vaginal cavity provides evidence of intercourse, important information regarding the time of sexual activity can be obtained from the knowledge that motile or living sperm may generally survive four to six hours in the vaginal cavity of a living person. However, a successful search for motile sperm requires that a microscopic examination of a vaginal smear be conducted immediately after it is taken from the victim. A more extensive examination of vaginal collections is later made at a forensic laboratory. Nonmotile sperm may be found in a living female for up to three days after intercourse and occasionally up to six days. However, intact sperm (sperm with tails) are rarely found 16 hours after intercourse but have been found as late as 72 hours after intercourse. The likelihood of finding seminal acid phosphatase in the vaginal cavity markedly decreases with time following intercourse, with little chance of identifying this substance 48 hours after intercourse (Davies, 1974). Hence, taking into consideration the possibility of the prolonged persistence of both spermatozoa and acid phosphatase in the vaginal cavity after intercourse, investigators should seek information to determine when and if voluntary sexual activity last occurred prior to the sexual assault. This information will be useful for evaluating the significance of a find of these seminal constituents in the female victim. Blood or buccal swabs for DNA analysis are to be taken from any consensual partner having sex with the victim within 72 hours of the assault.

Another significant indicator of recent sexual activity is protein p30. This semen marker is normally not detected in the vaginal cavity beyond 24 hours following intercourse. See Chapters 17 and 26 for complete discussions of sexual assault evidence collection.

Summary

An emergency hospital environment is not always controlled and organized. It does require that top priority be given to the immediate care and lifesaving interventions for the patient. In situations involving the medical treatment of victims and perpetrators of crime, physical evidence must be collected, documented, and preserved properly for subsequent laboratory examination. This book is testimony to the fact that relevant healthcare personnel, primarily the forensic nurse examiner, are becoming integral participants in the evidence collection process. Hopefully, the material contained within this chapter will provide useful guidance to the proper fulfillment of this objective.

Key Point *11-2*

It is vital that nurses be familiar with local and state guidelines regarding the collection and packaging of physical evidence.

Resources

Organizations

American Academy of Forensic Sciences

410 North 21st Street, Colorado Spring, CO 80904; Tel: 719-636-1100; www.aafs.org

American College of Forensic Examiners, Inc.

2750 East Sunshine, Springfield, MO 65804; Tel: 800-423-9737; www.acfei.com

Federal Bureau of Investigation

935 Pennsylvania Avenue NW, Room 7350, Washington, DC 20535; Tel: 202-324-3000; www.fbi.gov

Journals

Journal of Forensic Sciences

Journal of the American Academy of Forensic Sciences, Michael A. Peat, PhD, Editor, 7151 West 135th Street, PMB 410, Overland Park, KS 66223

Journal of Clinical Forensic Medicine

Journal of the Association of Police Surgeons, Journal Subscription Department, Harcourt Publishers, Foots Cray High Street, Sidcup, Kent DA14 5HP, UK

References

Davies, A., & Wilson, E. (1974). Persistence of seminal constituents in the human vagina. *Forensic Sci, 3*, 45.

Fisher, B. J. (2004). *Techniques of crime scene investigation* (7th ed.). Boca Raton, FL: CRC Press.

Kearsey, J., Louie, H., & Poon, H. (2001). Validation study of the Onestep ABAcard PSA Test Kit for RCMP casework. *Canadian Society of Forensic Science Journal, 34*, 63.

Ogle, R. R., Jr. (2004). *Crime scene investigation and reconstruction.* Upper Saddle River, NJ: Prentice-Hall.

Saferstein, R. (2004). *Criminalistics: An introduction to forensic science* (8th ed.). Upper Saddle River, NJ: Prentice-Hall.

Saferstein, R., ed. (2002). *Forensic science handbook , Vol. 1* (2nd ed.). Upper Saddle River, NJ: Prentice-Hall.

Saferstein, R., ed. (2005). *Forensic science handbook , Vol. 2*, (2nd ed.). Upper Saddle River, NJ: Prentice-Hall.

Sweet, D., Lorente, M., Lorente, J. A., et al. (1997). An improved method to recover saliva from human skin: The double swab technique. *J Forensic Sci, 42*, 320.

Chapter 12 Biological Evidence in Criminal Investigations

Henry C. Lee and Carll Ladd

Beginning in the 1960s, crime rates in the US rose dramatically. As a result, the public has become increasingly concerned about the impact of crime in our society. Americans place "crime and lawlessness" at the top of the list of national problems (Lee & Ladd, 1997). Crime rates, though decreasing significantly in the last decade, remain unacceptably high. The amount of violent crime is staggering. Nationwide, over 1 million aggravated assaults and sexual assaults are reported to the police each year. Justice department victimization surveys place the number even higher (Uniform Crime Reports, 2002).

During this time of growing public concern about crime, physical evidence has become increasingly important in criminal investigations. Courts often view eyewitness accounts as unreliable or biased. Physical evidence such as DNA, fingerprints, and trace evidence may independently and objectively link a suspect or victim to a crime or develop important investigative leads. Likewise, physical evidence may also prove invaluable for exonerating the innocent.

The natural consequence of its greater emphasis is increased legal scrutiny. Evidence integrity begins with the first investigator at the scene. Celebrated court cases (e.g., O. J. Simpson and Jon Benet Ramsey cases in the US) highlight standard challenges to the use of physical evidence in criminal investigations and suggest that even greater scrutiny of evidence collection, preservation, and handling is forthcoming. The entire case may be jeopardized if evidence is mishandled during the initial stages of the investigation. Indeed, physical evidence that is not properly recognized, documented, collected, and preserved may ultimately be of no probative value. Physical evidence is generally classified as biological, chemical, or pattern evidence (imprints, impressions, etc.). This chapter reviews the use of physiological evidence–recognition, collection and preservation, identification and individualization, and legal challenges–in criminal investigations.

Sources of Biological Evidence

Biological evidence has been associated with a wide variety of crimes, but is typically seen with violent crimes such as homicide, assault, sexual assault, child abuse, and hit and run accidents (Lee, Palmbach, & Miller, 2001). Common sources of biological evidence submitted to forensic laboratories can be found in Box 12-1.

Modes of Evidence Transfer

The sources of biological evidence (see Box 12-1) can be used to link one individual to another, to a piece of physical evidence, or to a crime scene. In addition, the evidence may substantiate or disprove an alibi, or may assist with crime scene reconstruction. In general, biological evidence can be transferred by direct deposit or by secondary transfer.

Box 12-1 Sources of Biological Evidence

- Blood and bloodstains
- Semen and seminal stains
- Tissues and organs
- Bones and teeth
- Hairs and nails
- Saliva, urine, and other body fluids

Direct Deposit

Blood, semen, body tissue, bone, hair, urine, and saliva can be transferred to an individual's body or clothing, to an object, or to a crime scene by direct deposit or direct contact. Once liquid biological materials are deposited, they adhere to the surface or the substratum and become stains. Nonfluid biological evidence, such as tissue, bone, or hair, can also be transferred by direct contact with the primary source.

Secondary Transfer

Blood, semen, tissue, hair, saliva, and urine can be transferred to a victim, suspect, witness, object, or location through an intermediary. With secondary transfer, there is no direct contact between the original source (donor of the biological evidence) and the target surface. For example, a rape victim's clothing bearing seminal fluid may rub against a car seat and subsequently be transferred to a second individual who sat in the same vehicle. Another example of secondary transfer is a person who picks up a victim's hair from the suspect's vehicle and then deposits the hair in another location. The transfer intermediary can be a person, an object, or a scene. The secondary transfer of physical evidence may, but does not *necessarily*, establish a direct link between an individual and a specific crime.

Collection and Preservation of Biological Evidence

Key Point *12-1*

Unless the evidence is properly recognized, documented, collected, packaged, and preserved, it will not meet the legal or scientific requirements for admissibility into a court of law.

The ability to successfully analyze biological evidence recovered from a crime scene, person, or object depends greatly on the types of specimens collected and how they are preserved. Thus, the technique used to collect and document such evidence, the quantity and type of evidence that should be collected, the way the evidence should be handled and packaged, and how the evidence should be preserved are some of the critical issues in a criminal investigation. Unless the evidence is properly recognized, documented, collected, packaged, and preserved, it will not meet the legal or scientific requirements for admissibility into a court of law. If the evidence is not properly documented prior to collection, its origin can be questioned. If it is improperly collected or packaged, cross-contamination may occur. Finally, if the evidence is not properly preserved, sample degradation may result. Therefore, it is extremely important to follow established procedures and use standardized techniques to collect and preserve biological evidence. Many publications discuss the collection and analysis of biological evidence in detail.

Collection of Sexual Assault Kit Evidence

The collection of the sexual assault kit warrants special consideration. Unlike most other crimes for which typically the police collect the evidence, victims of child abuse and sexual assault are examined by medical professionals in hospitals, clinics, or rape crisis centers. Critical biological evidence is subsequently collected by medical personnel who historically have been less familiar with the forensic legal issues pertaining to chain of custody and evidence collection. For the successful resolution of a criminal investigation, it is essential that all medical personnel attending sexual assault victims have the requisite knowledge and experience to recognize, collect, and preserve potential evidence for medical and forensic analysis. In addition, communication and cooperation between hospital staff, police, and the forensic laboratory is extremely important.

Body fluid evidence, especially seminal fluid, is commonly associated with sexual assaults and plays a particularly important role in the successful prosecution of these crimes (De Forest, Gaensslen, & Lee, 1983). For example, the identification of semen recovered from the vagina or other orifice is taken by the courts as proof of penetration–one possible element in proving that rape occurred. Other sources of biological material such as blood, hair, and saliva have also been very important in child abuse, assault, homicide, and sexual assault cases.

Best Practice *12-1*

The forensic nurse should describe and sketch on a body diagram and photograph the location of any possible injury, trace evidence, or blood/body fluid stains on the victim. Any bite marks, bruises, and abrasions should be included in this documentation process.

After the patient's health concerns are addressed, it is important that the examining physician or nurse thoroughly document all rape kit evidence upon collection to meet legal admissibility requirements. Describe and sketch or photograph the location of any possible injury, trace evidence, or blood and bodily fluid stains on the victim. Note potential bite marks, bruises, abrasions, and similar injuries. Whether the evidence is listed as a "stain on the victim's thigh" or documented as an "apparent bloody-seminal smear on the left inner thigh approximately 6 inches from the genital region," can significantly affect both the charges that are levied and the disposition of the case in court. It is also important to document (sketch and photograph) any pattern evidence on the victim's clothing such as cuts, tears, blood spatter, smears, and stains. Carefully collect the victim's clothing to minimize the loss of important trace evidence such as blood crusts, hair, and fibers and preserve any pattern evidence. It is often useful to have the victim disrobe over a large piece of clean paper. If clothing must be cut from the victim, avoid cutting or damaging any possible damaged areas, bullet or knife holes, and stained areas. All items of evidence be must be packaged *separately*. The evidentiary value may be seriously compromised if several articles of clothing or other evidence are packaged together. In addition, wet clothing must be air-dried prior to packaging in paper. Under no circumstances should the evidence be packaged in plastic or any airtight container; this causes samples to retain moisture, thus promoting bacterial growth.

Interview the victim and record a detailed account of the incident. Essential information includes when the assault took place and whether the victim changed clothes, showered, or otherwise cleaned up. The victim's recent sexual history (within the last 72 hours) should also be noted. References samples should be obtained from the previous consensual partner(s) for comparison purposes.

A number of sexual assault kits are commercially available that facilitate the evidence collection process. It is important that evidence be collected according to the instructions or other applicable guidelines. Typical specimens collected are listed in Box 12-2.

For each jurisdiction, a standardized collection protocol should be developed in conjunction with law enforcement, forensic scientists, and hospital staff. Routinely, vaginal and genital swabbings are collected. It is useful to place the swabs in a specially designed cardboard swab collection box (Fig. 12-1). Swab other areas as warranted by the examination, or as indicated by the victim. To minimize the recovery of skin cells from the body, collect any blood/body fluid stains as gently as possible. This collection can be accomplished by lightly swabbing the stained area. Pubic combings are regularly collected to identify evidence (foreign hairs, fibers) that could have been transferred from the perpetrator. Fingernail scrapings or clippings are collected where indicated by the assault. Here, too, it is important to avoid applying excessive force in this process to minimize collecting the victim's blood and skin. The victim's clothing (worn at the time of the assault) may have biological evidence or other physical evidence from the assailant. For example, seminal fluid may be deposited directly on the victim's clothing or may drain onto the undergarments. Drainage stains are relatively common. With time, it becomes progressively more difficult to detect semen within the vagina. Hence,

Box 12-2 Sexual Assault Kit Evidence Collected for Forensic Examination

- Swabs and stains (genital, vaginal, oral, anal)
- Clothing of the victim (or suspect)
- Foreign hair (head and pubic), fibers, other trace materials
- Known hair and fiber samples
- Reference blood and saliva samples (victim/suspect)
- Fingernail scrapings/clippings
- Other (specify)

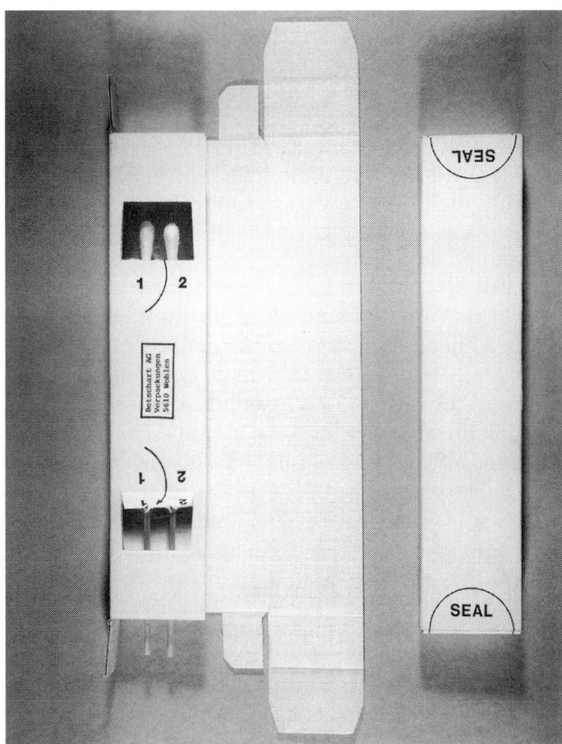

Fig. 12-1 Example of a swab collection box recommended for evidentiary examinations. (Courtesy of Dr. Manfred Hochmeister, Department Forensic Medicine, Uni Bern, Buehlstr. 20, Bern CH-3012, Switzerland.)

any drainage stains on the underpants can be pivotal evidence. Label all items accordingly.

Finally, to maintain the proper chain of custody, the evidence must be stored securely until it's transferred to a forensic laboratory. Refrigerate the evidence when necessary. A cool, dry environment is optimal for preserving biological samples. Moisture and heat can promote bacterial growth, which may seriously degrade the sample. All sexual assault kit evidence should be submitted for forensic testing as soon as possible.

Collection of Biological Evidence in Other Crimes

Many of the procedures described here apply to the recognition, collection, and preservation of biological evidence by medical personnel from victims (or suspects) of other violent crimes (e.g., homicide, assault, and child abuse) that often require medical attention. Furthermore, with these crimes, as with sexual assaults, biological evidence may be deposited on the body or clothing.

Key Point *12-2*

In a statutory sexual assault case, the products of conception can serve as proof of the crime. Samples include maternal and fetal blood and the aborted tissues.

Statutory sexual assaults, which have been vigorously prosecuted in recent years, may also involve evidence collection by medical personnel. Routinely, sexual assault kits are not collected because statutory sexual assaults may not be reported until weeks or months after the incident. However, because consent cannot be a defense, the product of conception is proof of the crime. Thus, the samples collected are typically blood (child and parents) or the abortus. In the event of an abortion, place the sample in a specimen jar and submit the evidence for forensic testing as soon as possible. It is vital that the specimen not be placed in any preservative, such as formalin, which will seriously degrade DNA. In addition, with termination of pregnancy early in the first trimester, it may be useful to send the sample to the medical examiner to identify tissue of fetal origin.

Best Practice *12-2*

When collecting the products of conception as evidence, they must be placed in a specimen jar without preservatives because preservative agents, such as formalin, seriously degrade DNA.

History of Biological Evidence Examination

Serological Testing

The identification of an individual by analyzing biological material such as blood, semen, hair, bone, and other materials has been reported in forensic science literature since 1904 (Gaensslen, 1983). Over the years, numerous red blood cell antigen systems, isoenzyme markers, red blood cell protein variants, serum protein markers, and human leukocyte antigens (HLAs) have been characterized and applied to forensic work (Lee, 1982; 1991; 1995). Historically, variation has been detected either by antigen-antibody reactions such as the ABO blood group system and secretor status, Rh blood typing system, HLA histocompatibility antigens, or by the electrophoretic separation of isoenzymes and proteins such as PGM, ADA, or GC variants (Gaensslen & Lee, 1984; Lee & Gaensslen, 1985; Gaensslen, Desio, & Lee, 1986).

DNA Testing

In the past decade, DNA typing procedures have become increasingly important in the fields of forensic science and forensic medicine (Lee, Gaensslen, & Pagliaro et al., 1994; 1998). Several DNA typing methods have been widely implemented for forensic use. If one adheres to applicable national guidelines and standards (DNA Advisory Board Standards, 1998), DNA analysis is generally considered reliable. DNA evidence and testimony are now accepted by the courts and greatly assist in the resolution of criminal and civil investigations.

Genetic variation can be detected by many DNA-typing techniques including restriction fragment length polymorphism (RFLP) analysis, polymerase chain reaction (PCR), and DNA sequencing. Developments over the past decade, such as more sensitive and discriminating PCR typing methods, the felon DNA data bank, and increased federal and state funding, have greatly enhanced DNA typing in forensic casework. Figure 12-2 offers an overview of methods utilized in forensic biology for the identification and individualization of biological evidence.

DNA typing was first used for criminal investigations in 1985 in the UK and was first applied to casework in the US by late 1986, with widespread use of DNA testing occurring in the 1990s. Today,

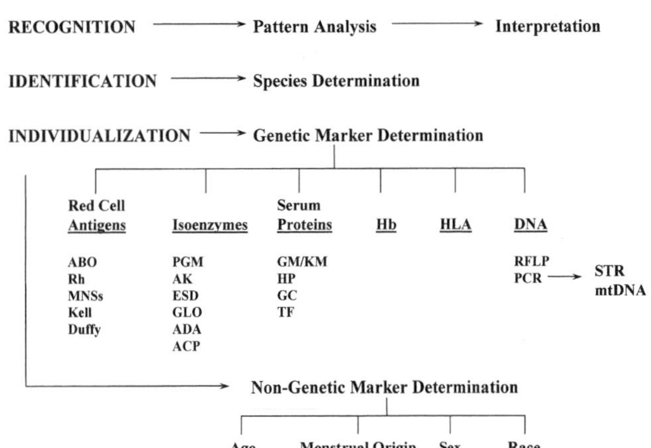

Fig. 12-2 Methods used to analyze biological evidence include recognition, identification, and individualization (genetic and nongenetic).

more than 130 laboratories in the US, both public and private, perform forensic DNA analysis. Each year, over 40,000 DNA cases are processed by these facilities (CODIS Statistics, 2003). The two major applications of DNA typing in forensic science are paternity testing and criminal investigation. The former application, because it deals with fresh blood samples, is relatively straightforward. However, because the quality of DNA samples from criminal cases is generally unpredictable, the latter application has been challenged more vigorously. Several national and international committees have been formed to address the use of DNA in criminal cases, and extensive studies have been conducted (US Congress, 1990; Committee of DNA Technology in Forensic Science, 1992; Committee on DNA Forensic Science, 1996).

Laboratory Analysis of Biological Evidence

Prior to the widespread use of DNA testing in crime laboratories, forensic serological testing was employed to identify the source of the biological evidence, to determine if the sample is of human origin, and then to include (or exclude) an individual as a potential source of the sample. As more forensic laboratories developed DNA testing capabilities over the past decade, serological methods (especially ABO blood grouping and isoenzyme typing) have been significantly scaled back or eliminated. Today, serological analysis is generally limited to identifying the type of biological evidence collected. Subsequently, the evidence is individualized–it is linked to (or excluded from) a particular person by DNA typing.

Serological Methods for Identifying Body Fluids

The process of examining items for the presence of biological evidence begins with recognizing and identifying likely candidates for further testing. Various screening tests can determine if a stain could be blood, saliva, semen, or other body fluid. Even if not diagnostic for a particular body fluid, evidence screening saves considerable time and money. Second, confirmatory tests conclusively demonstrate the presence of a specific body fluid. Last, the body fluid is individualized.

Screening tests for blood are based on the reaction of the heme component of hemoglobin with chemicals such as *o*-toluidine, phenolphthalein (Kastle-Meyer), luminol, and tetramethylbenzidine. These tests are extremely sensitive. However, false positive results are possible. A positive reaction with any of these reagents indicates that the sample *could* be blood. Microcrystal tests such as the Takayama test confirm the presence of blood but do not indicate the species of origin (could be animal blood). The presence of *human* blood can be determined using an immunological method that tests for human hemoglobin. This one-step procedure is the preferred method when sample quantity is limited.

A common screening method for semen is the acid phosphatase (AP) test. Acid phosphatase is present in high levels in semen but can also be found in other substances such as plant matter. In addition, lower levels of AP can be found in other biological samples (e.g., vaginal secretions, saliva, and fecal matter). The presence of semen can be confirmed by identifying sperm microscopically or by detecting the human seminal protein p30.

Detection of the enzyme amylase indicates the presence of saliva. Other tests may be conducted to identify biological substances such as urine, gastric fluid, and fecal matter. Hairs are examined microscopically and compared to reference samples from the victim and suspect.

DNA Testing of Biological Evidence

The forensic use of DNA constitutes a major advancement in the examination of biological evidence. DNA draws importance from its tremendous discriminating power and its stability. The ability to differentiate between individuals using genetic markers can be pivotal to the successful investigation of many crimes. This very strength is, though, also a prime reason that DNA has been challenged so vigorously in court.

Challenges to DNA Admissibility

Since their introduction into forensic science, DNA typing methods have been strenuously attacked in numerous protracted court battles. Initially, the general reliability of DNA typing procedures was questioned along with the statistical methods used to calculate DNA profile frequencies. In the last few years, legal challenges regarding the admissibility of DNA have clearly shifted their focus away from the general reliability of the methods. Although most courts accept the basic methodology behind DNA analysis, some defense objections regarding DNA evidence continue to be effective. Indeed, as with biological evidence generally, the few remaining challenges to the admissibility of DNA testing in court involve the initial collection, preservation, and subsequent handling of the biological evidence. A second type of challenge concedes that DNA typing methods are reliable *in theory*. Here, the defense argues that critical mistakes were made in testing which should invalidate the findings. With this strategy, typically the specific protocols and technical expertise of a particular laboratory or analyst are scrutinized.

Sources of DNA

Evidence that is suitable for DNA typing (with the exception of mitochondrial DNA, mtDNA) is limited to biological samples containing nucleated cells (see Box 12-1). Note that conventional DNA typing is possible only on hairs with roots. The hair shaft does not contain nuclei and can be typed only by mtDNA analysis. Other types of biological evidence, such as tears, perspiration, serum, and other body fluids without nucleated cells, are not amenable to standard DNA analysis. DNA has been isolated from materials such as gastric fluids and fecal stains. However, it is difficult to obtain sufficient DNA from these sources in case samples. It should also be noted that although DNA can often be recovered from the specimens mentioned in Box 12-1, in many cases the quality or quantity of the sample proves inadequate for DNA analysis.

Several factors affect the ability to obtain DNA typing results. The first issue is sample quantity. DNA typing methods (especially PCR-based tests) are very sensitive, but not infinitely so. The second factor is sample degradation. For example, prolonged exposure of even a large blood stain to the environment or to bacterial contamination can degrade the DNA and render it unsuitable for further analysis. It is important to note, however, that degradation will not change DNA profile "A" into profile "B." The third consideration is sample purity. Even though most DNA typing methods are robust, dirt, grease, some dyes in fabrics, and other elements can seriously inhibit the DNA typing process (Lee, Ladd, & Scherczinger et al., 1998).

Genetic Variation and Forensic DNA Typing

Two different classes of genetic variation are exploited by forensic DNA typing methods: sequence variation (single base changes) and length differences produced by variable number of tandem repeats (VNTRs). Important features of the two classes are illustrated in Figures 12-3 and 12-4.

VNTRs are currently the most common type of variation studied in forensic DNA analysis. Many well-characterized genetic regions (loci) contain core elements (sets of nucleotides) that are tandemly repeated. The number of these repeated units can vary from person to person. The size of the core repeat also varies between loci. Restriction enzyme recognition sites flank the repeats. Following restriction endonuclease digestion, which cuts the DNA molecules at specific sites, DNA fragments ranging in size from 500 to 22,000 base pairs (bp) long are resolved by agarose gel electrophoresis. This process is termed restriction fragment length polymorphism (RFLP) and is the oldest DNA typing method employed for both criminal and paternity cases.

Polymerase Chain Reaction

The ability to amplify small segments of DNA by PCR constitutes one of the more significant developments in molecular biology. PCR has facilitated revolutionary advances in many scientific disciplines and has proved an invaluable tool in biological research as well as in the diagnosis of genetic disorders and infectious diseases.

PCR was invented in 1985 and was subsequently adapted to forensic science. The procedure amplifies (duplicates) small segments of DNA and has been called "molecular photocopying." At the end of the process, the target DNA molecule has been amplified 1 million to 10 million times.

As a forensic tool, PCR-based strategies have several advantages over RFLP analysis. First, PCR requires only trace quantities of DNA. Typically, approximately 1 to 10 ng of human DNA is optimal for PCR, compared with 300 to 500 ng for RFLP typing. Consequently, PCR permits DNA typing of minute samples, even a single hair root or a cigarette butt containing epithelial cells. Second, PCR generates a large quantity of product in a very short period, considerably less time than that required for typing by RFLP analysis. Third, degradation of the DNA sample is less of a concern when using PCR because it amplifies small segments of DNA. In contrast, RFLP typing requires samples with predominantly high-molecular-weight DNA (relatively undegraded) because the DNA fragments analyzed by RFLP are much larger.

Type 1	AATTCGGAATTGC
Type 2	AATTCGG**T**ATTGC
Type 3	AATT**G**GGAATTGC

Fig. 12-3 Sequence variation. Variant bases are in boldface. Only one strand of the double helix is shown.

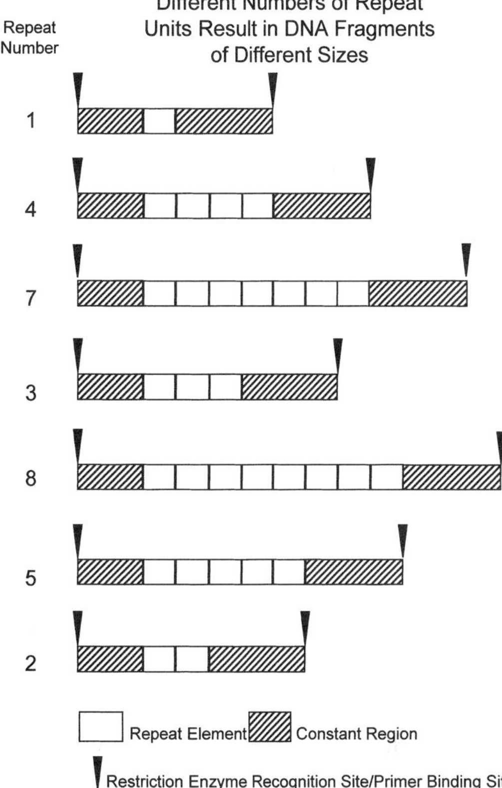

Fig. 12-4 Genetic variations at VNTR loci. With RFLP systems, restriction enzyme sites flank the repeats. With PCR tests, primers bind to flanking sequences in the constant region.

The first PCR tests routinely used for forensic purposes were DQA1, Polymarker (PM), and D1S80. Unlike RFLP tests, DQA1 and PM alleles display sequence variation that are detected by a colorimetric assay. DQA1 and PM DNA profiles are determined by a pattern of blue dots that develops. D1S80 typing, also called amplified fragment length polymorphism (AMP-FLP) analysis is a PCR-based DNA-typing strategy that detects length variation. D1S80 alleles contain different numbers of repeats, similar to RFLP. These three PCR systems are very sensitive; hence, they permit the analysis of minute samples. However, they are much less discriminating than RFLP.

Short Tandem Repeats

The primary DNA typing methods employed by the forensic community involves the analysis of short tandem repeats (STRs) by several fluorescent detection methods (Holt, Buoncristiani, & Wallin et al., 2002). Conceptually, STR analysis can be thought of as a combination of PCR and RFLP. As with RFLP, the different STR types exhibit variation in the number of repeated core

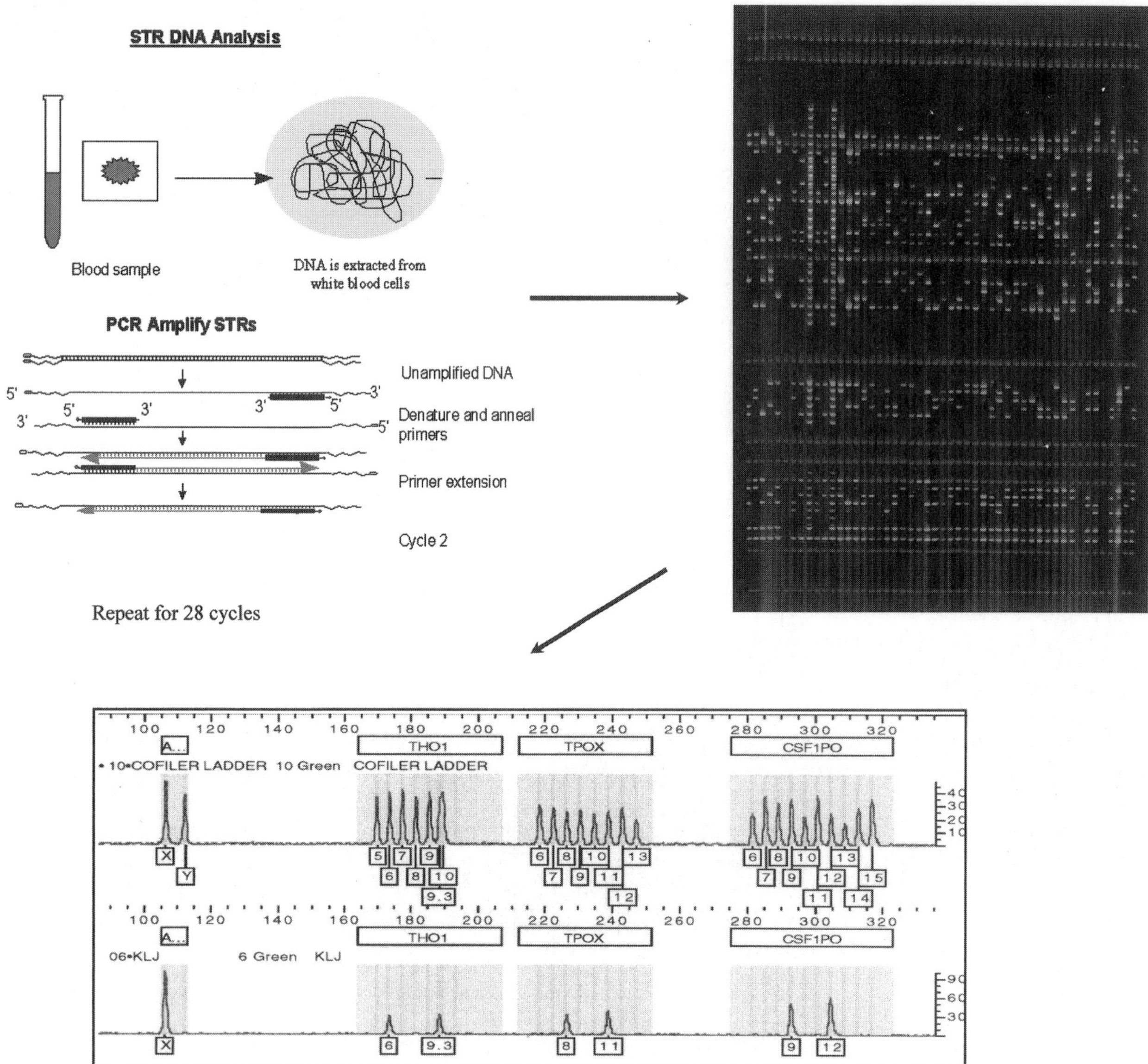

Fig. 12-5 DNA typing by STR analysis. Samples were amplified using the AmpFISTR COfiler kit (Applied Biosystems). The results for the green loci (XY, THO1, TPOX, CSF1PO) are shown for two samples. Fluorescent DNA profiles were detected using the ABI Prism 377 DNA Sequencer (Applied Biosystems). Open boxes indicate the STR profile for each sample.

elements they contain and have tremendous discriminating power. In addition, like other PCR methods, STR typing is also very sensitive. Furthermore, the use of different fluorescent dyes allows the analysis of multiple STRs in a single reaction with the aid of lasers and computers (Fig. 12-5). This saves considerable time and limits sample consumption. For these reasons, STRs has replaced the "traditional" PCR tests.

Y chromosome STR typing, in the early stages of implementation, constitutes an important new forensic method for processing sexual assault samples. Evidentiary samples in sexual assault cases are often mixtures of the victim and perpetrator. Y chromosome STRs are particularly well suited for resolving these mixtures because, generally, only the perpetrator has a Y chromosome.

Mitochondrial DNA Typing

Mitochondrial DNA analysis constitutes an important new forensic tool. The mitochondrial genome contains 16,569 bp of circular DNA. Mitochondrial (mt) DNA exists outside the nucleus and is present in multiple copies per cell. In addition, mtDNA is maternally inherited. Typically mtDNA typing involves PCR amplification followed by direct sequencing of the DNA. Mitochondrial DNA testing is particularly useful with two types of biological evidence: old/degraded skeletal remains and hair shafts, which contain only mtDNA. Given its inheritance, a mtDNA profile can be compared to anyone with the same maternal lineage. The procedure was first introduced in a US criminal trial in the summer of 1996.

Felon DNA Data Banks

One of the more significant developments in forensic science in recent years is the advent of felon DNA data banks. Given the high rate of recidivism associated with sexual assault, felon DNA data banks are particularly useful for solving these crimes; they will also assist in the investigation of many other violent crimes. Without a felon DNA data bank, if the sexual assault victim or police were unable to identify a possible suspect, little forensic testing was possible because the evidence must be compared to a known sample. These types of sexual assaults are called "no-suspect" cases. Today, it is possible to process no-suspect cases and compare the unknown DNA profile to a "library" of felon DNA profiles. All 50 states have felon DNA data bank statutes, and over 2 million felon profiles have been collected. Data bank technology has generated more than 9000 "cold hits," leading to numerous convictions (CODIS Statistics, 2003).

In addition, all 50 state databases can share information by connecting to the national DNA data bank system, CODIS (combined DNA index system), which now contains approximately 1.5 million felon profiles and 65,000 forensic unknown profiles. This database allows states to compare their no-suspect profiles to a national DNA repository and solve additional crimes.

Future Directions

DNA typing in forensic science has matured in the last decade and the field will continue to evolve rapidly. Greater use of robotics and the development of new DNA analytical tools are well under way. The number of STR cases will continue to grow, and mitochondrial and Y-STR DNA typing will be utilized on a much larger scale. Other developments such as SNP technology (single nucleotide polymorphism), mini-STRs, and phenotypic DNA profiling will provide new approaches for solving sexual assaults, homicides, and other violent crimes.

Regarding the database debate, the national trend is for states to expand their DNA data banks to include all felony convictions. As greater resources are provided for processing no-suspect cases, the number of "cold" cases solved, at both the state and national level, will continue to rise.

Yet, even though technological advancements in evidence processing are noteworthy, they are not enough. The biggest problems in forensic science, as in law enforcement generally, involve issues of judgment, ethics, and attitude, not inadequate technology or funding. Job performance failures prominently aired in high-profile cases (O. J. Simpson, Jon Benet Ramsey, Waco, Texas, Whitehurst, Rodney King, Ruby Ridge, etc.) may have significantly eroded public confidence.

Forensic scientists can correct these problems, but in many ways they have not moved effectively to do so, thus far. Accreditation and certification programs will not satisfy objections raised by defense attorneys. Efforts to impose analyst certification and laboratory accreditation are often seen by critics as self-policing. In addition, because the overwhelming majority of forensic analysts already know their trade technically, the discipline will not be significantly improved by formal certifcation measures.

The real challenge is in finding ways to maintain independence and impartiality within an *intentionally* adversarial system. Effective solutions may require "cultural change" (Bromwich, 1997). Forensic practitioners must place greater emphasis on dispassionate and professional evidence examination and testimony. They must avoid traps of emotion and advocacy. Furthermore, built around the expert witness, discovery, and cross-examination, the current system can be very effective; it deserves renewed appreciation. Finally, thorough "quality control" programs, including external proficiency testing of each analyst, are clearly the best vehicles for monitoring the technical skills of laboratory personnel.

Case Study 12-1 Sexual Assault and Crime Scene Evidence

A middle-aged nurse reported to a sexual assault clinic in California requesting an examination. She indicated that she had been sexually assaulted in the hospital parking lot as she left work after the evening shift. In addition to vaginal rape, the nurse was bitten several times on her neck and breasts. Although she could not describe her attacker in detail, she remembered that he was overweight and smelled of alcohol and tobacco. She mentioned that he had used a condom. The woman received a complete sexual assault examination and all evidence was collected according to the protocol designated by the State of California's Office of Criminal Justice. When law enforcement was notified, they searched the hospital parking lot in vicinity of the attack as recounted by the nurse. In addition to finding a recently used condom containing some apparent ejaculum, the investigators collected a cigarette pack and two cigarette butts. No other physical evidence was found in the immediate area where the woman had been assaulted. How could the evidence that was collected at the scene be used to eventually link a potential suspect with the victim and the crime?

Summary

Biological evidence has become increasingly important in recent decades, and its immense value in forensic investigations has been punctuated by high-profile cases. In addition to a new appreciation of its evidentiary value, law enforcement, forensic scientists, judiciary personnel and even the public have become aware of pitfalls or compromises in its collection and preservation that may impact the outcome of a case.

Physical evidence such as DNA, fingerprints, and trace evidence may independently and objectively link a suspect or victim to a crime or develop important investigative leads. It may also prove invaluable for exonerating the innocent.

Because evidence integrity begins with the initial investigators on the scene, often nurses, it is important that the forensic nurse examiner be skilled in regard to the collection, preservation, and transmission of such evidence. An entire case may be jeopardized if evidence is mishandled during the initial stages of the investigation.

Jay Miller, director of the CODIS project in 1997, recognized the forensic nurse examiner as the ideal clinician to provide sexual assault examinations, collect biological evidence, and coordinate this critical step with the CODIS system. Such recognition has served the IAFN and the Council of Sexual Assault Nurse Examiners well over the past years and has promoted the role of both the FNE and CODIS in developed and developing countries around the world.

To make a greater contribution to solving crime, the forensic community needs to enhance its standing in both the eyes of the public and the courts. Integrity and honesty are the cornerstones of public trust. Forensic scientists must submit to the discipline of the results and avoid anything that could be seen as a varnishing. If truth is served, justice will be well served.

Resources

Organizations

American Academy of Forensic Sciences

410 North 21st Street, CO 80904; Tel: 719-636-1100; www.aafs.org

American College of Forensic Examiners, Inc.

2750 East Sunshine, Springfield, MO 65804; Tel: 800-243-9737; www.acfei.com

Federal Bureau of Investigation

935 Pennsylvania Avenue NW, Room 7350, Washington, DC 20535; Tel: 202-324-3000; www.fbi.gov

Books

Handbook of forensic services. (1999). Washington, DC: US Department of Justice, Federal Bureau of Investigation.

Journals

Journal of Forensic Sciences

Journal of the American Academy of Forensic Sciences, Michael A. Peat, PhD, Editor, 7151 West 135th Street, PMB 410, Overland Park, KS 66223

Journal of Clinical Forensic Medicine

Journal of the Association of Police Surgeons, Journal Subscription Dept., Harcourt Publishers, Foots Cray High Street, Sidcup, Kent DA14 5HP, UK

References

Bromwich, M. R. (1997). Justice Department investigation of FBI laboratory: Executive summary, Department of Justice Office of the Inspector General. *Crim Law Reporter, 61*, 2017-2039.

CODIS Statistics. (2003). Washington, DC: US Department of Justice, Federal Bureau of Investigation.

Committee on DNA Forensic Science: National Research Council. (1996). *The evaluation of forensic DNA evidence. An update.* Washington, DC: National Academy Press.

Committee on DNA Technology in Forensic Science, National Research Council. (1992). *DNA technology in forensic science.* Washington, DC: National Academy Press.

De Forest, P. R., Gaensslen R. E., & Lee, H. C. (1983). *Forensic science: An introduction to criminalistics.* New York: McGraw-Hill.

DNA Advisory Board Standards. (1998). *Quality assurance standards for DNA testing laboratories.* Washington, DC: US Department of Justice, Federal Bureau of Investigation.

Gaensslen, R. E. (1983). *Sourcebook in forensic serology, immunology and biochemistry.* Washington, DC: US Government Printing Office.

Gaensslen, R. E., Desio, P. J., & Lee, H. C. (1986). Genetic marker systems for the individualization of blood and body fluids in forensic serology. In G. Davies (Ed.), *Forensic science.* Washington, DC: American Chemical Society.

Gaensslen, R. E., & Lee, H. C. (1984). *Procedures and evaluation of antisera for the typing of antigens in bloodstains: Blood group antigens ABH, RH, MNSs, Kell, Duffy, Kidd, serum group antigens GmlKm.* Washington, DC: National Institute of Justice, US Government Printing Office.

Holt, C. L., Buoncristiani, M. R., Wallin, J. M., et al. (2002). TWGDAM validation of the AmpFLSTR PCR amplification kits for forensic casework analysis. *J Forensic Sci 47*, 66-96.

Lee, H. C. (1982). Identification and grouping of bloodstains. In R. Saferstein (Ed.), *Forensic science review* (pp. 267-337). Englewood Cliffs, NJ: Prentice-Hall.

Lee, H. C., & Gaensslen, R. E. (Eds.). (1985). *Advances in forensic science.* Foster City, CA: Biomedical.

Lee, H. C., Gaensslen, R. E., Pagliaro, E. M., et al. (1991). *Physical evidence in criminal investigation.* Westbrook, CT: Narcotic Enforcement Officers Association.

Lee, H. C., & Ladd, C. (1997). Criminal justice: An unraveling of trust? *Public Perspective, 8*, 6-7.

Lee, H. C., Ladd, C., Bourke, M. T., et al. (1994). DNA typing in forensic science. *Am J Forensic Med Pathol, 15*, 269-282.

Lee, H. C., Ladd, C., Scherczinger, C. A., et al. (1998). Forensic applications of DNA typing: Collection and preservation of DNA evidence. *Am J Forensic Med Pathol, 19*, 10-18.

Lee, H. C., Palmbach, T. M., & Miller, M. T. (2001). *Henry Lee's crime scene handbook.* Boston: Academic Press.

Lee, H. C. (Ed.) (1995). *Physical evidence.* Enfield, CT: Magnani and McCormic.

Uniform Crime Reports. (2002). Washington, DC: US Department of Justice, Federal Bureau of Investigation.

US Congress, Office of Technology Assessment. (1990). *Genetic witness: Forensic uses of DNA tests.* OTA-BA-438. Washington, DC: US Government Printing Office.

Chapter 13 DNA and the CODIS Project

Patricia A. Loftus, Steven J. Niezgoda, and John J. Behun

The typing of DNA from biological evidence is one of the most important developments in forensic science. DNA analysis provides forensic scientists with a scientifically reliable means to eliminate from suspicion individuals falsely associated with biological sample and enables examiners to significantly reduce the number of potential contributors. Current DNA technology comprises genetic markers, multiple DNA typing strategies, powerful computers, and specialized software. These elements make the development of DNA profiles and the searching of DNA databases relatively rapid and easy. Because they can be generated much more rapidly than a decade ago, DNA databases are used to search DNA profiles in an increasing number of violent crimes.

After recognizing and demonstrating that DNA typing could support human identification in a forensic setting, the FBI developed a comprehensive DNA program with four major components. First, the FBI performs DNA analysis on cases submitted by local, state, and federal law enforcement agencies. Since the first case was submitted to the FBI in 1988, the DNA Analysis Unit has analyzed more than 30,000 cases. Second, the FBI has dedicated programs for applied research and development of DNA technology. For example, the FBI has pioneered many of the laboratory protocols used in forensic analysis throughout the US. Third, the FBI actively shares information with other law enforcement agencies through training, standards setting, publication, professional symposia, and technical consultation. In this vein, the FBI created the Scientific Working Group on DNA Analysis Methods (SWGDAM), a collaboration of local, state, and forensic scientists. Finally, the FBI created and continues to operate a national database of DNA profiles called the Combined DNA Index System, or CODIS. CODIS assists investigators in the identification of suspects of violent crimes and increases the efficacy of forensic laboratories by providing software to conduct DNA casework and perform statistical calculations.

According to statistics compiled by the Bureau of Justice Statistics, an average of 366,460 sexual assaults occurred annually in the US from 1992-2000. (BOJ, 2002). Recognizing the tendency of sex offenders to commit multiple crimes and the fact that biological evidence is often recovered from sex-related crime scenes, the FBI conceived CODIS. CODIS has been developed through the close cooperation and valuable input of the forensic community, particularly SWGDAM. By combining forensic DNA technology with computer software applications, CODIS can assist the law enforcement community in solving violent crimes that would not be solved through other means.

Best Practice 13-1

The forensic nurse will ensure that biological evidence collected from victims of sexual assault and other violent acts will be forwarded to a CODIS facility for DNA analysis to aid in suspect identification.

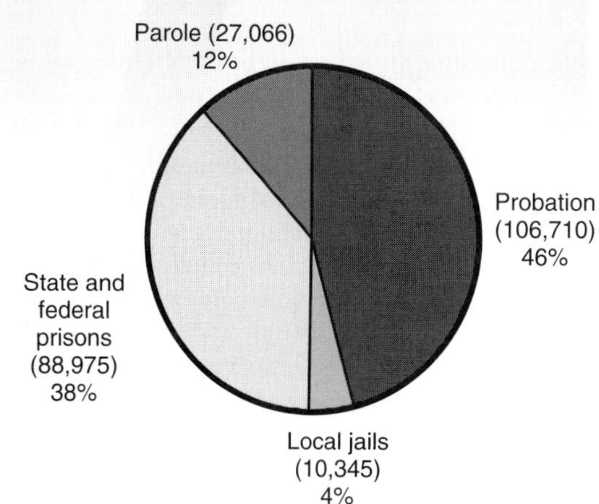

Fig. 13-1 Convicted sex offenders: care, custody, and control.

Another important fact relating to the need for CODIS involves the return of convicted offenders to their communities. Approximately 234,000 offenders convicted of sexual assault are under the control or care of correctional agencies, and nearly 60% of these sex offenders are under some type of conditional supervision in the community (Fig. 13-1) (Greenfeld, 1997). Furthermore, individuals convicted of sexual offenses return to society from incarceration in a relatively short time. The average period of incarceration served by a convicted rapist is about five years; those incarcerated for other sexual assaults typically serve less than three years (Greenfeld, 1997).

CODIS (Combined DNA Index System)

CODIS merges aspects of forensic science and computer technology to create an effective tool for providing investigative leads and solving violent crimes. To completely facilitate the comparison of DNA profiles nationally, CODIS must be a fully integrated network among crime laboratories. To this end, CODIS enables local, state, and federal law enforcement crime laboratories to exchange and compare DNA profiles (the set of genetic characteristics that result from forensic DNA analysis) electronically, link serial violent crimes, and identify potential suspects by comparing DNA profiles from crime scene evidence to those of convicted offenders.

The mission of CODIS is to facilitate the investigation of violent crimes where biological evidence is recovered. The mission is accomplished through the following initiatives:

- Utilizing leading edge information technologies to provide software tools for conducting DNA analysis
- Exchanging information between local, state, and federal law enforcement agencies
- Implementing improvements in forensic DNA analysis and testing methods, standards, and practices
- Exploiting advances in biological evidence collection, preservation, and tracking

DNA examiners rely on CODIS to develop DNA profiles during forensic examinations. CODIS organizes DNA profiles into several indexes according to the origin of the sample being analyzed (Box 13-1) :

1. Convicted Offender Index contains DNA records from individuals convicted of felony sex crimes and other crimes, depending upon state legislation. This index is used to generate investigative leads in official criminal investigations, create investigative leads in missing persons cases, and determine whether duplicate records exist in the index (i.e., alibi usage by repeat offenders).
2. Forensic Index contains DNA records attributed to individuals derived from lawfully collected specimens obtained during the course of a criminal investigation. This index generally contains DNA records from cases without a suspect.
3. Population File contains DNA types and allele frequency data from anonymous persons intended to represent major population groups found in the US. These databases are used to estimate statistical frequencies of DNA profiles.

Recently, additional indexes have been incorporated into CODIS. These indexes are as follows:

4. Unidentified Persons Index contains DNA from individuals whose identities are not known with certainty. This index includes unidentified body parts, human remains, and DNA from individuals who do not (or cannot) disclose their identity to the police.
5. Relatives of Missing Persons Index contains DNA records from missing persons and their close biological relatives. The Unidentified Persons Reference Index is searched against the Unidentified Persons Index to identify individuals or body parts.
6. Victims Index may be used to search DNA profiles found on, but foreign to, a suspect. The Victims Index will contain DNA records from victims, living or dead, from whom DNA may have been carried away by perpetrators.

When a crime laboratory develops a DNA profile through evidence collected from a crime scene, CODIS can be searched for potential suspects. If the DNA profile assembled from the collected evidence is searched against the Forensic Index and a match occurs, at the least, investigations are linked. Thus, police officers in at least two jurisdictions (or multiple cases in one jurisdiction) can coordinate their respective investigations. Matches resulting from this comparison provide investigators with a potential suspect's identity.

Box 13-1 Combined DNA Index System

- Convicted Offender Index
- Forensic Index
- Population File
- Unidentified Persons Index
- Relatives of Missing Persons Index
- Victims Index

The DNA identification records in CODIS contain limited information sufficient to enable profile searching. In general, the identification record contains (1) a laboratory identifier, (2) a specimen identifier, (3) DNA characteristics, and (4) information to classify and review the integrity of the DNA record. CODIS does not store criminal history information, case-related information, or social security numbers. If a CODIS search identifies a potential match, the laboratories connected to the matching profiles contact each other to validate or refute the match. After a match has been confirmed by qualified DNA analysts, the relevant laboratories may exchange additional information, such as the names and phone numbers of criminal investigators and other case details. In the case of a match against the Convicted Offender Index, the identity and location of the convicted offender is provided.

CODIS is implemented at three levels: local, state, and national (Fig. 13-2). Each tier contains the Forensic and Convicted Offender Indexes and the population database file. The Local DNA Index System (LDIS) is available at crime laboratories operated by police departments, sheriff's offices, or state agencies. All forensic DNA records originate at the local level and subsequently are transmitted to the state and national levels. Each state participating in the CODIS program maintains its own State DNA Index System (SDIS), which enables the comparison of DNA profiles within a state. Each SDIS also links the local and national levels and is typically operated by the agency responsible for maintaining a state's convicted offender DNA database program. The National DNA Index System (NDIS), which is administered by the FBI, is the single central repository of DNA records submitted by participating states. Participating state laboratories communicate via the FBI's dedicated, secure, high-speed, frame relay network known as the Criminal Justice Information Service Wide Area Network (CJIS-WAN).

The majority of data stored in CODIS is created and maintained by state and local crime laboratories. Federal convicted offender records are created by the FBI. The current version of CODIS software supports the storage and searching of both restriction fragment length polymorphism (RFLP) and polymerase chain reaction (PCR)-based DNA profiles. The CODIS software features include (1) computer-assisted analysis of RFLP profiles; (2) keyboard and computer-assisted entry of PCR analysis results; (3) batch entry of

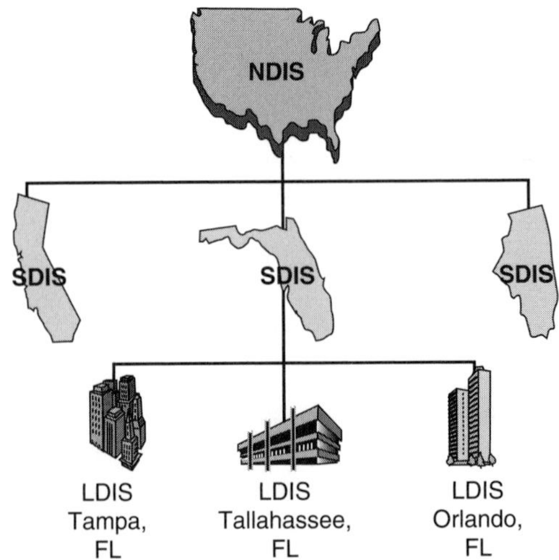

Fig. 13-2 National DNA Index System: National (NDIS), state (SDIS), and local (LDIS) CODIS implementation.

RFLP and PCR-based results produced by contract service laboratories; (4) intra- and interlaboratory searching of RFLP and PCR-based profiles; (5) searching the database of DNA profiles at the national level; and (6) calculation of DNA profile frequencies.

The foremost innovation of the CODIS program is the creation of a collaborative network among local, state, and federal law enforcement agencies. This collaboration occurs in the following ways:

- It creates a national standard for forensic DNA analysis. Historically, state and local governments operated independently. Realizing that there still may be an impediment to standardization, the FBI elected to carry the cost of development and to provide CODIS software free of charge. Additionally, through SWGDAM, standards were developed by peer-consensus for DNA analysis. The FBI also provides free help desk support and training.
- It provides legal guidance to states seeking to establish DNA databases of individuals convicted of violent crimes. The inclusion of all states creates a broader pool of profiles to search and promotes compatibility among states.
- It created NDIS to allow interstate comparisons of DNA profiles.
- Ultimately, the success of the CODIS program will be measured by the number and nature of crimes it helps solve. CODIS's primary metric, the "Investigation Aided," is defined as a case/investigation that CODIS assisted through a hit. A hit is defined as a match produced by CODIS that would not otherwise have been developed. As of September 2004, CODIS has aided 20,338 investigations across 47 states, two federal laboratories and Puerto Rico.

DNA Technology

The tools of molecular biology currently enable forensic scientists to characterize biological evidence at the DNA level. The methods presently available to the forensic scientist include (1) RFLP typing of variable number of tandem repeat (VNTR) loci (Wyman & White, 1980; Jeffreys, Wilson, & Thein, 1985a; 1985b); and (2) amplification of specified genetic loci by PCR (Saiki, Scharf, & Faloona et al., 1985) and subsequent typing of specified genetic markers (Budowle, Lindsey, & DeCou et al., 1995; Wilson, Polanskey, & Butler et al., 1995). Any material that contains nucleated cells, including blood, semen, saliva, hair, bones, and teeth, potentially can be typed for DNA polymorphisms.

The typing of VNTR loci by RFLP analysis has been the most discriminating, or individualizing, molecular biology technology for forensic identity testing. Although this approach is valid and reliable for forensic and paternity testing, it has certain limitations: (1) a sufficient quantity of high-molecular-weight DNA (usually at least 50 ng) is required for RFLP analysis; (2) samples that have been substantially degraded cannot be analyzed by RFLP typing; and (3) RFLP analysis is laborious, as well as time-consuming, requiring two to eight weeks to obtain results on six VNTR markers (Budowle & Baechtel, 1990).

An alternative strategy for forensic DNA typing is the use of PCR-based assays (Saiki, Scharf, & Faloona et al., 1985). Compared with the RFLP approach, the advantages of PCR-based technology include augmented sensitivity and specificity and decreased assay time and labor. Also, many degraded DNA samples can be amplified by PCR and subsequently typed, because amplified fragments generally are much smaller compared with fragments detected by RFLP analysis. These features make PCR a particularly useful tool for analyzing biological material found at crime scenes (Saiki, Scharf, & Faloona et al., 1985).

The ability to employ PCR has facilitated analyses of forensic biological samples. PCR is a sample preparation technique in which relatively large amounts of specific DNA sequences can be generated from relatively small (picogram or nanogram) quantities of DNA (Edwards, Hammond, & Jin et al., 1992; Report of a Symposium on the Practice of Forensic Serology, 1987; Budowle, Deadman, & Murch et al., 1988). A typical PCR is based on the annealing and extension of two short pieces of DNA (i.e., primers) that flank a specific target (template) DNA segment. Primers are single-stranded DNA oligonucleotides, usually 20 to 30 bases in length, that can be obtained commercially or synthesized in-house. The template DNA that is to be amplified by PCR is denatured into single-stranded DNA by heating the sample to approximately 95° C (203° F) using a thermal cycler. By lowering the thermal cycle temperature following denaturation (typically 37° to 72° C or 98.6° to 161.6° F), each primer anneals to a region of complementarity on one of the separated single strands. These three steps (denaturation, primer annealing, and primer extension) constitute a single PCR cycle. The newly synthesized strand can serve as a template for subsequent PCR cycles. Upon repeated cycles of denaturation, primer annealing, and primer extension (usually 28 to 36 times), an exponential accumulation of specific DNA fragments is generated, and millions of copies of target sequence can be obtained (Edwards, Hammond, & Jin et al., 1992; Report of a Symposium on the Practice of Forensic Serology, 1987; Budowle, Deadman, & Murch et al., 1988). PCR, in principle, is easy to accomplish and completed in one to two hours (Budowle, Deadman, & Murch et al., 1988).

Best Practice *13-2*

The forensic nurse will use impeccable techniques to obtain biological evidence to ensure against contamination that would create confusing and misleading results in the DNA profiling process.

The complex and sensitive procedures involved in DNA profiling make it susceptible to artifacts resulting from contamination of forensic tissue samples or the DNA extracted from those samples (National Research Council, 1992). For example, the power of PCR to afford identification of small amounts of DNA is also the cause of its likely problem. A sample contaminated with extraneous DNA that shares a sequence similar to the target DNA will result in amplification and detection of the contaminant as well as the desired region. This result may lead to an inability to distinguish one from the other. A potential source of impurity is tissue contamination (skin fragments, blood, or saliva) from healthcare professionals, laboratory personnel, or investigating officers. Strict procedures, such as donning gloves and quality assurance checks, are mandatory to minimize contamination (National Research Council, 1992).

Key Point *13-1*

DNA profiling is subject to flaws if the forensic tissue samples or extracted DNA is contaminated by extraneous DNA.

The short tandem repeat (STR) genetic markers appeared on the forensic scene only a few years ago but already have become the mainstay for forensic DNA testing (Demers, Kelly, & Sozer, 1998). STRs are tandemly repeating regions of DNA ranging in numbers from three to five nucleotides per repeat. As with VNTR loci, the number of times the succession is repeated varies among individuals. The STR regions are amenable to amplification by the PCR method; however, a greater number of loci (genetic markers) are needed to achieve comparable levels of discrimination compared with RFLP typing (Demers, Kelly, & Sozer, 1998).

In addition to DNA extracted from the chromosomes of the cell nucleus, small circular DNA molecules exist in the mitochondria outside the nucleus. Unlike the single nucleus where the nuclear DNA is found, cells may contain hundreds to thousands of mitochondria, each of which contain several copies of mitochondrial DNA (mtDNA). This fact is important in cases in which the amount of DNA in a sample is limited. Typical sources of DNA recovered from crime scenes, such as hair, bones, and teeth, are able to be characterized by mtDNA (Wilson, DiZinno, & Polanskey et al., 1995).

Another feature of mtDNA that can be advantageous to forensic scientists is the fact that mtDNA is inherited strictly from the mother. If known samples are obtained from maternally related individuals, the DNA sequences should, in absence of a mutation, exactly match each other. This technique is limited, however, in that it cannot discriminate between two individuals of the same maternal lineage, whereas nuclear DNA analysis can accomplish this (Wilson, DiZinno, & Polanskey et al., 1995).

Realizing the Full Potential of CODIS

It has been little more than 10 years since DNA analysis was first used for forensic identification purposes in the US. From a beginning in only a handful of local, state, and federal laboratories in the 1980s, DNA identification technology is now used by more than 140 forensic laboratories in 50 states.

All 50 states have passed legislation pertaining to the DNA database. More than half the states with an active collection program began their operations in the last seven years. The actual analysis of convicted offender samples has caught up with the legislation in 2001. In 1998, only 36 of the 42 states collecting samples analyzed those samples (Fig. 13-3).

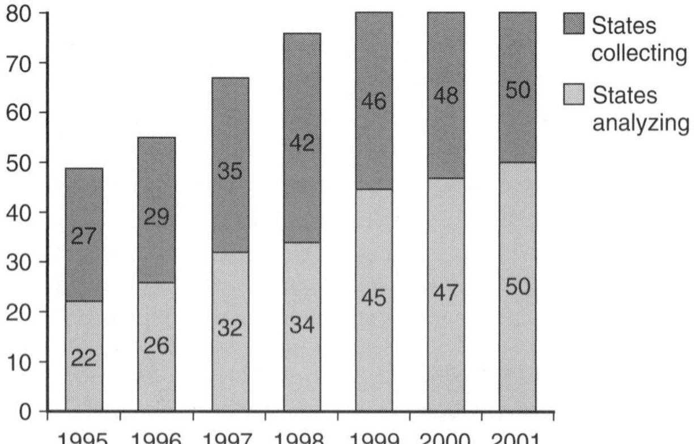

Fig. 13-3 Number of states collecting and analyzing offender samples from 1995 to 2001.

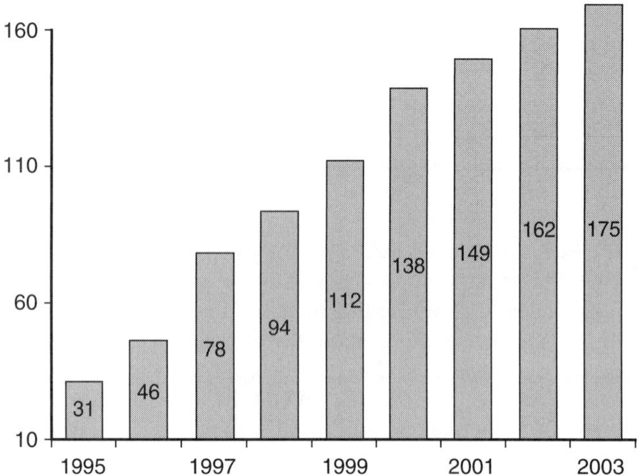

Fig. 13-4 Number of installed CODIS labs from 1995 to 2003.

As of January 2004, 175 US public crime laboratories are using the FBI-supplied CODIS software to support forensic and offender DNA work. Figure 13-4 shows the annual increase in the number of CODIS laboratories since 1995.

CODIS and DNA Casework Analysis

The term "DNA casework" includes two classes: cases with a known suspect and cases without a known suspect. The CODIS computer system supports investigations of both classes.

The first use of DNA identification techniques for forensic purposes in the US (1986) was for "known suspect" cases. In this type of case, the forensic laboratory is asked to compare the DNA profile of a known suspect to the DNA profile developed from evidence collected at a crime scene. The forensic examiner determines if the suspect's DNA matches the evidence DNA generally by making a "side-by-side" comparison of the profiles. In these known suspect cases, computer-based matching using the CODIS system increases the accuracy of the matching process and productivity of the examiner, allowing the laboratory to process more cases than would be possible with manual/visual matching alone.

The second class of DNA casework involves cases in which the police have not developed any suspects. These cases are called "unknown suspect" cases (also known as "unknown subject" or "unsub" cases). In unknown suspect cases, forensic laboratories attempt to match the DNA profile obtained from the crime scene evidence against DNA profiles from other cases, or against DNA profiles from convicted offenders. These cases also include those in which a suspect was originally developed, and upon DNA profile comparisons, the suspect is excluded as the source of the evidence. Linking unknown suspect cases together can provide investigators with new information that may lead to the development of a suspect.

In unknown suspect cases, a computerized DNA profile matching system, such as provided by CODIS, is critical. Without a computerized matching system, it would be extremely difficult to search for a match between the profile from a new unknown suspect case and hundreds, if not thousands, of profiles from previous unknown suspect cases. Similarly, effectively searching a profile against hundreds of thousand to millions of profiles from convicted violent offenders would be implausible without the assistance of computer technology.

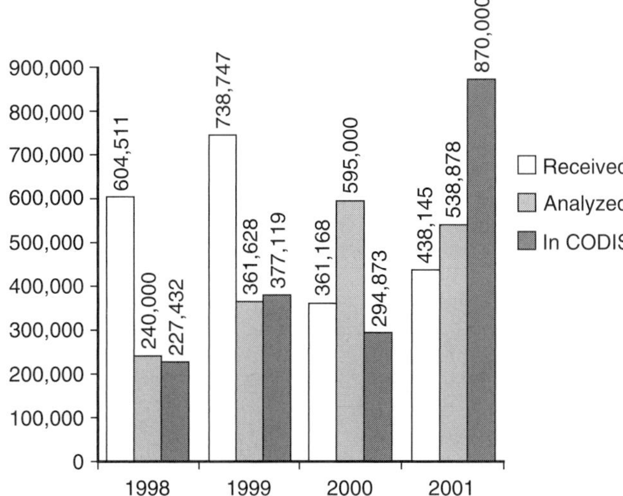

Fig. 13-5 Convicted offender samples received, analyzed, and stored in CODIS from 1998 to 2001.

Convicted Offender DNA Analysis

The complete coverage of state DNA database laws occurred in 1998, with all 50 states having enacted legislation. This legislation requires persons convicted of felony sex offenses (and other crimes, depending on each state's statute) to provide biological samples for DNA analysis. These samples are analyzed and entered into the CODIS database. Figure 13-5 provides a comparison of averages of the period 1998 to 2001 for offender samples received, analyzed, and stored in CODIS.

The backlog of unanalyzed samples (samples collected but for which DNA profiles have not yet been developed) increased in 1998, 1999, and 2000. However, the number of unanalyzed samples dropped in 2001, owing to increased analysis for DNA backlog elimination.

Offender DNA profiles must be entered into CODIS before they can be effectively used to aid the investigation of unsolved crimes. In 2001, an average of 30,000 offender profiles per month were entered into CODIS. The cumulative number of profiles stored in CODIS increased to 900,000 by the fall of 2001.

Aiding Investigations

As already noted, laboratory DNA activity of all types is increasing. The payoff of this increase was the number of investigations that were aided by computer matching of DNA profiles. As of January 2004, the 175 laboratories using CODIS had made 3004 forensic hits (occurs when CODIS matches two or more forensic profiles). Additionally, these laboratories made 7118 offender hits (occurs when CODIS matches one or more forensic profiles to an offender sample). As a result of these CODIS hits, the participating laboratories aided 11,220 investigations across 39 states and two federal laboratories.

Forensic Nursing and the CODIS Project

The work of the forensic nurse examiner has a direct impact on the success of the CODIS project. Forensic nurses are trained to facilitate the recognition, collection, and preservation of probative evidence (Lynch, 1991). The effectiveness of CODIS as a law enforcement tool lies in its ability to use evidence acquired from violent acts to solve crimes and prevent future violence. Unless the evidence collected by the forensic nurse is of high quality, the effectiveness of DNA profiling and the use of CODIS are immediately diminished. The success of a national DNA database truly depends on the efforts of the forensic nurse examiner.

The FNE provides direct and indirect services to the CODIS project and the FBI laboratory. The role encompasses the responsibilities following this section.

Liaison Between Medical Law Enforcement Communities

The forensic nurse functions as a liaison between the medical and law enforcement communities. In the past, separatism rather than cooperation marked the relationship between healthcare and law enforcement professionals. The FNE is in a position to bridge the gap and unite these two groups of professionals because this nurse uniquely understands the responsibilities of each discipline in the care for victims of violence. By serving as a liaison between these two disciplines, the forensic nurse examiner helps each profession view its role collectively and appreciate that its efforts help to advance the completion of another's work. The medical and law enforcement communities do not exist separately in a vacuum; the forensic nurse is a vital link in joining these disciplines (Lynch, 1991).

Weaknesses in communication hamper the ability of criminal justice officials and health professionals to disseminate and exchange vital information related to victims of violent crime. Interdisciplinary collaboration is required to provide competent and effective care for the survivor. The formation of a sexual assault response team (SART) is an important cooperative effort. Professionals who participate in the development of SART programs are responsible for assembling protocols specific to the community that will be served. The CODIS project directly benefits from standards that identify and outline a coordinated response to incidences of sexual assault and violence.

Collection and Preservation of Evidence

Through the proper recognition of probative evidence and identification of injury patterns, the nurse facilitates the collection and preservation of evidence. The proper starting point for a forensic nurse begins with the following inquiry: What constitutes forensic evidence? In answering this question, the forensic nurse must educate other medical professionals as to what is defined as evidence. This instruction can and will lead to the reevaluation of current healthcare practices and procedures. Although the health of the victim is of the utmost importance, there may be times when evidence collection can be achieved without additional harm to the victim. For example, a sexual assault victim may appear in the emergency department with bite marks on her breast. A healthcare professional's first priority is the health of the patient. However, more important forensic evidence may be recorded if the patient is properly cared for, thus preserving the evidence. Trace evidence such as hairs and fibers may inadvertently be brushed aside or overlooked during the removal of the patient's clothing or during the examination.

Community Education

The forensic nurse examiner educates the community on the role of the sexual assault nurse examiner (SANE) and SART program.

Key Point 13-2

In order to avoid the loss of critical evidence, the forensic nurse must instruct other healthcare professionals on the importance of evidence collection as it relates to the identification of the perpetrator, recognition of injury, and advances in DNA technology.

He or she must possess knowledge of the community's crime statistics. The members of the medical community need to be instructed on crime-prevention behavior, what occurs during a sexual assault examination, and the importance of seeking medical care following an assault.

The forensic nurse examiner interfaces daily with a multidisciplinary team of professionals, including stakeholders in the CODIS project. This includes victim advocacy groups, prosecutors, medical professionals, and law enforcement personnel. The primary goal of the CODIS program is to increase the arrest and conviction rates for violent criminals. The direct beneficiaries of CODIS's accomplishments are the victims or potential victim of violent crimes. The stakeholders are also impacted by the program's success. Because of the ability of the trained forensic nurse to collect evidence and educate the community, the CODIS program can meet its objectives. As a result, crime laboratories are able to provide high-quality DNA forensic services that are recognized by courts and are able to withstand legal challenges.

Case Study 13-1 DNA and CODIS at Work

On the morning of November 25, 1991, a masked man broke into the home of a newlywed couple in Ritchie, Illinois. The intruder shot and killed the husband and then raped and shot the wife. The attacker presumed the woman to be dead and drove away in the couple's car. The woman survived but was unable to identify her attacker, and the police were not successful in determining his identity. Two weeks later a man raped a 17-year-old girl. This victim was able to identify her assailant, and he was convicted of the crime. On April 6 of the following year, forensic scientists at the Springfield Crime Lab conducted a routine check of convicted offender DNA profiles against crime scene evidence in CODIS. The search produced a match between the DNA profiles of the suspect in the Ritchie, Illinois, murder/rape and the man convicted of raping the 17-year-old girl. The offender, Arthur Dale Hickey, was a neighbor of the couple in Ritchie. Hickey was sentenced by a jury to death in Joliet, Illinois, for first-degree murder, attempted murder, aggravated criminal sexual assault, and home invasion.

Summary

The CODIS project provides two significant benefits to society. First, CODIS facilitates the identification of serial offenders more expeditiously, thereby enabling law enforcement personnel to cut short a serial offender's crime spree and reduce the number of potential victims. By preventing the continued violent behavior of serial offenders, law enforcement will save time and resources, criminal investigations will be better focused and coordinated, and courts will have fewer cases to adjudicate. Second, incarcerated offenders who are linked to additional crimes by CODIS may face additional penalties that further delay or prevent their return to society.

Resources

Organizations

Federal Bureau of Investigation, 935 Pennsylvania Avenue NW, Washington, DC 20535; Tel: 202-324-3000; www.fbi.gov

Materials available from the Web site include the following:

CODIS Program Mission Statement and Background

National DNA Index System (Participating States and Statistics)

Quality Assurance Standards

Success Stories of Investigations Aided by CODIS

References

Budowle, B., & Baechtel, F. S. (1990). Modifications to improve the effectiveness of restriction fragment length polymorphism typing. *Appl Theor Electrophoresis, 1*, 181–187.

Budowle, B., Deadman, H. A., Murch, R., et al. (1988). An introduction to the methods of DNA analysis under investigation in the FBI laboratory. *Crime Lab Dig, 15*, 8–21.

Budowle, B., Lindsey, J. A., DeCou, J. A., et al. (1995). Validation and population studies of the loci LDLR, GYPA, HBGG, D7S8, and Gc (PM loci), and HLA-DQα using a multiplex amplification and typing procedure. *J Forensic Sci, 40*(1), 45–54.

Bureau of Justice Statistics Selected Findings. (2002). *Rape and sexual assault: Reporting to police and medical attention, 1992-2000.* Washington, DC: US Department of Justice.

Demers, D. B., Kelly, C. M., & Sozer, A. C. (1998). Multiplex STR analysis by capillary electrophoresis. *Profiles DNA, 1*(3), 3–5.

Edwards, A., Hammond, H., Jin, L., et al. (1992). Genetic variation at five trimetric and tetrametric repeat loci in four human population groups. *Genomic, 12*, 241–253.

Greenfeld, L. A. (1997). *Sex offenses and offenders.* Washington, DC: Bureau of Justice Statistics. Pub. No. NCJ-183931, pp. 1–3.

Jeffreys, A. J., Wilson, V., & Thein, S. L. (1985a). Hypervariable minisatellite regions in human DNA. *Nature, 314*, 67–73.

Jeffreys, A. J., Wilson, V., & Thein, S. L. (1985b). Individual-specific fingerprints of human DNA. *Nature, 316*, 76–79.

Lynch, V.A. (1991). Forensic nursing in the emergency department: A new role for the 1990s. *Criti Care Nurs Q, 14*(3), 69–86.

National Research Council. (1992). DNA technology in forensic science. Washington, DC: National Academy Press.

Report of a Symposium on the Practice of Forensic Serology, Method Evaluation (Topic 4). (1987). Sponsored by the California Department of Justice Bureau of Forensic Services, California Association of Criminalists, and the UNISYS Corporation.

Saiki, R. K., Scharf, S., Faloona, F., et al. (1985). Enzymatic amplification of beta-globin genomic sequences and restriction analysis for diagnosis of sickle cell anemia. *Science, 230*, 1350–1354.

Wilson, M. R., Polanskey, D., Butler, J., et al. (1995). Extraction, PCR amplification, and sequencing of mitochondrial DNA from human hair shafts. *Biotechniques, 18*, 662–669.

Wilson, M. R., DiZinno, J. A., Polanskey, D., et al. (1995). Validation of mitochondrial DNA sequencing for forensic casework analysis. *Int J Legal Med, 108*, 68.

Wyman, A. R., & White, R. (1980). A highly polymorphic locus in human DNA. *Proc Natl Acad Sci USA, 77*, 6754–6758.

Chapter 14 Forensic Toxicology

Sarah Kerrigan and Bruce A. Goldberger

Overview

Toxicological analyses are undertaken in clinical and forensic laboratories to facilitate medical intervention, diagnosis, or treatment, and as part of the criminal justice system. Toxicology also plays a fundamental role in determining the cause and manner of death and is widely utilized in the workplace to deter drug use. "Forensic" comes from the Latin word *forensis*, which means "forum," meaning a court or tribunal. Forensic toxicology is distinct from clinical toxicology in that it is often practiced within a legal domain for the purpose of upholding the law. However, clinicians and medical personnel do play an essential role in forensic toxicology. During medical treatment, they are often the first ones to make observations, diagnoses, and collect biological samples from injured persons who may be the subject of a legal investigation. Analyses of specimens without the context in which they were collected are generally of limited value. In order to properly evaluate these tests, the patient's or victim's history of drug usage is needed for proper interpretation. Furthermore, improperly collected specimens can yield improper or misleading results. Forensic nurses, because of their unique training, are in a position to aid clinicians, law enforcement officers, and legal personnel with investigations utilizing toxicological testing. They are familiar with the proper collection, storage, and testing of forensic specimens. In addition, they are experienced in conducting interviews and collecting histories, which will aid with the interpretation of results of the analyses.

Subdisciplines of Forensic Toxicology

The three major subdisciplines of forensic toxicology are human performance toxicology, postmortem toxicology, and forensic urine drug testing. Human performance toxicology is concerned with mental and physical effects of drugs that may, for example, impair judgment or coordination. Postmortem toxicology involves the investigation of drugs and poisons in circumstances of death. Forensic urine drug testing has become widespread in the military as well as in public and private sectors of the workplace.

Reasons for Drug Use

Unfortunately, in today's society, the ingestion of a drug or drugs in the absence of medical supervision is commonplace. One common motive for the misuse of drugs includes the pursuit of euphoric or psychedelic effects. Many times these drugs are used to enhance social situations, used as a result of peer pressure, used out of curiosity, or used for "fun" or to "get high."

Alternatively, drugs may be used to enhance mental, emotional, or physical well-being. For example, it is not uncommon for individuals to self-medicate for the relief of anxiety, depression, insomnia, or pain or to increase alertness or relaxation.

Toxicology Investigation

Toxicological findings may provide the necessary insight to explain behavioral or physiological effects (e.g., why a person drives off the road, attempts suicide, or unexpectedly falls unconscious). The use of prescription or over-the-counter (OTC) drugs in a manner inconsistent with accepted medical practice might be of relevance during a criminal investigation, particularly in a case involving driving a motor vehicle, operation of machinery, violent crime, or sexual assault.

As mentioned earlier, selection, identification, collection, and preservation of biological evidence have a profound impact on the quality of analytical data and the interpretation of toxicological findings. To this end, the toxicologist relies on a variety of analytical techniques, of which some may provide results in minutes or hours, and others may require several days.

There is considerable overlap between the subdisciplines of forensic toxicology, which are largely governed by the natural laws of pharmacology and chemistry. The most common questions asked of the forensic toxicologist are: Was a drug or chemical involved? If so, what was the drug or chemical? How much was taken and when? Was it responsible for the death or did it affect behavior? The key to answering these questions requires an understanding of pharmacokinetics, pharmacodynamics, and analytical techniques.

Trends in Drug Use

The 2002 National Survey on Drug Use and Health (NSDUH), conducted by the Substance Abuse and Mental Health Services Administration (SAMHSA), indicated that an estimated 19.5 million Americans (8.3% of the population ≥ 12 years old) were illicit drug users, 54 million participated in binge drinking, and another 15.9 million were heavy drinkers. Drug abuse, whether it involves illicit substances or the misuse of therapeutics, is nondiscriminatory in that it has permeated almost every level of society to some degree. Trends in drug use among the young are largely governed by the perceived risk of drug use. As perceived risk decreases, use increases, and vice versa. These findings offer the hope that comprehensive drug prevention efforts, based on drug education and risk assessment, can curb drug use among young people.

In 2002, marijuana was the most commonly used illicit drug in the United States (14.6 million) followed by nonmedical use of prescription drugs (6.2 million). Of these, an estimated 4.4 million used narcotic pain relievers, 1.8 million used antianxiety medications, 1.2 million used central nervous system stimulants, and 0.4 million used sedatives. In the same year, estimates for cocaine, hallucinogen, and heroin users were 2 million, 1.2 million, and 166,000, respectively (SAMHSA 2004).

According to the Drug Abuse Warning Network (DAWN), the number of cocaine-related emergency department (ED) visits increased 47% between 1995 and 2002 (from 135,711 to 199,198). Heroin-related visits increased 35% (from 69,556 to 93,519), and marijuana-related visits increased 164% (from 45,259 to 119,472). Although cocaine, marijuana, heroin, and alcohol in combination with other illicit drugs were the most commonly reported categories, significant increases in phencyclidine (25%) and inhalants

(187%) were also reported between 2001 and 2002. In addition to illicit drugs, nonmedical use of central nervous system and psychotherapeutic agents accounted for 37% of all drug-related visits to the ED. Statistics also indicate an aging drug-using population, many of whom have developed severe drug use and abuse problems. Projections suggest that the number of people over the age of 50 who require treatment for drug problems will increase fivefold in the next 20 years.

Drugs in the Military

In 1998, a worldwide survey of substance abuse and health behaviors among military personnel showed that drug use declined considerably between 1990 and 1998. This study, conducted by the Department of Defense every three to four years, showed that rates of substance abuse among male military personnel were significantly lower (2.8%) than in the general population (11.4%). This downward trend seems to coincide with the 1990 guidelines proposed by the Secretary of Defense and the Secretary of Transportation to regulate and implement a comprehensive drug-testing program of military personnel. This deterrent against drug use appears to have been extremely successful and has become widespread in both the public and private sectors. Incentives for a drug-free workplace are improved safety and a reduction in financial losses caused by absenteeism, adverse health consequences, and accidents.

Drugs and Crime

The 1997 survey of inmates in state and federal correctional facilities published by the Bureau of Justice Statistics indicates substantially higher rates of drug use among convicted inmates compared to the general population. Approximately 62% of women and 56% of men in state prisons reported having used drugs in the month prior to their offense. The number of male and female inmates who committed their offense while under the influence of drugs was reported to be 32% and 40%, respectively.

According to the Uniform Crime Reporting System of the Federal Bureau of Investigation, there were a total of 1,538,813 arrests for drug abuse violations and a further 1,461,746 arrests for driving under the influence. The 2000 annual report of the Arrestee Drug Abuse Monitoring (ADAM) program indicated that 64% of adult male arrestees had recently used one or more illicit drugs. The most commonly detected drug was marijuana (40.9%), followed by cocaine (30.9%), opiates (6.5%), methamphetamine (1.6%), and phencyclidine (PCP) (0.3%). Although only about one in five arrestees are female, 63% had recently used drugs. The most frequently detected drug in female arrestees was cocaine (33.1%), followed by marijuana (26.7%), opiates (7.2%), and methamphetamine (3.0%). Frequently, suspects and their victims are admitted to the ED for treatment, during which time biological specimens may be collected for medical management and toxicological analysis. These specimens not only provide essential information regarding the treatment of the patient but may also yield results of forensic significance–for example, the timely collection of blood from an inpaired driver or sexual assault victim.

Drugs and Driving

According to the Fatality Analysis Reporting System of the National Highway and Transportation Safety Administration (NHTSA, 2002), 41% of the 38,309 fatal traffic crashes in 2002 were alcohol-related. The exact number of traffic fatalities involving drugs other than alcohol is not known. However, NHTSA estimates that drugs are used by approximately 10% to 22% of drivers involved in accidents, often in combination with alcohol. A study of fatally injured drivers from seven states showed that alcohol was present in more than 50% of the drivers, and other drugs were present in 18% of the drivers. An ongoing NHTSA study of non–fatally injured drivers has shown that compared to the general population, the percentage of young drivers (under 21 years old) who test positive for drugs has almost doubled. The incidence of positive drug findings in injured drivers who receive medical treatment ranges from less than 10% to as high as 40%. The incidence of drug-use among drivers arrested for motor vehicle offences ranges between 15% and 50%. ED physicians may not have a legal obligation to report impaired drivers to the authorities, and as such, these drivers may not be held accountable for their actions.

In 2002, an estimated 11 million people reported driving under the influence of an illicit drug during the past year. This figure corresponds to 4.7% of the population aged 12 years or older (SAMHSA, 2004). Highest rates of drug use while driving were reported among 21-year-olds (18%) compared with those aged 26 or above (3%). One in seven Americans 12 years old and up report driving under the influence of alcohol at least once during the past year. Highest rates of alcohol-impaired driving were reported among 18- to 25-year-olds (26.6%), and males were nearly twice as likely as females to have driven under the influence of alcohol (SAMHSA, 2004).

Drugs and Health

According to the 2002 National Survey on Drug Use and Health, of the 19.5 million Americans who were illicit drug users in 2002, an estimated 7.7 million were in need of substance abuse treatment. A further 18.6 million were in need of substance abuse treatment for alcohol. However, only 1.4 and 1.5 million received treatment for drug- and alcohol-related problems. As many as 94% of people with substance abuse disorders did not receive treatment or did not believe they needed treatment. Dependence and suicide, followed by psychic effects, are the most frequently cited motives for drug use. Common reasons for drug-related admission to the ED are overdose, detoxification, unexpected reaction, chronic effects, or withdrawal. Unexpected reactions and overdoses were the predominant reasons for ED contact in episodes involving gamma-hydroxybutyrate (GHB), miscellaneous hallucinogens, PCP, inhalants, methylenedioxymethamphetamine (MDMA, Ecstasy), amphetamines, ketamine, marijuana (THC), lysergic acid diethylamide (LSD), and alcohol in combination with other drugs. Detoxification was the predominant reason for ED contact for episodes involving heroin and cocaine.

Despite being perceived as a low-risk drug, marijuana was the second most frequently mentioned illicit drug in the ED, composing 18% of the total episodes after cocaine (30%). Drug use remains somewhat regionalized, accounting for unrepresentative statistics in certain metropolitan areas and states. For example, LSD, GHB, and designer amphetamines such as MDMA are more prevalent in California, Florida, and New York, where the drug-culture associated with the "rave" scene is popular.

Club Drugs

"Club drugs," which are becoming increasingly popular with young people, are commonly encountered at nightclubs and "raves." These include the synthetic designer amphetamine MDMA, GHB, LSD, and methamphetamine, as well as illegally diverted and trafficked

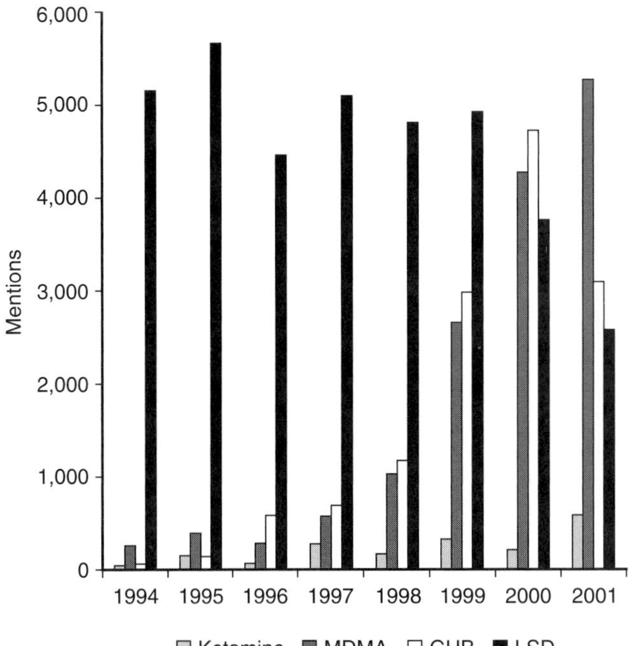

Fig. 14-1 Emergency department mentions for club drugs (1994-2001). (From Drug Abuse Warning Network. (2003). DHHS Publication No. (SMA) 03-3780. Rockville, MD.)

therapeutics, such as ketamine and Rohypnol (flunitrazepam). These drugs have been somewhat popularized by the rave culture and the false perception that they are not as harmful as mainstream illicit drugs such as cocaine and heroin. Statistics from DAWN show that ED mentions involving these drugs, notably MDMA and GHB, have increased at an alarming rate since the early 1990s (Fig. 14-1). Legislative efforts to curb this trend have included federal scheduling and inclusion of these drugs into the Controlled Substances Act. These legal efforts will be supported by a $54 million educational campaign, launched by the National Institute on Drug Abuse and partner organizations, to raise awareness of the dangers of GHB and other club drugs.

Pharmacokinetics

Pharmacokinetics describe the absorption, distribution, metabolism, and excretion of a drug. These factors influence the efficacy of the drug, its concentration at the active site, and the intensity and duration of the drug effect. Pharmacokinetic properties are used by pharmacologists, clinicians, and toxicologists to develop new therapeutics, understand the factors that govern use and abuse, determine how drugs can be detected in the body over time, and interpret their effects on human performance.

Routes of Administration

Onset of action, duration of effects, intensity, and the "quality "of the drug experience may vary, depending on the route of administration. Intravenous (IV) drug administration provides maximum drug delivery and rapid onset of effects. The injection of a drug bypasses the body's natural safeguards. Intravenous administration is complete and not affected by gastrointestinal absorption or intramuscular or subcutaneous absorption. In addition, IV drug administration also avoids the liver (first-pass metabolism) and is transported directly to the site of action without being

Box 14-1 Health Consequences of Intravenous Drug Use

- HIV
- Viral hepatitis (B and C)
- Sexually transmitted infection (gonorrhea, syphilis)
- Bone and joint infection
- Abscesses and cellulitis
- Endocarditis
- Tuberculosis
- Pneumonia
- Septic pulmonary emboli
- Septic arthritis
- Septic thrombophlebitis
- Mycotic aneurysm

inactivated by liver enzymes. Complications of intravenous drug use include infectious disease such as human immunodeficiency virus (HIV) and hepatitis as well as infection, emboli, blood vessel occlusion, thrombosis, and irritant effects (Box 14-1). For these reasons, inhalation and smoking are popular alternatives because these routes mimic IV administration. When a drug is smoked, it is rapidly absorbed in the lungs and transported to the brain via the arterial blood supply. Smoking is a preferred route of crack cocaine administration due to rapid onset, prolonged duration, intensity, and euphoria. However, pipes and smoking apparatus become hot and may burn the lips. The efficiency and speed of drug delivery increase the reinforcing effect of the drug and its abuse liability. However, not all abused drugs are amenable to all routes. The relative advantages and disadvantages of oral, inhalation, smoking, intravenous, intranasal, and dermal drug delivery are summarized in Table 14-1.

Absorption

For a drug to exert a pharmacologic effect, it must gain entry to the body by absorption and traverse biological membranes to its site of action. The route of entry determines the site of absorption: gastrointestinal, pulmonary, dermal, or parenteral. Unless the drug is administered intravenously, it is unlikely that all of it will be absorbed. The efficiency of this process, known as bioavailability, is the amount of drug that is absorbed relative to the amount that is administered. Physicochemical properties of the drug determine the efficiency of absorption, as well as the concentration of the drug, circulation, and surface area at the absorption site. Physical state, solubility, and formulation of the drug play important roles. Water-soluble liquids are absorbed more rapidly than oils, solids, or sustained-release formulations. Because absorption is largely dependent on diffusion, the greater the concentration gradient across the membrane (the higher the drug concentration), the faster the drug will be absorbed. A large surface area, such as the capillary-rich surface of the lungs or microvilli of the small intestine, facilitates absorption.

The pH and pKa of the drug determine how and where the drug gains entry to different compartments of the body. The pKa is the pH at which the drug is half ionized (Table 14-2). The majority of drugs can be classified as acidic, neutral, or basic. Phospholipid membranes within the body are selectively permeable, depending on size, charge, and lipid solubility of the drug. These membranes are effective barriers against passive diffusion of ionized drugs, which must undergo alternative methods of

Table 14-1 Common Routes of Administration for Abused Drugs

ROUTE	ADVANTAGES	DISADVANTAGES	DRUGS
Oral	Noninvasive	Slow absorption via GI tract First-pass metabolism Variable bioavailability Delayed onset Blunted reaction	Cannabinoids, opiates, LSD, mescaline, peyote, GHB, benzodiazepines
Inhalation	Noninvasive Rapid absorption	Limited to drugs with sufficient volatility	Solvents, gases, low boiling point alkaloids
Intravenous	"Rush" caused by bolus of drug Rapid onset	Invasive Deleterious health effects	Opiates, cocaine, methamphetamine, PCP
Smoking	Rapid onset Rapid absorption Noninvasive	Pyrolysis of drug Not all drugs heat stable Reduced bioavailability due to sidestream smoke	Marijuana, PCP, crack cocaine
Intranasal	Noninvasive	Irritation of the nasal mucosa Variable absorption	Cocaine, heroin, methamphetamine
Dermal	Noninvasive	Lipid-soluble drugs only Local irritation Delayed onset Blunted reaction, no "rush"	Fentanyl, nicotine

transport, such as filtration, phagocytosis, pinocytosis, and active or facilitated transport.

Strong acids have low pKa's (pH 1 through 5), which means that at physiological pH (7.2) they are mostly ionized. This state restricts the mobility of the drug because passive diffusion is not favored (Table 14-3). The pKa affects absorption and distribution of a drug. For example, the gastrointestinal tract varies widely in pH, from the buccal cavity (pH 7) to the stomach (pH 2), small intestine (pH 6), duodenum (pH 7), ileum, and colon (pH 8). As a result, uncharged acidic drugs tend to absorb well in the stomach. Strong bases, however, which have high pKa values, are predominantly uncharged at high pH. Even in the most alkaline regions of the gastrointestinal tract (pH 8), basic drugs like methamphetamine (pKa 9.9) are predominantly charged.

The pKa of the drug not only determines the absorption, but it also determines where the drug is most likely to reside. For example, when drugs are distributed into the sweat, which is slightly acidic (pH 5), basic drugs like cocaine and methamphetamine become charged and are trapped in the fluid in a process known as "ion trapping." This process becomes important during neonatal drug exposure, which will be discussed later.

Distribution

As soon as the drug is absorbed and enters the circulation, the distribution phase begins. Once more, depending on the physicochemical properties of the drug and the surrounding pH, passive diffusion, filtration, or transport mechanisms distribute the drug to surrounding tissues and organs. Upon entry into the circulation, plasma proteins may bind the drug. This bound state not only limits entry into the tissues, but also prevents interaction with receptors necessary to produce a pharmacological reaction. Simultaneous administration of multiple, highly bound drugs can inadvertently increase the free concentration of drug, resulting in an acute toxic reaction. Extensively protein bound drugs may have a delayed onset or prolonged duration of action (see Table 14-2). Highly perfused tissues, such as the heart, liver, kidney, and brain, come into contact with the drug much faster than muscle and fat, which are perfused at much slower rates and take much longer to reach equilibrium with circulating drug.

Drugs that are lipid soluble are distributed more readily into the tissues and may penetrate the blood-brain barrier. Tetrahydrocannabinol (THC), the active constituent of marijuana, is lipophilic. It is distributed and stored in tissues and fat depots within the body, accounting for its gradual release and long half-life (see Table 14-2). The extent to which a drug is distributed in the body is given by the volume of distribution (Vd), which is a function of lipophilicity, protein binding, and pKa. Highly water-soluble (hydrophilic) drugs, such as ethanol (Vd 0.5 L/kg), are distributed mainly in the body water and have low volumes of distribution (Vd $<$ 1 L/kg). Conversely, drugs with large volumes of distribution, for example, antidepressants (Vd 10–20 L/kg), are more likely to distribute throughout the body into the tissues. Heroin (Vd 25 L/kg) is capable of penetrating the protective endothelial and glial cells of the blood-brain barrier, whereas morphine (Vd 2–5 L/kg) does not.

Metabolism

Most drugs are highly metabolized by the body with only relatively small amounts being excreted unchanged (see Table 14-2). To facilitate the process of elimination and to prevent the accumulation of drugs, several different types of biological transformations occur that increase the water solubility of the drugs. Metabolism can affect the pharmacological activity of the drug, sometimes eliminating activity (e.g., cocaine metabolism to benzoylecgonine) or increasing it (e.g., heroin metabolism to 6-acetylmorphine and morphine).

During phase I metabolism, enzymes, such as cytochrome P450, monoamine oxidase, cholinesterase, and others, oxidize, reduce, hydrolyze, and dealkylate drugs, rendering them more hydrophilic by introducing polar moieties. This process occurs throughout the body, particularly in the liver, but also in the kidneys, blood, lungs, skin, and gastrointestinal tract. During phase II metabolism, water-soluble conjugates are formed between polar functional groups on the drug and endogenous ligands such as glucuronic acid, sulfate, and glutathione. Drugs that undergo

Table 14-2 Pharmacokinetic Properties of Commonly Abused Drugs

DRUG STREET NAME(S)	HALF-LIFE	DURATION OF EFFECT (H)	PROTEIN BINDING (%)	Vd (L/KG)	pKa	UNCHANGED IN URINE (%)	PRINCIPAL METABOLITE(S)
Cocaine *Blow, horn, nose candy, jelly beans (crack), rooster (crack), tornado (crack), moonrock (crack and heroin), wicky stick (crack, PCP, marijuana), snowball (cocaine and heroin)*	0.7-1.5 h	1-2	92	2-3	8.7	<10	Benzoylecgonine, ecgonine methylester, norcocaine
Fentanyl	3-12 h	0.5-1	79	3-8	8.4	1-5	Norfentanyl, hydroxyfentanyl
GHB *Goop, grievous bodily harm, good hormones at bedtime, max, soap*	0.3-1 h	2-5	0	0.4	-	<5	-
Heroin *Smack, hell dust , big H, thunder, nose drops (liquefied heroin), crop (low-quality heroin), dragon rock (heroin and crack), A-bomb (marijuana and heroin)*	2-6 m	3-6	40	25	7.6	<1	6-Acetylmorphine, morphine, glucuronide conjugates
Ketamine *Cat valium, K, jet, special K, super acid*	3-4 h	0.5-2	30	3-5	7.5	2-5	Norketamine, dehydronorketamine, glucuronide conjugates
Lysergic acid diethylamide (LSD) *Acid, acid cube, backbreaker, battery acid, doses, dots, Elvis, loony tunes, pane, superman, window pane, zen*	3-4 h	8-12	-	0.3	7.8	<1	NorLSD, 2-oxo-3-hydroxy-LSD
Marijuana (cannabinoids) *Bud, dope, ganja, herb, hydro, indo, Mary Jane, shake*	1-3 d (naive) 3-13 d (chronic)	2-4	97	4-14	10.6	<1	11-nor-Δ^9-carboxy-THC
Methamphetamine *Bikers coffee, chalk, chicken feed, crank, crystal meth, glass, go fast, ice, meth, poor man's cocaine, shabu, speed, stove top, trash, yellow bam*	6-15 h	2-4	10-20	3-7	9.9	43	*p*-Hydroxymethamphetamine, amphetamine, *p*-hydroxyamphetamine
MDMA *Disco biscuit, ecstasy, hug drug, go, X, XTC*	6-9h	2-4	-	5-8	-	65	Methylenedioxyamphetamine
Morphine	1.3-6.7 h	3-6	35	2-5	8.1	<10	Glucuronide conjugates, normorphine
Phencyclidine (PCP) *Angel dust, busy bee, cadillac, elephant tranquilizer, embalming fluid, hog, jet fuel, killer weed, tick*	7-46 h	2-4	65	5-8	8.5	30-50	4-Phenyl-4-piperidinocyclohexanol, 1-(1-phenylcyclohexyl)-4-hydroxypiperidine
Phenobarbital	2-6 d	10-20	50	0.5-0.6	7.2	20-35	*p*-Hydroxyphenobarbital, dihydrodiol, glucuronide conjugates

Data from Baselt, R. C. (2002). *Disposition of toxic drugs and chemicals in man* (6th ed.). Foster City, CA: Chemical Toxicology Institute; Wilson, J. M. (1994). *Abused drugs II.* Washington, DC: AACC Press.

extensive conjugation, such as morphine, may require enzyme hydrolysis prior to analysis, as will be discussed later.

Sometimes a drug may undergo biotransformation before entering the circulation. Enzymes in the gastrointestinal tract can metabolize orally administered drugs, reducing their pharmacologic activity and clinical utility. When the drug has been absorbed in the lower intestine, the portal circulation transports the drug to the liver, without it ever having reached the general circulation. This "first-pass" effect accounts for the reduced bioavailability of some orally administered drugs.

Table 14-3 Effect of pH and pKa on Acidic, Basic, and Neutral Drugs

	% IONIZED DRUG pH UNITS FROM pKa				
DRUG TYPE	−2	−1	pKa	+1	+2
Acidic drugs (e.g., acetaminophen, ampicillin, barbiturates, non-steroidal anti-inflammatory drugs, phenytoin, probenecid, THC metabolites)	1	9	50	91	99
Neutral drugs (e.g., carbamazepine, glutethimide, meprobamate)	0	0	0	0	0
Basic drugs (e.g., antiarrythmics, antidepressants, antihistamines, cocaine, narcotic analgesics, PCP, phenothiazines, sympathomimetic amines)	99	91	50	9	1

A great many variables can affect drug metabolism, including age, sex, genetic polymorphisms, health, disease, and nutrition. The expanding field of pharmacogenomics is beginning to elucidate the role of genes on drug metabolism. For example, differences in the abundance of certain isoezymes of cytochrome P450 account for differences in drug metabolism between ethnic populations. These factors are of scientific importance not only for the interpretation of drug findings but also for development of new therapeutic agents.

Elimination

Drugs and their metabolites are eliminated principally via the kidneys and liver, each of which is perfused with more than 1 L of blood every minute. Thus, the efficiency of drug elimination is dependent on hepatic and renal blood flow. During renal excretion of drugs glomerular filtration, reabsorption, and secretion occur. The resulting ultrafiltrate accumulates in the bladder via the collecting tubules. The fraction of drug bound to plasma proteins and the glomerular filtration rate determine the amount of drug that enters the tubular lumen of the kidney. Charged species are less likely to permeate the tubular cells and reabsorb, a process that significantly delays elimination of drug. In this way, the rate of elimination is variable, depending on the pH of the urine. The elimination of acidic drugs is enhanced by alkalinization of the urine using sodium bicarbonate. Conversely, basic drugs may be eliminated more readily by acidification of the urine using ammonium chloride. As much as 76% of a methamphetamine dose may be excreted unchanged in acidic urine, compared with only 2% in alkaline urine.

Hepatocytes in the liver secrete bile, which is stored in the gallbladder and is later excreted via the intestines in the feces. Biliary excretion is favored by large polar substances, but when metabolism renders a drug more lipid soluble, the drug may undergo reabsorption, a process known as enterohepatic recirculation.

When a fixed amount of drug is eliminated per unit of time (e.g., ethanol), the elimination is said to be zero order. However, most drugs follow a first-order elimination process, whereby a constant fraction of drug is eliminated over time. Half-life ($T_{1/2}$) is a measure of the rate of elimination. One half-life is the time it takes for the concentration of drug in the plasma to decrease by 50%. These values are dependent on volumes of distribution and clearance rates, which may vary with age, sex, disease state, or drug interactions. The lungs (for elimination of volatile substances) and even sweat, saliva, hair, nails, and breast milk are all relatively minor excretory pathways, but they may be of some forensic importance and will be discussed later.

Key Point *14-1*

The link between the amount of drug and its effect over time is the basis for establishing therapeutic and toxic drug concentrations for clinical management and intervention.

Pharmacological Effects

The pharmacological effect of a drug is a result of the drug's interaction at a given receptor site. The concentration of free drug circulating in the blood is in equilibrium with the concentration of drug at the receptor site. An increase in the concentration of free drug modulates the receptor response and enhances the pharmacological effect. The mechanism by which a drug modulates a receptor is described by pharmacodynamics. The link between the amount of drug and its effect over time is the basis for establishing therapeutic and toxic drug concentrations for clinical management and intervention. Such pharmacodynamic responses account for the pharmacological effect of a drug and are known as the dose-response relationship. However, pharmacological effect can be intrinsically dependent on the time passed since the dose was taken, rather than with the concentration of drug in the blood. A given concentration of drug may produce widely variable effects, depending on the time since administration. This phenomenon is referred to as hysteresis. For example, after consuming alcohol, a person tends to feel more excited and euphoric during the initial absorption phase than during the elimination phase, during which time the person may feel sedated and depressed. CNS stimulants such as methamphetamine follow a similar cycle. A concentration of 200 ng/mL methamphetamine in blood may coincide with euphoria, exhilaration, restlessness, and stimulation during the initial absorption phase. However, several hours later during the elimination phase, the same concentration of drug may coincide with confusion, depression, anxiety, dysphoria, and exhaustion.

The pharmacological effect experienced by the user may be apparent from vital signs or involuntary reflexes. For the purpose of determining impairment or acute or chronic toxicity, blood is the matrix of choice. The presence of the drug in the urine is only an indication of drug exposure, over a period of hours, days, or even weeks, rather than an indicator of impairment. With the exception of ethanol, there is no direct correlation between the concentration of a drug in the blood and the level of impairment for legal purposes. Any impairment by drugs is generally inferred by correlating the concentration of the drug with observations made by arresting officers or others involved with the impaired individual. Factors such as tolerance can have a profound effect on the pharmacodynamic response in an individual. A quantity of cocaine sufficient to produce a mild "buzz" in a chronic user could be acutely cardiotoxic in a naïve user, resulting in coma and death.

Drug Recognition

Drugs may affect normal behavior by enhancing or impairing human performance (e.g., cognition or psychomotor ability). The same drug may be capable of either enhancing or impairing performance, depending on the dose and pattern of drug use. Drug recognition is an important ability for clinicians, toxicologists, and law enforcement personnel. Recognition of abused substances, including illicit drugs and therapeutics, that may have been incorrectly administered or combined with other drugs, is a valuable skill.

Impairment may be observed and documented by either a trained clinician or a drug recognition expert (DRE). The DRE program was developed by the Los Angeles Police Department in the 1980s and is now used throughout the US and overseas. For law enforcement purposes, a series of physiological and psychomotor tests are used to determine the class of drugs that is likely present: CNS stimulants, CNS depressants, narcotic analgesics, hallucinogens, PCP, cannabis, or inhalants. Clinical characteristics such as blood pressure, pulse, respiration, body temperature, nystagmus, ocular convergence, pupil size, and pupillary reaction to light can be useful indicators of drug use (Table 14-4). Other observable effects, such as tremors, coordination, gait, muscle tone, perception, diaphoresis, emesis, lacrimation, and appearance of the conjunctivae may also provide valuable insight (Table 14-5). Abstinence syndromes resulting from chronic drug use produce effects that vary considerably from those caused by acute drug intoxication. These effects may be impairing and, in some instances, can be life-threatening (Table 14-6).

Drug and Disease Interactions

Certain disease states can affect the way in which a drug is absorbed, distributed, and eliminated. Clearance rates, protein binding, volume of distribution, and half-life may be affected in some individuals but not in others. Hepatic, renal, gastrointestinal, and respiratory disease have been shown to affect pharmacokinetic parameters in some populations, even though the underlying mechanisms are in many cases poorly understood. Drug interactions may occur when more than one drug is administered. The pharmacokinetics of one drug may change the pharmacodynamics

Table 14-4 Signs and Symptoms of Commonly Abused Substances

	MARIJUANA	NARCOTIC ANALGESICS	HALLUCINOGENS	CNS DEPRESSANTS	CNS STIMULANTS	PHENCYCLIDINE	INHALANTS
Blood pressure	Elevated	Low	Elevated	Low	Elevated	Elevated	Varies
Pulse rate	Elevated	Low	Elevated	Low	Elevated	Elevated	Elevated
Pupils	Dilated/normal	Constricted	Dilated	Normal	Dilated	Normal	Normal/dilated
Pupillary Reaction to light	Normal	Slow/none	Normal	Slow	Slow	Normal	Slow
Body temperature	Normal	Low	Elevated	Normal	Elevated	Elevated	Varies
HGN*	Not present	Not present	Not present	Present	Not present	Present	Present
VGN*	Not present	Not present	Not present	Possibly present	Not present	Usually present	Possibly present
Lack of Ocular convergence	Present	Not present	Not present	Present	Not present	Present	Present
30-second estimation	Distorted	Slow	Fast	Slow	Fast	Fast	Normal

*HGN, horizontal gaze nystagmus; VGN, vertical gaze nystagmus.

Table 14-5 Observable Signs and Symptoms of Commonly Abused Drugs

CNS DEPRESSANTS	CNS STIMULANTS	OPIOIDS	CANNABIS	PHENCYCLIDINE	HALLUCINOGENS
Poor coordination	Anxiety	Constipation	Ataxia	Agitated	Body tremors
Disoriented	Body tremors	Dry mouth	Body tremors	Ataxia	Dazed appearance
Decreased inhibitions	Bruxism	Dysphoria	Disorientation	Blank stare	Diaphoresis
Fumbling	Dry mouth	Euphoria	Eyelid tremors	Confused	Disorientation
Gait ataxia	Excited	Facial itching	Increased appetite	Cyclic behavior	Dysarthria
Ptosis	Euphoric	Low, raspy voice	Odor of marijuana	Diaphoresis	Hallucinations
Sluggish	Hyperreflexia	Poor coordination	Poor time and distance perception	Dissociative anesthesia	Memory loss
Slowed reflexes	Hypervigilance	Ptosis	Possible paranoia	Dysarthria	Muscle rigidity
Sedated	Insomnia	Puncture marks	Reddened conjunctiva	Hallucinations	Nausea
Slurred speech	Irritability	Mental clouding	Reduced inhibitions	"Moon walking"	Paranoia
	Muscle rigidity	Muscle flaccidity	Transient muscle rigidity	Muscle rigidity	Poor coordination
	Reduced appetite	Nausea			Poor time and distance perception
	Runny nose	Nodding off			Synesthesia
	Reddening of nasal mucosa	Sedation			
	Talkativeness	Slow reflexes			
		Vomiting			

Table 14-6 Withdrawal Symptoms of Commonly Abused Drugs

DRUG	WITHDRAWAL SYMPTOMS
CNS Stimulants	Muscular aches, abdominal pain, tremors, anxiety, hypersomnolence, lack of energy, depression, suicidal thoughts, exhaustion
Opioids	Dilated pupils, rapid pulse, piloerection, abdominal cramps, muscle spasms, vomiting, diarrhea, tremulousness, yawning, anxiety
CNS Depressants	Tremulousness, insomnia, sweating, fever, anxiety, cardiovascular collapse, agitation, delirium, hallucinations, disorientation, convulsions, shock
Marijuana	Anorexia, nausea, insomnia, restlessness, irritability, anxiety, depression

of the other, affecting therapeutic effect and toxicity. Although pharmacokinetics and pharmacodynamics of most drugs are relatively well known, very few studies have addressed the interactions of abused drugs or of abused and therapeutic drugs in combination with each other. For ethical and safety reasons, these studies may utilize healthy volunteers (drug experienced) who receive doses that are very much lower than those typically administered by chronic drug users. These studies provide limited data because they do not account for altered metabolism or possible health deficits associated with chronic drug use.

Interpretation

The duration and intensity of effects depend on the dose administered, individual metabolism, frequency of drug use, and the presence of other drugs. Because many of these factors are unknown, toxicological interpretation is often difficult. Questions regarding administration time can sometimes be answered using the pharmacokinetic principles, such as drug half-life. For a drug that is eliminated by first-order kinetics, 99% of the drug is eliminated by seven half-lives, with less than 1% of the drug remaining in the body. By ten half-lives, 99.9% of the drug has been eliminated. This information, together with the detection limit or cut-off concentration of the analytical technique, can be used to establish an approximate detection window. Although detection times for different drugs can be estimated, these vary with method of analysis, dose, frequency, metabolism, age, sex, or health (Table 14-7). Urinary detection times are even more difficult to predict, owing to differences in fluid intake, diuresis, and the effect of urinary pH on drug elimination. However, these values may be useful in determining an approximate time frame during which drug exposure took place. For example, the detection time of 6-acetylmorphine in urine is approximately two to eight hours, indicating recent heroin use.

Therapeutic, toxic, and lethal concentrations of illicit and therapeutic drugs are often useful, but must be interpreted with caution due to the differences among individuals, as previously discussed. Toxicological interpretation is usually based upon a combination of toxicological analyses and observations made by either clinicians or trained law enforcement personnel during medical evaluation, at autopsy, or at the scene of a crime.

Specimen Handling

Specimens for toxicological analyses are frequently collected in medical or emergency room settings. Appropriate selection, collection, preservation, and storage of biological evidence are essential during a toxicological investigation. Delays in specimen collection can also have a profound impact on the toxicological outcome, particularly in cases of driving under the influence or drug-facilitated sexual assault.

Selection and Collection of Evidence

The selection and collection of biological samples is often predetermined to some extent by the circumstances of the case and

Table 14-7 Therapeutic and Toxic Drug Concentrations of Commonly Abused Drugs

DRUG	THERAPEUTIC DOSE	THERAPEUTIC CONCENTRATION (NG/ML)	TOXIC CONCENTRATION (NG/ML)	APPROXIMATE DETECTION TIME IN URINE*
Methamphetamine	5-10 mg	20-60	100-1000	1-3 d
Cocaine	1.5 mg/kg	100-200	NA	1-3 d
Morphine	5-10 mg	10-80	>200	1-3 d
Tetrahydrocannabinol	NA	NA	50-200	1-3 d (naïve) several weeks (chronic)
Phencyclidine (PCP)	NA	NA	1000	3 d
Diazepam	5-30 mg	100-1000	>5,000	5-7 d
Propoxyphene	65-400	100-400	>500	1-2 d
Lysergic acid diethylamide (LSD)	NA	NA	2-30	<24 h
Phenobarbital	50-200 mg	10,000-40,000	>50,000	1-3 weeks
Methaqualone	150-500 mg	1,000-5,000	>6,000	1-2 weeks
Methadone	5-100 mg	100-400	>2,000	1-3 d

From Substance-Abuse Testing Committee, Therapeutic Drug Monitoring and Clinical Toxicology Division, American Association for Clinical Chemistry. (1988). Critical issues in urinalysis of abused substances: Report of the substance-abuse testing committee. *Clin Chem, 34*(3), 605-632; Baselt, R. C. (2002). *Disposition of toxic drugs and chemicals in man* (6th ed.). Foster City, CA: Chemical Toxicology Institute; Wilson, J. M. (1994). *Abused drugs II.* Washington, DC: AACC Press; Tietz, N. W. (1995). *Clinical guide to laboratory tests* (3rd ed.). Philadelphia: W. B. Saunders.

*Detection times of drug and/or drug metabolite(s) are dependent on dose, route of administration, frequency of use, health, and individual factors.

Table 14-8 Collection of Postmortem Specimens for Toxicological Analysis

SPECIMEN	AMOUNT
Blood, heart	10-25 mL
Blood, peripheral	10-25 mL
Urine	All
Bile	All
Vitreous humor	All
Gastric contents	All
Liver	25 g
Kidney	25 g
Spleen	25 g
Brain, fat	25 g
Lung	25 g
Hair	1/2 cm^2 area

the disposition of the donor, being either living or deceased. During postmortem examination, body fluids, tissues, and organs may provide insight into acute drug intoxication that could be highly relevant during a death investigation (Table 14-8). Femoral or subclavian blood should be collected if possible and the source of the blood should be clearly identified. Postmortem drug concentrations can be significantly affected by postmortem drug redistribution. Following death, drugs stored in fat or muscle may be released into surrounding blood. In the absence of a peripheral blood specimen, elevated drug concentrations in cardiac blood could be misleading during a death investigation if postmortem drug redistribution is not taken into account. The kidney and spleen may be especially useful in cases in which metals, carbon monoxide, or cyanide is suspected. Lipophilic drugs may be evident in brain tissue, and volatile substances may be detected in the lung, which should be collected in an airtight container. Collection of hair and nails may provide historical information on long-term exposure (months or years) to intoxicating substances.

Common Specimens for Testing

In the living person, blood and urine are the most common specimens for toxicological testing. Alternative matrices, such as hair, sweat, saliva (oral fluid), breast milk, and others, have been used, but analysis of these specimens is less common and has not yet gained widespread use. However, these specimens may offer distinct advantages over conventional samples and are highly applicable to toxicology. Examples of specific sample uses are sweat collection for probationary drug testing, amniotic fluid to determine prenatal drug exposure, and hair to determine a history of drug exposure (Table 14-9).

Containers Used for Specimen Storage

Glass or plastic containers are routinely used for specimen storage. Plastic containers should be evaluated prior to use, as they may contain plasticizers that may interfere with the analysis. Certain drugs may absorb onto the surface of the storage container, particularly if they are present at a low concentration. Drugs with polar moieties, such as morphine, may adsorb onto glass unless it is treated (silanized) to prevent adsorption. In a similar fashion, lipophilic or hydrophobic drugs, (e.g., THC) may adsorb onto the surface of plastic containers. Every attempt should be made to use a container of appropriate size and type to minimize adsorption or oxidative loss.

Preservation and Storage of Evidence

The use of appropriate containers, preservatives, and lowered temperatures can help minimize excessive drug losses as a result of exposure to light, oxidation, or hydrolysis. Blood is routinely preserved with sodium fluoride (2% weight per volume, w/v) to inhibit microorganisms and enzymes that can transform drugs in vitro. For example, cocaine is a basic drug with two labile ester moieties. In unpreserved samples, benzoylesterases in the blood rapidly convert cocaine to ecgonine methylester after collection and during storage. After 21 days as much as 100% of the cocaine may be lost at room temperature in the absence of preservative. Despite deactivation of some of the enzymes from using preservative, chemical conversions may occur as a result of the specimen pH. For example, cocaine spontaneously hydrolyzes to benzoylecgonine at physiological pH. The rate at which the drug undergoes enzymatic or chemical conversion is reduced by lowering the temperature. Specimens should be refrigerated (4°C or 39° F) for short-term storage for up to two weeks and frozen (–20°C or –4° F) for long-term storage. These temperatures inhibit bacterial growth and reduce reaction kinetics.

Preservatives Used for Specimen Storage

In addition to preservatives, anticoagulant agents such as potassium oxalate, sodium citrate, or EDTA (5 mg/mL) may be added for ease of sample handling. Sodium fluoride may be added to urine, but many postmortem specimens are stored without preservative in tightly sealed containers at low temperature. Some preservatives, such as sodium azide, can interfere with methods of analysis such as immunoassay. Antioxidants such as ascorbic acid or sodium metabisulfite (1% w/v) are sometimes used to prevent oxidative losses, but these agents can act as reducing agents toward some drugs. In a similar fashion, adjusting specimen pH is not generally favored, because just as some drugs are alkaline labile (e.g., cocaine, 6-acetylmorphine), others are acid labile.

Collection of Specimens

Commercial gray-top Vacutainer or Venoject blood tubes that contain sodium fluoride and potassium oxalate should be used for the collection of toxicological specimens. Urine collection should be observed by trained personnel to reduce the likelihood of donor manipulation, such as dilution, adulteration, or substitution. It is particularly easy for females to "dip" the urine container into the toilet bowl during collection. Direct observation and the addition of a coloring agent to the cistern will identify these cases.

Substitution of the urine specimen is less common, but commercial products including lyophilized drug-free urine are readily available for this purpose. In vitro or in vivo adulteration agents are widely available as common household products and OTC medications. In vivo adulteration involves the ingestion of a substance that may enhance elimination of a drug by either diuresis, acidification, or alkalinization of the urine. Commercial adulteration products are readily available, but their use is unlikely unless the subject has some advance notification. In vitro adulterants are added to the urine sample after collection. These substances may interfere with analysis by chemical degradation of

Table 14-9 Advantages and Disadvantages of Biological Specimens

SPECIMEN	ADVANTAGES	DISADVANTAGES
Hair	History of drug use (months) Readily available, easy collection Low potential for donor manipulation	New technology Not yet widely accepted Recent drug use not detected Environmental contamination Potential for ethnic bias
Saliva (oral fluid)	Readily available, easy collection Parent drug present Related to free drug concentration in plasma Minimal sample preparation Many drugs determined Indicates recent drug use	New technology Short drug detection time Small sample volume (1-5 mL) Potential for oral contamination Collection method influences specimen pH and drug content
Sweat	History of drug use (weeks) Cumulative measure of drug use Parent drug present Noninvasive collection Less frequent drug testing required Not readily adulterated	New technology Potential for environmental contamination High intersubject variability Requires collection device, expensive Skin irritation and discomfort Small sample volume No pharmacological interpretation possible
Nails	Easy collection History of drug use (months)	Limited data New technology Not yet widely accepted Recent drug use not detected Environmental contamination
Blood	Widely accepted matrix Determines recent drug use (hours-days) Related to pharmacological effect Not readily adulterated	Invasive collection Collection by medical personnel Drug not detected for extended periods
Urine	Widely accepted matrix Easy collection Longer detection window than blood (days-weeks)	Potential for donor manipulation Minimal parent drug Not related to impairment, pharmacologic effect
Amniotic fluid	Determination of prenatal drug exposure Not readily adulterated Minimal sample preparation Relatively few interferences	Invasive collection Risk of complications Limited data Collection by medical personnel
Breast milk	Determination of neonatal drug exposure Not readily adulterated Many drugs present	Privacy, invasive collection Limited data Interferences due to high lipid content Drug content varies with milk composition Variable matrix

the drug. Prevalence of adulterants, particularly in workplace urine drug testing, has led to dipstick tests and other diagnostic assays that can detect some of these agents. Common adulteration agents are listed in Table 14-10.

Evidence Security

The integrity of biological evidence is maintained at all times by tracking the handling and storage from specimen collection to final disposition. A chain-of-custody form is used to document the date, purpose, and name of the person handling the specimen. The four Ws of the chain of custody are as follows:

- Who handled the evidence
- What was handled
- Why it was handled
- Where it was located at all times

Specimen handling and disposition of evidence is scrutinized by the courts. Specimens must be stored in secure locations with limited access where they are not vulnerable to adulteration.

Toxicological Analysis

Typically, toxicological analysis involves a combination of two chemically and analytically distinct methodologies. Most commonly, a rapid screening test such as immunoassay or thin-layer chromatography precedes a more rigorous and labor-intensive analysis using gas chromatography–mass spectrometry (GC-MS) or liquid chromatography–mass spectrometry (LC-MS). Immunoassays and GC-MS are the most widely used techniques and will be discussed in more detail.

Screening Techniques

Immunoassays

Immunoassays are antibody-based tests that can provide toxicological results of a presumptive nature in a relatively short period of time (minutes to hours). Generally, these tests are amenable to automation, require very small sample volumes, require limited or no sample pretreatment, and are not technically demanding. Most

Table 14-10 Common In Vitro and In Vivo Adulterants

IN VITRO ADULTERANTS	DIURETICS
Ascorbic acid	**Prescription:**
Alcohols	Benzothiadiazines
Amber-13 (hydrochloric acid)	Carbonic anhydrase inhibitors
Ammonia	Loop diuretics
Bleach	Osmotic diuretics
Clear Choice (glutaraldehyde)	
Detergent	**Over the Counter (OTC):**
Drano	Aqua-Ban
Ethylene glycol	Diurex
Gasoline	Fem-1
Hydrogen peroxide	Midol
Klear (potassium nitrite)	Pamprin
Lemon juice	Premsyn PMS
Liquid soap	
Lime-A-Way	**Other:**
Mary Jane Super Clean 13 (detergent)	Alcoholic beverages
	Caffeine
Salt	Golden seal root
Stealth (peroxidase)	Herbal remedies
THC-Free (hydrochloric acid)	Pamabrom
UrinAid (glutaraldehyde)	
Urine Luck (pyridinium chlorochromate)	
Vanish	
Vinegar	
Visine	
Water	
Whizzies (sodium nitrite)	

immunoassays rely upon the competitive binding reaction that takes place between antidrug antibodies and either labeled or unlabeled drug. In an enzyme immunoassay, drug in a donor urine sample competes with enzyme-labeled drug for binding sites on an antibody molecule. If there is no drug in the urine, the enzyme-labeled drug binds to the antibody, unimpeded. However, if the urine sample contains a quantity of drug, the enzyme-labeled drug will not bind as readily; the more drug in the sample, the less enzyme-labeled drug will bind, and vice versa. The amount of enzyme that is bound can be determined colorimetrically and the intensity of the color is related to the concentration of drug in the sample.

Best Practice *14-1*

Specimens for toxicological analyses must be carefully controlled and stored in a secure location. A chain of custody must accompany all forensic specimens.

A wide variety of immunoassay technologies are commercially available, many of which rely on the use of enzyme-, radioisotope-, or fluorescent-labeled species for detection purposes. Some of these tests are highly automated, allowing high sample throughput on the order of several hundred tests per day, whereas others are more labor intensive and are less readily automated. Many of the highly automated assays are homogeneous in nature and can be performed in one step without the need for separation. Immunoassays that require a separation step to remove unbound from bound drug are called heterogeneous assays. These tests usually take longer to complete, are not readily automated, and are more technically demanding. However, because of the separation step that takes place prior to detection, heterogeneous immunoassays may be less susceptible to endogenous and exogenous interferences than their homogeneous counterparts. Heterogeneous assays are also less susceptible to matrix effects and are more amenable to blood and alternative fluids, often without sample pretreatment. Several commercial immunoassays used for drugs of abuse testing are summarized in Table 14-11.

Drawbacks of Immunoassay Testing. Because of the nature of the antibody-antigen reaction, immunoassays offer limited specificity. When the antibody recognizes a structural conformation, or

Table 14-11 Advantages and Disadvantages of Common Immunoassays

IMMUNOASSAY TECHNIQUE	ADVANTAGES	DISADVANTAGES
CEDIA (homogeneous) cloned enzyme donor immunoassay	Highly automated Long shelf-life Wide linear range	Susceptible to interferences Not amenable to all matrices
ELISA (heterogeneous) enzyme-linked immunosorbent assay	Sensitive Minimal matrix effects Potential for automation	Not adaptable to common automated analyzers Expensive
EMIT (homogeneous) enzyme multiplied immunoassay technique	Highly automated Long shelf-life	Matrix effects and interferences False negative results Not amenable to all matrices
FPIA (homogeneous) fluorescence polarization immunoassay	Highly automated More stable than enzyme reagents Highly sensitive	Expensive Endogenous interferences Sample pretreatment for blood
KIMS (homogeneous) kinetic interaction of microparticles in solution	Highly automated Inexpensive More stable than enzyme reagents	Special instrument maintenance Interferences may cause false positives Linear range is small
RIA (heterogeneous) radioimmunoassay	Highly sensitive Minimal matrix effects Amenable to blood and urine	Disposal of radioisotopes Limited shelf-life Limited automation potential

Table 14-12 Common Cross-Reacting Substances in Some Immunoassays

ASSAY	COMMON CROSS-REACTING SUBSTANCES
Amphetamine/methamphetamine	Benzphetamine, ephedrine, methylenedioxyamphetamine, methylenedioxyethylamphetamine, methylenedioxymethamphetamine, phenmetrazine, phentermine, phenylpropanolamine, propylhexedrine, pseudoephedrine
Benzodiazepines	Alprazolam, bromazepam, chlordiazepoxide, clonazepam, clorazepate, demoxepam, diazepam, estazolam, α-hydroxyalprazolam, lorazepam, nitrazepam, nordiazepam, oxazepam, prazepam, temazepam, α-hydroxytriazolam
11-Nor-Δ^9-carboxy-THC	Δ^9-Tetrahydrocannabinol, 11-carboxy-Δ^9-tetrahydrocannabinol, 11-hydroxy-Δ^9-tetrahydrocannabinol
Cocaine metabolite	Cocaine, cocaethylene, ecgonine, ecgonine ethyl ester, ecgonine methylester, norcocaine
Opiates	Codeine, dihydrocodeine, dihydromorphine, hydrocodone, hydromorphone, oxycodone, oxymorphone, morphine-glucuronide, nalorphine, norcodeine, normorphine
Phencyclidine	Diphenhydramine, dextromethorphan, PCP analogs, thiorizadine

epitope, on the drug molecule, it may bind, producing a positive result. Immunoassays are very rarely truly specific for the target drug because structurally similar molecules may also bind to the antibody to varying degrees. However, the degree of specificity may not necessarily limit the usefulness of the test. Some immunoassays are designed to be nonspecific in order to cross-react with several drugs within a given class. In contrast, the usefulness of a test may be severely limited by its specificity, for example, detection of methamphetamine. Endogenous phenethylamines or OTC decongestants or dietary supplements such as pseudoephedrine, ephedrine, phenylpropanolamine, and other structurally-related drugs may cross-react, producing false positive reactions. Common cross-reacting substances are given in Table 14-12. Because of the limitations of immunoassays, these results alone are not forensically defensible. Immunoassay screening tests are excellent tools to indicate which drug or class of drug is present, but a more rigorous and specific test must be performed to unequivocally confirm the presence of a particular drug for forensic purposes.

Effectiveness of Immunoassay Tests. The effectiveness of an immunoassay depends on the cut-off concentration, below which the sample is deemed negative. For the purposes of federal workplace drug testing, the Substance Abuse and Mental Health Services Administration (SAMHSA) has mandated cut-off concentrations for amphetamines, cannabinoids, cocaine metabolite, opiates, and PCP (Table 14-13). These cut-off concentrations are elevated in order to reduce the number of false positive results and to account for accidental drug exposure from dietary sources (e.g., poppy seeds) or passive smoke inhalation. However, for the purposes of death or criminal investigation, cut-off concentrations are typically much lower to reduce the likelihood of false negative results. Additional drug classes, including therapeutics such as benzodiazepines and barbiturates, are often included. The cut-off concentrations established by the testing facility are set at the lowest concentration of drug that can be reliably confirmed using other techniques (e.g., GC-MS). These low cut-off points are necessary to identify very low concentrations of drug that could be present after a single dose.

On-Site Drug Tests

A number of on-site drug tests now offer immediate results, without the need for sophisticated equipment or highly trained personnel. These tests rely on conventional immunoassay-based principles and utilize a chromatographic support to provide qualitative drug screen results. When blood or urine is added to one of these devices, capillary action allows any drug in the sample to migrate through the immunochromatographic medium. Unlike the instrument-based immunoassays, which rely upon measurement of absorbance, fluorescence, or radioisotopes, the progress

Table 14-13 Screening (Immunoassay) Cutoff Concentrations

		CUTOFF CONCENTRATION (NG/ML)	
DRUG	TARGET ANALYTE	SAMHSA[1]	FORENSIC[2]
Amphetamines	Amphetamine, methamphetamine	1000	50-100
Benzodiazepines	Oxazepam, nordiazepam	-	100-300
Barbiturates	Secobarbital	-	200-300
Cannabinoids	11-Nor-9-carboxy-Δ^9-THC	50	20-50
Cocaine	Benzoylecgonine	300	150
Lysergic acid diethylamide	Lysergic acid diethylamide	-	0.5
Methadone	Methadone	-	50-300
Methaqualone	Methaqualone	-	300
Opiates	Morphine	2000	10-100
Phencyclidine	Phencyclidine	25	25-50
Propoxyphene	Propoxyphene	-	300

[1]Urine
[2]Blood or urine

of the antibody-antigen reaction can be followed with the naked eye. Antibody molecules are often labeled with colored latex beads or colloidal gold, which may produce a concentrated blue or purple color in the test result window.

Although on-site tests are becoming popular in clinical and private sector toxicology screening, they are not yet widely used in medicolegal drug testing. On-site assays are largely designed for workplace or emergency room drug testing. These devices are less effective in forensic investigations owing to their elevated cut-off concentrations and the limited repertoire of drugs that are detected. However, the increasing popularity of on-site tests together with growing acceptance of alternative specimens, such as saliva, could have an impact on the criminal justice system in such arenas as highway safety and assessment of driving under the influence in the form of roadside drug tests.

Confirmatory Analysis

Because of the inherent uncertainty in immunoassay screening results due to cross-reactivity and interferences, positive drug screen results must be confirmed using a more rigorous technique. Gas chromatography-mass spectrometry (GC-MS) is the most widely used confirmatory technique in forensic toxicology. It can be used to specifically identify and quantify the drug or drugs present.

Prior to analysis, the drugs must be extracted from the biological matrix. Common isolation techniques are liquid-liquid extraction (LLE) and solid-phase extraction (SPE). During LLE, organic solvents such as chloroform or ether are used to isolate drugs from biological fluids by manipulation of pH. Partition of the drug between the two immiscible layers (e.g., buffered urine and solvent) depends on polarity, charge, lipophilicity, and the pKa of the drug. In a manner analogous to the distribution of drugs throughout the body, ionized drugs are more likely to partition into the polar aqueous layer (e.g., blood or urine), whereas uncharged or nonpolar drugs are more likely to partition into the solvent layer. In this fashion, drugs are extracted from biological fluids or tissues using solvents that are subsequently evaporated, concentrated, and analyzed.

Many of the same principles are utilized during SPE whereby the drug is adsorbed onto an immobilized solid support in a cartridge assembly. The affinity of the drug for the solid support allows the drug to bind temporarily. The mechanisms of attraction ("like attracts like") are analogous to those of LLE, with the added benefit of ion exchange, whereby a drug that is positively charged binds to a negatively charged chromatographic support and vice versa. A combination of polar, nonpolar, and ion exchange mechanisms can be used to isolate acidic or basic drugs that contain ionizable functional groups, such as carboxylic acids or amines. Once the drug is bound to the support, interferences are removed by washing and the drug is eluted from the cartridge using an organic solvent or by manipulating the pH to neutralize or reverse the charge.

Additional sample preparation steps may be necessary, depending on the matrix. This may include homogenization, sonication, dilution, centrifugation, protein precipitation, or hydrolysis. The latter of these is particularly important for polar drugs that are highly conjugated (e.g., cannabinoids, benzodiazepines, opiates). Chemical or enzymatic methods are used to hydrolyze the sample. Alkaline or acid hydrolysis is commonly used to release glucuronide conjugates of 11-nor-Δ^9-carboxy-THC and morphine, respectively. Chemical hydrolysis is efficient and reproducible, but acid or alkali labile drugs may degrade during the process. Enzymes such as β-glucuronidase can be used to hydrolyze drugs without the need for harsh chemical conditions, but these methods are more expensive, slower, and less reproducible.

Injection of the drug extract onto the GC/MS allows components of the mixture to be separated and identified. Upon entry to the GC inlet, vaporization occurs and the gaseous sample is transported by a flow of inert carrier gas (e.g., helium). The sample is transported through a heated capillary column, during which time separation takes place. The column, which is typically about 30 m long, is coated with a material which, depending on the physicochemical properties of the drug, allows it to adsorb. Depending on the extent of the interaction between the drug and the column, components of the extract will emerge from the end of the column at different times. The time taken for the drug to elute from the column, known as retention time, is the basis of chromatographic separation.

Drugs or components of the extract then pass through a heated interface and enter the mass spectrometer, where molecular identification takes place. First, the sample enters an ionization chamber. During the ionization process, each drug produces a characteristic selection of ions. Weak bonds in the drug molecule are broken and the resulting charged fragments are recorded by the mass analyzer. This array of ions, known as the mass spectrum, is like a molecular fingerprint of the drug, allowing it to be identified. GC-MS is a highly specific confirmatory technique because identification is based upon both the retention time of the drug and its characteristic spectrum.

Interpretation

Negative toxicology sometimes coincides with clinical signs and symptoms or a behavioral response that clearly indicates the presence of an intoxicating substance. These findings are often caused by limitations of the toxicological procedures. Common caveats in immunoassay testing includes the inability to detect drugs that may be present below the cut-off concentration or drugs that have low cross-reactivity with the antibody. Conjugated drugs do not always cross-react well in immunoassays and unless subsequent confirmatory analyses include a hydrolysis step, these drugs may be undetected. Inability to confirm positive immunoassay results may be the result of poor extraction efficiencies or detection limits. Detection of trace quantities of a drug (<10 ng/mL), such as THC, in blood samples may require highly sensitive and specialized techniques, such as negative ion chemical ionization gas chromatography mass spectrometry, that is not available in all laboratories.

Drug-Facilitated Sexual Assault

The majority of sexual assaults in the US are reported to be acquaintance rapes, "date rapes," and an increasing number may be drug-facilitated. Drug-facilitated sexual assault occurs when a chemical agent is used to assist or procure nonconsensual sexual contact. During a drug-facilitated sexual assault, a victim may be incapacitated or unconscious. Under these circumstances it may not be possible for a person to resist or consent to sexual contact. The CNS depressant drugs gamma-hydroxybutyrate (GHB) and Rohypnol (flunitrazepam) have received particular attention from the media as "date rape" agents. These reports however, have not been supported by the scientific literature, which suggests that more than 20 different drugs have been associated with this crime.

Alcohol and marijuana are the most commonly encountered substances in alleged cases of sexual assault, which supports the view that consumption of impairing substances is an important risk factor in sexual assault. The relationship between drug use and sexual assault is complicated: illicit drug use not only increases the risk of sexual assault, but sexual assault increases the risk of subsequent substance abuse. In a recent study of more than 2000 victims of sexual assault in California, nearly two thirds of the urine specimens contained alcohol or drugs: Alcohol (63%) and cannabinoids (30%) accounted for the majority of positive samples, and GHB and flunitrazepam accounted for less than 3%.

In a nationwide study of 1179 alleged victims of sexual assault, flunitrazepam metabolites were detected in only six urine specimens. A review of this study revealed that the prevalence of alcohol was high, followed by cannabinoids, cocaine, benzodiazepines, amphetamines, and GHB (Fig. 14-2). Nationwide, a total of 48 specimens tested positive for GHB (4.1%) compared with 8% in California alone, which highlights the importance of geographical and regional trends in drug use. Multiple drug use was evident in 35% of the cases, frequently in combination with alcohol.

Chemical submission applies to any drug that has the ability to render the victim passive, submissive, or unwilling or unable to resist. Potent, fast-acting depressant drugs that have amnesic properties are effective "knock-out drops." However, a variety of illicit and widely prescribed therapeutic agents, including benzodiazepines, barbiturates, muscle relaxants, hypnotics, and antihistamines, have been associated with drug-facilitated sexual assault (Box 14-2). Typically these agents are CNS depressants that impair consciousness, memory, or lower inhibitions. Others may have an anesthetic-type effect, causing unarousable sleep or produce an "out-of-body experience" whereby the conscious victim is powerless, paralyzed, or unable to move.

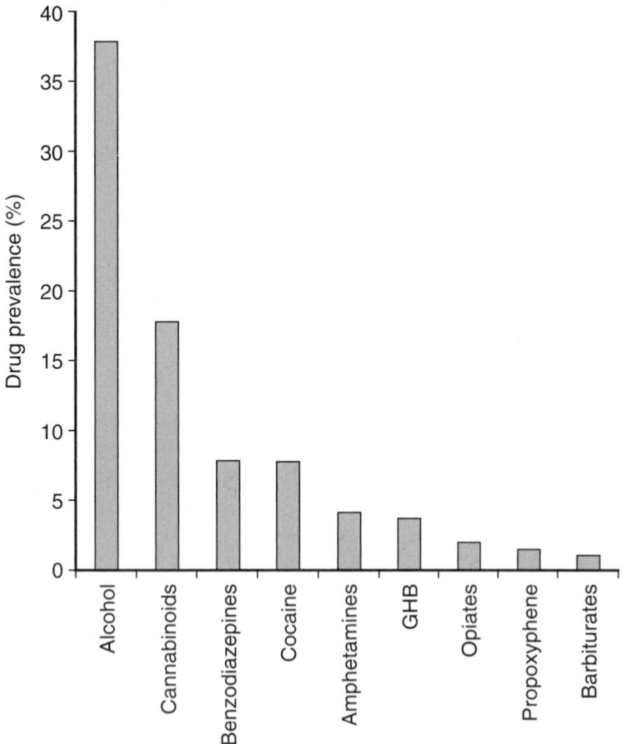

Fig. 14-2 Drugs prevalent in alleged cases of sexual assault. (Data from El Sohly, M. A., & Salamone, S. J. (1999). Prevalence of drugs in alleged cases of sexual assault. *J Anal Tox 23*, 141-146.)

Box 14-2 Substances Detected in Alleged Cases of Drug-Facilitated Sexual Assault

Alcohol	Flunitrazepam
Alprazolam	Gamma-hydroxybutyrate (GHB)
Amphetamine	Ketamine
Barbiturates	Lorazepam
1,4-Butanediol (BD)	Marijuana
γ-Butyrolactone (GBL)	Meprobamate
Carisoprodol	Methamphetamine
Chloral hydrate	Methylenedioxymethamphetamine (MDMA)
Chlordiazepoxide	Midazolam
Clonazepam	Opiates
Cocaine	Oxazepam
Cyclobenzaprine	Phencyclidine (PCP)
Diazepam	Scopolamine
Diphenhydramine	Triazolam
Ethanol	Zolpidem
Flurazepam	

GHB and Flunitrazepam

GHB and flunitrazepam have received particular attention in light of their rapid onset, extensive biotransformation, and detection difficulties. Flunitrazepam, which is seven to ten times more potent than diazepam (Valium), produces onset of actions within 15 to 30 minutes of administration. Disinhibition, passivity, lack of resistance, muscle relaxation, and anterograde amnesia have been reported as effects of flunitrazepam. Not legally available in the US, flunitrazepam was reformulated to turn blue or hazy in clear or colored beverages. However, illicit sources of flunitrazepam remain odorless, colorless, and tasteless. The effective dose of flunitrazepam is very low (1 to 2 mg) compared to that of GHB (2 to 4 g). Illicit formulations of GHB, which were placed into Schedule I of the Controlled Substances Act in April 2000, can take effect in as little as 15 minutes. This drug, which sometimes has a salty or soapy taste, can produce euphoria and disinhibition, as well as nausea, vomiting, respiratory depression, and coma.

Specimen Collection

Delay in specimen collection can profoundly affect the prosecutorial and toxicological outcome of the investigation. Coordination of law enforcement, medical, and scientific personnel is essential. Immediate action must be taken to preserve the evidence by collection of blood and urine by healthcare professionals, such as forensic nurses, with authority to initiate the evidence collection process and chain of custody. The victim should be urged not to urinate until the specimen can be properly collected. The rape/evidentiary examination should include collection of 20 mL of blood preserved with sodium fluoride and potassium oxalate (gray-top tubes). Inadequately preserved blood drawn into yellow- or lavender-top tubes may compromise the toxicological investigation or preclude toxicological analysis altogether. Collection of blood is essential if the ingestion of drug occurred within the last 24 hours. It may also provide valuable interpretive information regarding pharmacological response or impairment. It is possible that positive blood toxicology can be used to corroborate involvement of the drug in the sexual assault, whereas urine toxicology is only indicative of prior exposure to the drug.

Best Practice *14-2*

Because delays in specimen collection can profoundly affect the prosecutorial and toxicological outcome of the investigation, specimens should be promptly obtained, annotated with a precise time and date of collection, and refrigerated immediately to prevent degradation of the sample.

Samples should be refrigerated immediately and the date and time of specimen collection documented. Chain-of-custody procedure should be initiated. Supplemental information, such as symptoms exhibited by the victim, the suspected date and time of the ingestion, as well as alcohol, drugs, or medications ingested prior to the assault, should be fully documented. Prosecution of drug-facilitated sexual assault and interpretation of toxicological findings can be complicated in cases of multiple drug use by the victim. Incapacitation may be the result of a combination of substances, consumed both voluntarily and involuntarily. For example, voluntary ingestion of alcohol, combined with the surreptitious administration of other CNS depressants, may have a potentiating or synergistic effect that could impair the victim to a far greater extent.

Legislative Efforts

Legislative efforts to curb the growing trend in drug-facilitated sexual assault have included restricting drug access, federal scheduling, and increased sentencing. In particular, the Drug-Induced Rape Prevention and Punishment Act of 1996 (Public Law 104-305) increases penalties for those who use drugs to assist in the commitment of a violent crime. Under this law, administration of a controlled substance with the intent to commit a sexual assault or other violent crime is a federal felony, punishable by up to 20 years' imprisonment.

For this reason, it is important that the toxicological analysis is conducted by a forensic laboratory familiar with cases of drug-facilitated sexual assault. The use of appropriate cut-off concentrations and sensitive confirmatory testing procedures are required to identify single doses of drugs that may be present at very low concentration. Confirmatory analysis is usually necessitated in these instances, regardless of the screening results. Limitations include the poor cross-reactivity toward conjugated drugs and the absence of effective and reliable screening tests for drugs such as GHB. Drugs administered in low dose (e.g., alprazolam), those with short half-lives (e.g., GHB), or drugs that undergo rapid and extensive biotransformation (e.g., flunitrazepam) pose a particular challenge to drug detection agencies. Typically, detection limits of less than 10 ng/mL are necessitated in these instances. Urine is advantageous from the standpoint of detection time, although drugs with short half-lives may be undetectable within 96 hours or less (Table 14-14). GHB, which is administered in high doses, is detectable in blood and urine for approximately six to eight hours and 12 hours, respectively. Drug detection times vary considerably, depending on dose, metabolism, and the method of analysis.

Effects Experienced by Victims

Victims of drug-facilitated sexual assault may experience confusion, dizziness, psychomotor impairment, drowsiness, impaired judgment, reduced inhibitions, or slurred speech. Victims may lose their ability to ward off attackers, may develop amnesia, and may provide unreliable or confused recall of events. Drug-induced anterograde amnesia, whereby the drug temporarily disables the brain's ability to store information into memory, may cause the victim to be uncertain about the facts surrounding the assault. This uncertainty may procure an unwillingness to report the rape or provide biological samples for forensic testing. Because many of the depressant-type effects of drugs used to incapacitate the victim are similar to the effects of alcohol, it is probable that many incidents of drug-facilitated sexual assault are not recognized.

Table 14-14 Doses and Half-Lives of Selected Depressant Drugs

DRUG	DOSE (MG)	HALF-LIFE
Alprazolam	0.25-1	6-27 h
Barbiturates (short-acting, e.g., pentobarbital)	50-200	15-48 h
Barbiturates (intermediate-acting, e.g., butalbital)	50-100	30-40 h
Barbiturates (long-acting, e.g., phenobarbital)	50-200	48-120 h
Methaqualone	150-500	20-60 h
Chlordiazepoxide	10-25	6-27 h
Clonazepam	0.5-2	19-60 h
Diazepam	5-10	21-37 h
Diphenhydramine	50-100	3-14 h
Flunitrazepam	1-2	9-25 h
Flurazepam	15-30	1-3 h
γ-Hydroxybutyrate (GHB)	2000-4000	0.3-1 h
Lorazepam	0.5-2	9-16 h
Nitrazepam	5-10	17-48 h
Propoxyphene	65-400	8-24 h
Temazepam	15-30	3-13 h
Tetrahydrocannabinol	5-20	1-3 d (naïve) 3-13 d (chronic)
Triazolam	0.25	2-4 h
Zolpidem	5-10	1.4-4.5 h

Data from Baselt, R. C. (2002). *Disposition of toxic drugs and chemicals in man* (6th ed.). Foster City, CA: Chemical Toxicology Institute; Wilson, J. M. (1994). *Abused drugs II.* Washington, DC: AACC Press.

Warning Signs

Rape treatment centers provide educational material and tips to help identify and minimize the likelihood of drug-facilitated sexual assault. Women who feel unusually intoxicated and suspect that they may have unknowingly ingested a drug should seek immediate assistance. The following warning signs suggest a possible drug-facilitated sexual assault (Rape Treatment Center, 2004):

- If the victim recalls having a drink, but cannot recall what happened for a period of time after consuming the drink
- If the victim suspects that sexual contact has taken place, but cannot remember any or all of the incident
- If the victim feels more intoxicated than the usual response to the same amount of alcohol
- If the victim wakes up feeling hung over and experiences a memory lapse or cannot account for a period of time

Prevention of Drug-Facilitated Sexual Assault

Healthcare workers, educators, and public officials have developed a list of "don'ts" to increase awareness of the dangers of unknowingly ingesting substances such as sedating or incapacitating drugs. A national program supports the distribution of educational brochures and posters within high schools, colleges, bars and lounges, and other locations frequented by youth and older singles. The following guidelines have been developed to prevent drug-facilitated sexual assault:

- Don't drink beverages that you did not open yourself.
- Don't share or exchange drinks with anyone.
- Don't drink from a container that is being passed around.
- If someone offers to buy you a drink, accompany that person to the bar, watch the drink being poured, and carry the drink yourself.
- Don't leave your drink unattended.
- If your drink has been left unattended, discard it.
- Don't drink anything that has an unusual taste or appearance (e.g., excess foaming, salty or soapy taste, unexplained residue)

Infant Drug Exposure

Unfortunately, within recent years it has been suggested that as many as one tenth of all infants are exposed to illicit drugs during pregnancy. In a 2002 study of self-reported drug use, 6.8% of pregnant women aged 15 to 25 used an illicit drug within the past month (SAMHSA, 2004). The most frequently used drug was marijuana. Binge drinking (defined as five or more drinks on one occasion) was reported in 4.5% of pregnant women in the same age group. Although the American Academy of Pediatrics does not recommend universal screening of infants, it proposes prevention, intervention, and treatment services to pregnant women and their children. Cocaine, heroin, amphetamines, and nicotine are reported to cause impaired fetal growth and acute withdrawal syndromes. Higher rates of fetal distress, growth retardation, and abnormal neurodevelopment have been reported in babies when the pregnant mother commonly abused drugs. A 1997 study of gestational drug exposure in nearly 3000 newborns in Michigan indicated that as many as 44% of neonates tested positive for drugs. Of these, 30.5% tested positive for cocaine, 20.2% for opiates, and 11.4% for cannabinoids.

Drug Use in Nursing Mothers

Drug use in nursing mothers is also a concern. It is estimated that between 0.4% and 27% of nursing mothers in the US abuse drugs. Although the developmental effects of drug exposure as a result of nursing are largely unknown, acute toxicity and withdrawal effects are possible. Several difficulties are associated with the study of drug abuse during pregnancy or in nursing mothers:

- It can be difficult to recruit participants for the studies.
- Lifestyle of women abusing drugs may predispose them to adverse pregnancy outcome owing to poor nutrition, living conditions, general health, or socioeconomic status.
- Multiple-drug use, particularly in combination with tobacco or alcohol, can complicate assessment.
- Unreliability of subjects is often associated with reporting such factors as drug use, dose, and duration.

Effects of Drug Exposure on the Fetus or Neonate

Exposure of the fetus or neonate to intoxicating substances may cause deleterious effects, including higher rates of fetal distress, demise, abnormal neurodevelopment, and growth retardation. Chronic alcohol use during pregnancy has been long recognized to cause neonatal changes and the effects have been characterized as fetal alcohol syndrome. Cocaine, heroin, amphetamines, and nicotine have been associated with impaired fetal growth and withdrawal syndromes. During normal pregnancy, amniotic fluid is circulated, swallowed, and processed by the fetus at rates of up to 50 mL/hour. Encapsulation of the fetus in this "protective" fluid can actually prolong the exposure to harmful drugs or metabolites that cross the placental barrier. Small lipid-soluble drugs can rapidly diffuse across the placental barrier, yet large, polar drugs are transferred more slowly. The amniotic sac and its contents serve as a deep compartment with restricted, slow equilibrium between adjacent compartments. Basic drugs, such as methamphetamine, may accumulate in amniotic fluid as a result of ion trapping. This phenomenon can produce concentrations of drug that exceed those found in fetal or maternal plasma.

Drugs in Breast Milk

Drugs are also transported by passive diffusion across the mammary epithelium into the breast milk. The slightly acidic pH tends to trap basic drugs and the presence of emulsified fats tends to concentrate lipid-soluble drugs such as THC and PCP. Amphetamines have been detected in breast milk at concentrations three to seven times those of maternal plasma. THC can be eight times higher. In addition, drugs linger in the body; PCP was detected as long as 41 days following cessation of drug use. The transfer and accumulation of drugs in breast milk increases the likelihood of infant toxicity.

Determining Prenatal or Neonatal Drug Exposure

Prenatal or neonatal drug exposure can be determined using conventional analytical techniques mentioned earlier (e.g., immunoassay, GC-MS). However, interpretation of toxicological findings is often limited because drug dose, route, and time of administration are often unknown. Despite our understanding of the maternal consequences of drug abuse, fetal consequences remain poorly understood. Determining the long-term implications of prenatal drug exposure is a challenging area of maternal-fetal medicine.

Summary

Toxicology is an essential discipline within the forensic sciences. The three major subdisciplines of forensic toxicology are human performance toxicology, postmortem toxicology, and forensic urine drug testing. Because the results of various types of drugs testing are vital elements in the outcomes of many judicial proceedings, there is no room for error in the selection, identification, collection, and preservation of biological evidence.

Forensic nursing personnel have several important responsibilities in ensuring that tests provide precise and accurate data, beginning at the point of deciding which individuals should have toxicological analyses to support their clinical management and to serve as a database for subsequent judicial proceedings.

Case Study 14-1 Wrong Way Driver

Disposition

A 23-year-old male driving the wrong way on the highway at 90 mph crashed into oncoming traffic. The driver suffered only superficial injuries, but both passengers in the oncoming vehicle were killed. The driver exhibited muscle twitching and very rapid speech. A pipe, an off-white substance, and drug paraphernalia were found in the vehicle. A drug recognition evaluation revealed blood pressure of 162/111 mm Hg, pulse 145 bpm, pupils dilated (9 mm), slow reaction to light, no horizontal or vertical gaze nystagmus, and time estimation of 30 seconds was only 7 seconds.

Findings/Interpretation

Immunoassay of blood and urine taken from the suspect two hours after the accident indicated the presence of amphetamines. Symptoms observed by the officer were consistent with CNS stimulant use. Confirmatory GC-MS analysis revealed a concentration of 730 ng/mL methamphetamine in the blood, which is inconsistent with therapeutic drug use. The concentration of methamphetamine in the blood, which falls into the toxic range, is more consistent with a tolerant or chronic drug user.

Case Study 14-2 Asleep at the Wheel

Disposition

Drivers on a city street observed a 35-year-old female "nodding off" at the wheel while driving approximately 20 mph. The vehicle eventually stopped at a light post and caused minor property damage. At hospital, where the driver received treatment for slight injuries, vital signs indicated blood pressure of 112/60 mm Hg, pulse 42 bpm, pupils constricted (1.5 mm), unreactive to light, with horizontal gaze nystagmus, and lack of convergence. Eyelids were droopy and hands felt cold and clammy. The woman stated she had had two glasses of wine with lunch, 30 minutes earlier. Prescriptions for Vicodin and Xanax were found in her purse.

Findings/Interpretation

Blood alcohol concentration at the hospital, one hour after the accident, was only 0.02%. Immunoassay drug screen results were negative, but confirmatory GC-MS analysis revealed therapeutic concentrations of hydrocodone and alprazolam at 10 and 30 ng/mL, respectively. Drug signs and symptoms were consistent with the combined use of three CNS depressant drugs, which have an additive effect.

Case Study 14-3 Unexplained Coma

Disposition

A 15-year-old girl at a party suffers dizziness, vomiting, and falls unconscious after consuming a nonalcoholic drink. Upon arrival at the ED, she is comatose, hypothermic, and bradycardic. The girl, who had no history of drug or alcohol use, awoke from the coma several hours later, suffering amnesia. The following day, the girl claimed a sexual assault had taken place at the party.

Findings/Interpretation

In the ED, an immunoassay drug screen for common drugs of abuse was negative. Blood drawn at the hospital was consumed during medical management. Blood and urine collected at the police station 24 hours after the alleged sexual assault was analyzed for "date-rape" drugs. GHB was present in the urine (100 mg/L), but not in the blood, consistent with detection times of the drug. Clinical signs and symptoms were consistent with GHB administration.

Key Point *14-2*

Delays in specimen collection can also have a profound impact on the toxicological outcome, particularly in cases of driving under the influence or drug-facilitated sexual assault.

Resources

Books

Moffat, A. C. (2003). *Clarke's isolation and identification of drugs* (2nd ed.). London: Rittenhouse Book Distributors.

Ellenhorn, M. J. (1996). *Ellenhorn's medical toxicology: Diagnosis and treatment of human poisoning* (2nd ed.). Baltimore: Williams & Wilkins.

Haddad, L. M., Shannon, M. W., & Winchester, J. F. (1998). *Clinical management of poisoning and drug overdose* (3rd ed.). Philadelphia: W. B. Saunders.

Hardman, J. G., Limbird, L. E., & Gilman, A. G. (Eds.). (2001). *Goodman & Gilman's The pharmacological basis of therapeutics* (10th ed.). New York: McGraw-Hill.

Hawks, R. L. & Chiang, C. N. (Eds.). (1986). *Urine testing for drugs of abuse.* National Institute on Drug Abuse. Research Monograph Series. Number 73. Washington, DC: US Government Printing Office.

Karch, S. (Ed.). (1998). *Drug abuse handbook.* Boca Raton, FL: CRC Press.

Levine, B. (Ed.). (2003). *Principles of forensic toxicology* (2nd ed.). Washington, DC: AACC Press.

Liu, R. H. & Goldberger, B. A. (Eds.). (1995). *Handbook of workplace drug testing.* Washington, DC: AACC Press.

Mandatory guidelines for federal workplace drug testing programs: Final guidelines; notice. (1988). Federal Register, 53, 11970-11989.

Siegel, J. A. (Ed.). (2000). *Encyclopedia of forensic sciences.* London: Academic Press.

Physicians' Desk Reference. (2004). Thompson Healthcare.

LeBeau, M., & Mozayani, A. (2001). *Drug-facilitated sexual assault: A forensic handbook.* San Diego: Academic Press.

References

Baselt, R. C. (2002). *Disposition of toxic drugs and chemicals in man* (6th ed.). Foster City, CA: Chemical Toxicology Institute.

National Highway and Transportation Safety Administration (NHSTA), US Dept. of Transportation, Washington, DC.

Rape Treatment Center. (2004). Santa Monica-UCLA Medical Center, Santa Monica, CA. Retrieved from www.endrape.org.

Substance Abuse and Mental Health Services Administration (SAMHSA). US Dept. of Health and Human Services, Washington, DC.

Substance Abuse Testing Committee, Therapeutic Drug Monitoring and Clinical Toxicology Division, American Association for Clinical Chemistry. (1988). Critical issues in urinalysis of abused substances: Report of the substance-abuse testing committee. *Clin Chem* 34(3), 605-632.

Tietz, N. W. (1995). *Clinical guide to laboratory tests* (3rd ed.). Philadelphia: W. B. Saunders.

Wilson, J. M. (1994). *Abused drugs II.* Washington, DC: AACC Press.

Chapter 15 Air Bag–Induced Injuries and Deaths

William S. Smock and Catherine C. Smock

Overview

During the past decade the world has been shocked to learn that air bags, the much-touted safety device promoted by the automotive industry, is taking lives as well as saving them (The Air Bag Crisis, 1997; Smock, 2000; National Highway Transportation Safety Administration [NHTSA], 2004). In the US, over the last 15 years more than 250 men, women, and children have been fatally injured by deployed air bags (NHTSA, 2004). Thousands more have sustained serious but nonfatal injuries, including: amputations of fingers and hands, massively comminuted fractures of the forearms, closed-head injuries, and cervical spine fractures (Smock, 2000; NHTSA, 2004). The National Highway Transportation Safety Administration (NHTSA) has estimated that air bags have saved approximately 13,000 lives (NHTSA, 2004)–that is, one life sacrificed for every 52 saved. This ratio would be judged totally unacceptable if air bags were held to the same Food and Drug Administration (FDA) standards that are applied to other "lifesaving" drugs or medical devices. It is astonishing to note that the vast majority of these serious and fatal injuries were incurred in low- to moderate-speed collisions in which no serious or fatal injury would have been expected (NHTSA, 2004). Many of the accident victims were also properly restrained with shoulder harness and lap belt devices, supposedly providing even greater protection (NHTSA, 2004).

History of Air Bags

Ford and General Motors began experimenting with early air bag prototypes in the 1950s and 1960s. Data indicating the air bag's harming potential were quickly generated. Ford conducted crash simulations in the 1960s that demonstrated air bag deployment could traumatically eject a child from a vehicle and amputate a steel-hinged arm from a dummy (Grenier, 1997; Appendix to the Air Bag Crisis, 1997). When testing involved animal models, the list of severe and fatal injuries grew (Horsch, Lau, & Andrzejak et al., 1990; Mertz, Driscoll, & Lennox et al., 1982; Mertz & Weber, 1982, Prasad & Daniel, 1984; Viano & Warner, 1976). Atlanto-occipital dislocation, decapitation, cervical spine fractures, cardiac rupture, hepatic rupture, aortic and vena cava transection, splenic rupture, and severe closed-head injuries were induced by the mechanical forces inherent in air bag deployment (Horsch, Lau, & Andrzejak et al., 1990; Mertz, Driscoll, & Lennox et al., 1982; Mertz & Weber, 1982, Prasad & Daniel, 1984; Viano & Warner, 1976).

Ongoing testing has continued to demonstrate risk for injury induction. Testing by General Motors in the 1970s using baboons for models (comparable to a child's or small adult's stature) demonstrated that "if the head is in the path of the deploying air bag, it is concluded that injury is likely to occur in the form of brain or neck injury" (Patrick & Nyquist, 1972). Testing by Ford in the 1970s caused one engineer to compose a warning that "the right front seat should be used only by persons who are more than five feet [1.52 m] tall and are in sound health. Smaller persons and those who are aged or infirm should be seated and belted in the rear seat" (Appendix to the Air Bag Crisis, 1972). Research and testing have revealed several critical factors contributing to injury induction and severity, and they are the size of the individual and the physical proximity of the individual (whether whole body or body part, i.e., arm, hand, or finger) to the air bag at the moment of deployment.

Air Bag Design and Function

Between 1987 and 1997 (the effective date of the federal air bag mandate) the automobile industry voluntarily put 82 million air bags (56 million on the driver's side and 26 million on the passenger side) in cars on America's roadways. Different manufacturers chose different designs, but they all have some critical components in common.

The air bag is a canvas bag housed in a module that is constructed of a variety of materials. These materials include thermoplastic and rigid methane foam covered with polyvinyl or rigid metal plates covered with foam or vinyl. At the moment of deployment, the module cover splits along seams intentionally weakened in manufacture (which fracture outward), allowing the air bag to inflate.

Sodium azide is the explosive propellant used to initiate the deployment cycle in most air bag designs in use today. When it is ignited, the gaseous by-products of combustion fill the bag, propelling it toward the occupant at 336 kph (210 mph). The module cover is also propelled toward the occupant at this speed. Either of the two components, the air bag or the module cover, can cause serious or fatal injuries. The types of injuries incurred are relevant to the component inflicting them.

The air bag can maim and kill at any point during its deployment. Deployment can be broken down into three phases: initial, middle, and final phases. The different types of air bag–inflicted wounds seen can be correlated to the phase in which they were incurred. In the initial phase of deployment, punch-out wounds are observed. They include atlanto-occipital dislocations; cervical spine fractures and brain stem resection; cardiac, hepatic, and splenic lacerations; diffuse axonal injuries; subdural and epidural hematomas; and decapitation (Figs. 15-1 to 15-3). Catapult type injuries are seen when occupants impact the air bag during the midstage of its deployment. They are injuries consistent with the head and neck having been driven rapidly upward and rearward. Severe cervical spine hyperextension occurs with energy sufficient to rupture blood vessels and ligaments and to fracture cervical vertebrae. Bag slap type injuries are incurred during the final stage of air bag deployment when the bag is at the peak of

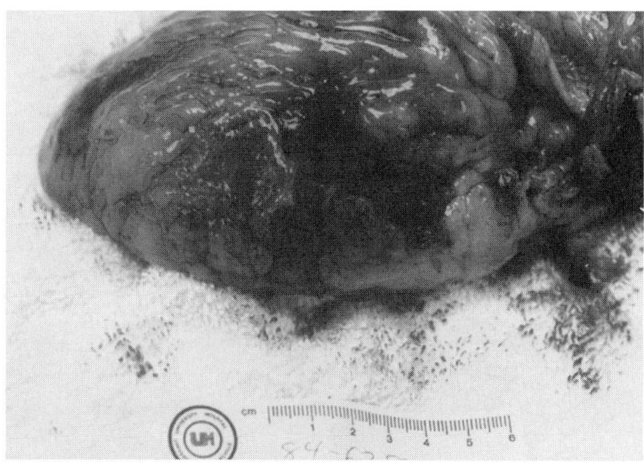

Fig. 15-1 Cardiac rupture can occur if the driver's chest is on or near the air bag module cover at the time of deployment.

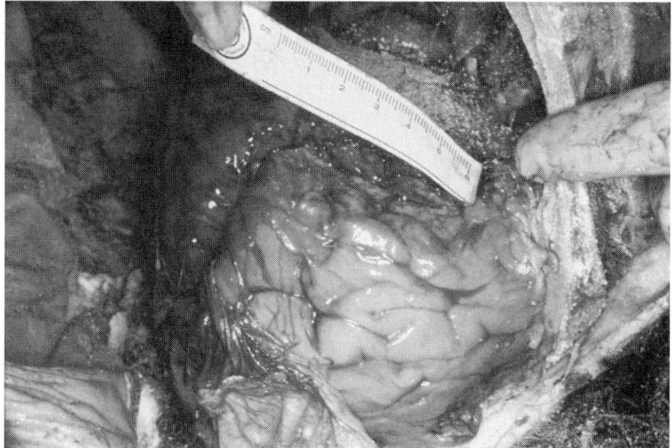

Fig. 15-2 Air bag deployment rapidly accelerated the victim's head rearward, causing bridging veins to tear and this resultant subdural hematoma.

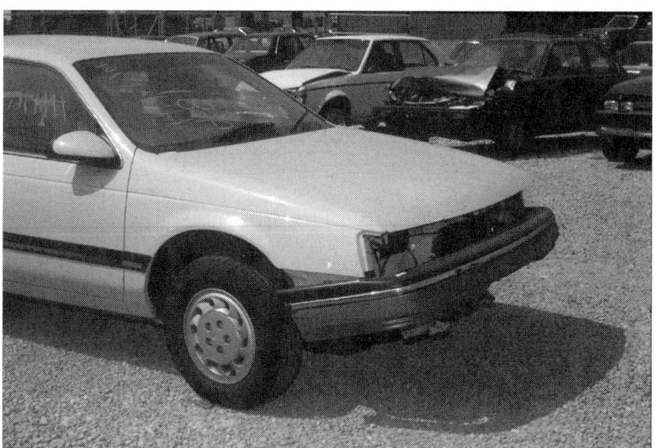

Fig. 15-3 A 5'1" restrained 35-year-old female sustained fatal head injuries in a minor collision involving a 1991 Ford Taurus. The short-statured driver sustained the fatal injuries from impact with the module cover.

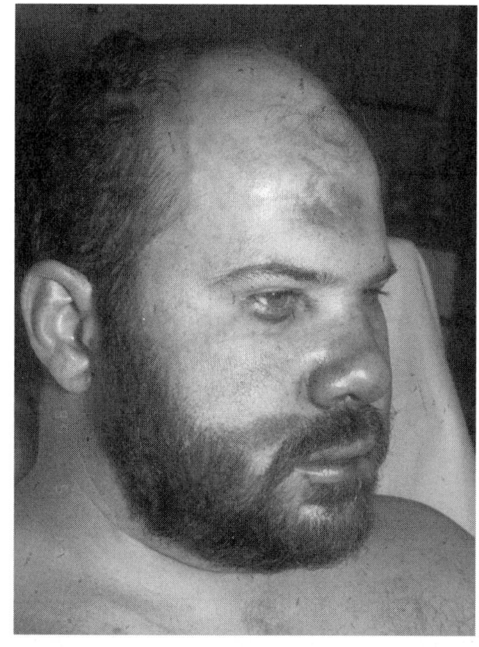

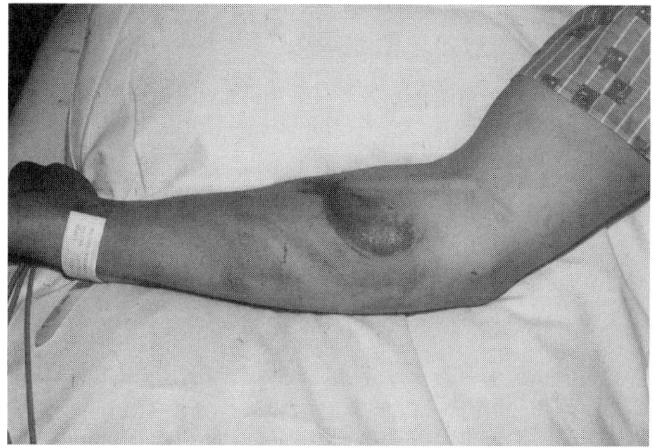

Fig. 15-4 Abrasions to the face (*A*) and arms (*B*) are common injuries and are typically sustained during the final or "bag-slap" state of deployment.

its excursion. When the canvas bag slaps the occupant's face, injuries to the eye and epithelium are commonly observed (Fig. 15-4, *A* and *B*).

The air bag module cover as well as the air bag can inflict severe injuries. The driver's side module cover is generally made of a rubberized plastic material, but the passenger side may have a metal housing (Figs. 15-5 to 15-8). One major problem with steering wheel–mounted air bags is the fact that the horn is usually also mounted in the steering wheel. Hand and arm injuries observed in individuals whose extremities were in contact with the module at the moment of its rupture include degloving, fracture dislocations, and amputation (partial and complete) of digits and forearms (Smock, 2000; Smock & Nichols, 1995; Huelke, Moore, & Comptom et al., 1994; Smock, 1992). If the module cover impacts the occupant's face, head, or neck, skull fractures and severe and fatal head injuries have been observed (NHTSA, 2004; Smock & Nichols, 1995).

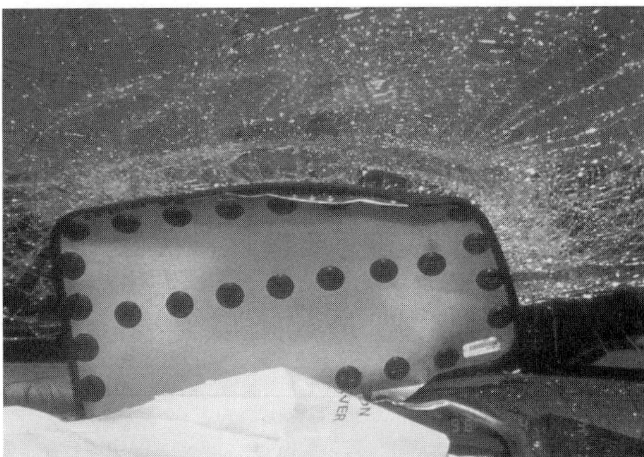

Fig. 15-5 Passenger-side air bag module covers may contain a metal housing. Placement of any extremity on the module cover, to brace oneself, will result in very severe traumatic injuries including amputations of hands, arms, fingers, and feet.

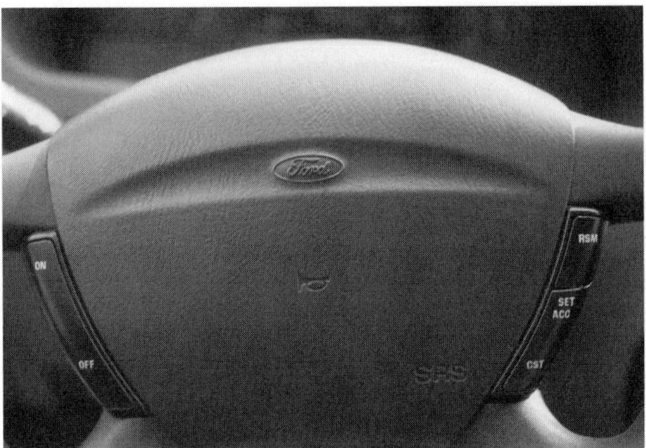

Fig. 15-6 The placement of a horn activation button on the module cover is an invitation to a traumatic upper extremity injury. Many severe air bag-induced hand injuries have occurred because drivers were attempting to blow the horn when the air bag detonated.

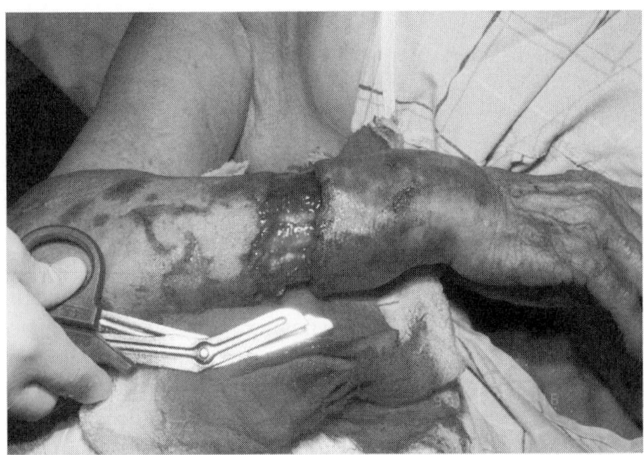

Fig. 15-7 A severe degloving, open fracture of the radius and ulna from forearm contact with the module cover of a 1989 Lincoln Continental.

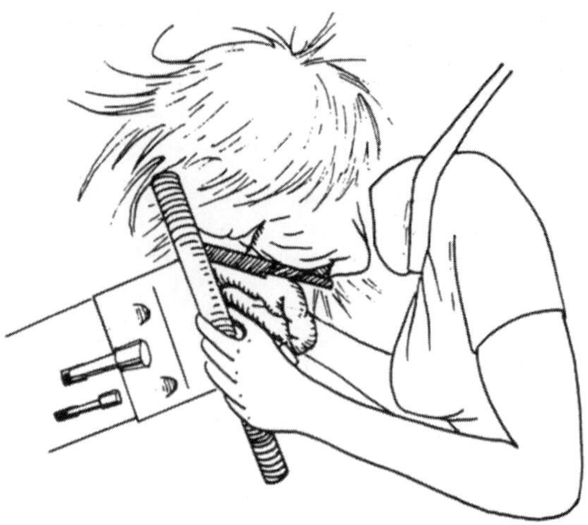

Fig. 15-8 Contact with the module cover can occur if the face is within the arc of the deploying cover. This contact will induce severe and fatal facial and cervical spine injuries.

Air Bag Injury Patterns

Injuries to Extremities

For obvious reasons, upper extremities are especially vulnerableto traumatic injury from deploying air bags and their module covers. The driver can expect to sustain multiple fractures or tissue degloving or amputation of fingers, hands, or forearms if the hand or forearm is on or near the module cover at the moment of deployment (Smock, 2000; Smock & Nichols, 1995; Huelke Moore, & Comptom et al., 1994; Smock, 1992). The horn located within the module cover appreciably increases the risk for injury because accident situations frequently compel drivers to blow the horn in an attempt to avert harm (see Fig. 15-6). Forces from air bag deployment may be transmitted up through the hand and arm all the way to the humerus. Comminuted fractures of the wrist, forearm, elbow, and distal humerus have been observed (Figs. 15-9 to 15-12).

Best Practice *15-1*

Emergency personnel should thoroughly assess all individuals who have been involved in a motor vehicle accident in which an air bag has deployed. Serious and even life-threatening trauma may have occurred, even though presenting injuries appear minor.

Passenger-side air bags have caused some of the most severe injuries because many of the module designs are nothing more than a thin plastic coating over metal (see Fig. 15-5). The placement of hands and feet on a passenger-side dashboard in a bracing maneuver can result in traumatic amputations (Fig. 15-13) and death. NHTSA reports that children in the front seat are more likely to be killed or injured in vehicles equipped with passenger-side air bags than in vehicles without them.

Injuries to the Face

The most common air bag injury is the facial abrasion (Fig. 15-14). The abrasions occur as a result of a sliding contact between the bag and the face.

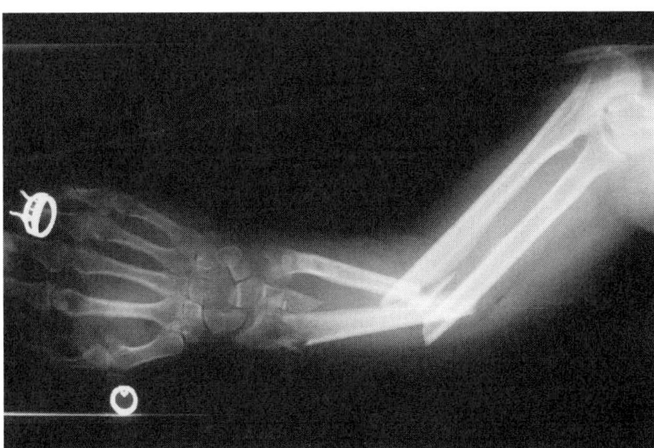

Fig. 15-9 Open comminuted fractures of the wrist and forearm from impact with the passenger module cover in a 1997 Chrysler minivan.

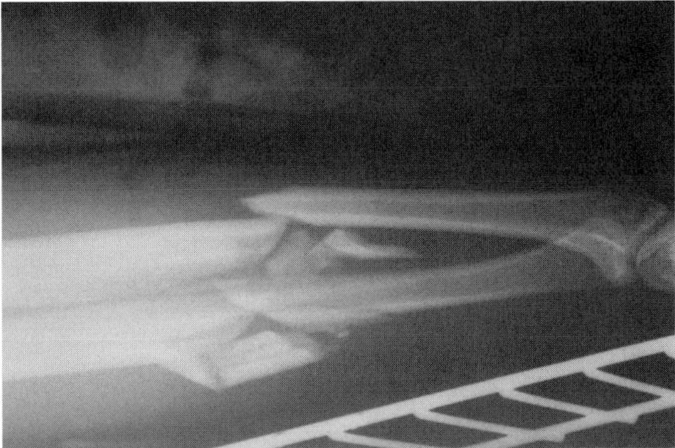

Fig. 15-10 Open comminuted fractures with tension wedging of the radius and ulna from impact with the driver's module cover in a 1993 Toyota Corolla.

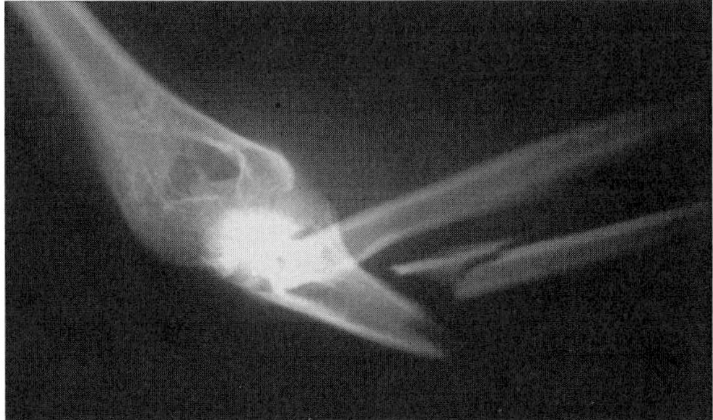

Fig. 15-11 Comminuted fractures of the proximal radius and ulna were sustained when the elbow was impacted by the driver's module cover in a 1994 Toyota Paseo.

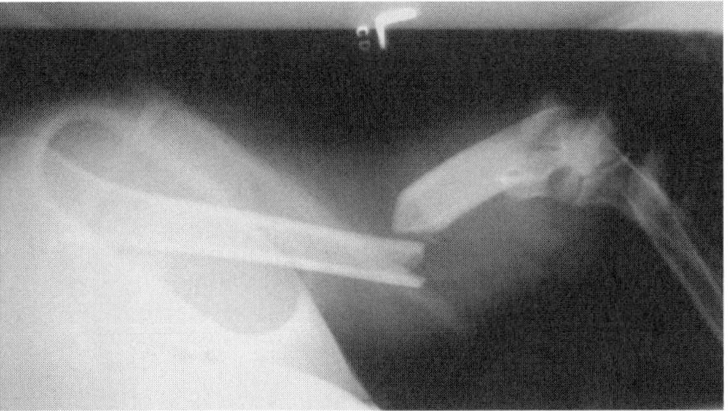

Fig. 15-12 A humeral fracture from impact with the passenger module cover in a 1997 Hyundai Sonata with no visible damage.

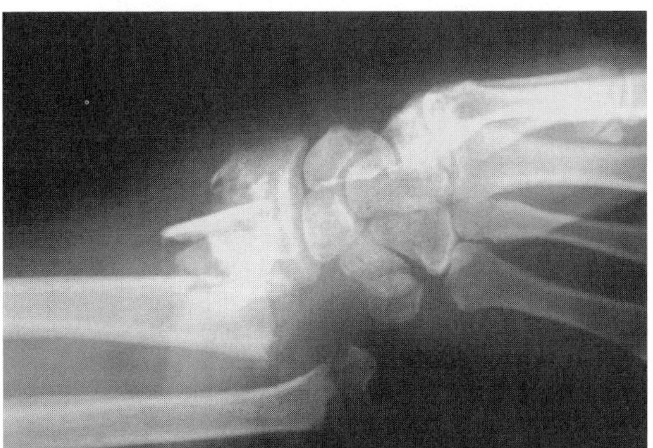

A

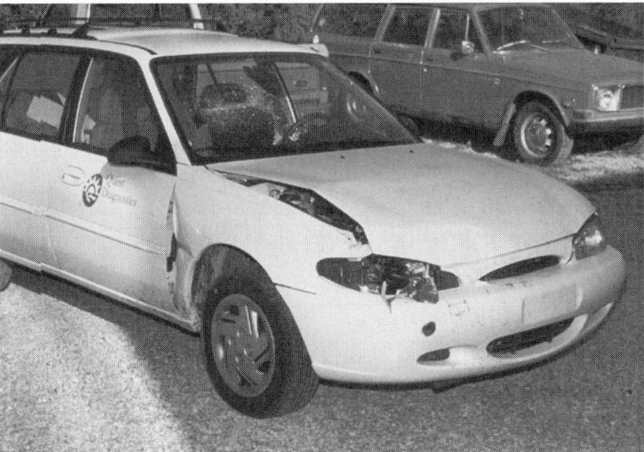

B

Fig. 15-13 *A*, This victim sustained a partial hand amputation from placement of a hand on the passenger module cover while bracing for a minor impact. *B*, The 1995 Ford Escort displays minor damage yet the restrained passenger sustained a permanently disabling hand injury.

Ocular Injuries

Eye injuries from air bags range in severity from corneal abrasions to chemical burns–basic (high pH), from contact with unburned sodium azide–to retinal detachment and globe rupture (Figs. 15-15 and 15-16) (Baker, Flowers, & Singh et al., 1996; Bhavasar, Chen, & Goldstein, 1997; Dumas Kress, & Porta et al., 1996; Gault, Vichnin, & Jaeger et al., 1995; Ghafouri, Burgess, & Hrdlicka et al., 1997; Han, 1993; Kuhn, Morris, & Witherspoon et al., 1993; Larkin, 1991; Lesher, Durrie, & Stiles, 1993; Manche, Goldberg, & Mondino, 1997; Rosenblatt, Freilich, & Kirsch, 1993; Scott, Greenfield, & Parrish, 1996; Scott, John, & Stark, 1993; Vichnin, Jaeger, & Gault et al., 1995; Walz, Mackay, & Gloor, 1995; Whitacre & Pilchard, 1993). In some cases, eye glasses appear to

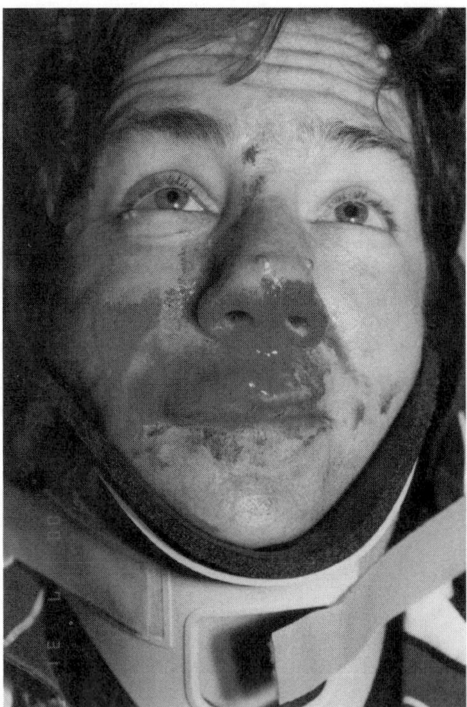

Fig. 15-14 Facial abrasions are the most common air bag-induced injury seen in the emergency department. This 34-year-old restrained driver estimated that her face was approximately 12 inches from the module cover at the time of deployment.

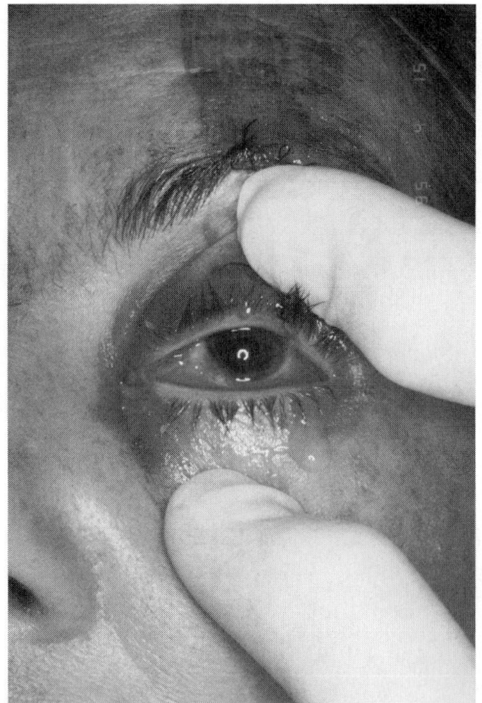

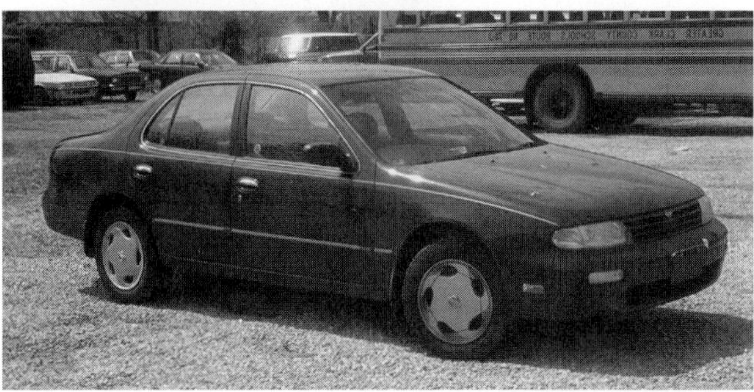

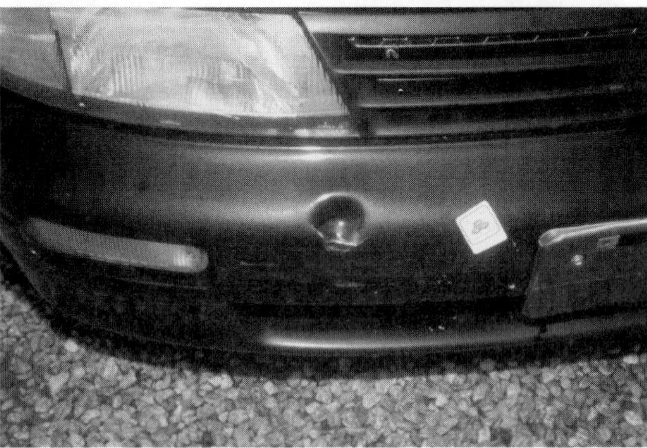

Fig. 15-15 *A*, This 33-year-old restrained passenger suffered a detached retina when her 1993 Nissan impacted, at very low speed, the trailer hitch of a stopped truck (*B*). Note minor damage on bumper from trailer hitch (*C*).

have afforded the wearer an appreciable degree of protection from these sequelae.

Cranial and Intracranial Injuries

Cranial and intracranial injuries may result from impact from either the air bag or the module cover (see Figs. 15-2 and 15-3). When the forces of acceleration are applied to the head, a variety of traumatic injuries can result, including subdural hematomas, cortical contusions, atlanto-occipital dislocations, skull fractures, and brain stem transections (Horsch, Lau, & Andrzejak et al., 1990; Mertz & Weber, 1982; NHTSA, 2003; Prasad & Daniel, 1984).

Cervical Spine Injuries

The blow from an air bag or its module cover, which catapults the head rearward, causing a rapid and violent hyperextension of the cervical spine, can have significant consequences for the cervical vertebrae. The cervical spine injuries more commonly seen from this kind of movement are atlanto-occipital dislocation, comminuted fractures of one or more vertebrae, rupture of the anterior and posterior longitudinal spinal ligaments, and cervical spine disarticulation with transection of the cervical cord (see Fig. 15-3) (Horsch, Lau, & Andrzejak et al., 1990; Mertz & Weber, 1982; NHTSA, 2004; Prasad & Daniel, 1984). Given the nature of how the air bag is mounted and therefore deploys, the majority of these injuries occur in the upper cervical vertebrae, although injuries to the lower cervical vertebrae have also been observed.

Airway Injuries

Chemical pneumonitis and asthma-type symptoms have been observed in individuals who have inhaled the gaseous by-products

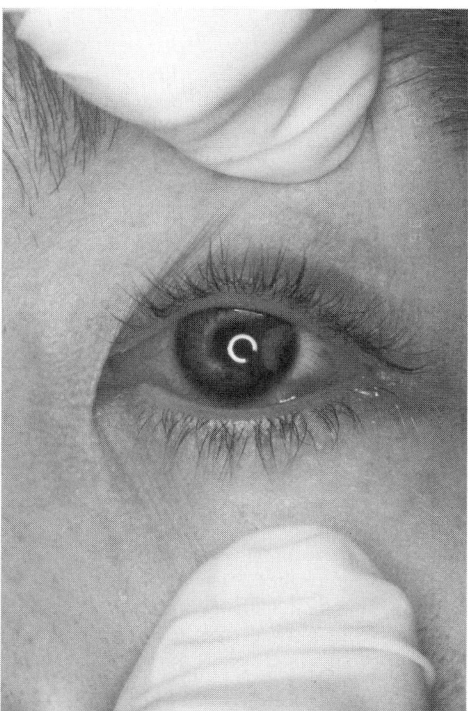

Fig. 15-16 Blunt force trauma to the eye from the late "membrane" phase impact can cause hyphemas.

of the combustion of the sodium azide propellant, as well as other inert materials (principally cornstarch and talc) in the air bag itself (Gross, Koets, & D'Arcy et al., 1995; Gross, Haidar, & Basha et al., 1994; Weiss, 1996). Air bag deployment is often associated with the simultaneous presence of a whitish cloud of these products that occupants frequently mistake for smoke from a vehicle fire. The gaseous products may cause chemical irritation to open wounds also.

The airway is also susceptible to direct trauma. Blows to the trachea or larynx from the module cover or air bag can fracture the hyoid bone and laryngeal structures and thus may compromise respiratory efforts (Perdikis, Schmitt, & Chait et al., 2000). Air bag–induced retropharyngeal hematomas have also resulted in fatal airway compromise (Tenofsky, Porte, & Shaw, 2000).

Forensic Issues and Air Bag Injuries

Examination of the air bag and the module cover will reveal evidence of impact with the injured occupant (Smock, 2000). Trace and gross evidence may give investigators valuable clues regarding an occupant's position at the time of the collision and the configuration of the steering wheel at the moment of the bag's deployment. Evidence transferred from occupant to air bag may take various forms. Of course, blood and epithelial tissue are the most common transfers but also common is make-up, such as lipstick, blush, and mascara.

Summary

If air bags take 1 life for every 52 they save, then doctors and nurses in the nation's trauma centers are encountering many more air bag–induced injuries than were previously expected. The forensic nurse examiner's index for suspicion of air bag involvement should be very high when emergency medical services brings in a patient with severe injuries and report mysteriously little damage to the vehicle. Equally high should be suspicion for air bag involvement when the injuries are principally isolated and involve exclusively the upper extremities, head, or neck.

Key Point *15-1*

Emergency staff members and forensic nursing personnel should consider air bag–associated trauma when the injuries are principally isolated and involve exclusively the upper extremities, head, or neck.

Millions of vehicles travel on highways today and will for many years to come, and their air bag technologies have the potential to kill or maim thousands of drivers and front seat passengers.

US physicians and nurses can expect to see thousands more injuries over the years, especially in the population of short-statured people and those who are not warned of the dangers associated with hand or arm placement over the module cover. The NHTSA will permit the installation of an air bag on/off switch for individuals that are at risk of injury or death due to their height or medical conditions (NHTSA, 2004). Until public awareness reaches such a pitch that these technologies are disabled or modified, this "lifesaving" device will continue to kill more children than it saves, amputate extremities, decapitate children, induce blindness, and never be approved "safe" if regulated by the FDA.

Case Study 15-1 Children and Air Bags

When a family with a two-year-old child purchased a new vehicle, the presence of safety devices, restraint systems, and other occupant protective devices were major issues in the vehicle selection decision. The first year was uneventful after the purchase of a sedan equipped with safety air bags. By now the child, three years old, had grown taller but had not yet met the requirements for being placed in the front seat of the vehicle.

During a visit from grandparents, the parents left for a weekend holiday with the grandparents in charge of caring for the child. The grandfather decided to take the child to a local park one afternoon in order to allow the grandmother a few hours of quiet and rest. The grandfather had placed the child's car seat in the front in order to keep a closer watch on the child and to be able to converse more easily because of his degenerative hearing loss. No one had explained the rationale for placing the seat in the back of the car, nor had anyone warned him of the dangers of air bags with small children.

As they approached an intersection only a block from the park, an oncoming vehicle failed to yield to a stop sign, colliding with the right passenger side of the car. The air bags demonstrated the instant protection for which they had been designed and detonated. Unfortunately, the child was too small and too close to the device and the sudden inflation and expulsion resulted in complete decapitation of the child.

Resources

Organizations

Air Bag and Seat Belt Safety Campaign

1025 Connecticut Avenue NW, Suite 1200, Washington, DC 20036; Tel: 202-625-2570; www.nsc.org/airbag.htm

American College of Emergency Physicians

Fact Sheets on Air Bag Safety, Seat Belts and Protecting Children in Motor Vehicles

1125 Executive Circle, Irving, TX 75038-2522; Tel: 800-798-1822 or 972-550-0911; www.acep.org

National Highway Transportation Safety Administration

www.nhtsa.dot.gov/airbags

Sensible Solutions LLC

7301 Brookside Drive, Frederick, MD 21702; Tel: 877-773-7908; www.airbagonoff.com

References

Appendix to *The air bag crisis: Causes and solutions.* (January 19, 1972). Ford Motor Company, Automotive Safety and Emissions Program, Product Development. APP 135-140.

Appendix to *The air bag crisis: Causes and solutions.* Parents for Safer Air Bags. (October 1997). Memo to R. Hauesler from L. L. Baker, Assistant Chief Engineer, Chrysler Automotive Safety and Security. APP 75-79.

Baker, R. S., Flowers, C. W., Singh, P., et al. (1996). Corneoscleral laceration caused by air-bag trauma. *Am J Ophthalmol, 121*(6),709-711.

Bhavasar, A. R., Chen, T. C., & Goldstein, D.A. (1997). Corneoscleral laceration associated with passenger-side airbag inflation (Letter to the Editor). *Br J Ophthalmol, 81*(6), 514-515.

Dumas, S. M., Kress, T. A., Porta, D. F., et al. (1996). Airbag-induced eye injuries: A report of 25 cases. *J Trauma, 41*(1), 114-119.

Gault, J. A., Vichnin, M. C., Jaeger, E. A., et al. (1995). Ocular injuries associated with eyeglass wear and airbag inflation. *J Trauma, 38*(4), 494-497.

Ghafouri, A., Burgess, S. K., Hrdlicka, Z. K., et al. (1997). Air bag-related ocular trauma. *Am J Emerg Med, 15*(4), 389-392.

Grenier, E. P. (October, 1997). The great air bag robbery. (Delivered to members of Congress.) in *Appendix to The air bag crisis: Causes and solutions.* APP 61-66.

Gross, K. B., Haidar, A. H., Basha, M. A., et al. (1994). Acute pulmonary response of asthmatics to aerosols and gases generated by airbag deployment. *Am J Respir Crit Care Med, 150*(2), 408-414.

Gross, K. B., Koets, M. H., D'Arcy, J. B., et al. (1995). Mechanism of induction of asthmatic attacks by the inhalation of particles generated by airbag system deployment. *J Trauma, 38*(4), 521-527.

Han, D. P. (1993). Retinal detachment caused by air bag injury (case report). *Arch Ophthalmol, 111*, 1317-1318.

Horsch, J., Lau, I., Andrzejak, D., et al. (1990). *Assessment of air bag deployment loads.* SAE Paper No. 902324. Detroit: Society of Automotive Engineers

Huelke, D. F., Moore, J. L., Comptom, T. W., et al. (1994). *Upper extremity injuries related to air bag deployments.* SAE Publication No. 940716. Detroit: Society of Automotive Engineers.

Kuhn, F., Morris, R., Witherspoon, C. D., et al. (1993). Air bag: Friend or foe? (editorial). *Arch Ophthalmol, 111*, 1333-1334.

Larkin, G. L. (1991). Airbag-mediated corneal injury. *Am J Emerg Med, 9*(5), 444-446.

Lesher, M. P., Durrie, D. S., Stiles, M. C. (1993). Corneal edema, hyphema, and angle recession after air bag inflation (case report). *Arch Ophthalmol, 111*, 1320-1322.

Manche, E. E., Goldberg, R. A., Mondino, B. J. (1997). Air bag-related ocular injuries. *Ophthalmic Surg Lasers, 28*(3), 246-250.

Mertz, H. J., Driscoll, G. P., Lennox, J. B., et al. (November 1982). Response of animals exposed to deployment of various passenger and portable restraining system concepts for a variety of collision severities and animal positions (pp 252-368). National Highway and Transportation Safety Administration, 9th International Technical Conference on Experimental Safety Vehicles, Kyoto, Japan.

Mertz, H. J., & Weber, D. A. (1982). *Interpretations of impact response to a three year old child dummy relative to child injury potential.* SAE Paper No. 826048. Detroit: General Motors.

National Highway Transportation Safety Administration. (2003). The Third Report to Congress on the Effectiveness of Occupant Protection Systems and Their Use and Air Bag Related Fatalities and Serious Injuries. Retrieved from www.nhtsa.dot.gov/airbags/.

National Highway Transportation Safety Administration (NHTSA). (2004). Sensible Solutions. Retrieved from www.airbagonoff.com.

Patrick, L. M., & Nyquist, G. W. (1972). *Airbag effects on the out-of-position child.* SAE Paper No. 720442. Detroit: Society for Automotive Engineers.

Perdikis, G., Schmitt, T., Chait, D., Richards, A. T. (2000). Blunt laryngeal fracture: Another airbag injury. *J Trauma, 48*(3), 544-546.

Prasad, P., Daniel, R. P. (1984). *A biomechanical analysis of head, neck and torso injuries to child surrogates due to sudden torso acceleration.* SAE Paper No. 841656. Detroit: Society of Automotive Engineers.

Rosenblatt, M. A., Freilich, B., & Kirsch, D. (1993). Air bag-associated ocular injury (case report). *Arch Ophthalmol, 111*, 1318.

Scott, I., John, G. R., & Stark, W. J. (1993). Air bag-associated ocular injury (case report reply). *Arch Ophthalmol, 111*, 1318.

Scott, I. U., Greenfield, D. S., & Parrish, R. K. (1996). Airbag-associated injury producing cyclodialysis cleft and ocular hypotony. *Ophthalmic Surg Lasers, 27*(11), 955-957.

Smock, W. S., & Nichols, G. N. (1995). Air bag module cover injuries. *J Trauma, 38*(4), 489-492.

Smock, W. S. Airbag related injuries and deaths. In Siegel, J. A., Saukko, P. J. & Knupfer, GC (Eds.). (2000). *Encyclopedia of forensic science.* London: Academic Press.

Smock, W. S. (1992). Traumatic avulsion of the first digit, secondary to air bag deployment. Proceedings 36 (p. 444). Des Plains, IL: Association for the Advancement of Automotive Medicine.

Tenofsky. P., Porter, S. W., & Shaw, J. W. (2000). Fatal airway compromise due to retropharyngeal hematoma after airbag deployment. *Am Surg, 66*(7), 692-694.

The air bag crisis: Causes and solutions. (1997). Washington, D.C.: Parents for Safer Air Bags.

Viano, D. C., & Warner, C. V. (1976). *Thoracic impact response of live porcine subjects* (pp. 733-765). SAE Paper No. 760823. Detroit: Society for Automotive Engineers.

Vichnin, M. C., Jaeger, E. A., Gault, J. A., et al (1995). Ocular injuries related to air bag inflation. *Ophthalmic Surg Lasers, 26*(6), 542-548.

Walz, F. H., Mackay, M., & Gloor, B. Airbag deployment and eye perforation by a tobacco pipe. *J Trauma, 38*(4), 498-501.

Weiss, J. S. (1996). Reactive airway dysfunction syndrome due to sodium azide inhalation. *Int Arch Occup Environ Health, 68*(6), 469-471.

Whitacre, M. M., & Pilchard, W. A. (1993). Air bag injury producing retinal dialysis and detachment (case report). *Arch Ophthalmol, 111*, 1320.

Chapter 16 Bite Mark Injuries

Gregory S. Golden

Forensic odontology is the branch of dentistry that deals with the collection, evaluation, and proper handling of dental evidence in order to provide assistance to law enforcement, civil, and criminal judicial proceedings. Three main areas encompass the scope of forensic dentistry:

- Identification of unknown deceased
- Documentation and analysis of bite mark evidence
- Examination of oral-facial structures for determination of injury, possible malpractice, or insurance fraud

Certainly in the field of nursing, health care personnel occasionally find themselves providing medical care for the recipient of single or multiple bites that have been inflicted by another individual or an animal. The practical aspects of collecting evidence from bites and documenting bite mark injuries falls under the purview of forensic nursing, because many of these injuries become important as evidence later in judicial settings. For this reason, recognizing bite marks and applying the clinical protocol for documenting and handling bite mark evidence are essential components for the forensic nurse examiner.

Psychological Aspects of Biting

Crimes with an element of violence (rape, homicide, battery, child and elder abuse), have been identified as those most associated with biting events. The psychological factors that motivate perpetrators of bites have been identified as varying themes of power, control, potency, and anger. The emotional overload and catharsis that occur can block any memory of the biting event and can suspend logical, rational behavior (Walter, 1985). Emerging research on domestic violence offenders who are prone to biting has identified numerous additional behavioral factors correlated with battery, abuse, alcohol use, emotional insecurity, and features of antisocial and borderline personality disorders (Murphy, 1994). In contrast to the previous situation is the event wherein the victim of the abuse bites the perpetrator. Although there are certainly fewer psychological implications in this situation, the act of biting nevertheless occurs as a response to motivational stimuli, especially in defending one's own life. Whatever the circumstances or the crime, bite mark evidence can contribute an integral part of the forensic investigation.

Animal Bites Versus Human Bites

The Center for Disease Control reports that more than 4 million dog bites occur every year in the US, and treatment for them usually occurs under the supervision of nurses in urgent care facilities and emergency departments. At first glance, animal and human bites can appear similar, but a closer evaluation will reveal some fundamental differences in their appearance.

Acknowledgment and thanks go to Linear Systems Inc. for reproduction of original images and figures presented in this chapter.

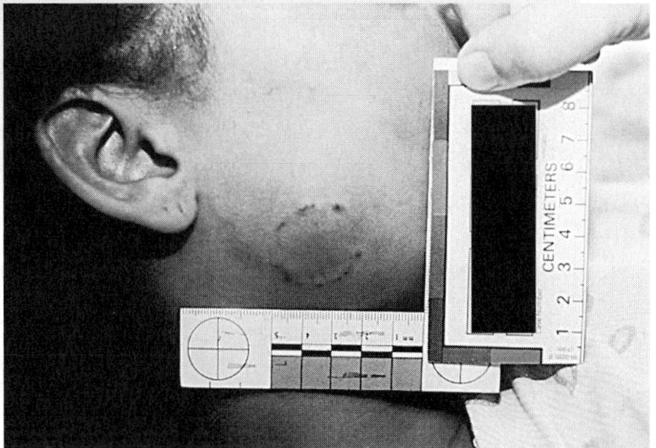

Fig. 16-1 Typical two-dimensional bite.

Bite Characteristics

The prototypical human bite is generally an ovoid or circular bruise pattern that consists of two opposing U-shaped arches separated at their bases by open space (Fig. 16-1). Frequently there is a central area of ecchymosis or contusion between the opposing arches. In many bite marks, individual tooth patterns or the "dental signature" left by the anterior teeth can be seen. If the injury meets these criteria, chances are excellent that it is, in fact, a bite mark. Many factors affect bite mark dynamics and appearance, with both the victim and the biter. Age and race of the victim play an important role in the variation of wound healing and visibility of bites. The location of the bite will affect its manifestation. Bites on unsupported tissue such as the breast usually are more diffused than bites on tissue that is well supported by muscle or bone. Thin skin such as one finds on the face will generally produce more class characteristics and individualizing characteristics of the biter's teeth than the thick skin found on the palms and soles of feet.

Factors linked with the perpetrator include the number of teeth, the strength of the biter, and movement during the act of biting. Bites made through clothing will result in a distinct bruise pattern. Additional variables to consider are time elapsed before the bite is documented and environmental factors such as temperature, humidity, and contamination.

It must be said at this point that there are other blunt force injuries from a variety of instruments that can mimic the appearance of a bite mark; however, in this chapter only examples of known bites will be shown. Ultimately the final determination should be made using the assistance of a qualified forensic odontologist.

Dog bites vary in degree of severity and can be more oblong and even "V"-shaped. In their least aggressive form they can appear as a superficial bruise (Fig. 16-2). Similarly, human bites seen and analyzed are often limited to damage of the surface epithelium, dermis, and muscle tissue; or they can appear to be only superficial

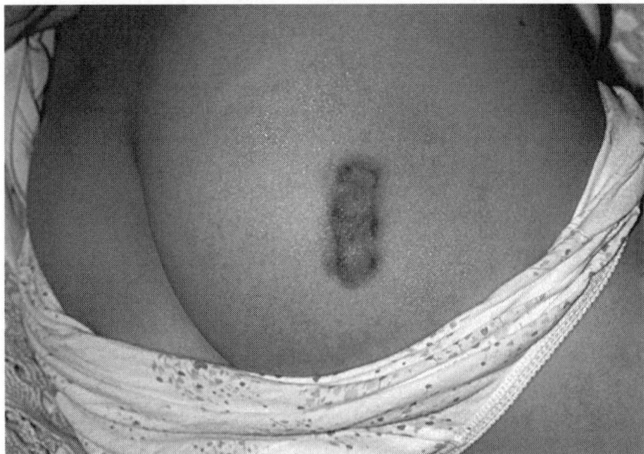

Fig. 16-2 Dog bite without laceration.

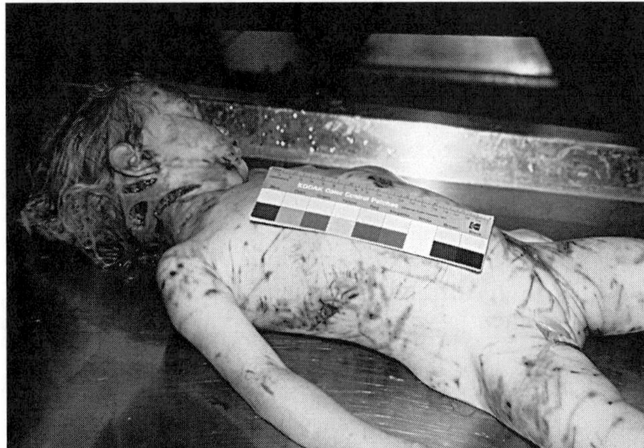

Fig. 16-3 Four-year-old decedent with multiple dog bites. Note the lacerations from canine incisors. (Photo courtesy of N. Sperber, DDS.)

or predominantly contusions and abrasions In contrast, the more severe dog bites typically involve punctures and laceration of the skin. Figure 16-3 shows a four-year-old with multiple dog bites who inadvertently climbed into a neighbor's back yard where several dogs lived and fatally attacked the youngster.

The most noticeable difference between animal and human bites occurs as a result of the canine teeth.

An examination of canine teeth in cats and dogs reveals that they are proportionally much longer, relative to the other anterior teeth, than are human canines to their adjacent anterior teeth. Figure 16-4 demonstrates the obvious size difference between the canines and anterior incisors in the mountain lion, which has been known to attack humans. Similar conditions exist in dogs, bears, snakes, and many other animals known to have bitten people. As the longest teeth, the canines create the most damage to the bitten victim. Animal canines typically produce telltale punctures and parallel linear abrasions or lacerations caused by movement of these teeth over the surface of the tissue as the bite occurs. Human canines, also typically the longest of the anterior teeth, do not usually inflict the same extent of damage or leave the same pattern as animal canines.

Both animal bites and human bites can take place either as single or multiple injuries. Some lacerations can be fatal, particularly in areas where large vessels are near the surface of the skin,

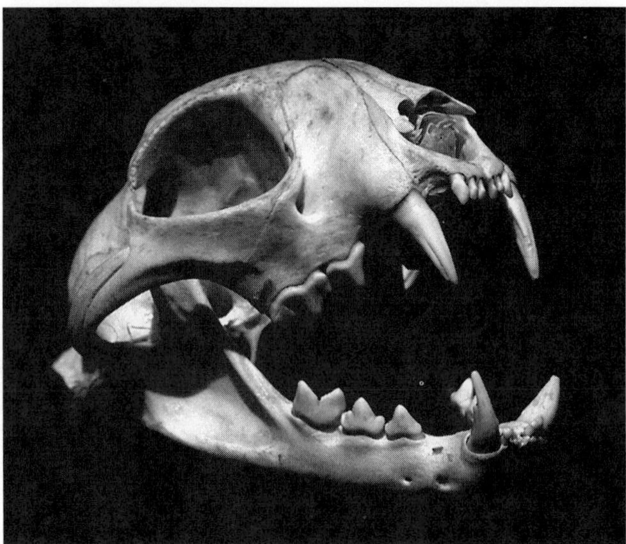

Fig. 16-4 Cougar skull: Note the length of the anterior canines in relation to other incisors.

such as in the neck. The crushing power of even a medium-sized dog's jaws has also been documented to cause multiple fractures in infant skulls and adult bones as well.

Whatever the severity of the bite, in any emergency department setting, concern for the patient is most important and pre-empts collection of the bite mark evidence. Only after the victim is stabilized and out of danger is attention to be directed to collecting evidence from the bite mark injury.

Key Point *16-1*

Penetrating bite wounds pose a serious risk for infection. *After* swabbing for DNA and photographic documentation, the bite mark wound should be thoroughly cleansed with a professional grade antimicrobial agent, and antibiotic therapy should be initiated.

Pathogenic Considerations

The most critical determinant for any animal bite, wild or domestic, is the possibility of rabies transmission. Although studies on maternal periparturient grooming and in licking wounds have shown dog saliva to have bactericidal effects against certain pathogens (*Escherichia coli* and *Streptococcus canis*) (Hart & Powell, 1990), other research has shown canine salivary bacterial content to often contain levels of *Pasturella multocida* and *Staphylococcus aureus*, both known human pathogens (Bailie, Stowe, & Schmitt, 1978). In any event, particularly deep bites contaminated by animal saliva frequently require antibiotic therapy (Peeples, Boswick, & Scott, 1980).

The human oral environment can support over 250 known gram-positive and gram-negative bacteria as well as viral components at any particular time (Leon Levy Center for Oral Health Research). A bite by a human is a much more serious injury than an animal bite from an infective standpoint. Likelihood of infection is virtually guaranteed if penetration of the skin has occurred and was left untreated. In the hospital emergency department or trauma care facility, after DNA sample collection and photographic documentation of a human bite has been completed, thorough cleansing of the wound with a professional grade antimicrobial detergent should be performed and antibiotic therapy should be initiated. Suturing is typically unnecessary in the majority of human bites, but the opposite is true in animal bites and in the most severe human bites. If left untreated, a penetrative bite to the hand or foot will often ultimately require surgical debridement, parenteral and oral antibiotics, and continued monitoring for cessation of infection.

Bite Mark Recognition

In order for a bite mark to be recognized as a bite, the injury should first meet the criteria previously mentioned that establish its validity as a bite pattern injury. Occasionally only a single arch is represented, such as in the case of a bite to a finger, hand, or foot (Fig. 16-5). If a nurse examiner is unsure whether or not an injury is in fact a bite mark, the assistance of a qualified forensic odontologist should be requested.

Within the classic bite pattern are individual "toothprints" generally created by the incisal or cutting edges of the six upper and six lower front teeth. Characteristics that may be used to individualize the dental signature to a particular suspect, or rule out others, are most important. Positional relationships of adjacent teeth, rotations, chips and fractures, spacing, and relative height in the dental plane of occlusion are all features that assist the forensic odontologist in the analysis of the bite mark. Some terms generally used to describe the extent of a bite mark injury are petechial hemorrhage, abrasion, contusion, erythema, ecchymosis, indentation, and laceration.

Types of Human Bites

Two-Dimensional Bite

A two-dimensional bite is the predominant type of injury that occurs during confrontational episodes. The typical two-dimensional bite has width and breadth but no penetration of the epidermis (see Figs. 16-1 and 16-5). Although one might misconstrue the pressure necessary to create such an injury to be minimal, usually the forces associated with the average human bite are significant and exceed normal pain threshold tolerances. The degree of subsequent bruising depends on a combination of factors, such as the age of the victim, elasticity of the skin, location of the bite including underlying structures, force applied, and morphology of the dentition.

Three-Dimensional Bite

A *three-dimensional bite* has all the components of the two-dimensional bite plus depth of penetration (Fig. 16-6). When appropriate and useful as evidence, when the skin surface has been broken during the act of biting, a reproduction of the injury may be obtained utilizing impression materials common to dentistry (Fig. 16-7). The impression should be taken by trained personnel and should be collected soon after the injury and before

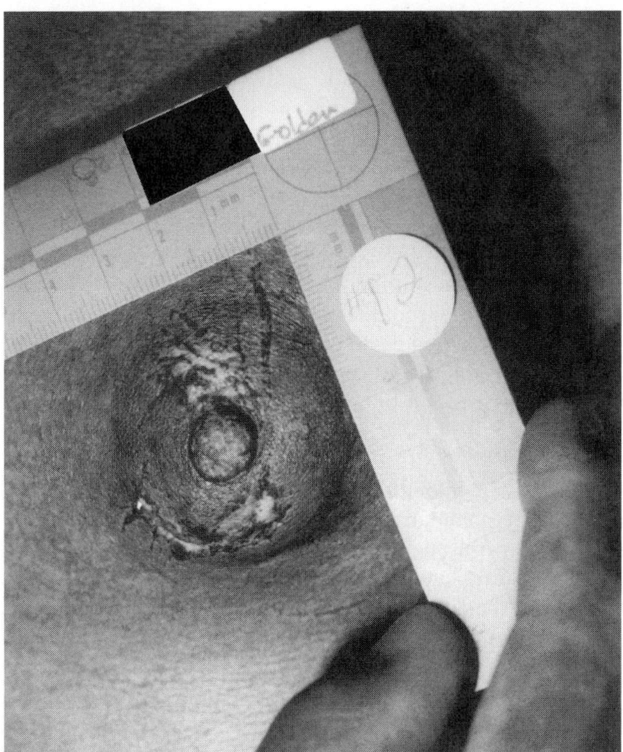

Fig. 16-6 Three-dimensional (penetrative) bite to breast. Reflective UVA photo.

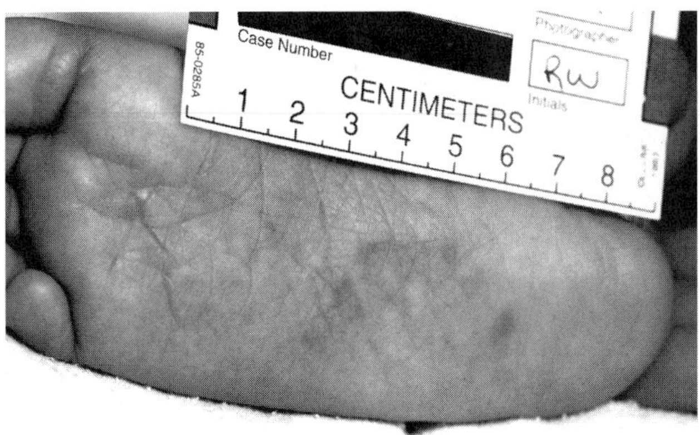

Fig. 16-5 Single upper arch bite on sole of foot.

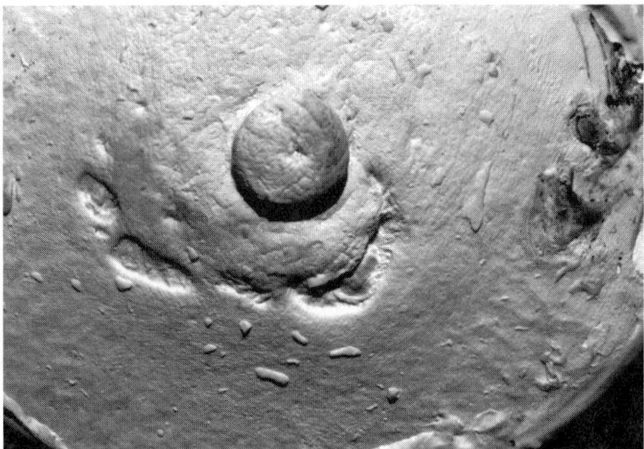

Fig. 16-7 Plaster cast of breast demonstrating three-dimensional bite with depth and penetration of tissue.

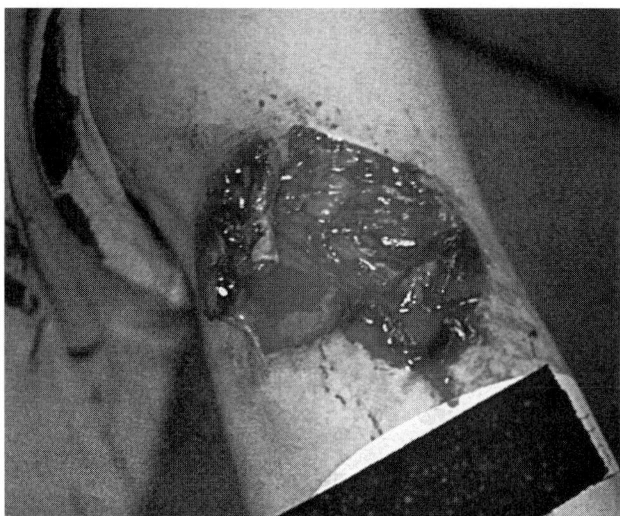

Fig. 16-8 Avulsed human bite on upper arm. (Photo courtesy of Colton Police Department, Colton, California.)

any long-term healing response occurs. The subsequent imprint of the damaged skin surface can then be used to create either a flexible or hard model of the injury that accurately represents the actual dimensions and depth of the bite. The replica of the injury may then be employed for comparison to suspects' teeth and later introduced as evidence or used as an exemplar in court.

Avulsed Bite

An avulsed bite is one that is so severe in force that the bitten tissue has been completely separated from the victim. Generally, avulsed bites result more frequently from large animals, although in rare instances avulsed bites have been produced by humans (Fig. 16-8). The avulsed bite is rarely useful as evidence because the actual dental information is lost in the process of forcible tissue removal. If recovered, the piece of tissue might be reattached surgically, but typically, no dental information exists after the suturing or surgical repair. For those people who are unfortunate enough to not survive an attack by animals such as bears, large cats and dogs, and sharks, supplementary information is usually available to confirm the source of the victim's demise. On some occasions, measurements of the teeth will be taken if a suspected animal is located so that a comparison for consistency can be made to the bite mark pattern injuries.

Bite Mark Analysis

A comparison of a suspect's teeth to the dental signature left on the skin of the victim can be accomplished by a variety of methods. For several decades the accepted protocol has included using transparent acetate overlays that indicate the biting edges of the six maxillary and six mandibular anterior teeth (Fig. 16-9). A 1-to-1 (life-sized) photographic print is then created from either a slide, negative, or digital image. The acetate overlay, traced from the biting edges of the suspect's teeth, is then compared to the pattern injury for consistent features or concordant points (Fig. 16-10). Some odontologists prefer to work at even larger magnifications such as 2-to-1 or even 3-to-1 for better visualization.

Recent technological advances have popularized the use of computers for bite mark analysis. Imaging software programs such

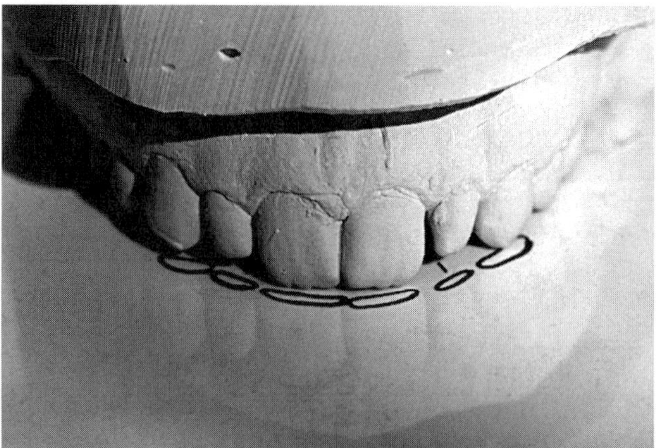

Fig. 16-9 Acetate overlay below model indicating outline of biting edges of teeth.

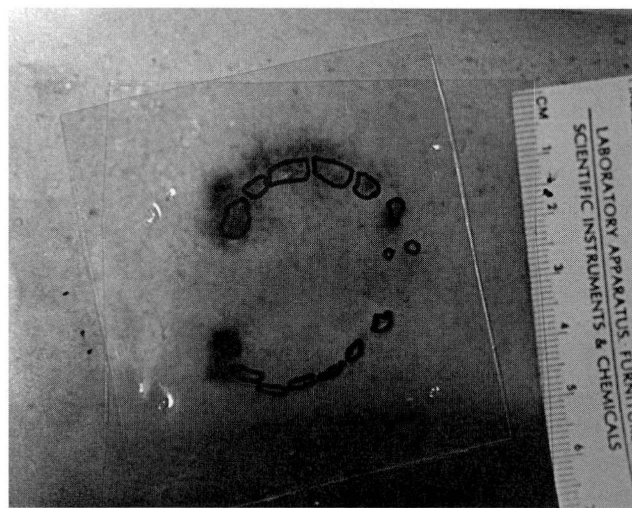

Fig. 16-10 Acetate overlay compared to life-sized photograph of bite mark.

as Adobe Photoshop allows the contemporary odontologist to employ a computer for *all* phases of bite mark comparison, especially generation of the overlays (Sweet, Parhar, & Wood, 1998), correction of photographic distortion of the bite mark (Johansen & Bowers, 2000), and the actual comparison of suspect's teeth to the bite.

It is of utmost importance to collect photographic evidence of the bite mark as soon as possible. As a bite mark ages and heals in the living victim, the intradental and interdental characteristics of individual teeth fade as the subcutaneous bruising diffuses into the surrounding tissues. The resultant amorphous bruise often looks like a "smoke ring" (Sperber, 1994) (Fig. 16-11). Extremely diffused bite marks usually contain minimal evidentiary value unless some measurement or determination can be made on gross features alone that would either rule out or implicate a suspect.

Collection of Evidence

Swabbing the Bite

The first and most important phase of evidence collection should be swabbing the bite for salivary residue. Recent research has

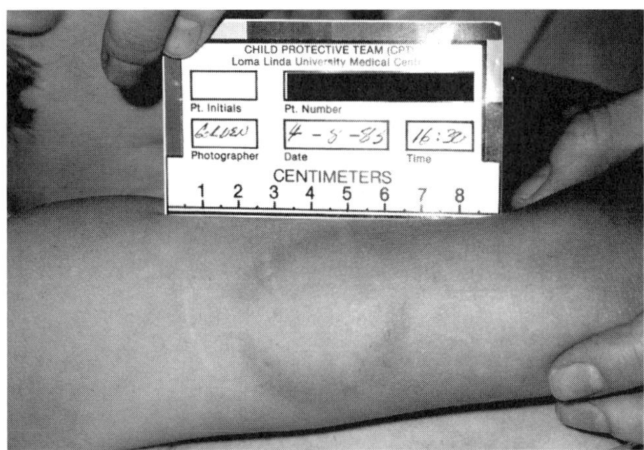

Fig. 16-11 Aging arm bite demonstrating the "smoke ring" phase of healing.

Best Practice *16-1*

Suspected bite mark wounds should not be cleansed until they have been swabbed for DNA evidence and photo-documented. The moistened, double-swab technique should be used and samples should be permitted to air-dry.

confirmed that bite marks frequently contain a salivary component and accompanying DNA microquantities that can be collected and identified through polymerase chain reaction (PCR) technique (Sweet & Lorente, 1997). Any secretory residue should be collected by employing the "double swab" method proposed by Sweet and colleagues (1998). Care should be taken not to touch the area of the bite before gloving so as to avoid cross-contamination. It is also important to refrain from washing the bite mark before this procedure is completed. In most instances, DNA swabbing is conducted by a crime scene technician or other qualified law enforcement investigator. If no criminalist is immediately available, the forensic nurse examiner should swab the injury. Prior to swabbing, the responsive victim should be asked whether or not the bite injury has been contaminated or disturbed in any way and whether or not the victim remembers biting the assailant. In this case, any suspects apprehended should also be examined for bite marks that can later be compared to the victim's dentition.

The first swab, usually consisting of a cotton-tipped swab (Q-tip) moistened with distilled or sterile water, is lightly rolled, (not scrubbed) over the bite mark, working from the outer area inward to the central portion of the bite. This moistened tip rehydrolizes the salivary sample. A second dry swab is then used to collect the moisture left from the first swab, moving in the same pattern from the outer edge of the bite to the central area where generally the tongue has left most of the salivary sample. The second swab routinely contains most of the biological specimen, although both should be submitted together.

Both swabs should be allowed to air-dry without coming into contact with anything before being offered for laboratory analysis. Heat-assisted drying is contraindicated, and the swabs should also be kept out of sunlight because heat and ultraviolet light degrades the DNA. If the samples are to be kept overnight before submission to an appropriate laboratory for analysis, they can be refrigerated but not frozen. Ideally if long-term storage is anticipated, the dried swabs should be maintained at cryogenic temperatures.

Key Point *16-2*

Accurate photo-documentation requires both orientation and close-up views of the bite mark. A series of high-quality photographs is crucial for establishing reliability of the forensic odontological evaluation process and will provide vital evidence for the criminal investigation and judicial proceedings.

Photography

The second and next important phase of evidence collection of bite marks is obtaining an accurate photographic image of the injury. Orientation and close-up photographs are routinely taken to document the pattern of the bite mark so that a record of the injury is obtained and the resultant photo can be used for indirect comparison to suspects at a later date. The photographic evidence is crucial to the investigation and judicial proceedings. Photographic accuracy in the documentation of evidence is exceedingly important in order to provide reliability in the forensic odontological evaluation process. Although numerous methods can be used to photograph injury patterns (digital, video, film), methods described herein will apply to the conventional film and digital techniques.

Photographic techniques have been standardized and a protocol established to ensure reliable, predictable results that will be acceptable as evidence (Stimson & Mertz, 1997, Dorion, 2005). Cameras and photographic equipment vary in their features, advantages, and benefits to the user, and all come with different price tags. Individual needs and the limits of one's budget usually determine the equipment one ultimately procures. If new equipment is out of financial reach, frequently excellent used and reconditioned camera bodies and close-up lenses are available from pawnshops and camera stores. With some basic knowledge of the requisites and a little professional help, one can find an acceptable outfit that fills all the requirements necessary for capturing a satisfactory close-up image on a slide, print film negative, or digital photo at a reasonable price.

With recent advances in and competition among manufacturers of digital cameras, these instruments have become affordable. Digital cameras provide a distinct advantage in that most of them have a liquid crystal viewing screen that enables the photographer to immediately see the image just taken. Another advantage of digital equipment is the ability to download images immediately to a computer and, if necessary, transmit them to other locations via electronic mail. The speed and ease of capturing and seeing the digital image immediately, combined with the elimination of additional costs for chemical photo processing and enlargement, will undoubtedly eventually bring an end to traditional film photography for practical purposes (Dorion, 2005).

Basic Equipment

Film (35-mm) Photography. If the photographer elects to employ traditional film photography, the 35-mm format is recommended for most forensic applications. A single reflex camera body with through-the-lens metering is preferable. A continuous focusing macro lens with a 60- to 105-mm focal length and good optical quality should provide excellent pictures. A point flash with a guide number of 40 to 45 should be mounted at the end of the lens via a mounting bracket. Ring flashes are also acceptable in most close-up applications, but they often leave reflective ghosts on wet surface specimens, and they are inappropriate for oblique, off-camera lighting angles. A sturdy tripod is also necessary. Several photographic equipment manufacturers make excellent tripods that have telescopic legs and three-axis tilt adjustment levers.

Instruction on basic camera familiarization and fundamentals of photography can be found through photographic supply stores, in books (Kodak Guide, 1989), at universities throughout the country, as well as in numerous independent photography courses. Ultimately, the goal of the photographer should be to get to know the camera and exposure settings well enough to be able to produce reliable and predictable results consistently and under any conditions. This level of expertise generally takes some practice and several test rolls of film, particularly because the fundamental principles of close-up photography are not always easily absorbed.

Digital Cameras. The forensic investigator or forensic nurse examiner who opts for digital format should make certain that the camera and lens are capable of taking close-up photographs (macrophotography) without any parallax or other distortion. Several mid-priced digital cameras now are manufactured with interchangeable lenses that allow the user to select the desired format under varying conditions.

The digital photographer who anticipates self-processing his or her images should have more than a basic understanding of how to download an image from the camera to a computer. One should also be able to open the file in an image management software program, print it life-size, and save it to storage media such as a disk, hard drive, or CD (compact disk). Numerous professional photo processing labs will provide these services if one prefers to use them instead, but this service is sometimes more expensive than straight film processing.

Digital photography involves numerous other factors that should be discussed with a knowledgeable person who can provide not only input about the hardware and software that goes with the camera but also technical support when problems arise.

Orientation Photos

Prior to close-up (macrophotographic) exposures, orientation photos should be taken to typically demonstrate exactly in what area of the body the bite exists. They are taken from a distance, usually without a scale, and are self-explanatory for information about the bite mark location. The camera need not be on a tripod, and there is little concern for angular distortion.

Shooting Close-Up Photographs

Some basic requirements apply for taking close-up pictures of bite marks. Use an appropriate scale with accurate millimeter markings. The scale should be placed adjacent to the bite mark without covering up the bite. The scale should also be positioned in the same plane as the injury in order to maximize the depth of field and to minimize photographic distortion. The scale can also be used to include information about the particular case. Data such as the case number, photographer's name, date, time, and agency can all be written on a label and placed on the scale at one end. One highly recommended scale is the ABFO # 2, which fulfills all the requirements for photographic accuracy (Fig. 16-12).

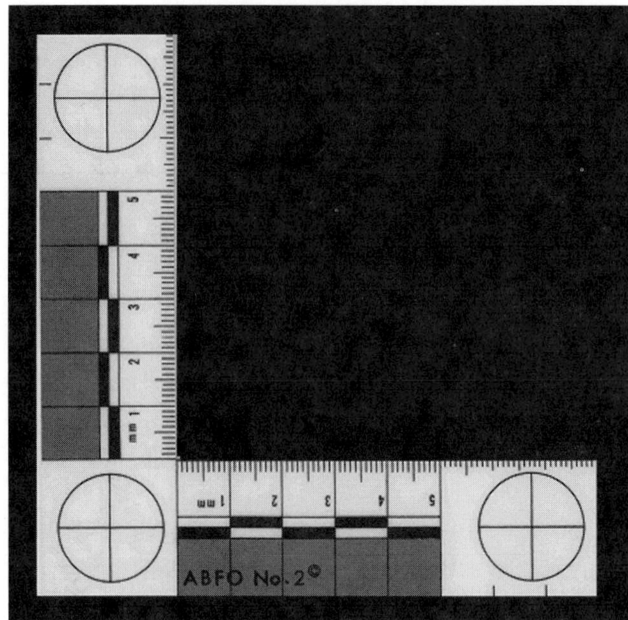

Fig. 16-12 ABFO No. 2 Scale. (Courtesy of Armor Forensics Co.; available from Lightning Powder Company, 1230 Hoyt Street SE, Salem, Oregon 97302.)

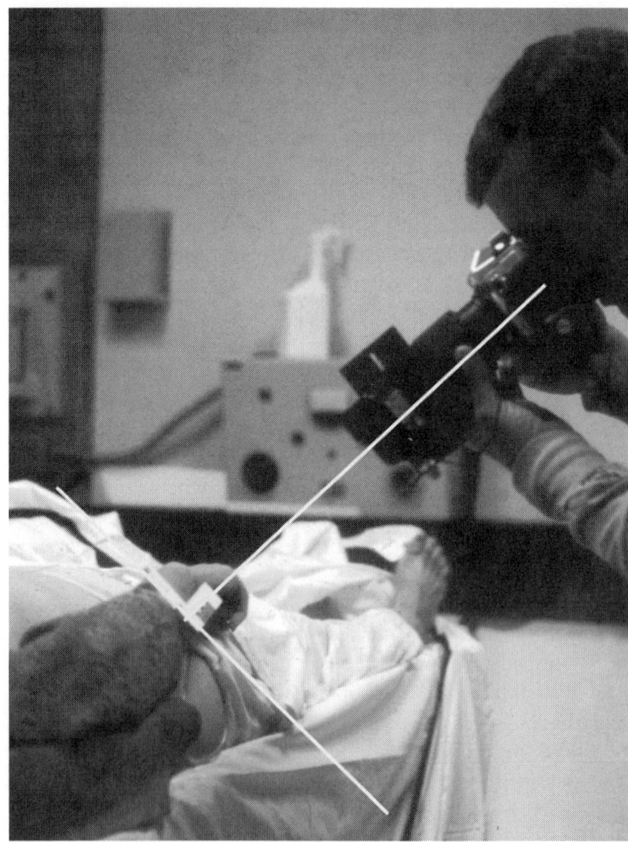

Fig. 16-13 Depiction of correct (perpendicular) angle position for close-up photography of bite marks.

Camera positioning relative to the injury should be perpendicular so that angular distortion is minimized (Fig. 16-13). Pictures taken at incorrect angles introduce errors in size and shape of the pattern injury. One way to determine whether or not the image coming through the lens of the camera is at 90 degrees to the plane of the bite mark is to use a small mirror placed immediately in front of the bite in the same plane as the injury. The photographer can then look through the viewfinder of the tripod-mounted camera and should be able to see his/her own eye looking back through the lens as it is reflected from the mirror.

A detachable flash with a coiled connecting cord will permit multiple shots at different angles of lighting (Fig. 16-14). The location of the incident illumination can be varied from directly over the bite mark to low angles. Additionally, the flash may be positioned at different reference points from the bite, as though moving around the face of a clock. Sometimes the depth of a three-dimensional bite can be highlighted at low incident illumination and shadows can be made to delineate individual teeth or spacing (Fig. 16-15). The low incident lighting angle image may look completely different than one taken from directly overhead (Fig. 16-16).

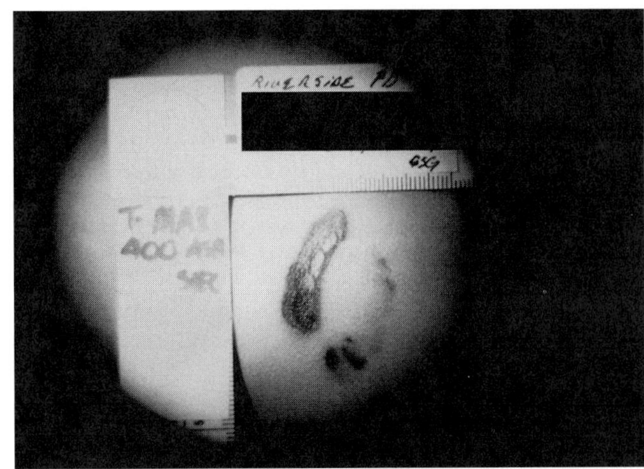

Fig. 16-16 Same bite mark shown in Figure 16-15, taken with overhead lighting angle. Note outlines of incisal edges of lower teeth.

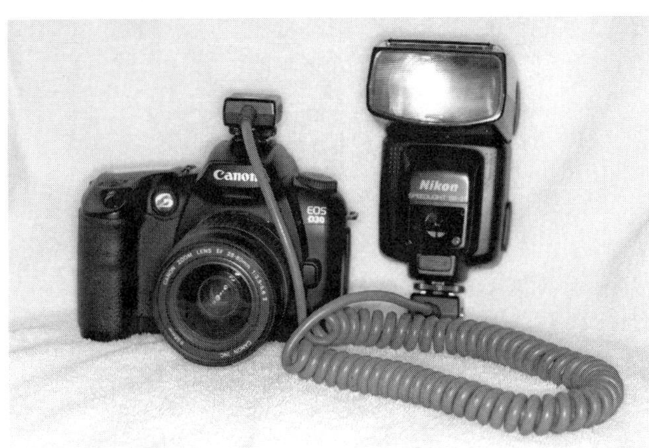

Fig. 16-14 Digital SLR camera demonstrating detachable flash for off-angle lighting.

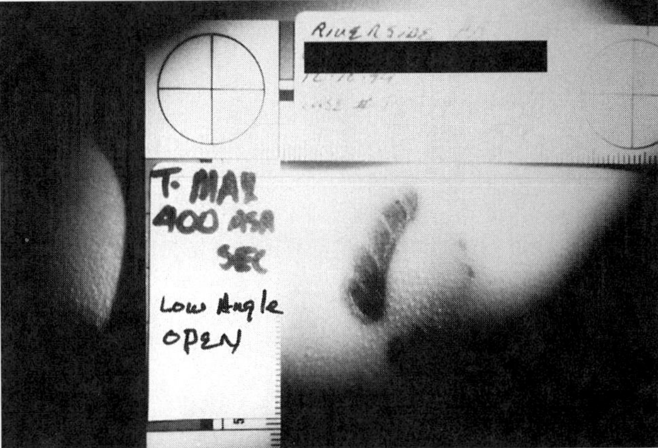

Fig. 16-15 Low incident angle of illumination showing injured tissue geography. Note raised areas where tissue was pinched between teeth.

Film types and armamentaria that are appropriate for bite mark and close-up photography differ with each technique. Advanced photographic techniques such as alternate light imaging, reflective ultraviolet, and infrared photography are available and typically conducted by experts who know the protocols for these techniques. For most situations applicable to photography in nursing care settings, digital cameras can be set at 100 ISO for most flash-accompanied forensic documentation. Color slide and print negative films with an ISO of 100 are also usually sufficient. "E-6" process slide film and "C-41" process print film from an established commercial manufacturer will suffice in most situations. Remember to take multiple shots and use the whole roll of film, bracketing for varied exposures. If employing the aforementioned advanced photographic techniques, higher speed color, special infrared, and panchromatic black-and-white films will be required, along with proper training. Typically for UVA photography a panchromatic film such as Kodak T-Max 400 is appropriate. Infrared photography requires specific film and special handling characteristics as well. Several additional equipment and training requirements apply for these advanced and non-visible light techniques. Periodic courses can be found in forensic continuing education venues where instruction on advanced photographic techniques are given. Two of these courses are the International Forensic Photography Course, given twice yearly in Miami through the Dade County Medical Examiner, and the Advanced Forensic Photography Seminar, sponsored by the University of Texas Health Sciences Center at San Antonio Dental School.

Summary

Forensic odontology can play an important role in identifying those suspected of committing violent crimes, specifically by the inclusion of bite mark evidence. For the bite mark evidence to become a useful part of the judicial process, serological swabs must be properly obtained for salivary deposition so that laboratory analysis for blood typing and DNA assessment can be performed. The bite must then be documented photographically with the scale and camera positioned correctly to eliminate angular distortion. An accurate image of the injury is mandatory for comparison to suspects and demonstration of findings during court proceedings and depositions.

The bridge between forensic odontology and forensic nursing crosses paths at bite mark recognition and documentation. It is imperative that the forensic nurse examiner has the ability to recognize bite marks and accurately document them as useful evidence. Meeting these requirements ensures competency that is vital to the leading role nurses perform as caregivers to the victims of violent crimes.

Case Study 16-1 Child Abuse/Homicide with Multiple Bite Marks

Karen Culuko and her boyfriend, Leslie Garcia, brought her seven-month-old infant, Jose Galindo Jr., to a family health center for respiratory distress. Following their arrival, the infant went into respiratory and cardiac arrest and expired, despite vigorous resuscitation efforts. Forensic nursing personnel noted extensive bruising on the infant and notified law enforcement officials.

A forensic expert in the field of child abuse examined the child and noted that the injuries were indicative of battering. There were numerous contusions, including hematomas to the forehead, left temporal area, cheek, lips, chest, lower abdominal area above the genitals, scrotum, arms, and legs.

The infant's mother, Ms. Culuko, stated that the injuries occurred as a result of the infant rolling off a bed onto the floor at the motel where they lived. Both Culuko and Garcia denied any involvement with the injuries. Homicide detectives were notified and an autopsy was conducted.

The actual cause of death was found to be internal bleeding from a ruptured artery within the posterior abdomen. The investigating pathologist stated that it would have taken a "major force, like a violent punch," to rupture this artery. There was also intracranial sub-dural bleeding, typically noted when infants have been violently shaken. Neither injury could have been caused by a fall from a bed.

Examination of other injuries revealed human bite marks to the right forearm, genitalia, and both feet (Figs. 16-17 to 16-21).

Search warrants for dental impressions and photographs of the teeth of both custodians of the child were obtained, and this evidence was collected (Figs. 16-22 and 16-23). One can observe from Mr. Garcia's teeth that he had significant canine wear, chipping, fractures, and rampant decay. Ms. Culuko's teeth on the other hand, exhibited sharp edges with no apparent wear, no abnormalities, and smaller arch width.

A comparison of dentitions to the bite mark injuries was conducted using life-sized prints of the injuries and revealed consistencies with the child's mother (Figs. 16-24 and 16-25). A significant aspect about this trial was that this was the first California case wherein alternate light imaging photos and reflective ultraviolet photos of bite marks were entered and accepted as evidence.

The two defendants were tried together in the Superior Court of Riverside County and convicted of second-degree murder, felony child endangerment, and aiding and abetting felony child endangerment.

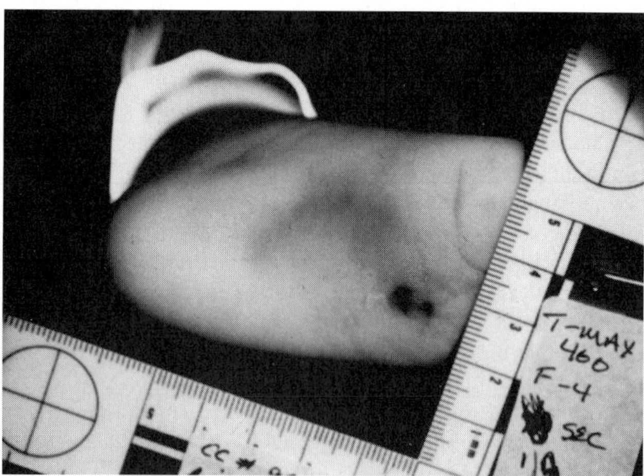

Fig. 16-17 Alternate light image revealing one arch of a bite mark on sole of left foot.

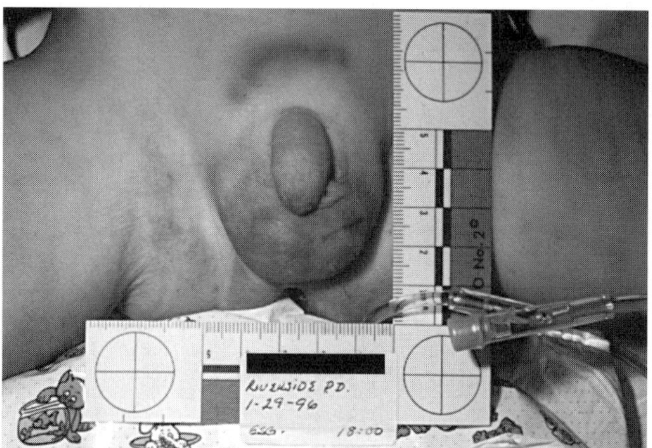

Fig. 16-18 Bite mark injury on genitalia of infant.

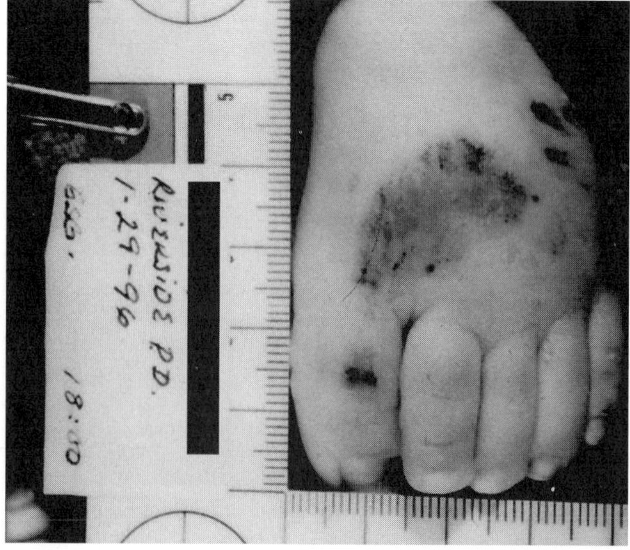

Fig. 16-19 One arch of bite injury to dorsum of left foot.

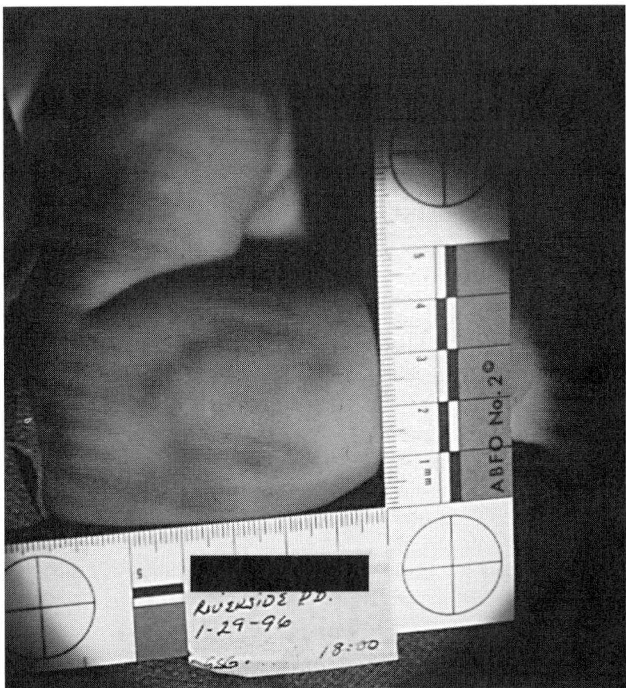

Fig. 16-20 Alternate light image of bite mark on right forearm.

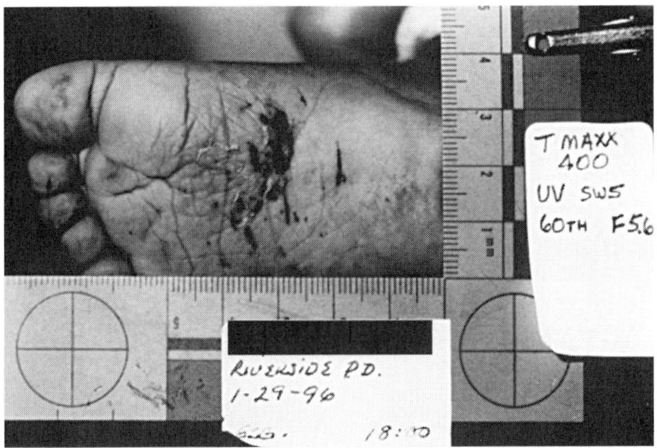

Fig. 16-21 Reflective UV photo of injury to sole of right foot.

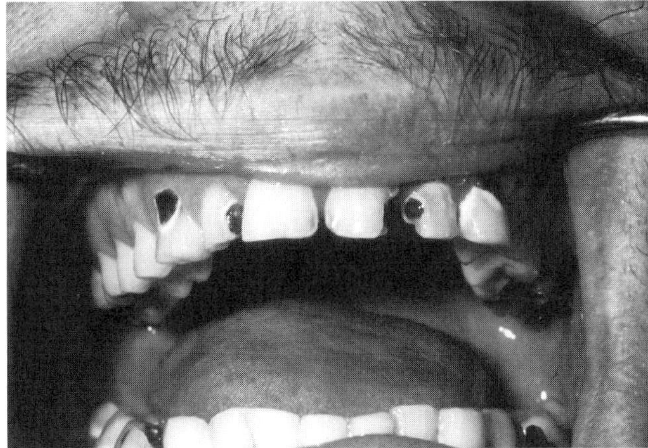

Fig. 16-22 Dentition of Garcia.

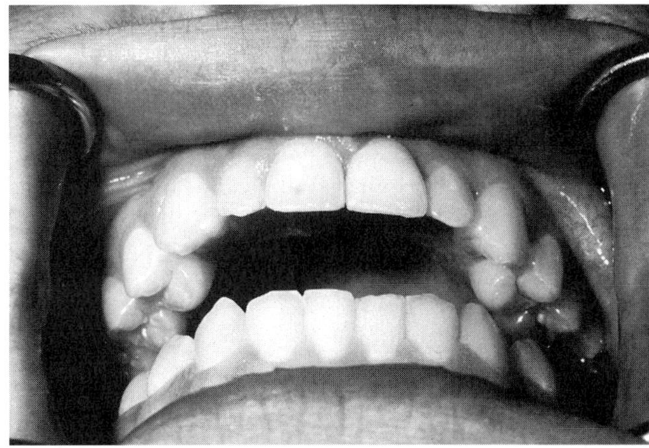

Fig. 16-23 Dentition of Culuko.

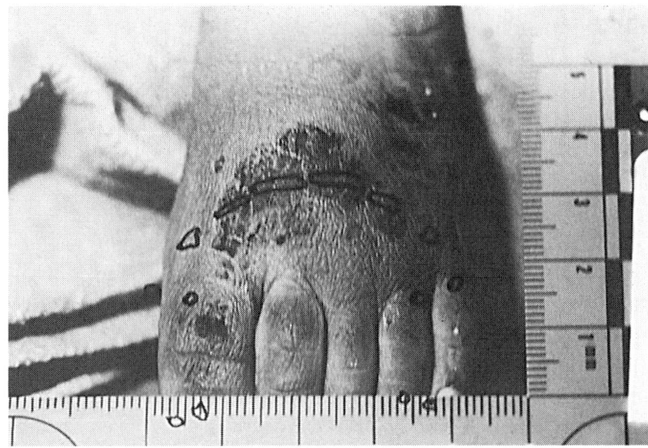

Fig. 16-24 Acetate overlay of Culuko's upper teeth placed on UV photo of bite injury to dorsum of left foot. Note consistent tooth width to abrasions on surface of tissue.

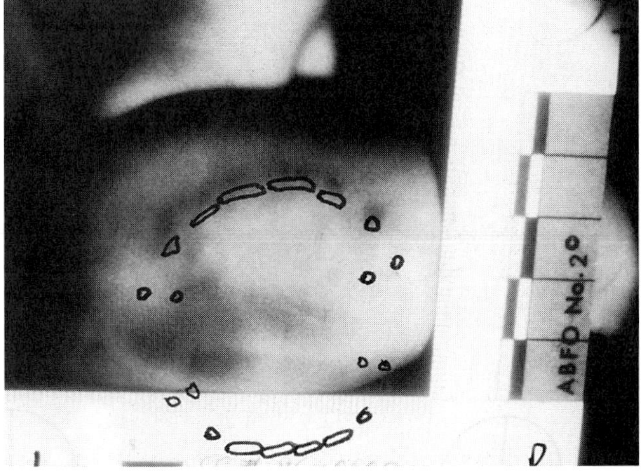

Fig. 16-25 Acetate overlay of Culuko's upper teeth placed immediately below bite mark on right forearm (alternate light image). Note consistency of arch shape and tooth position compared to bruise pattern.

Case Study 16-2 Dental Evidence

A 36-hour search for a 19-year-old college girl ended at 7:37 a.m. shortly after sunrise as the search and rescue team had started on the second day of an investigation for the missing student. Her body was discovered in a ravine near the railroad tracks in a small rural town where she was visiting relatives during a holiday from school. She had last been seen walking through the town with three other persons of about the same age, one girl and two boys.

On the afternoon of her disappearance several local townspeople reported they had seen her with her friends near the pizza and pool parlor where young people spend time during the weekends. One witness saw her get into a car with one of the boys as they parted from the other couple. No one remembered the type of car, just that it was a dark color and took off with a loud noise, bringing attention to the couple as they left.

As the search team came upon her body partially covered with grapevine and broken tree limbs it was obvious that she had fought furiously for her life. She had lost the fight when she was struck on the side of her head with a heavy blunt object. Although she had not been sexually assaulted, it was obvious that this had been the motive for the struggle. Her sweater and bra were pushed up toward her neck, and on her left breast was an oval patterned injury with abraded margins and bruising. Investigators photographed the injury, which appeared to be a bite mark, in detail using a variety of lighting angles.

Officers contacted the American Board of Forensic Odontology for a referral to one of the state's highly qualified forensic dentists. The investigation focused on a group of young men that regularly frequented the pool hall and were considered to be a rough crowd. Through the process of elimination, one suspect with a particularly unusual dental impression was identified as the perpetrator. The dental impression was notable for two teeth that had been broken in a fight with a pool cue. The uniqueness of the dental injury was specific to the sharp-edged tooth and the gaping space from the nearly missing tooth and matched the bite mark on the victim's breast exactly. Although the defense argued against the reliability of dental evidence, the suspect was found guilty of murder.

References

Bailie, W. E., Stowe, E. C., & Schmitt, A. M. (1978). Aerobic bacterial flora of oral and nasal fluids of canines with reference to bacteria associated with bites. *J Clin Microbiol, 7*(2), 223-231.

Golden, G. & Wright, F. (2005). Photography: Noninvasive analyses. In R. B. J. Dorion (Ed.). *Bitemark Evidence* (pp. 87-167). New York: Marcel Dekker.

Hart, B., & Powell, K. (1990). Antibacterial properties of saliva: Role in maternal periparturient grooming and in licking wounds. *Physiol Behav, 48*(3), 383-386.

Johansen, R., & Bowers, C. M. (2000). *Digital analysis of bite mark evidence using Adobe Photoshop*. Santa Barbara, CA: Forensic Imaging Services.

Kodak guide to 35mm photography (6th ed.). Rochester, NY: Eastman Kodak Co.

Leon Levy Center for Oral Health Research, University of Pennsylvania, School of Dental Medicine. Retrieved from http://biochem.dental.upenn.edu.

Murphy, C. (1994). Treating perpetrators of adult domestic violence. *Md Med J, 43*(10), 877-883.

Peeples, E., Boswick, J. A., Jr., & Scott, F. A. (1980). Wounds of the hand contaminated by human or animal saliva. *J Trauma, 20*(5), 383-389.

Sperber, N. (February 1994). Personal communication.

Sweet, D., & Lorente, J. (1997). PCR based typing of DNA from saliva recovered from human skin. *J Forensic Sci, 42*(3), 447-451.

Sweet, D., Parhar, M., & Wood, R. E. (1998). Computer-based production of bite mark comparison overlays. *J Forensic Sci, 43*(5), 1050-1055.

Walter, R. (1985). Anger biting. The hidden impulse. *Am J Forensic Med Pathol, 6*(3), 219-221.

Wright, F., & Golden, G. (1997). Forensic photography. In P. Stimson & C. Mertz (Eds.). *Forensic dentistry* (pp. 101-136). Boca Raton, FL: CRC Press.

Chapter 17 Binocular Microscopy in Sexual Assault Examination

Laura Slaughter

Historical Perspective

The use of microscopy in the evaluation of sexual assault victims began in the early 1980s in California (Slaughter & Brown, 1992). California was the first state to enact a law that created a uniform protocol for the examination of adult and child sexual assault victims in 1988. This movement grew from local organizations called sexual assault response teams (SART). The goals of these organizations were to improve services to victims of sex crimes by providing examinations using trained forensic nurse examiners and to encourage cooperation among the many agencies that interacted with these victims by having them come together under the umbrella provided by the SART team. The examination was moved from the emergency department, where victims were forced to compete in a medical triage system and had little privacy. Examiners were recruited and given specific training in sexual assault evaluation, including forensic evidence collection. In 1991, California developed a training curriculum for examiners of adult and child victims, recognizing both physicians and nurses as examiners. Following the publication of this document, nurses, who had always figured prominently in SART organizations, became the primary physical evaluators of adult and adolescent victims of sex crimes in California, with physicians serving as consultants. This model was soon adopted by other states, and in 1997, the American Nurses Association recognized the role of forensic nurse examiner (FNE).

It is not surprising that in this cooperative milieu, which brought together well-trained professionals, improvements to the current protocol began to occur. Colposcopy, which enhances visualization with magnification, began to be employed for children's examinations, because their genitalia are small and difficult to see. In adults the genitalia are difficult to see because of pigmentation, rugation, and hair growth. Compared to gross visualization, which detects genital injury in 10% to 30% of cases, colposcopy detects trauma in nearly 90% of rape victims (Table 17-1) (Slaughter & Brown, 1992). This technique represents a significant improvement over protocols relying on either gross visualization (Lenahan, Ernst, & Johnson, 1998) or toluidine blue dye (Table 17-2).

Table 17-1 Gross Visualization and Positive Genital Findings in Rape Victims

YEAR	AUTHOR	POSITIVE FINDINGS	%
2003	Sugar, M. F.	165/759	20
2000	Riggs, N.	388/736*	53
1999	McGregor, M. J.	31/95	33
1998	Biggs, M.	17/66	25.8
1997	Bowyer, L.	22/83	26.5
1992	Ramin, S. M.	23/129	18
1991	Satin, A. J.	24/114	17

*Victims include males and females, ages 1 to 85 years.

Table 17-2 Colposcopy versus Toluidine Blue Enhanced Visualization to Establish Findings in Rape Victims*

METHOD	NUMBER OF POSITIVE CASES PER TOTAL CASES	95% CONFIDENCE INTERVALS
Toluidine blue		
Lauber et al.	10/22 (45%)	0.242-0.658
McCauley et al.	14/24 (58%)	0.382-0.778
Colposcopy	114/131 (87%)	0.812-0.928

*All values are for patients who were seen within 48 hours and who experienced penile penetration.
From Slaughter, L., & Brown, C. R. V. (1992). Colposcopy to establish physical findings in rape victims. *Am J Obstet Gynecol, 166*, 83-86.

With a more detailed evaluation, the examiner can precisely identify the type of trauma present. Given this information, examiners have come to recognize a pattern of injury associated with sexual assault and to understand more completely the possible mechanisms of injury (Slaughter, Brown, & Shackleford et al., 1997). The ability to photodocument the examination is clearly important to the medicolegal process. Photography removes the need for lengthy technical descriptions of trauma to body parts that a lay audience does not understand. Additionally, it resolves the issue of possible hyperbole on the part of the witness, by allowing the court to view the evidence directly. These virtues also lengthen the window of opportunity to detect trauma or trace evidence (Box 17-1). In the past, conventional protocols recommended that victims who reported after 48 to 72 hours not be evaluated. These guidelines, based on the likelihood of recovery of trace evidence, excluded nearly 20% of sexual assault victims and were revised once examiners began to employ colposcopy. Over the last 20 years, colposcopy has become the standard of care for victims of sex crimes (see Table 17-2). As our understanding of genital trauma evolves, colposcopy will be only one of many technologies employed in the future.

Colposcopic Photography

Colposcopic photography should be used to document the genital, oral, and anal examination. Use a 35-mm camera to document lesions that are grossly visible, followed by colposcopy for detail. Photos of both normal and abnormal findings are essential. Not infrequently, a review of pictures may, in fact, reveal an area of abnormality that the examiner may have overlooked. Certain areas are particularly difficult to photograph and require special

Box 17-1 Advantages of Colposcopy

- Clarity of vision
- Precision of diagnosis
- Lengthening of the window of opportunity for the detection of trauma

Box 17-2 Facts about Toluidine Blue Dye

- General nuclear stain, used in a 1% aqueous solution
- Stain results depend on the presence or absence of a nucleated cell population at the exposed surface
- Positive staining occurs with trauma, cancer, or areas of inflammation with a nucleated cellular infiltrate
- 23 categories of benign disease, including columnar epithelium and mucous will take up this stain*
- Toluidine blue is nonspecific and should be used to enhance trauma seen with colposcopy
- Do not use TBD to date injuries
- Do not report patchy or diffuse uptake
- Do not report TBD uptake when no injury can be seen with colposcopy

*Data from Collins, C. G., Hansen, L., & Theriot, E. (1966). A clinical stain for use in selection biopsy in patients with vulvar disease. *Obstet Gynecol, 28*, 158-163.

Key Point *17-1*

Before colposcopy, sexual assault victims who presented 48 to 72 hours after the event were typically not examined. Colposcopy has lengthened the window of opportunity to detect trauma or trace evidence in these victims who do not promptly report the assault.

attention. Positioning the steep, narrow pelvis of some adolescents requires two hands, along with instruction in relaxation techniques, and with injury, the use of 2% lidocaine gel can be helpful. Of course, the use of these adjuncts must precede trace evidence collection. If an area is too painful and thus difficult to photograph, consider having the victim return in 1 or 2 days for reassessment. In this way, the injury can be followed from the outset and its nature and extent fully revealed. The interlabial folds must be carefully inspected for injury and trace evidence. Redundant hymens pose a challenge; careful documentation of the border and the attachment of the hymen to the introitus are needed.

Toluidine blue dye (TBD) is a nuclear stain that has been shown to enhance gross visualization of external genital (vulvar) injuries (Lauber & Souma, 1982; McCauley, 1986).TBD has some spermicidal activity (Lauber & Soma, 1982) and has been shown, in one small study, not to influence DNA analysis (Hochmeister, 1997). Stain results depend on the presence or absence of a nucleated cell population at the exposed surface. Therefore, a positive stain result can be seen with trauma, cancer, and areas of inflammation with a nucleated cellular infiltrate. Acutely, with tissue swelling and transudation, the dye may leach off quickly. Twenty-three categories of benign disease, including columnar epithelium, and mucus will take up this stain (Box 17-2) (Collins, Hansen, & Theriot, 1966). TBD is nonspecific and should be used to enhance trauma seen with the colposcope or as an adjunct for gross visualization. Recently, some examiners have advocated the universal use of TBD application to the posterior fourchette prior to speculum insertion to pick up preexisting injury and avoid confusion with iatrogenic injury (Jones et al., 2003a). While this is reasonable advice for those using gross visualization, a colposcopist should photograph the posterior genital area prior to instrumentation; sequential photos are faster, simpler, involve less tissue manipulation, and provide ample documentation. TBD should be applied with the smallest swab possible; it can be decolorized with 1% acetic acid or lubricating gel (Fig. 17-1) (Lauber & Souma, 1982). Specifically, do not use TBD to date injuries. Do not report diffuse

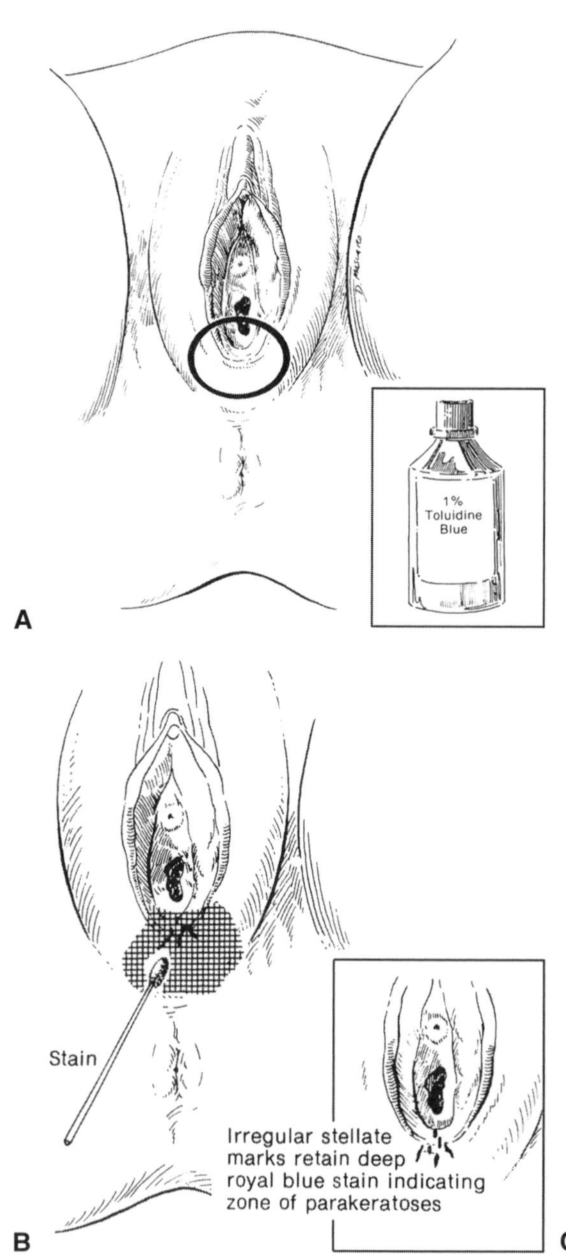

Fig. 17-1 Toluidine blue dye application procedure. *A,* Before. *B,* During. *C,* After. (From Lauber, A. A., & Souma, M. L. (1982). Use of toluidine blue for documentation of traumatic intercourse. *Obstet Gynecol, 60,* 644-648.)

Box 17-3 Photography of Injuries

- Use slide film or digital camera
  - Convenient
  - Magnification without distortion
  - Ease of storage
  - Inexpensive
- Make certain photos are correctly labeled
- Develop a standard technique for documenting the examination
- If a lesion can be seen grossly, start with 35-mm film
- Take lots of photos–include both the abnormal and the normal anatomy
- Photos must accurately reveal the nature and the extent of the injury
- Review all photographs for accuracy and clarity
- Be certain to take photographs at the follow-up examination

or patchy uptake (McCauley, 1987), Do not report uptake when no findings are seen with colposcopy (Slaughter & Brown, 1992).

The FNE will have this opportunity in time only once. Moreover, it should not be assumed that if one examiner did not see anything, no one else will. Comparisons between the abnormal and normal slides are excellent for teaching. Remember that this is exactly what forensic nurses are called upon to do for the court. Take lots of pictures and review them as a group for accuracy and clarity. A color gauge, measuring device, patient identification number, date, time, and examiner identification should be on each photograph or slide, as well as a method for determining the photograph's orientation. It is not uncommon for jurors to ask how slides are identified and how the examiner can verify that these slides were taken of a particular victim. The developer should number the photographs on each roll so that the order in which they were taken is preserved. This information is useful to rule out iatrogenic trauma or contamination. Moreover, if the pictures are sent for review, they are easily identifiable, thus facilitating discussion (Box 17-3).

Information and consent for photography and delivery of photographs, along with other evidence, to law enforcement are essential (Office of Criminal Justice Planning, 1998). Most victims and parents of child victims are very concerned with pictorial record identification and storage. Use of the patient record numbers (not the patient name) and maintenance of SART records separate from general patient information are common practice among hospitals. The precedent for this comes from the separation of mental health records from the general medical file. Any policy to separate SART records must take into account state laws governing the documentation of emergency visits in the general patient record. Generally, stamping the face sheet with "medical-legal examination" can satisfy this requirement.

Best Practice *17-1*

A color gauge, measuring device, patient identification number, date, time, and examiner's name should be on each photograph or slide, as well as a marker for determining the photograph's orientation. Consent for photography and delivery of photographs, along with other evidence, to law enforcement are essential.

Key Point *17-2*

Toluidine blue dye (TBD) can be useful for differentiating normal and traumatized tissue and will enhance trauma visualized by binocular microscopy. TBD will not pick up injuries not seen with magnification. A well-defined royal blue stain indicates a positive test.

Findings and Mechanism of Injury

When genital injury occurs in the course of a sexual assault, it generally involves the posterior aspect of the introitus. Using a clock face for reference, this region is located between 3-6-9 o'clock (Fig. 17-2) (Woodling, Evans, & Bradbury, 1977).

There are several reasons for this injury. Anatomically, the bony pelvis protects the anterior aspect of the genital opening. The position of the victim during the assault is also important, although this information is seldom an area of inquiry in most protocols. Most victims are subdued in the supine position and straddled by their attacker. This allows the attacker to restrain the victim with his body weight and frees the hands. The point of first contact of penis to vagina will then be in the area of the posterior fourchette (soft tissue) or perineal body, the juncture of the tendons of the superficial transverse perineal muscle and bulbocaveronsus muscles (Fig. 17-3) (Kaufman & Faro, 1994). These areas are inherently weak and continued force will cause tearing. Moreover, the position of restraint will effectively prevent the victim's ability to accommodate the erect penis. The angle of the erect penis is not the same as the angle the vagina makes with the vestibule (approximately 45 degrees). In consensual intercourse, the female partner must voluntarily tilt her pelvis by flexing the hips. Additionally, the vagina is considered a potential space. The lateral walls are more rigid (Fig. 17-4) (Kaufman & Faro, 1994) than the anterior and posterior wall so that in its normal state the anterior wall is collapsed onto the posterior wall, hence the use of the speculum to lift the anterior wall during the typical gynecological examination. Similarly, with sexual contact the real problem is intromission or getting the penis into the vagina. During voluntary sex, the changes that occur with sexual stimulation, the human sexual response, remove these normal anatomic barriers (Masters

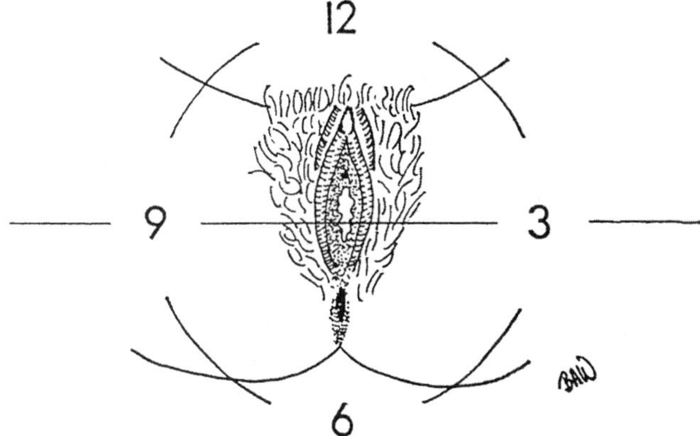

Fig. 17-2 The external female genitalia are visualized, using a clock face for orientation. Location of injury is indicated according to time settings on a clock. (From Woodling, B. A., Evans, J. R., & Bradbury, M. D. (1977). Sexual assault: Rape and molestation. *Clin Obstet Gynecol, 20*(3), 509-530.)

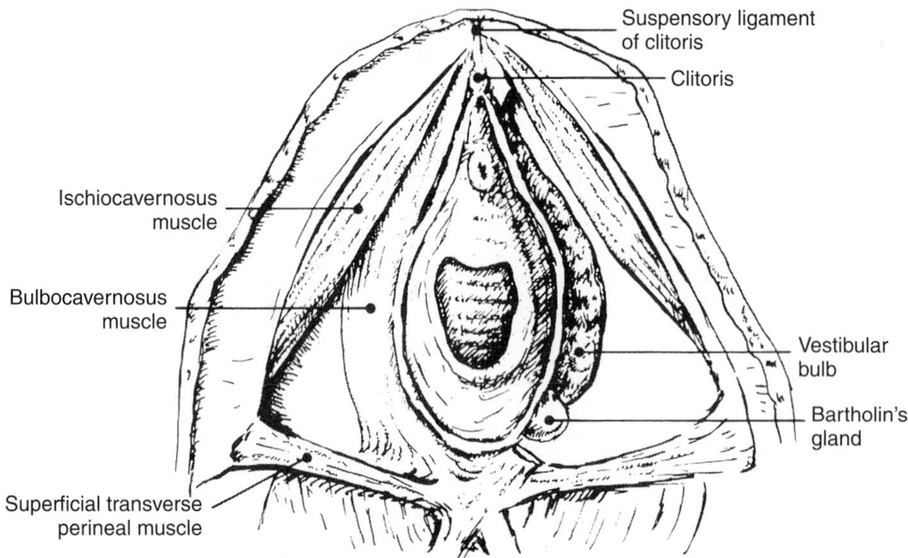

Fig. 17-3 Deeper structures of the vulva include formation of the perineal body, Bartholin's gland, and the vestibular bulb. (From Kaufman, R. H., & Faro, S. (1994). *Benign diseases of the vulva and vagina* (4th ed.). Chicago: Mosby-YearBook.)

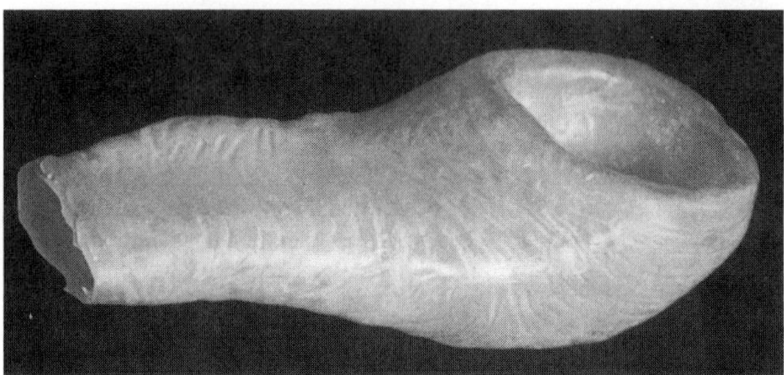

Fig. 17-4 Plastic mold of the vagina that was obtained from a live adult female. (From Kaufman, R. H., & Faro, S. (1994). *Benign diseases of the vulva and vagina* (4th ed.). Chicago: Mosby-YearBook.)

& Johnson, 1966). The two main physiological changes responsible involve an increase in blood flow to the pelvis, vasoconcentration, and an increase in muscle tone or myotonia. The entire human sexual response will not be reviewed in this chapter, but every sexual assault examiner should be thoroughly familiar with it.

The labia majora normally meet in the midline and are considered protective structures. These thin out and are pushed out of the way because of the influx of blood into the labia minora. The minor labia are responsible for adding at least a centimeter in length to the vaginal outlet. The vagina, with its rugations, lengthens and expands nearly twofold during this process (Fig. 17-5). The internal diameter of the vagina at its distal one third, sometimes referred to as the orgasmic platform, actually decreases as a result of engorgement or swelling. Additionally, to match the speed of penile erection (10 to 30 seconds), vaginal lubrication, occurs rapidly because it is a vascular phenomenon as well. The major source of vaginal lubrication during sexual stimulation is a transudate from the vasoconcentration in the pelvis. The vagina has no glands (Fig. 17-6). Other sources of vaginal lubrication include the cervical mucous glands and Bartholin's glands (Masters & Johnson, 1966). Cervical mucous glands do not alter output during sexual stimulation. Bartholin's glands are located at the vaginal outlet and produce only minute quantities of fluid late in the plateau phase. Their contribution is therefore considered negligible. The lubrication that these sources provide, combined with the natural distensibility of the vagina and mobility of the uterus, probably account for the relatively low rate of injury seen internally. The absence of these preparatory changes that alter the vaginal outlet for coitus is important to understanding the mechanism of injury in sexual assault (Box 17-4). Trauma occurs with attempts at entry (Jones et al., 2003b); it is external, and perhaps more appropriately termed a mounting injury (Table 17-3). When anterior injury is noted, the examiner should think of position changes, foreign objects, and inquire of the victim.

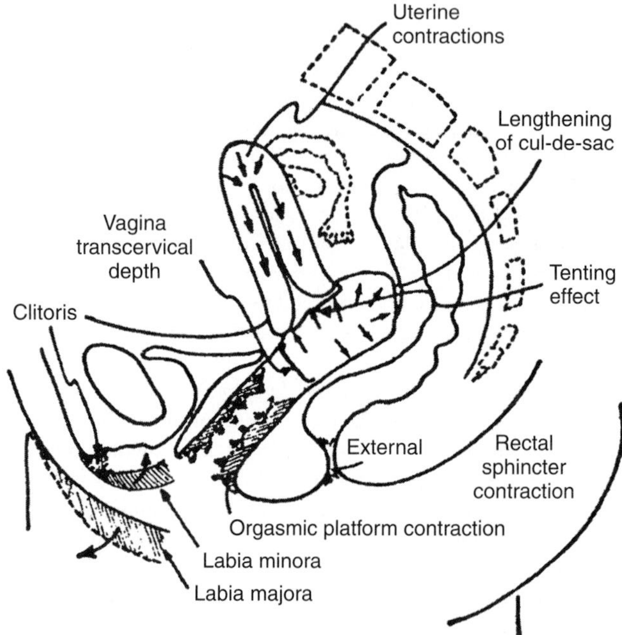

Fig. 17-5 Female pelvis: orgasmic phase. (From Masters, W. H., & Johnson, V. E. (1966). *Human sexual response*. Boston: Little Brown.)

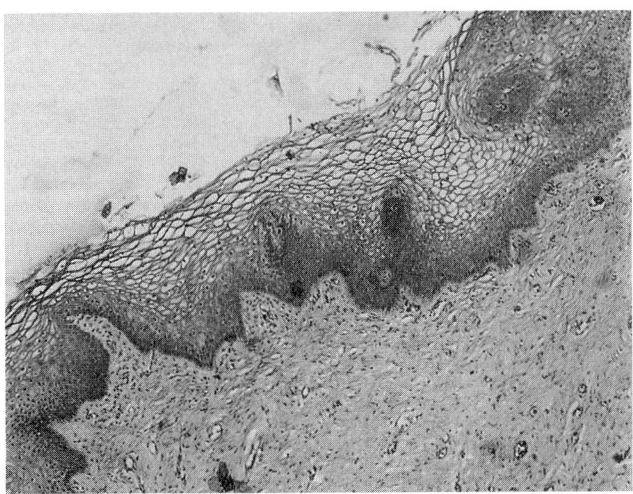

Fig. 17-6 Microscopic section of normal vagina. The lining consists of stratified squamous epithelium. The vagina itself contains no glands. (From Kaufman, R. H., & Faro, S. (1994). *Benign diseases of the vulva and vagina* (4th ed.). Chicago: Mosby-YearBook.)

Box 17-4 Mechanism of Injury in Sexual Assault

- Absence of the human sexual response
- Lack of cooperation/communication
- Lack of pelvic tilt
- Lack of partner assistance with insertion of the penis
- Lack of lubrication
- Increased force
- Male sexual dysfunction

Table 17-3 Substances Detected by Class in Sexual Assault Victims with One Positive Result (N = 793)

SUBSTANCE	NUMBER OF SPECIMENS	PERCENTAGE
Alcohol	546	69
Marijuana	145	18
Cocaine	40	5
GHB*	25	3
Other benzodiazepines	19	2
Opiates/propoxyphene	6	0.8
Barbiturates	6	0.8
Amphetamines	3	0.4
Flunitrazepam	3	0.4

*GHB = gamma hydroxybutyrate.
From Slaughter, L. (2000). Involvement of drugs in sexual assault. *J Reprod Med*, *45*(5), 425-430.

Typically, the most common site injured is the posterior fourchette, followed by the labia minora, hymen, and fossa navicularis (Table 17-4). More than 94% of victims have injury to one or more of the aforementioned sites. These sites account for nearly three quarters of all the injuries seen (Fig. 17-7) (Biggs, Stermac, & Dicinsky, 1998; Slaughter, Brown, & Shackleford et al., 1997; Adams, 2001; Jones et al., 2003b).

Table 17-4 Increasing Prevalence of Nongenital Trauma

YEAR	% NONGENITAL TRAUMA	STUDY AUTHOR
1987	40	Cartwright
1992	62	Satin
1997	57	Slaughter
1998	76	Lenahan
1998	81	Bowyer
2000	67	Riggs
2003	52	Sugar
2003	55	Jones

Table 17-5 Postmenopausal Women: Greater Risk for Genital Injury

STUDY	POSTMENOPAUSAL VICTIMS (%)	OTHER VICTIMS (%)
Tintinalli, 1985	63	32
Cartwright, 1989	52	N/A
Ramin, 1992	43	18
Sugar, 2003	36	20

The injuries are generally the result of blunt force and can be best described as tears, ecchymoses, abrasions, redness, and swelling (TEARS). Of particular note, the hymen is not the most common site injured in either adults or adolescents. The prevalence of hymenal tearing is statistically more common in adolescents than in adults. Age and sexual inexperience have been related to this finding (Biggs, Stermac, & Dicinsky, 1998; Slaughter, Brown, & Shackleford et al., 1997; Adams, 2001; Jones et al., 2003b; Sugar, Fine, & Eckert, 2004). Parity may be another factor, but has yet to be determined. Few protocols have information about these topics, and perhaps this lack should be remedied. Hymenal, vaginal, or combined tears are associated with a history of vaginal bleeding. Careful documentation of the source of any vaginal bleeding and a thorough menstrual history is therefore mandatory. In general, adolescents have more anogenital trauma than adults (Jones et al., 2003b; Sugar, Fine, & Eckert, 2004). However, once the patient is postmenopausal, injury rates increase (Table 17-5) (Cartwright & Moore, 1989; Ramin, Satin, & Stone et al., 1992; Sugar, Fine, & Eckert, 2004; Tintinalli & Hoelzer, 1985). Internal injury to the vagina and cervix is not as commonly (26%) reported as external trauma. Difficult to identify, even with colposcopy, these injuries may have simply been overlooked in the past. They are frequently associated with a history of lower abdominal or pelvic pain (Slaughter & Brown, 1992). Given the rich blood supply to the pelvis (Fig. 17-8) and findings at autopsy of deep pelvic contusion in some rape-homicide victims, the utility of additional imaging studies to evaluate these patients should be investigated.

Factors That Correlate with Genital Injury

Several other factors influence physical findings as well, making a thorough history and accurate documentation a critical element

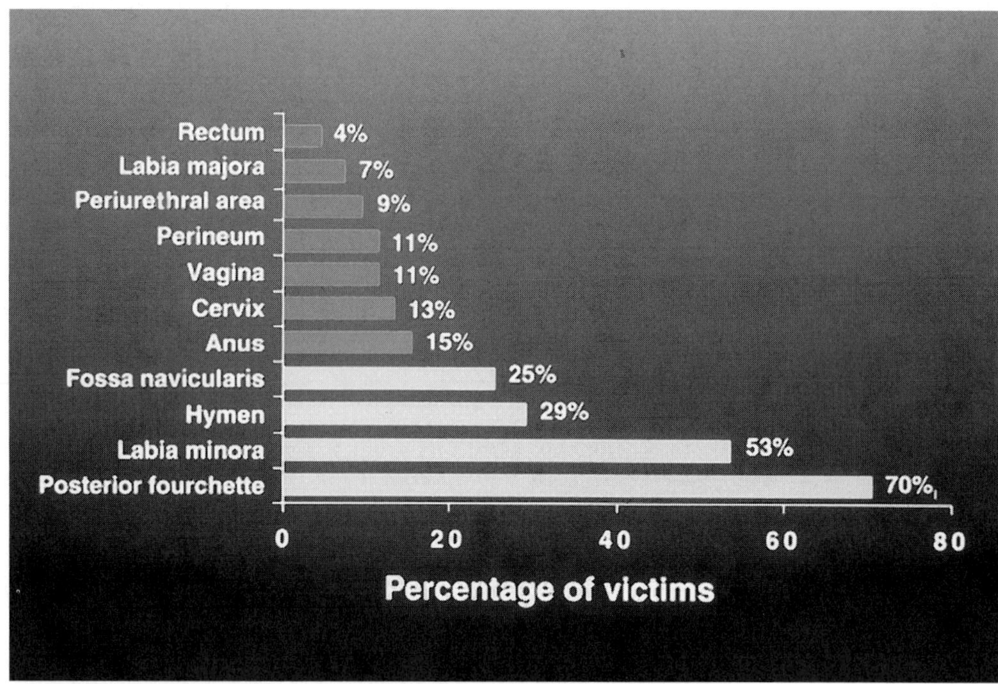

Fig. 17-7 Location and frequency of injury in 173 victims of sexual assault. (From Slaughter, L., Brown, C. R. V., Shackleford, S., & Peck, R. (1997). Patterns of genital injury in victims of sexual assault. *Am J Obstet Gynecol, 176*(3), 609-616.)

Box 17-5 Useful Information Not Routinely Asked on Sexual Assault Protocols

What positions were used during the sexual assault?
Was there repeated thrusting by perpetrator?
Did the victim assist with insertion of the penis?
Did the penis remain in the vagina after ejaculation?
What positions were used during the examination?
Was there alcohol or drug use by the victim and suspect?

- Use of drugs increases the risk of assault in the next two years.
- Drug use by victim escalates after assault.

Did the suspect have any sexual dysfunction? (e.g. ability to achieve or maintain an erection, etc.)
What was the gravity and parity? How many babies have you delivered?
Is there a history of prior victimization?

- Childhood abuse substantially increases the risk of revictimization in adulthood.
- Women who have experienced multiple childhood abuse are at most risk.
- Identification of women with abuse history is a prerequisite for prevention.

Are there any mental health problems?

- Patients are usually not forthcoming with this information.
- These patients make up about 25% of all patients seen.
- There is increased severity of sexual and physical attack.
- The perpetrator is more likely to be a stranger, the attack is more likely to occur outdoors, and usually greater than two orifices are assaulted.
- Attacks are associated with exacerbation of mental illness and higher rate of post-traumatic stress disorder (PTSD).

What medications are being used?
Is there tobacco use?
What is the medical history of the victim? What is the victim's prior sexual experience?
What trauma is noted without augmented lighting or magnification?
Were special examination techniques used?

- Toluidine blue dye
- Xylocaine gel

Was a separate evaluation done for each anatomical site?

Remember that the form to record sexual assault information was designed for the 20-year-old with no medical or mental health problems.

of the forensic examination. The protocol used by the FNE should be as complete as possible, but it should not limit the examiner (Box 17-5). The FNE should have a clear understanding of what events occurred and how they happened. Recording information that is nonsensical does not further the investigation or enhance understanding. Moreover, recognizing that certain details may be especially embarrassing or distressing to the victim, the examiner should always review the history when performing the physical assessment and carefully examine the mouth and anus. Additionally, in the course of the physical examination, the victim may experience pain that may elicit somatic memory and spontaneous statements. These statements along with the provoking circumstances must be preserved accurately by the examiner. A behavior-oriented interview of the victim is the best way to glean information about the suspect. The specific behaviors of interest to the FNE include the suspect's approach to the victim, methods of control, reaction to resistance, sexual activity (Hazelwood, Reboussin, & Warren, 1983), and specifically the presence of sexual dysfunction. In fact, sexual dysfunction, defined as erectile insufficiency, premature ejaculation, or retarded ejaculation, has been

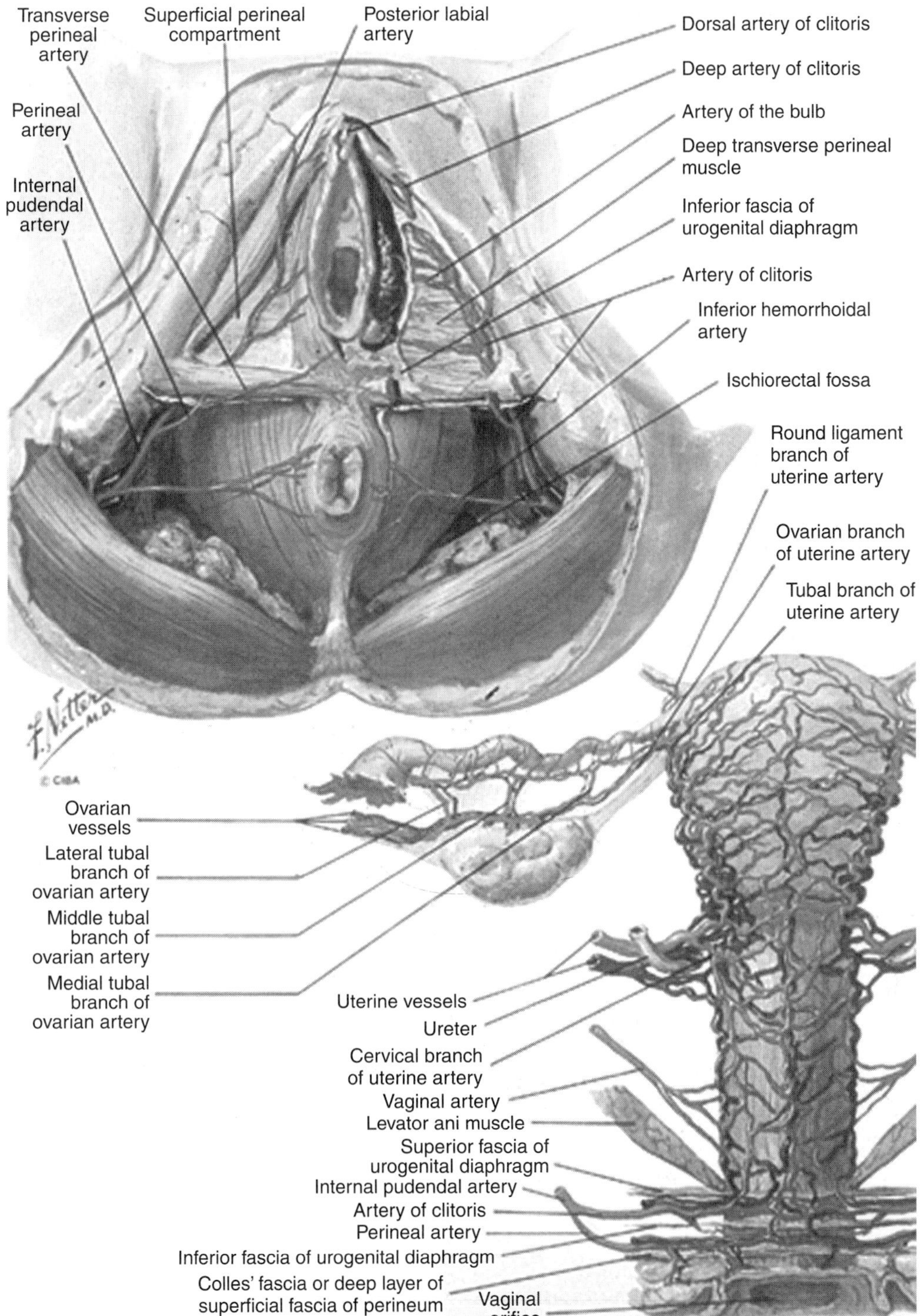

Fig. 17-8 Blood supply to perineum and uterus. (From Netter, F. (1954). The Ciba collection of medical illustrations: The reproductive system (Vol. 2). Summit, NJ: Ciba Pharmaceutical Products.)

shown to directly correlate with an increased incidence of both genital and nongenital injury, use of multiple sex acts, as well as decreased recovery of trace evidence (Groth & Burgess, 1977; Slaughter, Brown, & Shackleford et al., 1997). This is also a good time to inquire about any lesions, marks, or pathology of the perpetrator's genitalia. This information can be used for identification and confirmation of intimate contact (Reznic, Nachman, & Hiss, 2004). The examiner should always inquire about the use of strangulation. Victims seldom volunteer this information and case reports document cerebrovascular accidents up to two weeks following nonlethal strangulation. Moreover, strangulation occurs late in most situations of interpersonal violence, thus placing these victims at risk for increased morbidity and mortality (Funk & Schuppel, 2003; Wilbur et al., 2001).

The interval from assault to examination not only will affect the ability to visualize trauma but also will decrease the recovery of trace evidence. Communities must have the capability to examine victims 24 hours a day, every day. Even in communities with well-established protocols, nearly 20% of victims report late (greater than or equal to 72 hours). Consequently, continuing-education programs, which review the resources available to victims of sex crimes, are necessary, particularly for adolescents and young adults, who make up the majority of the victims seen (Jones et al, 2003a). Of interest, among late respondents, nearly 50% have genital injury. Surprisingly, these victims also had the same mean number of injury sites as those seen earlier. This finding indicates that time may enhance the visibility of some injuries or that the severity of injury may be a factor in delayed reporting (Slaughter, Brown, & Shackleford et al., 1997).

Penile penetration alone or in combination with other sex acts is significantly associated with genital injury. Stranger assault is associated with both more genital and nongenital injury (Stermac, Du Mont, & Kalemba, 1995). A history of a major psychiatric diagnosis is also associated with increased injury, and this is a topic that victims seldom volunteer. Recent studies have shown an increase in nongenital trauma from 40% to 80% in rape victims, suggesting that this crime has become more violent (Ramin, Satin, & Stone et al., 1992). Additionally, nongenital trauma should also alert the examiner to the likely presence of genital injury (Slaughter, Brown, & Shackleford et al., 1997; Adams, Girardin, & Faugno, 2001).

A history of anal contact carries special significance. The information itself may be difficult to obtain because of shame or guilt by the victim. Therefore, it is always important to evaluate the anus even if the history is initially negative. If no trauma is seen, it is prudent to re-inquire. Anal trauma occurs in about 50% of forced sodomy and this appears to have changed little with the use of colposcopy. Anoscopy should be done if the history is positive to rule out rectal injury. Studies now show that a report of anal contact is associated with an increase in anal trauma, genital trauma, or nongenital trauma (Slaughter, Brown, & Shackleford et al., 1997; Stermac, 1995; Adams, 2001; Sugar, Fine, & Eckert, 2004). The increased violence experienced by these victims has been related to offender preference for anal sex (Hazelwood, Reboussin, & Warren, 1989; Hazelwood & Warren, 1990) and sexual dysfunction (Hazelwood, 1983). Whereas this is valuable information about the rapist, it also provides a framework for understanding the nature of the injuries seen in the victim (Box 17-6).

Best Practice *17-2*

The anus should always be evaluated as a component of the sexual assault examination. If there is confirmation of anal contact, anoscopy should be done to rule out rectal injury

Drugs and alcohol play a major role in sexual assault (Muehlenhard & Linton, 1987; Koss, Dinero, & Seibel, 1988; Koss, 1989; Harrington & Leitenberg, 1994). Victims of sexual assault have a higher rate of drug and alcohol use than the general population (Johnston, O'Malley, & Bachman, 1993; Johnston, 1997). Moreover, there is no doubt that substance abuse influences jurors' decisions on issues such as responsibility and culpability (Hammock & Richardson, 1997; Scully & Marolla, 1984). Substance abuse is a medical problem, and much like a citation for driving under the influence (DUI), an encounter with the local SART may be the first warning sign of drug- or alcohol-related problems (O'Connor & Schottenfeld, 1998). A recent drug survey showed that the two most popular drugs used by victims of sexual assault are marijuana and alcohol (Slaughter & Brown, 1992; Slaughter, 2000). Of interest, the combination of benzodiazepines and alcohol has been implicated as a method to gain control of the victim and simultaneously erase the incident from her memory (Friend, 1998; Cohen, 1996). Other agents, such as gamma hydroxybutyrate (GHB), an anesthetic agent, can produce severe and even fatal effects. Because of its intensely disagreeable taste, this drug is usually not ingested voluntarily. Despite this information, there continues to be no routine surveillance of drug and alcohol usage among victims of sex crimes. Communities need to adopt protocols that routinely test victims and suspects. In this way, they will be able to spot trends in drug usage, provide a system of early warning, and make appropriate referrals for victims with drug- and alcohol-related problems. Despite the important role of substance use on the likelihood of sexual assault, it does not appear to affect genital injury (Cartwright, 1987; Adams, 2001; Sachs & Chu, 2002; Seifert, 1999; Jones et al, 2003a; Sugar, Fine, & Eckert, 2004). In fact, recent studies analyzing victims of drug-facilitated sexual assault have shown genital and nongenital injuries are less frequently encountered (McGregor et al., 2003).

Box 17-6 Factors That Correlate with Findings of Genital Injury

- Forensic training of examiner
- Completeness of protocol
- Use of colposcopy
- Time to examination
- History of penile penetration
- Age
- Sexual experience
- Presence of nongenital trauma
- History of anal contact
- History of sexual dysfunction of perpetrator
- History of a major psychiatric diagnosis
- Relationship between victim and suspect
- Environmental factors
- Tobacco use
- Tampon use
- History of nonconsensual sex

Coital injury is significantly associated with a history of nonconsensual intercourse. Three papers have appeared in the literature since 1981 directly comparing genital injury in rape victims with women who give a history of voluntary intercourse. Two used toluidine blue dye, gross visualization, and one genital site (posterior fourchette) to document trauma (Tables 17-6 and 17-7) (Lauber & Souma, 1982; McCauley, Guzinski, & Welch et al., 1987) and one used colposcopy, specifically trained examiners, and 11 genital sites (Table 17-8) (Slaughter, Brown, & Shackleford et al., 1997). Further investigation is needed to determine whether there is a finding or group of findings that can distinguish nonconsensual and consensual activity. One recent study looked at this topic in the adolescent population. While the number of anogenital injuries was not statistically significantly different between the consent and nonconsent groups, the localized pattern and severity of injury were (Jones et al., 2003a). Importantly, genital

Table 17-6 Toluidine Blue Documentation of Rape versus Consensual Intercourse: Lauber Study

FACTORS	VICTIMS	CONTROL SUBJECTS
Number	22	22
Nulliparous	10	7
Multiparous	12	15
Time to examination (hr)	48	1.5-45.5
Genital trauma present	10	1 *p=.004

From Lauber, A. A., & Souma, M. L. (1982). Use of toluidine blue in the documentation of traumatic intercourse. *Obstet Gynecol, 60*, 644-648.
*Fisher exact test

Table 17-7 Toluidine Blue Documentation of Rape versus Consensual Intercourse: McCauley Study

FACTORS	VICTIMS	CONTROL SUBJECTS
Number	24	48
Black	20	43
Caucasian	4	5
Nulliparous	9	8
Multiparous	15	40
Mean age	29	25
Genital trauma present	14	5 $P < 0.001$

From McCauley, J., Guzinski, G., Welch, R., et al. (1987). Toluidine blue in the corroboration of the adult rape victim. *Am J Emerg Med, 5*, 105-108.

Table 17-8 Relationship of Genital Injury and a History of Nonconsensual Sex

HISTORY	CONSENSUAL SEX	NONCONSENSUAL SEX
Total number	75	142
Number with injury	8	127
Percentage	11	88 $P = .0000$

From Slaughter, L., Brown, C. R. V., Shackleford, S., & Peck, R. (1997). Patterns of genital injury in victims of sexual assault. *Am J Obstet Gynecol, 176*(3), 609-616.

injury does not equal sexual assault. All examiners must be cognizant of the prevalence and type of coital injuries reported in the literature and knowledgeable about environmental factors that may also produce changes to the genitalia observable by colposcopy (Tables 17-9 to 17-11).

Trace Evidence Collection

Recovery, proper handling, storage, and documentation of trace evidence are mainstays of the forensic examination. About 10% of trace evidence can be seen only with colposcopy (Fig. 17-9). The evidence usually consists of hairs or fibers. Photodocumentation

Table 17-9 Genital Injury with Consenting Intercourse

AUTHOR	SITE	TIME PERIOD	CONSENTING SEX INJURY (N)
Sill, P. R.	Boroko, Papua, New Guinea	1983-1986	13
Smith, N. C.	Cape Town, South Africa	1976-1980	19
Rush, R.	Cape Town, South Africa	1964-1971	11
Wilson, F.	Washington, D. C.	1959-1968	37
Fish, S. A.	Dallas, Texas	1947-1954	14

Table 17-10 Distribution of Positive Findings after Intercourse (N = 18)

FINDING	NUMBER OF CASES
Telangiectasis*	7†
Broken capillaries	2
Microabrasions	2

*Dilated capillaries.
†Includes two women who had this same finding before intercourse.
From Norvell, M. K., Benrubi, G. I., & Thompson, R. J. (1984). Investigation of microtrauma after sexual intercourse. *J Reprod Med, 29*, 269-271.

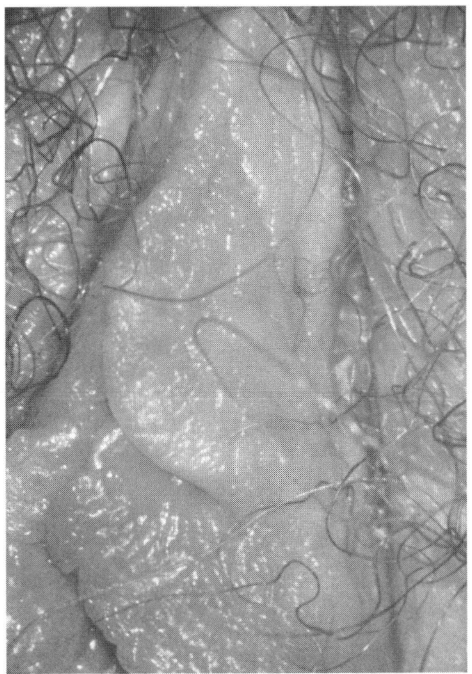

Fig. 17-9 Trace evidence seen only with the colposcopy. Note fiber on the clitoral hood. (Photo courtesy of Laura Slaughter.)

Table 17-11 Frequency of Consensual Intercourse in Relationship to Epithelial Changes

FREQUENCY OF CONSENSUAL INTERCOURSE	>2 WEEKS PRIOR TO EXAMINATION	1-4 TIMES / 2 WEEKS	>4 TIMES / 2 WEEKS
Epithelial changes/examinations	7/48	33/185	16/80
Percentage	14.6	17.8	20

From Fraser, I., Lahteenmaki, P., Elomaa, E., et al. (1999). Variations in vaginal epithelial surface appearance determined by colposcopic inspection in healthy sexually active women. *Hum Reprod, 14*(8), 1974-1978.

of the evidence in situ is recommended. Collection involves continuous observation through the colposcope while removing the evidence with tweezers. It is then placed on the sticky side of pregummed paper, carefully folded and placed inside a labeled evidence envelope. Naturally, each FNE must ascertain from the local crime laboratory whether the material used to make the paper sticky will interfere with testing. The inability to detect seminal product from the victim is frequently puzzling and depends on both victim and suspect factors. Most protocols ask whether ejaculation occurred; yet, many victims do not know. Sometimes they assume ejaculation did occur and so the history is simply incorrect. They make this assumption because the suspect stopped or another suspect started. It is always best to ask how the victim came to this conclusion. By employing this method, valuable information may be obtained. For example, the victim may have wiped and threw the tissue in a wastebasket. Additionally, during the human sexual response the vagina elongates and the uterus tilts up and back, deforming the posterior vaginal wall. With resolution phase, the anterior wall collapses onto the posterior, trapping semen deep in the vagina. Moreover, the engorgement of the distal one third of the vagina further prevents the escape of semen. If none of the changes that accompany the sexual response occur, the vagina is a fairly short straight tube (Masters & Johnson, 1966.) Therefore, changes of position, multiple episodes of thrusting, penis remaining in the vagina, or obstetrical trauma will all contribute to the loss of seminal product. This issue is further compounded by the fact that few protocols ask these salient questions. Suspect factors may also aggravate semen recovery. These factors include the use of drugs or alcohol and a history of sexual dysfunction (Boxes 17-7 and 17-8) (Groth & Burgess, 1977).

Box 17-7 Female Factors That Influence the Recovery of Semen

- Washing, douching, and wiping
- Semen will be lost upon withdrawal of the penis
- Changes of posture
- Earlier loss in the obstetrically traumatized patient
- Penis remains in the vagina after ejaculation
- Repeated thrusting will remove seminal product

Box 17-8 Male Factors That Influence the Recovery of Semen

- Sexual dysfunction: impotence, premature ejaculation, and retarded ejaculation
- Use of drugs and alcohol
- Use of condoms

Follow-Up Examinations

Follow-up of medical-surgical problems is a cornerstone of patient care. And the information derived here is extremely valuable to both patient and examiner. The care provider needs this feedback on problems and complications in order to derive strategies that really work. With time and diligence, the care provider can refine treatment methods and advice to better address and prevent common problems experienced by the patient. Unfortunately, this type of examination has been used little for victims of sex crimes despite nearly universal recommendations for doing so (Holmes, Resnick, & Frampton, 1998; Council on Scientific Affairs, 1992; Genecology, 1997). The use of oral prophylaxis for unwanted pregnancy and sexually transmitted infections, along with well-developed victim advocacy programs to support victims, have made the examiner less concerned about a second visit. Moreover, the forensic nurse examiner must maintain a certain degree of objectivity and, therefore, must not develop a long-term therapeutic relationship with the victim. However, this concern should never prevent a follow-up evaluation by a member of the forensic team. In fact, the ability to reevaluate the living victim is unique to clinical forensic medicine, and its advantages should not be overlooked (Box 17-9). With colposcopy, the follow-up examination is mandatory.

In particular, localized and generalized hypervascularity (Fig. 17-10) can be seen with colposcopy and have been reported in up to 11% of women (Slaughter, Brown, & Shackleford et al., 1997). These lesions may be confused with trauma (Hostetler, Jones, & Muram, 1994). Both women (Figs. 17-11 and 17-12) gave histories of digital penetration and both have single areas of apparent trauma to the cervix. The follow-up examination will exclude

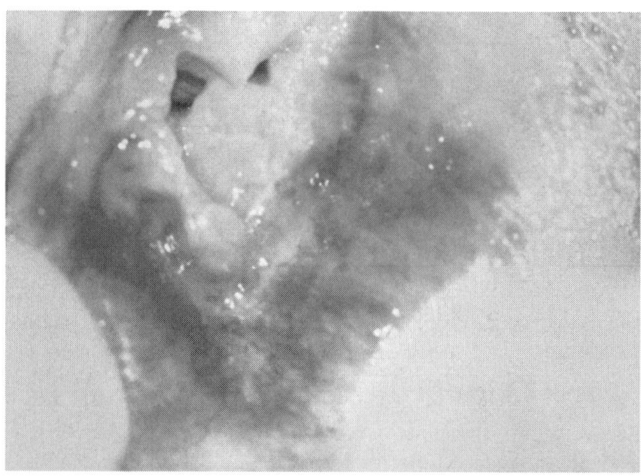

Fig. 17-10 Generalized hypervascularity surrounding the hymen is a normal variant. (Photo courtesy of Laura Slaughter.)

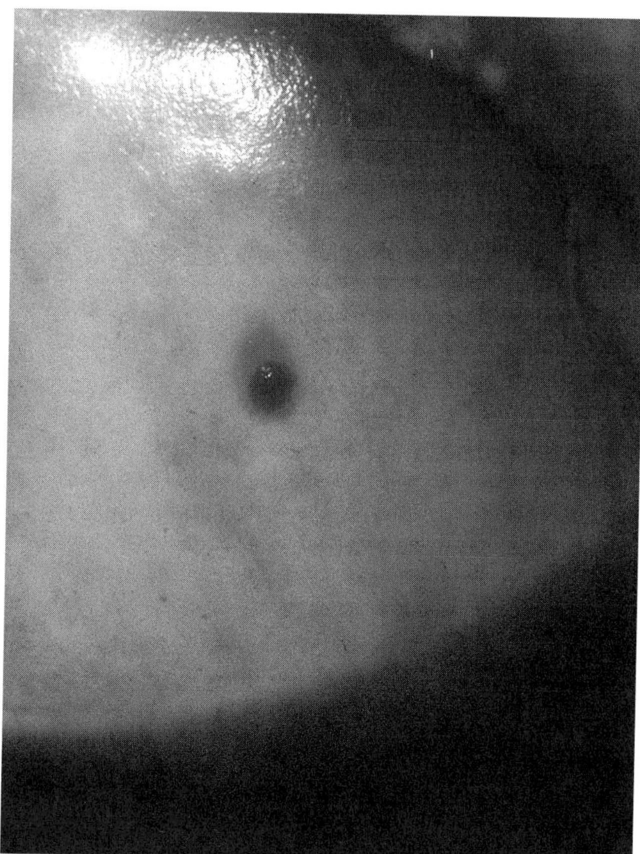

Fig. 17-11 Localized area of trauma to superior portion of the cervix; this was completely gone at follow-up.

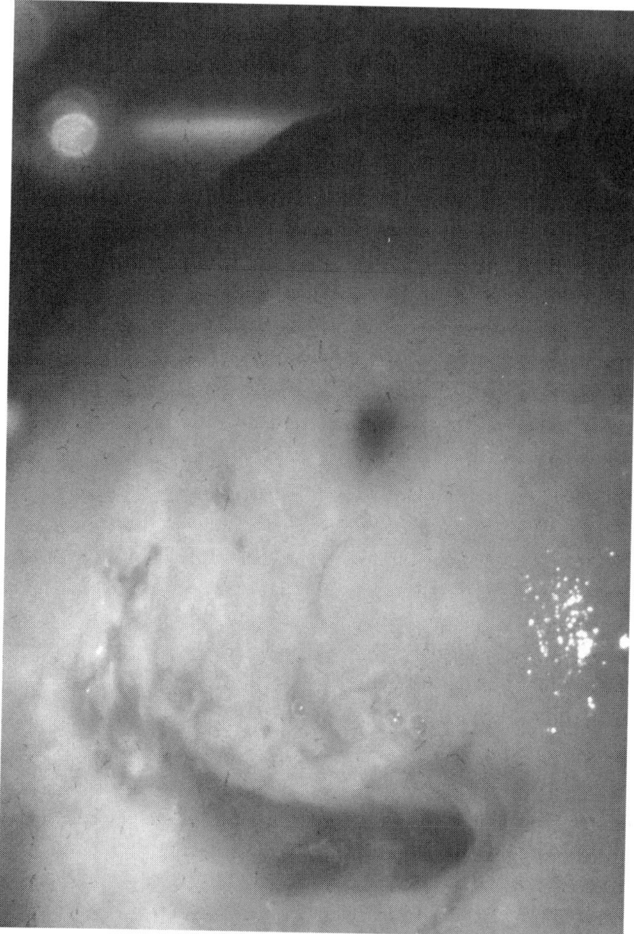

Fig. 17-12 Pigmented lesion of the cervix; seen at follow-up and referred for biopsy. (From Slaughter, L., Brown, C. R. V., Shackleford, S., et al. (1997). Patterns of genital injury in victims of sexual assault. *Am J Obstet Gynecol, 176*(3), 609-616.)

Box 17-9 Importance of the Follow-Up Examination

- Use the victim as her own control
- Clarify usual injuries (blunt-force trauma) in an unusual location (genitalia)
- Confirm the relationship of the injury to the assault
- Assess the severity of the injury by time to healing
- Rule out other gynecological conditions that might be confused with trauma
- Confirm the relationship of redness (nonspecific and increased interobserver variation) to injury
- Confirm the presence of swelling (difficult to see and increased interobserver variation) to injury

these gynecological conditions, allow the examiner an opportunity to evaluate healing, and provide a clearer understanding of the degree of genital injury (Adams, Girardin, & Faugno, 2001; Slaughter, Brown, & Shackleford et al., 1997).

Suspect Examinations

In many states, the suspect examination consists of the taking of swabs, smears, and clothing. There have been no publications about the benefits of colposcopy in the physical examination of suspects. However, colposcopy has improved the documentation and recognition of injury in male sexual assault victims (Ernst, Gree, & Gerguson et al., 2000).

The lack of attention to the suspect has been the turning point in many fiction novels by authors with keen insight into this area. In one of Patricia Cornwell's novels a serial killer is finally caught, but the DNA does not quite match; this mystifies his pursuers who find this fellow fits the profile in every way. Later, the killer meets his end and while on the medical examiner's table a surgical incision is noted. His medical records are obtained and they reveal that he has had a bone marrow transplant. The period of his illness corresponds to a time when no murders were committed. This series of events could never happen if the suspect had a history and physical examination by the same forensic team that evaluated the victim. How incredible that a woman can fight for her life with a suspect who later is subject to only the most cursory of examinations and evidence collection. The advantages of providing a careful history and physical examination by trained forensic examiners and colposcopy are inherent and should not be overlooked. Historical information not willingly provided by the suspect can be obtained from other sources. For the purposes of recording, the victim record is frequently used, but a specific history and physical examination form adapted to this specific task is really more appropriate and some communities have begun to use this format.

Deceased Victims of Sexual Assault

Despite the advances made in the development of sexual assault protocols for living victims, little has changed in the use of technology or documentation process for deceased victims. Although fewer than 1% of rape victims die, given the current method of screening (gross visualization) that figure is most certainly inaccurate. In some communities, the medical examiner (ME) and FNE have teamed up to rectify this situation. The FNE performs the examination of all orifices with colposcopic documentation, including trace evidence collection. After the sites of anogenital trauma and other suspicious areas are documented, the ME can then make sections and assess the exact nature of the injury and determine whether the injuries occurred pre or post mortem. Similarly, this partnership has proved valuable in the highly specialized area of child sexual abuse (Bays & Lewman, 1992). Certainly, joint examinations should be done whenever the investigating officer is considering a sexually motivated homicide. Additionally, joint examinations are appropriate for deceased victims in all child physical abuse cases, any suspicious deaths of children, adolescent suicides, and any female in which a sex crime is suspected. As with living victims, the historical information section of most protocols provides an excellent framework in which to analyze the information obtained from the physical assessment. Authorities should be directed to obtain this information from the victim's medical records. Physical examination should proceed as with living victims and TBD has been shown to be useful in this setting. Although TBD may not interfere with DNA testing, it should be used after all swabs and smears are completed. Because many of these deaths are not planned homicides, the FNE should be alert for signs of assault both before and after death. Moreover, there may be attempts to sanitize or clean up the crime scene and destroy physical evidence. Because of the anger and hostility involved in these crimes, one should also be alert to experimental or unusual sexual acts, particularly those involving foreign objects, multiple orifices, and especially abuse of the mouth and anus.

Because the ME's attention is often directed to the cause of death and most do not use a standardized format to record the sexual assault findings in an autopsy, discussion with the ME often elicits valuable, additional information. When a joint examination is not done, the FNE may be called upon to review 35-mm photographs and the autopsy report. Having slides made from the *original* negatives so they can be magnified without loss of quality is extremely helpful. Additionally, computerized photographic programs can improve overall picture quality and point to areas that deserve microscopic examination. These challenging and interesting cases demand accurate and thorough documentation (see Chapter 37).

Summary

The use of binocular microscopy to augment sexual assault examinations began in 1980 and has added an important new dimension to the forensic nurse examiner's documentation procedures.

Colposcopy, which enhances visualization with magnification, permits reliable identification of genital injury and enhances photodocumentation of injuries that previously had been difficult to visualize. This technique represents a significant improvement over former protocols using gross visualization either alone or enhanced with toluidine blue dye. Binocular microscopy is a state of the art technique that assists members of the forensic team in establishing convincing evidentiary photographs for courtroom exhibition during sexual assault testimony.

Case Study 17-1 Sexual Assault Evidence

During the investigation of a suspected rape/homicide case involving a 14-year-old girl the prosecution was in need of evidence that would confirm that the sexual assault had indeed occurred. This would be an important finding because it would permit the prosecution to add an additional criminal charge when indicting the suspect, a 24-year-old male with a history of violent behavior. It is also common within the forensic medical community that forensic pathologists cannot confirm evidence of sexual assault. A common practice in autopsy procedures has been to remove the internal genital organs and to dissect the vaginal canal observing for signs of injury within the tissues. However, because the most frequent injuries related to sexual assault are microscopic and superficial in nature, it is difficult to identify them without magnification. Unfortunately, dissecting the internal organs has a tendency to also destroy the very evidence that needs to be seen and documented. In this specific case the pathologist was aware of the work of the local forensic nurse examiners who specialized in sexual assault examination with the use of the colposcope as well as chemical markers to enhance photography. Although the body had been released for burial, and the only evidence the pathologist had at this point was the 35-mm photographs of the genital area, which had been taken before the autopsy, and before any dissection was performed. The pathologist contacted a forensic nurse examiner (FNE) and requested forensic consultation regarding the matter of sexual assault on the victim. Without magnification, the injuries were undetermined. The FNE asked permission to evaluate them with colopscopic magnification and to rephotograph them from this perspective.

Using colposcope magnification with the camera attached to this binocular microscope device, the new photographs provided significant evidence of injury consistent with forced sexual contact. Later at trial the FNE, as well as the forensic pathologist, testified, relating the importance of the new photographs, which were shown to the jury. The colposcope photographic corroboration presented persuasive evidence and resulted in a successful conviction. The jurors who were interviewed after the trial stated that it was the forensic nurse's testimony and photographic documentation that convinced them that the sexual assault had undeniably occurred.

Resources

Organizations

American Academy of Forensic Sciences

410 North 21st Street, Colorado Springs, CO 80904; Tel: 719-636-1100; www.aafs.org

American College of Obstetricians and Gynecologists

409 12th Streeet SW, P.O. Box 96920; Washington, DC 20090-6920; Tel: 202-638-5577; www.acog.org

International Association of Forensic Nurses

East Holly Avenue, Box 56, Pittman, NJ 08071-0056; www.forensicnurse.org

Journal of Forensic Sciences

Journal of the American Academy of Forensic Sciences; Michael A. Peat, PhD, Editor, 7151 West 135th Street; PMB 410, Overland Park, KS 66223

References

Adams, J. (2001). Evolution of a classification scale: Medical evaluation of suspected child abuse. *Child Maltreatment, 6*(1), 31-36.

Adams, J., Girardin, B., Faugno, D. (2001). Adolescent sexual assault: documentation of acute injuries using photo-colposcopy. *J Pediatr Adolesc Gynecol, 14*(4), 175-180.

Bays, J., & Lewman, L. (1992). Toluidine blue in the detection at autopsy of perineal and anal lacerations in victims of sexual abuse. *Arch Pathol Lav Med, 116*, 620-621.

Biggs, M., Stermac, L., & Dicinsky, M. (1998). Genital injuries following sexual assault of women with and without prior sexual intercourse experience. *Can Med Assoc J*, 159 (1), 33-37.

Cartwright, P. (1987). Factors that correlate with injury sustained by survivors of sexual assault. *Obstet Gynecol, 70*, 44-46.

Cartwright, P., & Moore, R. (1989). The elderly rape victim. *South Med J, 82*(8), 988-989.

Cohen, J. S. (June 20,1996). Drugs may be used in sexual assaults. *USA Today*, 1.

Collins, C., Hansen, L., & Theriot, E. (1966). A clinical stain for use in selection biopsy in patients with vulvar disease. *Obstet Gynecol, 28*, 158-163.

Council on Scientific Affairs. (1992). Violence against women: Relevance for medical practitioners. *JAMA, 268*, 3184-3189.

Ernst, A. A., Gree, E., Gerguson, M. T., et al. (2000). The utility of anoscopy and colposcopy in the evaluation of male sexual assault victims. *Ann Emerg Med, 36*(5), 432-437.

Friend, T. (July 30, 1998). Date rape drug. *USA Today*, 46.

Funk, M., & Schuppel, J. (2003). Strangulation injuries. *Wisconsin Med J, 102*(3), 41-45.

Groth, A., & Burgess, A. (1977). Sexual dysfunction during rape. *N Engl J Med, 297*, 764-766.

Hammock, G. S., & Richardson, D. R. (1997). Perceptions of rape: the influence of closeness of relationship, intoxication and sex of participant. *Violence Victims, 12*, 237-246.

Harrington, M. T., & Leitenberg, H. (1994). Relationship between alcohol consumption and victim behaviors immediately preceding sexual aggression by an acquaintance. *Violence Victims, 9*, 315-324.

Hazelwood, R., Reboussin, R., & Warren, J. (1989). Serial rape: Correlates of increased aggression and the relationship of offender pleasure to victim resistance. *J Interpersonal Violence, 4*, 65-78.

Hazelwood, R., & Warren, J. (1990). The criminal behavior of the serial rapist. *FBI Law Enforcement Bull, 59*, 11-16.

Hazelwood, R. (1983). The behavior-oriented interview of rape victims: The key to profiling. *FBI Law Enforcement Bull, 52*, 8-15.

Hochmeister, M., et al. (1997). Effects of toluidine blue and destaining reagents used in sexual assault examinations on the ability to obtain DNA profiles from postcoital vaginal swabs. *J Forens Sci, 42*(2), 316-319.

Holmes, M., Resnick, H., & Frampton, D. (1998). Follow-up of sexual assault victims. *Am J Obstet Gynecol, 179*(2), 336-342.

Hostetler, B., Jones, C., & Muram, D. (1994). Capillary hemangiomas of the vulva mistaken for sexual abuse. *Adolesc Pediatr Gynecol, 7*, 44-46.

Johnston, L. (1997). Contributions of drug epidemiology to the field of drug abuse prevention. *Substance Use Misuse, 32*, 1637-1642.

Johnston, L. D., O'Malley, P. M., & Bachman, J. G. (1993). National survey results on drug use: College students and young adults from the monitoring the future study, 1975-92. National Institute on Drug Abuse. Bethesda, MD: National Institutes of Health.

Jones, J., et al. (2003a). Anogenital injuries in adolescents after consensual sexual intercourse. *Acad Emerg Med, 10*(12), 1378-1383.

Jones, J., et al. (2003b). Comparative analysis of adult versus adolescent sexual assault: Epidemiology and patterns of anogenital injury. *Acad Emerg Med, 10*(8), 872-877.

Kaufman, R., & Faro, S. (1994). *Benign diseases of the vulva and vagina*. Chicago: Year Book Medical Publishers.

Koss, M. P., Dinero, T. E., & Seibel, C. A. (1988). Stranger and acquaintance rape: Are there differences in the victim's experience? *Psychol Women Q,12*, 1-24.

Koss, M. P. (1989). Discriminant analysis of risk factors for sexual victimization among a national sample of college women. *J Consult Clin Psychol,57*, 242-250.

Lauber, A., & Souma, M. (1982). Use of toluidine blue for documentation of traumatic intercourse. *Obstet Gynecol, 60*, 644-648.

Lenahan, L., Ernst, A., & Johnson, B. (1998). Colposcopy in evaluation of the adult sexual assault victim. *Am J Emerg Med, 16*, 183-184.

Masters, W., & Johnson, V. (1966). *Human sexual response*. Boston: Little, Brown.

McCauley, J., Gorman, R., & Guzunski, G. (1986). Toluidine blue in the detection of perineal lacerations in pediatric and adolescent sexual abuse victims. *Pediatrics, 78*, 1039-1043.

McCauley, J., Guzinski, G., Welch, R., et al. (1987). Toluidine blue in the corroboration of rape in the adult victim. *Am J Emerg Med, 5*, 105-108.

McGregor, M., et al. (2003). An exploratory analysis of suspected drug-facilitated sexual assault seen in a hospital emergency department. *Women & Health, 37*(3), 71-80.

Muehlenhard, C. L., & Linton, M. A. (1987). Date rape and sexual aggression in dating situations: Incidence and risk factors. *J Counsel Psychol,34*, 186-196.

Netter, F. (1954). *The Ciba collection of medical illustrations. The reproductive system* (Vol. 2). Summit, NJ: Ciba Pharmaceutical Products.

O'Connor, P. G., & Schottenfeld, R. S. (1998). Patients with alcohol problems. *N Engl J Med, 338*, 592-600.

Office of Criminal Justice Planning. (1988). California medical protocol for the examination of adult and child victims of sexual assault. Sacramento, CA.

Office of Criminal Justice Planning. (1991). California medical protocol for examination of sexual assault and child sexual abuse victims: Training curriculum. Sacramento, CA.

Ramin, S., Satin, A., Stone, I., et al. (1992). Sexual assault in postmenopausal women. *Obstet Gynecol, 80*, 860-864.

Reznic, M., Nachman, R., & Hiss, J. (2004). Penile lesions–reinforcing the case against suspects of sexual assault. *J Clin Forensic Med, 11*(2), 78-81.

Sachs, C., & Chu, L. (2002). Predictors of genitorectal injury in female victims of sexual assault. *Acad Emerg Med, 9*(2), 1146-1151.

Scully, D., & Marolla, J. (1984). Convicted rapists' vocabulary of motive: Excuses and justifications. *Social Problems, 31*, 530-544.

Seifert, S. (1999). Substance use and sexual assault. *Substance Use & Misuse, 34*(6), 935-945.

Slaughter, L., Brown, C., Shackleford, S., et al. (1997). Patterns of genital injury in victims of sexual assault. *Am J Obstet Gynecol, 176*, 609-916.

Slaughter, L., & Brown, C. (1992). Colposcopy to establish physical findings in rape victims. *Am J Obstet Gynecol, 166*, 83-86.

Slaughter, L. (2000). Involvement of drugs in sexual assault. *J Reprod Med, 45*, 425-430.

Stermac, L. E., DuMont, J. A., & Kalemba, V. (1995). Comparison of sexual assaults by strangers and known assailants in an urban population of women, *Can Med Assoc J, 153*(8), 1089-1094.

Sugar, N. F., Fine, D. N., & Eckert, L. O. (2004). Physical injury after sexual assault: findings of a large case series. *Am J Obstet Gynecol, 190*, 71-76.

Tintinalli, J., & Hoelzer, M. (1985). Clinical findings and legal resolution in sexual assault. *Ann Emerg Med, 14*, 447-453.

Wilbur, L. et al. Survey results of women who have been strangled while in an abusive relationship. *J Emerg Med, 21*(3) 297-302.

Woodling, B., Evans, J., Bradbury, M. (1977). Sexual assault: Rape and molestation. *Clin Obstet Gynecol, 20*, 509-530.

Chapter 18 Forensic Photography

Georgia A. Pasqualone

Historical Background

Alphonse Bertillon (1853–1914) was the first criminalist to use photography in an identification system called *bertillonage.* His photograph cards of criminals and suspects, representing the foundations of our present-day "mug shots," contained demographic information suitable for use in criminal investigations. This new concept of using photography in police work spread from Paris throughout the world. In 1859, photographic enlargements of questioned documents were introduced to the court system. The case involved questioned and known samples of handwriting in a dispute about the signature on a land grant (Moenssens, Starrs, & Henderson et al., 1995). The first record of the photograph as crime scene evidence dates back to June 1871, when the world viewed incriminating photodocumentation of the Paris police massacring the Communards at the end of the Franco-Prussian War (Sontag, 1977).

Nurses, by virtue of their job descriptions, are all occupational photographers. In other words, the camera has become a valuable tool, as serviceable as the stethoscope or syringe. The camera has now become an extension of the nurse's eyes. Through photodocumentation, time can be stopped and history captured. Forensic nurse examiners are in the position of being objective scientists, and photography is fast becoming a supplemental form of documentation that must augment our work responsibilities. There is no question that the nurse's first duty is to provide lifesaving treatment for the trauma victim, but the patient and society are ultimately best served when the nurse can also recognize and preserve evidence that may later be used in a forensic investigation.

Exigent Evidence

Along with performing the ABCs of cardiopulmonary resuscitation, forensic nurses must realize that photography should become an automatic function of all trauma protocols. It is not only the trauma victim who needs this instant attention. Certain forensic situations aside from trauma require the immediate responsiveness of photodocumentation. These situations are called "exigent." Exigent and exigency are terms used by the legal system and are interpreted to mean that, for whatever reasons, information must be obtained now, and not at a later time. Exigent evidence can be lost in seconds. It can be washed off, thrown away, flushed, or it may leave with a patient, friend, or family member. A nurse must quickly come to the realization that evidence is exigent. For this reason, nurses may have to justify their decision to photodocument without prior consent in court. If the nurse can justify that the photodocumentation of evidence had to be done immediately because the evidence could have been destroyed or lost, no judge should find that nurse liable.

One of the foremost examples of exigency and liability is child abuse. Nurses may become suspicious of a parent's or other caretaker's story, wanting to photograph injuries on the child. When consent is requested, parental refusal can create a very uncomfortable and difficult situation. Photographing the injuries is critical because the surface wounds will heal or, worse, the child may die as a result of those wounds. Lack of proper photodocumentation could allow claims that the event never occurred, allowing the perpetrators to go uncharged. Documentation must lock events into a proper chronological sequence for litigious review. The observed injuries and the caretaker's story may not match, producing cases in which photographs and x-rays alone have been the focal point of a child abuse trial, demonstrating injuries in various stages of healing. If a nurse acts in good faith in photographing a child's injuries, yet the court determines that no exigent circumstances were present, the photographs will usually not be allowed and there should be no repercussions against the nurse.

Key Point 18-1

> The principle of exigency of evidence allows the forensic nurse to photograph evidence that would be lost if altered with the passage of time without obtaining prior consent.

Justice is best served by objectivity. When attorneys, judges, and juries can evaluate photographs, along with the proper accompanying written documentation, the entire medical system is better protected from wrongful accusations. Photographing injuries in litigious situations protects healthcare givers from allegations that patients or clients never received the proper care. For example, if a person claims to have slipped and fallen on a patch of ice or in a tangle of wires, the environment must quickly be photodocumented before changes occur to that primary scene. Photography captures time and events for a very long time.

Camera Basics

The word *photography* comes from two Greek words meaning "writing (*graphe*) with light (*photos*)." It is the process by which light is used to create a picture. Four basic elements are required in order to make that picture: camera, lens, film, and light. All four of these components can be built into one unit in which they are preadjusted to a single setting and activated by pushing the shutter button. However, the four separate entities can also act individually so that every factor can be controlled independently. These components will be discussed, as well as some other important photodocumentation concepts, to explain how they contribute to the taking of a photograph.

The Camera

The camera is nothing more than a light-tight box with a round hole in the front for the lens and a hinged door in the back for the film. Understanding the simplicity of this concept should ward off any fears about handling new photographic equipment. Any further mystery surrounding the camera can be explained by reading the operator's manual and keeping it at hand for ready reference.

Healthcare professionals need use only two distinct camera systems in the forensic setting. These systems are distinguished by their viewing system, or the way in which they visualize the subject. All other systems tend to be either too complicated, too large, or otherwise inappropriate for the purpose of medical or crime scene photodocumentation.

The first system is the single-lens reflex camera, commonly known as the "SLR." The SLR allows the photographer to look through the viewfinder to "see" exactly what will be reproduced on the film. It has a "what-you-see-is-what-you-get" viewing system. The second visualization system is found in the rangefinder or point and shoot (P&S) cameras. In this system, the viewfinder is placed *near* the lens so that the photographer's view and the camera's view are close but not exactly the same. There is the potential for chopping off the top, bottom, or one side of the subject in the photograph. The problem becomes worse as the camera gets closer to the subject and becomes actually crucial when photographing close-up images of injuries. For this reason P&S cameras are not preferred for photodocumentation in the emergency department (ED) clinical setting. Unfortunately, most people prefer a P&S camera because of its ease and simplicity of operation. However, with a P&S camera, the necessary adjustments must be made on a specific geometrical plane while composing the image in the viewfinder. In the clinical setting when time is critical, it is desirable to use the SLR viewing systems in which the parameters in one's field of vision are precisely what is captured on film.

These two camera systems are further subdivided by the film formats they use. One type is the 35 mm. In this system, the film canister must be removed from the camera to be processed. A negative is produced and any number of prints and enlargements can be made from that negative with further processing. The second type is the "instant," self-developing film. The photograph is produced within minutes of exiting the camera. There is no negative, and any copies and enlargements must be created by other means outside the system.

The instant camera system is an almost foolproof method for certain crime scenes and clinical situations. When only a few photographs are needed to document an injury, the instant photograph is the perfect solution. Known by its proprietary name, Polaroid, the instant camera system made its debut in 1947. After more than 50 years of innovative improvements, Polaroid provides the closest thing to the P&S camera concept without the parallax error. Thus, the combination of the Polaroid Spectra and the Macro 5 cameras will produce a set of photographs ranging from full body to 5× magnification (Figs. 18-1 and 18-2).

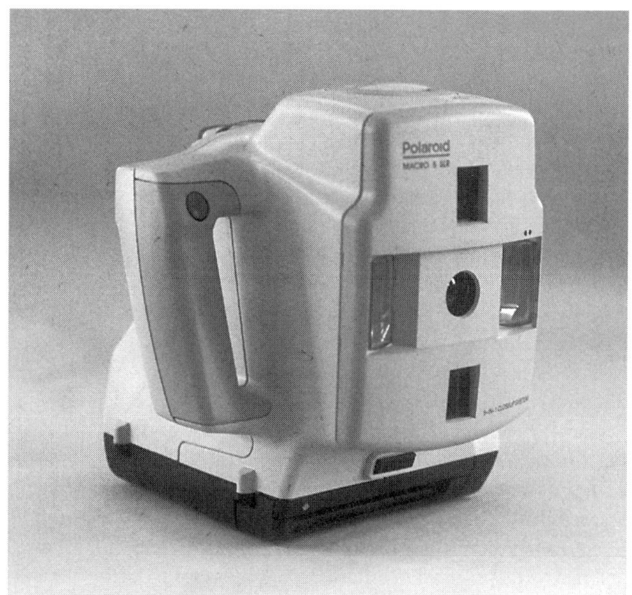

Fig. 18-1 Polaroid Macro 5 SLR camera.

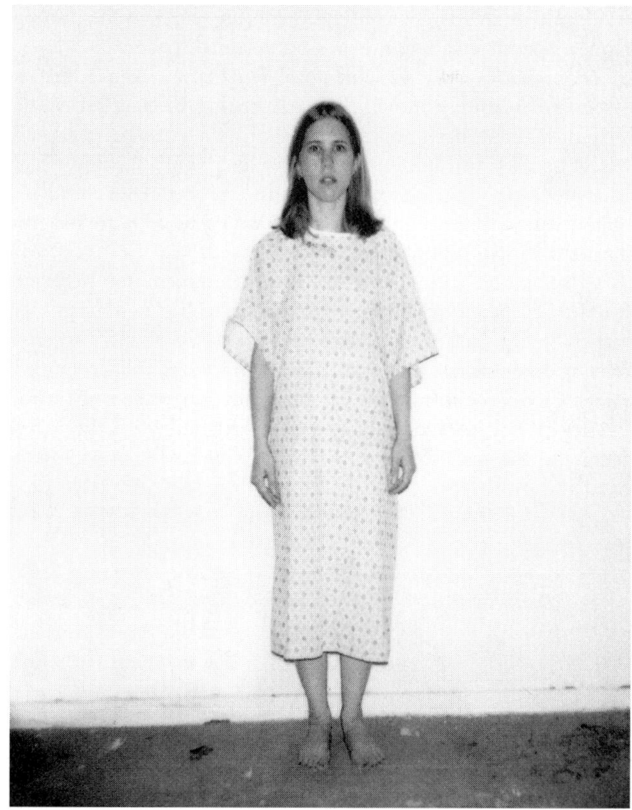
Fig. 18-2 Full-body view. (Polaroid Spectra camera.)

The Lens

The human eye is the equivalent of the lens on a camera. The lens is the window of the camera through which light and the image of the subject travel before imprinting on the film. The quality of the glass and the optics in the lens determine the quality of the resulting photograph. There are two basic types of lenses: fixed and interchangeable.

Fixed Lenses

Fixed lenses are usually available on the simpler cameras such as the P&S and most instant cameras. They cannot be removed from the camera body and the photographer has little or no control over how that lens is used. Fixed lenses also have a preset focal plane. This means that one usually cannot focus on any subject closer than $2\frac{1}{2}$ to 4 feet away. This severely limits the capability to take close-up photographs. When one must back up 4 feet from the subject, the composition of photograph is changed, resulting in more background than the intended subject.

Interchangeable Lenses

Interchangeable lenses are most commonly used on SLR cameras and allow the operator to pick various lenses to suit the situation or need. The basic reason for this would be to allow for changes in focal length and to accommodate depth of field and various lighting situations. Interchangeable lenses can be removed or attached to the camera with both a threading and screwing mechanism, or with a bayonet system. The bayonet mounting system attaches a lens to the camera by first aligning marks on both, inserting the lens, and then twisting the lens to lock it in place.

Lenses are categorized by a number expressed in millimeters and which represents the lens' focal length. Focal length is the distance measured from the center of the lens to the film plane and determines the field of vision seen through the lens. The most common lens is the 50 mm, or *normal* lens. The normal lens has a perspective similar to that of the human eye.

Lenses less than 50 mm are known as wide-angle lenses. The 28-mm lens is one of the most common. Wide-angle lenses give a wider view of things than only scanning one's eyes or moving one's head from side to side would provide. Wide groups of people, an entire room with its contents, and greater portions of crime scenes are better photographed with wide-angle lenses.

Lenses greater than 50 mm are known as telephoto lenses. Telephoto lenses work similarly to a telescope, enabling the subject to be closer to the photographer without moving him/her or the camera closer to the subject. They also make certain close-up tasks easier to achieve, especially when photographing injuries on an assault victim. The lens brings the injury closer to the photographer without invading the victim's personal space.

Zoom lenses have variable focal lengths and can adjust to distances by simply moving the telescoping mechanism of the lens forward and back. An excellent choice for a one-lens purchase would be a 24- to 140-mm zoom. This lens would accomplish all wide-angle through telephoto needs in one step. If expense is a major issue, a more economical range would be a 28- to 105-mm lens or a 35- to 70-mm lens.

Close-up and macro lenses are both convenient and necessary for detailed work by allowing the photographer to focus a few inches or centimeters away from the subject. For most forensic nursing applications, the terms *close-up* and *macro* will be synonymous. Close-up photography can mean anything from one quarter life-size (1:4 or .2×) to 5× enlargement, depending on the equipment and the available attachments. A 2× enlargement will give a head and shoulders view of the subject (Fig. 18-3). An example of

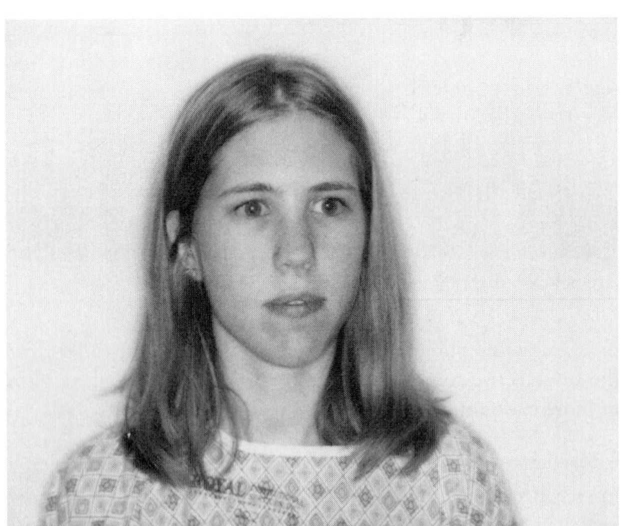

Fig. 18-3 Head and shoulders view. (0.2×, Polaroid Macro 5 SLR.)

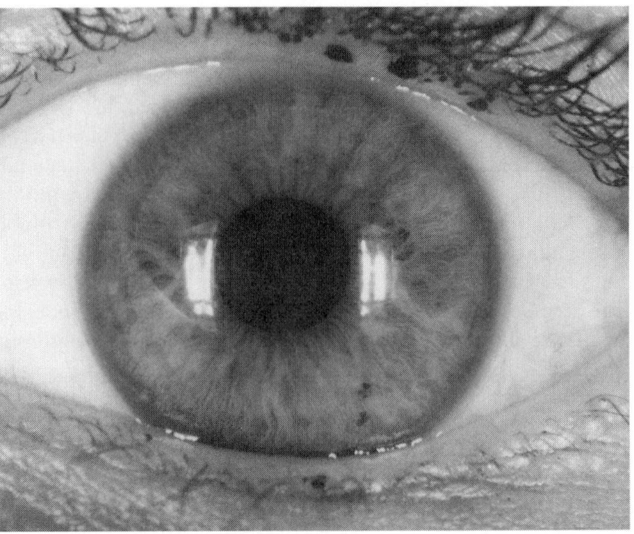

Fig. 18-4 Close-up. (5×, Polaroid Macro 5 SLR, with close-up attachment.)

a 5× enlargement would be a photograph of an eye magnified large enough to enable one to count the eyelashes and the blood vessels on the sclera (Fig. 18-4). With colposcopy, the subject matter is magnified up to 30×. (See page 175 for more on colpophotography.)

The Film

Film is the medium used to record the image of the subject. There are many film types on the market and there are specific films for specific functions. The two main categories of film are those that must be processed outside the camera and those that are processed internally, within the camera. Within both categories of film, photos can have color or be black and white, along with being developed as either prints or slides.

Color negative film has been the most versatile and, therefore, the most popular. Slide film may be referred to as transparency film or color reversal film. Additionally, the marketing name for this film type will sometimes end with the suffix "chrome." Read the package carefully before making a choice.

There are various sizes and types of film, corresponding to the size of the camera in which it will be used. A forensic nurse will be using predominantly 35-mm film in the SLR camera. The number of exposures per canister roll can vary from 8 to 36. The reproduction ratio of pictures is 2:3. This means that the dimensions of the resulting photograph should reflect the same ratio: 4 × 6, 6 × 9, 8 × 12, 16 × 24, and so forth. Prior to the "jumbo print" phenomenon, the older version of the print size was 3{1/2} × 5 inches. This means that for many years a good portion of the photo was being trimmed off. Therefore, in order for the photo to be enlarged to the proper proportions without cropping any edges, request that the negatives be printed "full out" or "full frame." The popularly accepted 8 × 10 loses 2 inches off the 10-inch edge of the photograph. "Full frame" will produce an 8 × 12 print with the subject intact.

In order for film to produce an image, it must be exposed to light. Light sensitivity is commonly referred to as film speed and represents the amount of light that is required to hit the film in order to properly expose it. The amount of light is regulated by a combination of lens opening, shutter speed, and light source. If the camera has a fixed lens, then the only thing that can be regulated is the brightness of the light source. Films are categorized as "slow-speed," "medium-speed," and "high-speed," also known as "fast" film.

Films are selected deliberately to perform a particular job. Color clarity and sharpness must not be compromised. Choose films that are sensitive and balanced for all colors. This will require a small comparative research study of the various manufacturers' products. Experiment with as many types of film as possible to discover the qualities best suited to the purpose. Photographs must have a reasonably fine grain, which is the element allowing the prints to be enlarged without seeing minute black spots throughout the enlargement. The best all-purpose film speed range for clarity in color and texture for medical photography is 100 to 400.

Best Practice *18-1*

Film to be used for forensic photographs should be stored in a cool, dry place and consumed prior to the expiration date. If film has been stored in a refrigerator, it should be allowed to attain room temperature before it is loaded into the camera. Process the film as soon as possible after it is exposed.

Film has an expiration date stamped on the outside of its box. Do not use expired film for photodocumentation of injuries when color is a crucial matter. Keep film stored in a cool, dry place. Personal experience has proved that, if stored correctly, there is a safety net of 6 months to 1 year for most films. If storing film in the refrigerator, maintain humidity at a minimum. Allow the film to stand and attain room temperature before loading it into the camera. Process the film as soon as possible after it is exposed. If this is not possible, simply continue to keep the film cartridge cool and dry. Never store film of any kind in a hot car during the summer months. Heat changes the chemical emulsion and greatly affects color. Polaroid instant films store best at room temperature. Polaroid film stored in a hot trunk or glove compartment for only a few hours will turn photographs orange-red and prolonged storage at cold temperatures will turn them blue.

Light and Flash

There are two physical aspects concerning light that one must remember. The first is that light travels in a straight line. The second is that there are varying intensities of light. Therefore, to use light to the best advantage, it must be provided, controlled, reflected, and bounced. The goal is to produce a photograph that accurately duplicates reality. The photographer must be able to testify that a photograph is a true and accurate depiction of the original scene as it was on the day in question.

There are two basic types of light: available and artificial.

Available Light

Available light, also known as ambient light, is the surrounding, existing light that is illuminating a particular room at a particular time, *no matter what the source.* It is the lighting inside a room, store, restaurant, train station, tunnel, or examination cubicle. The disadvantage of photodocumenting using only available light is that it is usually much dimmer than outdoor sunlight. Without the use of high-speed, low-light films, the photographer might have to rely on a tripod and slower shutter speeds in order to obtain correct exposure of the subject.

Artificial Light

Artificial lighting, which is illumination produced by other than natural sunlight, may also affect the color quality of the film used. Fluorescent lighting, frequently found in hospitals and medical examiner's offices, tends to give photographs a yellow to green hue. This can be eliminated only with the use of a light source brighter than the fluorescent lighting itself, or the electronic flash. In the majority of contemporary flash units, there are special sensors called *thyristors*, which are part of the electrical circuitry of the flash unit itself. Thyristors electronically calculate the amount of light that is required to correctly illuminate a subject. For instance, if the subject is close, the flash will not be used to its fullest intensity. This results in a faster recycle time for the next shot and conserves the life of the battery.

Under most circumstances the photographer must supply artificial lighting. This can be done via a flash unit built into the camera or an external light source. Flash units built into a camera are very limited with respect to any photographer control. Most consist of a direct flash that goes from the camera straight toward the subject. In some instances the flash may be turned away to bounce off another object such as the wall or ceiling. An external flash or light source usually gives the photographer more control of both intensity and direction of the light. With the ability to control the various aspects of lighting, subsequent photographs are usually better exposed. The only drawback is that it also makes the equipment bulkier.

Specialized lighting sources are available to be used with some cameras. Ring-light flashes are utilized with close-up photography to provide even lighting for dimensional subjects as opposed to harsh illumination or washouts. Ring-lights are usually standard equipment on the colposcope and are invaluable in lighting anogenital injuries.

Most contemporary autofocus 35-mm SLR cameras have a dedicated flash sensor built into the camera. It is not necessary to set the shutter speed to accommodate the flash because the camera automatically measures the light that reaches the film. On contemporary cameras with liquid crystal displays (LCD), verify that the camera is set for this type of automatic metering. In fact, always check the settings on all manual, digital, and LCD panel cameras before photographing any assignment.

Direct Flash. Direct flash can be harsh, especially if its too close to the subject. The flash can wash out detail, creating a "white out" or "hot spot" in the middle of the photograph. By bouncing the light from the flash, it becomes less harsh and still illuminates the subject adequately. This technique also makes it possible to document fine detail in scars, tool marks, and anything that mandates recording depth or dimension.

Bouncing Flash. Bouncing flash relies heavily on the color and height of the ceiling, affecting both subject lighting and color accuracy. There is a simple solution to this problem. Place a white card on the back of the flash so it faces the subject. It can be secured with a rubber band. When light is bounced off the ceiling, the cards reflects some of it forward into the dark recesses of shadow, whether on a face, around a fine scar, in a tire impression, or on tool marks made by a screwdriver to pry open a window. This bounce technique will be successful because the autoexposure mode of the flash is still working to determine the correct amount of light necessary for proper exposure (Fig. 18-5).

There are several ways to solve lighting issues in the clinical setting such as using secondary flash units or additional lights to

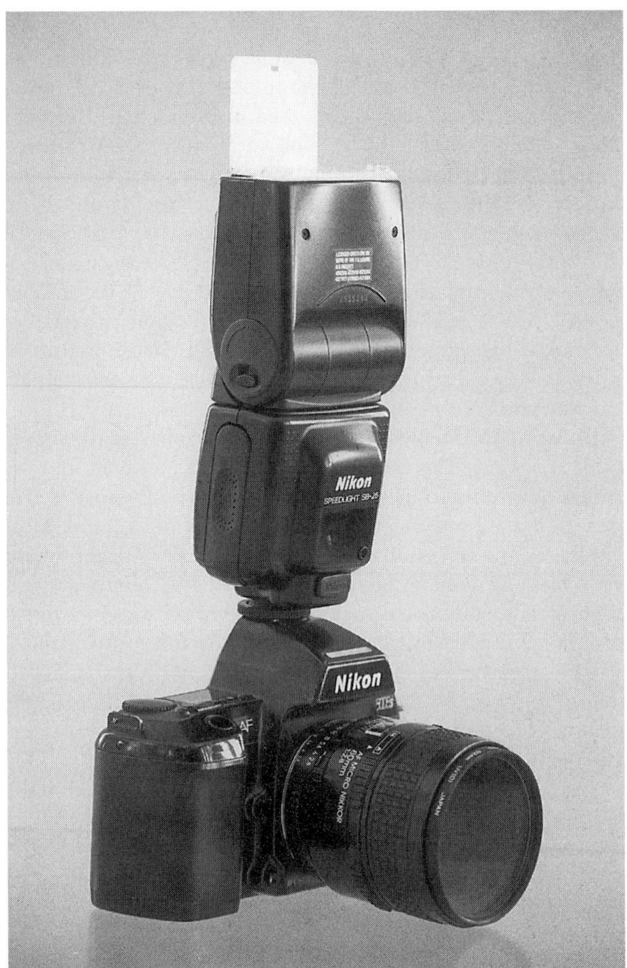

Fig. 18-5 A 35-mm SLR camera with flash attachment and white reflector card pointing upward in order to bounce the light off the ceiling.

prevent shadows. Use of a faster film speed will also help to accommodate for some lighting problems.

When taking full-length and intermediate photographs of patients in the clinical setting, the availability of equipment may be at a minimum. To increase control of the light from the flash and in order to eliminate harsh shadows behind the patient, place the patient in a corner. The light will bounce off the two opposing walls and illuminate the sides of the patient's face as well as eliminate the dark shadows behind the head that are created when shooting directly into the patient's face.

"Red eye" can be prevented by increasing the distance between the flash and the camera lens. This is one of the applications for an off-camera flash unit, synchronized to the opening of the camera's shutter with an extension cord.

Shutter Speed

The shutter of a camera is the mechanism that opens, closes, and determines the amount of time that light is allowed to reach the film. Setting the camera on "B" for *bulb* will allow the photographer to take a timed exposure. This means that the shutter is left open for any period of time over one second. Today, some cameras have an equivalent "T" for *time* setting.

Aperture

The beam of light that enters the camera and reflects on the film is controlled by an adjustable opening in the lens called the aperture. The aperture is known by many other names such as lens opening, iris, diaphragm, *f*-number, or *f*-stop. The aperture is an iris-like diaphragm, similar to the pupil of the human eye, which provides a variable-sized hole that regulates the amount of light passing through the lens. A lens is identified according to the *f*-number that corresponds to its widest lens opening. The widest lens opening has the optimal light-admitting capacity. The *f*-stop is controlled manually by a movable ring surrounding the lens (Figs. 18-6 through 18-8).

Depth of Field

Depth of field refers to an area both in front of and behind the subject that is in acceptably sharp focus, usually 7 through 13 feet. The depth of field can be increased by decreasing the size of the lens aperture. By closing the aperture, a longer shutter speed will be required to produce the same amount of light needed to reflect on the film.

Three principles of depth of field should be used as a reference:

1. The depth of field doubles if the *f*-stop is doubled (i.e., from *f*/8 to *f*/16).
2. Doubling the subject distance will increase the depth of field fourfold. Triple the distance, and depth of field will increase ninefold. Decreasing the camera to subject distance will decrease depth of field.
3. Reducing the focal length by one half will increase the depth of field fourfold (Fyffe).

One of the greatest challenges requiring depth of field knowledge is a situation in which the community health nurse must photodocument vast quantities of both prescription and OTC medications in the home of a client who has just expired. It is imperative to focus clearly on the patient's name, the names of the medications, and the names on the pharmacy labels. Stopping down to *f*-22 is not unusual, remembering that the shutter speed

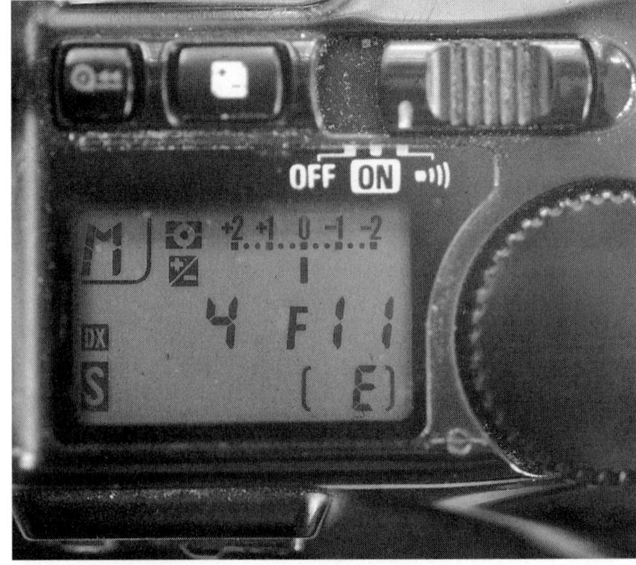

Fig. 18-6 LCD panel on a 35-mm SLR Nikon N8008s indicating shutter speed and aperture (f/11). The number "4" indicates ¼-second shutter speed.

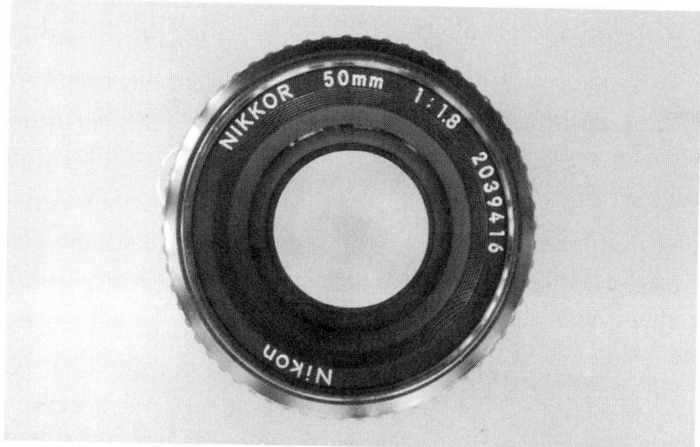

Fig. 18-7 Aperture of a Nikon 50-mm lens, wide open at f/1.8.

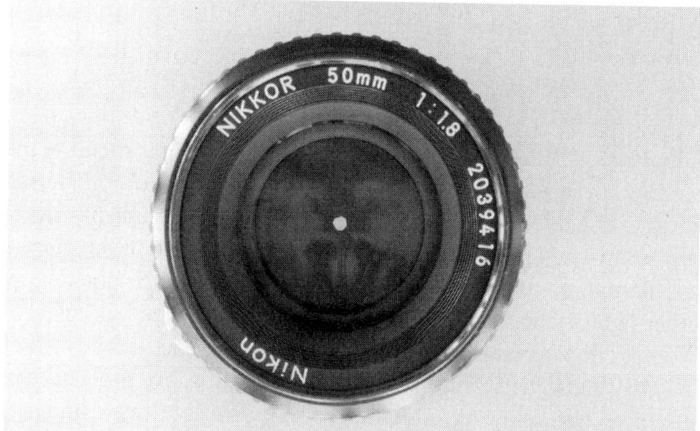

Fig. 18-8 Aperture f/22, stopped down all the way.

must also be readjusted to a slower speed to accommodate the diminished light coming through the lens. It might be necessary to use a tripod in order to ensure stability for those longer shutter speeds. A shutter speed of 1/15 second is also not unusual in these instances. Remember, too, that flash attachments might not be synchronized for the slower shutter speeds and, therefore, may not be an option in this particular case if close-up identification is to be made of the bottles (Figs. 18-9 and 18-10).

Filters

The lens on a camera is placed in some potentially hazardous positions. It may collide with objects or even get dropped on the floor. The most economical way of protecting the lens is by purchasing an ultraviolet (UV) filter (also known as a skylight, or haze filter). The UV filter is fitted over the lens and absorbs only ultraviolet rays; it does not affect the photographs and should be kept on at all times.

The second lens necessity is a circular polarizing filter. Polarizing filters reduce glare and haze and remove distracting reflections from nonmetallic glossy surfaces including water, glass, plastic, leather, and wood. The filter attaches directly to the front of any interchangeable lens. This type of polarizer consists of two rings, one that threads onto the lens, and another that spins to control the degree of polarized effect. Using the viewfinder, rotate the filter until the reflection or glare on the subject disappears. Be careful to rotate only the distal end of the filter to avoid accidental detachment.

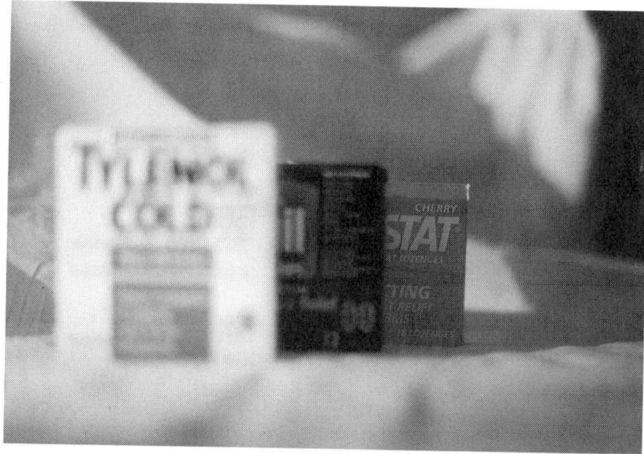

Fig. 18-9 Depth of field for OTC medication packages using a shutter speed of 1/125 with an f-stop of 4.

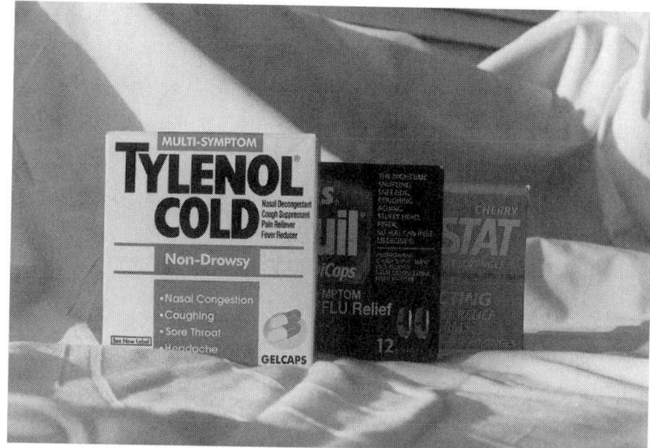

Fig. 18-10 Depth of field increases considerably with a shutter speed of 1/15 and an f-stop of 16.

Proper use of the polarizing filter includes knowing when to use it. If standing at an angle to a body of water or a store window, the reflections can be removed enough to be able to see beyond and under the surface of the water or through the window. Photographing the vehicle identification number (VIN) of an automobile requires shooting through the windshield. However, the sun may be reflecting on the window or one's own reflection may appear in the glass. Using the polarizer will eliminate the unwanted glare as well as reflections in the photograph.

Colpophotography

Colposcopy is another technique used in investigation and photodocumentation. The colposcope is an instrument consisting of a light source, variable magnification binoculars, and a camera. It was developed initially for visualization of the adult cervix, but has become invaluable in the detailed examination of both adult and child genitalia in incidences of sexual abuse (see Chapter 17). An accurate photographic record of the examination will provide invaluable evidence and may eliminate the necessity for a victim to be reexamined because a second opinion is needed.

One of the first forensic applications of the colposcope was documented in 1981 by a Brazilian physician, Dr. Wilmes Teixeira,

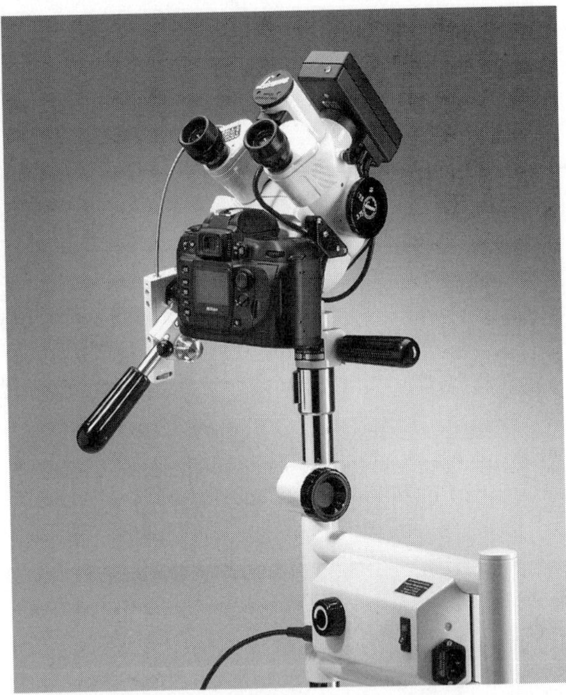

Fig. 18-11 Colposcope with Nikon 35-mm camera attachment. (Courtesy of CooperSurgical/Leisegang.)

who utilized it as part of the examination of adult sexual assault victims. Five years later, in 1986, Woodling and Heger reported their findings on colposcopy use during examinations of pediatric sexual abuse patients. Although colpophotography is traditionally a gynecological and sexual assault technique, there are other alternative uses. It most certainly can be and should be used in the photodocumentation of bite marks anywhere on the body, or any other microscopic or questioned injury (Fig. 18-11).

The colposcope provides illumination and magnification for the examination of the lower anogenital area of both adults and children. It is a stereoscopic or binocular device with variable features, which include magnification from 5× through 30×; up to a 150-watt halogen ring-light source for bright illumination; a 300-mm objective lens; and 35-mm photographic capabilities. The objective lens is surrounded by the ring-light flash. The magnification systems have multiple settings or may have zoom capability. The 35-mm camera is an SLR, usually with a data bank, which automatically imprints the time, date, and an identification number directly on the photograph. The camera may remain mounted on the scope even when photodocumentation is not desired.

In colposcopic photography, the light meter should show the photograph as being somewhat underexposed. This underexposure is necessary to compensate for ambient light and to ensure the highest quality photographs possible. With practice, the examiner can perfect the techniques needed for optimal photographs. The following guidelines may be helpful:

- The colposcope has a limited depth of field. The colposcope should be no more than 10 to 12 inches from the subject. Most 35-mm pictures should be taken at 6× and 10× for the best depth of field and field of view.
- What is seen in the monitor and through the scope is not what the 35-mm camera sees. Before snapping the picture, look through the viewfinder to ensure the subject is in focus and the field of view is correct. Don't forget to look through the camera with the dominant eye. The dominant eye is the one in which the best focus and clarity are seen.
- The higher the magnification, the more light is needed.
- Bracket each picture to allow for over- and underexposure.
- Be certain to document the magnification level for each picture.
- Not all film is equal! The brand of the film may affect the quality and color balance of the photograph.
- Photographs should contain an 18% gray scale with color guide in at least one picture per roll of film (Price, 1999).

Color scales and 18% gray rulers are available to both healthcare professionals and law enforcement officials through evidence collection and equipment supply companies. An 18% gray card reflects approximately 18% of the light to which it is exposed. Use of the gray card and color scale helps determine a comparison of true color and also the tones of gray between black and white in the photographs being entered as evidence.

Ultraviolet Light Photography

Ultraviolet (UV) light photography can significantly increase the amount of evidence obtained in child abuse, homicide, sexual assault, and bite mark cases. There are two types of UV photography techniques: fluorescent and reflective. Fluorescent photography will illuminate the phosphates found in semen. By eliminating all other light sources and shining an ultraviolet lamp, black light, or Wood's lamp on the surface in question, the presence of body fluids may be determined. This technique is an investigative tool and presumptive test, allowing establishment of probable cause and not proof of the presence of specific evidence. Laundry detergents also contain phosphates and produce a fluorescence on clothing and linens. It requires a certain degree of skill to make the determination as to what is evidence and what is not. An even distribution of fluorescence is more than likely detergent, while small stains or droplets could indicate the presence of semen or other protein matter.

Reflective UV photodocumentation will produce an image that is otherwise not seen nor photographed by conventional techniques. Reflective UV photography records the reflection and absorption of long-wave UV light by the subject matter, excluding exposure of the film by all other visible light (Krauss, 1985). Human skin contains melanin, a substance that absorbs UV radiation. This absorption process protects skin from sunburn. Trauma to the skin and underlying tissues causes a release and spread of melanin throughout the injury area. During the healing process, melanocytes congregate around the edges of the wound, creating an outline of the tissue injury pattern. UV photography is possible because, with the increase of melanin around the injury site, absorption of long-wave UV is greater there than in the surrounding area. Injuries have been photodocumented with reflective UV as long as 5 months post trauma.

Reflective UV photography can be accomplished using high-speed black and white film. Most applications will require hand-held camera situations. Because of the dimness of the light source in combination with the smaller apertures, the high-speed films will allow faster shutter speeds. Optimal results are obtained when using a red filter on the camera, which requires a filter frame holder and an adapter ring to secure the filter on the camera lens. The primary light source must be UV lighting. Move the UV light source around the site until the best visualization of the injury is achieved. This UV illumination should permit visualization of the injury with the naked eye. Photographs are taken perpendicular, at a 90-degree angle to the subject. In other words, the *film plane* must be parallel to the injury site. The patient should remain absolutely still. Stop down to increase the depth of field. The entire injury encompasses areas of tissue below the skin surface. If only the skin surface is focused, the lower levels of injury could be blurry. Use of an ABFO No. 2 scale for two-dimensional measurement of the injury will enhance the evidentiary value of the photographs.

Digital Photography

Digital photography electronically captures an image through the use of a filmless camera. Other than the absence of film, the physical features of the digital camera are relatively similar to the SLR 35-mm camera. It still utilizes lenses, aperture, and a shutter at varying speeds, depending on the availability of light. Instead of film, the camera records an image on a CCD, or *charge coupled device.* The CCD chip has a light-sensitive surface. The light-sensitive surface can be equated to the ASA or ISO of film. The sensitivity of the chip can be increased just as the sensitivity of film can be increased.

The image, once it is recorded, is then stored inside the camera on a computer disk or storage device. It can then be transferred, or downloaded, at a later time through the use of a computer and electronic technology. One of the storage devices can be the computer's hard drive. If a disk is used for storage, the disk can be removed from the camera, installed into a personal computer (PC) or laptop, and instant images are available. The images themselves can be downloaded to a color printer; they can be Emailed to other computers; or they can simply be viewed on the computer screen or a television set in a matter of minutes.

Even without benefit of a digital camera, traditional photographs and illustrations can be scanned either onto the hard drive of a computer, onto a disk, or onto a photo CD (compact disk). This electronic format can be stored in the computer for future viewing or transmission. When recording an image in the digital camera, the camera stores it. It will continue to store pictures until the storage capacity is filled. Then, the storage device must be cleared by downloading the images into a computer or replaced with a blank storage device. Other ancillary equipment to support digital photography includes a photoediting program, scanner, a removable hard drive or CD recorder to store the digital images, and a photo-quality printer laser or inkjet printer. Also needed is premium picture paper that is compatible with the printer. Laser prints are preferable to inkjet, but both are acceptable. High-gloss, ultrasmooth finish paper produces the greatest detail.

Resolution of Images

The digital photograph consists of tiny squares called picture elements, or pixels. The number of pixels in a photograph can vary from hundreds to millions. The quality, or resolution, of the image depends in part on the number of pixels used to create the image. Resolution is one of the most important factors to be considered in digital photography. Resolution is the determining factor when considering an appropriate size of the completed image. As with traditional photographs, the larger they are reproduced, the grainier they become. In other words, with each enlargement, resolution decreases and the photograph loses detail. The greater the number of pixels, the greater the detail within the image.

Resolution is expressed in the numbers of horizontal versus vertical pixels. There should be at least 200 ppi (pixels per inch) in an image to sustain a minimally acceptable standard of quality. Low resolution is approximately 640 × 480 pixels, which is the resolution of many standard computer monitors and television screens (640 pixels/200 ppi equals 3.2 inches and 480 pixels/200 ppi equals 2.4 inches, or the equivalent of a wallet-sized photograph). An 8 × 10 enlargement from this low resolution would result in a poor quality, degraded image. To obtain an optimal 8 × 10 enlargement, the number of pixels would need to be at least 2000 × 1600. As technology advances, the number of pixels will increase significantly, resulting in finer resolution for the maximum amount of enlargement.

The numbers can become very confusing, but the most important thing to remember is that the higher the resolution, the higher the quality of the images. Therefore, the camera, monitor, and color printer must all have high-resolution qualities. The objective is always the perfect photograph, and the perfect photograph still requires good technique and quality equipment. The techniques used with conventional cameras remain the same in digital photography.

There are advantages to using digital photography over conventional methods. It saves both time and resources. There is no film to be processed. Chain of custody is simplified because images can be instantaneous. Images can also be transmitted instantly as long as there is an electronic signal and someone with a computer to receive it. The camera and computer combination is now the photo processing laboratory.

The *Federal Rules of Evidence* fully defines the admissibility of digital photographs. Article X, Rule 1001 (1) addresses "writings and recordings or their equivalent (such as) mechanical or electronic recording, or other form of data compilation." Rule 1001 (3) states, "if data are stored in a computer or similar device, any printout or other output readable by sight, shown to reflect the data accurately, is an 'original.' " Rule 1001 (4) states "a 'duplicate' is a counterpart produced by the same impression as the original, or from the same matrix, or by mechanical or electronic re-recording, or by other equivalent techniques which accurately reproduces the original." Rule 1003 states, "a duplicate is admissible to the same extent as an original unless (1) a genuine question is raised as to the authenticity of the original or (2) in the circumstances it would be unfair to admit the duplicate in lieu of the original." In brief, the existence of digital photographs is acknowledged; the storage of digital images in a computer is acceptable; a digital image stored in a computer is considered an original; and any digital image or duplicate may be admissible as evidence.

There have been several court cases setting precedence with regard to the acceptance of digital imaging as legal evidence. In the case of the *State of California v. Phillip Lee Jackson*, in 1995, the defense asked for a Frye hearing on the use of digital image processing on a fingerprint in a double homicide case in San Diego. A Frye hearing establishes the general acceptance of a scientific technique by the scientific community. The Frye test must be utilized to guarantee reliability of any new or novel scientific evidence and the presiding judge must determine that the basic underlying principles of the scientific evidence have been sufficiently tested and accepted by the relevant scientific community.

The court ruled the hearing to be unnecessary owing to the fact that digital processing is an accepted practice in forensic science and that the integrity of the image had been maintained (Staggs, 2001). In the case of the *State of Washington v. Eric Hayden*, also in

1995, a homicide case was taken through a Kelly-Frye hearing in which the defense specifically objected on the grounds that the digital images were manipulated. The court authorized the use of digital imaging and the defendant was found guilty. In 1998, the appellate court upheld the case on appeal (90 Wash. App. 100, 950 P.2d 1024).

The major objection to digital photography by attorneys and other criminal justice personnel is the fact that the images can be altered or "manipulated" with the assistance of any number of photoediting software computer programs. These programs enable the photographer to enhance and crop the images; change colors; straighten lines or create curves; eliminate scratches or red eye; and even add or eliminate objects or people. This manipulation makes it difficult to rely on the image as an accurate depiction of the crime scene when viewed as photographic evidence in a court of law. In the past, images were controlled in the traditional darkroom with lighting techniques, burning, dodging, and processing chemicals. Essentially, other than the lighting effects, the original subject matter remained unchanged. Today, a simple computer software program can totally change, add, eliminate, or distort an original image.

Authenticity

One of the primary issues to be considered with regard to digital photography is that of determining authenticity. Testimony must be given that the image entered as evidence accurately portrays the scene as viewed by the photographer at the time the photograph was taken. In view of the ease with which digital photographs can be altered, there must be safeguards in place to uphold the integrity of the images. First, a particularly secure audit trail from the initial image through to the copy produced in court must be established. Two computerized authentication methods are known as *encryption* and *watermarking*. Encryption is a way of mathematically breaking an image down, transmitting it, and reconstructing it at the receiving end with the appropriate authorization coding. This does not prevent manipulation, but it does help prevent interception of the transmitted images. Encryption also helps to maintain confidentiality, as well as specifying origins and destinations. Watermarking is an operation that places an arbitrary image in the background of a document or photograph in order to corroborate its legitimacy, such as the watermarks on finer stationery and paper money.

Safeguards against Tampering

One of the newest technologies being utilized to safeguard digital photography as legal evidence is called cyclic redundancy checking (CRC). Originally used as a method for tracking errors in data that had been transmitted on a communication link, it is now being used successfully to establish authenticity and ensure integrity of digital images. The CRC authentication software has three major components: digital signature firmware on the camera; authentication software for the host computer; and a public key management system to enable a trusted third party or third-party proxy to have custody of the public key, ensuring authenticity (Eastman Kodak Company, 2000).

The technology behind CRC can be likened to the information found in the genetic codes of DNA's VNTRs (variable number of tandem repeats). Digital color images contain three primary colors: red, green, and blue. There are two bits of information in each pixel. There are 256 levels of color (8 bits) contained within each of the three colors. Eight bits are required for each of the three colors to maintain a continuous "photorealistic" image. Each pixel can contain 256 values for the red component, 256 for the green, and 256 for the blue. Therefore, any one pixel can have 24 bits associated with it, or $256 \times 256 \times 256 \times 2^{24}$, or 16,777,216 possible values (Davies & Fennessy, 1999).

CRC technology applies a proprietary algorithm to the data sets that are derived from the pixels. The manufacturer of the image-capturing software usually has the proprietary algorithm, as it is protected for security reasons. The encrypted algorithm is a means of improving the integrity of the validation process. A computation should be performed the moment the photograph is taken into the software. The computation produces a unique, discreet value, a series of numbers and letters. If any discreet value in a pixel is changed, even by one digit, or fraction thereof, which causes an increase or decrease in the number of the red, green, or blue color components, the result is a completely different CRC number when the algorithm is applied (Davies & Fennessy, 1999).

Rather than arguing that an image has not been altered, it is an accepted fact during a trial that an image can be altered to make something more apparent to a juror or trier of fact. The original image, however, can be verified through the CRC numbers. Frye challenges will not arise because an image has been altered, but will be based on certain technological disputes regarding the algorithm or the source code or any other aspect of the computerized electronic media and data storage. It has not been questioned as yet, primarily because most states simply have an authentication statement in their rules of evidence.

There will also be attempts by attorneys to question the authenticity of images transmitted to a forensic professional for review. The challenge would be in the fact that the reviewer is not actually seeing the authentic image due to changes caused by transmission of the image. *"What you were looking at was not the actual photograph. Therefore, wouldn't your opinion be different because it wasn't the original?"* With CRC technology in place, the image transmitted is the image received and, therefore, the image reviewed. The New Jersey Division of Criminal Justice has been one of the first organizations to accept colposcopic digital imaging capability in its sexual assault cases due to the security of the images and the CRC method of validating that the image was in fact the one that was taken on a particular date and time.

On October 21, 2002, a ruling in favor of forensic digital imaging was signed into effect in Broward County, Florida, after a Frye hearing was requested in the case *State of Florida v. Victor Reyes*. Digital images had been made of photographs of latent fingerprints. The original fingerprints were unreadable and therefore found to be of "no value." The latent prints were enhanced digitally in order to be readable. After extensive evidence and expert witness testimony was presented, the ruling was made to accept the forensic digital imaging as an established discipline in the field of forensic science.

With the acceptance of digital imaging in US courts of law, standards and protocols must be established in order to govern and validate our practices, as well as build confidence in a new technology. The mission statement of the Scientific Working Group on Imaging Technologies (SWGIT), in conjunction with the Department of Justice and Federal Bureau of Investigation, is "to facilitate the integration of imaging technologies and systems within the Criminal Justice System (CJS) by providing definitions and recommendations for the capture, storage, processing, analysis, transmission, and output of images." SWGIT has written "Definitions and guidelines for the use of Imaging Technologies in the Criminal Justice System" (Version 2.1–June 8, 1999) and is one of the best sources to reference for standardized policies and procedures acceptable in courts of law. Although there is a certain sentimentality regarding 35-mm film and the ways in which we have traditionally captured our past, inevitably digital imaging will dominate our future.

Consent

There is little reason why photography should not be included in the general consent signed by a patient or victim when he or she registers at the hospital or ED. After all, the patient consents to treatments, tests, medications, transfusions, x-rays, release of information, and reimbursement. It is reasonably prudent to allow photographic recording of injuries and findings that are likely to help in the evaluation, treatment, and the prosecution of those responsible. As with any medical, surgical, or invasive procedure, the patient must give permission to photograph his/her injuries. The nurse is acting as patient advocate, but it is the patient's body being photographed. After death, a consent is not required to take forensic photographs. Medical examiners and police departments make the decisions and follow their own protocols for accepted procedures with photography. In life, the victim does have control over these procedures, and individuals must give consent for photographs to be taken. If the victim is unconscious, however, and the injuries are linked to a potentially litigious situation, it is advisable to photograph them because one could reasonably assume that the patient would have given consent for this documentation of the trauma.

Most trauma centers and emergency departments have treatment consent forms that also contain statements such as "patient consents for treatment and documentation of injuries with photography." Consent forms can also be presented to the patient or client when it has been determined that there are forensic issues involved. If the permission is already blanketed in the facility, allow the patient the option of refusing photography. Some patients may be uncomfortable with the concept. Stress that this is part of the advocacy program and can benefit the patient if the case goes to litigation. However, some facilities' permission for treatment forms include a request for permission for photography and use for educational material. This can be most beneficial to the patient if he or she later wishes to file charges or prove extent of injury for insurance or survivor's benefits, and to professional educators who are responsible for providing illustrations that reflect exact duplication of injuries and evidence.

A well-thought-out and printed policy and procedure must precede the situation. Get the legal department of the facility involved and discuss the various issues with the hospital attorneys. Sit down with department managers and local police departments and establish protocols, policies, and procedures regarding photography. Discuss various consent forms. A simple form merely states the patient's name, giving permission to either the institution or the clinician to photograph the injuries listed. Note any objections the patient might have. For example, the patient may only agree to the photographs being used for litigation and not for educational purposes. It is then signed by the patient and the clinician, dated, stamped with the patient's plate and identification number, and included in the medical record. Give attention to the "exigent circumstances" that may occur throughout the clinical areas. These are the critical situations when the nurse must have the institution's legal support.

If a *consent to photograph* is not included in the *consent for treatment*, Figure 18-12 provides an example of some consent statements for consideration by the legal department of an institution.

Guidelines for Photodocumentation in the Clinical Setting

Before initiating any photodocumentation process in the clinical setting, establish a written photography protocol. Work closely with the nurse manager, medical director, and staff as well as the chief nursing executive, the risk manager, and hospital attorney. It is desirable to have at least one or two nurses on each shift who have been trained in forensic photography and evidentiary documentation.

Simple injuries, such as facial wounds, singular animal or human bites, or injuries not due to multiple trauma, domestic violence (DV), or sexual assault, require only an identifying photograph of the face and of the injury. Multiple trauma, DV, and sexual assault cases require a series of photographs depicting both presence and absence of injuries.

A full-body photograph of the patient must be taken, with the face included. Take a full-body photo of the back of the patient to show both presence and absence of injuries. Have the patient turn the face toward the camera for identification purposes. To preserve the patient's modesty, supply a blanket or sheet to use as a robe or cover. Gently maneuver the cover to reveal the injuries that must be photodocumented. The cover will provide the patient with a sense of control over the situation.

Take mid-distance images of each injury, also including the face for identification purposes. Include the patient's face in at least one of these photos to establish that the documented injuries were, in fact, found on this patient. Mid-distance photographs provide more detail and relativity than full-body photographs.

Take close-up images of each injury, one with a standard (ruler) to show injury size and another without to show the standard did not obscure information. Standards get their name from objects that are of a standard size or shape. It is something universal that is recognized by everyone for what it is. Standards are usually rulers, called scales, but can also be a familiar object or coin, such as a quarter. Always place the standard on the same surface level with the injury so that the focus will be sharp and perspective will not be altered. Photograph dimensional injuries by using an ABFO No. 2 reference scale. This scale will also serve as a reminder to photograph all injuries parallel to the film plane (i.e., camera at a 90-degree angle to the injury surface). When the injury is parallel to the film, the circles on the scale will appear circular, not elliptical (Fig. 18-13).

Best Practice *18-2*

All forensic photographs should have affixed labels that contain the subject's name and/or hospital number, the date, the time, and the name of the photographer. Never write directly on the photograph or use paper clips or staples to attach it to other documents.

Label all photographs separately. Never write directly on the back of a photograph, as this can create an indentation on the front, altering the image in the photo. Write all information on a self-adhesive label–patient's name or hospital number, the date, time, and the name of the photographer. Adhere the label to the back of the photograph. Photographs are a part of the patient record and should be kept in the patient's file at all times. Do not keep photos separate from regular patient records. Photographs can be adhered to special sheets with either self-adhesive strips or

Consent to Photograph

I authorize ____________________ Hospital and the staff of the Emergency Department to photograph or permit other persons employed by this facility to photograph ____ (name of patient) while under the care of this facility. I have been informed and understand that:

Photographs taken for medical purposes will become part of my medical record and will be subject to subpoena with my record.

Photographs in my medical record may be released if they are requested by a person authorized to obtain my medical record. If I do not want photographs released with my medical record, I must specifically exclude them in any authorizations that I sign.

I do not authorize any other use to be made of these photographs.

______________________________ ____________________

Patient's signature (Parent or guardian if under 18) | Date

______________________________ ____________________

Street Address | Witness

____

City | State | Zip Code

Deposition of Photographs: To be completed by Facility Staff

__________ Photographs were placed in a sealed envelope marked with the patient's name and medical record number and sent to Medical Records

Fig. 18-12 Consent to photograph form

slits that have been precut to accommodate a specific size (e.g., 4 × 6 or Polaroid instant). Photographs are to be kept as confidential as the written patient record.

If the patient requests a set of photos and a Polaroid camera was used, a set may be provided after obtaining the photodocumentation needed. Use the close-up copy stand provided in the camera kit to duplicate the photos requested by the patient. Be sure to advise the patient that if she or he is a domestic violence victim, the photos may place the patient in danger if found by the batterer. If the patient was provided with a set of photographs, note this on

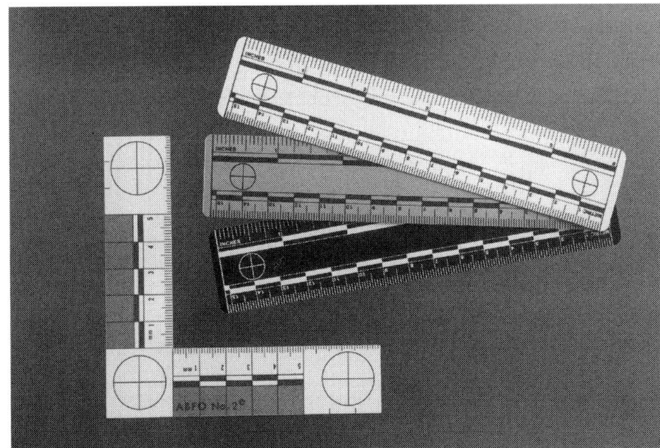

Fig. 18-13 Standards and the ABFO No. 2 scale. (Courtesy of Armor Forensics Co.)

the patient's chart. Include the quantity and date the images were provided.

Generally, if patient's photographs are subpoenaed, the medical records department need only provide a copy of the images. The original photographs will require a separate, more specific court order. Check the state laws for further information.

The photographs taken by the forensic nurse or other staff members should not be released to the police, but retained with the patient's record to maintain chain of custody. The local police departments are equipped with their own camera systems and photographs taken by their personnel will include not only physical appearance, but also pieces of hard evidence. They will be photographing weapons, such as knives and guns, and bullets and other projectiles removed from the patient by the emergency department physician. It is perfectly acceptable to be asked by the police to take the photographs for them with their own equipment. It is often easier for the nurse to accomplish this task due to the rapport that has been established between care provider and patient.

Foreign material removed by surgeons in the operating room (OR) should be photographed by forensic nurses in the OR. These photographs also belong to the permanent patient record. The projectiles will be turned over to the police as evidence, but if not photographed, their existence can be disputed if lost along the way.

When forensic nurse examiners are outside the clinical area in a patient's home or at a crime scene, the geographical location must be established with the initial photographs, called *orientation shots*. In order to establish the actual location of the scene, it may be necessary to begin photographing from the street sign inward. Moving from the outside in, photographing from the general to the specific, and indicating the relationship of one object to another are mandatory for reconstruction of the crime scene. After the scene is released by the police, there is no way to preserve the scene as it was when it was secured.

Photograph "north, east, south, west." In other words, photograph the entire scene in a clockwise manner in order to create 360-degree coverage. Just as the photographer takes full-length, intermediate, and close-up views of the patients, other crime scenes are photographed in the same way. Long views establish geography, location, entrances, exits, and escape routes. Intermediate views establish relationships between people and objects. Close-up views show fine detail, dimensions, and measurements. When taking close-up views of any subject matter, always take one photograph with and one without the standard. Keep the standard on the same plane with the subject. Compose photographs carefully. Be aware of anyone or anything standing in the viewfinder that will distract from the final product. Upon completion of the photodocumentation, rewind the film and process it as quickly as possible. Do not mix more than one crime scene on the same roll. A photographic log should be maintained with each roll of film and for each exposure made (Fig. 18-14).

Remember that photographers tell a story without words through photodocumentation. The full-body and orientation photographs are the introduction. The intermediate and relativity photographs contain the core. The close-up views can be considered the conclusion, the punch line, or the *coup de grâce*. Combined, the entire set of photographs describes a historical event that cannot be portrayed simply with the written word.

Establish a business relationship with a professional photography lab. Inform the key personnel of the lab that they will be processing crime scene photographs and that the strictest chain of custody and confidentiality must be maintained. Consider the use of a chain of custody form with the lab if there is ever a question about the possession of the film or the length of time the film is out of one's possession. Delegate drop-off and retrieval of the film and photographs to as few individuals as possible. When the photographs are processed, insert them into the patient's record or institutional report immediately. It is important to understand the exact procedure for storage of photographs within the medical records department.

When photodocumenting with 35-mm film in a hospital setting, it is imperative that all the intricacies of transport concerning the film are considered in the writing of the policy and procedure. Chain of custody will be scrutinized and the timing of an event may not be convenient for expeditious film processing. If an event occurs at change of shift at midnight, determine where the film will be secured until it can be processed, who the courier will be, and who will retrieve both the processed photographs, negatives, and then the medical record for insertion of the photographs (Fig. 18-15).

Key Point *18-2*

A forensic photograph is demonstrative evidence and is a legal document considered part of the medical record. Photographs are generally admissible if they demonstrate content and information of value to legal proceedings. Photographs will not be admissible if they convey unfair prejudice, confuse issues, or might be misleading to the jury.

Photographs as Legal Documents

In today's litigious society, the more evidence that exists to support the truth, the greater the advantage for healthcare workers who advocate for their patients. Although there are certain concerns about photodocumentation within hospitals, documentation of injuries of abuse, traumatic wounds, and other situations may serve to protect the hospital and its staff members by ensuring precise documentation. There is no simple way to document accurately with written words alone the distribution of 53 stab wounds on a victim's body. The same is true for documenting the existence of bridging in a laceration, blood spatter or body fluid drainage patterns, stippling, or

PHOTO LOG

Photographer	Event or Case
Camera (Make & Model)	Location
Film (Type & ISO)	Date/Time
Other	

Exp	Subject	Lighting	Lens	Notes
1				
2				
3				
4				
5				
6				
7				
8				
9				
10				
11				
12				
13				
14				
15				
16				
17				
18				
19				
20				
21				
22				
23				
24				
25				
26				
27				
28				
29				
30				
31				
32				
33				
34				
35				
36				
37				

Fig. 18-14 Photo log.

Chain of CUSTODY

Received from:

By:

Date: Time: AM/PM

Received from:

By:

Date: Time: AM/PM

Received from:

By:

Date: Time: AM/PM

Received from:

By:

Date: Time: AM/PM

Received from:

By:

Date: Time: AM/PM

Received from:

By:

Date: Time: AM/PM

Received from:

By:

Date: Time: AM/PM

Received from:

By:

Date: Time: AM/PM

Fig. 18-15 Chain of custody form.

an abrasion ring around a gunshot wound. The completion of the forensic examination of a sexual assault victim includes not only the collection of forensic evidence but also photographs of the evidence, as well as both external and internal trauma.

A forensic photograph is a legal document and must be considered part of the record. In many instances, it completes the record, and, at the very least, it supplements it. Mechanism of injury can often be demonstrated with one photograph. The truth or falsehood of a statement may be proved with a photograph. Photography can capture the tiniest detail that the eye does not see until the photograph is developed. The photograph captures valuable information that may link a victim to the perpetrator, or the perpetrator to the crime scene. Photographs also refresh the memories of victims, law enforcement officials, and witnesses as to the events, conditions, and facts of a matter as they actually existed when the photograph was taken.

Under the *Federal Rules of Evidence*, a photograph is generally admissible if it demonstrates content and information of value to legal proceedings. Photographs will not be admissible "if their probative value is substantially outweighed by the danger of unfair prejudice, confusion of the issues, or misleading the jury, or by considerations of undue delay, waste of time, or needless presentation of cumulative evidence" (*Federal Rules of Evidence,* Rule 403). "It has become well settled that color photographs are admissible, provided (1) what they depict is relevant to the issues in the case; (2) they have been shown to be true and accurate representations; and (3) their probative value is not outweighed by gruesomeness or inflammatory character" (Moenssens, Starrs, & Henderson et al., 1995, p. 148).

Photographs are demonstrative evidence. Demonstrative evidence illustrates, demonstrates, or helps explain oral testimony. The *Federal Rules of Evidence*, Rule 1001, states "a 'duplicate' is a counterpart produced by the same impression as the original, or from the same matrix, or by means of photography, including enlargements and miniatures. . .which accurately reproduces the original." Also, the "best evidence rule" can be interpreted as "the best evidence that the nature of the thing will afford." Therefore, because large objects, situations, conditions, or history cannot be brought into the courtroom, the photograph is the next best evidence utilized to demonstrate the original.

Photographs are not likely to be admitted as evidence if there is no reference to them in the medical record. Nor are they likely to be admitted if there is no reference to the injuries in the medical record that the photographs themselves document. The photographs and medical record supplement and corroborate each other.

If photographs are admitted as evidence, the photographer may be called upon to testify to the circumstances under which the photographs were taken. Discuss this situation with the attorney handling the case. When called as a fact witness, remember that photography is a tool that amplifies nursing documentation. The court will not consider you to be an expert witness in photography. Testimony will include verification that the photograph is a fair and accurate depiction of the scene as it appeared at the time it was taken.

Beyond the Medical Setting

In addition to assault and trauma cases, photography must be considered for those settings outside the hospital. All nurses must be aware of the opportunities that present themselves in alternative settings and be prepared to photodocument factual information. Industrial injuries, injuries resulting from faulty appliances, the homeowner whose furnace explodes in his face, the facial injuries resulting from motor vehicle crashes, and bruises on the child who makes frequent visits to the school nurse will require adjudication and should be photographed to complete the record.

There are many categories of forensic patients. Any medical incident that the nurse or physician feels will eventually end up in an attorney's office or a court of law is a forensic case and necessitates the gathering of as much evidence as possible. What better way to provide the truth? In addition to those cases already mentioned, there are multiple categories of forensic patients who require photography as part of their documentation and history-taking process: assault and battery; abuse of children, elders, and the disabled; sexual assault; transportation injuries; suicide attempts, which include ligature and hesitation marks; resultant injuries from medical malpractice; product liability including injuries sustained from unsafe products, toys, and tools; physiological abuse from transcultural medical practices, cults, and religious groups; human and animal bites; and any other suspicious, unrecognized, and unidentified trauma. These photos should be taken and retained as part of the medical record.

All healthcare providers in all clinical settings must be alerted that it is to their benefit to use photography as a documentary tool. Forensic nurses are aware of the injuries and trauma inflicted upon the victims of violence. They are becoming astute in recognizing that photodocumentation is one of the prime tools in the pursuit of justice. One does not need to be a professional photographer to photograph injuries. The equipment does not have to be expensive or sophisticated. Cases have been won on the basis of poor quality photographs. If a nurse or physician captures the handprint around a little girl's neck or the bruises on a woman's back, blurry but unmistakably there, the case can be won. Essential equipment is listed in Box 18-1.

Summary

Photography is an essential skill for the forensic nurse examiner. Photodocumentation illustrates and supplements written records

Box 18-1 Essential Equipment for the Clinical Setting or Crime Scene

- 35-mm SLR camera and/or a Polaroid Spectra and/or a Polaroid Macro 5 and/or digital camera equipment
- Appropriate film, adequate exposures, extra memory cards for digital cameras
- Thyristor flash unit (as well as a second slave unit if appropriate for the department)
- Ring flash
- Synchronization cord at least three feet long (to allow it to be held at arm's length)
- 50-mm lens and/or a telephoto zoom lens
- Various filters (polarizer, UV light)
- Scales, standards, ABFO No. 2 scale
- Tripod
- Cable release
- Various appropriate-sized extra batteries for all camera equipment
- Various boxes of film appropriate for camera equipment (12-, 24-, and 36-exposure rolls for 35 mm)
- Securable carrying case or transportable cart for all photographic equipment
- Large flash umbrella (Caution: This does not double for a large rain umbrella, though, if working in precipitation.)
- Slotted pages and/or manila envelopes for 35-mm negatives and prints and Polaroid photographs. (Have necessary forms within easy access, including consent to photograph, chain of custody, photography log.)

and preserves images or injuries and other evidence that can change over time. Photographs also act as an aid to memory, preserving important details of a situation that might have otherwise been overlooked or forgotten. Photos are of great value in the courtroom because they permit the jurors to view injuries and crime scenes, helping them to determine if testimony being presented makes sense in context of the documented details. In order to support intelligent, dispassionate legal deliberations, photographs for the courtroom must accurately depict a scenario without being unduly gruesome or inflammatory (Box 18-2).

The FNE does not need to be a professional photographer. However, the nurse must possess basic knowledge and skills of forensic photography to ensure that the resultant images are high quality and can withstand the legal scrutiny for courtroom admissibility. The nurse must be prepared to answer technical questions regarding photodocumentation procedures, maintenance of chain of custody, and authenticity of the images used.

Case Study 18-1 Ted Bundy

During the 1970s, some of the most heinous cases of human violence occurred involving the infamous serial killer Ted Bundy. In one particular scenario during his final rape and murder spree in Tallahassee, Florida, forensic photography provided the most crucial evidence for the prosecution. Because of the number and breadth of atrocities committed by this sexual predator, as well as his ability to escape from high-security detention facilities, the recovery of forensic evidence was essential. Apprehension and identification of Bundy became the priority of all law enforcement agents in Florida and across the US. There was no doubt that he would kill again.

On January 15, 1978, Bundy struck again, attacking and killing Lisa Levy and Martha Bowman in the same room in their sorority house at Tallahassee's Florida State University. Police stated they had never seen such a brutal attack. Lisa Levy was raped, strangled, and beaten. Margaret Bowman was strangled with a pair of pantyhose and severely beaten. Two other girls in the sorority house had been attacked and less than an hour and a half later; the man assaulted a fifth victim, who survived. Just a few weeks after that, he abducted, raped, and killed a 12-year-old girl.

No fingerprints were found at the crime scene. The attacker had taken his weapon with him so that item of evidence was also missing from the crime scene collection. Authorities had a blood type, a few print smudges, and sperm samples, but all proved inconclusive. DNA was not yet available. However, a particular piece of evidence was to become a centerpiece during the trial: an odd bite mark on the left buttock of Lisa Levy. One officer laid a yellow ruler against the patterned abrasion and then stepped back for the photographers. His presence of mind might have made all the difference between conviction and acquittal for Bundy because the tissue specimens were lost by the time of the trial, destroyed in all the analyses. However, the application of forensic photography had memorialized the physical evidence of the bite mark that was to become the world's most famous patterned injury and the crucial evidence needed to convict Ted Bundy.

Box 18-2 Suggested Policy for Photodocumentation of Injuries

The staff person who is most competent in photographic technique should be responsible for photodocumentation. When the easiest adherence to chain of custody is an issue, it is recommended that an instant camera system be utilized for these services. Use a 35-mm SLR camera if an appropriate policy ensuring chain of custody of film and photographs is in place.

Policy

Photodocumentation of injuries is the accepted standard of care. Photodocumentation is an extremely important service that should be offered to the patient. Photographs require written informed consent and become part of the medical record.

Purpose

The purposes of photodocumentation are as follows:

1. To record and communicate that which cannot be communicated with the written word alone.
2. To serve as objective witnesses by providing photographic evidence for purposes of adjudication.
3. To protect healthcare providers against claims of inappropriate care or failure to accurately document physical appearance, condition, or injuries.

Procedure

Follow proper procedures when considering photodocumentation.

1. Determine the need for photodocumentation. Forensic categories of patients potentially requiring photographs include, but are not limited to, the following:
   - Abuse of children, elders, disabled
   - Domestic violence
   - Negligence and malpractice
   - Transcultural medical practices (e.g., cupping, coining, tribal scarring)
   - Environmental and toxic hazards
   - Forensic psychiatric situations (e.g., suicide attempts, hesitation marks, burns, self-mutilation)
   - Transportation injuries (motor vehicle, motorcycle, boating, airplane, railroad)
   - Sexual assault
   - Assault and battery
   - Personal injury
   - Occupation-related injuries
   - Questioned death
   - Product liability
   - Human and animal bites
   - Sharp force injuries (stabbing, puncture)
   - Burns over 5% body surface area
   - Firearm injuries
   - Gang violence
   - Acts of terrorism resulting in mass destruction of property or injuries of victims
   - Any other suspicious, unrecognized, or unidentified trauma
2. Informed consent must be obtained. Signature is required on the consent for photography or in the general consent for treatment, and signed by the patient, guardian, or caretaker upon arrival to the ED. In emergent cases when a signature is unobtainable, consent will be implied.
3. Steps in photodocumenting injuries
   - Take "before" and "after cleaning" photographs of all injuries. This is most important in recording blood spatter patterns, gunshot residue, and dirt.

(Continued)

Box 18-2 Suggested Policy for Photodocumentation of Injuries—Continued

- Some jurisdictions require that essential identifying data, such as the patient's name, date, and case number, be written legibly on a piece of paper and photographed on the first exposure of any given roll of film.
- Take a full-length photograph that captures both the patient's face and injuries so that it is clear that the trauma was sustained by the victim in the photograph. Also take a full-length photograph of the back of the patient with the head turned toward the camera. This objectively records both presence and absence of injuries. Respect a patient's privacy. Allow the patient to cover up with a blanket or sheet, moving it to expose only the areas and injuries that need to be photographed.
- The four principal anatomic positions that photodocumentation should consider, but not be limited to, are anterior/posterior, posterior/anterior, right lateral, and left lateral.
- If the location of the injury does not allow for such a photograph, a picture of the face should be included in the set of photographs and an identifying document (e.g., the patient's driver's license) can be included in a picture with the injury.
- Take an intermediate-view photograph, including the patient's face, and a closer view of as many injuries as possible in the same photograph. Have the patient sit in a chair or on a stretcher in a sitting position, exposing the injuries with a sheet or blanket draped over the patient to maintain modesty.
- Take a close-up photo of each of the injuries. The face is not required in these photographs. Identification has already been established with the full-length and intermediate views. Take this view both with and without a standard (ruler) in place. For other than linear injuries, in order to document dimension, photograph both length and width of the injury.

4. Label each photograph with the date and time taken, the name of the hospital, the medical record number, and the name of the photographer. Do not write on the back of the photograph. Place this information on a self-adhesive label and affix the label to the back of the photograph.
5. Photographs are to be kept in the patient's medical record in a sealed envelope with the written statement "photographs of patient's injuries" or placed in slotted pages specifically for the purpose of inclusion in the medical record. If the prints are obtained from negatives, the negatives are considered the primary evidence. They must be kept with the record along with the prints.
6. If extensive bruising is expected to appear at a later date, and the patient is anticipating litigation, the patient should be advised to return to the emergency department, police department, attorney's office, or insurance company within 72 hours to have additional photographs taken.
7. Assure chain of custody for film processing and retrieval.
8. Assure that final photographs and negatives are placed in the medical record.

Resources

Books and Articles

Girardin, B., Faugno, D., Seneski, P., et al. (1997). *Color atlas of sexual assault.* St. Louis: Mosby.

Krauss, T. (1993, February). Forensic evidence documentation using reflective ultraviolet photography. *Photo Electronic Imaging,* 18-23.

Miller, L. (1993). *Sansone's police photography* (3rd ed.). Cincinnati: Anderson.

Otoupalik, S. (1999). Bringing the crash scene into the emergency department. *J Emerg Nurs, 25*(5), 388-391.

Pasqualone, G. (1996). Forensic RNs as photographers: Documentation in the ED. *J Psychosoc Nurs Ment Health Serv, 34*(10), 47-51.

Redsicker, D. (1991). *The practical methodology of forensic photography.* New York: Elsevier.

Ricci, L. R. (1994). *Draft guidelines for photographic documentation of child abuse.* Chicago: American Professional Society on the Abuse of Children.

Storrow, A. B., Stack, L. B., & Peterson, P. (1994). An approach to emergency department photography. *Acad Emerg Med, 1*(5), 454-462.

Warlen, S.C. (1995). Crime scene photography: The silent witness. *J Forensic Ident, 45*(3), 261-265.

References

Davies, A., & Fennessy, P. (1999). *Digital imaging for photographers.* Oxford, England: Focal Press.

Eastman Kodak Company. (June 7, 2000). Press release: Authentication software for Kodak DC5000 and DC280 digital cameras provides alert when images are manipulated or tampered with.

Fyffe, J. E. *Practical crime scene photography. Reference manual.* Public Agency Training Council.

Krauss, T., & Warlen, S. (1985). The forensic use of reflective ultraviolet photography. *J Forensic Sci, 30,* 262-268.

Moenssens, A., Starrs, J., Henderson, C., et al. (1995). *Scientific evidence in civil and criminal cases* (4th ed.). New York: The Foundation Press.

Price, B. (1999). Forensic colposcopy: Getting the most from your equipment. Colposcopy photograph hints. Proceedings of the International Association of Forensic Nurses, Seventh Annual Scientific Assembly.

Sontag, S. (1977). *On photography.* New York: Anchor Doubleday.

Staggs, S. (2001). *The admissibility of digital photographs in court.* Retrieved from www.crime-scene-investigator.net/admissibilityofdigital.html.

State of Washington v. Eric H. Hayden. 90 Wash. App. 100, 950 P.2d 1024.

Teixeira, W. R. (1981). Hymenal colposcopic examination in sexual offenses. *Am J Forensic Med Pathol, 2,* 209-214.

Woodling, B. A., & Heger, A. (1986). The use of the colposcope in the diagnosis of sexual abuse in the pediatric age-group. *Child Abuse Neglect, 10,* 111-114.

Unit Four

Mechanisms of Injury

Chapter 19 Blunt and Sharp Injuries

Patrick E. Besant-Matthews

The forensic nurse examiner must thoroughly understand the multiple characteristics of blunt and sharp force injuries or wounds and be able to predict the types of mechanical forces that might have caused them. This includes, in some cases, a specific weapon or wounding instrument. To make accurate annotations in the medical records, or to convey pertinent information to members of law enforcement or the judicial system, it is essential that precise, nonambiguous descriptive terms are used in both oral and written communications. In addition, for known or potential forensic cases, photo-documentation is a vital element to record the size, location, and nature of blunt or sharp force injuries. The ability to relate this information to accident or crime scene reconstruction can assist in the identification of the wounding instrument and eventually the perpetrator.

This chapter introduces wound identification, classification, and documentation by focusing on the details that will contribute to appropriate medical care and later to a credible forensic investigation.

Wound Terminology

In the English language, many words have multiple meanings, which gives rise to the misuse of words, even common ones. A good example is the word *fire*, which has at least nine common meanings:

1. The phenomenon of combustion manifested in heat and light
2. To inspire a person
3. Liveliness of imagination
4. Brilliancy, luminosity
5. To discharge or let off
6. To discharge from a position, dismiss from employment
7. To process by applying heat
8. To fuel or tend a boiler or furnace
9. To eject or launch a projectile

Almost any large, unabridged dictionary will list several other less common meanings.

In the healthcare and law enforcement fields, doctors, nurses, paramedics, emergency medical technicians, and police officers devote considerable time during training to mastering necessary technical phrases. Failure to continue this education into description of injury often results in reduced quality of documentation, even though reports may be lengthy. The surgeon's report after an operation may contain numerous statements about an injury and what was done to it, yet this report often fails to specify where on the body surface the wound was located or to include other characteristics such as its size and appearance, which may be of great importance when a lawsuit is filed.

Anyone working in the medical or law enforcement fields may be called on to interpret injury patterns; to write reports concerning the condition of someone, dead or alive; and sometimes to testify concerning the appearance of an injured party. Proper use of descriptive terms greatly enhances one's ability to write effective reports and to provide meaningful information in depositions or testimony. This also applies to day-to-day progress notes. Skill and effort will be wasted if descriptions are not absolutely clear and meaningful.

Documenting Wound Characteristics

A common failing of treatment and surgical reports is that they do not mention the specific place, depth, and direction of force related to the identified injuries. After a critical surgery, the location of wounds should be included in the dictated report. For example, in the case of a single stab wound, failure to note that it entered the abdomen at a point located about 3 inches diagonally above and to the patient's right of the umbilicus, penetrated for a maximum depth of about 3 inches, and was directed from front to back and slightly downward, is a significant omission. What was injured and repaired will almost always be mentioned, but without a location this information will not be much use. Courtroom questions will inevitably be centered on the location, depth, and direction, because it is these features that will fit or discredit the allegations and circumstances.

Body Diagrams

Outline diagrams of the human body and body parts can be very useful Simply draw the findings on these outlines and add notations. It is fast, accurate, helps to prevent right/left errors, and makes it easier to document angles and patterns. Body diagrams are excellent supplements to other documentation. (See Appendix C for body diagram samples.)

Clock Face Orientation

The clock face is sometimes used to document the angulation or inclination of a feature or wound. For instance, if a person is standing at attention (in the standard anatomical position) and has a streak of dirty material running from the inner part of the left eyebrow to the lower right corner of the mouth, then this might be described as being oriented from 1 to 7 o'clock when viewed from the front. If the standard anatomical position is not used, additional documentation is needed, such as "when viewed from the right, with the patient lying face up, the wound is angled from 10 to 4 o'clock."

Track and Tract

A *track* (spelled with a "k") is detectable evidence that something has passed, a vestige or trace, or the course along which something has moved. Note that the word *tracks* is also used to describe the linear scars overlying veins resulting from repeated intravenous injections associated with drug abuse.

A *tract* (spelled with a "t") is a series of bodily parts that collectively serve a combined anatomical purpose. There are more than 50 tracts within the body.

So unless someone swallows or inhales a bullet, it will pass down a track, not a tract. Failure to distinguish between track and tract is a reliable indicator of the amount and quality of training received, as well as the care, or lack of it, in producing reports.

Instrument and Weapon

An *instrument* is something with, or through which, something is done or effected (i.e., a tool, implement, or utensil). Namely, it is an object with a primary function other than use as an offensive or defensive weapon. A *weapon* is an instrument of offensive or defensive combat; something to fight with; an object of any kind used in combat to attack or overcome others. A weapon is essentially an object whose primary function is as an offensive or defensive device. An object such as a kitchen knife, while manufactured as an instrument, can be used as a weapon. Proper use of the terms will depend on the circumstances and fashion of use (e.g., to cut bread or to cause injury).

Following are many of the terms used to describe injuries. It is suggested that anyone who treats patients, evaluates injuries, or works in the fields of law or law enforcement be exposed to and be aware of these terms, not only for personal benefit but also to protect the interests of the institutions and individuals they serve.

Key Point *19-1*

Forensic nurse examiners may be requested to testify or to give a deposition; therefore it is important to use appropriate and precise terms when describing injuries or wounds in forensic cases. The failure of a report to be completely accurate may cast doubt on one's credibility as a witness or testifying expert.

Documentation and Legal Proceedings

An injury that is of little consequence medically may be extremely important to family members, investigators, insurance companies, attorneys, and the courts. For example, suppose there's an L-shape abrasion (graze) about 1¼-inch in greatest dimension, on the inner aspect of the left lower leg near the bony prominence of the ankle joint. The wound is reported to be the result of an automobile collision, is not life threatening, and will soon heal. Later it turns out that both occupants of the vehicle are unconscious, the brake pedal is bent, and the main issue is determining who was driving. If the leg is in a cast, and nothing was noted in the chart, the wrong person may be charged with negligent driving, manslaughter, or even vehicular homicide.

There are several routes to good documentation. Here are some points to ponder:

- Describe wounds in logical sequence, such as from head to foot, or from front to back, or from wrist to elbow. Organization is important in court
- Use landmarks that cannot easily be challenged by a skilled attorney. Good landmarks include the midline of the body, the notch at the top of the breastbone, the centerline of a limb, the base of a heel (provided the ankle is at 90 degrees), the top of the head, the external ear canals, or the Frankfort plane (the horizontal line between the bottom of the eye socket and the top of the external ear canal). The best choice depends on the case and even on the direction of force.
- When dealing with stab wounds (and bullet holes), measure from the body landmark to the center of each. This is important when there are many irregular wounds, or else the distances between them will not add up.
- If measurements are made around a body curvature, make it clear in the description. Failure to do so will cause a wound that's recorded as 12 cm to the left of the front midline of the face to sound as though it is out in space somewhere, instead of 5 cm in front of the ear canal.
- Do not locate one injury and then say that another was at a certain distance from it. Doing this will accumulate measurement errors. This rule does not apply if injuries are obviously paired (e.g., carving fork) or grouped (e.g., dinner fork).
- Do not split up or disperse parts of a single injury within the notes. If there is no choice but to examine the outside before the inside, then "Subsequent examination of . . ." will get the narrative back on track
- When describing marks that encircle or partly encircle the wrists, ankles, or neck, pick a starting point, and begin with "For descriptive purposes, the marking commences at a point . . . "; continue on, until returning to the starting point.
- Use national standard or internationally accepted abbreviations. A common error is to use cc for fluid volumes, when fluids are measured in liters not centimeters. Thus, ml is technically correct. In many important cases, consultants will read the report, note minor errors, and bring them to the attention of the defense.
- If someone misinterpreted a birthmark as a bruise, but injuries were not substantiated, it will help to make notations such as "Not found–evidence of injury to the face" or "Incidental findings–birthmark ("port wine" stain) on face."

Good forms and a notation system (using arrows and lines with clock face numbers at each end) make notes easier to read during a deposition or courtroom testimony.

Mechanics of Blunt and Sharp Injuries

From a medical perspective, the ability to distinguish between the various types of injuries is extremely important because it provides valuable information about causation and, in some cases, will determine treatment. For example, a confused young female patient is admitted to the emergency department with a linear injury to her upper forehead. If this injury was due to a sharp instrument such as a straight razor, there is little to be done except to suture the wound and then explore how it was incurred. Did it occur as an accident? Was it the result of interpersonal violence? Was it self-inflicted? Answers to these questions will be extremely important to the healthcare team and to law enforcement. Perhaps the patient had been drinking or taking drugs? However, if the linear injury was caused by being struck forcefully by the edge of a coffee table or a piece of angle iron, then the clinical problem is quite different and involves wound contamination, blunt force injury, potential for skull fracture, and neck injury, plus the need to consider brain injury with or without intracranial bleeding. Sharp force injury rarely contains trace evidence.

Proceeding appropriately requires distinguishing a sharp injury from a blunt injury. However, these are the two most frequently mistaken for one another in those areas of the body surface that have bone beneath them, including the skull.

The forensic nurse examiner must actively be involved as an investigator when providing wound care in a clinic or within the hospital emergency department. If the wound occurred as an industrial accident (on-the-job) rather than while the individual was engaged in recreation, workers' compensation and other insurance coverage may be relevant. If the victim of injury subsequently has extended complications or dies from the wound, there may be issues of liability and criminal negligence. The cause of death or permanent disability also impacts the payment of claims on disability policies or life insurance. If the wound was self-inflicted, there are important mental health implications to explore. If an assailant caused the wound, there is the need for law enforcement to find the perpetrator. Forensic responsibilities cannot be taken lightly because they may make a huge impact on law enforcement, the judicial system, and the overall economy. Taking time to carefully remove clothing, to photograph and measure the wounds, and to precisely document the patient's statements regarding how the wound was incurred will become extremely important if there are subsequent judicial proceedings.

Symmetry of abrasion, bruising, and undermining of tissue is consistent with a more perpendicular application of force. An example would be on the scalp, over the curved surfaces of the skull, if an individual were struck with the flat surface of a 2-by-6-inch piece of wood. Because lacerations result from blunt impact, shearing, or tearing, they are likely to be contaminated with foreign material such as road gravel and dirt, headlight glass and paint chips, or clothing fibers indicating the kind of surface that was contacted. For example, examination of a traffic accident victim may reveal the presence of small fragments of paint within a tear on the side of the head, indicating that the head contacted part of a vehicle; or it might contain gravel and greasy dirt, which is more in keeping with contact with the underside of a vehicle.

Improper description and interpretation of injuries may lead the police on a lengthy search for a knife or sharpened object when in fact they should be looking for a brick, angle iron, or other such angular object with a definite edge to it. Experience shows that sharp injuries (cuts and stabs) are better understood than blunt injuries (scrapes, bruises, tears, and fractures).

Pattern of Injury

A *pattern of injury* is a combination or distribution of external or internal injuries that suggest a causative mechanism or sequence of events, indicating infliction of wounds over a period of time versus those occurring simultaneously. A pattern of injury may be indicative of repetitive abuse whereas injuries occurring from a single incident are generally associated with nonintentional injury.

Pattern Injury

A *pattern injury* is one that possesses features or configuration indicative of the object(s) or surface(s) that produced it (Smock, 2001). For instance, it may bear the imprint of clothing, an object such as the radiator grill of a car, or the head of a specific type of hammer.

Penetrating and Perforating

A penetrating injury is one that enters but does not exit, whereas a perforating injury passes through-and-through. Thus, confusion may arise because a knife that entered the front of a thigh and stopped just short of the bone represents not only a penetrating injury of the thigh as a whole but also a perforating, through-and-through wound of the skin. It is necessary therefore to specify what was or is penetrated or perforated. Use *penetration* as the common term for the majority of injuries that enter and do not exit, and refer to all others as *through-and-through* injuries.

Blunt Force Injury

There are four main subdivisions of blunt injury:

1. Scratches and grazes–abrasions
2. Bruises–contusions
3. Tears–lacerations
4. Fractures of bone

These types of injury often occur in combination, but each will be reviewed separately.

Abrasions

An abrasion represents the removal of the outermost layer of the skin by a compressive or sliding force. Usually the skin is not perforated, but this can occur if the force and severity are sufficient or if the injury is great enough for areas to be physically worn away. Abrasions are seldom life threatening, but they are of great importance in interpreting what happened because they must, by their very nature, mark the exact point at which contact occurred (Fig. 19-1). Thus, the presence, form, and distribution of abrasions may need to be recorded in considerable detail. As blunt force is applied to the surface of the body, two vectors of force come into play. One is directed primarily inward and the other primarily longitudinally or parallel to the skin surface. The magnitude of each may differ, producing characteristics that allow subdivision into pressure or sliding types. It is well to consider abrasions in these terms, because it makes one think about the mechanism of

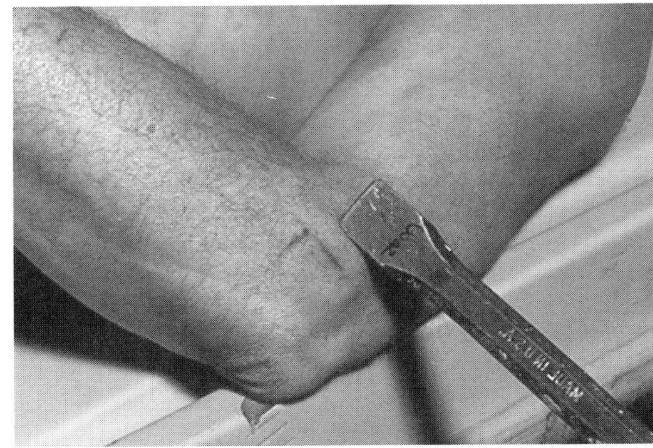
A

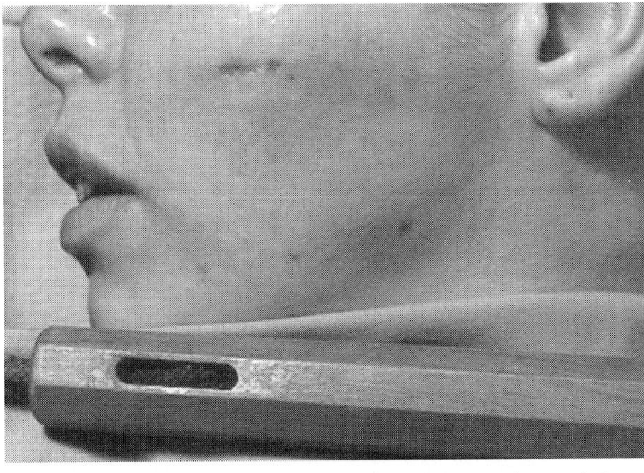
B

Fig. 19-1 *A*, Patterned abrasion. Note the contact point and the mirror image of the pry bar. *B*, Wounding instrument and resultant pattern abrasion and slight contusion.

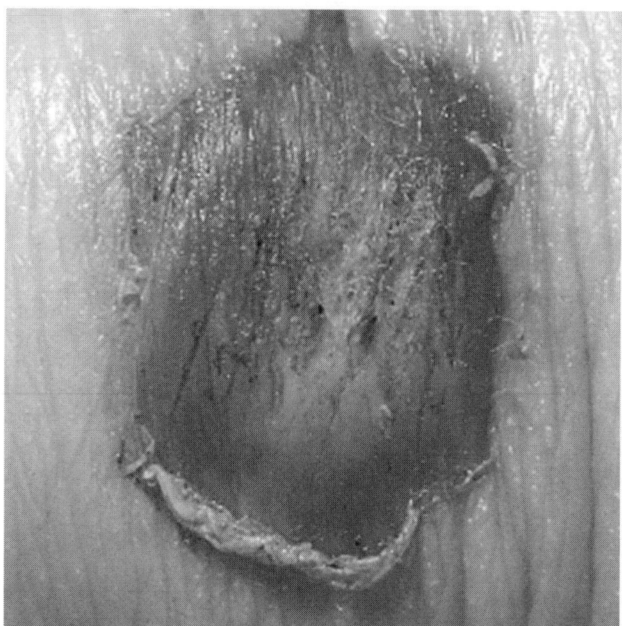

Fig. 19-2 Knee abrasion of pedestrian struck by auto. Note the skin roll on bottom wound edge that indicates the direction of the impact force.

injury and direction of force. The surface tissues may be pushed toward one end of a sliding abrasion, like dirt moved to the far end of the "push" by a bulldozer or road grader, in which case tags and tissue fragments frequently indicate the direction toward which the force was applied (Fig. 19-2).

Similar to most wounds, abrasions tend to darken as the tissues dry. In most instances, this is noted first at the edges of the wound or in more shallow areas of the abrasion. After death, when there is no longer circulation or body movement to keep them moist, abrasions will dry and darken. This may lead to the false interpretation that the injury resulted from burning, bruising, or even that a hot object contacted the tissues.

Abrasions are sometimes classified according to their shape. If long and narrow, as from contact with thorns, they are called *scratches*. If wider areas are involved, they can be called *grazes*. The claws of a cat will leave scratches. The knee of a child who fell from a tricycle onto blacktop will be described as grazed. The direction of force is useful in evaluating the patient's statement of how the injury occurred. For instance, are the abrasions due to being struck on the thigh or buttock by the front of a car or due to the victim's sliding along the road surface after being knocked down? The form and appearance of the injury should be noted because it may help interpret the mechanism and circumstances of injury.

In summary, abrasions

- indicate contact with a rough surface or object.
- indicate the exact site of contact or impact.
- will eventually crust over or scab (i.e., dry and darken).
- may reveal the direction of the force of injury.
- may exhibit characteristic patterns (e.g., knurled tool handles, motorcycle drive chains).
- may be seen in conjunction with bruises and lacerations because forces sufficient to produce scraping may distort the underlying soft tissues enough to tear vessels.

Contusions

A contusion, or bruise, results from leakage of blood from vessels into the tissues after sufficient force has been applied to distort the soft tissues and tear one or more vessels–hence the term *extravasation* (*extra* = outside; *vasa* = vessel). The vessels involved are usually small (such as capillaries), but they may be larger and on occasion, when a larger vessel is involved, leakage can occur quite rapidly. An abrasion may be observed nearby, and if present, it may signify the exact point of contact or application of force. Fresh bruises may be slightly raised above the adjacent surfaces, if enough blood escapes and, even when a large bruise is deeply seated, swelling may be apparent when the size of a limb or body part is compared to its opposite member.

Contusions result when blunt forces distort the soft tissues to an extent sufficient to result in disruption and leakage of blood vessels. Escape of blood from the blood vessels is what produces the discoloration. The amount of blood that escapes from the vessels will depend on features such as the size of the contusion and the pressure within it, the ability to clot, the space available for blood to leak into, and so on.

The subcategories of contusions include the following:

- Deep seated, such as in the internal organs, often in the form of hematomas
- Beneath the skin, where contusions give the discolorations commonly know as bruises
- In the skin itself, where the contusions give rise to patterned bruises

There are two other meanings of the word *contusion,* both of which relate to the brain:

1. The clinical meaning of contusion describes a somewhat imprecise clinical diagnosis of a patient who, after a blow to the head, suffers prolonged loss of consciousness with appearance of clinical signs of brain injury. Note that the expression "contusion of the brain" is not typically used in the presence of dramatic and definite clinical signs such as paralysis. In such circumstances, the description becomes "head injury with hemiplegia."
2. Contusion of the brain substance occurs when forces are exerted on the head, sufficient to cause the crests of the gyri (surface ridges of the brain) to contact the inner surface of the skull. This results, in the early stages, in small linear hemorrhages resembling splinters of wood under a fingernail. These hemorrhages may become larger and more confluent if injury is more severe.

Fresh Bruises and Color of Bruises

A fresh bruise usually begins with the reddish color of oxygenated blood, from the arterial side of the circulation, but like superficial vessels they may appear blue. This is because blue light bounces (e.g., blue light bouncing off dust particles in the atmosphere gives blue skies) and red penetrates more deeply (e.g., restaurants use infrared lights over the food to keep it warm). Also think in terms of varying depths of skin and yellow fat. Later bruises turn a more purplish hue and ultimately, as the blood pigments break down, the sequence of colors passes through those of a ripening banana, through greens, yellows, and browns, at which point the coloration fades. A closed bruise with only a scrape on the skin above it will not behave the same as a bruise forming in distorted or torn fat, or one that can leak out through a defect in the skin.

The persistence of discoloration varies with age, location of the bruising on the body (circulatory efficiency), and the amount of blood released. Some individuals bruise more easily than others of the same age and sex do; others seldom bruise. Bruising can be masked by natural coloration of the overlying skin and may be almost invisible if the skin is heavily tanned or naturally dark. At very late stages, long after injury, discoloration may remain. However, this remaining discoloration may well be more of a response to injury (scar formation, breakdown products of blood pigments, and melanin) than true bruising.

Best Practice *19-1*

When recording information about bruising, do not attempt to predict the age of the bruise based on coloration. Describe the characteristics of the bruise in terms of location, color, and pattern. Color photography provides the optimum documentation of bruising.

Estimating the Age of a Bruise

The rate at which a bruise appears and disappears depends on many factors, including the quantity of blood originally released, the effectiveness of the local circulation, age, location of the bruised area on the body, and the general physical activity and condition of the individual. Some textbooks and journal articles suggest the rate at which bruises fade is fairly predictable; however, the various authors disagree on the rate. Any opinion concerning the age of a bruise based on its color is extremely difficult and should be attained and stated with the greatest caution and circumspection (Smock, 2001).

Estimating the age of bruises based on appearance or coloration is difficult, both before and after death. To prove the difficulty during life, simply observe bruises of *known age*. In postmortem tissues, age estimation is difficult with both the unaided eye and the microscope. The pathologist should obtain a set of tissue sections to ensure a truly average and representative sampling. During testimony, it is prudent to admit that there is every reason to be both cautious and skeptical when trying to match changes in injured soft tissues in a person who may have been in shock and organ failure or undergone treatment (including advanced life support, transfusions, antibiotics, and dialysis), and then try to draw a parallel with results from studies in humans and experimental animals, taken in the days before modern-day techniques were even thought of.

The forensic nurse examiner should make detailed annotations about the size and appearance of the bruise rather than attempt to estimate the age of the bruise based on literature. Photographs of bruises taken immediately upon examination are also helpful as a means of documentation because the characteristics of the affected area change gradually over hours and days.

Distribution of Bruises

Distribution of bruises may be important. Small bruises around the neck or on a limb may be the only external signs of violence. Indeed it is possible to have massive internal injury with very little evidence on the body surface, and on occasion there may be no evidence whatsoever. Sometimes superficial patterned bruising may be of value in identifying a particular instrument or weapon such as a whip or cane in which the bruises may have a linear or double line configuration. When called on to examine the victim of an alleged assault, remember that bruises may not become visible immediately and therefore may not be visible at the time of an examination performed soon after the event. Recent advances in technology using alternate light sources aid in detecting bruised tissue, even before the skin reveals any type of discoloration. Later on, even without special adjuncts, bruises are likely to become visible on the body surfaces. Reexamination of a victim, updated annotations in the medical record, and careful photo-documentation may provide helpful comparisons with the original observations. This is particularly true with cases of alleged abuse of an elderly person in a nursing home. Bruising may be found in the areas around the eyes and within the soft tissue of the eyelids themselves, particularly in the elderly who sustain minor impacts to these regions when they collapse or fall. Discolorations do not necessarily appear at the place(s) at which force was applied because the coloration may result from blood that has tracked around muscles and flowed in the tissue fluids on route to the surface. For example, hitting the ankle sometimes results in discoloration of the toes. Only an abrasion or a pattern in or near the bruising itself will indicate the actual point of contact.

Bruiselike discoloration can appear many inches away from the point at which force was applied and look just like bruising when it was not involved in the force and remains the same color until it fades. Bruises of many colors are seen simultaneously as a result of a single episode of injury. This should confirm that bruises do not develop at the same speed or progress and resolve in a uniform fashion. In addition, there are cases in which several bruises result from accidents such as a fall or walking into a door. Yet these bruises disappear at different rates, some taking far longer than others. The forensic nurse examiner should consider that one or more bruises of different ages may be adjacent to or overlapping one another, confusing the assessment.

Advanced Assessment Techniques

Because color tends to be an unreliable indicator for the age of the bruise, the forensic pathologist may need to use advanced techniques of tissue study to determine the timing or duration of the injury that caused the bruising. Subspecialists may also be used to provide additional information about certain body tissues such as the heart, brain, or liver. It is imperative, however, that representative tissue samples are obtained and that reference tissues from other body parts are used for comparison, especially when there are complicating factors such as cardiopulmonary resuscitation procedures, blood administration, or the use of mechanical ventilation.

Best Practice *19-2*

If someone states the exact age of a bruise based on its color, continue to evaluate the case because there is a high probability that the estimate of age will be wrong. Arrests of suspects should not be based on bruise coloration alone, but on the result of a comprehensive investigation of all pertinent factors.

Patient Populations with Easy Bruising

Bruising is accentuated in the presence of blood dyscrasias such as leukemia or any impairment of the blood-clotting processes, including hemophilia. Bruising is also commonly noted in patients who are on anticoagulants or antiplatelet drugs. Selective serotonin reuptake inhibitors, a class of antidepressants (e.g., Zoloft), inhibit blood platelet activity and may be associated with bruising in unusual locations.

It is generally easier for blood to escape into loose tissues and fat; therefore, bruising is more common:

- In certain parts of the body
- At the extremes of age
- After weight loss
- In obesity
- If there is disease of the blood vessels

Relationship between Blunt Forces and Bruising

The intensity and duration of forces associated with bruising are difficult or impossible factors to estimate unless other features such as abrasions or lacerations are also present. Significant blunt forces do not necessarily result in the formation of bruises. Not every blow a boxer strikes results in a bruise, and many such blows are forceful. Tissues exposed to repeated trauma may firm up and scar, making it harder for blood to enter and for bruising to occur. The forceful distortion of tissues necessary to result in bruising may itself selectively alter the ability of blood to make its way through injured tissue, such as fat, to the body surface to produce discoloration. If a vessel is lacerated, any blood that escapes will tend to depart through the open wound rather than permeate into the adjacent tissues. Thus, a laceration may have less bruising adjacent to it, not more, even though the force was greater. Likewise if fat is slightly torn beneath a closed wound, the blood will pass more easily into some parts than others.

In the living, a bruise may appear more or less prominent, according to the amount of peripheral vasoconstriction (standing out in the cold) or vasodilatation (just after a hot bath) of adjacent and overlying skin.

Postmortem Bruising

The question often arises as to whether it is possible to produce bruising at and around the time of death or even after death. Limited bruising can be produced immediately following death if the body is mishandled or struck, assuming enough blood is present and is free to move (not set, sludged, fixed, clotted, or otherwise altered) under the influence of gravity. Therefore, everyone who handles the recently deceased should be cautious.

Postmortem bruises are, however, usually small, few in number, and localized, and they do not usually pose much of a problem. Bruises are easily overlooked in areas into which blood has been forced or has settled (including postmortem lividity), or in areas in which circulation is failing. In some instances of very severe injury accompanied by rapidly falling blood pressure, bruises that are still forming at the time circulation ceases may assume colors that are more commonly associated with greater age. These often have a subtle, almost grayish appearance.

After death, it may be necessary to cut into the skin to demonstrate subtle or concealed bruising, especially if there is any significant degree of natural coloration of the overlying skin. In some European countries, where open-casket funerals are relatively rare, it is not uncommon to demonstrate the presence of bruising at autopsy by completely removing selected areas of skin. In the US, where open-casket funerals are common, only the minimum number of incisions necessary to properly define the nature and extent of bruising are made.

Focal bleeding within the soft tissues of decomposed or decomposing bodies is difficult to interpret, requiring considerable experience on the part of the forensic specialist. Decomposition makes it much harder to tell antemortem from postmortem bruising. Bruising is harder to see in areas of postmortem lividity.

Case Study 19-1 Postmortem Bruising

A body (following death from head injuries) was first examined in the autopsy room and had a normal color, normal face, and unswollen eyelids. Photographs that included the face were taken of injuries on the front of the body, and other photos were taken for identification purposes. After the examination of the front was completed, the body was turned facedown for examination, documentation, and photography of injuries on the back. By the time the body was once again turned faceup for opening and internal examination, both upper eyelids had swollen and turned blue-gray from leakage of blood from fractures of the supraorbital plates, the thin bone between the frontal lobes of the brain and eyes. Although uncommon, under the right circumstances, if blood is present and free to move, such effects can and do occur.

Keep these points in mind when assessing bruising:

- Bruises may not become visible for minutes, hours, or even a few days. This is possible because it may take time for blood leaking from vessels located beneath fat or behind other structures such as fascial planes to wend its way to the surface. Furthermore, in the presence of shock, the extravasation of blood may be retarded until adequate perfusion pressure has been restored.
- Bruises are often larger than the area of impact or the causative object because of the flowing and spreading of blood as it makes its way to the body surface (Box 19-1).

Lacerations or Tears

The term *laceration* is commonly misused when describing injuries. Blunt objects produce lacerations, and sharp objects produce cuts, incisions, or incised wounds (Wright, 2003). A surgeon may make an incision with a surgical knife (scalpel) and call it an incision, then walk into the emergency department, examine a knife cut on a patient's face, and call it a laceration. This misuse is not only incorrect, but it can also cause confusion with legal implications.

Key Point *19-2*

Lacerations are blunt force injuries resulting from tearing, ripping, crushing, overstretching, pulling apart, bending, and shearing soft tissues.

Strictly speaking, lacerations are defects in soft tissues resulting from tearing, ripping, crushing, overstretching, and shearing. Soft tissue defects should be described as tears (lacerations) or cuts (incised wounds) to indicate if an injury was blunt or sharp when a medical record is reviewed.

In the boxing community, a tear near a boxer's eyebrow is referred to as a cut. The tear in the skin near the eye occurs when the heads of the two boxers collide so that the soft tissues between the bony ridges and surfaces are forced aside. To illustrate, lay a line of toothpaste along the edge of a bathroom sink and then press a finger into it. The paste will escape from either side of one's finger.

Box 19-1 Studying Bruising Patterns

To learn more about the practical aspects of bruising, use 3-by-5 file cards or make forms on a computer. Put the following headings on the cards or forms, and fill in the data whenever bruises of exactly known age are observed. Be extremely selective, and include only those cases in which the time of injury is absolutely known and is therefore the true time since injury.

- Identifying information, such as hospital, ambulance, or dispatch number
- Date and time of observation
- Ambient/prevailing lighting
- Age, sex, skin color
- Location and size of bruise/bruises
- Bruise color in your own words
- Cause of the injuries and bruising (e.g., motor vehicle collision, bar fight, fall)
- Ambient/prevailing temperature and prior activity (vasoconstriction or vasodilatation)
- Any medications or conditions that would affect the clotting process

Look for injuries that occurred at the same time but that developed different colors (for instance, if someone falls and the bruise on the face is yellow while another on the trunk is purple).

Another worthwhile study is to make a note of the date and minute when you accidentally hit yourself hard enough to notice it. If a bruise appears, you will know the time of injury to a minute and be able to record any discolorations that result. If you do not bruise, you will be able to state that when you hurt yourself to the point of discomfort you only get a bruise a certain percentage of the time. Whether you do or do not bruise easily, the results may surprise you.

So it often is with soft tissues and, to be technically correct, lacerations do not result from sharp objects. *Use of the term* laceration *should be strictly reserved to those wounds that result from blunt force.*

Compressive shearing force applied to a tissue or organ may cause an internal tear without external tearing; the impact site in such instances may only be denoted by an abrasion or nearby bruise. Because overstretching of tissue is an important factor in the production of lacerations, the plasticity or potential mobility of the tissues will influence the occurrence of this type of blunt injury. Therefore, skin lacerations are frequently found overlying bony prominences of the body where the skin is relatively fixed and less able to move when stressed. Similarly, laceration of the aorta or other organs occurs most frequently at points of relative immobility or mechanical disadvantage, particularly if the energy of impact is conducted to a point at which the vessel or organ is fixed to an adjacent structure.

Typical Skin Lacerations

The typical skin laceration has an irregular margin that may be scraped or bruised, especially if there was an impact with an object or rough surface. Because the tissue is torn apart, there is frequently an incomplete separation with stronger tissue elements (such as little blood vessels, nerves, and connective tissue strands) surviving to bridge or span the gap from one part or side of the wound to the other. This bridging of tissue is particularly evident deep within a wound or at its corners and is helpful in accurately differentiating blunt from sharp force injury. Closer inspection of lacerations may reveal characteristics that are useful in interpreting the mechanism of wound production. For example, if one side is scraped/abraded and the opposite margin undermined, partly crushed, or pushed aside, these findings suggest that the force was directed at an angle over the surface, which was scraped and directed toward the side that is crushed, undermined, or pushed back (Figs. 19-3 and 19-4).

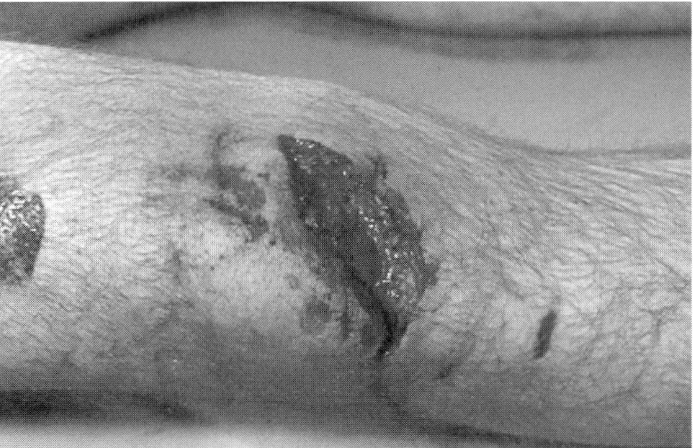

Fig. 19-3 Laceration from blunt force trauma incurred by the knee of an unrestrained passenger hitting the dashboard in a motor vehicle crash. Note the grazes, which illustrate the direction of the forces of impact.

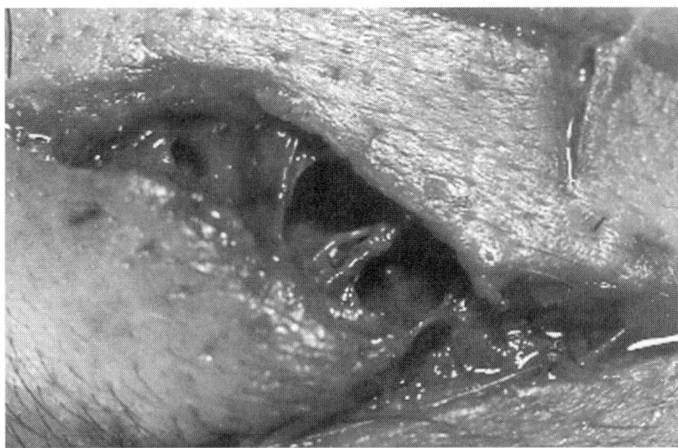

Fig. 19-4 Homicide victim with multiple stab wounds and a large laceration with tissue bridging.

Internal Organ Lacerations

Lacerations of internal organs are a relatively common result of blunt force or impact applied to the exterior of the body. Classical injuries involve the liver, spleen, and kidneys, all of which tear with relative ease if the force is sufficient. The lungs may be torn by inwardly displaced ends of broken ribs or result from very severe forces. It is noteworthy that it is possible to have serious internal blunt injures without surface manifestations such as abrasions and bruises. If this were not so, surgeons would never have to undertake exploratory procedures to rule out injury. Surface indications are often present, but they do not have to be, and their absence does not rule out the possibility of internal injury. The following list identifies key points to remember when assessing lacerations:

- Lacerations result from blunt force, crushing, tearing, ripping, shearing, overstretching, bending, and pulling apart of soft tissues.
- They have ragged, variably irregular margins.

- They will, in most cases, have scraping and bruising of the wound margins.
- They may bleed less and become infected in crushed tissues (especially if the victim survives).
- Lacerated tissue may survive the force and be observed "bridging" or "spanning" within parts of a wound if it is a stronger tissue component, such as blood vessels, nerves, tendons, and connective elements. Hair roots and other skin structures may be seen protruding from the margins, having been torn out of their supporting tissues.
- They frequently contain foreign materials including trace evidence such as glass, paint chips, bark, fibers, and grease.
- Their overall size and shape vary widely by virtue of their blunt, tearing, shearing, or crushing origin. When attempting to reapproximate the edges of a blunt torn injury, the examiner may notice that the wound still looks ragged, whereas most sharp injuries are more easily restored for suturing.
- Tears resulting from forceful contact with angular objects can, if there is underlying bone, lead to the formation of linear injuries which may be mistaken for cuts due to sharp objects.
- Lacerations may indicate direction of force when, for instance, the bent knee of a vehicle occupant hits the lower part of the dash in a frontal collision. Some people use the expression *trapdoor laceration* to describe the directional nature of such an evulsion injury, an inverted U- or V-shaped flap of skin that remains attached at its upper margin.

Fractures

The fourth major variant of blunt injury is bone fracture. Bone may fracture in different ways according to the amount of force and the fashion in which it is applied. The classical transverse or V-like fracture of the lower leg due to being hit by a car bumper is likely to be different from the spiral twisting of the fracture sustained by a falling skier. Most of the time it is not easy to tell what happened because most of the bones are covered by tissue and the fracture sites may have been dressed to prevent infection. An observant, well-trained orthopedic surgeon, nurse, or paramedic may see features at the time of treatment that can help solve the classic "hit from the front, back, or side" question. It may be easier at autopsy because tissue can be removed and there is less blood to impede the examination, but even then detection may not be possible.

Summary of Blunt Force Injuries

The four major varieties of blunt injuries have been reviewed. The principal points to note are the following:

- Abrasions, although not life threatening, can be of great assistance in working out what happened.
- Assessing the age or duration of bruises is difficult and unreliable.
- *Laceration* is a term that is widely misunderstood and misused. Lacerations result from blunt injuries and may be contaminated with foreign material or contain trace evidence. Lacerations of soft tissue, brought about by contact with angular objects in areas that overlie bone, may be mistaken for cuts.
- Directional characteristics are frequently present in abrasions and lacerations, and occasionally in fractures, although broken ends of bone are seldom examined with direction of force in mind (with the exception of bullet wounds).

Sharp Force Injuries

There are two main subdivisions of sharp injuries: cuts (which include slashes and slices) and stab wounds.

Cuts

In cuts, a sharp object comes against the skin with sufficient pressure to divide it. The force is usually directed mainly along the surface while some inward pressure is applied. Thus, such wounds are, by definition, longer than they are deep. Cuts may tail off at one end and be more superficial at one end than the other. The characteristics of the cutting instrument are usually not well reflected by a cut. After all, did a cut result from the last inch of a long blade or most of a short one? If only one edge did any cutting, how can one possibly tell anything about the edge that never made contact? It is also difficult to assess the amount of force required because this largely depends on the sharpness and configuration of the instrument and the resistance offered by clothing, if any (Fig. 19-5).

Two similar terms that refer to sharp injury are *slash* and *slice.* Slash means cutting or wounding with strokes or in a sweeping fashion with a sharp instrument or weapon: to gash, to strike violently or at random, to move rapidly or violently, to cut slits in, or to deliver cutting blows.

A slice is a relatively thin, flat, broad piece cut from the primary object; a sharp cut or to cut cleanly.

Thus, these terms are commonly used in two circumstances:

1. When describing cuts on the wrists, neck, and other body parts of a person attempting suicide and as a descriptive term (e.g., "she slashed her wrists")
2. In reference to reckless savage cutting, with overtly malicious intent, often forcefully and in a sweeping manner without careful aim. Such injuries are associated with gang wars, vendettas, crimes of passion, sex murders, control of prostitutes, and retaliation against suspected informants.

A slash, or slice, is a special variant of cut. Keep the following factors in mind when evaluating cuts:

- Cuts result from sharp objects coming against the skin with pressure to cause an injury.
- Cuts are longer than they are deep (in contrast to stab wounds).

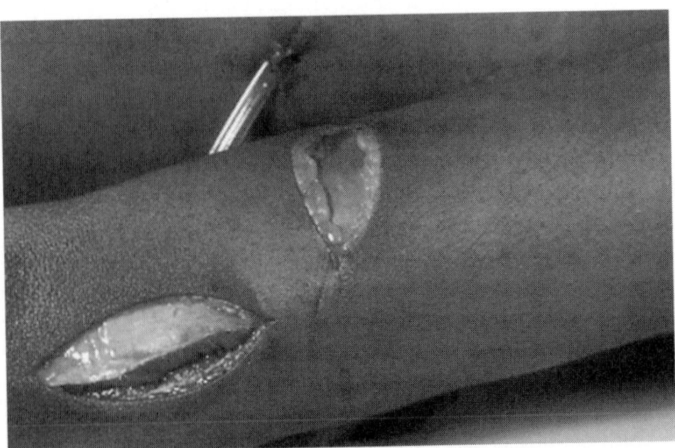

Fig. 19-5 Characteristic sharp force injury.

- Cuts have clean-cut edges, usually without abrasion or bruising.
- In cuts, there is no bridging, spanning, or selective sparing of tissues.
- Overlying hair, the hair roots, and other small structures within the skin will be cut if the object is sufficiently sharp.
- There is scarcity or total absence of foreign material and trace evidence unless something such as glass is present.
- Cuts tend to bleed freely unless vessels are completely divided and able to retract. There is no scraping or bruising at the edges.
- Cuts may be irregular if the skin was creased, wrinkled, or affected by clothing at the moment of cutting.
- Cuts may be deeper at one end than the other. This can give rise to questions of right or left-handedness.
- A cut can be irregular if the skin was moved between the time of injury and examination.

Stab Wounds

Stab wounds result whenever a sufficiently sharp and narrow object is forced inward. This is not necessarily due to a thrust but can occasionally result when one falls onto something sharp. Relative motion and enough force to cause the object to pass through the skin are conditions that are required for stabbing to result. The skin does offer most of the resistance, and once it has been penetrated the amount of force required will diminish unless tissues such as cartilage or bone are encountered. Although there is a great deal of deliberate stabbing with knives, other less sharp objects may be used such as metal rods, ice picks, and screwdrivers. If a penetrating object is not truly sharp, or if it tapers and becomes thicker as it enters then it is possible to see some stretching of the wound margins with resulting abrasion; however, stab wounds are primarily sharp in character. Occasionally, force is so great that really blunt objects are driven into the body, in which case these injuries are best classified and described as lacerations.

Stab wounds are more likely to reflect information of forensic importance–such as the causative instrument or weapon–than are cuts, because a rounded object tends to cause a rounded hole, a square object a squarer hole, and so forth. For example, a fairly thick knife blade that is sharpened only on one of its two edges will tend to leave a defect that has a cleanly cut acute angle at one end and a more squared-off or slightly torn, angular appearance at the other. A cross-shaped Phillips screwdriver may produce wounds, which have a subtle, but definite cross-shaped configuration when examined carefully. Unless a known stabbing object is present for examination, the exact depth of penetration must remain unknown until the body is opened at surgery or autopsy. For this reason, many surgeons elect to explore the internal situation following stab wounds. Occasionally stabbing instruments (tips of cast blades or big pieces of glass) may break off in the depths of a wound, especially if bone is encountered. Recovery and retention of such fragments may be vital to effective prosecution of a criminal case or even to prove the cause of an accidental injury. Always look for evidence that a knife or tool was forced in as far as its handle (Smock, 2001). Areas of abrasion near the entry defect may signify this. Regardless of the length of the blade, such features indicate that it went in all the way, and generally this is not favorable to the patient as it increases the potential for deep-seated injury.

This classification into cuts and stabs is simplified for clarity and instructional purposes. Classic stabs and cuts represent opposite ends of a spectrum of injuries. For example, one may wonder what to call a wound that is about as deep as it is long. The important thing is to recognize it as a sharp injury and be able to separate it from the results of a blow (blunt injury). Stabs and cuts are often seen together in a single patient or victim. Decide if the force was primarily inward or transverse with respect to the skin, and describe the injuries as best as possible. Photography remains the best method of documentation.

If criminal activity is involved, try to document the surface dimension, depth, and direction of wounds. Cuts that are inflicted across the natural lines of tension (Langor lines) in the skin tend to gape open. Those inflicted parallel to the lines of tension tend to remain closed and relatively undistorted (i.e., the "Ziploc" bag effect). Surgeons are familiar with these lines of tension and endeavor to make their incisions parallel to them. Members of the street scene do not worry about such subtleties, so the injuries inflicted are often distorted by the effects of tension in the skin combined with body movement. This means one must consider how the injury looked before skin tension and body movement led to a change of shape. Beveling or shelving of wound margins are again clues to the internal direction of a wound track. Tracks should never be probed indiscriminately. In the event a chest tube or other device should be placed through a fortuitously located injury, this should be clearly indicated in the treatment or operative report. Otherwise, if the victim dies, the pathologist may not be in a position to properly interpret the features and wounds inflicted by an assailant (Figs. 19-6, 19-7, 19-8, and 19-9). However, it is preferable to never insert a chest tube into a bullet wound or stab wound.

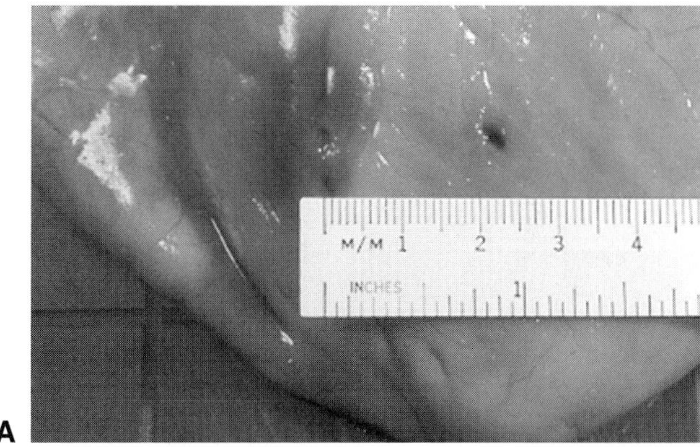

A

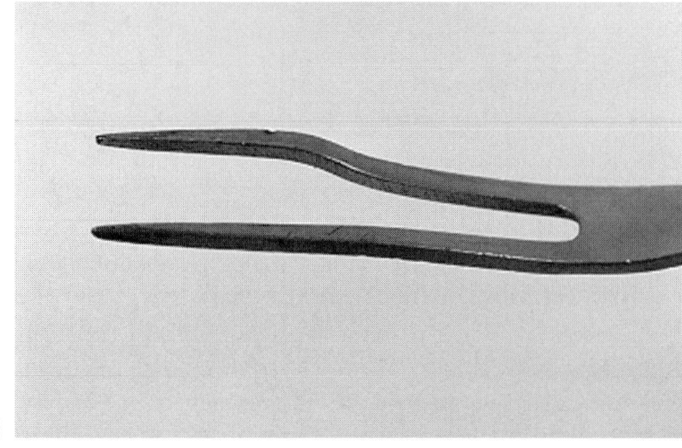

B

Fig. 19-6 *A*, Stab wound of heart with a meat fork. *B*, Meat fork used in the stabbing episode.

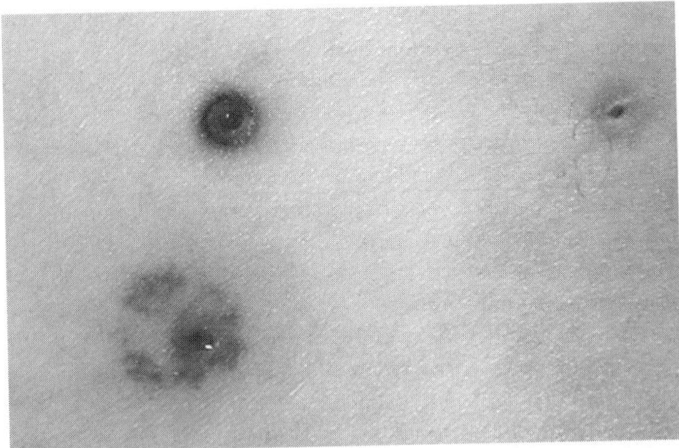

Fig. 19-7 Stab wounds inflicted by an ice pick. Note the lower left entry illustrating the contusion from the ringed-collar of the pick's handle.

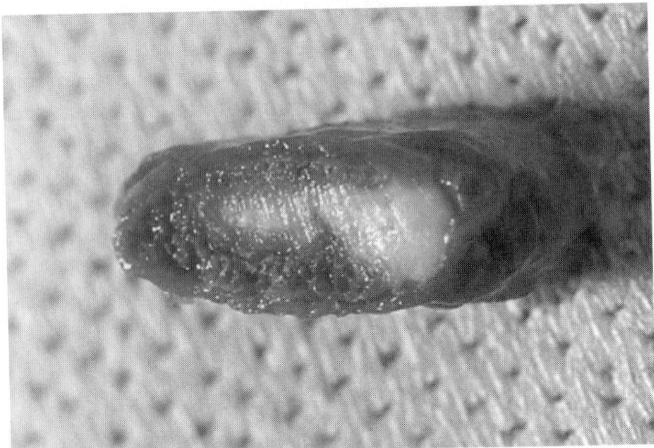

Fig. 19-8 Stab wound involving a rib that reveals a multilinear pattern, suggesting the type of knife used in the assault.

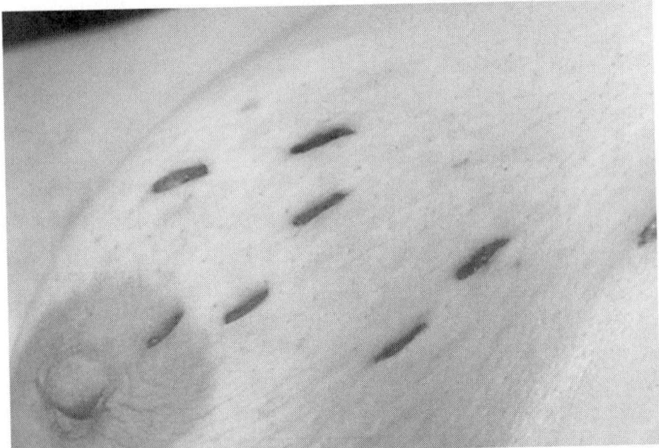

Fig. 19-9 Multiple stab wounds of the chest clearly distinguishing the sharp *(left)* and dull *(right)* edges of the knife

Not infrequently, autopsy or surgical exploration reveals a wound track that extends inward for a distance greater than the length of the weapon alleged to have caused it. This is because when someone is struck with a blow, the body wall may compress with momentary indentation of the tissues, which may even be combined with a subsequent change in the position of the body by the time the internal examination takes place. Even the chest wall can be compressed. This is why modern CPR can effectively squeeze the heart between the momentarily depressed sternum and the forward projection of the vertebral bodies and overlying structures. A short, stubby knife is certainly capable of inflicting a wound an inch or two longer than its greatest dimension, especially in the abdomen or when there is little muscle to resist momentary indentation.

Exactly how much increase is possible in these cases is not clear because of a lack of controlled circumstances. By the time of surgical exploration, the living patient has been repositioned, the bowel has gone completely or partially into a state of ileus (mechanical or adynamic obstruction), blood and gas have collected, and the intestine has rearranged itself. This leads to estimates of weapon size that are often significantly in error. In an elderly person with reduced abdominal musculature and a sagging, relaxed abdominal wall, a relatively short blade can easily reach the aorta and inferior vena cava if a forceful blow is struck. In addition, tangential injuries may appear larger at the surface than those directed radially inward.

Summary of Sharp Force Injuries

Keep the following points in mind when evaluating sharp force injuries:

- Stab wounds result from variably sharp or pointed objects forced inward by a thrust, movement, or fall.
- Depth exceeds width in stab wounds.
- With stab wounds, there is danger to vital internal structures and the risk of delayed incapacitation, exemplified by cardiac tamponade (blood in the sac surrounding the heart) or tension pneumothorax (air trapping between a lung and the chest wall).
- Stab wounds may begin with internal bleeding, then later blood may appear when the victim "overflows" or collapses. This often confuses inexperienced or untrained individuals.
- Stab wound may reflect the causative instrument or weapon (single edge, double edge, square, round, etc.).
- There is relatively little abrasion of stab wound margins unless the weapon is tapering and wedges/stretches the skin on its way in.
- Occasionally fragments of a penetrating object will break off in a stab wound. Remnants should be recovered and retained whenever practicable and handled as potential evidence.

Other Wounds

There are other wounds with characteristics that do not necessarily fit well into either blunt or sharp force injuries. The weapon or instrument, as well as the forces involved, will determine the type of resultant injury.

Mixed Blunt and Sharp Injuries

Mixed blunt and sharp injuries exist and are frequently observed because people are attacked and injured by semisharp, semiblunt objects. Examples include old axes, machetes, meat cleavers, roofing hatchets, being ejected onto crushed rock, or falling onto scrap metal. However, understating the basic subtypes of blunt and sharp injury will allow one to recognize a mixture of injuries.

Chop Wounds

Chop wounds are deep, gaping wounds often involving major structures and resulting from the use of relatively heavy and sharp objects such as meat cleavers, axes, machetes, and brush hooks. If the instrument is fairly sharp, wounds may show a mixture of both sharp and blunt characteristics. One key to recognizing them is the combination of force and depth.

Blister or Friction Blister

The friction blister is not usually of medicolegal significance, but blisters may be observed on the feet of those who have been walking a lot. This is especially true if the person is not used to much walking or has new, unsuitable, or ill-fitting footwear. Blisters cause high rates of disability in the military services, especially during training and on the march. Occasionally, the associated ulceration (when the surface layer separates) and secondary infection can be significant and may even become life threatening, especially in diabetics and the elderly when there is poor circulation to the area. Research has shown that dry and extremely wet skin affords less friction than slightly moistened surfaces.

The friction blister is not due to heat and does not represent second-degree burns, even though it may feel hot. Research has never shown a temperature rise of more than a few degrees, even under extreme experimental conditions. Blisters are formed by a shearing between the more superficial and deeper skin structures, resulting eventually in a split or cleft into which fluid flows or transudes. Blisters are most frequent in the skin of the hands (palms) and feet (soles, heels, sides of the feet, and tops of the toes). The cleft almost invariably occurs above the basal cells, in or below the granular layer of the skin. The fluid within blisters contains most of the proteins of blood serum, but in lesser concentration and usually with little or no fibrinogen. It is important to remember that there are other possible causes of skin blistering, including burns, exposure to chemicals, prolonged immersion, and decomposition.

Defensive Injuries

Defensive injuries are incurred in attempts to ward off blows of a weapon or assailant or in trying to grasp a sharp weapon. Injuries resulting from blunt attack can be in the form of scrapes, bruises, tears, and even fractures. In the case of a sharp attack, defensive injuries could be cuts and stabs. Defensive injuries are likely to be found on the arms and hands, but they may be seen elsewhere. They are usually found on those parts of the body that a victim tends to interpose between himself or herself and the assailant and including the backs of the hands, wrists, forearms, and to a lesser extent the shoulders and elbows (Sheridan, 2001).

Defense wounds are helpful since they indicate that the victim was, regardless of drugs and alcohol, aware, conscious, and able to resist. They also indicate if the weapon was sharp or blunt. On occasion, the type of weapon may be evident and the sequence of events apparent (Fig. 19-10).

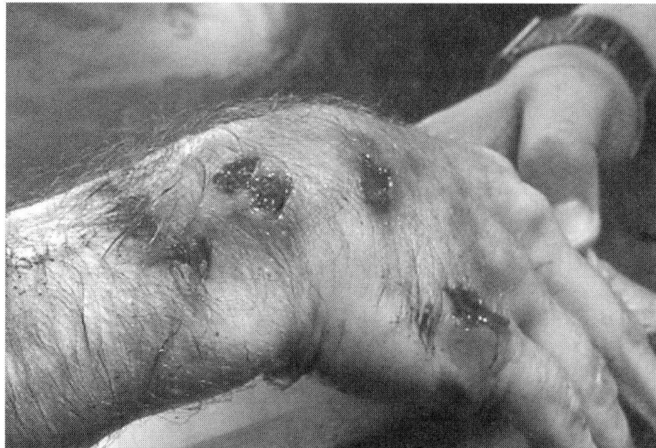

Fig. 19-10 Defensive wounds of the hand used to protect the body during a stabbing scenario.

Diversionary Wounds

Although not a common a term, the phrase *diversionary wounds* is sometimes used to describe those wounds inflicted in the course of an attack, in order to promote a response that will facilitate the exposure of previously guarded, less exposed, or more vital areas. Diversionary wounds merge into, and may be indistinguishable from, defensive injuries.

Factitious Injuries

Factitious injuries (i.e., injuries that have been fabricated, forged, or invented) are self-inflicted, not with the intent of suicide but with the intent of accusing or blaming someone else, obtaining money or reward by false pretenses, or avoiding unpleasant duty. They are not particularly common in North America but are more common elsewhere; nevertheless, factitious injuries occur often enough that the possibility should not be ignored. Factitious injuries are often superficial or relatively minor in nature, usually located on readily accessible parts of the body, and they may be encountered in disturbed or mentally ill persons or in those who bear a grudge. These injuries are usually superficial, blunt, not too painful, and usually located in those areas where self-infliction is easy. Injuries on the face are likely to be vertical and more oblique on the left in a right-handed individual, and they do not show the irregularity associated with a fight or the movement in struggle. Another clue is often that the person with self-inflicted wounds is very open about them and wants them to be noticed. To experiment with possible angles and marks, have a nonmedically trained person inflict imaginary injuries using a marker or water-soluble dye on a swab.

Hesitation Marks

Hesitation marks (trial, tentative, decision cuts) are the superficial, often somewhat parallel cuts made in the course of attempting suicide, in an attempt to gain courage or attention, or arising from vacillation. For instance, a person bent on self-destruction by cutting may try the blade on the wrists and neck to see how painful it is before inflicting deeper wounds. The significance is that these wounds strongly support the conclusion that they are self-inflicted and help to separate suicide from homicide. In any suspected suicide it is always worth looking for well-healed, faint, and barely visible parallel cuts on the wrists, arms, and neck (from a previous episode of self-inflicted injury).

Paired or Grouped Injuries

It is essential to keep in mind the possibility that more than one injury may be inflicted simultaneously by instruments such as scissors, shears, and forks. Some medieval weapons also produced injuries in this fashion. The same thinking applies today with irregularly shaped objects such as tools and gear wheels. Some of these injuries may have an obvious pattern to them. An important aspect is that the number of wounds observed may exceed the alleged/reported number of thrusts or blows.

Scrimmage Wounds

Scrimmage wound or *scrimmage enlargement* are terms that have been used to describe the enlargement by tearing of a wound as a consequence of relative motion between the tissues and a weapon before it is completely withdrawn. Sometimes it is used to refer to a partially double track, for instance, when a stab wound was inflicted, the victim moved, and the assailant promptly pressed the knife in again to its fullest extent. This usually applies when the penetrating weapon enters and is then withdrawn in a forceful manner to one or other side of the plane in which it entered. Such wounds show features of both the initial stab and the subsequent reinsertion component.

Wrinkle Wounds

The term *wrinkle wound(s)* is sometimes used to describe a situation wherein a single sweeping cut or motion of a sharp instrument contacts the skin several locations in sequence as it passes by. This may occur if the skin is folded or deeply creased, if the individual is obese, or if clothing intervenes, produces folds, or offers a variable amount of resistance.

The importance of identifying wrinkle wounds is that the number of cuts, slashes, or thrusts reported by witnesses may not match the number of wounds on the body. A similar result may occur in relation to anatomical landmarks or positions. For instance, two cuts sustained when the arm was bent at the elbow may appear distinct and separate when the patient or victim later comes to assume the arms-at-the-side position during treatment or autopsy examination.

Summary

Preservation of evidence in the clinical setting requires planning, attention to detail, and precise adherence to established policies and procedures (Hoyt, 1999). Because everyone makes mistakes, the aim is to make as few as possible and become proficient as soon as possible. Documentation failure usually has a variety of causes, including inadequate training, excessive workloads by personnel, a lack of photographic resources, and inattention to detail.

The location, size, and appearance/character of injuries must be documented before they are altered by treatment, passage of time, inflammation, and the healing process. Usually there is only one chance for accurate documentation. By the time of trial there will probably be nothing except scars on living victims, the records relating to the case, and perhaps an autopsy report reflecting postmortem findings.

Resources

Books

Anderson, W. R. (1998). *Forensic sciences in clinical medicine: A case study approach*. Philadelphia-New York: Lippincott-Raven.

Knight, B. (1997). *Simpson's forensic medicine* (11th ed.). New York: Oxford University Press.

Other Resources

Blunt force, sharp force and pattern injuries, examination, interpretation, documentation (video instruction). ANITE Group, P.O. Box 375, Pinole, CA 94564; www.projectile.com

References

Hoyt, C. A. (1999). Evidence recognition and collection in the clinical setting. *Crit Care Nurs Q*, *22*(1): 19-26.

Sheridan, D. J. (2001). Treating survivors of intimate partner abuse: forensic identification and documentation, In . J. S. Olshaker, M. C. Jackson, & W. S. Smock, *Forensic emergency medicine* (pp. 203-228). Philadelphia: Lippincott Williams & Wilkins.

Smock, W. S. (2001). Forensic emergency medicine. In J. S. Olshaker, M. C. Jackson, & W. S. Smock, *Forensic emergency medicine* (pp. 63-84). Philadelphia: Lippincott Williams & Wilkins.

Wright, R. K. (2003). Investigation of traumatic deaths. In *Forensic science: An introduction to scientific and investigative techniques*. (pp. 27-44) Boca Raton, FL: CRC Press.

Chapter 20 Gunshot Injuries

Patrick E. Besant-Matthews

Firearms

Ever since gunpowder was invented, firearms have operated faster than the eye can readily see. This has led to misleading statements and mystique, which confuses healthcare providers and hinders the evaluation of injuries. In addition, the entertainment industry often portrays people being thrown several feet and through windows by a single bullet, while the person shooting them does not move, which defies the laws of physics. The general level of understanding of missile-tissue interaction is poor.

Although there may seem to be an immense variety of weapons, for practical purposes, they can be divided, more or less, into three types: (1) handguns and submachine guns, (2) shotguns, and (3) rifles and machine guns. All firearms use gunpowder, which propels one or more missiles at a high rate of speed.

Handguns and Submachine Guns

Handguns include revolvers, semiautomatic pistols, derringers, and single-shot weapons (which accept only one cartridge at a time). Submachine guns utilize handgun ammunition, but do so in a fully automatic fashion rather than firing once for each pull of the trigger.

Shotguns

Shotguns require a separate review because of the many different wads, shot metals, shot sizes, filler materials, and components within their cartridges.

Forensic personnel must understand the basics of firearm injuries if they expect to participate in crime scene documentation and associated evidence collection. When there is a small, well-demarcated area of powder markings on the skin, and the suspect says the victim was shot from the other side of the street, one should know that the suspect is wrong or not telling the truth. Conversely, if a man comes in for treatment of a bullet graze wound on one side of the chest and has a few small stipple marks scattered over the adjacent skin after he dropped his gun on the floor, his story is believable.

Bullet Characteristics

A cartridge consists of a formed metal cylinder (commonly of a brass alloy) that is more or less closed at one end with primer mixture at the rim of the base (rimfire cartridge) or a primer cap in a recess in the center of the base (centerfire cartridge). A specified weight or charge of gunpowder is introduced through the open end. Finally, a bullet is inserted to close the opening, prevent the powder from falling out, and rendering the cartridge a self-contained unit.

When a firing pin strikes the rim of a rimfire cartridge or the centrally located primer of a centerfire cartridge, the primer mixture explodes, resulting in a small burst of flame, hot gas, and particles; this causes the main powder charge to undergo chemical change, thereby generating the gas pressure necessary to force the bullet down the barrel. It is doubtful that any normal smokeless powder charge ever burns completely. Therefore, a small, and somewhat variable, but significant percentage of the powder charge in any given cartridge is not consumed. These unburned grains, and remnants of others in various stages of consumption, follow the bullet out of the barrel, accompanied by the gray, sooty products resulting from the gunpowder that was consumed in the process of making gas.

Therefore, what an observer sees on the body surface and clothing will depend on the range of fire unless objects such as doors, furnishings, and clothing are interposed.

Following injury or death by firearms, three main items need to be evaluated and documented:

1. Range of fire
2. Relative angle of impact
3. Interposed factors (between the firearm and tissue)

Range of Fire

Range of fire is the factor that considers the distance from the barrel or muzzle of a firearm to the target. It can be considered contact (or near contact), close/short range, medium range, or long range.

The estimation of range depends on reproducing the diameter, distribution, and density of the powder marks or soot observed and described at the start of the case. Exact distances do not need to be known.

Near Contact and Contact Range

In a near contact or contact range, the weapon is very close to touching or makes actual contact with the skin and clothing. In addition to the bullet hole, powder, and soot, other features may be seen, such as the following:

- Evidence of transient heating
- Tearing of soft tissues by the gases escaping behind the bullet under pressure
- A marking to indicate that the barrel itself touched the skin as the tissues, expanded by in-rushing gases, came back on to the muzzle of the weapon. Such barrel markings may be complete enough to indicate or characterize a type of weapon (e.g., revolver versus pistol) and on rare occasions a specific make or model of weapon. Exactly what one finds will depend on a multitude of factors including barrel length, muzzle configuration, type of weapon, amount of gas (itself a function of caliber and load), and presence or absence of bone just beneath the skin (Smock, 2001) (Fig. 20-1).

Key Point 20-1

The presence of powder or soot, in addition to a bullet hole, indicates a near-contact or contact-range injury.

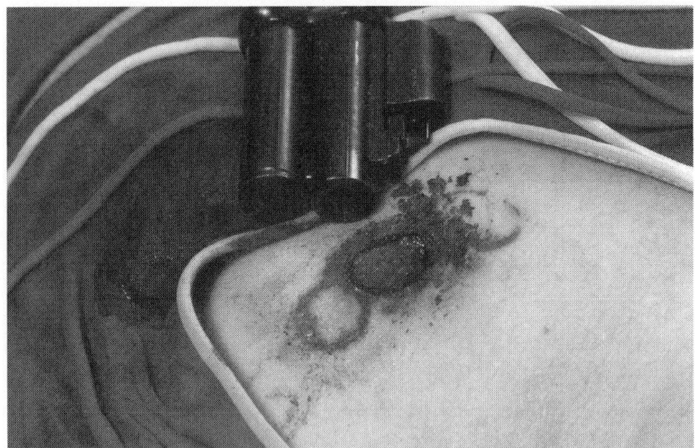

Fig. 20-1 Muzzle marking with soot and outline of tubular magazine and foresight cover, indicating that the weapon was in direct contact with the skin.

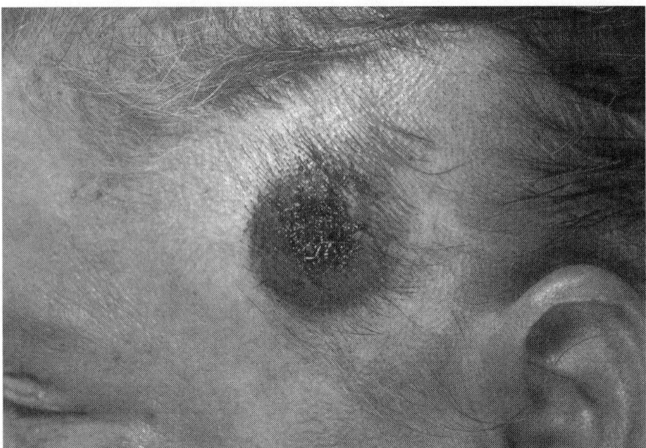

Fig. 20-2 When the muzzle of a weapon is very close to the target, a sooty residue from burned gunpowder will be deposited.

Short or Close Range

When the muzzle of the weapon comes within a few inches of the skin or clothing, one will find the bullet wound, the powder grains or powder markings called *fouling*, and an additional feature, namely the powder soot (or simply soot) produced by combustion of the gunpowder itself. The powder that was consumed in the process of producing gas gave rise to a gray sooty residue. Just as powder grains vary in size and shape, so they also vary in their burning characteristics. Some give rise to very little soot and others to far more. So it is not possible to state the exact range from an examination of soot near a wound. One can only say that it was a few or several inches, or soot would not be found. Once again, additional information and a test firing are usually required (Fig. 20-2).

Medium Range

Within the medium range, the weapon is within a few feet of the victim and not only is the bullet wound found, but there is also evidence that some gunpowder grains struck the skin or clothing with sufficient force to leave small impact marks or even to be driven partly or completely into the surface if they strike with sufficient force. Although gunpowder grains are capable of traveling many feet from a gun after firing, it is only for the first 2, 3, or sometimes 4 feet that these particles retain sufficient energy to mark the skin or stick in the weave of clothing materials. The marks will be varied, but dependent on the size and shape of the individual particles. When the gunpowder grains strike the skin with sufficient force to make marks, the aggregation of impact markings is usually called *tattooing* or *stippling*. *Speckling* or *peppering* are less frequently used but acceptable terms. Those who are detail minded may elect to use the term *stippling* for impact marks and *tattooing* for actual indriving of grains. While either term is understood, it may be an important distinction when it comes to deciding if an injury was the result of an attempted homicide or suicide (Fig. 20-3).

Modern single base (nitrocellulose) and double base (nitrocellulose with nitroglycerin) smokeless gunpowders are manufactured in discrete grains of various shapes and sizes (Rowe, 2003). There are many shapes, but for any given size and weight of grain, some will have better aerodynamic properties than others and fly more readily through the air as they leave a barrel behind a bullet. Flake powders were very common until the early to mid-1930s when ball powders were developed. With several different shapes on the market, it is desirable to know which are prevalent within a specific area. One reason is that older textbooks inaccurately state that powder from handguns is incapable of marking skin beyond about 18 to 24 inches. Generally, flake powder is still unlikely to mark skin at distances greater than about 2 feet, but ball powders may do so out to about 4 feet, with the maximum distance for

Key Point 20-2

Stippling or tattooing of the skin by gunpowder residue is characteristic of medium-range firearm injuries.

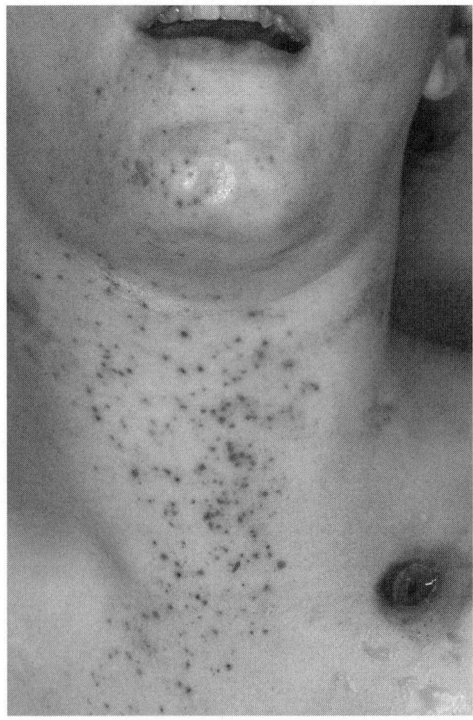

Fig. 20-3 This wound is consistent with a range of fire that is greater than 8 inches but less than 18 to 36 inches, characterized by *stippling* (small abrasions and hemorrhages) created when unburned or partially burned gunpowder strikes the skin.

flattened ball falling somewhere between. A second reason is that one must look critically at the shape and size of the markings on the skin, as they generally reflect the size and shape of the grains that made them. It is a simple mirror image or impression phenomenon. Small more or less spherical grains leave rather numerous, uniform rounded markings, whereas larger flakes give rise to fewer, larger, and more variable markings. Some grains, especially from the 22-caliber rimfire cartridges, may be small enough that the distances at which they will mark are less than might be predicted from their shape alone. Size, shape, and weight are the major determinants of their ability to fly and to strike with sufficient force to leave marks (Rowe, 2003).

Long or Distant Range

At this range, only the bullet will reach the skin and clothing. As the bullet makes contact with the skin, it causes a momentary indentation, like pressing the tip of the little finger into the soft, fleshy front part of the forearm. This is important because, for an instant, there is friction between the front and side of the bullet and those parts of the skin that are going to constitute the margins of the entrance wound. Thus, when the bullet continues inward and the surface returns to the former, nonindented, position, one should anticipate a hole, slightly smaller than the bullet, because of inherent tissue elasticity, surrounded by a narrow rim of superficial abrasion or scraping commonly called the abrasion ring or margin. The abrasion margin is due to the forward, pushing motion of the bullet–it does not result from rotation of the bullet about its longitudinal axis imparted by rifling, nor is it due to the bullet being red hot. Bullets are warm after firing, but they can be picked from the floor of a range with the fingers and they are regularly recovered by shooting into cotton wool, which is only occasionally set on fire, and even then, only by friction.

Another myth is that bullets enter with a rotary, screwlike, drilling motion. In fact, the average handgun bullet makes about 1 turn in 10, 12, 14, or 16 inches of forward movement, so even if a bullet is making 1 turn in 10 inches it will only complete $1/10 \times 1/16$ or 1/160th of a turn while passing through skin that is 1/16th of an inch thick. If an entry wound happens to lie in skin that has bone closely underlying it, the abrasion margin may be narrower and harder to see, especially with certain shapes of bullet, because the skin is not so easily indented as the bullet enters.

If the bullet is made of lead alloy, has lubricant on its surface, or if it picked up any sooty dirt as it passed down the barrel, then an additional feature known as bullet wipe or bullet wipe-off (particularly if the bullet enters through light color clothing) may be seen (Fig. 20-4). A detailed examination of skin wounds occasionally reveals the presence of traces of such dark foreign material toward the periphery of the abrasion margin where it may be known as gray ring or gray rim, but obviously bullet wipe or bullet wipe-off are sound, descriptive terms. Naturally such remnants are far less commonly present if a bullet has a clean, hard metallic jacket and came from an unsoiled barrel.

Presence of an abrasion margin or bullet wipe-off indicates that a wound is one of entry until proven otherwise. If a bullet enters a surface at right angles, then the zone of abrasion will be more or less symmetrically developed around the wound; but if it should enter at an angle, there will be far more abrasion on the side where the bullet first made contact. This knowledge is useful because unless a victim was very obese or is in a different position than when injured, the abrasion margin gives a useful preliminary and generally reliable indication of the direction in which the bullet was traveling.

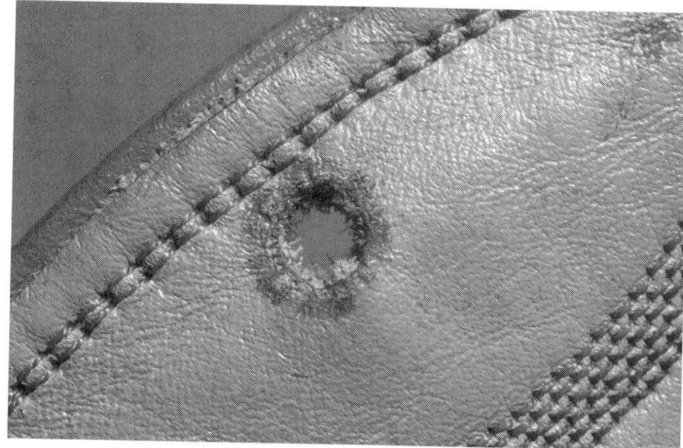

Fig. 20-4 This defect is characterized by bullet wipe or wipe-off, which appears as a grayish discoloration surrounding the perforation on the shaft of a boot.

Therefore, healthcare personnel should appreciate that the estimation of range depends on reproducing the diameter, distribution, and density of the powder marks observed and described at the start of the case.

Relative Angle of Impact

The relative angle of impact refers to the relative angular directions from/at which the bullet entered the body. Direction is best described with respect to the standard body position: standing at attention with hands open, palms to the front, and thumbs to the outside. The relative angle can be influenced by many factors, including the position of the weapon, the type of ammunition, interposed objects, and protective clothing. A wider margin of abrasion usually indicates the direction of travel from the firearm (Spitz, 1993) (Fig. 20-5).

Interposed Factors

Interposed factors refer to any observations or evidence that provides information about the weapon and the ammunition or

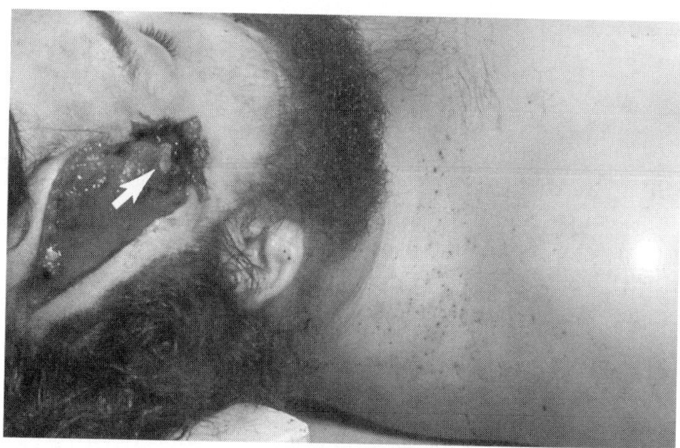

Fig. 20-5 Contact wound of head (with revolver suicide); angulation of weapon and injection of gas created scalp laceration and irregular clavicular stippling.

about any objects that may have been interposed between the gun and the victim at the time of shooting. Some are surprisingly easy to see, such as bits of clothing, wood, plaster, or metal, indicating that the bullet hit some other object before reaching the intended target.

Myths and Realities

There are many examples of inaccurate and poorly documented accounts of shooting incidents. In order to put things into perspective, it is important to understand the basics of the energy forces involved in firing a weapon, the bullet's travel to the target, and the ultimate impact upon the victim's body.

Ballistic experts and enthusiasts usually think and speak in units such as feet per second, grains of weight, and foot-pounds of energy. Unfortunately most healthcare workers are unfamiliar with these measurements. In order to appreciate the basic concept of velocity and impact force, here are some examples. Across a street or room, bullets from handguns and 22-caliber rimfire weapons typically travel about the speed of, and up to about a third faster, than a jet airliner at cruise. The kinetic energy they possess, roughly equating to 2 to 4 "ace" serves by a top tennis professional.

Clearly such bullets will not have what it takes in terms of potential to throw people off their feet, into walls, or cause individuals to behave as depicted in motion pictures. This is important because these images give false expectations, particularly if gunshot wounds are relatively uncommon in a given jurisdiction or unfamiliar to the jurors.

In general, when hit by commonplace "street" bullets, the victim will do one of the following three things:

1. Continue in the direction in which he was previously moving, less a small fraction of a foot per second
2. Fall in the direction in which he was leaning, until such time as his legs give way or muscular action of any kind, deliberate or not deliberate, causes him to do otherwise.
3. Go down immediately and perhaps exhibit some transient muscular twitching if struck in the spinal cord or most parts of the brain

Wounds: Assessment and Documentation

When watching movies, people often get a false impression of what happens when a firearm hits someone. This fact can be demonstrated in several ways. Let's look at some contrived and actual scenarios of what might happen when a bullet impacts a person to appreciate how the human body responds to the forces generated by the weapon being fired.

Some real-world examples follow:

- If a researcher were to place approximately 170 pounds of sand (the equivalent of average adult weight) into a bag, cover it with body armor, and suspend it from a rope or coil spring so that it could swing free when struck by a missile, one would be unlikely to see much action. In actuality, after the firearm is discharged and contacts the sandbag target, very little happens, perhaps a slight swinging motion of about ½ to 1 inch.
- An average-sized man floating in microgravity within an orbiting spacecraft will take about 7 to 8 seconds to drift backward 1 foot, should he absorb the entire energy of a medium-caliber handgun bullet such as from a 9-mm semiautomatic pistol. If he is heavier, it will take longer. One can calculate the momentum involved: Mass × Velocity = Mass × Velocity.
- If action and reaction are indeed equal and opposite, as taught in school, a victim should no more be thrown about or propelled by the bullet striking him than the person who was holding the weapon.
- When debriefing personnel who have shot others in the course of military or police duties, nearly all express surprise at how little effect their bullets often seemed to have, unless they have struck the brain or spinal cord.
- One needs to merely watch what happens when actual shootings are recorded on videotape during times of war and in terrorist incidents. For example, soldiers storming the beaches of Normandy on D-day were not thrown back into the English Channel by rifle and machinegun bullets. They continued to walk or run up the beach or stumble forward before they collapsed. The bullets that struck them carried far more energy of motion that the bullets commonly dealt with today.

Other false impressions perpetuated by motion pictures include the following:

- Excessive damage produced at the time of bullet impact, such as doors and walls falling down, when the usual is a small hole.
- Too much blood too soon and over too big an area. Many shooting victims have less blood on them 15 minutes after injury than in the next frame following a motion picture "shooting."
- Bullets causing great showers of sparks on impact when, in fact, production of sparks is a rarity in average circumstances. Most bullets are made of lead and copper alloys, which do not give rise to sparks.
- Incorrect relationships between the sounds of weapons discharging and the arriving bullet. For instance, a military rifle is shown being fired some distance away, but the sound is heard before the bullet arrives, when in real life it is the reverse. Wouldn't it be interesting if a hunter shot at an animal, the animal heard the sound of the rifle, and moved before the bullet arrived; or if an infantryman could take cover after he heard a shot! The reality is that the speed of sound in air at sea level standard temperature is about 1116.45 feet per second (1120.27 feet per second is used for ballistic calculations), so rifle bullets at 2800 feet per second are moving 2 to 2½ times faster than sound!

Learn to evaluate gunshot wounds means first seeing through the layer of misinformation that covers and surrounds them, blocking clear vision. Blunt injuries on a gunshot victim resulted from the fight that preceded the shooting, or from the fall, vehicle crash, or blows that followed the shooting, not from the bullet physically throwing the victim around. Other things can occur with heavy weapons in military combat, but that is not the ordinary course of events.

These facts offer several lessons:

- Books written before the 1940s are outdated when it comes to the maximum distances at which gunpowder from handguns and similar weapons is capable of marking skin. Two feet was about the maximum when powder was only made in flakes, but today one is likely to encounter newer and more aerodynamic shapes with better flight characteristics. These may mark the skin or get stuck in the clothing at distances up to 3 or 4 feet.
- Careful examination of the markings on the skin may help to determine the shape of the grains that were involved. The

situation is much the same as the sliding scraping marks of bulged, laminated windshield glass, and the small cuboid, dicelike fragments from the tempered side and rear windows that produce the markings often referred to as dicing.

- With any powder grains or particles on the skin or clothing, a sample should be collected and retained. One way to do this is to hold a strip of self-adhesive masking tape, adhesive side out, over the thumbs, and use this to pick up grains. Then, these grains should be placed over a glass slide to assist experts in subsequent range determination and other tests.
- If there were two assailants, both or several bullets exited, and the assailants used different cartridges loaded with different powders, the powder remnants may help distinguish one type of ammunition from another.
- The 2- to 4-foot range is a distance at which people struggle for control and possession of weapons.
- Something must be known about the caliber before making range estimates because there may be an associated change in grain size, especially in some of the small calibers.
- It is not possible simply to look at a zone of powder markings and estimate the exact range of fire until one has considerable experience. More information or a test firing is usually required, even by experts who are familiar with the many variables.

Entrance Wounds

A number of unfamiliar terms, although they may appear complicated, are simply an attempt on the part of a prior observer to convey the perceived relationship between the barrel and the skin or clothing at the moment of discharge. If it was concluded that the muzzle was very close to, but not actually touching, then words such as *near, close,* or *impending contact* may be used. If the barrel actually made contact, then the terms *full, tight, firm, hard,* or *press(ed) contact* are appropriate. If the barrel was not held at right angles but was inclined to the surface, words such as *angled* may appear. It is the combination of these expressions (e.g., *angled near contact* or *inclined hard contact*) that generates the apparent complexity, but in practical terms they all mean that the gun was so close to the skin and clothing that the details become largely a matter for the forensic expert. The care provider deals with a bullet traveling at top speed, plus some residues and gas under pressure.

If a partial or complete outline of the muzzle is present, this may be called *muzzle stamp, muzzle imprint, barrel abrasion,* and similar terms. It is often relatively easy to distinguish a contact wound due to a revolver from one due to a semiautomatic (auto loading) pistol. Outlines of foresights, ejector rods, slides, and similar gun parts may be clearly visible at the margins of the entry wound, either continuous with or adjacent to the barrel marking itself. Obviously such findings are highly significant and should be recorded with care, commonly by means of a diagram or sketch. They may be overlooked beneath blood and dressings.

So although the features one may see are subject to considerable variation in terms of the distance at which they occur, and not all authors use this simple system of range classification, the fundamental thing is to understand the sequence of events: at a distance bullet only, at a few feet bullet and powder, at a few inches bullet powder and soot, then finally the realm of contact. For instance, a bullet hole surrounded by a slightly enlarged and irregular abrasion with slivers of wood on the overlying shirt is in keeping with the victim standing next to a wooden door when a bullet came through it. Absence of residues on the skin combined with absence of clothing during the cold season means that the whereabouts of the clothing must be determined before any conclusions concerning range can be drawn. A gray zone resembling soot on a white T-shirt, but without a trace of gunpowder, may in fact be lead dust because a lead bullet passed through a car door as the victim stood behind it and became sprinkled with lead particles. Some bullets emitting particles or small metal fragments (e.g., copper-jacketed bullets) may be mistaken for powder particles and their impact marks.

It is not particularly significant if an investigator prefers to use a given number of inches as the dividing line between medium and close range or to subdivide the range into all sorts of complicated zones provided the proposed system makes sense and is applicable to the weapon and situation. In real life, the weapon is often unknown at the time a patient is examined or an autopsy performed, which is why a general system, which makes allowance for variation from weapons to weapon, is so practical.

If a weapon is in contact with soft tissues when it is discharged, there may be actual tearing by the propulsive gases as they leave the barrel and enter the tissues behind the bullet. How much tearing occurs will vary according to powder charge, gas volumes, gas pressure, caliber, elasticity of the tissues, how much soft tissue there is to cushion the shock, presence or absence of underlying bone, and similar factors (Smock, 2001). Contact wounds may not be torn at all or may be the width of a hand. Parts of the head may even come away if the weapon is powerful enough and the conditions are right. Exact figures for the gas pressures behind bullets as they exit the muzzle are not readily available for handguns but certainly many hundred to a few thousand pounds per square inch are reasonably common figures according to caliber, barrel length, type of powder, and powder load. Wildly exaggerated figures are often quoted for gas volumes, such as "thousands of gallons." If such fantasies were true (1) elite naval personnel would not be able to fire their weapons under water without emptying the swimming pool, dying of blast injuries, and causing great spouts of water during training exercises and (2) firing a gun in a room would result in departure of the windows, doors torn off their hinges, and eardrums ruptured by overpressure. These phenomena do not usually occur.

Suppose a person commits suicide by means of a powerful handgun (such as a .357 Magnum revolver with relatively short barrel and one of the higher-pressure cartridges). Suppose further that the barrel is held just in front of and slightly above the right external ear canal and the gun is aimed from right to left, and upward at about 30° with respect to the horizontal axis–what should one expect to see? Probably a hole in the soft tissues at the entry site about 1 to 1¼ inches diameter and extending upward from this a somewhat Y-shaped laceration of the skin extending into the scalp, measuring as much as 3 to 4 inches vertically. Sooty residues and powder grains will be visible in the entry wound with some focal pink coloration due to carbon monoxide. On the left side of the head, the exit wound will be located about 3 inches higher than the corresponding point of entry but will appear sharp edged and about ¾ inch to 1 inch in greatest dimension. Such observations are very important because this is a case in which the gas-torn wound of entry is far larger than the wound of exit, and many people wrongly believe that exit wounds are always larger than entry wounds.

Indeed, an entry wound may be larger than an exit wound for several reasons:

- Situations, such as the one discussed earlier, in which the soft tissues at the entry are torn by in-rushing gases and the exit wound is of average size, relatively far smaller.

Key Point *20-3*

Wound size should never be used as the sole determinant of entry or exit.

- When a bullet is yawing as it enters, perhaps because of striking something en route to the target or very occasionally because of insufficient longitudinal rotation imparted by rifling
- When an entire bullet enters but only a portion of it exits
- Tangential entry wounds with focal avulsion of tissue and bone
- Bullets entering through folded or creased skin but exiting through a less complicated surface
- Tangential entry wounds but less angled exits
- Combinations of the above

Wound size should never be used as the sole determinant of entry or exit. Size alone is totally unreliable and potentially very misleading. Size is just one many features that should be considered. Record the size of wounds, but decide if they are entries or exits based on their characteristics and by the "company they keep."

Entrance wounds vary widely and should be described in terms of location and appearance (Figs. 20-6 and 20-7). From a clinical standpoint, the important factors are the type of bullet and how that bullet interacts with the tissue it encounters (Silva, 1999).

Exit Wounds

Assume that a bullet is coming through the tissues and approaches a body surface. As it reaches the skin, it pushes from within and, if it has the necessary energy of motion, it will burst the skin outward producing a sharp-edged, slightly irregular wound. Such wounds are sometimes called stellate because many have a somewhat star-shaped configuration. There will be no marginal abrasion because the bullet pushed its way out, not in. The majority of simple handgun and submachine gun exit wounds are less than 1 inch in greatest dimension, some a little larger. Rotation of bullets about their longitudinal axes, induced by rifling, is only sufficient to make them stable in air and unless the bullet hits something or the circumstances are exceptional, bullets remain pointed forward and do not tumble in flight. However, it would require about 25 to 35 times (the square root of the density ratio between tissue and air) more axial/longitudinal twist to stabilize bullets in tissue, which is impractical. This means that most bullets are potentially unstable in tissue, and they will yaw and tumble eventually unless they exit before doing so, or unless the distribution of weight or their shape prevents it from happening.

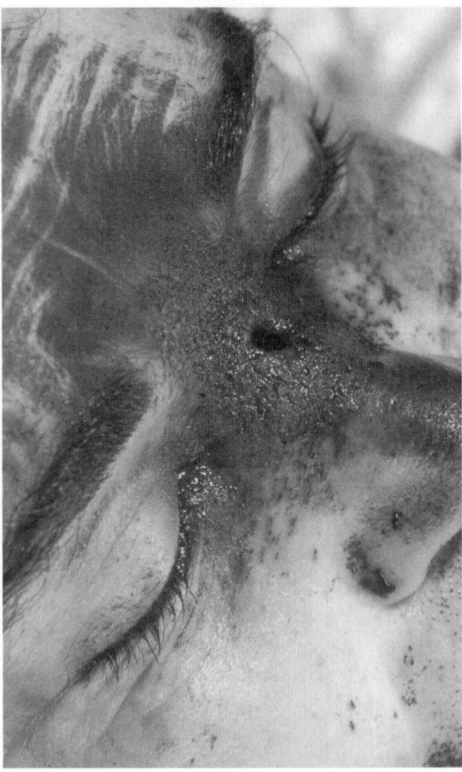

Fig. 20-6 Entrance wound at the bridge of the nose. Note heavy soot deposits and indriving of gunpowder, indicative of an entrance wound.

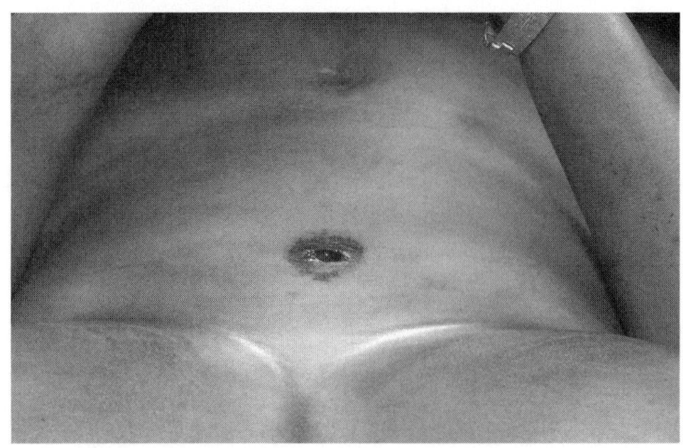

Fig. 20-7 Suicide victim with entrance wound between breasts. Notice the cylinder flare evident on both forearms.

If (1) an exit wound is produced by a bullet that was tumbling, or (2) for any reason the bullet is coming sideways through the tissues, or (3) the exit wound happened to be in a part of the body in which the skin has a fold or change of direction (buttock crease, parts of the face, underarm, groin, or umbilical areas), then the exit wound may appear elongated and slitlike. After examining gunshot wounds on a regular basis, it will only take a few weeks before one encounters an exit that appears remarkably like a stab or incised wound. This resemblance occasionally gives rise to mistaken impressions during clinical care.

Skin is tough, resilient, and equivalent in resistance to a greater thickness, perhaps a few inches, of muscle or liver, so it is not uncommon to find bullets beneath the skin, more or less on the opposite side of the body from which they entered. It is always worth scrutinizing and actually making a point of feeling the body surface for any signs of slight bulging, fluctuant bleeding into the subcutaneous tissues, or a hard lump that may represent a bullet. This can be very helpful both during clinical treatment and in making initial assessments before x-rays have been taken because the vast majority of "street" bullets pass through the body in a slightly curved or more or less straight line path unless they ricochet due to striking bone or other obstructions in their pathway.

A typical entry wound, then, is rounded or elliptical with marginal abrasion, sometimes with bullet wipe, whereas a typical exit wound has sharp edges, is outwardly bursting in nature, and is sometimes elongated (Fig. 20-8).

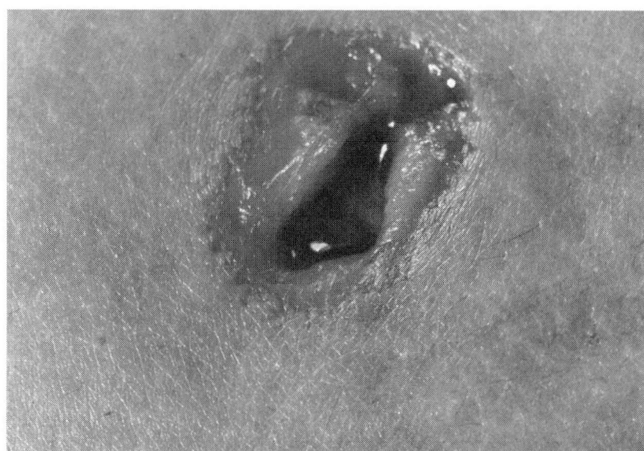

Fig. 20-8 Atypical "shored up" exit wound. Note the irregular pattern abrasion and elongated wound.

Shored or Supported Exit Wounds

There are circumstances and conditions that can cause confusion and are exceptions to these guidelines–for example, whenever a bullet emerges through an area of skin that is sufficiently supported by something. Chairs, car seats, mattresses and bedding, clothing, articles in pockets, floors, walls, and doors are common supporting objects. In such circumstances, the skin surrounding the exit wound is apt to be forced outward, in effect squeezed or slapped against the supporting surface by the emerging bullet, which often leads to the formation of a zone of abrasion at the margins of the exit. Any such abrasion results from a cause totally unrelated to a bullet having forced its way inward; however, such features may be mistaken for wounds of entry. In fact, when such wounds are examined critically, many will exhibit a mixture of entry and exit characteristics with entry often appearing to predominate at first glance.

Identification

The usual indication that the wound was a shored (as in shored-up or supported) exit is that the abrasion is irregular at its edges, lopsided, too large, or simply doesn't make sense because it is not in keeping with the shape of an entering bullet (even one that is distorted or tumbling). Such features help forensic experts and other skilled observers to ascertain that a victim was on or adjacent to a surface such as a floor or seat when shot. Occasional shored exits can be difficult to distinguish from entry wounds, for instance, when it is cold and many layers of clothing are being worn, but then the situation should immediately be clarified by examining the clothing. It is possible to have more than one exit defect associated with a single bullet entry because of fragmentation, separation of bullet jacket from core, displacement of bone fragments, and so on.

Fortunately there is yet another directional characteristic–the fashion in which bone chips or breaks when struck by a bullet. The appearance is similar to the behavior of glass when it is chipped by a bullet or small stone. If glass remains sufficiently intact to examine, the entry side will appear sharp edged and relatively small whereas the exit side will be sloping and larger. That is, a cone-shaped chip is produced and the defect tapers, becoming larger in the direction in which the bullet was traveling (the apex or point of the cone points back to the origin of the bullet). There are many areas within the body where this works consistently and well, including the skull, sternum, pelvis, ribs, and almost any relatively flat bone of sufficient thickness. Unfortunately, there are some locations (including parts of the facial bones, supraorbital plates, metacarpals, and metatarsals) where it may not prove helpful because the bone in these locations is so thin that it is often impossible to read the bevel even with the aid of a dissecting microscope. The same chipping, beveling effect may also be observed in teeth, dentures, thumbnails, and other items of suitable consistency on and about the body (Rowe, 2003).

The Skull

There are, as is so often true, a few initially perplexing situations such as when a bullet makes tangential contact with a curved surface such as the skull. If this occurs, one may observe chipping in both directions because the bone that is struck first chips inward, then the surface subsequently contacted chips outward, producing what some refer to as a keyhole wound. Likewise, when a bullet passes through windshield glass, separation of fragments at the margin of the outer or inner glass layer can simulate reverse beveling. One must look closely and correlate all the findings.

Unusual Situations

In addition to these basic rules, the occasional difficult or unusual situation may crop up. For instance, a bullet might pass through something substantial (window, vehicle, door, crate, plywood, drywall, furniture, thick shoe sole) en route to the body or exit one body part and reenter another that was in contact with it. In such circumstances, the usual guidelines may appear to have failed, even if they have not. In the latter case, the slapping of skin against skin can produce abrasions around the primary exit and the reentry, or one or other may appear like a slit. However, as soon as the basics are understood, one knows when something doesn't look right.

It is also possible to encounter cases in which a surgeon altered bone at the entry or exit wounds while trying to save the victim's life. Most surgeons will not notice, and therefore fail to document the direction of chipping. Generally, however, bone is very helpful. Fractures propagate through bone much faster than all common bullets travel, therefore it is occasionally possible to determine which of two holes was made first (or if the victim was struck and then shot in contradistinction to shot and then struck) because of the way in which the fractures associated with each injury intersect.

Best Practice *20-1*

Do not determine that wounds are entrance wounds or exit wounds. Confine the description to the location and characteristics of the wound

Examination and Documentation of Clothing

Preservation, examination, and retention of the clothing must be emphasized and regarded as a priority in all gunshot cases. Without clothing, it may not be possible to ascertain the range of fire. If a weapon is discharged in the vicinity of thick clothing during cold weather, the residues are most likely to be on the outermost clothing, not on the skin (in the course of which it is common for clothing to be indiscriminately cut off or torn away). Clothing should not be cut away or torn through the bullet hole if it can be avoided; instead clothing should be cut between, around, or at a distance from the bullet hole. Improper handling makes subsequent examinations in the crime laboratory that much more difficult. Likewise, if part of the head hair adjacent to a wound is removed during treatment, it should be preserved for gunshot residue analysis.

Best Practice *20-2*

Save all body tissue fragments, hair, clothing, and physical debris associated with gunshot wounds and preserve them in the same manner as other forensic evidence.

Gunshot Residues

The previous discussion brings us to the various residues and how they are used in range determination. Firearm or gunshot residues fall into two main categories: those normally visible and those that are not. The basic understanding of visible residues associated with gunpowder was discussed earlier. If nothing can be seen with the unaided eye or with a magnifier, then state so. It does not mean that the police laboratory cannot, by means of sophisticated instrumentation or methodology, find some minute traces of something at a later time. The statement "absence of visible residues" means to the best of one's ability, in the prevailing circumstances, no residue was discernable. If powder grains, grain markings, or a combination of these with soot were found, then they should be documented by the character, distribution, and size of the areas involved in relation to the point at which the bullet entered. Only then (perhaps weeks, months, or even years later) will it be possible for the laboratory staff to compare their test patterns to these findings and thereby estimate the range of fire. The better and more informative the description, the more accurate the conclusion can be.

As distances increase, the grains lose their ability to strike with sufficient force and they may just remain capable of marking skin but not the paper, cardboard, or other target substituted for skin in the laboratory. Thus, there is a danger that, if there is insufficient mutual understanding and communication between the examining clinician or pathologist and the lab personnel, significant and potentially embarrassing differences of interpretation can arise, which may not become apparent until trial. If a person is shot into a certain type of clothing, an identical material is tested; however, skin cannot be tested the same way. So testers resort to target enhancement, using carbon paper, thin layers of plastic, or other such means, in selected cases. Gunpowder grains can mark skin through clothing in certain instances. For example, when heavier weapons are fired at fairly short distances (up to a foot or so) with certain powders, grains may be driven through thin clothing (e.g., a single layer of a blouse or a shirt) or mark the skin through it.

Primer Mixture

Important but invisible residues are derived from the primer mixture, not from the gunpowder. Modern primers contain a number of substances, and in the momentary intense heat of detonation, minute particles containing lead, barium, and antimony are formed, resolidify, and come to rest on the skin or clothing. These can be seen and photographed, even analyzed, with a scanning electron microscope. Most of these minute particles only travel short distances in the gas cloud and beyond about 3 to 6 inches are seldom present in sufficient numbers for anything but a scanning electron microscope to detect. They may be removed from the skin by any action or process that would remove talcum powder, such as wiping, rubbing, washing, putting the hands in pockets, or doing ordinary things for a few hours. It is for this reason that a paper bag (not plastic because of subsequent internal condensation of skin moisture) should be carefully placed over the hands of any victim of recent gunshot wound to protect them until the police or a forensic scientist can obtain specimens for primer residue tests by whatever method is in use.

Because scanning electron microscopy is relatively time consuming and expensive, other methods may be used whenever large numbers of gunshot cases are being processed. For instance, one effective technique is swabbing the appropriate portions of the backs and palms of both hands with 5% analytical grade nitric acid and then quantitating the trace metals by means of flameless atomic absorption spectrophotometry. Firearm examiners must use special techniques to visualize gunshot residue on dark, bloodstained clothing (Rowe, 2003).

The methods vary according to needs, budgets, demands, skills, and available technology. Remember that a positive finding is meaningful but that a negative only means that no metals characteristic of primer residues were detected.

Absence of primer residues may imply the following:

- Residues might never have been present.
- Residues might have been present but then removed or reduced below the critical threshold of methodology.
- Residues were not sought out in timely fashion.
- The cartridge primer might not have contained all three metals, especially in the case of some 22-caliber rimfire primers. Because of attempts to reduce the amount of lead in the environment, other metals such as zinc and manganese may be found in some primer mixtures.
- Residues might have been deliberately removed.
- Not all those who fire a weapon will test positive for primer residues even if tested immediately after firing. The type of weapon has considerable bearing on the probability. In lab tests, only about half of those firing handguns might be negative for residues by flameless atomic absorption spectrophotometry (FAAS). All things being equal, those who shot revolvers should test positive more often than those who operated pistols because of cylinder flare (gases leaking between the cylinder and barrel of a revolver). With rifles and shotguns, only a few might test positive according to the condition of the weapons and the methods used.

For these and other reasons, gunshot residue tests may not be performed as often or in the way they once were. However, prompt, careful examination of the hands is essential in any case of injury by firearms because the circumstances of injury are often unknown at the time of treatment.

Other chemical and physical tests are used to detect invisible metal particles and nitrogen compounds on clothing, bedding, and other objects. Most good books on criminalistics are likely to contain information about them with their practical applications and limitations.

Powder Burns

A potential source of misunderstanding is the expression *powder burns*. In fact, the term is outdated and should not be used on a regular basis. From the time of its invention until about 1890, gunpowder was made of entirely different ingredients than it is today. Black powder, as the old kind is commonly known, is a mechanical mixture of about 15 parts charcoal, 75 parts potassium nitrate, and 10 parts sulfur. It is still used in punt guns, line throwers, signaling flares, blank rounds, and antique weapons, but is almost never used in modern cartridges and firearms of the kind used on the street. When a weapon charged with black powder is fired there is considerable muzzle flash and large amounts of white smoke appear.

In the days when clothing consisted entirely of natural fibers, it wasn't unusual to sear or focally ignite the clothing at shorter distances. This is how the term *powder burns* originated. Today, small arms are usually loaded with single (about 90% to 99% nitrocellulose), double (about 50% to 85% nitrocellulose plus 20% to 45% nitroglycerin), or even triple base smokeless powders.

Bullet Design and Types of Guns

Bullet Design

Weapons generally discharge bullets that are made of lead or of a lead core partially or completely covered by a jacket that is almost always made of a harder metal than the core itself. Jackets are often made of a copper alloy, but many other alloys and materials have been used ranging from aluminum to steel and plastic. Some bullets that appear jacketed are not made by forcing a lead core into separately formed jackets but instead are made of lead that is then plated with quite a thick layer of copper or brass material known as a "wash" or "coat," which serves the same function. Many designs and types of bullet exist, and therefore the type of bullet recovered is potentially meaningful to the firearm expert and to the disposition of justice. It is important to keep bullets from different wounds separated from one another, unless this is impossible by virtue of two bullets coming to rest side by side in the same location, perhaps in an accumulation of blood in part of a body cavity.

Centerfire Rifles

Centerfire rifles operate in the same general fashion as rifles but are more powerful. The numbers, including gas pressures, bullet weights, and velocities, are significantly greater, and rifles are effective at far greater distances than are handguns and submachine guns. Accurate shooting at several hundred yards is commonplace. Muzzle velocities in a few commercial calibers are as much as 4000 feet per second from the muzzle, but initial velocities in the range of 2100 to 3700 feet per second are more usual. Bullet weights range between about 0.05 to 1.15 ounces with a few even greater. Exit pressures are often approximately several thousand pounds per square inch and sometimes far more. The momentum and kinetic energy of a bullet varies according to its mass (weight in our daily terms) and velocity, so higher velocity mean that rifle bullets possess considerably more energy of motion than do bullets from handguns and submachine guns, therefore inflicting more injury.

Intermediate Weapons

Between handguns and submachine guns, there are weapons that are intermediate in terms of their power and performance. Some are known as carbines, a rifle of short length and light weight originally designed for mounted troops. A modern example of such a weapon is the US 30-caliber M1 carbine, which was developed in World War II as a combat improvement to the 45-caliber semiautomatic pistol. There are also a few special-purpose, single-shot handguns, some of which are chambered for a variety of large handgun and rifle cartridges, which fall into this intermediate group. Although firearms and their injuries tend to fall into categories according to type and caliber, there is a continuum from the smallest to the largest, and injuries do not increase in a stepwise fashion.

Rifle injuries are not radically different from other gunshot wounds. In fact, it is the different wounding mechanisms and the addition of features such as a considerable amount of bullet fragmentation that make the difference.

Firearm Wounds: Mechanics and Characteristics

The internal effects of bullets are frequently misunderstood. The potential of a bullet goes into many things including the following:

- Crushing, punching, and tearing
- Stretching and splashing
- Friction
- Heating
- Various combinations of bullet distortion, expansion, and fragmentation
- Imparting slight motion to the target
- Generation of sound waves
- Exiting and striking something else
- Rotation about the longitudinal axis

Therefore, most of the energy eventually ends up as heat and the potential of a bullet cannot all be devoted to producing injury. This simple fact is all too often ignored.

In practical terms, there are two major interactions between bullet and body:

1. *Crushing, punching, and tearing of tissue due to physical passage of the bullet itself.* This corresponds approximately to the size, configuration, and attitude of the bullet as it penetrates. The inherent elasticity of some tissues results in some measure of restitution of the walls of the track along which a bullet passed, but it is the crush/punch/tear combination that produces most of the so-called permanent cavity seen at the time of surgery or autopsy.
2. *Stretching or splashing.* As a bullet passes through tissue, it leaves a momentary wake or splash, akin to a boat speeding across, or a stone thrown into, water. This effect is also known as temporary cavitation.

Water closes in behind a boat or a stone as the ripples spread. Tissue behind a bullet behaves in similar fashion; however, tissues are not perfectly elastic and the end result of momentary stretching depends largely on the nature of the tissue involved. Momentarily stretch a loop of small intestine containing only gas and the result is usually a hole about the size of the bullet, but stretch a congested friable spleen and the result will be a zone of shattered, mushy tissue. Other tissues behave in accordance with their structure and consistency. Lung and muscle often exhibit bullet holes surrounded by zones of bruising and hemorrhage.

Therefore, when looking at a wound, two things should be kept in mind: (1) the path along which the bullet passed and (2) the variable amount of splashing and stretching along the tissue margins where the bullet is passing. Wound ballistics (a part of terminal ballistics) is the study of the combination of these two effects, in other words, a study of the missile-tissue interaction.

Sonic Pressure Waves

When a bullet strikes tissue, a sonic pressure (sound) wave travels ahead of the bullet in the tissues. Various ill effects have been ascribed to this reaction, but the duration is exceedingly short, so short that there is no time for significant tissue displacement to occur. It has not, to the knowledge or satisfaction of many experts, been proven that this produces any significant ill effects. After all, medical science uses concentrated sound waves for diagnosis (ultrasound) and many minutes of focused shock waves (from a lithotriptor) to break up kidney and gallstones without soft tissue damage. Part of this disagreement may be because some articles confuse and fail to distinguish between (1) splash/stretch, known as temporary cavitation, and (2) sonic pressure/sound waves.

Correlation between Type of Gun and Injury Caused

Then, of course, differences in injuries are brought about by bullet behavior and in particular by the occurrence or nonoccurrence of fragmentation. The damage caused by a bullet is directly associated with its intended purpose. For example, most military bullets are intended to remain intact and cause casualties. These bullets are better able to pass through doors, windows, and vehicles. Casualties are desirable from the standpoint of an opponent. Civilian hunting ammunition, however, is intended to stay within the game animal, not only for safety, but to induce maximum damage and kill the animal.

There are exceptions both ways–for instance, the M-193 bullets from the US M-16A1 combat rifle, which often fragment, and bullets for elephant and cape buffalo, which must remain relatively undistorted if they are to penetrate deeply enough. The very fact that some bullets fragment in tissue and others do not is the source of part of the confusion and is potentially hazardous in the ballistic and medical literature in the last quarter of the twentieth century. The forensic nurse should remain skeptical and apply strict scientific methodology.

Classic Errors and Myths

Some classic errors are summarized below:

- *Believing that velocity is the sole determinant of injury.* If this were true, the initial portions of wounds would be larger and more significant than the parts produced after bullets have slowed down.
- *Relying on scientific articles that have been centered around loss of bullet energy, based on the difference between velocity at entry and exit, but which ignored loss of weight due to bullet fragmentation.* Thus, the presumed weight(s) at exit and the calculations based on them are invalid.
- *Drawing conclusions concerning fragment behavior and position based on studies using x-rays taken only in a single plane.* Fragments were assumed to lie in one part of a wound when in fact they were somewhere else altogether.
- *Concluding that bullets above a certain speed are unstable in flight and tumble end over end.* If this were so, weapons would lack accuracy, many military bullets would be unable to enter their targets, streamlining bullets by making them pointed would be a total waste of time, and thin "witness" sheets placed along their flight paths would show elongated as opposed to rounded holes.
- *Assuming that energy delivery equates to severity of injury.* It cannot because the specified amount of bullet energy might be delivered into clothing, a thick layer of body wall fat, or muscle, with a far lesser amount to vital areas such as the heart and great vessels.
- *Expecting the human body to react the same way other objects would react to impact.* Shooting bullets into watermelons and cans of water may look impressive, but neither relate to, or constitute part of, the human body. The body does not contain as high a percentage of water, as do melons, and does contain a large amount of connective tissue, which prevent the human body from splattering all over the floor.
- *Forgetting that terms often have different meanings in parts of the world.* For instance, "high velocity" may mean faster than sound in one country but imply 2000 feet per second elsewhere. Simply stating the velocity in feet or meters per second avoids the problems arising from nonscientific terms.

Unfortunately, the dissemination of such erroneous information can also be to the disadvantage of injured patients. A victim may be brought in saying he has been shot with a rifle whereupon a surgeon, largely unfamiliar with such wounds, immediately envisions dire internal consequences and proceeds to remove more tissue than is actually justified. Fortunately, medical and surgical treatment are well covered elsewhere in the literature.

Bullet-Tissue Interaction

The injuries found in a patient or a victim at autopsy depend largely on the bullet-tissue interaction. Therefore, the particular combination of crush/punch/tear (permanent cavity) and splash/stretch (temporary cavity)–unless propulsive gases happen also to be involved–is crucial for correctly understanding injuries. All bullets tear a track, but some, by virtue of different energy of motion, construction, and behavior after impact, produce more temporary cavitation than others. Most handgun and submachine gun bullets cause injury mainly by crush/punch/tear with some stretch/splash. Rifle bullets also crush/punch/tear but often have significantly more splashing/stretching, plus fragmentation to take into account. This is why some rifle calibers have at times been regarded as unduly injurious. Indeed, when the effects of cavitation were first encountered, some armed forces were even accused of using exploding bullets (Fig. 20-9).

To be effective for law enforcement or combat purposes, there must be the following:

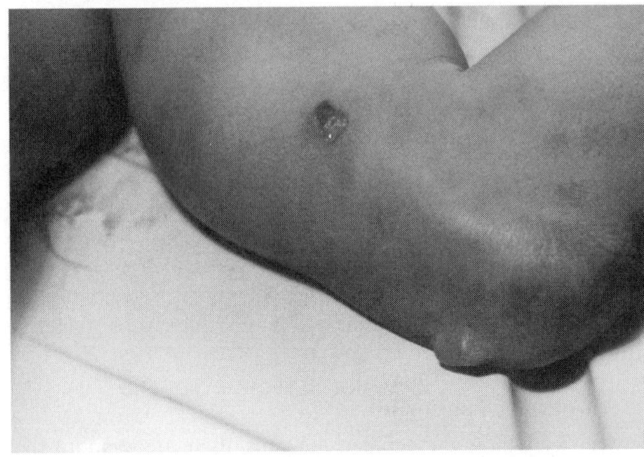

Fig. 20-9 Wadcutter bullet lodged just under the skin at the elbow.

- Sufficient depth of penetration to reach a vital organ
- A large enough hole in a vital organ
- Suitable placement of the shot

Guns Fired into the Air

Guns fired into the air constitute yet another cause of speculation and source of misinformation. The key is to distinguish clearly between two situations:

- Guns are fired upward at very steep angles, so that the bullets eventually come to a halt and then fall back to earth. Common handgun bullets take about 9 to 14 seconds to go up and about 16 to 26 seconds to fall. When they approach the ground, they are only falling at about 130 to 250 feet per second, which is close to the speed at which bullets are able to penetrate skin. Thus, some will bounce off and others will cause a superficial wound. Serious injury seldom results from shooting handguns into the air. Rifle bullets, however, fall faster and thus stand a slightly greater chance of causing injury, but they are not particular threatening.
- Guns are fired at high angles but at an elevation such that the bullets move in a high arcing trajectory and retain some of their forward velocity. This can and sometimes does cause serious injury or death.

Radiological Examination

Always x-ray gunshot victims if equipment and circumstances permit because x-rays diminish chances of error in wound assessment and prediction of resultant organ and tissue injury. X-rays constitute part of the documentation and show the situation existing before the victim was opened or altered surgically. At least one lateral view is needed to show depth of penetration and distribution of fragments if there are any (Fig. 20-10). X-rays are vital adjuncts to wound evaluation because they demonstrate the following:

- How many bullets or fragments there are
- Where bullets and fragments came to rest
- The nature and extent of injuries

By accurately showing the exact site of a resting bullet, x-rays reduce inadvertent and further tissue damage induced by probing for a bullet that may have been lodged in deep tissue or have impacted bone. X-rays also locate bullets, or parts thereof, that may have traveled in the flow of blood and lodged at a different location (bullet emboli).

X-rays also reveal any separation of jackets from cores. Taking x-rays is particularly important if something exited. It could have been a core by itself, meaning that the jacket, which bears the land and groove impressions from the rifling, can still be present inside the victim. Radiographic films also characterize some types of bullets by their terminal behavior. About 10 to 20 types of ammunition have fairly typical appearances, and in some instances, x-rays may also characterize or suggest certain weapons.

Other benefits of x-rays are that they help to do the following:

- Reveal unsuspected ("old") bullets from previous shooting episodes, both wartime and civilian.
- Locate occult or unsuspected wounds if, for instance, a bullet should enter through the open mouth or ear canal.
- Reveal injuries when the body surface is altered or obscured. It is not unusual for criminals to kill, rob, and then set fire to a building. If the body surface is hard to examine for any reason, be sure to take x-rays.

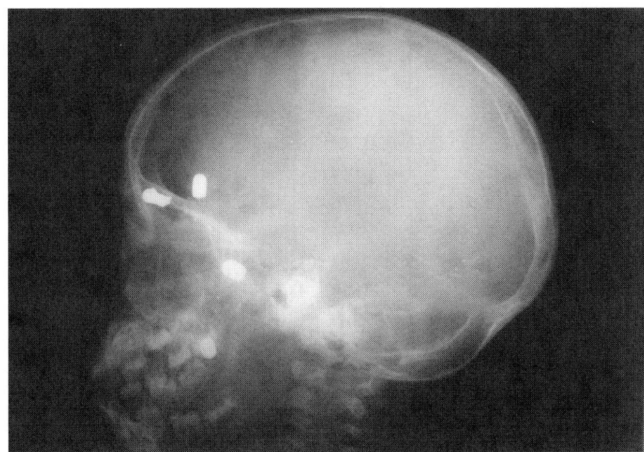

Fig. 20-10 X-ray of a skull showing bullets lodged in the frontal region.

- Reveal the presence of intervening objects when bullets enter through objects such as zip fasteners, jewelry, and spectacle frames, or drive small coins into the tissues.
- Locate bullets and bullet fragments in bloody clothing.
- Disclose how many significant fragments are present if a bullet is no longer intact.

There are rare instances when a bullet is almost stopped by the edge of body armor and produces a superficial wound that looks serious enough, but then the bullet may be pulled out by some remaining strands of Kevlar. A small piece of metal in the x-ray, on the underlying bone or in the tissue, proves how the injury was produced, even though the treating physician may be unable to explain what happened.

Simple x-rays, however, will not permit immediate determination of caliber (because of projection distortion or possible bullet deformation) and will not prove the direction of travel of a bullet (possible internal deflection without fragmentation). In addition, certain alloys such as aluminum bullet jackets may show up poorly or not at all. Likewise, the direction in which a bullet is pointing after it has come to rest is not a reliable indication of its initial direction because of the inherent instability of most bullets in tissues and the tendency of many to come to rest in the reversed position.

In the autopsy setting, if getting x-rays proves difficult (for instance, through inability to take a decomposed body into the local hospital), don't overlook local veterinarians. They are highly skilled and often equipped to x-ray large animals in difficult circumstances.

Healthcare personnel should do the following:

- Always look carefully at the hands of any shooting victim for features such as abrasions, visible gunpowder, or soot
- Be sure to maintain a legally sufficient chain of custody, possession, or evidence for all bullets
- Always glance at bullets before packaging them in case they show something helpful. For example, if one appears to have struck bone and the preliminary examination only disclosed a flesh wound of the thigh, something was overlooked.
- When removing bullets from tissues, use only gloved fingertips or forceps with tips protected by rubber tubing or pads to prevent making any marks on the bullet that might interfere with crime lab procedures. Metal on metal can

unintentionally leave markings that can confuse ballistic specialists when they attempt to determine the exact weapon used in the crime under investigation. Bullets should be placed in a padded, clean receptacle to avoid additional defects. Do not wash the bullet or place it into formalin or other fluids because this is likely to displace any hair, fiber, or other evidence from the bullet's surface.

- If the patient dies soon after being injured, cover the hands with paper bags to protect any primer residues or other evidence that might be present.
- Be sure to save the clothing for the medical examiner, coroner, or police, as the case may be. If it is wet or bloody, air-dry it before packaging. Obtain packing instructions from the medical examiner, coroner, or police laboratory.
- Do not cut away clothing through the gunshot holes unless absolutely necessary. Doing so makes the job of the forensic pathologist and criminalist more difficult.

Best Practice *20-3*

Care of the living always comes first, but while attempting to save life, see to it that a minimum of damage is done to the evidence that other care providers and agencies (state and local police, medical examiner/coroner, federal agency) will need if they are to do their job effectively.

Wound Documentation

The documentation of wounds is a vital detail for the forensic nurse to understand. Following is a checklist that, if properly completed, should ensure the gathering of all necessary information. Note that this is the full list, such as would be used in the course of an autopsy, and it must therefore be modified for use in the case of a living patient. Nevertheless, this is the kind of information that experts will require if they are to help make interpretations or back up the findings when legal action or a trial begins. The fact is that much of the information can be obtained in the course of treatment or during surgery. Don't worry if one or more of the following items must be omitted in a living person. Simply do the best in the prevailing circumstances. At the very least, for each wound, note the following:

- Location
- Dimension
- Character

Location and Dimension of Wound

Note the location of the center of the entry wound with respect to fixed landmarks such as the midline, the top of the head, the base of the heels, the external ear canal, and so on. Report these dimensions in whichever units are most familiar to police, judges, and jurors. Some countries use centimeters and others inches. If in doubt, consider using both. If measuring around any curvature of the body, be sure to make this clear or else a wound reported as being 5.5 inches to the left of the front midline of the face may sound as if it is somewhere in space to the left side of the head. Measure to the center of wounds, not to their edges because as soon as more than one wound is present the distances from one to another won't add up without extraordinary organizational and mathematical effort. It's also easier to calculate angles.

Character of Wound

The size and description of the entrance wound and any adjacent features other than stippling and powder soot must be recorded. Make annotations regarding the condition of clothing at the site. Note any visible gunshot residues, stippling, and soot on the skin or clothing. If there is none, state this in the documentation. If present, specify the character, overall dimensions, and distribution in relation to the line along which the bullet entered. If powder particles are seen, they can be picked up with an adhesive aid such as a Post-It note and placed in a sealed envelope.

The x-ray appearance of the involved body parts should be documented, noting bullets or significant fragments. To appreciate anything beyond simply the location of an intact bullet, obtain x-rays in two or more planes.

The track and resulting injuries, best described in the direction and sequence in which the bullet traveled, are vital factors to be recorded. Include the amount of blood evacuated from cavities and other findings that will inevitably be relevant, such as major nerve damage and the size of holes in critical organs such as the heart and great vessels. Without these data, it will be difficult, if not impossible, to answer questions at a later date concerning incapacitation, rate of loss of consciousness, pain and suffering, chances of survival if treated sooner, and so forth. Be sure to integrate the description into a coherent whole. Avoid making classic errors such as putting parts of injuries elsewhere under some other description. For instance, putting the entry wound at the beginning of a report and the injury to the liver elsewhere allows easier comprehension if there are several wounds in a single victim. Fragmented description also creates problems when testifying. Having the wound description in proper order in one part of the report, under a heading such as "Evidence of Injury" or simply "Injury," makes things easy when asked to describe the findings. Another error in simple cases is to assign different numbers to each entry and exit wound or to call the first bullet recovered "number one" even though it was recovered from the second wound described. A few such organizational errors and nobody will understand. The essence of good report writing is to recognize that almost no one who reads it will have medical training. Therefore, the clearer the report is, the fewer phone calls and requests for clarification there will be.

In the early stages of documenting internal features of injury, it is preferable to err a little on the side of detail because this will help an expert to assist with wound interpretation at a later date should the need arise. This usually occurs when the prosecution claims a deliberate shooting and the defense an accidental stray shot. With good reporting, the details of injury permit evaluation of bullet behavior, from which velocity and thereby estimates of probable range can be derived. If in doubt, draw the wound profile on a piece of squared paper (in approximate diameters and features along the length of the wound track).

The place(s) at which the bullet or its major parts were recovered and the greatest depth of penetration should be documented too. Be certain to mention any fragments that were recovered, their appearance, and how they were preserved or conveyed to the police or responsible agency. Do not state an exact caliber or manufacturer. Simply measure, weigh, or photograph the bullet for documentation. Do look at the bullet for the possible presence of foreign material or unusual markings such as evidence of ricochet before handing it over. Learn how to mark and package a bullet. Establish and preserve legal chain of custody/possession of the evidence, noting the date and time and obtaining a signature with each transfer. Any failure or procedural error or omission will be brought out in court, in almost theatrical fashion, with impressive flourish.

Annotate the location and description of the exit wound, if any, and the approximate distance, if it can be measured, from entry to exit. Indicate the condition of the clothing at the exit.

Check for the possibility of residues in, on, or adjacent to the exit wound and clothing. Occasionally residues are blown from a contact wound along the entire length of a wound track, especially in smaller body parts and in children. It is also possible for the entry of another wound to be located near the exit being described, when a comment to ensure clarity and separation of unrelated features is called for.

The direction from which the bullet entered and traveled is vital to investigations. This is best recorded with respect to the standard anatomic position in all three axes. If a bullet entered the front of the right shoulder and continued in virtually a straight line to exit the back of the left shoulder, the trajectory would be described as being from right to left, slightly from front to back and horizontal. In the event the bullet should have entered in one direction and then after some distance deviated for any reason, the initial angle of entry should be noted and distinguished from the subsequent direction.

Forensic examiners seldom know what position a person was in at the moment of injury and it is only later, perhaps in court, that various possibilities and scenarios will be proposed by council. Good notes allow the examiner to state if the findings are consistent with theories or otherwise.

Add any other notes that are necessary. For instance, if numerous spotty skin lesions or petechial hemorrhages (or, on the dead victim, marks made by insects) are found adjacent to an entry wound, a comment regarding their presence and specifically that they do not represent powder grain impact markings is essential. Such information is easy to document at the time; otherwise, in the event that the photographs don't turn out too well or that the color film was inadvertently developed as black and white, there could be a problem explaining the markings at trial. Mark the various wounds on an outline diagram of a body, and it is a good idea to make a simplified diagram part of the chart. In this way, police, attorneys, judges, and jurors will be able to understand the essentials of the case at a glance. If unskilled with a camera, see to it that photographs are taken for the record.

If unsure whether the wound was one of entry or exit, or if it isn't necessary to make such a determination, simply call each a "wound" or "perforation" of the skin, and record its location, dimension, and appearance, leaving the direction unspecified (Smock, 2001). Good notes provide the data for someone who understands the subject.

Summary

Forensic personnel must realize that oversimplification and assumptions regarding ballistics may compromise legal proceedings. Preservation of evidence and documentation are vital responsibilities of healthcare personnel (Russell & Noguchi, 1999). It may not be possible to obtain every item of information, even when the clinician is highly trained and experienced. The forensic nurse must simply do the best job possible, following guidelines for assessment and documentation of all forensic evidence, with considerable attention paid to the wound itself, noting the location, dimensions, and characteristics.

Case Study 20-1 Determining Range of Fire

An individual, under the influence of crack cocaine, starts a fight with two law enforcement officers and ends up being shot in the back. Questions are asked, an inquiry held, and someone asks that his shirt be examined for gunshot residues. Both visible (gunpowder and soot) and invisible (primer) residues should be examined in order to estimate the range of fire. One version of events was that he was shot deliberately from about 8 feet after he had given up and had raised his hands above his head. The other story is that he was just getting up off the ground holding a gun wrested from one officer when he was shot at close range by the other. If his arms were raised in surrender, the hole should be relatively lower in the shirt than in his back.

Resources

Books

Gunshot Wounds

Anderson, W. R. (1998). *Forensic sciences in clinical medicine: A case study approach* (pp. 71-94). Philadelphia-New York: Lippincott-Raven.

DiMaio, V. (1985). *Gunshot wounds.* New York: Elsevier Science.

Knight, B. (1997). *Simpson's forensic medicine* (11th ed., pp. 66-71). New York: Oxford University Press.

Olshaker, J., Jackson, C., & Smock, W. (2001). *Emergency forensic medicine* (pp. 64-73). Philadelphia: Lippincott Williams & Wilkins.

Shotgun Wounds

Anderson, W. R. (1998). *Forensic sciences in clinical medicine: A case study approach* (pp. 89-791, 211-213). Philadelphia: Lippincott-Raven.

DiMaio, V. J. M. (1999). *Gunshot wounds: Practical aspects of firearms, ballistics, and forensic techniques* (2nd ed.). Boca Raton, FL: CRC Press.

Knight, B. (1997). *Simpson's forensic medicine* (11th ed., pp. 66-68). New York: Oxford University Press.

Additional Reading

Fackler, M. L. (1986).Ballistic injury. *Ann Emerg Med, 15,* 1451-1455.

Fackler, M. L. (1987). Bullet performance misconceptions. *Int Defense Rev, 20,* 369-370.

Fackler, M. L. (1988), Handgun bullet performance. *Int Defense Rev, 21*(5), 555-557, and *J Assn Firearm Toolmark Examiners, 20,* 446-448.

Fackler, M. L. (1987). Physics of penetrating trauma. In McSwain, J. L., & Kerstein F. (Eds.), *Evaluation and management of trauma* (chap. 2). Stamford, CT: Appleton-Century-Crofts.

Fackler, M. L. (1992). Police handgun ammunition selection. *Wound Ballistics Rev, 1*(3), 32-37.

Fackler, M. L. (1988). Wound ballistics: A review of common misconceptions. *JAMA 259,* 2730-2736.

Fackler, M. L. (1992). Wound ballistics research of the last twenty years: A giant step backwards. *Wound Ballistics Rev, 1*(3), 19-24.

Fackler, M. L. (1992). The wound profile and the human body: Damage pattern correlation. *Wound Ballistics Rev, 1*(4), 12-19.

Fackler, M. L., & Lindsey, D. (1988). Missile-caused wounds. In T. E. Bowen, & R. F. Bellamy, *Emergency war surgery: NATO handbook* (chap. 2). Washington, DC: US Government Printing Office.

Fackler, M. L., & Malinowski, J. A. (1985). The wound profile: A visual method for quantifying gunshot wound components. *J Trauma, 25,* 522-529.

Fackler, M. L., Breteau, J. P. L., Courbil, L. J., et al. (1989). Open wound drainage versus wound excision in treating the modern assault rifle wound. *Surgery, 105,* 576-584.

Other Resources

Deadly effects (wound ballistics), deadly weapons (firearms and firepower), gunshot wounds (examination, interpretation, documentation) and forensic firearms evidence (video instruction). ANITE Group, P.O. Box 375, Pinole, CA 94564.

References

Rowe, W. F. (2003). *Firearm and tool mark examinations in forensic science: An introduction to scientific and investigative techniques.* Boca Raton, FL: CRC Press.

Russell, M. A., & Noguchi, T. T. (1999). Gunshot wounds and ballistics: Forensic concerns. *Top Emerg Med, 21*(3), 1-10.

Silva, A. J. (1999). Mechanism of injury in gunshot wounds: Myths and reality. *Crit Care Nurs Q, 22*(1), 69-74.

Smock, W. S. (2001). Forensic emergency medicine. In J. S. Olshaker, M. C. Jackson, & W. S. Smock (Eds.), *Forensic emergency medicine* (chap. 4). Philadelphia: Lippincott Williams & Wilkins.

Spitz, W. U. (1993). *Spitz and Fisher's medicolegal investigation of death.* Springfield, IL: Charles C Thomas.

Unit Five

Special Forensic Issues in Healthcare

Chapter 21 Organ Donation

Teresa J. Shafer

Other than a few papers in medical journals during the 1970s and early 1980s (after cadaver kidney recovery became more commonplace), little has been published concerning the effect of a medical examiner/coroner (ME/C) on organ retrieval efforts since kidney transplantation began in the US in the late 1950s. Only since the early 1990s and the decade that followed has the issue of medical examiner/coroner cooperation and its effect on organ donation been examined with a critical eye Organ donation and transplantation has changed substantially during the past 20 years. In the past, bodies were transported to the medical examiner's office following death and the autopsy was conducted unencumbered by requests for organs. Today, however, the organs from heart-beating, brain-dead individuals are desperately needed for the thousands of people in our communities waiting for organ transplants. Nearly 10% of those waiting for a heart or liver will die before an organ becomes available. A person dies every two hours waiting for an organ (United Network for Organ Sharing [UNOS], 2004).

Nationwide, more than 80,000 people are waiting for lifesaving or life-enhancing organ transplants, yet only approximately 22,000 organs from 6200 organ donors have been available each year (UNOS, 2004). The organ donor shortage is the foremost challenge faced by the transplant community. Organ recovery has not significantly increased in recent years, despite the fact that the transplant community has attempted to maximize organ donation by doing the following:

1. Studying methods to increase public acceptance of organ donation (Ganikos, McNeil, & Braslow et al., 1994)
2. Understanding and implementing best practices to increase family consent for donation (Ehrle, Shafer, & Nelson, 1999)
3. Understanding and implementing methods to increase consent rates and donation within the minority populations (Shafer, Wood, & Van Buren et al., 1997)
4. Focusing on and improving organ procurement organization (OPO) and hospital processes and collaboration to increase donation (Beasley, Capossela, & Brigham et al., 1997)
5. Studying healthcare professionals' attitudes and their effects on organ donation (Siminoff, Arnold, & Caplan, 1995)
6. Exploring the possibility of using financial incentives to increase organ donation (Council of Ethical and Judicial Affairs, 1995)
7. Implementing required request legislation (US Code Annotated, Title 42, 1987)
8. Exploring public policy initiatives such as presumed consent and mandated choice (Council of Ethical and Judicial Affairs, 1994)
9. Studying, proposing, or implementing other major legislative, regulatory, and policy initiatives (Siminoff, Arnold, & Caplan et al., 1995)
10. Increasing the use of "marginal" or older donors and expanding donor medical suitability criteria, including the use of organs from non-heart-beating donors (Kauffman, Bennett, & McBride et al., 1997)

Compared to the growth in the waiting list each year, the number of organ donors has remained relatively flat since 1986 (UNOS, 2004). In fact, the growth in organ donors has averaged only about 3.5% per year (Table 21-1). In contrast, the recipient waiting list has grown at 10 times that rate, significantly and steadily increasing during that same time (Fig. 21-1). Put simply, the number of organ donors continues to lag far behind the number of people waiting for a life-saving organ.

Despite numerous local public education activities, legislative actions–such as required request and contractual requirements between hospitals and OPOs mandated by federal law, involvement of the surgeon general and the US General Accounting Office (US Department of Health and Human Services [DHHS], 1991; US General Accounting Office [GAO], 1993), and nationwide public awareness campaign themes–there were no significant increases in organ donation in the 1990s.

Medical professionals sometimes mistakenly believe that only young, healthy individuals can be organ donors. While the *ideal* organ donor has an irreparable brain injury, is relatively young, is a trauma victim, is otherwise medically well, and has excellent multiorgan function, donors dying under these circumstances are becoming more and more uncommon due to demographic changes regarding age in the country's population (Morrissey & Monaco, 1997). Transplantation professionals look at *all* brain-dead patients, regardless of age or current medical condition, as potential organ donors. Nonetheless, the shortfall of organ donors has continued, despite the fact that donor criteria have been greatly relaxed in order

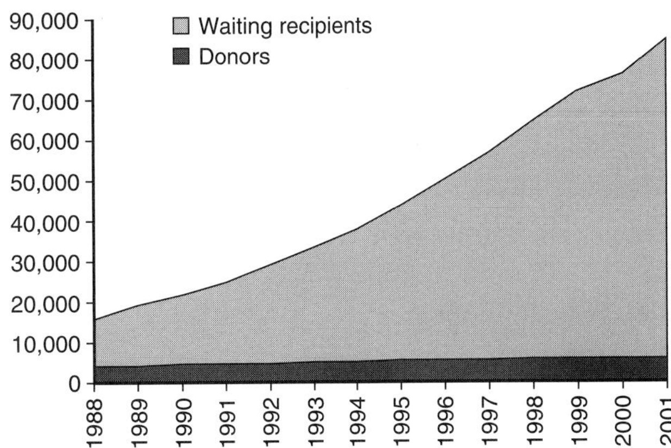

Fig. 21-1 Organ donors waiting for potential recipients, 1988-2001.

Special thanks to the United Network for Organ Sharing, particularly for the excerpts from *Donation and transplantation: Medical school curriculum*. Richmond, VA: United Network for Organ Sharing, LCCN: 92-60708.

Table 21-1 Organ Donors, Waiting List, and Cadaveric Organ Transplants in the US

YEAR	PERSONS ON WAITING LIST	PERCENTAGE INCREASE IN PATIENTS ON WAITING LIST	CADAVERIC ORGAN DONORS	PERCENTAGE INCREASE IN ORGAN DONORS	CADAVERIC ORGAN TRANSPLANTS	PERCENTAGE INCREASE IN ORGAN TRANSPLANTS
1980	5072‡	–	2138†		NA	
1981	NA	–	2141†	0.1	NA	
1982	NA	–	2300†	7.4	NA	
1983	NA	–	2705†	17.6	NA	
1984	NA	–	3290†	21.6	NA	
1985	NA	–	3637†	10.6	NA	
1986	NA	–	3990†	9.7	NA	
1987	13,115	159	4000†	.3	NA	
1988	16,034	22.3	4084	2.1	10.783	
1989	19,169	19.6	4019	−1.6	11,208	3.9
1990	21,914	14.3	4509	12.2	12,858	14.7
1991	23,901	9.1	4526	0.4	13,318	3.6
1992	28,987	21.3	4520	-0.1	13,471	1.1
1993	33,181	14.5	4861	7.5	14,635	8.6
1994	37,365	12.6	5100	4.9	15,083	3.1
1995	43,333	16.0	5360	5.1	15,780	4.6
1996	49,445	14.1	5418	1.1	15,784	0
1997	55,751	12.8	5479	1.1	15,044	−4.7
1998	62,740	12.5	5798	5.8	16,748	11.3
1999	69,054	10.1	5810	0.21	16,810	0.4
2000	76,115	10.2	5985	3.0	17,081	1.6
2001	84,798	11.4	6081	1.6	17,591	3.0

All data are from the United Network for Organ Sharing (UNOS) unless otherwise indicated. US Scientific Registry of Transplant Recipients and the Organ Procurement Transplant Network: Transplant Data 1989-2000. (2001, February 16). Rockville, MD and Richmond, VA: HHS/HRSA/OSP/DOT and UNOS.

† 1980-1987. From Evans, R. W. (1992, June). The national Cooperative Transplant Study. United Network for Organ Sharing/Health Care Financing Administration. Health and Population Research Center, Battelle-Seattle Research Center, Seattle, WA. BHARC-100-91-020, Control Number 01.

‡ From Southeastern Organ Procurement Foundation, Richmond, VA.

to recover more organs for those who wait. Given this shortage of organs, every suitable donor from whom organs are not recovered results in the loss of lives.

Actual recovery of organ donors falls far short of the potential donor pool for a number of reasons, chief among them being (1) denied consent from families for organ donation when asked to donate and (2) nonreferral of the potential donor by the hospital to the organ procurement organization (OPO) (Fig. 21-2). Additionally, to some extent, downward trends in motor vehicle accidents, gunshot wounds, and other traumatic brain injuries play a role (Sosin, Sniezek, & Waxweiler, 1995). Decreased speed limits as well as helmet and seat belt laws have greatly decreased the number of motor vehicle accidents, with a concomitant decrease in organ donors who have died under these circumstances. Organ donors whose circumstance of death was motor vehicle accident *decreased* 31%, from 34.3% in 1988 to 23.5% in 2002. Over the same period, organ donors with the diagnosis of cerebrovascular death rose 52%, from 27.7 % to 42% of all deaths (Fig. 21-3).

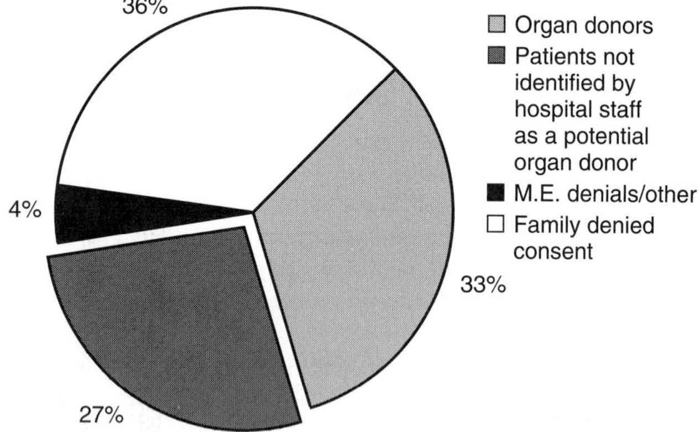

Fig. 21-2 Outcome of total US potential donor pool: medical examiner and nonmedical examiner cases, 1998.

Key Point *21-1*

Healthcare personnel should view *all* brain-dead patients, regardless of age or current medical condition, as potential organ donors.

Further, with age being greater in the population of individuals dying of cerebrovascular accidents (CVAs), along with the relaxed restrictions on donor criteria, recovery of organs from donors older than 65 grew an astounding 900% for the same period, from 0.9% in 1988 to 9% of all donors in 1999 (UNOS, 2002). In fact, maintaining recovery levels along with the minor increases in donors has only been achieved through the recovery of older, more marginal donors.

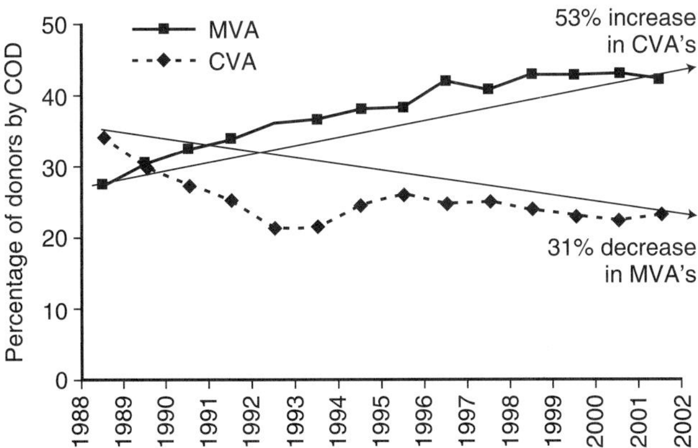

Fig. 21-3 Percentage of donor deaths by circumstances/cause of death: motor vehicle accident versus cerebrovascular accidents.

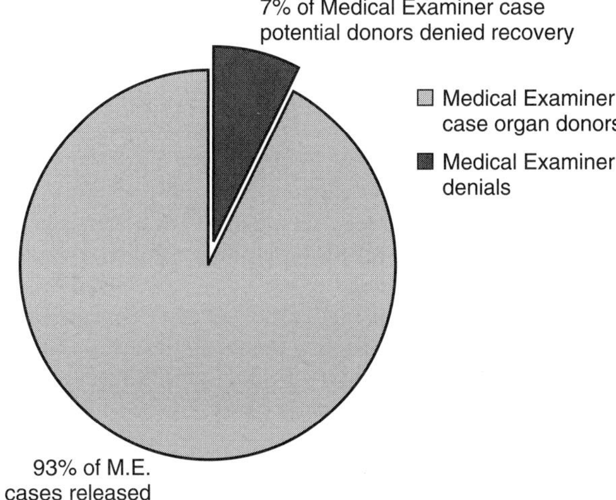

Fig. 21-4 Percentage of medical examiner cases released/denied organ recovery, 1994-2001.

Impact of the Medical Examiner on Organ Donation

Another reason for the organ shortage lies directly in the sphere of forensic death investigation. Despite widespread attention in 1994 to organ donor losses due to medical examiner denials, many areas of the country still needlessly lose significant numbers of organ donors because a local medical examiner refuses to release the organs of potential donors. In this chapter, the term *medical examiner* will be considered in the legal sense the same as coroner and justice of the peace. Medical examiners are the physicians who are trained to do autopsies. Coroners and justices of the peace may have a background in law enforcement. In counties that do not have medical examiners, coroners or justices of the peace may give authorization for organ and tissue recovery. In some instances, the justice of the peace or a coroner may possess the legal authority to release such organs, so this information on organ recovery also applies to these officials except when a reference is made to specific medical duties such as performing an autopsy (see Chapter 33; "Medical Examiners," 1994; "Organ Releases," 1994; Shafer, Schkade, & Warner et al., 1994; "Study Finds," 1994; Voelker, 1994). The most recent study on this issue indicates that the loss of transplantable organs due to medical examiner refusals remains close to the 1992 level, about 7% (Shafer, Schkade, & Evans et al., 2004) (Fig. 21-4).

This is particularly a problem with potential pediatric organ donors who have died due to suspected child abuse or sudden infant death syndrome (SIDS). Nonrecovery of organs in this age group is a significant contributing reason for the pediatric death rate on the waiting list for a liver transplant in children age five and under. In 1990-1992, 22% of all medical examiner/coroner denials were from child abuse cases, compared with 25% in 2000-2001. In 1990-1992, 73% of child abuse potential organ donors were denied, compared with 44% in 2000-2001. In one report of loss of pediatric organs for transplantation due to ME/C denials, 20.1% of all ME/C denials involved children less than one year old increasing to 41% of all denials involving children age 10 and less. Because there were only 183 actual organ donors in 2000-2001 less than one year old, it followed that nearly one third (31.1%) of these potential donors were denied recovery (Shafer, Schkade, & Evans et al., 2004). Denials associated with pediatric potential organ donors remain a serious issue.

Medical examiners play a vital role in organ transplantation and could significantly increase organ recovery in the US if cases falling under their jurisdiction, after appropriate examination, were routinely and expeditiously released for organ recovery and transplantation. Because litigation in general has increased over the years, the development of protocols detailing procedures used in recovering evidence before organ recovery might assist ME/Cs in releasing cases for organ donation. If such protocols as well as firm public policy requiring organ release in ME/C cases were put into place throughout the US, a truly significant increase in organ donors would be accomplished. Such firm public policy would mandate that medical examiners and transplant professionals collaborate to satisfy mutual needs.

Therefore, medical examiners and forensic nurse examiners (FNEs) have a key role in the US public health in working with the dead–and the living–in a number of ways. The role of the FNE in death investigation puts him or her in an ideal position to affect the lives of patients throughout the US waiting for an organ that will give them their second chance at life. The FNE works directly with medical examiners and organ procurement specialists to ensure that all forensic evidence is collected and that all medically suitable organs are recovered. With close cooperation between the FNE and OPO, the expectation should be that in cases in which the family has consented to donate and the potential donor is medically suitable, organs for transplantation will be recovered 100% of the time.

The FNE role in tissue donation will be discussed separately in this chapter, following the discussion on organ donation.

Best Practice *21-1*

The forensic nurse examiner should work directly with medical examiners and procurement specialists to ensure that all forensic evidence is collected and that all medically suitable organs are recovered 100% of the time when the family has consented to donate.

Impact of the Forensic Nurse on Donation

As a public policy issue, it is crucial that the supply of organs and tissues for transplantation be maximized. Congress acknowledged this public policy goal by mandating hospital protocols that offered organ donation as an option in appropriate cases and, in 1997, by mandating by regulation that all US hospitals participating in the Medicare and Medicaid Program refer every death occurring within the hospital to an organ procurement organization [42 U.S.C.§ 273(b)(2)(k)]. One source of donated organs that can be tapped immediately is the group of organs lost from ME/C denials of organ recovery. Because of this, nurses practicing in the emergent field of forensic nursing are in an ideal position to assume a leadership role in improving the public health crisis in the US due to the desperate shortage of organs.

Nurses have longed served the public through the many roles they have assumed, and the roles they have been asked to assume, throughout the history of nursing. No other healthcare professional so touches the basic human needs of people. Nurses are accustomed to dealing with a variety of clients, including patients, their families, and the communities in which they live; nurses do this while juggling many priorities and tasks. It is cliché to attribute this quality to a feminine nature, but, nonetheless, this cooperative and sometimes "nurturing" quality can be attributed to nurses–male or female–who have historically demonstrated, through practice, the caregiving role in the greatest sense of the word. Historically, when entering specialty-nursing roles, nurses have not given up their nurturing, caring side; they have not become more circumscribed, elevated, and less accessible to their patients and community. Nurses never abandoned their generalist, their Nightingale image. The ability to see the larger picture is what enables FNEs to look beyond the important but unidimensional need of death investigation and see the waiting recipients, the potential donor families and their families, and the community at large. The FNE, by keeping the big picture in view, ensures that organ donation is accomplished in all cases simultaneously with competent death investigations, a primary responsibility of the FNE.

It is reasonable and appropriate to expect a forensic nurse examiner to ensure that the forensic investigations are grounded, thorough, and expedient, and that they work in harmony with the recovery of lifesaving organs intended for transplantation. Such a holistic approach of care to a variety of individuals (waiting potential transplant recipients, donor, donor family crime victim, crime victim's family, police, attorneys, transplant team, community members from both the donor and the recipients respective communities) involved in the organ donation and forensic examination process is certainly not foreign to the nursing profession. It is here where the FNE can excel–in investigating the death of the potential donor using the highest possible standards of forensic death investigation, ensuring the transplantation of the potential donor's organs, and resolving any conflicts between the two in the process.

The resolution of any perceived conflicts between organ recovery and death investigation has been referred to as a win-win situation in that forensic evidence is collected and organs are recovered. The term *win-win* is certainly an oversimplified description of the interdisciplinary process through which an FNE works to ensure, in a holistic approach to care, that the community is served.

The National System

The National Organ Transplant Act (1984) mandated the establishment of both the national Organ Procurement and Transplantation Network (OPTN) and the national Scientific Registry of Transplant Recipients (SRTR). The OPTN and SRTR were to be administered by a private, nonprofit entity through contracts with the US Department of Health and Human Services. The United Network for Organ Sharing (UNOS) administers the OPTN, and the University Renal Research and Education Association (URREA) administers the SRTR. UNOS is responsible for promoting, facilitating, and scientifically advancing organ procurement and transplantation throughout the US while administering a national organ allocation system based on scientific and medical factors and practices. URREA is responsible for ongoing evaluation of the scientific and clinical status of transplanted organs and organ procurement organization performance for recovery of organs for transplantation.

Policies governing the transplant community are developed by the OPTN membership through a series of regional meetings, national committee deliberations, a public comment period, and final approval by a board of directors that includes both physicians and nonphysicians. The OPTN has adopted policies to ensure equitable organ allocation to patients on the national waiting list. These policies forbid favoritism based on political influence, race, sex, or financial status; they rely, instead, on medical and scientific criteria (Bowers & Servino, 1992).

Procurement Organizations

Organ procurement organizations (OPOs) are nonprofit, government-certified agencies that facilitate organ recovery services in designated areas of the US. OPOs are the link between the organ donor and the transplant center and recipient. Highly specialized and trained OPO staff members, who normally come from nursing backgrounds, provide these major services:

- Assist hospitals with procedures and education on donation
- Receive all organ and tissue donor referrals
- Evaluate potential donors
- Discuss and obtain consent for donation from families
- Medically manage patient for organ preservation
- Coordinate surgical organ and tissue recovery
- Allocate organs
- Transportation of organs to transplant centers
- Arrange importing/receiving/procuring of distant organ (imports)
- Enter and maintain recipient waiting lists
- Provide professional education for nurses, physicians, and other healthcare professionals
- Provide public education about donation and increase public awareness of the need for organ donation
- Provide public policy advice and assist in public policy formulation
- Maintain extensive data base on organ donation and provide data to UNOS and other governmental agencies

OPOs can also facilitate tissue recovery either directly or indirectly by referring the potential donor to a tissue, skin, or eye bank. OPO and tissue personnel are available 24 hours a day, 365 days a year, to assist physicians, nurses, and families as needed (Bowers & Servino, 1992).

Box 21-1 Process of Organ Donation

1. The patient
   - is admitted to hospital.
   - does not respond to efforts made to save the patient's life.
   - has sustained head injuries, bleeds, or anoxic events severe enough that patient will not recover.
   - is pronounced brain dead after evaluation, testing, and documentation.
2. Referral is made to the organ procurement organization (OPO) to evaluate the patient as an organ/tissue donor.
3. The patient is evaluated by the OPO and the family is approached about donation.
4. Consent for donation is requested to initiate the recovery process.
5. The medical examiner's (ME) cases need the ME's authorization to proceed with donation.
6. The donor is maintained on a ventilator, stabilized with fluids and drugs, and undergoes numerous laboratory and diagnostic tests.
7. Recipients are identified for the placement of organs.
8. Surgical teams are mobilized and coordinated to arrive at donor hospital for removal of organs and tissues.
9. The donor is brought to the operating room on the ventilator once the surgical teams have arrived at the local hospital where the donor is located.
10. Multiple organ recovery is performed with organs being preserved through special solutions and cold packaging. Ventilator support is discontinued following cross-clamping of the aorta.
11. Tissue donation occurs once the vascular organ donation is completed.
12. The donor's body is reconstructed and surgically closed.
13. The donor's body is released to the funeral home.

Note: Confidentiality is maintained for the donor family and recipients.

The Donation and Death Investigation Process

The organ donation process is complex. Box 21-1 provides a general overview of the steps involved during the donation process. The major steps always occur, but the sequence and time frame between events vary depending on the individual circumstances. Once the family consents to organ or tissue donation, the time frame for this process will vary from a few hours up to 20 or more hours. Coordinated teamwork between the physicians, nurses, hospital staff, surgical recovery teams, and the procurement coordinator are critical for assuring the viability of the transplant graft. Four major steps generally define the donation process: potential donor identification and referral, consent, donor evaluation and maintenance, and organ and tissue recovery (Seem & Skelley, 1992).

Donor Criteria

More than 20 different organs and tissues can be transplanted or used in research. Each potential donor's options for organ and tissue donation are assessed by a procurement specialist. Criteria have expanded, so it is essential that an organ or tissue procurement organization be referred to every single hospital death for evaluation as a potential donor.

Organ donors are previously healthy individuals who suffer irreversible and catastrophic brain injury resulting in brain death with sustained cardiac function (heartbeat). To sustain cardiac function, they are maintained on a ventilator and clinically managed with appropriate fluids and medications until the organs are removed. Transplantable organs include heart, kidney, liver, lung, pancreas, and small bowel. Some physicians accept non-heart-beating donors as organ donors.

Tissue donors, on the other hand, are non-heart-beating. That is, tissue is most commonly obtained from a person who has died of cardiopulmonary arrest or from a solid-organ donor after removal of transplantable organs. Transplantable tissues include dura, eyes, corneas, skin, fascia, cartilage, tendons, ligaments, bones (e.g., ribs, femurs, tibias, fibulas, and ilium), saphenous veins, and heart valves. Tissues are recovered within 24 hours after death if the donor's body has been refrigerated (6 hours or less preferable for eyes) (Seem & Skelley, 1992).

Brain Death

Brain death is a medically and legally valid declaration of death and is defined as the complete and irreversible loss of brain and brain stem functions. Brain death is determined by considering the following factors:

- There is a known etiology for the brain death.
- Reversible conditions, such as hypothermia, drug intoxication, or metabolic abnormalities, must be excluded.
- The patient must be clinically examined to demonstrate (1) absence of cerebral function, (2) no spontaneous movements, (3) no response to stimulation, (4) no brain stem reflexes, and (5) apnea.
- Diagnostic tests, such as CT scans, EEGs and cerebral blood flow (CBF) studies, may be performed in conjunction with a clinical exam.
- CBF studies may be used as a confirmatory test for the diagnosis of brain death
- Brain death can be diagnosed in full-term newborns older than seven days, provided that confirmatory tests are employed.
- When brain death is diagnosed, the patient is declared dead and appropriate documentation is made in the patient's record.
- If the brain-dead patient is to be an organ donor, organ donor management interventions must be continued until the time of organ recovery.
- If the patient is not to be an organ donor, mechanical support of the body functions can be terminated (Seem & Skelley, 1992).

Donor Identification and Referral

First, the hospital staff identifies a potential donor and makes a referral to the local OPO. This may be done by an attending or consulting physician, a staff nurse, or designated hospital staff. Organs are recovered from individuals declared dead on the basis of brain death criteria (98% of all US organ donors) or individuals who have sustained a severe neurological injury, the family chooses to withdraw life support, and cardiac death occurs in such a manner that organ recovery can proceed immediately (5 to 10 minutes) after cessation of cardiac function (less than 5% of US organ donors) (UNOS, 2004).

The physician determines death according to neurologic criteria and informs family members of the patient's death. The decedent's family members in most cases are not approached about donation until it has been determined that they understand that "brain death" is death. Family members often raise the issue of donation themselves prior to this time and hospital or OPO staff may make a premention of donation as the futility of care becomes evident to all involved. The OPO procurement coordinator is able to provide specific information about donation to the family in a way that ensures informed consent is accomplished and the benefits of donation for both the donor family and the waiting recipients is fully explained. If the family wishes to donate, a consent form, supplied by the hospital or OPO coordinator, is completed and signed (Seem & Skelley, 1992).

Up until this point, the medical examiner's office has usually not been contacted. It is normally only after the official declaration of death that the medical examiner is notified. However, the OPO coordinator is normally on the scene much earlier than this point and ensures that the medical examiner is notified immediately following pronouncement of death. At this time, the forensic nurse examiner might join the OPO coordinator at the hospital, whether that be in the emergency department or intensive care unit, and begin collecting forensic evidence.

Table 21-2 lists items that may be provided to the medical examiner's office by the hospital or OPO staff. In some circumstances, the FNE might facilitate collection of such evidence by going directly to the hospital in which the potential organ donor is located and speaking directly with the OPO and hospital staff. This provides for enhanced communication between the medical examiner's office and hospital/OPO staff serving not only the purposes of collection of evidence and establishment of chain of custody, but also the reinforcement of the role of the FNE in the healthcare community. Additionally, it allows the FNE to examine the body in the hospital, soon after death, so that an exam by a trained forensic examiner is conducted before organ recovery, and that, in addition to organ recovery in all situations in which there are one or more organs suitable for transplant in a brain-dead patient, more tissues (bone, skin, eyes) might be released for donation. The FNE's role is to collaborate with medical examiners, hospital staff, and organ procurement professionals.

Family Consent

Acute care hospitals are legally obligated to offer families of potential organ donors the option of organ and tissue donation. Approaching a grieving family about donation can be difficult. But research reveals that when the conversation is sincere and sensitive, the majority of families experience important short- and long-term benefits whether or not they choose to donate. In fact, families can become angry and frustrated when denied the opportunity to donate. Research on public attitudes and family experience of donation repeatedly have come to the same conclusion: the manner in which the donation request is made is the main factor in a family's ultimate decision, regardless of preexisting attitudes.

Approaching a family about donation requires coordinated efforts among the physician, hospital staff, and the OPO coordinator. The physician has the responsibility to inform the family of their relative's death. Time must be allowed for the family to accept the reality of death before raising the question of donation. The person who is most comfortable and knowledgeable about donation should discuss donation with the family, and that individual is usually the OPO coordinator. OPO coordinators bring knowledge, experience, and a confidence in their ability to handle all aspects of the donation process. They know first hand the benefits that the process offers the family (Ehrle, Shafer, & Nelson, 1999). Donation is a process. Obtaining consent does not consist of simply asking the family if they wish to donate, in

Table 21-2 Items That May Be Provided to Medical Examiner's/Coroner's Office by Hospital/OPO Staff*

ITEM	COMMENT
Two red-top tubes of blood	Labeled with the donor's name, medical examiner case number, date and time of collection, and initials of the collecting party. All should be sealed inside of a protective container with evidence tape. (Whenever possible, a pretransfusion serum sample, so labeled, should be provided.)
Urine sample	Labeled with the donor's name, medical examiner case number, date and time of collection, and initials of the collecting party. All should be sealed inside of a protective container with evidence tape and admission. (Whenever possible, an admission urine sample, so labeled, should be provided.)
A copy of the OPO medical record	In a plastic bag.
Polaroid photos of the body	To be taken prior to any preoperative procedures, with the date and medical examiner case number written in black on a white sheet of paper, which is to be displayed in the foreground of the photo. (The medical examiner is responsible for training OPO staff in the appropriate techniques for obtaining such photographs.)
Additional photos of the body will be taken preoperatively, using a 35-mm camera and with the medical examiner case number and date displayed as above	Each roll of film is to contain photos of only one donor. No photos of any other subject will be included on the roll. The roll of film will be placed in a film-processing envelope provided by the medical examiner, labeled with the date and medical examiner case number, and delivered by OPO staff to the medical examiner's office.
An operative note dictated by one of the transplant surgeons in attendance noting all operative findings.	Delivered to the medical examiner in a timely manner.
Written reports of any organ biopsies performed by OPO or transplant centers	To be submitted upon request of the medical examiner's office.
X-rays or reports of x-rays	In child abuse cases, a CT or MRI of the head may be useful.

*Each office and OPO is different and has its own arrangement. This is a list of those items that may prove useful to the medical examiner in certain circumstances.

essence, "popping the question." Informed consent takes time; OPO staff members have the time that busy physicians and nurses do not have. OPO staff spend significant time, often many hours, with families during the donation process (Shafer, Schkade, & Evans et al., 2004). An investment of the time of bedside nurses and physicians is not possible in today's environment of limited healthcare resources.

Best Practice *21-2*

The forensic nurse examiner can reinforce with the family the value of organ and tissue donation, in cases in which hospital and OPO staff are making the request for donation. If the FNE is making the request for tissue donation in a case that has not yet been consented by hospital or OPO staff, the FNE should ensure that the family is fully informed about the value of tissue donation before requesting their consent.

The family should be provided sufficient information to make an informed decision about whether or not they wish to donate organs or tissues. The positive benefits of donation help families cope with their loss by helping to save the life of someone else, by having their loved one live on in a sense, and by fulfilling the implicit and explicit wish of their loved one.

Concerns of the family should be anticipated and addressed in a forthright manner. A person's reluctance to donate is most often rooted in misinformation or a lack of information. Prior to beginning the donation discussion, OPO coordinators assess families as to their knowledge and acceptance of brain death as death. Families are informed that (1) all costs involved with donation are paid by the OPO, (2) there is no disfigurement of the body and that an open-casket funeral is possible, (3) their loved one will feel no pain because their loved one is dead and the brain has no ability to sense or convey pain, and (4) all major religions and religious traditions allow organ donation. Some families have questions about how the organs are distributed and to whom they are given. They are informed that there is a national Organ Procurement and Transplant Network that monitors and regulates organ distribution to assure fairness. Buying and selling of organs is illegal (Seem & Skelley, 1992).

Once the OPO coordinator has obtained consent for donation, the FNE can confer with the family, answering any questions they might have regarding the process that will occur following donation with the autopsy. Families often have questions about the autopsy process, which, by default, nurses and OPO coordinators answer because there is no representative of the medical examiner's office present. This is another role the FNE could fill in a more informed manner than hospital or OPO staff.

Donor Evaluation

Evaluation begins at the time of referral. The referring physician or nurse provides specific information about the donor, such as age, sex, race, date and time of admission, diagnosis, and vital signs (admission and current). The donor's hemodynamic stability is maintained through mechanical ventilation until the time of organ removal. Individuals who have died from cardiopulmonary arrest may be acceptable donors of corneas, skin, bone, heart valves, and other tissue. Other initial criteria for donor suitability include age limits specific to each organ and tissue and an absence of metastatic cancer or unresolved systemic infections.

Once the procurement coordinator arrives at the donor hospital, he or she begins with a thorough chart review. A review of the emergency department admission record and the emergency medical services run report is essential. Information regarding the cause of admission, including details such as a cardiac or respiratory arrest, ejection from a vehicle, and submersion in water, is vital to the multiorgan donor workup. Knowledge of such events may help indicate whether the organs have suffered significant damage. A review of physician and nursing notes provides an overall picture of the patient's status. A complete assessment of blood pressure and temperature curves, use of vasoactive drugs, and episodes of hypotension, hypertension, bradycardia, and tachycardia are noted. Progress notes should provide documentation of the patient's brain death determination. Brain death laws vary from state to state, as do determination and criteria policies from hospital to hospital.

The coordinator conducts a thorough assessment of the social and medical history of the donor. The social profile includes occupational history, sexual habits and preferences, marital and family status, and substance use or abuse. History of foreign service or travel of the donor in the previous 12 to 18 months may need to be reviewed with the donor's family, due to possible exposure of the donor to malaria, typhoid fever, acquired immune deficiency syndrome, or other serious illnesses. Past medical history includes recent and past illnesses, previous operations, and blood transfusions. The donor's family usually can answer the social and past medical history questions.

The laboratory studies from admission are important in the establishment of a baseline of individual organ systems and in preparation for donor management. Blood samples for cytomegalovirus, HIV I/II, HTLV I/II, hepatitis B and C, and syphilis (VDRL) are tested. Box 21-2 includes laboratory and other diagnostic tests that are normally performed in donor evaluation (Mendez & Phillips, 1992). The FNE can collect all of these findings and put them together in the assessment of this individual's life and death.

Donor Management and Organ Placement

Donor management should be considered the beginning of organ preservation for transplantation. The ultimate survival of the transplanted organs depends heavily on the pre- and intraprocurement management of the cadaveric organ donor, as well as organ preservation after removal. Ideally, medical management should begin as soon as death is pronounced. Irreversible cardiac arrest usually ensues within 48 to 72 hours of brain death in adults despite all efforts to maintain hemodynamic stability.

After death has been declared by neurological criteria and proper consent has been obtained from the family, the procurement team needs to maximize the function of the various organs being considered for transplantation. Teamwork and coordination between the intensive care, surgical, and anesthesia staffs are paramount in assuring graft function following transplantation.

The donor is managed medically by an OPO coordinator with the assistance of the nurse caring for the patient. The coordinator, under the guidance of the OPO medical director, usually writes hospital orders for donor management. Donor management is aimed at maximizing the function of organs prior to surgical removal. Hemodynamic and oxygenation status is monitored and laboratory studies initiated.

Hemodynamic instability begins prior to the diagnosis of brain death. Intracranial hypertension secondary to the brain becoming

Box 21-2 Laboratory and Diagnostic Tests Done on Organ Donors

CHEMISTRY PROFILE

Chem 7, Chem 6
Electrolytes
Na
K
Cl
CO2
Ca
Serum Osmo
Cr
BUN
Glu
Amylase
Lipase
Bili-tot
Bili-direct
Bili-direct/indir
Liver Profile
ALT
AST
GGT
Tot protein
Albumin
LDH
Alk phosphatase
CK
CK-isoenzymes and/or MB
ABG
Mg
PO4
Drug screen (i.e., Pentobarbital)

HEMATOLOGY

- CBC/platelets
- Diff
- H/H
- PT
- PTT
- Fibrinogen
- Fibrin split products

MICROBIOLOGY

- Blood culture
- Urine culture
- Sputum culture
- Urinalysis
- Gram stain
- Microsensitivity (Kirby-bauer)

ischemic and necrotic results in severe system hypertension. A low cardiac output state secondary to ventricular dysfunction characterizes the brain dead patient. Associated pulmonary changes, due to hemodynamic instability, might contribute to the frequent acute failure of lung function following lung transplantation.

Following the diagnosis of brain death, the most important cause of hemodynamic instability is hypovolemia. Cerebral resuscitative measures prior to the declaration of brain death generally incorporate diuresis and dehydration. Marked increases in serum osmolality occur in the majority of brain-dead patients. This increase occurs in spite of accurate central venous pressure (CVP) monitoring of fluid balance and attempts at replacement therapy with vasopressin for diabetes insipidus.

Subsequently, other factors compound the tendency toward hypotension. Extremely rapid fluctuations in blood pressure may occur in brain-dead patients due to instability of the brain stem vasomotor center. Complete brain stem herniation can occur at any time, even after the diagnosis of brain death. Pontine and medullary structures are destroyed, leading to a breakdown of all central regulatory mechanisms and resulting in the loss of spontaneous respiration and circulatory regulation, as well as hypothermia.

Electrolyte status at the initiation of donor management dictates fluid replacement. Donors frequently become hypernatremic, hypokalemia, and hypomagnesemic secondary to free-water loss from both diabetes insipidus (DI) and diuretics. Hypocalcemia and hypophosphatemia can also occur and, when severe, cause myocardial depression.

An important determinant of organ viability is the maintenance of an adequate systemic perfusion pressure. Volume expansion and replacement of urinary losses stabilize the hemodynamic status of many brain dead patients. CVP monitoring facilitates volume repletion and is recommended by many transplant centers for all organ donors. Arterial lines are also strongly recommended for moment-to-moment vigilance of blood pressure and the effects of agents employed to normalize hemodynamic function. Pulmonary artery catheters in certain donors prove useful.

The ideal hematocrit for a multiorgan donor ranges from 25% to 35%; if necessary, transfusion is required to obtain this level. Fluid resuscitation to a CVP of 15 mm Hg may be all that is needed to normalize hemodynamic status in many initially unstable kidney donors. However, for multiple organ donors, institution of dopamine when the CVP is greater than 10 mm Hg and the systolic pressure remains below 100 mm Hg may be required. Low-dose dopamine increases systemic pressure while dilating the renal vasculature increasing renal blood flow. The mesenteric and coronary vessels are also dilated with doses below 5 mcg/kg/minute.

All donors are maintained on mechanical ventilators. Management of pulmonary status varies little from the living patient in that arterial blood gases determine ventilator settings. Positive-end expiratory pressure (PEEP) of 5 cm H_2O helps prevent atelectasis, as do tidal volume of 15 ml/kg. To ensure cardiovascular stability, the donor's core temperature should be maintained above 34° C.

The list of patients waiting throughout the US for an organ is maintained by UNOS. The UNOS computer must be accessed to obtain a national donor identification number and to identify potential recipients for extra-renal (heart, liver, lungs, pancreas) organs. The procurement coordinator contacts prospective extra-renal transplant teams and relays donor information. This information includes the donor's medical status, including past medical and social history.

While awaiting the transplant surgical teams, the procurement coordinator manages donor care. Following the diagnosis of death, hypovolemia is the most frequent cause of hemodynamic instability resulting from the following (Boyd, Diethelm, & Phillips, 1992):

- Cerebral resuscitative measures
- Instability of the brain stem vasomotor center
- Nonfunction of the sympathetic nervous system
- Diabetes insipidus (77% to 98% develop diabetes insipidus)

Surgical Recovery of Organs

Once all recipients are identified, the coordinator schedules the operating room for organ and tissue removal. The procurement coordinator arranges the arrival and departure times of the surgical teams for removing extra-renal organs. Local surgical teams remove kidneys. The teams typically consist of transplant surgeons, their assistants, and organ procurement or preservation coordinators. When the surgical teams arrive, the donor is taken to the operating room. Vital signs are monitored en route to the operating room, usually by portable monitor. The operating room is staffed by the donor hospital surgery staff and consists of scrub nurses, circulating nurses, and anesthesia. An anesthesiologist or nurse anesthetist is present to assist in donor ventilation, monitoring hemodynamic status, and administering fluids and medications (Mendez & Phillips, 1992).

The medical examiner may, in selected cases, attend the donation surgery in order to view the organ recovery. This affords the medical examiner physician a direct view of the organs in the oxygenated and perfused state, an opportunity obviously not available on the vast majority of his or her cases. Because time constraints rarely allow for the medical examiner to do this, attending surgery is reserved for the most unusual cases in which the physician feels that his or her attendance in the operating room might allow for observation of something that the transplant surgeon might miss. The medical examiner might also feel that, on selected cases, attendance in the operating room would leave little room for questions from a future defense attorney about the thoroughness of the autopsy. However, the medical examiner's attendance in surgery occurs rarely to never in most jurisdictions, primarily because it is not needed, even in homicide and other high-profile cases, to obtain the required forensic evidence. The medical examiner or the FNE would more likely view the patient in the intensive care unit in the hospital. This is more convenient because it can be done any time prior to the surgical recovery of the organs.

In most situations, the medical examiner simply requests a copy of the operative notes or an organ donor operative assessment sheet, the structure of which has been agreed on in advance by both the medical examiner's office and the OPO. OPOs and medical examiners' offices routinely work out such procedures in order to assure that the mutual goals of organ recovery and collection of forensic evidence are met. An example of such a donor operative assessment sheet is included in Appendix F. Forms such as these can be used to document the condition of the organs intraoperatively. (This is information the medical examiner would *not* obtain in the vast majority of cases because they are not organ donors.) Additionally, the FNE will already have documented through notes as well as photography the outward appearance of the body.

Prior to the actual removal of the organs, the aorta is cross-clamped and mechanical ventilation as well as monitoring devices are discontinued. Tissue recovery occurs after organ recovery is completed (if permission for tissue recovery was obtained). Eye banks and tissue banks do not always require the operating room for tissue recovery. Once tissue recovery is completed, the body is reconstructed and surgically closed. Disposition of the body takes place according to hospital guidelines. An open-casket funeral is possible, as the decedent should have a normal appearance after organ and tissue donation.

The recovery teams return to their transplant hospitals with the organs maintained hypothermically in special preservation solutions. The recipients are taken to surgery and the organ transplants are performed. Recovered corneas are processed and transplanted within days following recovery. Other tissues, such as bone segments and heart valves, may be stored for many years, depending on preservation techniques (Mendez & Phillips, 1992).

Follow-Up of Transplanted Organs

The OPO coordinator follows up with the healthcare professionals involved in the donor case by writing a letter regarding the disposition of the organs. This normally includes information such as whether or not the organ was transplanted and, if not, the reason it was not transplanted, as well as the general location of the recipient and the initial function of the organ following transplantation. Patient identifiers are omitted. Medical examiners have found this information useful in the past when testifying as to the cause of death in a trail. Should the defense attorney bring up the heart, for example, as possibly involved in the cause of death (instead of the gunshot wound to the victim's head), the medical examiner can refer to and enter into evidence the letter from the organ procurement organization documenting the medical condition of the heart and its function in the recipient.

Child Abuse Cases: Special Attention

In 1992, roughly 30% of the cases that were denied were child abuse cases. For every child abuse or suspected child abuse case released by the medical examiner for organ recovery, approximately two cases were denied. This is the most frequently denied circumstance of death in medical examiner cases that are potential organ donors. This is especially unfortunate for two reasons: first, pediatric organs are in critically short supply and are essential for needed transplants in young recipients where size is crucial; second, nonfatal child abuse cases are routinely prosecuted with evidence that can be gathered through external physical examination, lab results, x-rays, CT scans, and so on. In the case of organ donation, all this medical data can still be provided, and in addition, direct examination and photography of internal organs and tissues can be offered as further evidence (Shafer, Schkade, & Warner et al., 1994).

The FNE can be instrumental in interfacing with the pediatric intensivist, the child's physician and nursing staff, to ensure that photographs are taken early in the hospitalization prior to death. If the child is hospitalized for some time, some crucial evidence may be lost that may have proven useful. OPO staff will become involved in the case after it has been determined that the child has had a devastating head injury but well before the declaration of death. The OPO can work with the FNE to ensure that the appropriate specimens are obtained and may actually facilitate doing some needed diagnostic tests prior to organ removal and cessation of circulation. Such documentation is more likely to occur when the OPO is evaluating the cases for organ donation than when the child does not have the potential to become an organ donor. This is another reason for the medical examiner to cooperate with organ recovery from child abuse cases: he or she will obtain more diagnostic information about the nature of the child's injuries, which can be invaluable in the death investigation.

Therefore, there is greater chance for more information to be collected, which may prove useful to the medical examiner if the child becomes an organ donor, not vice versa. Actual visualization of the organs in vivo is accomplished, whereas this would not be the case if the child were not an organ donor. The FNE could either take such information in the form of a written report from the transplant surgeon (see Appendix F) or request that the medical examiner attend surgery to view the actual operative recovery, noting the condition of the organs at the time of surgery. Biopsy specimens, if needed, could easily be obtained for the ME/C.

Case Law Related to Organ Donation

Theoretically, a criminal investigation or prosecution could be impaired by evidence that is lost, damaged, or altered by virtue of the removal of the crime victim's organs for donation. There has been no case in which a state was unable to adequately investigate a crime or prosecute a criminal defendant because necessary evidence had been impaired by organ donation. Further, no reported case was found that demonstrated that the removal of organs for donation rendered a subsequent autopsy so deficient that the cause of death could not be determined (Strama, Burling-Hatcher, & Shafer, 1994). To the contrary, several cases demonstrate that an autopsy performed after organ donation was sufficient to determine the cause and/or time of death (*People v. Bonilla,* 1983; *People v. Eulo*, 1984; *People v. Wilbourn*, 1978; *State v. Morrison*, 1989).

Key Point *21-2*

Case review to determine whether any reported case demonstrated that a criminal investigation or prosecution has been impaired or adversely affected by organ donation reveals that no such incident has ever occurred.

Although no reported cases indicated that a criminal investigation or prosecution was impaired or adversely affected by organ donation, the removal of a crime victim's organs has been asserted as a defense by defendants. Penal laws define homicide in terms of conduct that *causes* the death of another person. Therefore, in order to convict a defendant for murder or manslaughter, a state must prove beyond a reasonable doubt that the defendant's conduct caused the victim's death. Accordingly, defendants in homicide cases have asserted that the removal of the victim's organs or the termination of life support systems was the cause of the victim's death, not the defendant's actions (Strama, Burling-Hatcher, & Shafer, 1994).

Case Study 21-1 **People v. Bonilla and People v. Lai**

In *People v. Bonilla* (1983), the court addressed the question of whether a defendant who inflicted a mortal wound on another person can escape a homicide conviction because of the acts of physicians in removing the victim's organs for transplant and thereafter disconnecting life support systems. The defendant, who had been convicted of manslaughter, alleged on appeal that because the victim's organs had been donated, the state had not proven beyond a reasonable doubt that the defendant had caused the death of the victim. The defendant contended that, therefore, he could not be found guilty of murdering the victim because organ retrieval was an intervening cause of death.

The court expressly rejected defendant's assertion, finding that "the bullet wound to the brain was the proximate cause of death and the homicide was properly attributed to the defendant" (*People v. Bonilla* at 608-809, 1983). Thus, although the defendant alleged that the declaration of brain death and the removal of organs were intervening causes of the victim's death, the court rejected the argument and affirmed the guilty verdict. This same claim was unsuccessful in *People v. Lai* (1987) when the defendant's conviction for murder was affirmed despite the defendant's assertion that the victim's death was not caused by the gunshot wound inflicted by the defendant but was caused by surgery to remove the victim's organs for transplantation and the subsequent disconnection of the respirator (*People v. Lai*, 1987).

Case Study 21-2 **State v. Matthews**

In *State v. Matthews* (1986), the defendant was convicted of the murder of a 16-year-old girl. The victim's kidneys were donated after she had been pronounced dead. On appeal, the defendant asserted that the doctors prematurely declared the victim dead and that the removal of her kidneys created a superseding cause of death that relieved the defendant of liability for murder. The court rejected defendant's assertion. South Carolina law provided that negligent medical treatment by a physician would not relieve a defendant from liability. The court held that the decision to declare a patient dead and to harvest organs for transplantation is clearly part of the care or duty that a doctor is responsible for providing. Therefore, the physician's actions were not a superseding cause of the victim's death.

Case Study 21-3 **People v. Wilbourn**

In *People v. Wilbourn* (1978), the defendant appealed his conviction for murder. The defendant asserted that the decedent/victim had died as a result of cardiac arrest following the removal of his kidneys on the day of his death, and that therefore the operation to remove decedent's kidneys was the cause of death, supervening the effect of the gunshot wound delivered by the defendant. The court disagreed, finding that the evidence in the case demonstrated beyond a reasonable doubt that the gunshot wound to decedent's head was the cause of death.

Case Study 21-4 **People v. Eulo and State v. Shaffer**

In *People v. Eulo* (1984), a homicide defendant asserted that his conduct did not cause the victim's death where the victim's respirator was turned off after the victim's vital organs were removed. In assessing the defendant's criminal responsibility, the court stated that if a victim's death is prematurely pronounced due to a doctor's negligence, the subsequent procedures may have been a cause of death, but that negligence would not constitute a superseding cause of death relieving the defendant of liability. The court in *Eulo* found that there was sufficient evidence for a rational juror to have concluded beyond a reasonable doubt that the defendant's conduct caused the victim's death and that the medical procedures were not superseding causes of death.

Similarly, in *State v. Shaffer* (1977), the court affirmed the defendant's appeal from a conviction for first-degree murder. After the victim was pronounced dead, his kidneys were removed and the respirator was turned off. In affirming the defendant's conviction, the court stated that "[w]here a person inflicts upon another a wound which is calculated to endanger or destroy life, it is not a defense to a charge of homicide that the alleged victim's death was contributed to or caused by the negligence of the attending physicians or surgeons."

Although the fact that the victims' organs were donated did provide the defendants in the above cases with an additional defense, in none of the cases was the defense found to be valid. Therefore, these cases do not support an assertion that organ donation has adversely affected the investigation or prosecution of a criminal case.

Legal Cases Involving Removal of Life Support

Although there have not been many cases in which a defendant has asserted that the donation of his victim's organs was a supervening cause of death relieving the defendant of liability, there have been numerous cases in which defendants have asserted that the removal of a victim from life support systems constituted an intervening cause, relieving the defendant of criminal responsibility. The defendants have been equally unsuccessful in such cases (Strama, Burling-Hatcher, & Shafer, 1994).

For example, in *State v. Velarde*, the defendant was convicted of second-degree murder. On appeal, the defendant asserted that the termination of decedent's life support systems was the cause of victim's death, not the injuries inflicted on the victim by the defendant. The court rejected this assertion, stating that the victim was brain dead before the respirator was removed. The court stated that the head injuries inflicted by the defendant were the cause of the victim's death, not the removal of the respirator. The court noted that even if the support systems were removed prematurely, the defendant still would be responsible for the victim's death since intervening medical error is not a defense to a defendant who has inflicted a mortal wound upon another (*State v. Velarde*, 1986).

Similarly, in *State v. Meints*, the court affirmed the defendant's conviction for vehicular homicide. The court held that the trial court properly instructed the jury that the withdrawal of life support from the victim was not an intervening cause of death. The court found that the fact that some other agency combined with the act of the defendant to cause the victim's death is not a defense unless the other agency is an efficient intervening cause. The court held that proof of brain death is sufficient as proof of the victim's death in a homicide case, and removal of life support systems is not an efficient intervening cause of death in such cases (*State v. Meints*, 1982). Numerous other cases have reached the same conclusion (*Commonwealth v. Golston*, 1977; *Commonwealth v. Kostra*, 1985; *People v. Saldana*, 1975; *People v. Vaughn*, 1991; *State v. Brown*, 1971; *State v. Fierro*, 1979; *State v. Inger*, 1980; *State v. Olson*, 1989; *State v. Watson*, 1983; Strama, Burling-Hatcher, & Shafer, 1994).

Evidentiary Issues Presented by Organ Donation

Defendants in criminal cases also have attempted to use the removal of the victim's organs to preclude the admission of photographs into evidence. For example, in *Green v. State*, the defendant was found guilty of murder. On appeal, the defendant alleged that the trial court erred in admitting into evidence a photograph of the victim taken after several of his organs had been removed for transplantation. The court rejected defendant's assertion, stating that the gruesome nature of the photo was not grounds to exclude it if it shed light on the issue being tried (*Green v. State*, 1991). Similarly, in *State v. Bock*, the appellate court rejected the defendant's assertion that photographs of the victim taken after his organs had been removed for donation had been admitted into evidence improperly. The court found that although the admission of the photographs may have been prejudicial, such error was harmless (*State v. Bock*, 1992; Strama, Burling-Hatcher, & Shafer, 1994).

Immunity from Liability

All 50 states have enacted a statute governing anatomical gifts. These state acts are based largely on the Uniform Anatomical Gift Act ("UAGA"), which provides immunity for those participating in organ donation. The UAGA insulates from civil and criminal liability those involved in the organ donation process who act in good faith. Section 11 of the UAGA provides that a person who acts in accordance with the UAGA or with the applicable anatomical gift law of another state (or a foreign country) or attempts in good faith to do so is not liable for that act in a civil action or criminal proceeding. Thus, it is likely that the anatomical gift acts in individual states contain provisions that provide immunity to those who participate in the organ donation process in good faith, including hospitals, physicians, and medical examiners (Strama, Burling-Hatcher, & Shafer, 1994). "Good faith" is defined as an "honest belief, the absence of malice and the absence of design to defraud or to seek an unconscionable advantage" (*Black's Law Dictionary*, 1979). In one case, the court held the eye bank acted in good faith in removing eyes from the decedent because it relied on facially valid permission form and did not have actual knowledge that the woman who signed the form was not formally married to decedent (*Nicoletta v. Rochester Eye & Human Parts Bank, Inc.*, 1987).

Some states have expanded on the liability provisions of the UAGA. For example, the Texas statute pertaining to declared donors pursuant to a driver's license signification of donation provides the following:

> *A person who carries out this section is not civilly or criminally liable. The legislature recognizes that because swiftness of action is required in organ and tissue donation situations, good-faith errors are preferable to delay as a matter of public policy. Medical examiners are encouraged to permit organ and tissue removal at the earliest possible time consistent with their duties regarding the cause and manner of death. (Strama, Burling-Hatcher, & Shafer, 1994, p. 21)*

Summary of Case Law Discussion

Although case law on legal issues related to organ donation is relatively scarce, the cases that have been reported generally give great deference to the encouragement of organ donation procedures and uphold the immunity provisions of the UAGA. Good faith decisions with respect to organ procurement should not subject OPOs, physicians, or medical examiners to civil or criminal liability (Strama, Burling-Hatcher, & Shafer, 1994). (See Box 21-3 for legal notes.)

State Legislation

Two states have legislation requiring medical examiner release on organ donors: New York and Tennessee. Three other states require medical examiner release unless the medical examiner or his or her designee is physically present in surgery, viewing the organ in question: New Jersey. Texas, and California. (Boxes 21-4 and 21-5). In December 1993, the New Jersey Assembly and the Senate voted unanimously to allow the medical examiner to deny organ recovery only if the medical examiner or his or her designee attended the surgical procedure. Similarly, in 1995 the Texas legislature also unanimously passed legislation requiring medical examiner release of organs unless the medical examiner was present in surgery, viewing the organ in question, and then denied the recovery due to concerns (Tex. Rev. Civ. Stat. Ann. art. 6687b). Finally, in 2003, California passed essentially the same legislation. These laws prevent the denial of an organ recovery without doing everything possible to gather the information needed by the medical examiner. They allow the medical examiner to make a decision relative to release or nonrelease of organs after viewing the organ in its undisturbed state during surgery, which might prove helpful in child abuse cases. This can be done by personally attending

Box 21-3 Legal Notes

Commonwealth v. Golston, 366 N.E.2d 744, 750 (Mass. 1977), *cert. denied*, 434 US 1039 (1978). In affirming the defendant's conviction for murder, the court found that the physician's disconnecting the respirator was not a superseding act that was the sole cause of the victim's death.

Commonwealth v. Kostra, 502 A.2d 1287 (Pa. Super. Ct. 1985). In affirming the defendant's conviction for homicide by motor vehicle, the court rejected the defendant's argument that the direct cause of the decedent's death was not the car accident but the removal of life support systems.

People v. Bonilla, 467 N.Y.S.2d 599, 602 (N.Y. App. Div. 1983), *aff'd sub nom.*

People v. Eulo, 482 N.Y.S.2d 436 (1984) (superseded by statute). The medical examiner performed an autopsy the day after the victim's organs were removed and determined the cause of the victim's death.

People v. Saldana, 121 Cal. Rptr. 243 (Ct. App. 1975). In affirming the defendant's murder conviction, the court rejected the defendant's assertion that the removal of the victim from a respirator removed the defendant's criminal responsibility for the victim's death; rather, the court concluded that the victim was already dead when he reached the hospital and when the artificial life support systems were removed.

People v. Vaughn, 579 N.Y.S.2d 839 (Sup. Ct. 1991). The defendant is not relieved of criminal liability, even if the victim's life support system was turned off by an unauthorized act of a third party.

People v. Wilbourn, 372 N.E.2d 874 (Ill. Ct. App. 1978). Based on postmortem examination, the medical examiner testified as to cause of decedent's death.

State v. Brown, 491 P.2d 1193 (Or. Ct. App. 1971). In affirming the defendant's conviction for murder, the court rejected the defendant's assertion that disconnecting the victim's respirator was the act that terminated the victim's life, not the bullet wound delivered by the defendant.

State v. Fierro, 603 P.2d 74, 77 (Ariz. 1979). In affirming a conviction for murder, the court stated that the removal of life support systems did not alter the natural progression of the victim's physical condition (from the gunshot wounds in the head) to his death.

State v. Inger, 292 N.W.2d 119, 124-125 (Iowa 1980). Even if the victim's respirator was stopped prematurely, the defendant remains liable since intervening medical error is not a defense to a defendant who inflicts a mortal wound upon another.

State v. Morrison, 437 N.W.2d 422 (Minn. Ct. App. 1989). An autopsy was performed the day after a child abuse victim's organs were donated, and the coroner testified about the condition of the child's internal organs and injuries.

State v. Olson, 435 N.W.2d 530, 534 (Minn. 1989). The doctor's conduct in removing the infant from life support was not a superseding, intervening cause; rather, the medical intervention was a normal, foreseeable consequence of the defendant's shaking the child, and removal of life support did not produce a death that would not otherwise have occurred.

State v. Watson, 467 A.2d 590 (N.J. Super. Ct. App. Div. 1983). Death resulted not from turning off the victim's respirator but from the acts of defendant, which undeniably caused the victim's brain to die.

Box 21-4 Autopsy and Tissue Organ Analysis

State of New Jersey

Introduced March 15, 1993, by Senator Bassano

An ACT concerning autopsy and tissue or organ analysis and supplementing Title 52 of the Revised Statutes. BE IT ENACTED by the Senate and General Assembly of the State of New Jersey:

1. Notwithstanding any provision of law to the contrary, if a deceased person whose death is under investigation pursuant to section 9 of P.L. 1967, c.234 (C.52:17B-86) is a donor of all or part of his body as evidenced by an advance directive, will, card or other document, or as otherwise provided in the "Uniform Anatomical Gift Act," P.L. 1969, c.161 (C.26:6-57 et seq.) , the State Medical Examiner or the county medical examiner, or his designee, who has notice of the donation shall perform an examination, autopsy, or analysis of tissues or organs only in a manner and within a time period compatible with their preservation for the purposes of transplantation.
2. A health care professional authorized to remove an anatomical gift from a donor whose death is under investigation pursuant to section 9 of P.L. 1967, c.234 (C.52:17B-86), may remove the donated part from the donor's body for acceptance by a person authorized to become a donee after giving notice to the State Medical Examiner or the county medical examiner or his designee, if the examination, autopsy, or analysis has not been undertaken in the manner and within the time provided in section 1 of this act. The State Medical Examiner or the county medical examiner or his designee shall be present during the removal of the anatomical gift if in his judgement those tissues or organs may be involved in the cause of death. In that case, the State Medical Examiner or the county medical examiner or his designee, may request a biopsy of those tissues or organs or deny removal of the anatomical gift. The State Medical Examiner or the county medical examiner or his designee shall explain in writing his reasons for determining that those tissues or organs may be involved in the cause of death and shall include the explanation in the records maintained pursuant to section 15 of P.L. 1967, c.234 (C.52;17B-92).
3. The health care professional performing a transplant from a donor whose death is under investigation pursuant to section 9 of P.L. 1967, c.234 (C.52:17B-86) shall file with the State Medical Examiner a report detailing the condition of the part of the body that is the anatomical gift and its relationship to the cause of death. If appropriate, the report shall include a biopsy or medically approved sample from the anatomical gift. The report shall become part of the Medical Examiner's report.
4. This act shall take effect immediately.

the surgical recovery of the organs or having another do so. Colorado attempted unsuccessfully in 2000 to pass the Texas and New Jersey medical examiner laws while California, in 2003, passed the legislation through both houses (California State Leg AB 777, 2003; Vaughn, 2000).

On November 19, 2002, the Advisory Committee on Organ Transplantation, appointed by Tommy G. Thompson, Department of Health and Human Services, unanimously agreed on a series of recommendations concerning various aspects of organ donation and transplantation. One of the recommendations directs the secretary to use his good standing with the National Governor's Association, the National Association of State Legislatures, the Uniform Commissioners of State Laws, or with individual states to amend the Uniform Anatomical Gift Act (UAGA) to add a new subsection that mirrors the Texas and New Jersey laws. The amendment, which would appear at the end of Section 4 of the act, would insert language nearly identical to that of the Texas medical examiner law. Further, the secretary has been asked to

Box 21-5 Texas Legislation Regarding Organ Donation and Medical Examiner Cases

Introduced January 27, 1995, by Senator Moncrief

AN ACT relating to clarifying procedures for the removal of organs or tissues from decedents when an inquest is required.

693.002. Removal of Body Part or Tissue from Decedent who Died Under Circumstances Requiring an Inquest

(a)(1) On request from a qualified organ procurement organization, as defined in Section 692.002, the medical examiner may permit the removal of organs from a decedent who died under circumstances requiring an inquest by the medical examiner if consent if obtained pursuant to Section 693.003.

(2) If no autopsy is required, the organs to be transplanted shall be released in a timely manner to the qualified organ procurement organization, as defined in Section 692.002, for removal and transplantation.

(3) If an autopsy is required and the medical examiner determines that the removal of the organs will not interfere with the subsequent course of an investigation or autopsy, the organs shall be released in a timely manner for removal and transplantation. The autopsy will be performed in a timely manner following the removal of the organs.

(4) If the medical examiner is considering withholding one or more organs of a potential donor for any reason, the medical examiner shall be present during the removal of the organs or during the procedure to remove the organs. In such case, the medical examiner may request a biopsy of those organs or deny removal of the anatomical gift. If the medical examiner denies removal of the anatomical gift, the medical examiner shall explain in writing the reasons for the denial and shall provide the explanation to the qualified organ procurement organization.

(5) If, in performing the duties required by this subsection, the medical examiner is required to be present at the hospital to examine the decedent prior to removal of the organs or during the procedure to remove the organs, the qualified organ procurement organization shall on request reimburse the county of the entity designated by the county for the actual costs incurred in performing such duties, not to exceed $1,000. Such reimbursements shall be deposited in the general fund of the county. The payment shall be applied to the additional costs incurred by the medical examiner's office in performing such duties, including the cost of providing coverage beyond the regular business hours of the medical examiner's office. The payment shall be used to facilitate the timely procurement of organs in a manner consistent with the preservation of the organs for the purposes of transplantation.

(6) At the medical examiner's request, the health care professional removing organs from a decedent who died under circumstances requiring an inquest shall file with the medical examiner a report detailing the condition of the organs removed and their relationship, if any, to the cause of death.

encourage individual states to adopt state laws to the same or similar effect (Department of Health and Human Services, 2003).

Organ Procurement and the Medical Examiner

Approximately 7% of organs were denied recovery in 1992, and Shafer et al. (2003) documented that 7% of medical examiner cases were denied each year in 2000-2001 in this country. Best estimates based on this study revealed that likely 1451 individuals did not receive a second chance at life during 2000-2001 due to medical examiner denials. There are, however, many areas of the country, including large metropolitan areas, where there are no, or zero, medical examiner denials of organ recovery.

The issue of nonrelease of organs for recovery and transplantation from medical examiner cases has become increasingly controversial ("Medical Examiners," 1994; "Organ Releases," 1994; "Study Finds," 1994; Vaughn, 2000; Voelker, 1994) as the number of deaths on the transplant waiting list has increased.

Release/Nonrelease Patterns

Trends have appeared from the data. In 1992, 29.3% of all the cases that were denied were child abuse cases, and 22.8% of the cases involved a gunshot wound (GSW) to the head. Seventy-one percent of all denied cases were possible homicide cases. In 1992, for every child abuse case that was released for organ donation, two were denied; for every SIDS case that was released, one was denied. Other than these obvious trends, no other common threads to medical examiner denials were reported in this study (Shafer, Schkade, & Warner et al., 1994). In the narrative comments received during the 1992 study, several respondents noted that release for organ donation could depend on which examiner is on call, whether or not the request was made during daylight hours, and whether or not the case was a homicide or high-profile case.

Successful Collaborations among Medical Professionals

It is clear that numerous models exist throughout the US where death investigation and organ transplantation occur in harmony. Most of the strategies reported by organ recovery professionals that are used in assisting release of donors from the medical examiner's office are strategies designed to protect the collection of forensic evidence, provide more clinical data for the medical examiner's investigation, and foster positive communication. The forensic nurse examiner is in an ideal position to figure prominently in making these strategies successful in accomplishing both goals of collection of forensic evidence and recovery of lifesaving organs.

These strategies include the following:

- Obtaining blood, urine, and other specimens for the medical examiner at or before the time of organ recovery and locate admission specimens in the hospital
- Inviting the medical examiner or his or her designee to attend the surgical procedure
- Obtaining additional exams that the medical examiner would not be able to obtain, such as CAT scans, MRIs, echocardiograms, cardiac catheterizations, and other diagnostic and laboratory tests
- Videotaping the operative recovery of the organs
- Providing follow-up to the medical examiner/coroner on the organs recovered and the progress of the recipients; additionally, transplant surgeons may offer to provide testimony at any later trial as to the condition of the internal organs at the time of organ recovery

It is the responsibility of the organ procurement and transplant community to represent the potential recipient, just as it is the responsibility of the medical examiner to represent the community in successfully concluding death investigations. It is their joint responsibility to the community to do them together–saving lives. Even one life lost is tragic; forensic nurse examiners can play a pivotal role in the health of the communities in which they work, if they help resolve these situations where duties overlap.

There is a balance between protecting forensic evidence and protecting recipients and potential donor families. Medical examiners routinely release donors in some areas of the country, so it can be done. Medical examiners have often changed their ruling and allowed donation to proceed after someone, usually a transplant or organ procurement professional, has questioned the decision and personally conferred with the medical examiner. The forensic nurse examiner can provide this communication early in the organ donation process so that organ recoveries are not delayed.

ME/C denials vary by geographic area. During 2000-2001, in New York, Houston, and Philadelphia–three of the five largest cities in the US–and in four states, there were no (0) potential organ donor denials by ME/Cs (Shafer et al., 2003). The absence of any donor denials in these large cities and states begs the questions: (1) Shouldn't we work toward zero donor denials in all areas of the country? (2) Should potential recipients, those people waiting on the national waiting list, be dependent on the good working relationships between medical examiners' offices and organ recovery organizations? (3) Should there be appropriate state and federal statutes that ensure that organs are recovered whenever family consent is obtained, while ensuring that steps are taken to preserve valuable forensic evidence for the medical examiner in order that he or she may fulfill all legal obligations? (4) Finally, how best can the forensic nurse examiner serve the community in fulfilling his or her role in death investigation while working with organ and tissue donation healthcare professionals?

Dr. Edmund Donoghue, chief medical examiner of the Office of the Medical Examiner of Cook County in Chicago, during his year as president of the National Association of Medical Examiners (NAME), presented an abstract at the annual NAME meeting in 1999, noting:

> *Medical Examiners may have a conflict of interest between their duty to criminal justice in prosecuting homicide cases and their duty to public health in making organs available for transplantation. Difficulties arise when they weight their duty to one sector more heavily than another. First comes the recognition that multiple obligations exist. Next come solutions that allow forensic pathology, criminal justice, and public health to each fulfill their responsibilities.*
>
> *Events in Illinois have led us to review policies for organ transplantation in Cook County. Recently, a coroner in another part of the state imposed a ban on organ transplantation in all homicide cases. Based on our experience in Cook County, this clearly seemed unreasonable.*
>
> *When we examined our own denials, we realized that they might not be entirely reasonable. We found that refusals were based on irrational fear and the false belief that organ transplantation might interfere with the prosecution of homicide cases. Thirty years' experience with organ transplantation in the US offers absolutely no evidence that this is true.*
>
> *A 1994 JAMA study of regional organ procurement organizations revealed ten areas of the country with no donor denials and five other areas with only one donor denial. Areas cited for outstanding performance included St. Louis, MO; New York City; Tennessee; North Carolina; Hawaii; Hartford, CT; Long Island, NY; Fort Worth, TX; and Indiana.*
>
> *If colleagues in other areas could do this without difficulty, we began to wonder whether we might match their performance. As a result, we are making changes in policy that will attempt to make Cook County a no denial area. We would be very pleased if our remaining colleagues would examine their policies and see if they might also attempt to become no denial areas. (Donoghue & Lifeschultz, 1999)*

Forensic nursing examiners and medical examiners play a vital role in organ transplantation and therefore play a vital role in the public health. They are involved in 50% to 60% of all organ donor cases. If situations such as those seen in New York City, Houston, Texas, and other successful cities in which organ donation and death investigation occur in tandem could be replicated, this would undeniably result in the largest overall increase in organ donation in the past several years. The donor pool has not been maximized, and there is room for improvement. Medical examiners, coroners, and forensic nurse examiners may be the sole group with the ability to increase organ donation.

Tissue Donation

An estimated 450,000 Americans receive tissue transplants each year, ranging from sight-saving corneas to hip replacements and bone repair to heart valves. The availability of donated bone, tendon, and ligament tissue for transplant has revolutionized the practice of sports medicine–and extended the playing careers of athletes from sandlot to Olympic stadium.

But the average American can be forgiven for not knowing about the benefits of tissue transplantation. Although 25 tissue transplants are performed for every organ transplant, the lion's share of attention has been garnered by the inherent drama of organ transplantation. When a celebrity receives an organ transplant, it is headline news. When an equally popular public figure receives a tissue transplant, the action receives little attention. Patients and their families may not even realize that donated tissue made their recovery possible.

With the exception of blood and bone marrow, virtually all allograft tissue (a transplant from one individual to another) is donated after death. As with organs, the need for donated tissue is growing at a much faster rate than donation. In part, this supply-demand problem is due to rapid advances in the science and practice of transplant medicine and the increase in medical applications for tissue. Population shifts also contribute to demand, especially the maturing of the baby boom generation and the improving health and longevity of older Americans. The availability of donated tissue helps Americans of all ages to recover from a growing list of debilitating conditions.

Many healthcare professionals know little or nothing about tissue donation. Whereas the donation of solid organs–the heart, lungs, kidneys, pancreas, and liver–can occur only when a patient is declared brain dead and dies in a hospital where mechanical support/ventilation is available to keep the organs viable, tissue donation can occur in a much wider range of circumstances.

Transplantable tissue does not require a blood supply, so brain death and artificial support are not essential criteria (although organ donors can donate tissues as well). This means that individuals who die of cardiac (heart) failure or who die away from a hospital can be tissue donors. Even when an autopsy is required, as for homicides and some accident victims, tissue donation is a realistic possibility. Because tissue can be donated under such varying conditions, the potential pool of tissue donors is significantly larger than for organ donors.

Another important distinction between tissue and organ donation is that most tissue, after it is processed, can be stored for later use. Organs, on the other hand, must normally be transplanted within 48 hours of donation. Donated tissues are subjected to rigorous testing and processing procedures before they are made available to transplant surgeons by bone banks, eye banks, and skin banks. There is no single national waiting list for tissue comparable to the United Network for Organ Sharing (UNOS), the nonprofit body contracted by the federal government to manage the matching and allocation of organs. The nation's tissue banks are, however, regulated by the Federal Food and Drug Administration.

Tissue donation affects so many lives. A single tissue donor, depending on the extent of the donation, can provide tissue for as many as 50 people. From the child with the congenital heart-valve defect to the cancer victim facing loss of a limb, from the promising athlete with a potentially career-ending injury to the older citizen with crippling arthritis, from the burn patient to the visually impaired–the gift of just one tissue donor holds the promise of faster healing, improved function, restored mobility, and the return to healthy and productive living ("Tissue Donation," 2000).

The recovery of tissues should begin as soon as possible once the evaluation and consent process is completed in order to minimize the overgrowth of skin organisms. If retrieval must be delayed, it is imperative that the body of the donor be refrigerated at 4° C. Both the American Association of Tissue Banks (AATB) and the Southeastern Organ Procurement Foundation (SEOPF) standards require that tissue must be retrieved within 24 hours of death, provided that the body of the donor has been refrigerated. Otherwise, the maximum postmortem period for safe tissue recovery is 12 hours (Leslie & Bottenfield, 1989).

Surgical recovery of tissue may be performed in a standard operating room environment using routine sterile technique or in a clean environment using nonsterile technique. It should be noted that all tissues recovered by the latter method will require some means of terminal sterilization. Most large tissue banks have teams available at all times to travel throughout their region to perform tissue recovery. Teams generally consist of two to three technicians or nurses who are specially trained in operative procedures and techniques specific to tissue recovery. The recovery teams are self-contained, providing all supplies, packs, and instruments necessary to recover donated tissues in a sterile manner. The donor hospital operating room staff is not usually required to assist. These procedures are not deemed to be emergency in nature and can be scheduled so as not to interfere with normal operating room cases.

The donor is brought to the operating room, shaved, prepped, and draped in standard surgical fashion. Because of the extent of the incisions to be made, additional bactericidal solution my be left on the skin for additional protection from contamination by normal skin flora. The extent of the prep will be determined by the specific tissues donated. If vascular organs are also being donated, tissue recovery will follow excision of the organs. In this case, the donor will be reprepped and draped prior to initiation of tissue recovery (Leslie & Bottenfield, 1989). See Box 21-6.

Box 21-6 Process for Tissue Donation Only

1. The patient dies from a cardiac arrest.
2. A referral is made; local organ or tissue banks are notified.
3. An evaluation for tissue donation is made (i.e., eyes, skin, bone).
4. The family is approached regarding donation.
5. The consent for donation triggers several activities.
6. The medical examiner's (ME) cases need the ME's authorization to proceed with donation.
7. Extensive chart reviews and laboratory testing are done for communicable diseases and infection.
8. Tissue recovery is performed in the operating room, morgue, or ME's office.
9. The donor's body is reconstructed as needed and surgically closed.
10. An autopsy is performed when required or requested.
11. The donor's body is released to funeral home.

Note: Confidentiality is maintained for the donor family and recipients.

Bone Recovery

The actual excision technique for each tissue will vary somewhat according to individual tissue bank procedures. In general, with bone recovery, long incisions are made along the lateral aspect of the legs with the long bones and iliums removed. Occasionally a rib or ribs will be removed, which obviously requires a chest incision. Also, occasionally, the humerus and humeral heads are removed from the arms, requiring a long incision on the lateral aspect of the upper arm and shoulder. Mandibles are also occasionally removed in bodies that are scheduled for cremation.

Crucial to the recovery process is an attitude of respect for the donor. After all donated tissues are removed, the donor's body is carefully reconstructed to restore natural form and appearance. Prosthetic devices are placed in the surgical incisions to restore form where large bones have been removed. Finally, the incisions are tightly closed using heavy silk suture. It is important for the OPO or tissue bank to develop close working relationships with the funeral home professionals in their area to avoid any interference with funeral arrangements because of tissue donation.

The bone may be used with little processing (simple hypothermia or fresh frozen) or it may be processed and sterilized using chemical (ethylene oxide) or physical (radiation) methods. It may be stored using, again, simple hypothermia, deep freezing, cryopreservation, or lyophilization (freeze-drying). Care is taken to maintain the biological integrity of the allograft.

Skin Recovery

Using a dermatome, skin is removed from the front and back of the torso and the front and back of the upper legs. It is removed in strips .015 to .030 inch thick. After removal, the body might look as if the cadaver had a sunburn. A body suit is put on the body following recovery to prevent seepage of serous fluid following recovery. Procured skin is placed in a sterile solution to be transported to the tissue bank, where it will either be stored fresh (unfrozen), frozen and stored at −70°, frozen and stored at −170°, or freeze-dried. The length of time skin can be stored varies greatly from seven days for fresh skin to an indefinite time period for fresh frozen skin. Next to autografts, allogeneic skin continues to be the most effective coverage for the burn wound. Because of this and a growing number of other uses for dermal grafts, skin donation remains insufficient to meet increasing clinical needs (Alexander, Plessinger, & Robb, 1992).

Heart Valve Donation

Cryopreserved allograft valves have been shown to have impressive long-term durability and low reoperation rates, lasting up to 10 to 12 years. It is also known from past experience that they have low thromboembolic, hemorrhagic, and infectious complication rates, which allow these valves to compare favorably with mechanical valves and porcine bioprostheses.

The heart itself is removed without clamping the aorta and with the entire arch, part of the descending aorta, and the main branches of the pulmonary artery included. Caval and pulmonary veins are divided at their entry to the heart. In contrast to hearts retrieved for immediate transplantation, those used for valve donation do not require the use of cardioplegia solutions. In fact, it is important to avoid needle punctures in the aorta of hearts recovered for valves.

Once removed from the donor, the heart is placed in cold saline solution, double-covered in sterile plastic bags, packaged in ice, and sent to the processing lab. Explanted hearts must arrive for processing within 16 hours of recovery. They are immediately dissected to salvage pulmonary and aortic valves and the accompanying valved conduits–the arterial stems. In over 70% of cases, both valves are usable. The valves are incubated for 8 to 24 hours in an antibiotic-containing medium and, following incubation, placed in a tissue culture medium with 10% dimethyl sulphoxide (DMSO) solution and frozen at a regulated rate in a microprocessor-controlled liquid nitrogen freezer (Miller & Moreno-Cabral, 1992).

Eye or Corneal Donation

The cornea is the 12-mm "clear window" in the front part of the eye. Corneal transplantation, such as penetrating keratoplasty, penetrating corneal transplant, and penetrating corneal graft, is a surgical procedure in which abnormal, full-thickness corneal tissue is removed from a patient and substituted with full-thickness donor corneal tissue.

Two methods are used to obtain donor cornea. One method involves whole-eye enucleation. The eyes are placed in a sterile, moist chamber in a cool transporting box and transported to the eye bank. There, the eyes are placed in a storage-viewing chamber containing preservation media. The enucleated eyes are then examined carefully with a slit-lamp microscope to identify any abnormal endothelial cells that would make the cornea tissue unsuitable for corneal transplantation. The second method of tissue recovery entails removing the cornea with a rim of sclera (in-situ) and placing the tissue directly into preservation media. The corneal tissue also is examined with a slit lamp by the eye bank in the storage containers. Eye caps are placed in the eye socket of the donor following the recovery of the eyes or corneas (Shapiro, 1992).

OPOs who recover tissue as well as freestanding tissue and eye banks also work closely with the medical examiner/coroner in requesting consent for release of tissue in cases falling under the jurisdiction of the medical examiner. For obvious reasons, tissue donors are far more numerous than organ donors. For this reason as well as the fact that tissue transplantation is not lifesaving (in most instances), there are more circumstances in which tissue donation is not authorized by the medical examiner than organ donation, particularly in homicide cases, child abuse or SIDS cases, and occasionally accidental deaths or apparent suicide cases. The FNE could greatly aid in increasing release of tissue donors in these ME/C cases as the medical examiner or coroner's concerns largely rest with fear that the evidence may be altered with the recovery of tissue. In most cases, the medical examiner's concerns could be allayed if the FNE examined the body and documented her or his findings prior to the actual tissue recovery. Particularly with eye donors, if the medical examiner is not looking for retinal bleeding as is seen with some deaths, and because eyes should be recovered within six hours after cessation of heartbeat, the FNE could travel to the hospital or morgue within six hours of death, and, as part of the initial examination, examine the condition of the head, face, and neck and review the cause of death. More likely, the FNE could do the examination in the medical examiner's/coroner's office when the body arrives, allowing for eyes to be removed in a timely manner.

If the cause of death fell within certain protocols, the FNE could examine the condition of the eyes and eyelids and then, after conferring with the medical examiner, authorize eye donation. Three broad categories in which the FNE could assist would include the following: (1) deaths from homicide or suspicion of homicide; (2) asphyxial deaths, a broad category including death by manual or ligature strangulation, hanging, overlays (heavy object on chest), drowning, noxious fumes, and so on; and (3) deaths from unknown causes. In all cases, the nurse could document that condition of the eyes by looking for and photodocumenting any subconjunctival hemorrhage. The protocols might exclude authorization of eye donation in cases where retinal hemorrhage needs to be documented. For example, in situations such as shaken baby syndrome, in which the pediatrician may already have documented these hemorrhages, the medical examiner will section the eye and further document them.

Summary

The FNE can serve as a bridge between families of the bereaved and the medical examiner. Time spent with grieving families, helping them to cope with the events surrounding the death of their loved one, is certainly a role in which the forensic nurse examiner, as a nurse, would excel. Organ and tissue donation are often the only comfort that a family gains in an otherwise tragic situation. The FNE works closely with the organ recovery coordinator by coordinating information in donation situations, and she or he works jointly with other healthcare professionals by assisting families in moving forward through their loss.

The FNE plays a vital role in organ and tissue donation and transplantation and, therefore, in the health and welfare of the community. The FNE is a catalyst in forging positive and lasting relationships among the medical examiner, healthcare professionals (including OPO staff), and the community, ensuring that death investigations and organ donation proceed in harmony. His or her background is ideal for such a role. In more ways than one, the FNE plays a lifesaving role in the community. The FNE, who often conducts the preliminary death investigation, serves as a bridge between the medical examiners' offices, law enforcement agencies, OPOs, and tissue and eye banks. Collaborative practice between the FNE and organ recovery coordinators offers the greatest opportunity and reward, both for the professionals involved and the community. It is a lifesaving and life-honoring collaboration.

Resources

Organizations

American Society of Transplant Surgeons

1020 North Fairfax Street, Suite 200, Alexandria, VA 22314; Tel: 888-990-2787; www.asts.org

National Kidney Foundation

30 East 33rd Street, Suite 1100, New York, NY 10016; Tel: 800-622-9010, 212-889-2210; www.kidney.org

North American Transplant Coordinators Organization

8310 Nieman Road, Lenexa, KS 66214; Tel: 913-492-3600; www.natco1.org

United Network for Organ Sharing

700 North 4th Street, Richmond, VA 23219; Tel: 804-782-4800; www.unos.org

World Kidney Fund

National Kidney Foundation, Singapore, 81 Kim Keat Road, Singapore 328836; Tel: +65 251-7555; www.worldkidneyfund.org

Web Sites

Transweb.org
www.transweb.org
Map of organ procurement locations and contact information for the US.

Organ Donation

www.organdonor.gov
Umbrella government site for organ and tissue donation issues. Lists all US organ procurement organizations and provides contact information.

US Department of Health and Human Services, Division of Transplantation

www.hrsa.gov/osp/dot/dotmain.htm

References

Alexander, J. W., Plessinger, R. T., & Robb, E. C. (1992). Skin transplantation. *Donation and transplantation: Medical school curriculum.* Richmond, VA: United Network for Organ Sharing, LCCN: 92-60708.

Beasley, C. L., Capossela, C. L., Brigham, L. E., et al. (1997). The impact of a comprehensive, hospital-focused intervention to increase organ donation. *J Transpl Coord, 7*(1), 6-13.

Black's Law Dictionary. (1999). 7th ed., 623.

Bowers, V. D., & Servino, E. M. (1992). An overview of organ and tissue donation. *Donation and transplantation: Medical school curriculum.* Richmond, VA: United Network for Organ Sharing, LCCN: 92-60708.

Boyd, G. L., Diethelm, A. G., & Phillips, M. G. (1992). Donor management. *Donation and transplantation: Medical school curriculum.* Richmond, VA: United Network for Organ Sharing, LCCN: 92-60708.

British Transplantation Society. (1975). The shortage of organs for clinical transplantation: Document for discussion. *Br Med J, 1*(5952), 251-255.

California State Legislature. (2004). Concurrence in Senate Amendments AB 777 (Dutton). As amended July 15, 2003. As passed ASM floor May 29, 2003, Senate July 21, 2003.

Chinnock, R. E., & Bailey, L. L. (1995). Letter to the editor. *JAMA, 273*(20), 1578.

Commonwealth v. Golston. (1977). 366 N.E.2d 744, 750 (Mass.).

Commonwealth v. Kostra. (1985). 502 A.2d 1287 (Pa. Super. Ct.).

Coroners and transplant. (1977). Letter: From our legal correspondent. *Br Med J, 1,* 1418.

Council on Ethical and Judicial Affairs, American Medical Association. (1995). Financial incentives for organ procurement: Ethical aspects of future contracts for cadaveric organ donors. *Arch Intern Med, 155,* 581-589.

Council on Ethical and Judicial Affairs, American Medical Association. (1994). Strategies for cadaveric organ procurement: Mandated choice and presumed consent. *JAMA, 272*(10), 809-812.

Davis, J. H., & Wright, R. K. (1977). Influence of the medical examiner on cadaver organ procurement. *J Forensic Sci, 22,* 824-826.

Department of Health and Human Services. (2003). *Secretary's advisory committee on organ transplantation (ACOT) interim report, recommendations and appendices;* ACOT authorized by section 121.12 of the amended final rule of the Organ Procurement and Transplantation Network (OPTN) (42 CFR Part 121).

Dixon, D. S., & Blackbourne, B. D. (1987). Letter to the editor. Clinical forensic medicine and organ transplantation. *Am J Forensic Med Pathol, 8*(1), 88-91.

Donoghue, E. R., & Lifschultz, B. D. (1999, October 20). "Every organ, every time" Could we do it? Special session–organ and tissue donation and effective death investigations: Tensions and resolutions. Abstract presented at the annual meeting of the National Association of Medical Examiners, Minneapolis, MN.

Duthie, S. E., Peterson, B. M., Cutler, J., et al. (1995). Successful organ donation in victims of child abuse. *Clin Transplant, 9,* 415-418.

Ehrle, R. N., Shafer, T. J., & Nelson, K. R. (1999). Determination and referral of potential organ donors and consent for organ donation: Best practices–A blueprint for success. *Crit Care Nurse, 19*(2), 21-33.

Ganikos, M. L., McNeil, C., Braslow, J. B., et al. (1994). A case study in planning for public health education: The organ and tissue donation experience. *Public Health Reports, 109*(5), 3256-3257.

Goldstein, B., Shafer, T., Greer, D., et al. (1997). Medical examiner/coroner denial for organ donation in brain-dead victims of child abuse: Controversies and solutions. *Clin Intensive Care, 8,* 136-141.

Green v. State (1991). 591 So. 2d 576 (Ala. Crim. App.).

Hanzlick, R. (1995). Letter to the editor. *JAMA, 273*(20), 1578

Hauser, J. E. (1969). The use of medical examiner-coroner cases as transplant donors. *J Forensic Sci, 14,* 501-506.

Hegert, T. F. (1995). Letter to the editor. *JAMA, 273*(20), 1578-1579.

Jason, D. (1994). The role of the medical examiner/coroner in organ and tissue procurement for transplantation. *Am J Forensic Med Pathol, 15*(3), 192-202.

Jaynes, C., & Springer, J. W. (1996). Evaluating a successful coroner protocol. *J Transpl Coord, 6*(1), 28-31.

Jaynes, C. (1995). In reply. *Am J Forensic Med Pathol, 16*(3), 259-260.

Jaynes, C. L., & Springer, J. W. (1994). Decreasing the organ donor shortage by increasing communication between coroners, medical examiners and organ procurement organizations. *Am J Forensic Med Pathol, 15*(2),156-159.

Kauffman, H. M., Bennett, L. E., McBride, M. A., et al. (1997). The expanded donor. *Transplant Rev, 11*(4), 165-199.

Kramer, J. L. (1995). Letter to the editor. *Am J Forensic Med Pathol, 16*(3), 257.

Kurachek, S. C, Titus, S. L., Olesen, M., et al. (1995). Medical examiners' attitudes toward organ procurement from child abuse/homicide victims. *Am J Forensic Med Pathol, 16*(1), 1-10.

Lanz, P. E. (1995). Letter to the editor. *Am J Forensic Med Pathol, 16*(3), 257-259

Lescoe, R. J. (1973). Why not take the beating heart? *J Leg Med (NY), 1*(1), 26-27.

Leslie, H., & Bottenfield, S. (1989). Donation, banking, and transplantation of allograft tissues: Organ and tissue transplantation. *Nurs Clin North Am, 24*(4), 891-905.

Mendez, R., & Phillips, M. G. (1992). Donor evaluation. *Donation and transplantation: Medical school curriculum.* Richmond, VA: United Network for Organ Sharing, LCCN: 92-60708.

Miller, D. C., & Moreno-Cabral, C. D. (1992). Heart-valve allografts. *Donation and transplantation: Medical school curriculum.* Richmond, VA: United Network for Organ Sharing, LCCN: 92-60708.

Miracle, K. L., Broznick, B. A., & Stuart S. A. (1993). Coroner/medical examiner cooperation with the donation process: One OPO's experience. *J Transpl Coord, 3,* 23-26.

Morrissey, P. E., & Monaco, A. P. (1997, August 15). A comprehensive approach to organ donation. *Hosp Pract,* 181-196.

Nicoletta v. Rochester Eye & Human Parts Bank, Inc. (1992). 519 N.Y.S.2d 928 (Sup. Ct.).
Organ releases needlessly delayed. (1994, November 23). *San Francisco Examiner.*
People v. Bonilla. (1983). 467 N.Y.S.2d 599, 602 (N.Y. App. Div.).
People v. Eulo. (1984). 482 N.Y.S.2d 436.
People v. Lai. (1987). 516 N.Y.S.2d 300 (App. Div.).
People v. Saldana. (1975).121 Cal. Rptr. 243 (Ct. App.).
People v. Vaughn. (1991). 579 N.Y.S.2d 839 (Sup. Ct.).
People v. Wilbourn. (1978). 372 N.E.2d 874 (Ill. Ct. App.).
Seem, D. L., & Skelley, L. (1992). The donation process. *Donation and transplantation: Medical school curriculum.* Richmond, VA: United Network for Organ Sharing, LCCN: 92-60708.
Shafer, T. (1995). In Reply. *JAMA, 273*(20), 1579.
Shafer, T. J., Schkade, L. L., Evans, R. W., et al. (2004). The vital role of medical examiners and coroners in organ transplantation. *Am J Transplant, 4,* 160-168.
Shafer, T. J., Schkade, L. L., Siminoff, L. A., et al. (1999). An ethical analysis of organ recovery denials by medical examiners, coroners and justices of the peace. *J Transpl Coord, 9*(4), 232-249.
Shafer, T. J., Schkade, L. L., Warner, H. E., et al. (1994). The impact of medical examiner/coroner practices on organ recovery in the United States. *JAMA, 272*(20),1607-1613.
Shafer, T. J, Wood, R. P., Van Buren, C. T., et al. (1997). A success story in minority donation: The LifeGift/BenTaub General Hospital in-house coordinator program. *Transplant Proc, 29*(8), 3753-3755.
Shapiro, M. B. (1992). Cornea transplantation. *Donation and transplantation: Medical school curriculum.* Richmond, VA: United Network for Organ Sharing, LCCN: 92-60708.
Sheridan, F. (1993). Pediatric death rates and donor yield: A medical examiner's view. *J Heart Lung Transplant, 12*(6), 179-186.
Siminoff, L. A., Arnold, R. M., & Caplan, A. L. (1995). Health care professional attitudes toward donation: Effect on practice and procurement. *J Trauma, 39*(3), 553-559.
Siminoff, L. A., Arnold, R. M., Caplan, A. L., et al. (1995). Public policy governing organ and tissue procurement in the United States: Results from the National Organ and Tissue Procurement Study. *Ann Intern Med, 123,* 10-17.
Skegg, P. D. G. (1974). Liability for the unauthorized removal of cadaveric transplant material. *Med Sci Law, 14*(1), 53-57.
Sosin, D. M., Sniezek, J. E., & Waxweiler, R. J. (1995, June 14). Trends in death associated with traumatic brain injury, 1979-1992. *JAMA, 273*(22), 1778-1780.
State v. Bock. (1992). 490 N.W.2d 116, 123 (Minn. Ct. App.).
State v. Brown (1971). 491 P.2d 1193 (Or. Ct. App.).
State v. Fierro. (1979). 603 P.2d 74, 77 (Ariz.).
State v. Inger. (1980). 292 N.W.2d 119, 124-125 (Iowa).
State v. Matthews. (1986). 353 S.E.2d 444 (S.C.).
State v. Meints. (1982). 322 N.W.2d 809 (Neb.).
State v. Morrison. (1989). 437 N.W.2d 422 (Minn. Ct. App.).
State v. Olson. (1989). 435 N.W.2d 530, 534 (Minn.).
State v. Shaffer. (1977). 574 P.2d 205 (Kan.).
State v. Velarde. (1986). 734 P.2d 449 (Utah).
State v. Watson. (1983). 467 A.2d 590 (N.J. Super. Ct. App. Div.).
Stickel, D. L. (1970). Medicolegal and ethical aspects of organ transplantation. *Ann N Y Acad Sci, 169*(2), 362-375.
Strama, B. T., Burling-Hatcher, S., & Shafer, T. J. (1994, Summer). Criminal investigations and prosecutions not adversely affected by organ donation: A case law review. *Newsletter of Medicine and Law Committee.* Tort and Insurance Practice Section, American Bar Association, 15-21.
Study finds examiners sometimes delay organ release for no reason. (1994, November 23). *Northwest Herald,* Woodstock, IL.
Thorne, C. (1999, February 18). Doctors want access to organs of crime victims. Associated Press.
US Department of Health and Human Services: Public Health Service. (1991, July 8-10). The surgeon general's workshop on increasing organ donation. Proceedings report.
US General Accounting Office. (1993, April). Organ transplants: Increased effort needed to boost supply and ensure equitable distribution of organs. Washington, DC: US General Accounting Office; Publication GAO/HRD-93-56.
US Code Annotated. (1997, December 22). Title 42: The public health and welfare 273: Organ procurement organizations and organ procurement and transplantation network [42 U.S.C.§ 273(b)(2)(k)].
Vaughn, K. (2000, April 17). Battle looms over organ donations. *Rocky Mountain News,* Denver, CO.
Voelker, R. (1994). Can forensic medicine and organ donation coexist for the public good? *JAMA, 271*(12), 891-892.
Wick, L., Mickell, J., Barnes, T., et al. (1995).Pediatric Organ Donation: Impact of medical examiner refusal. *Transplant Proc, 27*(4), 2539-2544.
Zugibe, F. T., Costello, J., Breithaupt, M., et al. (1999). Model organ description protocols for completion by transplant surgeons using organs procured from medical examiner cases. *J Transpl Coord, 9*(2), 73-80.

Chapter 22 Research with Vulnerable Participants

Louanne Lawson and Cynthia Cupit Swenson

Violence is a complex, sometimes deadly experience that leaves surviving victims at risk of physical, emotional, and social difficulties. Effective prevention and intervention strategies are key to resolving these difficulties. Unfortunately, interventions for victims and those accused or convicted of committing crimes are still in their infancy. As forensic nurse examiners who are committed to evidence-based practice develop and test new interventions, it will be important to maximize the protection of the victims and those accused or convicted of committing crimes who participate in our research. In addition to an obligation to learn and teach, forensic nurses must protect those from whom they learn, especially when they become a subject of attention due to personal adverse situations.

This chapter examines the risks and benefits of conducting research with victims and those accused or convicted of committing crimes who are vulnerable because of their safety needs and lack of autonomy (Lutz, 1999). This discussion (1) defines vulnerable research participants; (2) presents principles guiding human participants research; (3) reviews protections for vulnerable participants, in addition to those requiring extra protection via Title 45; (4) discusses issues in protecting vulnerable participants; and (5) presents practical steps for researchers to assure protection and compliance with Institutional Review Board (IRB) regulations.

Who Are Vulnerable Research Participants?

Although the utmost care should be taken to protect the privacy and well-being of all human participants, the Federal Policy for Protection of Human Subjects, commonly referred to as the Common Rule, in the Code of Federal Regulations (CFR), Title 45, Part 46, identifies populations that are considered vulnerable and in need of additional protection when participating in research. These populations include children, prisoners, pregnant women, mentally disabled persons, and economically or educationally disadvantaged persons. They are considered vulnerable because due to life circumstances, age, or disabilities, participation in research brings elevated risk. Prisoners, along with children and mentally infirm adults, are considered vulnerable because of the potential for their exploitation (Brody, 1998).

The risk to vulnerable participants is especially great when identification as a potential participant can in itself be dangerous. In the interest of safeguarding these participants, it may be tempting to exclude them from studies. However, this mechanism for protecting vulnerable participants from the risks posed by research has the unintended effect of also excluding them from potential direct and indirect benefits. Direct benefits may include access to services such as treatment programs. Indirect benefits may include knowing that they have made an important social contribution even if there is no direct benefit to them personally. Investigators must consider the benefits to participants themselves and to the social good, along with the risks of participation. The conflict is intensified when the research being conducted is critically important to the very population of vulnerable participants under study. The Nuremberg Code suggests that risks are warranted if the results of research provide useful information that cannot be developed in any other way (*Trials of War Criminals before the Nuremberg Military Tribunals under Control Council Law No. 10*, 1949). If the risks are warranted, however, then researchers must be especially mindful of guarding the safety of participants. To do so, guidelines for applying the principles of informed consent, assessing risks and benefits, and selecting participants for research with vulnerable subjects have been developed (Department of Health, Education, and Welfare, 1979).

Key Point 22-1

The forensic nurse investigator must carefully consider the risks and benefits of research in regard to the vulnerable participants themselves and to the social good of the larger society.

Principles Guiding Human Participants Research

Current laws and ethical principles provide guidelines for procedures researchers should follow to minimize the risk of research to vulnerable populations. Conducting ethical research for the social good challenges individuals to think carefully about the ethical principles of respect for persons, beneficence, and justice. The laws and principles that guide the ethical conduct of research with human participants are outlined in the Nuremberg Code (1949), the Belmont Report (1979), and Title 45–Public Welfare, Part 46–Regulations on Protection of Human Subjects (1999). Subparts B, C, and D of Title 45, Part 46, also outline specific guidelines for conducting research with vulnerable participants, defined in these subparts as pregnant women, fetuses, neonates, children, and prisoners. These principles guide the actions of IRBs, which are the committees within research institutions that approve and monitor research conducted by the scientists in that institution.

The Nuremberg Code

The Nuremberg Code was published in 1949 in response to the atrocities committed by Nazi physicians when they conducted biomedical experiments on concentration camp inmates (Shuster, 1997). According to the Nuremberg Code, potential research participants must have the legal capacity to consent, the freedom to decline, and the information needed to make an informed decision. The principal investigator of a study is responsible for ensuring that these conditions are met. Human beings are to be used in research only when there is substantial reason to think that the study will yield results for the public good and there is no other way to gather the necessary information. Unnecessary physical and mental suffering should be avoided and studies should not be conducted that carry substantial risk that participants will die or be disabled as a result of their participation. The risk to an individual participant should not exceed the social benefit. Only qualified scientists should conduct research, and they should be willing to terminate an experiment when necessary to protect participants from injury, disability, or death. Participants should be free to withdraw at any point for any reason (or for no reason) without fear of reprisal.

The Belmont Report

The National Commission for the Protection of Human Subjects of Biomedical and Behavioral Research wrote the Belmont Report in 1979 (Department of Health, Education, and Welfare, 1979). It expands the principles outlined in the Nuremberg Code to define the boundaries between research and clinical practice, develop risk-benefit criteria, provide guidelines for selecting human participants, and define the concept of informed consent.

Research and practice are distinguished based on the purpose for the activity and the expectation of results. Research is generally considered to be any activity designed primarily to develop new knowledge. Scientists who conduct research recognize that experiments are as likely to fail as they are to succeed. Practice, on the other hand, is designed to enhance the well-being of persons and carries with it a reasonable expectation that the clinician's efforts will be successful.

The basic ethical principles used to develop risk-benefit criteria, provide guidelines for selecting participants, and define informed consent are respect for persons, beneficence, and justice. When applied to vulnerable persons, the principle of respect for persons requires that two sometimes-competing standards be applied. Prisoners, for example, should not be "deprived of the opportunity to volunteer for research" (Department of Health, Education, and Welfare, 1979, p. 4). On the other hand, prisoners are subject to coercion and undue influence in ways that free citizens are not, and their right to decline to participate in research should be carefully protected.

The principle of beneficence requires that researchers go beyond the minimal obligations to other human beings and include acts of kindness and charity on behalf of vulnerable participants. That is, it is not enough to "do no harm." Researchers must also do their best to ensure that the benefits of participation in research are maximized and risks are minimized.

The principle of justice is particularly important when planning and conducting research with vulnerable participants. This principle requires that the advantages to society accrue as much to people in the participant's circumstance as they do to society at large. The investigator cannot select participants simply because they are accessible, perhaps by virtue of being confined to institutions or being treated in a charity ward of a hospital. In some instances, the burden borne by the poor has been maximized in research, whereas the benefits of the results have been enjoyed by people with greater financial or social advantages. The most famous example is the Tuskegee syphilis study, which ran from to 1932 to 1972 (Rothman, 1982).

The three principles noted above are applied to human participants research through the process of assessment of risks and benefits, selection of participants, and informed consent. First, the investigator assesses the risk to benefit ratio by determining whether it is necessary to involve human participants at all. It is appropriate, for example, to use human participants in conducting research on socially deviant acts such as rape because deviance is a human construct. Whereas other species create social order and, presumably, social disorder, the social construction of reality is a uniquely human phenomenon because it is based on language (Berger & Luckman, 1966). Some animals may have language, but it is not accessible to humans, at least for now, so studying deviance from a non-human perspective does little to answer questions about how and why rapists do what they do.

Case Study 22-1 Tuskegee Syphilis Study

In 1932, a study was designed to determine the progression of syphilis in human subjects. Three hundred ninety-nine disadvantaged, rural, African-American men were deliberately infected with syphilis and then monitored over time to identify the course of the disease. They were not informed as to what disease they were suffering but were told they were being treated for "bad blood." Even when effective treatment was developed, these research participants were left untreated and were even prevented from receiving appropriate treatment. Moreover, they were not given the information they needed to make an informed decision about their continued participation in the study. This study violated the principle of justice by selecting participants and maintaining their involvement on the basis of their disadvantaged social position.

Best Practice *22-1*

The three principles noted in the discussion are applied to human participants' research through the process of assessment of risks and benefits, selection of participants, and informed consent.

On the other hand, it is not necessary to use human participants in experiments about the nature and extent of wounds inflicted by violent acts such as rape because computer models or photographs are sufficient to answer the questions. For example, it would not be appropriate to conduct a randomized controlled trial of genital injury inflicted during sexual assault. Instead, questions about the nature and extent of genital injury under conditions of rape can be answered by having photographs of genital findings examined by blinded reviewers. This process allows investigators to identify genital injury associated with unwanted sexual contact without exposing people to unnecessary risk. When research is being conducted, if researchers are determining that the treatment increases risk of harm to participants or if they see a beneficial effect, participants have a right to this information.

Key Point *22-2*

The procedures used to select participants should ensure fairness; subjects who might be vulnerable to manipulation or coercion should be carefully protected.

The procedures used to select participants should ensure fairness and people who are vulnerable to manipulation or coercion should be carefully protected. Prior to an individual's involvement in a study, researchers should protect a person's right to choose what will happen to him or her by providing participants with information in language they can understand and by preventing coercion, thereby ensuring that consent is informed and voluntary. Title 45, Part 46, of the federal regulations governing research with human participants, which is outlined in the next section, specifically defines procedures for assessment of risks and benefits, selection of participants, and informed consent.

Title 45–Public Welfare, Part 46–Protection of Human Subjects

Regulations

In 1974, the Department of Health, Education, and Welfare issued regulations governing the protection of human research participants. In 1991, Part A of 45 CFR 46 was adopted by a number of federal agencies and is known as the Common Rule. The Common Rule requires research institutions receiving federal support to establish institutional review boards and delineates requirements for informed consent. The Department of Health and Human Services (DHHS) provides guidelines for additional protections not included in the Common Rule in research conducted with pregnant women, human fetuses and neonates, children, and prisoners (subparts B through D). In general, these special protections are designed to ensure that research activities with vulnerable participants, as with all human participants, are conducted ethically and address socially important questions. In particular, they outline the mechanisms for managing participant selection and informed consent, with the special considerations that IRB's use to protect vulnerable participants.

Pregnant Women and Fetuses

The IRB is required to ensure that preliminary studies are conducted with animals and nonpregnant women before pregnant women are exposed to the risks associated with research. The risk to the fetus must be as minimal as possible, and the investigator should not be involved in decisions to terminate the pregnancy or in the process of establishing the viability of the fetus. When conducting research with a fetus, the investigator's primary aim must be to meet the health needs of the fetus, and the investigator must establish that there is no alternative mechanism for gathering the needed information. In general, the father as well as the mother must give consent before the research is conducted, except under specific conditions.

Children

Children are considered vulnerable participants because they have not reached the legal age for consent. To include them in research, the investigator must establish the potential for discovering effective methods for treating disease and promoting development. Greater than minimal risk must be justified by the anticipated benefit to the individual child or be no greater than the risks associated with alternative treatments.

Often, researchers and referral sources worry that risk is increased because a child is assigned to a comparison treatment and not the treatment being studied. There may be an automatic faith in the experimental condition because it is hypothesized to be a better treatment. However, when there is no empirical evidence that the experimental treatment is superior to the control treatment at the outset of a study, this worry is unfounded. The risks associated with current treatment or no treatment at all may be greater than the risks associated with the research, and the balance among the relative risks must be taken into consideration.

For example, a clinician may incorporate research-based strategies that are commonly used in treating adult intrafamilial sexual offenders against girls. Because the treatment is well known and generally thought to be effective, therapists working with adolescent offenders might use a modified form of the treatment with their patient population. It would be quite appropriate to modify the intervention using theories of adolescent development and resilience and then carefully monitor patient-specific outcomes. Trying the new intervention does not constitute research, but systematically evaluating the intervention and generalizing the results of the study for use with other patients does constitute research and should be approved and monitored by an Institutional Review Board.

Best Practice 22-2

Subject referrals should not involve fax or Email because these communication modes can compromise confidentiality and privacy.

When determining how to recruit children, researchers must carefully define the population to be studied and set up a specific screening procedure to correctly select participants. Care should be taken in how referrals come in so as to protect confidentiality. An example is referrals for abused and neglected children coming from a child protective services (CPS) agency. If the child is in the parent's custody, CPS cannot give out phone numbers or addresses of families without permission from the legal guardian. To address this confidentiality protection, CPS can have parents sign a release that allows the agency to give to the researcher information on the family that the agency wants to refer. Researchers need to be careful about taking referrals over a fax machine or Email, however, as these methods do not protect confidentiality. Once a referral is made, a member of the research team must carefully review the specifics of the study with the parent or legal guardian and ensure that the potential participant has the information needed for informed consent. If parents are giving information about themselves or answering questions about their child, they must sign an informed consent form for themselves as research participants before they participate in the study. Then, if research data are being collected on the child, the parent must sign permission for their child's participation (see example in Box 22-1). In addition, the IRB responsible for approving the study determines whether the child is capable of assenting, taking into account the "ages, maturity, and psychological state of the children involved" (Title 45, part 46, §46.408). In cases where custody of the child changes during the study, the new legal guardians must sign a consent for themselves and the child before they participate in the research. For example, if a child enters CPS custody during the study, the CPS caseworker or supervisor must give informed consent before the child can participate because the caseworker is *in loco parentis* (legally serving as the parent). A copy of the consent form should be given to each legal guardian or other adult who gives informed consent, for his or her own personal records.

Box 22-1 Sample of Parent/Legal Guardian Consent Form

MEDICAL UNIVERSITY OF SOUTH CAROLINA
Informed Consent Agreement for Home-Based Multisystemic Therapy versus
Parent Group

I, ____________________, do hereby consent for my child, ______________, to participate in a research project studying ways to help families with children who have been physically abused. Researcher ____________ has explained to me the information described below.

PURPOSE: This study will compare two treatments (home-based multisystemic therapy [MST] and parent group [PG]) to see which is better at (1) improving a child's behavior and ability to get along with other children, (2) improving a parent's ability to manage his or her anger, discipline his or her child, and handle stress, (3) reducing a parent's physical abuse of his or her child, and (4) improving family relationships.

PROCEDURES: Families who participate in the study will either be treated in their home by an MST therapist, or they will attend a parent group at the Charleston/Dorchester Mental Health Center office. This will be decided by random choice (much like flipping a coin). Families participating in home-based MST will receive visits in their home several times a week for four to six months. The MST therapist will work with the family on better ways to handle problems with the child and in the family. Families participating in the parent group will meet seven (7) times, each for about 1 to 1½ hours, at the Mental Health Center and receive help on handling problems with the child or in the family. All meetings of home-based MST will be audio taped.

All families, regardless of whether they participate in MST or PG, will be asked some questions by our trained researchers and be given some written questions to answer. The questions will be about your child's behavior, your behavior, and how you and your child get along with each other and with other people. The assessments will be done at the beginning of treatment and again 2, 4, 10, and 16 months later. Each of these assessments will take about 2½ hours.

Your family's therapist, Department of Social Services (DSS) caseworker, and other agencies with whom you are involved will be contacted once a month to help us gain information on problems with child abuse, the services you have received, and how much these services have cost.

DURATION: Your participation in the study will last about 16 months. You will be interviewed five times during that period.

POSSIBLE DISCOMFORTS OR RISKS: The physical, social, legal, and economic risks to your family are very small. The major risk of participation in the study is the release of personal information, and the researchers have taken steps to make that risk very small. There is some loss of privacy with any treatment; however, your therapists are trained to keep information private and to ask about only information that is needed. A certificate of confidentiality that has been obtained to protect your privacy is described in section L.

POSSIBLE BENEFITS: Both home-based MST and parent group are expected to reduce family problems and to help children and parents. The information from this study may help other families in which a child has been physically abused.

OTHER WAYS TO GAIN TREATMENT: If you and your child decide not to participate in this study, your child will still receive services that he or she would otherwise have received. Alternatives include, but are not limited to, referral to other agencies that treat children and families.

COST OF PARTICIPATION: There will be no charges to you for participating in this study.

COMPENSATION: You and your child will receive a total of $50 for each assessment you complete. That is a total of $250 for completing all five assessments.

STUDENT PARTICIPATION: If you or your child is a student of MUSC, no record of your participation, or your decision not to participate, will be part of your or your child's academic record at MUSC. Neither will your participation, or your decision not to participate, be part of any decisions in your or your child's academic performance.

EMPLOYEE PARTICIPATION: No record of participation, or decision not to participate, will be part of your or your child's personnel record if you or he or she is an employee of MUSC. Neither will your participation, or your decision not to participate, be part of any decisions in job performance or evaluation.

NEW INFORMATION: Any new information that is developed during the course of this study that might influence you or your child's willingness to continue participation in this study will be given to you or your child.

CONFIDENTIALITY: To help us protect your privacy, the investigators have obtained a confidentiality certificate from the Department of Health and Human Services (DHHS).

With this certificate, the investigators cannot be forced (for example, by court subpoena) to disclose information that may identify you in any federal, state, or local civil, criminal, administrative, legislative, or other proceedings. Disclosure will be necessary, however, upon request of the DHHS for audit or program evaluation purposes.

You should understand that a confidentiality certificate does not prevent you or a member of your family from voluntarily releasing information about yourself or your involvement in this research. Note, however, that if an insurer or employer learns about your participation and obtains your consent to receive research information, then the investigator may not use the certificate of confidentiality to withhold this information. This means that you and your family must also actively protect your own privacy.

Finally, you should understand that the investigator is not prevented from taking steps, including reporting to authorities, to prevent serious harm to you or others. All cases have been investigated by the DSS, and this information is already known to legal authorities. If any information about new or unreported abuse is learned during the course of this study, a new report will be filed with child protection authorities. Also, if you or your child reports suicidal or homicidal information, services will be sought to protect you, your child, and others.

Results of this research will be used for the purposes described in this study. This information may be published, but you will not be identified. Any information that is obtained concerning this research that can be identified with you will remain confidential to the extent possible within state and federal law. The investigators associated with this study, the sponsor, and the MUSC Institutional Review Board for Human Research will have access to identifying information. The certificate of confidentiality will help protect your records if they are subpoenaed by a court of law.

In the event that you are injured as a result of participation in this study, you should immediately go to the emergency room of the Medical University Hospital, or in the case of an emergency, go to the nearest hospital and tell the physician on call that you are in a research study. The hospital will call your study doctor who will make the arrangements for your treatment. If the study sponsor does not pay for your treatment, the Medical University Hospital and the physicians who render treatment to you will bill your insurance company. If your insurance company denies coverage or insurance is not available, you will be responsible for payment for all services rendered to you.

Your participation in this study is voluntary. You may refuse to take part in or stop taking part in this study at any time. You should call the investigator in charge of this study if you decide to do this. Your decision not to take part in the study will not affect your current or future medical care or any benefits to which you are entitled.

The investigators and/or the sponsor may stop your participation in this study at any time if they decide it is in your best interest. They may also do this if you do not follow the investigator's instructions.

VOLUNTEER'S STATEMENT

I have been given a chance to ask questions about this research study. These questions have been answered to my satisfaction. If I have any more questions about my participation in this study or study-related injury, I may contact Dr. ________________. I may contact the Medical University of SC Hospital medical director concerning medical treatment.

If I have any questions about my rights as a research subject in this study, I may contact the Medical University of SC Institutional Review Board for Human Research at ________________.

I agree to participate in this study. I have been given a copy of this form for my own records.

If you wish to participate, please sign below.

______________________________ ____________
Signature of Person Obtaining Consent Date

______________________________ ____________
Printed Name of Participant* Date

______________________________ ____________
Signature of Legal Guardian (if applicable) Date

*For participants 12 to 17 years old: "My participation has been explained to me, and all of my questions have been answered. I am willing to participate."

Signature: ____________________

Age: _____ Date of Birth: ____________

Prisoners

Prisoners are also offered special protection because their incarceration puts them at risk for coercion. The IRB that approves and monitors the study must include a prisoner or prisoner representative. Any benefits associated with the research, including more or better quality food, more comfortable living space, or opportunities for earning money or privileges, should not be so great that they would induce an otherwise reluctant prisoner to participate. The risks to prisoner-participants should not be greater than the risks to nonprisoner-participants, and selection procedures should be impartial. Parole boards may not use participation or nonparticipation in their decisions about release. Follow-up monitoring, where warranted, should be planned with variability in the length of sentences in mind. Teams conducting research with prisoners related to their status as prisoners or the actions that resulted in incarceration should include an expert in criminology, either as a member of the team or as a consultant. If researchers are going to study individuals who are incarcerated or who could potentially be incarcerated during the study, they must state this in their research plan for the protection of human participants that is reviewed by the IRB.

Prisoners are vulnerable to coercion in ways that free citizens are not (Bach-y-Rita, 1974). They live in a controlled society, with limited access to information, support, and counsel. The level of risk a prisoner is willing to accept may be higher than that acceptable to a free person because the benefits of participation in research may be more immediate and tangible than potential risks. Also, prisoners are vulnerable to coercion because the environment they live in can produce dependence, depersonalization, helplessness, and anonymity. Any financial inducements attain a level of worth out of proportion to their dollar value because prisoners have limited access to gainful employment. The living conditions on a research unit may be considerably more pleasant than those in the general prison. Indeed, researchers who conduct their studies in prison settings may consider themselves responsible for improving the living conditions of the inmates who live there and participate in the research. At the same time, attention to potential exposure to unfamiliar risks is a measure of the investigator's personal integrity and is an important component of project planning. In particular, investigators should guard against taking advantage of the prisoner's situation because to do so would be to inappropriately remove themselves from the observer role (Rothman, 1982).

When they enter a prison setting, researchers should recognize that they are entering an unfamiliar environment, with its own rules, boundaries, and social contracts (Rubin, 1976). Prisoners may challenge the investigator's commitment to the research and attitudes toward criminals. The investigator should be cautious about an overzealously cooperative attitude. Instead, honest discussions about the investigator's beliefs and values, coupled with accepting responsibility for limiting coercion, promote successful research.

Other Vulnerable Participants

In addition to these identified by the Department of Health and Human Services, vulnerable participants may include those people who are at risk for decreased autonomy (Tyson & Fleming, 1999). Forensic nurse investigators address the concept of vulnerability from the perspective of those accused or convicted of crimes, as well as those who are victims of crimes. For victims, vulnerability is associated with limited access to social and environmental resources, which puts them at risk for poor health and higher morbidity and mortality rates (Flaskerud & Winslow, 1998). For those accused or convicted of committing crimes, vulnerability is associated with the potential for coercion and unfair distribution of the risks and benefits of participating in research (Brody, 1998). Socially responsible research must carefully address the special issues facing these vulnerable participants in order to improve outcomes and promote scientific integrity (Lutz, 1999).

Victims as Research Participants

Victims of crimes are considered vulnerable because they have special safety needs (Parker, Ulrich, & NRCVA, 1990). Battered women, for example, are vulnerable to further violence from their abuser. Research with a woman who is being battered exposes her to retaliation from an abusive spouse or to the stigma associated with being labeled a victim. The person who is doing the battering may be hypervigilant about the victim's answers in research interviews or concerned that the woman will disclose the abuse. In such cases, safety plans should be established with the victim because participation alone can increase stress and the risk of harm, regardless of the answers given in the interview. Certain characteristics of conducting research may increase risk for victims, and these include recruitment from a small population, investigator biases, and recruitment from sites representing unique groups

Research conducted with samples from small populations can lead to "deductive disclosure," by which a person can be identified by demographic information alone (Morris, Sales, & Berman, 1981). For example, once a study involved treatment in a relatively small community. People from the community knew about the project and therefore could deduce that families interacting with the researchers or therapists were research participants. The study involved both substance-abusing youth and youth who were doing well, in order to look at resilience in a high-crime neighborhood. Because the researchers were meeting with most families in the neighborhood who had children, the identity of those receiving treatment was less obvious. In such cases, researchers must work closely with families to protect their identity as research participants. When research participants are presented in case studies, extra care should be taken to conceal the identity of participants. Researchers may do this by changing or leaving out some demographic information, using case numbers or names of trees or flowers rather than typical person names, and assuring that the results of the research are disseminated through professional peer-reviewed journals or books, not in community-wide papers or newsletters (J. Schaller-Ayers, personal communication, April 14, 1999).

There are also risks to victims from investigator biases (Lutz, 1999). For example, sometimes investigators with an unexamined philosophical bias are tempted to over- or underreport a problem. Although the intent of overreporting may be to galvanize support, there is danger in distorting the magnitude of a problem. Conversely, if the problem is underreported, perhaps to avoid "pathologizing" participants (Kurz, 1987), there is a risk of decreasing the resources and support available to true victims. For example, society's response to research that challenges beliefs about marriage and violence may cause concern for potential participants. Research protocols include protections against biased interpretation of data in order to safeguard scientific integrity. Consent forms should outline how the data will be used so potential participants have the information needed to make an informed decision.

Participant recruitment is another sensitive topic (Parker, Ulrich, & NRCVA, 1990). Participants who are recruited from agencies serving unique groups, such as battered women's shelters, women's health centers, and legal aid clinics, are likely to be in a reasonably safe situation. However, these unique groups may not represent the entire population being studied. Battered women who are recruited by public advertising are more reflective of the entire population, but they may inadvertently put themselves at risk because of inexperience with disclosure. To protect both the participant and the researcher from retaliation by the batterer, the researcher should create specific procedures for contacting the participant, conducting the initial interview, handling copies of the consent form, and providing ways to contact the researcher (Parker, Ulrich, & NRCVA, 1990).

Decisions about how to balance care with research should be made prior to data collection. Nurse researchers are ethically bound to intervene in particularly dangerous situations, even if interventions contaminate the research, because the principle of beneficence (as outlined in the Belmont Report) requires that the benefits of participation are maximized and the risks are minimized. The possibility that a forensic nurse investigator may have to choose between providing immediate assistance and continuing to collect data from a participant should be fully explored prior to instituting the study.

Issues in Protecting Participants

Confidentiality

Assurances of confidentiality are a critical component of research. The current approach to confidentiality began with the Nuremburg trials, which emphasized confidentiality as a way to prevent or minimize physical and psychological harm. Confidentiality is used to protect the participant's privacy and to enhance the credibility of the research process itself. Not only is protecting privacy the fair thing to do, but it increases the likelihood that people will participate in research and will provide honest answers to the researcher's questions (Blanck, Bellack, & Rosnow et al., 1992).

There is certain information that is not kept confidential. Research participants must be correctly informed as to what information will be kept confidential and what information is not confidential (see the sample consent form in Box 22-2). For example, child and adult participants must be told at the time of giving informed consent that if a child or adult discloses abuse, a mandated report will be made to the appropriate protective services department. If a participant was referred to the study because of a history of abuse, it should be made clear that past abuse that has already been reported will not be reported again. However, abuse not previously reported will be reported to CPS. Also, disclosure of suicidal or homicidal intent must be openly discussed with individuals who can help provide safety for the participant or intended victim. The obligations imposed on clinicians by the Tarasoff ruling, which requires that public policy protecting confidentiality between patients and psychotherapists must yield, at least to the extent to which disclosure is essential to avert danger to others, operate in research situations as well. That is, disclosure of homicidal intent must be reported to the police and the intended victim. When participants learn that there are limits to confidentiality, they may opt to give incorrect responses to sensitive questions. However, they may be more honest if the behavior in question (e.g., abuse of a child) is already out in the open.

Privacy

In December 2000, the DHHS issued regulations to carry out the mandate of the Health Insurance Portability and Accountability Act of 1996 (HIPAA) to establish federal standards for safeguarding the privacy of individually identifiable health information (National Institutes of Health, 2003). The Privacy Rule was amended on August 14, 2002, and most covered entities were required to comply with this rule by April 14, 2003. Protected health information (PHI)

Box 22-2 Sample of Subject Form from Medical University of South Carolina

MEDICAL UNIVERSITY OF SOUTH CAROLINA
Informed Consent Agreement for Home-Based Multisystemic Therapy versus
Parent Group

I, ____________, agree to participate in a research project studying ways to help families with children who have been physically abused. Researcher ____________ has explained to me the information described below.

PURPOSE: This study will compare two treatments (home-based multisystemic therapy [MST] and parent group [PG]) to see which is better at (1) improving a child's behavior and ability to get along with other children, (2) improving a parent's ability to manage his or her anger, discipline his or her child, and handle stress, (3) reducing a parent's physical abuse of his or her child, and (4) improving family relationships.

PROCEDURES: Families who participate in the study will either be treated in their home by an MST therapist, or they will attend a parent group at the Charleston/Dorchester Mental Health Center office. This will be decided by random choice (much like flipping a coin). Families participating in home-based MST will receive visits in their home several times a week for four to six months. The MST therapist will work with the family on better ways to handle problems with the child and in the family. Families participating in the parent group will meet seven (7) times, each for about 1 to 1½ hours, at the Mental Health Center and receive help on handling problems with the child or in the family. All meetings of home-based MST will be audio taped.

All families, regardless of whether they participate in MST or PG, will be asked some questions by our trained researchers and be given some written questions to answer. The questions will be about your child's behavior, your behavior, and how you and your child get along with each other and with other people. The assessments will be done at the beginning of treatment and again 2, 4, 10, and 16 months later. Each of these assessments will take about 2½ hours.

Your family's therapist, Department of Social Services (DSS) caseworker, and other agencies with whom you are involved will be contacted once a month to help us gain information on problems with child abuse, the services you have received, and how much these services have cost.

DURATION: Your participation in the study will last about 16 months. You will be interviewed five times during that time.

POSSIBLE DISCOMFORTS OR RISKS: The physical, social, legal, and economic risks to your family are very small. The major risk of participation in the study is the release of personal information, and the researchers have taken steps to make that risk very small. There is some loss of privacy with any treatment; however, your therapists are trained to keep information private and to ask about only information that is needed. A certificate of confidentiality that has been obtained to protect your privacy is described in section L.

POSSIBLE BENEFITS: Both home-based MST and parent group are expected to reduce family problems and to help children and parents. The information from this study may help other families in which a child has been physically abused.

OTHER WAYS TO GAIN TREATMENT: If you decide not to participate in this study, your family will still receive services that you would otherwise have received. Alternatives include, but are not limited to, referral to other agencies that treat children and families.

COST OF PARTICIPATION: There will be no charges to you for participating in this study.

COMPENSATION: You and your child will receive a total of $50 for each assessment you complete. That is a total of $250 for completing all five assessments.

STUDENT PARTICIPATION: If you are a student of MUSC, no record of your participation, or your decision not to participate, will be part of your academic record at MUSC. Neither will your participation, or your decision not to participate, be part of any decisions in your academic performance.

EMPLOYEE PARTICIPATION: No record of participation, or decision not to participate, will be part of your personnel record if you are an employee of MUSC. Neither will your participation, or your decision not to participate, be part of any decisions in job performance or evaluation.

NEW INFORMATION: Any new information that is developed during the course of this study that might influence your willingness to continue participation in this study will be given to you.

CONFIDENTIALITY: To help us protect your privacy, the investigators have obtained a confidentiality certificate from the Department of Health and Human Services (DHHS).

With this certificate, the investigators cannot be forced (for example, by court subpoena) to disclose information that may identify you in any federal, state, or local civil, criminal, administrative, legislative, or other proceedings. Disclosure will be necessary, however, upon request of the DHHS for audit or program evaluation purposes.

You should understand that a confidentiality certificate does not prevent you or a member of your family from voluntarily releasing information about yourself or your involvement in this research. Note, however, that if an insurer or employer learns about your participation, and obtains your consent to receive research information, then the investigator may not use the certificate of confidentiality to withhold this information. This means that you and your family must also actively protect your own privacy.

Finally, you should understand that the investigator is not prevented from taking steps, including reporting to authorities, to prevent serious harm to you or to others. All cases have been investigated by DSS and this information is already known to legal authorities. If any information about new or unreported abuse is learned during the course of this study, a new report will be filed with child protection authorities. Also, if you or your child reports suicidal or homicidal information, services will be sought to protect you, your child, and others.

Results of this research will be used for the purposes described in this study. This information may be published, but you will not be identified. Information that is obtained concerning this research that can be identified with you will remain confidential to the extent possible within state and federal law. The investigators associated with this study, the sponsor, and the MUSC Institutional Review Board for Human Research will have access to identifying information. The certificate of confidentiality will help protect your records if subpoenaed by a court of law.

In the event that you are injured as a result of participation in this study, you should immediately go to the emergency room of the Medical University Hospital, or in the case of an emergency, go to the nearest hospital and tell the physician on call that you are in a research study. The hospital will call your study doctor who will make the arrangements for your treatment. If the study sponsor does not pay for your treatment, the Medical University Hospital and the physicians who render treatment to you will bill your insurance company. If your insurance company denies coverage or insurance is not available, you will be responsible for payment for all services rendered to you.

Your participation in this study is voluntary. You may refuse to take part in or stop taking part in this study at any time. You should call the investigator in charge of this study if you decide to do this. Your decision not to take part in the study will not affect your current or future medical care or any benefits to which you are entitled.

The investigators and/or the sponsor may stop your participation in this study at any time if they decide it is in your best interest. They may also do this if you do not follow the investigator's instructions.

VOLUNTEER'S STATEMENT

I have been given a chance to ask questions about this research study. These questions have been answered to my satisfaction. If I have any more questions about my participation in this study or study-related injury, I may contact Dr. _______________. I may contact the Medical University of SC Hospital medical director concerning medical treatment.

If I have any questions about my rights as a research subject in this study, I may contact the Medical University of SC Institutional Review Board for Human Research at _________________.

I agree to participate in this study. I have been given a copy of this form for my own records.

If you wish to participate, please sign below.

________________________________ ____________

Signature of Person Obtaining Consent Date

________________________________ ____________

Signature of Participant Date

________________________________ ____________

Signature of Legal Guardian (if applicable) Date

pertains to an individual's past, present, or future physical or mental health condition or the provision of healthcare, and payment. HIPAA regulations apply to privacy both in practice and in research. HIPAA establishes conditions under which covered entities can provide researchers with PHI when it is necessary to conduct research. The DHHS Web site provides information on HIPAA. Researchers must develop a HIPAA authorization form regarding the PHI that will be disclosed from the research. On this form, information should be presented regarding the purpose of disclosure, what will be disclosed, who will disclose, and who will receive the information. Research participants are not required to sign the HIPAA authorization, but if they choose not to sign, they cannot be allowed to participate in the research. An example of an IRB approved HIPAA authorization form is found in Box 22-3.

Threats to Confidentiality

Subpoena

Assurances of confidentiality are not absolute. Although the participant has a right to privacy, the public has an equal right to certain types of information. Subpoenas can be issued for reasons that have nothing to do with research. For example, a prosecuting attorney may issue a subpoena for research data if there is reason to believe it contains evidence of illegal activity. Information obtained by subpoena becomes part of the public record and is accessible through the Freedom of Information Act (Melton & Gray, 1988), unless it is protected from disclosure by a protective order, or a court places it under seal (J. Myers, 2000, personal communication). Researchers are advised to check with the attorney for the Institutional Review Board approving the study if jurisdiction-specific questions arise.

The threat of subpoena may tempt researchers to destroy data, especially if the data put a vulnerable participant at risk. However, deviating from accepted data archiving procedures is considered scientific misconduct, even when it is done to protect a vulnerable participant. Data archiving procedures, established by institutional regulations, should be followed, and any deviation from the procedures should be directly addressed. At a minimum, the data should be securely locked, identifying information should be separated from the data, and public disclosure of identifying information should be prevented. Further, computer files should be password protected.

Best Practice *22-3*

Research data should be securely locked with any information that could identify the subject separated from the data, and public disclosure of identifying information should be prevented. Computer files should be password protected.

An example of a method for assuring anonymity in an individual's decision about research participation is an instrument development study being conducted with prisoners convicted of child sexual assault. A unique feature of this project is the option for anonymous withdrawal from the study. A postcard with the protocol number stamped in the upper right-hand corner is left with each participant. Participants who change their minds about participating in the study can drop the postcard in the mail, and the study staff will destroy all associated study materials. The consent forms remain in the site coordinator's files because no notification of withdrawal from the study is made to the site coordinator. This procedure ensures that none of the officials responsible for registering, screening, or treating offenders are informed of a participant's withdrawal from the study, safeguarding his or her right to withdraw from the study without penalty.

Freedom of Information Act

The federal Freedom of Information Act, passed in 1966, raises issues about confidentiality. The act is designed to provide public access to public records. Prior to 1974, people had to justify their attempts to access records. After the Watergate scandal, the rules were changed. According to Montgomery (1979), with this law, any person is entitled to unlimited access to public records, regardless of the demands placed on employee time or the expense of paperwork and photocopying. A public record is accessible if it contains information that is required by law. An agency is considered public if the government funds it.

Additional Protection of Confidentiality

Certificates of Confidentiality

One way to protect against unwarranted intrusion into the research process is to obtain a certificate of confidentiality. In the 1970s, a need arose to protect information collected on illegal drug use. The solution was to create legal protection against disclosure of participant information in research on the use and effects of drugs. This was granted by the secretary of Health, Education, and Welfare under the Comprehensive Drug Abuse Prevention and Control Act of 1970. An amendment in 1974 (Comprehensive Alcohol Abuse and Alcoholism Prevention, Treatment, and Rehabilitation Amendments of 1974) expanded protection of information to mental health, including information on alcohol use. A 1988 amendment expanded the protection to mental health in general (Health Omnibus Extension Programs Extension of 1988).

At present, the confidentiality protection comes in the form of a certificate of confidentiality, and federal funding is not required for this. Researchers must apply for the certificate, and protection is granted only when the research is of a sensitive nature and protection is necessary to meet the research objectives. Certificates of confidentiality may be obtained from the Public Health Service, as well as from other agencies, and can help balance the interests of the individual with the interests of the state by protecting participants from harm and promoting research integrity. However, they protect only the names and identities of participants in the research, not the data (Blanck, Bellack, & Rosnow et al., 1992; Lutz, 1999). There are seven areas of research to which the certificate can be applied:

1. Information relating to sexual attitudes, preferences, or practices
2. Information relating to the use of alcohol, drugs, or other addictive products
3. Information pertaining to illegal conduct
4. Information that if released could reasonably be damaging to an individual's financial standing, employability, or reputation within the community
5. Information that would normally be recorded in a patient's medical record, the disclosure of which could reasonably lead to social stigmatization or discrimination

Box 22-3 Privacy Act

MEDICAL UNIVERSITY OF SOUTH CAROLINA
Health Insurance Portability and Accountability Act (HIPPA)

Authorization to Use or Disclose Protected Health Information (PHI) for Research Purposes

Home-Based Multisystemic Therapy versus Parent Group

HIPPA is a federal law that requires the protection of information that can identify you. Protected health information includes information that pertains to your past, present, or future physical and mental health conditions or the provision of healthcare. You are being asked to sign this authorization because you are in the research study listed above.

The researchers and the National Institute of Mental Health agree to protect your protected health information by using and disclosing it only as permitted by you in the authorization and as directed by state and federal law.

WHAT IS THE PURPOSE OF DISCLOSING YOUR PROTECTED HEALTH INFORMATION?

The purpose of this project is to develop and evaluate the clinical and cost-effectiveness of multisystemic therapy (MST) as a treatment modality for families being followed by child protection because of a report of child physical abuse. MST will be compared to parent group services offered in the community. The protected health information you will be asked to provide about your child as part of this study is solely for research purposes. You and your child's protected health information may be used to determine if one treatment model is more effective and will only be disclosed to regulatory agencies for audit purposes.

WHAT PROTECTED HEALTH INFORMATION WILL BE USED OR DISCLOSED?

You and your child will be asked to provide health-related information detailed in the informed consent agreement. Researchers will also generate new information about you as a result of the research procedures, tests, visits, and questionnaires/interviews. The information that will be used or potentially disclosed during an audit includes data from interviews.

WHO WILL DISCLOSE MY PROTECTED HEALTH INFORMATION?

The regulatory agencies whose role is to protect the safety of research participants occasionally conduct audits of research studies. In the event that this study is audited, your protected health information will be disclosed by the researchers of this study to the auditing agency. The researcher authorized to release your information is the principal investigator (Dr. Cynthia Cupit Swenson). Dr. Swenson is on faculty at the Medical University of South Carolina.

WHO WILL RECEIVE YOUR PROTECTED HEALTH INFORMATION?

Possible disclosure of your protected health information could be to one of the following:

- Committees with oversight or quality improvement responsibilities
- Institutional Review Board of the Medical University of South Carolina
- Institutional Review Board of the South Carolina Department of Mental Health
- National Institute on Mental Health (the sponsor of this research study)
- Office of Human Research Protections (a federal agency with oversight of research investigations)

Parents of minors younger than 16 years old may receive protected health information without authorization from the child.

Once this information leaves MUSC, we cannot guarantee that it will be protected by this authorization.

DO YOU HAVE TO SIGN THIS AUTHORIZATION?

You do not have to sign this authorization. If you choose not to sign the authorization, it will not affect your treatment, payment, or enrollment in any health plan or affect your eligibility for benefits. You will not be allowed to participate in the research study.

IF YOU SIGN THE AUTHORIZATION, CAN YOU CHANGE YOUR MIND?

You have the right to withdraw your authorization to allow MUSC to use or share your protected health information collected for this research study. Protected health information that has already been used or disclosed cannot be withdrawn. Your protected health information may still be used and disclosed if you have an adverse event. Once authorization is withdrawn and you are no longer participating in the study, no more protected health information will be collected. If you want to withdraw your permission, you must do so in writing to the investigator. The investigator's address is

[Fill in investigator's name and contact address]

If you withdraw your authorization, you will not be allowed to participate in the research study.

You will not be allowed to see or copy the information described on this form as long as the research is in progress. When the study is over, you will have the right to see and copy the information described on this authorization form.

AUTHORIZATION

You authorize Dr. __________ and her staff to use and disclose your and your child's protected health information for the purposes described above.

PRIVACY NOTICE

You have been given a copy of the privacy notice that describes the practices of MUSC regarding your protected health information. Please initial here: ________.

If you have any questions or concerns about your privacy rights, you should contact MUSC's privacy officer at ______________.

You will be given a signed copy of this form.

There is no expiration date for this authorization.

______________________________________ __________
Signature of Research Participant Ages 16 and Above* Date

______________________________________ __________
Research Participants' Personal Representative** Date
(if applicable)

____
Printed Name of Research Participant or Research Participants' Personal Representative (if applicable)

____
Representative's Relationship to Research Participant

*If research participants are between the ages of 16 and 18, signatures of both the research participant and the personal representative are required.

**A personal representative is someone authorized under state or other law to act on behalf of the individual in making health-related decisions. Examples include court-appointed guardians with medical authority, healthcare agents under a healthcare proxy, and parents acting on behalf of an unemancipated minor.

6. Information pertaining to an individual's psychological well-being or mental health
7. Genetic information

Certificates of confidentiality do not prevent disclosure of sensitive material such as threats of self-harm or evidence of ongoing child abuse, but those limits are expected to be included in a consent form. An application for a certificate should include the title of the project, any funding sources, the sponsoring institution, and documentation of approval by the institutional review board. The dates of the study, a description of the project, including the characteristics of potential participants, and the reasons for requiring confidentiality should be included. The Public Health Service (PHS) reviews the consent/assent forms and the qualifications of the investigator, as well as the means for protecting the identity of the participants, before it issues a certificate of confidentiality.

Tests of Drug Act of 1970

Two tests of the 1970 act have been documented in case law. Each case has a different outcome. In June 1972, an individual was shot and killed in Manhattan. A witness to the shooting reported that she had seen the killer previously at a methadone maintenance treatment clinic. A subpoena was served to Dr. Robert Newman, director of the New York City Methadone Maintenance Treatment Program, requiring him to give to the courts photos of African-American male patients of the clinic who were between the ages of 21 and 35. Dr. Newman refused to honor the subpoena based on the supposition that the 1970 act prevented him from releasing the photographs and that doing such would be a violation of patient confidentiality. The attorney general had granted absolute confidentiality to records of patients in Dr. Newman's program. A motion was made to quash the subpoena. The motion was denied; Dr. Newman was found in contempt of court and sentenced to 30 days in jail. The district attorney argued that the Drug Abuse Office and Treatment Act of 1972 required Dr. Newman to produce such documents. The 1972 act maintained that identity, diagnosis, prognosis, or treatment of patients seen due to substance abuse were confidential, subject to disclosure upon authorization by a court of competent jurisdiction. Upon appeal, the court was tasked with determining if the 1972 act repealed the 1970 act. The case was decided on May 31, 1979, and the decision was to reverse the order. The 1972 act did not repeal the 1970 Act (*People v. Newman,* 1979).

In a second case (*People v. Still,* 1975), a patient at St. Mary's Methadone Maintenance Clinic was arrested and charged with criminal possession of a controlled substance, methadone. He reported that he was authorized to carry the methadone with him because he was a patient at St. Mary's program and this was his weekend supply. He produced a letter from St. Mary's signed by the project director that declared he was indeed a patient of this program and that he had received take-home medication on the day of his arrest. The district attorney subpoenaed St. Mary's clinic to produce its books and records related to this client. A motion was made to quash the subpoena based on *People v. Newman* and the 1970 act. The subpoena for records was quashed but a subpoena of employees to serve as a witness was permitted. This motion was then modified allowing subpoena of books and records pertaining to this client to be delivered to the trial court to allow the People to make limited inspection and disclosure of portions of these records that are relevant to the guilt or innocence of the client on the charge at issue. The difference in this case and the *Newman* case is that in *Newman,* the 1970 act protected the identification of the defendant as a participant in the treatment program. In the *Still* case, the client had voluntarily disclosed his identity as a patient at the treatment program and had used this fact as a defense. He had thus waived his statutory right to anonymity. Under the court's supervision, the records would be used to either aid the defendant in his case or serve the public interest by refuting his claims.

Key Point *22-3*

The first step in conducting ethically and legally compliant research is to develop a plan for protection of human participants and an informed consent process.

Practical Steps to Ensure Protection and Compliance

Protection Documents and Procedures

The first step in conducting ethically and legally compliant research is to develop a plan for protection of human participants and an informed consent process. If the research involves vulnerable participants, protection must be well thought out. Universities maintain research and compliance offices, and working with someone in those offices from the start can help researchers set up protection correctly and save time. IRBs at agencies and universities typically have forms that must be completed and guidelines for informed consent that can help a researcher get started. The informed consent must be in language understandable to the participant. When participants do not speak English, an informed consent document must be provided in a language they understand. Alternatively, an oral presentation of informed consent can be made in conjunction with a short written consent document stating that the elements of the consent have been given orally, along with a written summary of what was presented orally. A witness to the oral presentation must be present, and the participant must be given copies of the short document and summary.

The requirements for the informed consent document are outlined on the Web site for the National Institutes of Health (www.nih.gov) and typically include the following:

- A statement that the study involves research
- An explanation of the research
- Expected duration of the individual's participation
- Descriptions of the procedures and identification of those that are experimental
- A description of foreseeable risks or discomforts
- A description of expected benefits
- Disclosure of alternative procedures or courses of treatment that might be advantageous
- A statement describing how confidentiality of records will be maintained
- An explanation of whether compensation or medical treatments will be available if injury occurs
- Names of the person(s) to contact for answers to questions about the research or participant rights
- A statement that the research is voluntary and refusal to participate will not carry a penalty or loss of benefits
- A statement that the individual can discontinue participation at any time without penalty or loss of benefits

When appropriate, the following elements should be included:
- A statement that the research may involve risks that are unforeseeable
- Circumstances under which the individual's participation may be terminated by the investigator
- Additional costs to the participant
- A statement that new findings that may affect the individual's willingness to continue the research will be provided
- The approximate number of participants expected.

In addition to setting up the informed consent and plan to protect human participants, the institution conducting the research must provide written assurance of compliance with the requirements outlined in Title 45. When the research is supported by a federal agency, a statement is required certifying that each application or proposal has been reviewed and approved by an IRB. The agency obtains a Federal Wide Assurance (FWA), a document assuring compliance that is on file with the Office for Human Research Protection (http://ohrp.osophs.dhhs.gov/index.html). When the study is being conducted at another agency, it must determine whether or not that agency is engaged in the research (see http://ohrp.osophs.dhhs.gov/humansubjects/assurance/engage.htm). If it is "engaged," that agency must file for a FWA. However, the agency may still use the university IRB for oversight of the human participant's requirements while the FWA holds the agency responsible for the conduct of the research. If the agency uses the university IRB, it must name the designated IRB in the FWA and enter into an interinstitutional agreement that outlines the responsibilities of each agency.

Developing the Data Safety and Monitoring Plan

Research funded by the NIH requires a plan showing how the researcher will monitor and protect the integrity of the data and confidentiality. The data safety and monitoring plan is filed with the NIH. An example is shown in Box 22-4.

Box 22-4 Sample of Data Safety and Monitoring Plan

DATA SAFETY AND MONITORING PLAN

Grant Title: Community-Based Treatment for Child Physical Abuse: Costs and Outcomes

PI: Cynthia Cupit Swenson, PhD

PROCEDURES FOR MONITORING THE SAFETY OF SUBJECTS WITHIN THE STUDY

Monitoring of subject safety is paramount in a study where participation is a result of a family already coming to the attention of child protective services. Monitoring of subject safety occurs within the context of research assessments and clinical services.

Research Assessments

Research assistants are trained to red-flag critical items on the assessment that indicate a child or parent is experiencing suicidal or homicidal ideation or intent or that unreported child abuse has occurred (e.g., sexual abuse). In cases where the research assessment reveals risk of suicide, homicide, or child maltreatment, the principal investigator, who is also the project coordinator individually interviews the child or parent, further assesses the risk, and recommends a course of action. If unreported abuse is disclosed, a report is filed with the proper authority (i.e., child protective services if abuse is by a parent or institution [*in loco parentis*], law enforcement if abuse is by an individual other than a parent).

Other risks to safety of subjects involve confidentiality. Research assessments are conducted in the home or in places that the family chooses. The risk involved is that individuals in the neighborhood can see that unknown people are coming to the house and the researcher could potentially be recognized by someone in the neighborhood. Also, data are collected at the child's school. To protect others from learning that the family is involved in treatment due to abuse of their child, the project was given a name not related to violence or abuse and this name is known in the community as PEACE, Betta Fuh Fambly (Project Empowering Adults, Children, and Their Ecology, for the Family). Betta Fuh Fambly is the Gullah language, which is a regional language. Researchers are trained regarding the limits of confidentiality. No data are gathered from the school without a signed release from the parent or legal guardian. No contacts are made with the schools without a signed release by the parent or legal guardian. Schools are not told that the child is in treatment due to abuse. Researchers are also trained to not give information to anyone in the home or neighborhood who is not a parent or guardian.

Clinical Services

Clinically, if suicidal or homicidal ideation or intent is indicated, the therapist conducts an assessment and then either works to hospitalize the child if needed or works with the family to set up protection. If no previously reported maltreatment of a child or older adult is revealed, a report is filed with Child Protection if the abuse is by a parent or person working in an institution *(in loco parentis)* or with law enforcement if the person is not a parent. All families are under the supervision of a child protective services caseworker, and the caseworker is given a report of progress on each family every two weeks. As with the research staff, the clinical staff is trained to only release information to an individual who the parent or legal guardian deems appropriate via a signed release or exchange of information.

PROCEDURES FOR MONITORING THE SAFETY OF DATA

All data are collected on scanable forms. A participant's name is never recorded on the teleform. Participant ID numbers are used. Assessments are conducted in the home and community. Upon completion of the assessment, all forms are returned to a locked desk until they are ready for scanning. Once scanned, all forms are filed in a locked filing cabinet. Computerized data will be maintained in a limited access, password-protected hard drive or on floppy disks locked in the research office.

Adverse Events

Seven potential adverse events have been identified that could possibly happen to study participants or staff. These include (1) minor physical abuse of a child (e.g., striking the child leaving a mark) by a parent, (2) moderate assault of a child by a parent (e.g., burning, tying up, or striking with an object), (3) severe assault of a child by a parent (severe beating, shooting, stabbing, choking), (4) child fatality, (5) illicit drug overdose of a child or parent, (6) accidents involving study participants (e.g., car accident) being transported by a staff member, and (7) allegations of abuse against a staff member.

If any of these adverse events occur, they will be reported according to the guidelines set forth in the informed consent and according the policy of the university IRB. In keeping with the university IRB requirements, events that are **not considered severe** are reported to the IRB in writing no later than 10 working days after the investigator learns of the event. Potential project events that fall under this category include numbers 1 and 2 above.

(*Continued*)

Box 22-4 Sample of Data Safety and Monitoring Plan—Continued

Alarming events are reported via a telephone call to the IRB chair or vice chair as soon as the investigator learns of the event. Potential project events that fall under this category include numbers 6 and 7 above.

Fatal or life-threatening events or those in which a participant is at immediate risk of death from the event are reported via telephone call to the IRB chair or vice chair as soon as possible but no later than three working days after the investigator first learns of the event. A written report is also submitted no later than three working days following the telephone report. Potential project events that fall under this category include numbers 3, 4, 5, and potentially 6.

Events that require inpatient hospitalization, that prolong existing hospitalization, or that result in persistent or significant disability/incapacity, cancer, overdose, or is a congenital anomaly/birth defect are reported in writing to the IRB as soon as possible but no later than 10 working days after the investigator first learns of the event. Potential project events that fall under this category include numbers 3, 5, and potentially 6.

In addition to reporting the adverse event to the IRB, those events that involve maltreatment of a child will be reported to child protective services if the person committing the violence is a parent or guardian or to law enforcement if the person committing the violence is not in a parent role. For accidents or injuries that require hospitalization, the investigator or clinical team will work with the family to assure that the participant receives needed services.

Current Status of Adverse Events

To date we have reported one adverse event to the IRB. This event involved a child being kicked by a grandparent who came to pick him up from school. We reported this event to the Social Services caseworker and to the appropriate police jurisdiction. In addition, we worked with the family and caseworker to create safety for the child by eliminating unsupervised contact between the child and grandfather.

To date, no children in the study have suffered injuries as a result of maltreatment.

Out-of-Home Placements

All children and families in our study are monitored by a child protective services caseworker. Many children in the project will be in foster care, kinship care, residential care, or other out-of-home placements. In cases where risk for potential maltreatment is increasing, the MST therapist will staff the case with the child protective services caseworker to determine an immediate plan for safety. In some cases, children will be placed temporarily with a relative or friend, or if those resources do not exist, a child may be taken into protective custody and placed in foster care.

In all cases, when a child is moved to an out-of-home placement, the move is made by the caseworker. The MST therapist may recommend respite care or a move out of the home if risk is increased. This action is not an adverse event but instead is preventing an adverse event. An example of an MST therapist recommending a move out of the home is as follows:

In one of our cases of a 10-year-old client, the mother had a history of psychosis that was controlled by medication. The psychosis became active and mother was hearing voices telling her to push the children down the stairs. She contacted the MST therapist. The therapist worked with the child protective services caseworker to move the children in with relatives until the mother's psychotic symptoms were under control. This was accomplished in a week and the children were safely reunited with their mother.

STUDY ADVISERS ON ETHICAL ISSUES AND PROTECTION OF SUBJECTS

The program director for Charleston County's child protective services, Eugene Caldwell, serves as an adviser on child and family safety. On a weekly basis, Caldwell and the principal investigator (PI) meet to staff all open cases. The staffing involves a discussion of progress and issues such as safety, adverse events, confidentiality, and application of reporting laws. When an adverse event occurs, Caldwell is informed at the weekly staffing and advises on the appropriate action to be used.

REVIEW OF DATA TO IDENTIFY POSSIBLE SAFETY ISSUES

Trends for unwanted outcomes (e.g., dropouts due to lack of efficacy, hospitalization, suicidal behaviors) are monitored via research rounds and clinical supervision on a weekly basis and as these problems occur. Once a week, the research team meets with the PI (who is also the project coordinator) to discuss each open research case. A review of the specifics of a family who has dropped out of the research or never engaged is conducted. If there is a safety risk involved (e.g., suicidal, homicidal, new reports of child maltreatment), the PI contacts the family or appropriate authorities to determine how to keep the child and family safe. Families are contacted on a monthly basis by the research team to assess service utilization for the child and family. If safety issues are uncovered during this contact, the PI is immediately informed and as project coordinator contacts the family or proper authorities to keep everyone safe.

Clinical supervision for the MST condition is conducted two times per week, and any unwanted outcomes are reported to the PI as they are discovered. The data manager for the project meets with the therapist for the parent group condition on a weekly basis. Any reports of unwanted outcomes are conveyed to the PI from the data manager as they are reported.

Rather than looking to an analysis of data and trends in the data to determine unwanted outcomes, each individual case is monitored carefully each week as long as the family is in the project. This close scrutiny is necessary due to the violent and vulnerable nature of the family situations with which our project deals.

Setting Up Research Files

When the project begins, the researcher should act as if he or she is preparing for an IRB audit from the start. All correspondence with the IRB or research office should have the date of receipt recorded and be systematically filed in a regulatory binder. An IRB correspondence binder should include copies of the following: assurances; all letters, Email, and documentation of phone calls with IRB or research office staff; original copies of consent documents; copies of all paperwork submitted to the IRB; and copies of all amendments. Files should also be kept that contain all memos and documentation of training of research staff, including certificates or other documentation of training on compliance and human participants protection. If someone other than the principal investigator (PI) is obtaining consent, there should be a record of formal delegation of authority and training of those so delegated.

Study participant files include documents containing names or other identifying participant information and should be kept separate and stored in a locked filing cabinet. A checklist of all documents required for each study participant should be kept in the files. All signed consent documents should be kept together in a locked file. Along with signed consents, research staff should keep progress notes tracking phone calls and contacts and explaining delays or problems in obtaining informed consent. Data computer files should be password protected and backup copies should be maintained in a locked location. Finally, when research participants are paid for their participation, careful records should be kept of those payments. A separate file or binder is needed with receipts for payments, and participant signatures must be on those receipts.

In addition to setting up audit-ready research files, researchers should conduct periodic internal audits of files. Doing so will enable a researcher to catch common errors and correct those practices. In addition, audits that compare computer files to raw data will help catch errors that may be taking place in data entry or scanning.

Summary

Conducting research with vulnerable participants requires sensitivity to the risks participants face as well as respect for the public's right to know. Victims and those accused or convicted of committing crimes, in particular, may be endangered by the very act of participating in research. Assuring confidentiality to participants, however well intended and ethically defensible, is not always enforceable, especially if a judge subpoenas the information. The Freedom of Information Act requires that the public's business is conducted publicly and any citizen, regardless of the reason, is able to access information about federally funded research. Certificates of confidentiality protect the participant's name and identity in the event of a subpoena, but researchers must also help with protection.

The best advice for beginning investigators is to take time to read the laws on human participant protection, take courses to learn how to comply with regulations designed to protect participants, keep records organized and in places where only people with a need to know (i.e., auditors, research staff) can access data, and work closely with IRB office staff to set up the project. In addition, working with seasoned researchers may help to identify potential risks to vulnerable participants. Advocacy groups are acutely sensitive to the risks their constituents face and are excellent sources of counsel. Institutional review boards are required to include a prisoner or a prisoner representative in their deliberations. Professional organizations can help with legislative efforts to protect the rights of participants in research and to disseminate ethical standards. The best protections for the participant, for the investigator, and for the public are sensitivity, public deliberation, and a close working relationship with the institution's IRB.

Resources

Web Sites

Belmont Report

http://ohsr.od.nih.gov/guidelines/belmont.html

Collaborative IRB Training Initiative (CITI)

www.miami.edu/citireg

Michigan State University's Center for Biomedical Research: Responsible Conduct of Research

www.msu.edu/~biomed/rcr

President's Council on Bioethics

www.bioethics.gov

National Institutes of Health

www.nih.gov

National Science Foundation

www.nsf.gov

Nuremberg Code

www.ushmm.org/research/doctors/Nuremberg_Code.htm

US Department of Health and Human Services: Office of Research Integrity

www.ori.dhhs.gov

US Department of Health and Human Services

www.os.dhhs.gov

World Health Organization

www.who.int/en

References

Bach-y-rita, G. (1974). The prisoner as an experimental subject. *JAMA, 229*(1), 45-46.

Berger, P. L., & Luckman, T. (1966). *The social construction of reality.* Garden City, NY: Doubleday.

Blanck, P. D., Bellack, A. S., Rosnow, R. L., et al. (1992). Scientific rewards and conflicts of ethical choices in human subjects research. *Am Psychol, 47,* 959-965.

Brody, B. A. (1998). *The ethics of biomedical research: An international perspective.* New York: Oxford University Press.

Comprehensive Drug Abuse Prevention and Control Act of 1970. (1970). Pub. L. No. 91-513, ~3(a). Washington, DC: US Government Printing Office.

Comprehensive Alcohol Abuse and Alcoholism Prevention, Treatment, and Rehabilitation Amendments of 1974. (1974). Pub. L. No. 93-282, ~122(b). Washington, DC: US Government Printing Office.

Department of Health, Education, and Welfare. (1979). *The Belmont report: Ethical principles and guidelines for the protection of human subjects of research.* Washington, DC: US Government Printing Office.

Flaskerud, J. H., & Winslow, B. J. (1998). Conceptualizing vulnerable populations health-related research. *Nurs Res, 47,* 69-78.

Health Omnibus Programs Extension of 1988, Pub. L. No. 100-607, ~163. Washington, DC: US Government Printing Office.

Kurz, D. (1987). Emergency department responses to battered women: Resistance to medicalization. *Soc Probl, 34(1),* 69-81.

Lutz, K. F. (1999). Maintaining client safety and scientific integrity in research with battered women. *Image: J Nurs Scholarship, 31*(1), 89-93.

Melton, G. B., & Gray, J. N. (1988). Ethical dilemmas in AIDS research: Individual privacy and public health. *Am Psychol, 43(1),* 60-64.

Montgomery, B. J. (1979). Abuses of Freedom of Information Act. *JAMA, 242,* 1007-1009.

Morris, R. A., Sales, B. D., & Berman, J. J. (1981). Research and the Freedom of Information Act. *Am Psychol, 36,* 807-818.

National Institutes of Health (NIH) (2003). Retrieved from www.nih.gov.

Parker, B. Ulrich,Y., & Nursing Research Consortium on Violence and Abuse (NRCVA). (1990). A protocol of safety: Research on abuse of women. *Nurs Res, 39,* 248-250.

People v. Newman. (1979). 32 NY 2d 379. Decided May 31.

People v. Still. (1975). 80 Misc 2d 881, modified. June 23.

Regulations on Protection of Human Subjects. (1999). 45 CFR Part 46

Rothman, D. J. (1982). Were Tuskegee & Willowbrook "studies in nature"? *Hastings Cent Rep, 40,* 5-7

Rubin, J. S. (1976). Breaking into the prison: Conducting a medical research project. *Am J Psychiatry, 133,* 230-232.

Shuster, E. (1997). Fifty years later: The significance of the Nuremberg Code. *N Engl J Med,* 337, 1436-1440.

Trials of War Criminals before the Nuremberg Military Tribunals under Control Council Law No. 10. (1949). Vol. 2, pp. 181-182. Washington, DC: US Government Printing Office.

Tyson, S., & Fleming, B. (1999). Conceptualizing battered women as a vulnerable population: A case study report. *Nurs Clin North Am, 34*(2), 301-312.

Chapter 23 Child Abuse and Neglect

Kathleen B. LaSala and Virginia A. Lynch

Child abuse and neglect have occurred throughout history, but for many years no laws existed to protect young victims or to ensure their human rights. In the late 1800s, a group of church workers in New York state had to use laws written by the Society for the Prevention of Cruelty to Animals to protect a young child from an abusive home situation (Holter, 1979). In 1961, Dr. Henry C. Kempe spoke of the child abuse problem to the American Academy of Pediatrics, providing clear data on what he termed the battered child syndrome (Kempe, Silverman, & Steele, 1962). Dr. Kempe's presentation had such a significant impact, legislation to protect the battered child was developed in all 50 states within the next four years. In 1973 a Senate hearing resulted in the Child Abuse Prevention and Treatment Act (CAPTA).

Carol Bellamy, executive director of UNICEF, stated in the United Nations Intervention on the Rights of the Child, "A century that began with children having virtually no rights is ending with them having the most powerful legal instrument that not only recognizes but protects their human rights" (Moorhead, 1997, p. 151).

The role of the pediatric forensic nurse examiner (PFNE) in child abuse and neglect cases is to ensure that child abuse and neglect are promptly identified and that appropriate interventions and referrals are initiated to ensure the child's welfare and safety. Detailed documentation of the child's appearance and behavioral interactions with parents or other caregivers is imperative, and photographs and other evidence should be obtained according to standard procedures of the PFNE.

Best Practice 23-1

Infants and children encountered in any healthcare setting should be assessed for indications of abuse and neglect; documentation, reporting, and referrals should be promptly accomplished.

Definitions

Child abuse and neglect are defined at both US federal and state levels. The federal Child Abuse Prevention and Treatment Act is the federal legislation that outlines minimal guidelines the states must follow (National Clearinghouse on Child Abuse and Neglect, 2004). CAPTA defines the term *child abuse and neglect* to mean the physical or mental injury, sexual abuse, negligent treatment, or maltreatment of a child under the age of 18 by a person who is responsible for the child's welfare under circumstances that indicate that the child's health or welfare is harmed.

State statutes of what is considered abuse may vary in terms of "harm or threatened harm" in a child's health (National Clearinghouse on Child Abuse and Neglect, 2003a). In addition, the states may differ on exemptions, for instance, a religious exemption, cultural practice, corporal punishment, and poverty. Many states have begun to include the term *abandonment* in their definitions of child abuse and neglect.

Although statutory laws and definitions vary from state to state, there are concrete areas of agreement (Giardino, Christian, & Giardino, 1997; National Clearinghouse on Child Abuse and Neglect, 2003b). Child abuse may include acts of omission or commission, usually found to be on a continuum rather than an isolated incident. Although each state has its own precise delineations and definitions for various types of neglect and abuse, laws typically consider four broad categories: neglect, emotional abuse, sexual abuse, and physical abuse. For example, the Commonwealth of Virginia includes abandonment in its definition of maltreatment; Rhode Island defines mental injury to include failure to thrive, loss of ability to think or reason, loss of control of aggressive or self-destructive impulses, acting out or misbehavior, including incorrigibility, ungovernability, or habitual truancy. Each state's unique definitions and interpretations of what constitutes abuse and neglect determine reporting requirements for that state.

An epidemic of global violence, the effects of recent changes to the US Citizenship and Immigration Services (USCIS) law, and the need to review state laws governing crime and victimization are bringing forensic patients from each corner of the world into nursing practice. Immigrants and refugees bring with them the traditional and cultural healthcare practices that are often misunderstood, misinterpreted as abuse or neglect, and thus impact healthcare delivery. The expected results include developing models, tools, best practices, and ethical guidelines for global planning and interventions.

Models and Theory

Over the past few decades several child maltreatment models (Cowen, 1999) have presented the multiple facets involved in the maltreatment issue, including the model that examines the complex nature of the interactions between the parent and the child, the stressors within and outside the family, and the broader social and cultural system (Howze and Kotch, 1984). This model expanded on earlier models to include familial, social, and cultural aspects, as well as the impact of these relationships with stress, social support systems, and child maltreatment. These authors recognized that stress in the maladaptive abusive family may be situational, acute, or chronic. Milner (1993) worked to develop a physical child abuse risk assessment tool that could be used to assess demographic, social, cognitive/affective, and behavioral risk factors. He based his work on Belsky's (1980, 1993) organizational model that described four ecological levels found in other models of child abuse: (1) the ontogenic level (individual factors in the child); (2) the microsystem (refers to family factors); (3) the ecosystem (reflecting the community); and (4) the macrosystem (identified as the culture). Belsky (1993) asserted that his model and assessment tool helps predict the risk of maltreatment behaviors, but not actually maltreatment. Additional models and theories are developing, but they appear to have similar concepts. Milner (1993) has refined his own work to include sociocultural, family system, and learning paradigms and sublevels of understanding of each concept, including such details as understanding the social information processing in the abusive parent. The review of literature reveals a complex etiology for child abuse and neglect.

Incidence

In 2003, according to the National Child Abuse and Neglect Data System (NCANDS) annual report of reported child maltreatment cases in the US, an estimated 2.9 million referrals alleging child abuse or neglect were reported and accepted by the state and local child protection agencies (US Department of Health and Human Services, 2004). Of these cases, approximately 906,000 children were identified as actual victims of child abuse and neglect. Childhood neglect was responsible for 60% of the cases, physical abuse equated 20%, sexual abuse accounted for 10%, and the remaining 5% were emotional maltreatment cases. Data reveals infants and children age birth to 3 years old are the most common victims of maltreatment, and females are slightly more likely to be abused than males (US DHHS, 2004). In addition, race and ethnicity studies showed the highest rates in Pacific Islanders (21.4 per 1000 children); American Indian or Alaska Natives (21.3 per 1000); African-Americans (20.4 per 1000 children); and whites (11.0 per 1000 children). In 2003, an estimated 1500 child fatalities were the result of maltreatment, a rate of 2 deaths per 100,000 US children. Documentation of specific cases remains difficult to quantify due to various reporting criteria and definitions among states, as well as underreporting.

Of the documented NCANDS cases in 2003, approximately 57% of the victims received some sort of services following the assessment and investigation (US DHHS, 2004). Services included in-home and foster care services. Child victims of multiple types of maltreatment were more likely to receive treatment than those with physical abuse alone.

In 2003, NCANDS reported approximately 80% of the perpetrators were parents; 16% were other family members or unmarried partners of parents; and the remaining 4% were "others" (US DHHS, 2004). Women were more common perpetrators than men (58% to 42% respectively) and were generally younger than male perpetrators. For sexual assault, approximately 76% of the perpetrators were friends or neighbors, with the remaining 30% being family members (only 3% of these were parents).

Dynamics of Child Abuse and Neglect

Experts in child maltreatment have identified a dynamic interrelationship of three types of characteristics that must exist for child abuse to evolve (Milner, 1993; Belsky, 1980). These three characteristics involve the parent or adult (perpetrator), the child (victim), and environmental context. The interaction of all three groups is deemed necessary for predicting high risk for abuse.

Parental or Adult Characteristics (Perpetrator)

Parental characteristics associated with child abuse include parents who had serious difficulties in the parent-child interactions when the parents were children, for example, they were either abused themselves or observed abuse in their family. The parent may have poor social contacts, be isolated, and have little social support. These parents often have inappropriate expectations of the child, with a poor understanding of normal growth and development, intellectual status, and physical abilities of the child. They may lack necessary parenting skills or be aware of the physical and emotional needs of the child, as with adolescent parents and low-income parents (Houxley & Warner, 1993). In their own relationships, their dependency needs have not been met, and they are frequently unable to develop close, trusting relationships with others. Perpetrators generally display a low self-esteem with poor impulse control and poor coping mechanisms. Other risk factors include adolescent parents, single parents, and military personnel. Less than 10% of these adults have severe mental disorders such as psychosis.

Child Characteristics (Victim)

Characteristics of the abused child include being considered "special" or "different." For example, the child may be the result of an unwanted pregnancy, may be the "wrong" sex, or may simply look like a "wrong" person. The intensity of the "special child" or "different" characteristics is defined in the parent's eyes. In more obvious cases, the child may have an acute or chronic illness or a limiting disability (mental or physical) or be preterm, requiring a great deal of time and attention (Hobbs, Hanks, & Wynne, 1993). Poor mother-infant attachment or bonding has been associated with prolonged separation at birth (high-risk infants) and even with multiple births (Sachs & Hall, 1991). Theorists assert it is difficult for a mother to bond or attach with more than one infant at a time; therefore, one or more children in a multiple birth are left with potential delayed bonding.

Environmental Characteristics

Environmental characteristics associated with child abuse include a family that is in stress. This may be acute, chronic, or situational stress, or a series of crises such as serious illness, death, divorce, extramarital affairs, financial problems, and unemployment. Inadequate housing or substandard living conditions characterized by crowding, lack of privacy, and disrepair are also contributing elements. Repeated relocations may mean social isolation and a lack of support systems, which leaves the adult with no one to turn to for help, advice, or caregiving relief from the child (Ricci & Botash, 2002). Children who witness domestic violence can suffer severe emotional and developmental issues similar to those who have been direct victims (National Clearinghouse on Child Abuse and Neglect Information, 2004).

Parent-Child Interactions

Parent-child interactions may present themselves in a parent not comforting a child or being detached from the child. The parent may demonstrate a lack of control or impulsive behaviors. A child or parent may have inappropriate expectations of the child based on age and development stage. Some clinicians report observing conflicts that more closely resemble parent-parent (adult-adult) interactions than child-parent.

Key Point *23-1*

Nurses need to be knowledgeable of possible indicators of abuse and neglect, especially those that are manifested *before* a child suffers a serious injury, emotional impairment, or developmental delay. Early recognition and intervention are the keys to preventing subsequent abuse and negative sequelae.

Categories of Child Abuse and Neglect

Physical Abuse

Physical abuse is defined as a situation in which the offender inflicts physical injury to the child, ranging from bruises to multiple fractures and brain damage. Physical abuse is not usually a controlled, planned action. It is generally an impulsive reaction to stress that involves a cycle of stages, including a tension-building stage, the actual abusive act, and periods of nurturing in between. As with other forms of abuse, it is considered a family problem and reflects a dysfunctional family. All family members suffer when abuse occurs, even those not being physically harmed. Physical child abuse is seldom an isolated incident.

Emotional Abuse

Emotional abuse is defined as a maladaptive parent-child interaction. In emotional neglect there is a failure to meet the affection, attention, and nurturing needs of the child (Hockenbery, Wilson, Winkelstein et al., 2002). An additional form of emotional abuse occurs when the adult purposely attempts to destroy or hamper the child's self-esteem (Nester, 1998). This form of abuse is seen when a parent rejects, isolates, terrorizes, or verbally assaults the child. Frequently in emotional abuse inappropriate expectations or demands are placed on the child. For example, toilet training may be expected too early. A child may also be expected to carry out more adult functions, such as childcare for siblings, cooking, and cleaning. A parent may place a heavy emotional burden on the child or have adult expectations that result in a reversal of the child-adult roles.

Sexual Abuse

Sexual exploitation can range from noncontact indecent exposure to fondling and genital contact to actual adult-child sexual intercourse (National Clearinghouse on Child Abuse and Neglect, 2004). The Child Abuse and Prevention Act states sexual abuse is the "use of persuasion or coercion of any child to engage in sexually explicit conduct, or the producing of visual depiction of such conduct, or rape, molestation, prostitution, or incest with children." A child does not have the knowledge, emotional maturity, or social skills necessary to enter into a sexual relationship of any nature on an equal basis with an adult. Therefore, it is legally concluded that a child cannot be held responsible for a sexual relationship with an adult.

There are two primary forms of sexual abuse. The first is when an adult initially pressures a child into a nonsexual liaison based on a long-term trusted relationship. As the relationship grows, the child eventually participates in the sexual activity to maintain the rewards, attention, approval, or recognition provided by the adult who essentially uses the child to meet his or her unfulfilled needs. The second type of sexual abuse is the forced relationship in which the offender intimidates the child by threatening harm or actually harming the child or someone else they care about. The adult has no emotional investment in the child, but rather uses the victim to meet short-term sexual needs. Authorities believe that most offenders do not actually desire to harm the child; however, a few of the perpetrators seem to obtain vicarious pleasure from harming the child (Hockenbery, Wilson, Winkelstein et al., 2002).

Neglect

Child neglect is defined as the failure to provide adequate care. Neglect is considered an act of omission and accounts for over half of the reported child maltreatment (Cowen, 1999; Helfer, 1990; Hockenbery, Wilson, Winkelstein et al., 2002). Situations of neglect may include inadequate supervision, which may lead to accidents and injury. Overall lack of attention to food, shelter, and medical needs are also considered neglect and can quickly endanger the well-being of a child. In addition, the lack of providing education at both the grade school and high school levels is deemed neglect. Many of these factors are closely related to poverty, single parenthood, and unemployment, leading to a multifaceted social problem. The 1974 Child Abuse Prevention and Treatment Act deemed neglect a form of abuse and required medical attention. Although reporting has improved, actual cases of neglect remain high.

Neglect can result in malnutrition, poor dental care, and a generally poor health status. Children left unattended are at a high risk for injury. Over 75% of neglect victims were reported to have a serious injury or illness within three years of documented neglect (Green & Kilili, 1998). Neglected children can be extremely passive, withdrawn, undisciplined, or disabled (Cowen, 1997). More extreme neglect can lead to failure to thrive syndrome (FTT). Manifestations of FTT include withdrawn affect, decreased and agressive social interactions, and fewer positive play behaviors such as offering, sharing, accepting, and following (Peterson & Urquiza, 1993). Additionally, the child may experience impaired or delayed growth, delayed language development, and maturational and behavioral difficulties in achieving developmental milestones (Schmitt & Mauro, 1989). It is not uncommon for a child with FTT to die from secondary metabolic defects or other illnesses. Their deaths may also be the result of intentional or nonintentional trauma and neglect. The differential diagnosis of FTT may include a wide range of possible organic conditions (inborn metabolic disorders, congenital viral infections, chromosomal syndromes) and external factors including criminal acts.

Forensic pathologists determine if a child's death is natural or unnatural. If abuse and neglect are the determined cause or contribute to the cause of death, criminal charges can be filed. Since there are important consequences, the diagnosis must be confirmed. This may be difficult when there may be several underlying causes such as organic FTT, cystic fibrosis, abuse, and neglect. A detailed forensic investigation is required.

Case Study 23-1 Power Windows

A three-year-old girl became trapped in a power window of her mother's car and was killed. She was left in the car while her mother went inside a friend's house. The girl apparently removed her seat belt and lowered the window of the running car. The mother told investigators she found the girl caught in the window when she returned after about five minutes. Emergency crews found the girl was not breathing when they arrived at the scene. She was pronounced dead about an hour later at the medical center.

Other Abuse and Neglect Issues

Sibling Abuse

Sibling abuse is among the most overlooked forms of child abuse. Sibling abuse takes the form of physical, sexual, and emotional abuse and has devastating consequences to victims. Sibling abuse victims often suffer long-term social and psychological disturbances and perpetuate cycles of family violence. Numerous familial and environmental factors have been identified as predicted risk factors for sibling abuse. Forensic investigation of suspicious circumstances concerning child injury, behavior, or death is paramount to changing historical cultural neglect of child abuse cases and to initiate prevention strategies to help eliminate sibling abuse in society.

The murder of a child by his or her sibling is categorized as *siblicide*. From animal research on killing of siblings, one can hypothesize that sibling abuse occurs as a result of a deficiency in the family or parental structure that will cause children to exhibit abusive behaviors toward siblings to gain more resources. However, not enough is known about sibling abuse to draw firm conclusions. Despite the lack of attention that sibling abuse receives from parents and society at large, it can have detrimental long-term effects in children and can result in premature death in some cases.

Statistical information reveals that child abuse committed by siblings is a prevalent social problem that has previously been ignored. In a Canadian study (2001), siblings were perpetrators of 28% of sexual offenses and 24% of physical assaults in child victims less than 12 years of age (Johnson & Au Coin, 2003). Research results are particularly shocking when examining incidences of sexual abuse. The National Society for the Prevention of Cruelty to Children indicates that siblings are twice as likely to be abused by brothers than by fathers or stepfathers (Spenser, 2000). Incidences of sibling abuse differs somewhat from that of adult abusers. Unlike parental child abuse where the most vulnerable age for maltreatment is 12 months to 5 years, children of any age can be targets of sibling abuse. Younger children have a higher mortality rate whether the perpetrator is an adult or a sibling.

Physical and emotional neglect is quite commonly associated with parental child abuse, whereas phenomena such as bullying are more often related to sibling abuse. Dominance and control appears to be a common link among most types of child abuse and is especially apparent in different forms of sibling abuse.

Sibling abuse is often mistaken as "sibling rivalry," a seemingly harmless and playful interaction, which parents tend to ignore or join in with the supposed playfulness. However, survivors of this type of abuse report their parent's reaction to sibling violence of one of nonchalance, denial, or blame (Wiehe, 1997). Parents commonly trivialize the event or do not believe such reports, and often accuse victims of deserving or perpetuating maltreatment. For example, when a child is verbally degraded, retaliatory self-defense may be seen by the parent as the initial cause of the child being teased. Unfortunately, if parents do not address sibling abuse, they are essentially condoning abusive behaviors.

Teasing

Teasing is a common form of emotional abuse. Emotional abuse has been found to be the most destructive force among all types of abuse with the most damaging long-term effects (Wiehe, 1997). Teasing and other forms of emotional abuse often accompany physical and sexual abuse. According to Wiehe, 7% of his sample indicated emotional abuse alone, compared to 71% that indicated experiencing emotional, physical, and sexual abuse.

It may be difficult to distinguish abuse from playful interaction between siblings, parents, or other adults or children. Social interaction that revolves around negative verbal communications directed at a child can be considered emotionally abusive. This differs from joking because it is conducted at the victim's expense (Wiehe, 1991). Fear and intimidation are often used against victims as a means of control and dominance. Older siblings may be able to inflict more emotional damage because they are often idolized by the younger and have developed more hurtful behaviors (Simonelli, Mullis, Elliott et al., 2002). Victims often internalize hurtful comments, which produce feelings of low self-worth. Conversely, some victims externalize emotional abuse, which manifests itself as negative behaviors (Hart & Brassard, 1987).

Bullying

A prime example of the integration of emotional abuse with other forms of sibling abuse is bullying. Bullying is primarily emotional but can also lead to physical intimidation and violence. Bullying is emotional intimidation perpetrated by a person who is stronger than or in a position of power over the victim. The bully child often has high dominance needs, lacks empathy, and has a positive view of aggression. Bullying can take on many forms and often occurs between peers or siblings.

Research reveals that children involved in sibling bullying are more likely bullies or victims at school (Duncan, 1999). According to Duncan, 53% of 210 college freshmen reported bully victimization during their childhood. Yet society continues to underestimate the potential emotional damage of bullying. Research statistics indicated that 22% of participants who were bullied were pushed, hit, or shoved, and 81% reported being beaten up (Duncan, 1999). Bully victimization has been linked to psychological difficulties such as depression, anxiety, and low self-esteem.

Identification of Abuse and Neglect

The FNE with pediatric expertise, working with other members of a multidisciplinary team, provides an effective strategy for identifying, confirming, and confronting child abuse and neglect. This requires a planned, objective, and coordinated response with defined policies and procedures that can be put into effect the moment abuse or neglect is suspected (Pasqualone & Fitzgerald, 1999). If these are in place, the child's safety is assured and staff can promptly involve other healthcare services, community agencies, and systems of advocacy.

Intervening on the child's behalf may prevent further injury or death. Some hospitals and long-term institutions for children are developing positions for advanced practice nurses such as the forensic pediatric nurse practitioner (FPNP) or forensic clinical nurse specialist (FCNS). As an in-house forensic clinician, these specialists are considered an essential part of the multidisciplinary team who are qualified to detect, assess, and manage cases of child abuse and neglect.

History

Obtaining and documenting a thorough history is a critical step in the assessment of child abuse. The child may be accompanied by a nonabusive parent or adult, the abusive offender, or a child protection services worker (Ricci & Botash, 2002). It is important to interview the child and the adult separately. If an adult tries to prevent the child's privacy, the nurse may need to intervene on the child's behalf. The pediatric forensic nurse examiner should use open-ended questions that do not lead the child. The interview should include questions not only about actual abuse (physical, sexual, emotional, or neglect) but also domestic violence and witnessing abuse (Ricci & Botash, 2002).

Red-flag findings in the history include the absence of an adult, poorly explained histories, or conflicting histories from different sources. Histories that are inconsistent with physical findings or inconsistent with the child's growth and development stage may reflect a false story or an inappropriate expectation for the child

(Lynch, 1997). The caregiver may be reluctant to explain, may blame others for the injury, or may refuse additional tests or treatments. Sometimes the caregiver reflects an inappropriate level of concern or is absent altogether. With sexual abuse, the child will often speak of a special relationship or convey that he or she is keeping a secret. When there are delays in seeking medical treatment and a history of repeated injury or unmet medical, physical, and emotional needs, child abuse should be considered.

Often, adults will bring the child in for complaints other than those directly related to the abuse, or have either increased or decreased level of concern related to the actual problem presented. The child or adult may be reluctant to explain the injury, may blame someone else, or may refuse additional tests or treatments. In sexual abuse, the child may refer to a "special relationship" or a "secret" they have with an adult. These children should be specifically asked about sexual abuse issues. If they are threatened, disclosure may be very difficult.

Occasionally the historian will be an eye-witness to the abuse; however, in the absence of a witness, the nurse should never ignore subtle or overt "cries for help" from either the child or the adult. Child abuse is seldom an isolated event. The history should be compared to the physical findings as well, including the child's appearance and behavior, parent-child interactions, and physical clues. Laboratory, radiographic, and body scan testing may be necessary, and careful documentation through charting and forensic photography is essential (see Appendix D for sexual abuse forms).

Child's Appearance and Behavior

A child may display hostility or appear to be fearful of the adult. In other cases, the child may actually cling to or go to the abusive person for protection or comforting. Other typical behaviors displayed by the child include social withdrawal, aggression, depression, and helplessness. Some children may demonstrate inappropriate infantile-type or adult behaviors inconsistent with their age, growth, and development. With older children, some of the sequelae of child abuse may already begin to exhibit themselves in such behaviors as poor school performance, poor social interactions with peers, fantasies, phobias, eating and sleeping problems, drug and alcohol abuse, sexual promiscuity, running away from home, suicidal thoughts and attempts, and specific psychiatric disorders (Green & Kilili, 1998; Hockenbery, Wilson, Winkelstein et al., 2002).

Physical Evidence of Abuse and Neglect

Children of abuse often will present with physical clues that are well-defined and others that are more vague or hidden. Signs of neglect and emotional abuse are less clearly presented than those of physical abuse. Sexual abuse may be completely missed if a sexual history or examination is not performed as part of routine visits.

Some signs of neglect include poor skin care, grooming, and oral hygiene, or malnutrition and dehydration without a medical cause (Hockenbery, Wilson, Winkelstein et al., 2002). Repeated accidents reflecting improper supervision, poor health maintenance (e.g., no immunizations), and failure to thrive symptoms, which improve with hospitalizations, all reflect potential neglect. Emotional abuse is more difficult to pinpoint; it may result in failure to thrive, feeding disorders, enuresis, sleep disorders, and developmental delays.

Sexual abuse indicators can be found in any genital, rectal, oral, or buttocks trauma, bleeding, or discharge. Sexually transmitted infections, pregnancy, recurrent urinary tract infections, or general somatic complaints are commonly associated with sexual abuse. Physical abuse should be suspected in any injury to a child less than 12 months old. Other suspicious injuries include injuries of the soft tissue, such as hematomas, bruises, lesions, and scars in different stages of healing or injuries reflective of an inflicting implement (e.g., ropes, buckles, cigarettes). Multiple fractures, bleeding (including retinal bleeds), burns, neurological damage, convulsions resulting from poisoning, coma, and abdominal distention or injury may be seen in child abuse and warrant investigation.

Immersion Burns

Immersion burns are those that result from a child being placed in scalding liquid, most often tap water. These first-, second-, and third-degree burns are identified as "forced immersion" burns. With most forms of burn injuries, a pattern is present or develops, enabling medical and investigative personnel to determine how the injury might have occurred. There are significant patterns recognized in forced immersion burns. For instance, the face and neck are generally spared. When the child is held, dipped, or plunged into hot liquid, the child will react by flexing that portion of the body contacting the hot liquid, thus sparing the flexion crease areas. Clinically, three characteristic burn patterns result from immersion:

- "Donut" pattern (central sparing): produced when the body is held against the bottom of a heated container such as a large metal pan or porcelain tub of hot water.
- "Stocking or Glove" pattern: produced by the waterline when the child's feet, hands, or legs are held in hot liquid (Fig. 23-1).

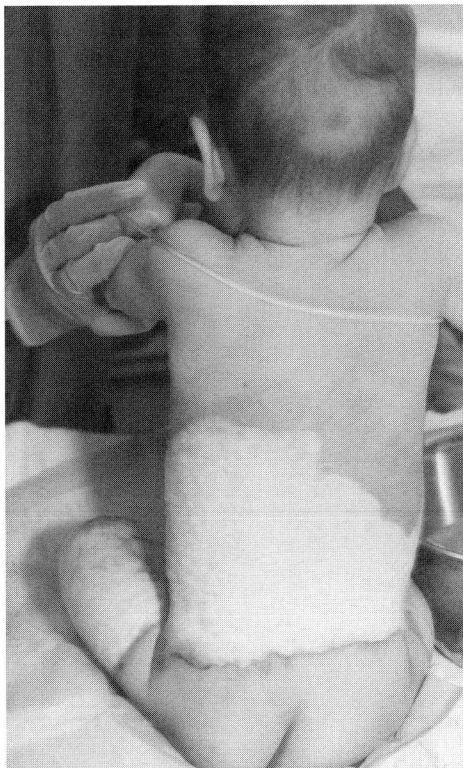

Fig. 23-1 Immersion burn. Note sparing in diaper area and bald area on head, which sometimes indicates prolonged lying in one position.

- "Tripod" pattern: induced by a child raising up on his hands and feet to protect his buttocks and perineum from burning in a shallow-filled container of hot water.

On the other hand, the child who is accidentally burned by falling or climbing into or turning on hot water presents a burn injury consistent with the action. The waterline may be blurred and there are likely to be splash burns. A splash pattern injury, however, cannot be used as a single factor in determining whether the burn is accidental or intentionally induced, since they are sometimes noted in association with forced immersion.

Best Practice *23-2*

It is essential that nurses gain an understanding of the immersion burns as a form of physical child abuse and be able to differentiate accidental from intentional burns.

Patterned Burns

Intentional burns occur primarily in the high-risk child age range of 12 months to 5 years of age. There are more male victims than female, and when extensive burns occur, younger children have a higher mortality rate than older children. The majority of burn injuries associated with abuse resemble the pattern of the object involved. Common patterns noted by forensic experts have been inflicted by hairdryers, irons, cigarettes or a car cigarette lighter, or hot cooking or eating utensils (Fig. 23-2). Patterned burns commonly are seen on the dorsum of the feet or hands, and occasionally on the face or neck.

Bite Marks

The FNE may note wound characteristics of a bite on any body surface and must differentiate human bites from animal bites (see Chapter 16). Since both adults and children can inflict bites, the wound must be photographed, diagrammed, and precisely measured for evidentiary purposes (Fig. 23-3). Serial photographs may be required on subsequent days postinjury to fully appreciate the wound characteristics. Distances of greater than 3 cm between canine teeth typically indicate an adult bite (Suggs, Lichenstein, McCarthy et al., 2001). Because human bite marks are most frequently indicative of sexual abuse, wounds should also be swabbed for DNA to assist in identification of the perpetrator. Serial photographs may be required on one or more subsequent days post-injury to fully appreciate the wound characteristics, since redness and edema can interfere with visualization of subtle marks useful in pinpointing the individual that inflicted the bite.

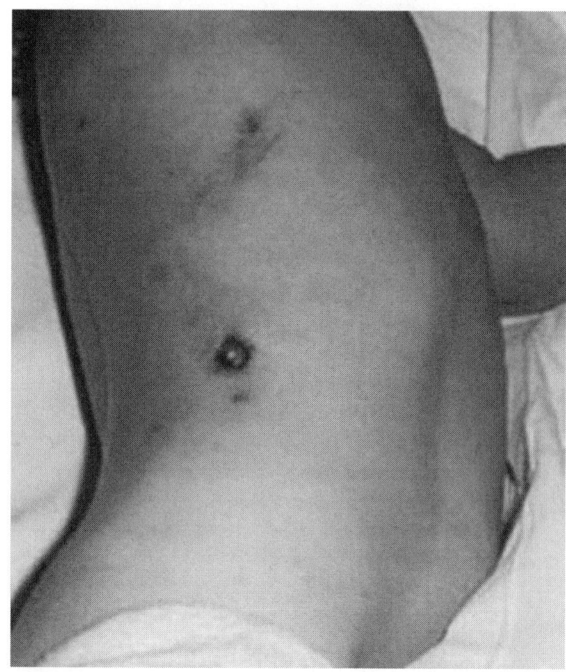

Fig. 23-2 Cigarette burn; location strongly supports an intentional injury by a perpetrator.

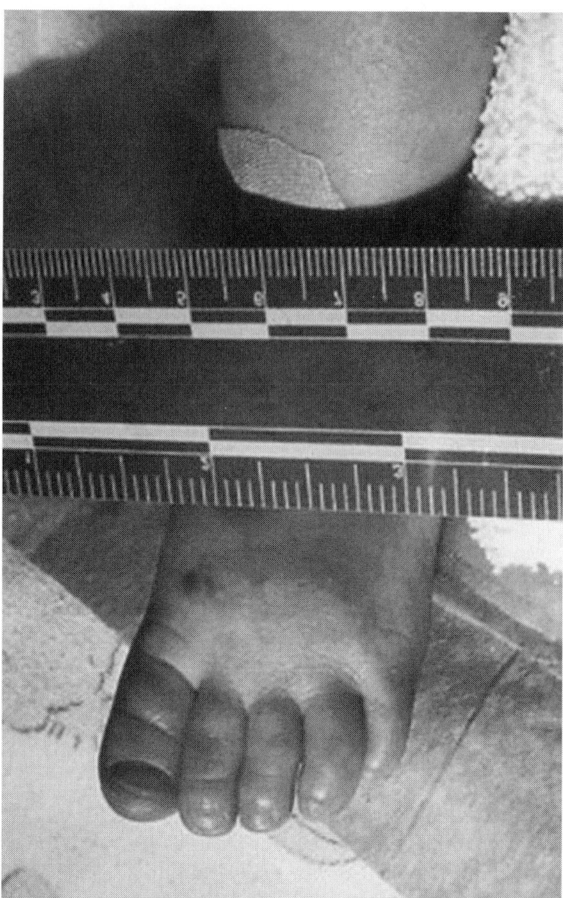

Fig. 23-3 Bite mark on foot of an infant.

Munchausen Syndrome by Proxy (MSBP)

A curious category of child abuse, known as Munchausen syndrome by proxy (MSBP), is rarely recognized and uncommonly seen. MSBP, also known as factitious illness by proxy, is a dangerous form of child abuse in which a parent or caregiver induces or fabricates numerous illnesses and falsifies medical history that results in unnecessary medical evaluation and treatment leading to prolonged or repeated contact with the healthcare system. The deception is usually repeated on numerous occasions, resulting in hospitalizations, morbidity, and death. The perpetrator injures their victims in order to gain sympathy or attention for her- or himself.

It is not uncommon for the abuse to continue during periods of hospitalization. Pediatric FNEs can provide an important role in the observation and surveillance with video cameras to monitor and document the abuse. The use of covert video surveillance (CVS) has been tied to some legal issues involving the Fourth Amendment of the US Constitution and is subject to some controversy. However, visual evidence is often required to convince the courts that parents could do such things to their children (Brown, 1997).

Shaken Baby Syndrome (SBS)

Shaken baby syndrome (SBS) is a significant cause of infant morbidity and mortality, most often involving children younger than 2 years, but may be seen in children up to 5 years of age. The hallmark of SBS findings is the absence of any external trauma to the head, face, and neck, along with massive intracranial or retinal hemorrhages. Because the child is most often nonverbal or unable to tell what occurred, one must be aware of the signs and symptoms associated with SBS. In less severe cases, there is typically a history of poor feeding, vomiting, lethargy or irritability, hypothermia, failure to thrive, and increased sleeping with difficulty arousing. In more severe cases, there may be seizures, a full or bulging fontanel, bradycardia, respiratory distress, and eventually coma and cardiovascular collapse. MRI and CT imaging are required to substantiate repeated SBS injuries that point to abuse.

Sudden Infant Death Syndrome (SIDS)

Sudden infant death syndrome (SIDS) is defined as a sudden, unexpected death of an infant less than one year of age, which remains unexplained after an autopsy, toxicological studies, and a thorough investigation of the scene and the circumstances surrounding the death. This term is used to describe a deceased infant and not a condition or disease. Most SIDS deaths occur in infants between two and four months of life. Although intensive studies have been implemented to ascertain the causes of SIDS, the etiology is still unknown. There is no test for SIDS. Conditions that may be associated with child abuse must be thoroughly considered such as facial fractures and vertebral artery compression. Without evidence of underlying trauma, however, suffocation is indistinguishable from SIDS at autopsy. Emergency physicians or pediatricians cannot legally diagnose SIDS, which constitutes an ME/C case and is only determined after the exclusion of any other possible cause.

Seat Belts and Child Restraints

The law requires the use of vehicular seat belts and child restraints because they are considered one of the most protective devices for infants and children in the event of vehicular collisions. Children up to four years old or 40 pounds in weight are required to use a child safety seat.

By current laws, the adult driving is responsible for the safety of the child and will be charged with negligence or vehicular homicide if the child is killed under the specific circumstances of the law related to child safety. Adults have the right to choose whether they will be in violation of state seat belt laws; children do not. The child's fate is partly decided by the adults who care for him or her. Experts in the investigation of transportation collisions are responsible for the accurate interpretation of evidence and accident reconstruction, which may determine the outcome of charges filed.

Child Prostitution

Throughout history children have been sexually victimized and child prostitution remains one of the most ignored forms of child abuse. Although prevalent across centuries, the US documented an increase in child prostitution in the late 1970s due to the Juvenile Justice Delinquency Prevention Act passed in 1974 that forbade law enforcement to detain runaway children, therefore allowing them to exist on the street. A study released in 2001 reported that between 300,000 and 400,000 US children are victims of some type of sexual exploitation each year (Estes, 2001). According to Estes, child exploitation is the most hidden form of child abuse in North America. It is estimated that 75% of the child sex trade victims are white and from middle-class families; boys are victimized as often as girls (see Chapter 30).

Sequelae of Child Abuse and Neglect

The physical, psychosocial, and economic sequelae of child abuse and neglect can potentially damage generations. Results may include physical disfigurement, neurological damage, and major emotional and psychological trauma (Cowen, 1999; Green & Kilili, 1998; US DHHS, 2004; Ricci & Botash, 2002). The abuse teaches violence in the family and society, resulting in victimization and future potential abuse cycles. Child maltreatment can interrupt the physical and emotional development potential of a child, resulting in a lack of trust, feelings of helplessness, poor peer relationships, sexual promiscuity, and potential alcohol and drug use (National Center of Child Abuse and Neglect Data, 1997). Children also manifest with frequent complaints of illness and discomfort, sleep and eating disorders, and an inability to concentrate or short attention span, delaying their potential cognitive and emotional development (Schuster, Wood, Duan et al., 1998). McCauley, Kem, and Kolonder (1997) agree with the previous problems, and identify in addition anxiety disorders, depression, interpersonal sensitivity, and suicidal thoughts and attempts.

Case Study 23-2 A Lifetime of Abuse

Long before Lydia was old enough to start school, she was a victim of both physical and psychological abuse by an alcoholic father as well as a dependent and frustrated mother. Lydia was the youngest of five children and the only girl. Her family lived far from town in an isolated rural area with no neighbors within sight. During the day, her mother assigned chores beyond Lydia's physical and mental development, punishing her at any opportunity to maintain power and control. Her father tied her to a tree in the front of the house and left her there through the night. This terrorized Lydia and instilled an unnatural fear of the dark as well as fear of both parents and a fear of being punished. Because her three older brothers were gone from home, Lydia also became the target of teasing, bullying, and sexual abuse by the one older brother who remained at home.

Lydia looked forward to starting school and escaping the continued abuse. On her first day at school, she carefully prepared to make a good impression on her teacher, wearing her best dress and carrying wildflowers as a gift. Her mother had given Lydia a stick of chewing gum as a favor on this day, telling her to behave and learn well. When Lydia approached the teacher with the flowers, the teacher suddently reached up, slapped her face so hard the gum flew from her mouth, and said, "Don't you ever come into my room chewing gum again!" Lydia never recovered emotionally from this day and subsequently felt that there was no place where she was safe.

Over the next years, she submitted to various abuses with expectation. As an adolescent she became promiscuous. As a young adult, she married a dominant man who controlled her just as her parents had. She continued to reach out to men for attention. As she inadvertently sought conversation, her best friend's husband raped her. Afterward, she became the victim of numerous incidents and sexual assaults in various settings. Depression, guilt, and hopelessness led to suicide ideations. Lydia never escaped her childhood abuse and those who victimized her.

Mimicking Injuries

The PFNE makes vital assessments that help to determine if the child requires specific healthcare, protective custody, or other interventions. The evaluation of physical injury in children requires a team approach, and common sense must be used when evaluating the injury and correlating it with the history. These phenomena may be confused with child abuse.

Mongolian spots are slate blue, dark brown, or blue-black patches of skin commonly seen in pigmented skin. Approximately 90% of African Americans have such spots. These spots can also be found in Asian, Hispanic, and other children with pigmented skin. These darkened areas are congenital and commonly found on the lower back and buttocks, but may occur anywhere. They often fade early in life, usually by age five. They do not sequentially change colors as bruises tend to, but often are mistaken to be the result of trauma when initially observed.

Impetigo contagiosa is a bacterial, inflammatory skin disease, characterized by the appearance of pustules in which the developing vesicles do not rupture, put progress to form bullae, which collapse and become covered with crusts. Sometimes occurring epidemically in hospital nurseries and schools, it may mimic cigarette burns and be suspected as abuse.

Osteogensis imperfecta (OI) is another congenital abnormality that causes bones to break, sometimes for no apparent reason. This disease is often misunderstood and misdiagnosed as child abuse. Signs may include a tendency to bruise easily; hearing impairment; excessive laxity of joints (Silence, 1988); sclera with a blue, purple, or gray tint; and a tendency toward spinal curvature. A punch biopsy of the skin for analysis of collagen synthesis will be an important test to rule out or confirm OI (Bays, 1994).

Coining. This Southeast Asian healthcare practice is commonly misinterpreted as child abuse outside of the countries that practice it. It is a cultural healing method where warmed oil is applied and then rubbed with the edge of a coin or spoon in a linear fashion, usually on the chest or back. The repetitive rubbing causes bruises and welts (Yeatman & Dang, 1980).

Key Point *23-2*

There are conditions that mimic abuse and these must be carefully differentiated during the examination processes in order to prevent false accusations of child abuse.

Laws and Regulations

Laws Requiring Report of Suspicion

All 50 states have laws that require the reporting of suspected child abuse or neglect by all healthcare professionals practicing in their professional or official capacity and employed by a private or public hospital, institution, or facility caring for children. Others mandated to report include school personnel, childcare providers, social workers, law enforcement officers, and mental health professionals. Healthcare professionals must be informed of the laws governing their state practice, as each state has its own definitions and particular reporting protocols. Generally states require the practitioners report directly to the local health department child protection services.

Purpose of the Report

Despite mandatory reporting laws in all 50 states, some professionals claim reasons for not reporting, such as patient-provider confidentiality protection. All states have eliminated the right of confidentiality when child abuse is suspected (National Clearinghouse on Child Abuse and Neglect Information, 2003b, 2003c). The report helps protect the child and society from any future harm, and initiates the process to help the family. Other providers are concerned about alienating or angering the parent. The provider must recognize the report is the beginning step to helping the child and family and should tell the accused there will be a report submitted, not an allegation of abuse. The decision to wait and see or give the parent another chance puts the child in jeopardy for additional harm and does not help the parent.

Content of the Report

An oral report of the suspected child abuse or neglect is made by telephone or in person within 24 hours to the appropriate agency. A written report is then made within 72 hours. Reports should be as inclusive and objective as possible, including but not limited to the description of the nature and extent of the injury or condition and any evidence that would support it (see Appendix D for sexual assault forms). Most state laws allow the reporter to take photographs (color and black-and-white recommended) and roentgenologic studies (to rule out unsuspected old and recent fractures) without the consent of the parent or persons responsible for the child when the abuse or neglect is suspected.

A thorough examination by a trained sexual assault nurse examiner (SANE) should be done in the case of suspected sexual assault, including objective data collection of gonorrhea cultures, serologic tests for syphilis and DNA samples, Wood's light exam to detect seminal fluid, and pregnancy testing. Other testing might be necessary to rule out abuse, such as coagulation studies to test for clotting disorders and neurological examinations.

Descriptions of the child and parent behaviors and interactions are strongly recommended. Documentation needs to focus on objective observations, rather than drawing conclusions. Hearsay is a legal term referring to one individual saying what another person said. If a child's statements are properly documented as part of a medical examination, they may be admissible in a later court proceeding. Experts recommend documenting the questions ask, the direct verbal responses (quotations are useful), and any nonverbal communication. Most states have an exception to the hearsay rule for certain statements provided to healthcare professionals during diagnostic and treatment sessions.

Documentation is essential from the very beginning of any contact with the child or parent. Each visit or event should be documented carefully during or immediately following the contact. Records are allowed in court as admissible evidence only if they are recorded at or near the time of the contact. Describe behaviors, rather than labeling them. Inconsistencies in facts need to be documented, especially when history and physical examination findings do not match.

Forensic nurse examiners are in a prime position to help healthcare professionals learn what data is needed for collection and how to best document findings. Most professionals are not aware of the legal ramifications of poor charting. Documentation is also important in cases handled out of court, as it provides a baseline for the child protective agency work.

Penalty for Failure to Report

All but five states have laws that include penalties for failure to report suspected child abuse and neglect (National Clearinghouse on Child Abuse and Neglect Information, 2003b). Penalties are a criminal offense with fines up to $1000 and can evoke prison sentences up to one year. Criminal charges are basically nonenforceable, but there have been some cases that proved a conscious choice by the reporter to break the law.

Under civil law, two California cases have supported the right of the victim or parents to sue and receive awards for damages due to the practitioner's negligence to report. In *Landeros v. Flood* (1976), an eleven-month-old child was taken to a hospital for diagnosis and treatment of a leg fracture, and presented with other injuries including multiple bruises and a skull fracture. The child was treated and released home to her mother, with no explanation provided. Later the child was seen again for nonaccidental injuries. The child's subsequent guardian sued the doctor for negligent failure to diagnose and report battered child syndrome. The guardian won the case, and the mother and common-law husband were convicted in a criminal action of child abuse.

In the second California case, *Robinson v. Wical, M.D. et al* (1970), a young boy was brought to a hospital twice with severe injuries by his mother and her boyfriend. In neither incident did the hospital report suspicion of abuse. A day later the child was diagnosed at a different hospital with permanent brain damage. The father, who was divorced from the mother, sued the first hospital and doctors for negligence in failure to report suspected abuse. The case was settled out of court for $600,000 awarded to the father.

Laws That Provide Immunity Protection

All states provide some type of immunity, if only qualified immunity for protection from legal liability for those who file a report of suspected child abuse (National Clearinghouse on Child Abuse and Neglect Information, 2003b). Most states provide immunity to those reports submitted in good faith, meaning that the reporter believed that there were reasonable grounds to suspect child abuse or neglect. It is important to remember the law does not require proof of abuse; reporting is required when a professional has evidence that would lead any reasonable professional to suspect abuse or neglect. Delaying a report until all doubt is eliminated violates the intent of the law.

Approximately half the states have a clause in the law that presumes good faith. In the case of immunity, the plaintiff would have to prove the child abuse report was filed with malicious intent, or possibly with gross negligence (National Clearinghouse on Child Abuse and Neglect Information, 2003b). This immunity clause generally covers health professionals who take the child into temporary custody.

Temporary Holding Custody

State laws provide the right for a physician, child protective service personnel, or law enforcement official to take a child into custody for up to 72 hours without prior approval of the parents or guardians, when it is believed that the continued residence or care by that individual puts the child's life or health in imminent danger.

The Investigation

Except in specific cases, the local child protection services agency is responsible for receiving and investigating complaints and reports. The investigation, viewed as a fact-finding mission, is to be initiated within 72 hours of the complaint (National Clearinghouse on Child Abuse and Neglect Information, 2003b).

DeShaney v. Winnebago County Department of Social Services (1989) questioned whether aggravated negligence by the state in failing to protect a child from physical abuse can amount to an unconstitutional deprivation of liberty for that child under protection of the 14th Amendment (Reidinger, 1989). The lower courts were questioned regarding the state's duty to protect a four-year-old child from his abusive father, even though the state had not assumed custody of the child (a caseworker was closely following the case, but had not removed the child from the home). The US Supreme Court ruled in 1990 that the state agency's failure to protect the child from the violence did not violate the child's rights under substantive component of the due process clause.

At the time of investigation, the child protection services is not required by law to inform the accused perpetrator of the charges being made, and no state law requires that the investigation be limited to the reported charge (National Clearinghouse on Child Abuse and Neglect Information, 2003b). However, if an individual has been placed under criminal arrest under charges of child abuse or neglect, no information gathered (including statements or evidence) can be used in a court of law unless the individual has been advised of his or her rights. The members of the military are an exception, as information can be shared.

Testimony and Judicial Hearings

Forensic nurses and other healthcare professionals can best prepare themselves for court with an accurate understanding of the state and federal laws associated with child abuse and neglect. Proper collection and documentation of evidence is essential. Healthcare professionals are frequently called to testify as expert witnesses because they have special skills to assess and work with children and families. Thorough review of documents, as well as guidance of an attorney, is recommended prior to testifying (see Chapters 42 and 43).

In the Pennsylvania case *Commonwealth v. Haber* (1989), the court deemed that judicial creation of the tender years hearsay exception, which provided for the admission of hearsay testimony of sexually abused children, is unjustified on evidentiary and constitutional grounds. The courts may order psychological, psychiatric, and physical examination of a child or parent.

The US Supreme Court ruled in the case *Coy v. Iowa* (1989) that a defendant has a constitutional right in the Sixth Amendment to confrontation with the accuser (the case specifically dealt with sexual assault). Several other cases have been related to the *Coy v. Iowa* case, including *Kenteek v. Stiner* (1986), in which the US Supreme Court held that a defendant suffered no confrontation clause violation when excluded from in-chambers competency hearings of two minor witnesses. In *Louisiana State v. Murphy* (1989), the court ruled that the state's statute, which generalized the presumption that a child victim or sexual abuse victim would suffer trauma as a result of testifying in the presence of the accused, does not outweigh the criminal defendant's right to confrontation.

In criminal cases, the evidence must establish by preponderance of evidence that the abuse was the fault, by either omission or commission, of the accused at the time the injuries occurred. In civil cases, the law requires evidence to support the abuse allegation beyond a reasonable doubt. The forensic nurse needs to understand the types of evidence that will be required and have guidance in that direction.

Summary

The United Nations Convention on the Rights of Children (1989) states "Mankind owes to the child the best it has to give." Without early identification and intervention to interrupt the cyclical nature of abuse, the surviving child will be most often damaged in the overt or covert results of human abuse. Often, this cyclical behavior is referred to as the three-generational pattern of abuse; perpetuating abuse of one generation onto the next, from child abuse to intimate partner abuse and into the most recent phase of interpersonal crime, abuse of the elderly. Forensic specialists in nursing will promote the necessary expert skills and insight to the eradication of abuse against children. The sequelae of childhood abuse incorporate a variety of consequent symptoms in the living and validation of suspected overt or covert violence in the deceased.

Health professionals must understand federal and state laws in order to protect children and avoid negligence charges against themselves. Forensic experts are in a key position to educate healthcare workers on appropriate assessment, collection, and documentation techniques.

Resources

Organizations

National Center for Missing and Exploited Children

Charles B. Wang International Children's Building, 699 Prince Street, Alexandria, VA 22314-3175; Tel: 703-235-3900, 800-THE-LOST; www.missingkids.com

References

Bays, J. (1994). Conditions mistaken for child abuse. In R. M. Reece (Ed.), *Child abuse: Medical diagnosis and management.* (Pp. 358-385). Philadelphia: Lea and Febiger.

Belsky, J. (1980). Child maltreatment: An ecological integration. *American Psychologist, 35,* 320-335.

Belsky, J. (1993). Etiology of child maltreatment: A developmental-ecological analysis. *Psychological Bulletin, 114,* 413-434.

Brown, M. (1997). Dilemmas facing nurses who care for Munchausen syndrome by proxy patients. *Pediatric Nursing, 23*(4), 416-421.

Cowen, P. S. (1999). Child neglect: Injuries of omission. *Pediatric Nursing, 25*(4), 401-430.

deMause, L. (Ed). (1974). *The history of childhood.* New York: Harper Torchbooks.

DeShanney v. Winnebago County (109 S. Ct. 998).

Duncan, R. D. (1999). Peer and sibling aggression. An investigation of intra- and extra-family bullying. *Journal of Interpersonal Violence, 14*(8), 871-886.

Estes, R. J. (2001) *The sexual exploitation of children: A working guide to the empirical literature.* Philadelphia: University of Pennsylvania, School of Social Work.

Giardino, A. P., Christian, C.V., & Giardino, E. R. (1997). *A practical guide to the evaluation of child physical abuse and neglect.* Thousand Oaks, CA: Sage Publications.

Green, B. F., & Kilili, S. (1998). How good does a parent have to be? Issues and examples associated with empirical assessments of parental adequacy in cases of child abuse and neglect. In J. R. Lutzker (Ed.) *Handbook of child abuse research and treatment.* New York: Plenum Press.

Hart, S. N. & Brassard, M. R. (1987). A major threat to children's mental health: psychological maltreatment, *American Psychologist, 42,* 160-165.

Helfer, R. (1990). The neglect of our children. *Pediatric Clinics of North America, 37*(4), 923-942.

Hobbs, C. J., Hanks, H. G. I., & Wynne, J. M. (Eds). (1993). *Child abuse and neglect: A clinician's handbook.* Edinburgh, Scotland: Churchill Livingston.

Hockenbery, M. J., Wilson, D., Winkelstein, M.L, et al. (2002). *Wong's nursing care of infants and children.* St. Louis: Mosby Company.

Holter, J. C. (1979). Child Abuse, Nurse Clin North Am 1979 Sept:14(3): 417-427

Houxley, P., & Warner, R. (1993). Primary prevention of parenting dysfunction in high risk cases. *American Journal of Orthopsychiatry, 63*(4). 582-588.

Howze, D. C., & Kotch, J. B. (1984). Disentangling life events, stress and social support: Implications for the primary prevention of child abuse and neglect. *Child abuse and neglect, 8*(4), 401-409.

Johnson, H., & Au Coin, C. (Eds). (2004). Statistics Canadian Center for Justice Statistics, Family Violence in Canada: A statistical profile, 2003. Published by the authority of the minister responsible for statistics in Canada. Minister of Industry 2003. June 2003. Ottawa.

Kempe, C. H., Silverman, F. N., & Steele, B. P. (1962). The battered-child syndrome. *JAMA,* (1), 105-112.

Landeros v. Flood (51 P. 2nd 3889)

Lynch, V. A. (1997). *Clinical forensic nursing: A new perspective in trauma and medicolegal investigation of death.* Fort Collins, CO: Bearhawk Consulting Group.

McCauley, J., Kem, D.E., Kolonder, K. (1997). Clinical characteristics of women with a history of childhood abuse: Unhealed wounds. *JAMA, 227,* 1362-1368.

Milner, J. (1993). Social information processing and physical child abuse. *Clinical Psychology Review, 13,* 275-294.

Moorhead, C. (1997). All the world's children, *Index on Censorship,* 2, 51-160.

National Child Abuse and Neglect Data System. (2003). Services to prevent child maltreatment. Retrieved on April 18, 2005, from www.acf.dhhs.gov/programs/cb/ststs/ncands97/s11.htm.

National Clearinghouse on Child Abuse and Neglect. (2003a). *Definitions of child abuse.* U.S. Department of Health and Human Services. http://nccanch.acf.hhs.gov/general/legal/statutes/define.cfm

National Clearinghouse on Child Abuse and Neglect. (2003b). *2003 Child abuse and neglect state statute series statutes at a glance: Mandatory reporters of child abuse and neglect.* http://nccanch.acf.hhs.gov

National Clearinghouse on Child Abuse and Neglect. (2003c). *2003 Child abuse and neglect state statute series ready reference: Reporting laws: Immunity for reporters.* U.S. Department of Health and Human Services. http://nccanch.acf.hhs.gov.

National Clearinghouse on Child Abuse and Neglect. (2004). *Children and domestic violence.* http://nccanch.acf.hhs.gov/general/legal/statutes/domviol.cfm

Nester, C. (1998). Prevention of child abuse and neglect in the primary care setting. *The Nurse Practitioner, 23*(9): 61-73.

O'Keefe v. Osoui (Cook County Circuit Court, N. 70L-14884.)

Pasqualone, G. & Fitzgerald, S. (1999). Munchausen by Proxy Syndrome: The forensic challente of recognition, diagnosis, and reporting. *Crit Care Nurs Q, 22*(1): 52-64.

Peterson, M. & Urquiza, A. (1993). The role of mental health professionals in the prevention and treatment of child abuse and neglect. Washington, DC: US Department of Health and Human Services.

Reece, R. M. (1994). *Child abuse: Medical diagnosis and treatment.* Philadelphia: Lea & Febiger.

Reidinger, DeShaney V. (1989). Winnebago County Department of Social Services, 489 U.S. 189. 812 F.2d 298 (7th Cir., 1987).

Ricci, L. R., & Botash, A. S. (2002). Pediatrics, child abuse. *eMedicine, 3*(4). Retrieved April 17, 2005, from www.emedicine.com/emerg/topics368.htm.

Robinson v Wical (3 Cal. S. Ct.)
Sachs, B., & Hall, L. (1991). Maladaptive mother-child relationships: A pilot study. *Pub Health Nurs, 8*, 226-233.
Schmitt, B., & Mauro, R. (1989). Nonorganic failure to thrive: An outpatient approach. *Child Abuse & Neglect*, 13, 235-248.
Schuster, M., Wood, D. L., Duan, N., et al. (1998). Utilization of well-child services for African-American infants in a low-income community. *Pediatrics, 101*, 999-1005.
Silence, D. (1988). Osteogenesis Imperfecta nosology and genetics. *Annals of the New York Academy of Science*, 543, 1-15.
Simonelli, C. J., Mullis, T., Elliott, A. N., et al. (2002). Abuse by siblings and subsequent experiences of violence within the dating relationship, *J Interpersonal Violence,* 17, 2, (February 2002):103-121.
Spenser, D. (2000). Sibling abuse. *Times Educational Supplement*, Issue 4405, p.20.
Suggs, A., Lichenstein, McCarthy C et al. Child Abuse/Assault. In J. S. Olshaker et al. (2001), *Forensic emergency medicine* (p. 161). Philadelphia: Lippincott Williams & Wilkins, Philadelphia.
U.S. Department of Health and Human Services (2004). Administration for children and families: Summary: Child Maltreatment 20:03.
Wiehe, V. (1997). *Sibling Abuse: Hidden, Physical, Emotional, and Sexual Trauma* (2nd Ed.). Thousand Oaks, CA: Sage Publications, Inc.
Yeatman, G. & Dang, V. (1980). Cao gio (coin rubbing): Vietnamese attitudes toward healthcare. *JAMA, 244*, 2748.

Chapter 24 Domestic Violence

Barbara A. Moynihan

Experiencing violence transforms people into victims and changes their lives forever. Once victimized, one can never again feel quite as invulnerable. Violence between intimates is often referred to as spousal abuse, domestic violence, family violence, or intimate partner abuse. Domestic violence includes abuse or battering as a pattern of psychological, economic, and sexual coercion of one partner in a relationship by a current or former intimate partner (Fulton, 2000; Hayward & Weber, 2003; Schwarz, 1999) and is often punctuated by physical assaults or serious threats of bodily harm. Domestic violence is seen as a learned, controlling behavior and attitude of entitlement that is often culturally supported. Many victims of domestic violence are unaware that it is a crime.

In addition to being at increased risk for physical injury or death, victims of domestic violence have an increase in a variety of medical problems such as depression, anxiety disorders, eating disorders, and alcohol and substance abuse. For those who try to leave, it may take many years to break completely free of the relationship, during which the degree of abuse can escalate and escape becomes more dangerous.

This chapter addresses the forensic considerations integral to the holistic care of victims of domestic violence and will be developed in gender-specific terms. Although violence can occur in any intimate relationships, the focus of this chapter will be limited to partners in heterosexual relationships. Domestic violence can be a problem in same-sex relationships, and there are reported cases of men being beaten by women (Eisenstat & Bancroft, 1999). Violence in gay and lesbian relationships is rarely discussed, and violence against men in heterosexual relationships even less so (Straus & Gelles, 1986).

Violence against another person is a violation of the law as well as contrary to the moral and ethical standards that guide human behavior. Studies indicate that the primary targets of abuse are women and children. Approximately 90% of abuse involves women who are abused by men. Men are also abused by their spouses and partners, yet they most often do not report due to embarrassment and fear of disbelief. As a result, insufficient information is available regarding male domestic abuse. Barriers exist in identifying individuals involved in domestic violence that result in greater numbers of unrecognized and untreated victims of human abuse. Victims or batterers often do not seem to fit a distinct personality or socioeconomic profile. Often the perpetrators are charming to others but use intimidation to keep their victim in line (Eisenstat & Bancroft, 1999). People who know the batterer are generally not aware of their friend or colleague's dark side. The victim is often afraid to talk to anyone about the abuse for fear of retaliation or that the person they trust will actually tell the abuser, which can lead to another violent episode.

With the increasing emphasis on the impact of domestic violence in society, healthcare organizations have developed guidelines for improved identification and treatment of victims with injury related to domestic violence. Hospitals nationwide have enacted programs to reduce and prevent further abuse. Domestic violence is recognized as preventable trauma. The Joint Commission for Accreditation of Healthcare Organizations (JCAHO, 2004) has specific guidelines that require all healthcare professionals to routinely screen for this syndrome. Some suspected barriers in screening include the lack of clinical guidelines and the brevity of healthcare visits, clinicians' discomfort with the subject, lack of access to services that deal with the perpetrator, and misconceptions about who are the typical victims of abuse (Ellis, 1999).

Most victims of domestic violence indicate that they had hoped that the clinician would ask if they were being abused, and that if asked in a caring manner, they would have discussed their abuse history (Ellis, 1999). Some clinicians may not have been trained on the procedures for screening for abuse. They may not know how to identify relevant historical and physical findings, document such findings clearly in the medical record, refer for appropriate services, and assess whether the individual is in immediate danger. It is essential for clinicians to be aware that the victim's statement about the cause of injury may be inconsistent with the physical findings, and thus they must maintain their suspiciousness of abuse, despite the victim's account of injuries.

The role and responsibility of the forensic nurse examiner (FNE) intersect with the victim as a result of the forensic needs of the patient. Safety issues as well as consultation with other medical providers and with the legal system are within the purview of the FNE. As a clinical investigator, the FNE joins and collaborates with other providers to protect and preserve the patient's rights, facilitating their journey to autonomy and safety and at times testifying on their behalf. This specialized level of response ensures that intervention, treatment, and documentation will be accurate and follow-up services are comprehensive.

In another important role, the FNE serves as a clinical educator and forensic consultant to all hospital departments when a forensic consult is requested. In this capacity, the FNE can emphasize the structured protocols and procedures that have been designed to optimize care for such victims. By educating other members of the healthcare team and the community, the FNE will assist in eroding stigma that compromise and interfere with objective and unbiased treatment.

Scope of the Problem

The Senate Judiciary Committee in 1990 stated, "If every woman victimized by domestic violence were to join hands, the string of women would span from New York to Los Angeles and back again." The extent and prevalence of domestic violence is of major concern in the US. The scope and dynamics associated with domestic violence not only compromise the health, well-being, and quality of life of the victim, but also directly or indirectly compromise the health and well-being of any children involved in the relationship.

Battered women are representative of the population at large (Stark & Flitcraft, 1996). The following facts illustrate the far-reaching dimensions and the severity of domestic violence. It is estimated that 20% to 50% of all females presenting to hospital emergency departments are battered women (Ellis, 1999). In most populations, one in four women may be physically or sexually abused. Battering is now recognized as the single most common cause of injury to women in the US (Kircher, 1996). Battered women range in age from adolescents to the elderly. The US surgeon general reported that domestic violence is the leading cause of injury to women in America between ages 15 and 44 and accounts for more injuries than muggings, stranger rapes, and motor vehicle accidents combined (Fulton, 2000). The rate at which women separated from their spouses suffer violent victimization was 128 per 1000 or over 12 times that of never-married women, approximately twice that of divorced women, and more than six times the rate of married women (Feminist Majority Foundation, 1998).

Every year six million women are victims of abuse by someone they know, and every three of four female homicide victims are killed by their husbands or lovers (Cook, 1997). Approximately 25,000 individuals die annually as a result of intentional homicide, and millions of Americans suffer emotional and physical scarring from nonfatal violence (Ellis, 1999). Statistically, more women who leave their batterers are killed than those who stay. The risk of homicide increases by 75% when women leave (CADV Voice, 1989).

Informal studies suggest that if a women's history reveals a pattern of canceled medical appointments and the person canceling the appointments is a male, 90% of these women are victims of domestic violence (McAfee, 2001). Each year medical expenses from domestic violence total at least $3 million to $5 million; businesses forfeit another $100 million in lost wages, sick leave, absenteeism and nonproductivity (Colorado Domestic Violence Coalition, 1991).

Research (Steinmetz & Luca, 1998; Straus & Gelles, 1986) and a host of other self-report surveys, such as data collected from the National Crime Victimization Survey (Bureau of Justice Statistics), consistently find that no matter what the rate of violence or who initiates the violence, women are seven to ten times more likely to be injured in acts of intimate violence than are men.

Male Victims of Spouse Abuse

For centuries the public has focused on abuse of women. Although women are eight times more likely than men to be victimized by an intimate partner (Lamberg, 2000), 1.5% of men are victims of domestic abuse by their female partners (Scott-Tilley, 1999). Victimization occurs regardless of gender. Male battering is not a recent trend resulting from contemporary society. In the eighteenth century, men who were abused by their wives were made to wear inappropriate clothing and ride a donkey backward through their villages (Steinmetz & Lucca, 1988, p. 233). Statistics published in *Time* magazine stated "282,000 men are beaten by their wives each year" (Pagelow, 1985, p. 179).

The failure to report and the lack of statistics result in the public's disbelief in relation to the dimensions of the problem. Consequently, the issue of male victims has been neglected. The size and strength of men make it hard for many people to believe that they can be victims of abuse. Male battering is, however, as much a complex domestic violence issue as female battering; and, unfortunately, it is unfairly ignored. Battering of the male spouse is the most underreported type of family violence (Pagelow, 1985).

According to Herzberger (1996), a social psychologist, "many reports suggest that women and men are about equally likely to aggress against a partner" (p. 10), and women tend to be more abusive in almost all categories except for pushing and shoving. One nationwide study on spouse abuse in 1980 indicated that 27% of violent abuse was by men and 24% was abuse by women (Herzberger, 1996). Another research project conducted in 1985 indicated that there were 124 assaults by wives per 1000 couples and only 122 assaults by husbands (Price, 1994). It is important to emphasize that in light of the number of men who batter, there are men who would never hit a woman. These men, when put into a violent situation with a woman, will grab her fists to keep her from hitting him or push her away, but will not hit her.

Herzberger (1996) reported that battered men are also less likely to seek help from social service agencies or the police. Men fear the public humiliation of being beaten by a woman. Another reason they remain silent is that they fear rejection from friends and families. Unfortunately, when a male victim does call for help, the usual response is, "What did you do to provoke her?" (Beaupre, 1997). Where, then, do male victims go for help? Laws have been made, shelters formed, and special services are available to female victims, but in reality there are "virtually no programs, shelters or support groups aimed at helping abused men" (Beaupre, 1997). Contrary to evidence, the public still has difficulty believing male battering is a genuine problem

In 2000, a Colorado Springs man, Jerry Miranda, experienced these identified responses from law enforcement and friends when he had to testify in court against his abusive and alcoholic wife. Afterward he told a friend he had never been so embarrassed in his life and that the jury made him feel like a liar. Although he had experienced domestic violence for 22 years, he had never hit his wife. As the abuse began to escalate, he attempted to confide in others, his colleagues and commander at work. However, no one seemed to believe him until his wife entered his office at the US Air Force Academy and assaulted him with a knife, stabbing him in the back. The police did not appear to believe him, but she was arrested and jailed. Yet, Miranda was required to provide funds to bond her release. While awaiting trial, she had a gun; she entered his residence, destroyed his furniture, threatened to kill him, and stalked him. He feared for his life. During this period, Miranda sought help and counseling. The local domestic violence resource did not seem to believe him. They did not know what to do and had no immediate help for him. Only when his case was addressed on national television did many of the professionals or acquaintances believe him. At trial, Miranda's two grown sons testified against their mother regarding the years of violence and abuse that had been directed not only at their father, but also to them as children.

The FNE must be aware of these statistics and be able to recognize signs of male battering. Observe for wounds on men that may seem unusual and inconsistent with the history given, such as defense wounds, patches of missing hair, black eyes, a bloody lip, groin injuries, bruises, scratches, burns, and bite marks. Gender biases are often the reason male victims do not disclose and remain untreated. Forensic nurse examiners need to feel comfortable approaching these biases and must be able to provide a caring, open, and understanding environment for male victims (see Chapter 31).

Risk Factors

The risk factors or circumstances that place women at risk for abuse are broad and unique. Women are legitimate targets for violence, particularly male violence. Although men can be, and at

Key Point *24-1*

If the batterer is sincere in his determination to end his violent behavior, he must commit to taking responsibility for his behavior, engage in programs designed for batterers, and learn appropriate strategies for anger management and conflict resolutions.

times are, the targets for battering, women are the most frequent victims. Women who at some level pose a threat to their partner educationally, financially, or socially often become the targets for male/intimate partner rage. The pattern of injury is suggestive of the male's attempt at control. Head, trunk, and torso injuries are consistent with domestic violence. What better mechanism to increase isolation and withdrawal than through the infliction of obvious and embarrassing injuries? Other triggers for violence in intimate relationships may be dependency, financial stresses, substance abuse, low self-esteem on the part of the perpetrator, and pregnancy. There is no particular risk profile for battering other than pregnancy. Domestic violence affects pregnant women and their unborn children. The problem of men battering their partners during pregnancy is not well understood. Abuse at this time may be a conscious or unconscious attempt by the perpetrator to terminate the pregnancy or may even be a form of prenatal child abuse.

Battering of adult and teenage women during pregnancy is now recognized as a frequent and serious health problem with links to low infant birth weight, miscarriages, stillbirths, preterm deliveries, birth defects, and multiple maternal risk factors such as poor weight gain, increased infections, anemia, higher rates of first and second trimester bleeding, smoking, alcohol use, and drug abuse. All women abused during pregnancy are at a serious risk for increasing degrees of physical and psychological abuse, which can ultimately lead to homicide, such as in the high-profile case of Lacy Peterson where both mother and fetus were murdered in 2003. This case has brought the attention of the public to abuse during pregnancy as the Nicole Simpson case did to domestic violence in general. Psychological problems, such as drug abuse, alcohol abuse, and depression may result from the pain of being battered. Pregnant women are more likely than nonpregnant women to use tobacco, alcohol, and drugs during pregnancy, often because the perpetrator demands it of her or as a method of dulling the pain of the situation. Abuse and violence occur more often in pregnancy than do hypertension, gestational diabetes, or any other major antepartum complication.

Like abused women, men who batter come from all walks of life–all types of racial, ethnic, religious, socioeconomic, and educational groups. One common factor does exist with abusive men–the majority come from homes where they witnessed the abuse of their mothers or were themselves abused as children. Men who batter women when they are not pregnant will continue battering in spite of pregnancy. During pregnancy, violence may escalate. The prevalence of women experiencing violence during pregnancy is estimated to be between 0.9% and 20.1% (Ballard, Saltzman, & Gazmararian et al., 1998). Pregnancy is a high-risk period for increasing violence as 23% of pregnant women are in violent relationships. Injuries are usually seen on the genitals, breast, and abdomen.

Abused pregnant women usually do not receive prenatal care until the third trimester. During pregnancy, the health consequences of abuse-related problems involve not only the woman's health but that of her unborn child as well. Complications that arise from violence toward pregnant women include vaginal bleeding, preterm labor, low birth weight, *abruptio placentae*, fetal injury, or death (Fulton, 2000). Blunt abdominal trauma during pregnancy may result in fetal injury or death, either as a direct consequence of trauma to the fetus or indirectly from uterine trauma that results in *abruptio placentae*, uterine perforations, rupture of the bladder, amniotic fluid embolus, hemorrhage, disseminated intravascular coagulation, rupture of membranes, or premature birth. Patterns of injury may be suggestive of abuse, particularly injuries to the breast, abdomen, head, neck, multiple injuries, bilateral forearm injuries (suggestive of self-defense as the result of raising of one's arms), and injuries in various stages of healing.

After delivery, consequences from domestic violence may continue. Mothers have a risk for postpartum depression. Infants from abused mothers have a risk for feeding problems and failure to thrive. Abused mothers often have trouble relating with their own children. Some babies start to turn away from their mothers; in turn, their mothers display frustration and neglect. These children experience emotional shutdown after repeated abandonment from their mothers and do not recognize their feelings and the feelings of others (Lamberg, 2000). Because there is no "fail proof" risk profile other than pregnancy, universal screening is of the utmost importance in identifying and assessing this, at times invisible, population.

The social image of pregnancy must be reevaluated and recognized as a trigger for abuse and battery that includes kicking, slapping, punching, shoving, and sexual assault accompanied by psychological and emotional cruelty. Statistics indicate that one in six pregnant women is a victim of domestic violence (McFarland, Parker, & Sodken, 1996). Routine assessment of abuse with a planned intervention for all pregnant women is essential. The population most vulnerable to battering is pregnant women who have increased physical, social, emotional, and economical needs. Yet pregnancy is a time when physical and sexual abuse often begins or escalates.

As with any form or type of abuse, the abuser desires power and control over the victim and, with pregnancy, often sees the fetus as an intruder or competitor. For some men, jealousy or ambivalence about the pregnancy, growing financial pressure, increased dependency by the woman, or decreased sexual availability may increase risk of abuse. In a study of women in their third trimester of pregnancy recruited from a prenatal clinic in a large private teaching hospital, the battered group of 65 victims offered explanations to why their partners abused them, which included (1) denying fatherhood of the child, (2) opposing views on wanting a child, (3) anger due to normal pregnant illness, (4) jealousy of the unborn child, (5) anger toward the unborn child, and (6) "business as usual." Although no theory to date can fully explain a causal relationship between pregnancy and risk of abuse, abuse prior to pregnancy usually continues or escalates during pregnancy. The more severe and frequent a woman is beaten before pregnancy, the more likely she will be beaten during pregnancy. Abuse in pregnancy is also associated with an increased number of pregnancies, marriage because of pregnancy, and the abuser being violent outside the home.

The FNE provides a specific function through the application of the nursing process in assessing (identification), diagnosing (validating), planning (resources, safety), implementing (treating, counseling), and evaluating (follow-up). The forensic nurse utilizes this entire process to intervene with abused pregnant women seen in primary care health facilities. Routine assessment cannot be overemphasized and initiates and maintains contact for women who are diagnosed with abuse. A battered pregnant woman is often in denial, believing she can make the violence stop (Davy & Davy, 1998).

These interventions will help to reduce and prevent further abuse during pregnancy. The FNE in the emergency department (ED) environs can function as a portal to the healthcare system for women involved in the cycle of abuse, isolation, and victimization (Abbott, 1997). Often, the first contact this population of abused women has had with the healthcare professionals during their pregnancy is in the emergency department. By routinely screening for injured pregnant women presenting to the ED, the forensic nurse examiner can assess for abuse situations, counsel, and provide resources for the safety of the woman and her unborn child.

Dynamics of Intimate Partner Violence

The central focus of this chapter is violence against intimate partners. Women battering or domestic violence exists within the greater societal context because it is rooted in the historical oppression of women. The politics of female abuse speak to their socialization within our culture. It has been only a little over a hundred years since Massachusetts became the first state in the US to legally repudiate "wife-battering." In 1871, it was declared that the "privilege, ancient though it be, to beat her with a stick, to pull her hair, choke her, spit in her face, or kick her about the floor, or to inflict upon her other indignities, is not now acknowledged by our law." The expression "rule of thumb" is directly related to English law that allowed the beating of one's wife with an instrument no thicker than a man's thumb. Domestic violence is a pattern of coercive control. Battering encompasses the range of behaviors that hurt, intimidate, coerce, isolate, control, or humiliate another, most commonly an intimate partner and most frequently a woman. Although the prevalence may be viewed as greater in certain populations (i.e., patients who utilize emergency departments or police services), there are those who may endure incredible abuses, exploitation, or deprivation without reaching out for assistance. Presentations may be masked by inaccurate or plausible histories and thus may be missed by an uninformed or busy specialist.

Clinical Presentation

The battering of female partners is a significant health problem that affects at least 4.4 million women in the US each year according to a national survey (Campbell, 1997). Women physically abused by a spouse or live-in partner were more likely to define their health as fair or poor, may have been diagnosed with sexually transmitted diseases, or describe having medical needs that were not met (Campbell & Lewandowski, 1997.) Battered women present for treatment in a variety of settings, such as women's healthcare clinics, primary care centers, emergency departments, and private physician's offices. Injuries as the aftermath of domestic violence may result in the specialist limiting his or her assessment of domestic violence to this population.

The FNE is a central figure in broadening the scope of knowledge regarding clinical presentations to include nonphysically traumatic complaints as well. Battering involves physical, sexual, and emotional abuse. Thus, clinical presentations are representative of these abuses. Battered women may be at increased risk for gynecological problems, HIV/AIDS, and dysmenorrhea due to forced and unprotected sex (Campbell & Lewandowski, 1997). The psychological and emotional sequelae of domestic violence often result in battered women developing depression, post-traumatic stress disorder, or attempting suicide.

Best Practice *24-1*

It is essential that women being treated for substance abuse are screened for domestic violence. Substance abuse and battered women are a dangerous combination often unrecognized and undertreated.

Battered women also present for treatment with vague somatic complaints. Psychosomatic disorders are signs of abuse. They include headaches, difficulty sleeping, abdominal/pelvic pain, chest pain, and a variety of gastrointestinal disorders (appetite changes and dysphagia) that are frequently associated with domestic violence (Ellis, 1999; Fulton, 2000). Battered women with histories of loss of consciousness or head injury may manifest symptoms of traumatic brain injury and may require extensive and comprehensive rehabilitation. Physical abuse may manifest in bleeding injuries, bruising, malfunction of internal organs, skeletal damage (cracked ribs and vertebrae, skull and pelvic fractures and broken jaws, arms, and legs), burns (cigarettes, hot appliances, stoves, irons, chemicals, and boiling liquids), and human bites (Fulton, 2000; Scott-Tilley, 1999). These injuries are usually located in the central part of the body (breast, genitals, abdomen, chest, or back) where the victim can easily conceal them. Peripheral injuries also occur in domestic violence (Fulton, 2000).

Children as Victims and Witnesses

The risk of child abuse is extremely high in families in which domestic violence occurs, as 35% to 75% of spouse batters also abuse their children (Fulton, 2000). Children who see their mothers abused regard violence as normal. In the US, at least 3.3 million children between the ages of 3 and 17 years old witness parental violence annually. Children of battered women are much more aware of the violence than their parents are aware of or imagine (Attala, Bauza, & Pratt et al., 1995). Boys are more aggressive, threatening, and destructive. Girls are more withdrawn. Abused children also demonstrate significant behavioral or emotional problems: post-traumatic stress disorder (flashbacks, difficulty with concentration or sleep, attachment problems, sudden startling or hypervigilance, and at-risk behaviors based on a sense of a limited future); psychosomatic disorders, stuttering, anxiety and fears, excessive crying and school problems (Elliot, 2000). Battered women often delay seeking help because they fear losing their children. The partner may also use this as a threat to deter the woman from disclosing abuse. In some ways, children are more vulnerable than the primary victim, because they have less ability to seek help and significant dependency needs. Children who grew up in violent homes often experience aggression, guilt, and violence in their own relationships. These children are 18 times more likely to commit suicide, 26 times more likely to commit sexual assault, 57 times more likely to abuse drugs, and 74 times more likely to commit crimes toward other people (Lamberg, 2000). Mandated reporting statutes in cases of risk or abuse of children must be clearly adhered to, and the woman must be presented with additional sources of assistance rather than implying loss of custody or a statement of poor parenting skills.

The FNE is in a unique position to help to make a difference in the lives of these children through identification, access to services, and coordination with child protective services. Many abusers were abused as children or witnessed violence against their mothers. Thus, the need for early intervention with children who witness violence is of critical important in interrupting the cycle of violent behavior.

The FNE located within the school-based clinic is in a prime position to intervene and advocate for children who are experiencing the significant distress associated with domestic violence. In planning for the safety and well-being of children involved in domestic violence situations, the FNE should consider the risk of the batterer kidnapping the child and should work with the mother to alert school and day care personnel regarding the dangerousness of the home situation. In addition, alerting school personnel to the home situation allows them to understand the predictable consequences for the children in terms of school performance and socialization. With comprehensive planning, multidisciplinary coordination, and appropriate follow-up, a cushion of safety for children will be established. Specific and long-term strategies are necessary in order for these children to build on their strengths and look forward to a brighter future.

Men Who Batter

There are a multitude of factors associated with male perpetrators of domestic violence. Batterers are also representative of the population at large. There does not appear to be one characteristic that is consistently found in male batterers. The majority of batterers are violent only with their female partners or wives; many batterers are responsible citizens outside of their homes. This increases the difficulty when the female partner thinks, plans, or hopes to leave. The contradiction between violent behavior in the home and responsible citizenry in the community often increases confusion and self-doubt and delays or interferes with help-seeking behaviors. Abusers manipulate, control, and hurt their victims through physical abuse, emotional abuse, isolation, economic abuse, intimidation, and using children to manipulate control. Victims are vulnerable when their children are involved. Knowing this, abusers use children to make their victims feel guilty, have children relay messages, use visitation to harass the victim, and even threaten to take the children away.

Physical abuse develops injuries from punching, kicking, slapping, biting, or being pushed or strangled. As violence becomes more severe, the mechanism of injury becomes more harmful and injuries become more severe (Fulton, 2000). Emotional abuse produces low self-esteem and poor self-image. Abusers accomplish this by making their victims feel bad about themselves, calling them names, playing mind games (making them think they are crazy), humiliating them, placing guilt on the victim, and blaming the victim for the abusive behavior. The abuser degrades victims by treating them as servants, making all the decisions, determining the roles, and acting like the head of the household (Metropolitan Nashville Police Department, 2000). Abusers perceive their victim's family and friends as a threat, so they keep them away (Scott-Tilley, 1999).

Victims are abused economically. Their abusers prevent them from getting or keeping a job, taking their money, and not letting them know about or have access to family income. Batterers make their victims ask for money or give them an allowance. By controlling the money, the perpetrators decrease the independence of their victims. All abusers use intimidation. They make their victims afraid by using looks, gestures, or actions; smashing things, abusing pets, and displaying weapons. Abusers make or carry out threats to hurt the victim. Through intimidation, abusers coerce victims to do illegal things and drop charges filed against them. (Metropolitan Nashville Police Department, 2000). Abusers share several traits: excessive jealousy, overpossessiveness, impulsiveness, controlling behavior, low frustration levels, and drug or alcohol abuse. Research has shown that batterers generally rate high on borderline and antisocial personality disorder scales (Scott-Tilley, 1999).

Many batterers have themselves witnessed or experienced violence in their own homes, so they learn to resolve conflict through violence, coercion, and control. Battering is learned behavior and is often overlooked or in some way condoned.

Key Point *24-2*

Many batterers have themselves witnessed or experienced violence in their own homes, so they learn to resolve conflict through violence, coercion, and control. Battering is learned behavior and is often overlooked or condoned.

Elder Abuse

Domestic violence in earlier relationships often does not end until the abuser is no longer physically or mentally able to inflict intimidation or injury. Elder abuse constitutes a significant risk to a very vulnerable population. Statistics indicate that more than 2 million older adults are or have been abused by a caretaker, either a relative, friend, or individual upon whom the elderly patient is dependent (Sampselle, 1991). Abuse to the elderly is manifested in several ways, including physical or sexual abuse, financial abuse or exploitation, neglect, and emotional or psychological abuse. Withholding of medications or treatment is a more subtle form of abuse and neglect and may be harder to identify. The dynamics of elder abuse are similar and yet subtly different from abuse of younger patients. The elder patient may be reluctant to ask for help, acknowledge the maltreatment, and identify the abuser who may be a son, daughter, or close relative or friend. There have been too many instances in which abuse has occurred in settings that should have been safe (medical or custodial facilities). An assessment for safety should be routine for every patient.

Elder abuse may be represented in various ways. Physical neglect, inappropriate dress for the time of year, signs of poor personal hygiene, and malnutrition are causes for concern and raise the index of suspicion that proper care and treatment are not being delivered. Mismanagement of funds is more difficult to identify unless during assessment the patient indicates that he or she is unable to purchase groceries, toiletries, and other necessities due to lack of funds, which someone else controls. Demeaning, humiliating, and degrading verbal abuse can result in depression, withdrawal, and suicide attempts by an elder patient who begins to believe that he or she is worthless and is a burden for the family or caregiver. Erickson (1963) has identified this stage of development as "late adulthood" with the task of "integrity versus despair." When task accomplishment is positive, the patient identifies life as meaningful; when interference or mistreatment occurs, the outcome is a life viewed as meaningless. Assessment, intervention, and referral conducted for each patient regardless of age or presentation will help to clear the path to the bridge of safety.

It is in this area that the special skills of the FNE can make the difference between safety and increased risk. Legal protections for the elderly should be included in the planning of any intervention. Mandated reporting statistics were developed to assist and protect the elder person. Familiarity with these mandates will enhance protection for the victim. There is a myriad of risk factors confronting the elder victim. Dependency needs, failing health, isolation, stressed caregiver, and transgenerational violence contributes to the abuse of the elderly individual. Discharge planning for the elder victim of abuse involves linking and networking with appropriate home care or residential treatment facilities. If caretaker stress is a causative factor, service for the caretaker, including respite services, support groups, and ongoing monitoring, is required to decrease the potential for further abuse. Relocation of the elderly victim may be necessary to protect her or him from further harm.

Best Practice *24-2*

The FNE with the education and expertise to identify these issues and needs is a vital link to additional services. His or her skills, critical thinking ability, and partnerships with community services contribute to holistic care and empowerment for the victim.

The Nurse's Role

The Interview

The importance of the interview cannot be overemphasized. The skills of the interviewer can make the difference between disclosures and continued imprisonment. The FNE with sensitive and nonjudgmental communication skills can open the door to freedom for those entrapped in violent relationships. The interview should be conducted in a private area, which affords the victim the opportunity to disclose the precipitating factors resulting in her or his symptoms. The interviewer should be suspicious of abuse when the partner refuses to leave the room and answers questions that were directed toward the injured. The nurse should notice if the victim is reluctant to speak or disagree with his or her partner (Fulton, 2000; Scott-Tilley, 1999). The following guidelines should be used for structuring the medical/forensic interview:

1. Ask simple, direct questions in a safe, confidential area removed from the general population area.
2. Avoid asking direct questions regarding abuse or violence when the partner is present. Ask the partner to leave. However, should the partner insist on remaining and becomes problematic, contact a hospital security officer to assist with removal; if the patient wants a partner to stay, however, these wishes must be respected. Oftentimes, the victim is well aware that the abuse can increase if the partner is excluded from the interview. If this is the case, the FNE should create a realistic pretense that will allow the patient to see the nurse alone (e.g., obtain a urine specimen).
3. Inform the victim that he or she has the right to be safe and free from harm.
4. Identify community and legal resources.

The FNE will rely on verbal and nonverbal cues to identify situations that involve domestic violence. Relying only on the presence of injuries or the evidence of trauma deprives victims who are being severely abused of any remote possibility of relief. Anxiety, depression, or noncompliance with medications or appointments may suggest that violence or intimidation in some form is interfering with the individual's ability to function. Establishing follow-up appointments, either in person or via the telephone, will provide the individual with a continued source of relief and protection. Establishing a safe time for the appointment or being available on the telephone is essential for the success of these interventions. This also fosters and promotes a sense of control and participation by the victim in establishing a safety net that works. Sensitive and direct questions validate and confirm the seriousness of the situation and the availability of help.

Assessment

Assessment begins with the first contact that the individual has with the medical system and includes identifying the need for immediate medical care. Additional assessment and planning can occur once the victim is stabilized. Universal screening for domestic violence is essential if appropriate services are to be utilized. Each time a battered person presents for care, the window of opportunity opens. Abuse escalates and increases in severity over time, thus the pattern of repeated visits to healthcare systems, in and of itself, can be an indicator of domestic violence.

Key Point *24-3*

When battered women are not identified, they and their children experience increased health problems, which result in increased emergency department visits, hospitalizations, and use of outpatient facilities. (Campbell, 1997)

Studies revealed that most victims who present at emergency departments as a result of domestic violence are there for minor medical complaints rather than trauma (Campbell & Lewandowski, 1997). Screening limited to those who present for injuries will exclude a major population of battered victims. The key to comprehensive assessment includes insight and knowledge of the various presentations that are consistent with domestic violence. Individuals who present with a history of trauma should be carefully assessed for injuries that are not consistent with the history of the injury. Injuries to the face, head, trunk, and upper extremities are the areas most consistent with battering. Nontrauma-related presentations include vague somatic complaints, depression, suicide attempts, substance abuse, and gynecological or genito-urinary problems.

An essential component of any coordinated effort to reduce, preserve, or eliminate domestic violence is to develop a unified and uniform assessment tool. An important responsibility for the FNE is to establish a mechanism for primary prevention through community education. Unfortunately, by the time the victim sees the FNE, it may be too late for primary prevention. However, secondary and tertiary prevention models are both realistic and essential in terms of safety planning. A model-screening program piloted in Connecticut in 1995 is Project SAFE. A safety assessment must be accomplished for everyone, regardless of the nature of the chief complaint. All staff should be made aware of the most frequent location of injuries, consistent with domestic violence. Complaints of general malaise, fatigue, depression, sleep and appetite disturbances, dysphagia, noncompliance with medications, and suicide attempts are also consistent with domestic violence. Other indicators include sexual assault, forced pregnancy, and coerced abortions. Knowledge, expertise, and multidisciplinary collaboration inherent in the role of the FNE contribute to the identification of victims and open the door for interventions. Relief and rescue are not limited to the victim, but are also for the children, both born and unborn.

Key Point *24-4*

Abuse during pregnancy contributes to complications including maternal or fetal death and stillbirths.

One area often unrecognized is the severe isolation imposed on victims and children because of the violence in their home. They may be prohibited from maintaining family relationships, friendships, and even access to spiritual or religious practices. Although the discussion of domestic violence in this chapter has focused on the heterosexual couple, it is important to note that domestic violence occurs in intimate relationships, which include both heterosexual and homosexual partners. Because the identification and self-reports of violence within same-sex couples are inconsistent at best, assessment for domestic violence should not be overlooked because the couple is not heterosexual. Safety assessment can make the difference between life and death in these highly volatile and extremely dangerous situations. Assessment must also include screening for substance abuse (alcohol, street drugs, and prescription drugs). In a desperate attempt at seeking relief, battered persons may turn to drugs or alcohol, which then could become the focus of treatment. Therefore, it is of critical importance that substance abuse treatment facilities screen for domestic violence, or the cry for help will be neither heard nor addressed.

Although many perpetrators of domestic violence show no signs of a mental health condition or of having a criminal background, one must consider that either the victim or the perpetrator, or both, may have mental disorders. The batterer may provide unreliable information about the victim's state of mental health. A batterer may state that his or her partner is mentally ill and a danger to herself or himself as a way to maintain control. It is important to confirm or rule out domestic abuse in those who are being assessed for psychological disorders.

Best Practice *24-3*

The forensic nurse should consider compliance with follow-up appointments as a realistic outcome.

Interventions

Domestic violence is a crime, and subsequently the legal system should be involved in the investigation, examination of evidence, protecting the victim, and holding the offender accountable. The FNE is eminently qualified to meet the responsibilities inherent in situations involving the legal system. First and foremost, the process must be explained in detail to the victim, and permission is required before any legal action can be undertaken.

In situations in which the victim is unable to give permission either due to physical and or psychological condition or due to a language barrier, appropriate administrative and policy guidelines must be followed. Once the patient has been informed regarding the forensic issues and understands the benefit of permitting these procedures to be conducted and has agreed, the FNE can then complete appropriate tasks. Evidence in cases of domestic violence may include the following:

- The medical record. The victim must understand that the medical record can be subpoenaed and will prove to be important in court
- Photographs–bruises, cuts abrasions. Because wounds generally heal within a reasonable time, should a court appearance occur there would usually be no visible evidence of trauma. The photographs can provide powerful documentation of the violence that occurred. All photographs must be labeled with the patient's name, date of photograph, and name of the photographer; refer to policy manual for specific protocols regarding photographs. The victim should be given a photograph and one should be stored safely with the medical record. Note that if the victim has a copy of the photograph, advise the victim to store it in a safe place; should the batterer locate the photograph, the violence could escalate.
- Clothing that is torn or stained with blood or other body fluids should also be preserved and examined as evidence of violence.

Evidence of domestic violence in nontraumatic situations exists within the presentation, victim complaint, and awareness by the FNE. Objective criteria in terms of assessment and documentation of findings will provide the victim with the most effective response by the legal and medical systems.

Any situation that includes the legal system and the healthcare system falls into the realm of the FNE. His or her expertise will benefit the patient as well as the systems and agencies involved. Developing partnerships with community agencies and services is crucial to effective intervention with battered women and men and their children.

Discharge Planning

The planning and coordination of services extend beyond the usual medical follow-up considerations. Safety planning, referral to community services, linkages with legal systems (if appropriate), and, most important, collaboration with the victim throughout this process and all activities related to care must all be given careful consideration. Realistic planning for discharge and safety includes situations in which the victim decides to return home. The FNE working in concert with the victim and in coordination with appropriate resources can enhance the victim's belief in himself or herself as competent. In addition, maintaining a relationship will allow the victim to return to the system when necessary. Safety planning should also include advising the victim to do the following:

- Develop a backup plan should she or he need help to leave home.
- Establish a code or signal with family, friends, or a neighbor to alert them to call the police.
- Have a safe place to store extra money, car and house keys, clothing, important papers, and so on.

These steps can decrease a sense of isolation and helplessness and provide options other than remaining in a dangerous, violent situation.

A major concern in any situation involving domestic violence is the effect that the violence in the home has had or will have on children. Children in homes where domestic violence occurs suffer both emotionally and physically. Discharge planning concerns must also include concerns about the children.

It is essential to assess the level of violence in the home and work with the victim to protect children from further harm. The FNE has a professional, ethical, and legal responsibility to report to the proper child protection agencies any situation that results in minor children being at risk for neglect or abuse. This responsibility must be carefully explained to the victim as an additional resource rather than a prerogative action based on his or her decision to return home. The thought of losing one's children could result in the healthcare system being viewed as an extension of the powerlessness experienced at home and consequently may result in the patient cutting herself or himself off from services.

The decision to return home may trigger negative responses by staff members who may have little or inaccurate information or understanding regarding the dynamics of domestic violence. Staff may communicate disapproval of the victim's decision and further contribute to feelings of anxiety and insecurity regarding the victim's decision. The patient wants the abuse to stop but does not necessarily want to leave home. It is here that the FNE can be the conduit for staff education and enlightenment. The forensic nurse examiner must work closely with the individual to develop safety plans that will work, should the violence resume. It is essential that a follow-up appointment be scheduled at a time when the victim can return. Continuous assessment of the level of violence must be conducted each time the victim returns for follow-up.

Outcomes

Establishing realistic outcomes can be difficult when dealing with a population as unpredictable and powerless as battered women or men. In establishing nursing practice interventions, protocols, and outcomes, the FNE must rely on his or her knowledge base regarding the dynamics of domestic violence, the impact on the family system, the goals for the response to seeking help, and the unique components of the family unit.

Best Practice *24-4*

The FNE should collaborate with mental health professionals to ensure that their assessments and intake interview include a thorough screening for domestic violence.

Advocacy and Legal Issues

The forensic nurse examiner represents a variety of roles to both the victim and the community and legal system. Knowledge of the legal system and familiarity with legal terms and other protocols provide patients with accurate information regarding other systems and allows them access to these services. This can effectively reduce the feelings of isolation and uncertainty that contribute to the victim's inability to reach out for help. It is essential that the FNE maintain an unbiased and professional role throughout his or her interventions. The nurse must be viewed as knowledgeable, nonjudgmental, and as an expert.

Consultation within the Medical Center

Staff training and education throughout the medical center is as important as direct intervention with victims of domestic violence. Thus, staff training in all clinics and care areas will benefit those victims who disclose upon entry in to the medical system and those whose presentation is less obvious. The FNE as consultant within the medical center enhances the legitimacy and credibility that the medical center places on the issue of domestic violence.

Key Point *24-5*

The forensic nurse should assume responsibility for developing and updating agency policies and protocols in compliance with accrediting agencies and recommendations of experts in domestic violence.

Working in conjunction with administration, nursing, and medical providers, as well as with ancillary services (admitting, radiology, ultrasound, etc.), contributes to maintaining standards of excellence throughout the medical center.

As consultant, researcher, and resident expert, the FNE sets the tone for holistic care. Another important role that the FNE fulfills is in the area of primary prevention. Community education, including education within the medical system, is vital for educating the public regarding the circumstances that contribute to domestic violence and for identifying appropriate strategies to reduce the risks of violence. Stress management techniques, self-esteem building, and conflict resolution skills are as important as evidence collection and handling. Universal screening for domestic violence through the efforts and endeavors of the FNE could result in a multisystems response to the development of similar procedures. As a consultant within the medical center, the FNE conducts case reviews and peer reviews on a regular basis. Monitoring the accuracy of documentation is vital to the continuity of care for the individual identified as a victim of domestic violence. The documentation in the medical record serves several purposes: (1) to meet the requirement of nursing practice and policy, (2) to accurately record any and all findings, and (3) to alert the next provider to the existence or suspicion of domestic violence.

The development of tools to assess risk and danger fall within the responsibilities of the FNE. Case review on various units throughout the medical center provides staff with the opportunities to problem-solve and update existing policies and procedures on a regular basis. The direct benefit to this approach is to improve and broaden care interventions. The indirect benefit is to increase awareness, educate staff, and heighten critical thinking approaches to treatment.

Forensic nursing is a relatively new area of specific expertise; however, nurses have long been involved in the forensic evaluations of victims, yet, without the specialized knowledge and skills necessary for effective and efficient practice. In cases of domestic violence, the FNE is extremely qualified to function in this role based on his or her completions of the educational and clinical requirements as established by the International Association of Forensic Nurses (IAFN) and the American Nurses Association (ANA) Scope and Standards of Practice for Forensic Nurses.

Expert Witness

An additional benefit that the FNE brings to the holistic care of the patient who has experienced domestic violence is expert witness testimony in court. To qualify as an expert, the FNE must be able to identify his or her area of expertise, education, experience, and credentials (American Association of Nurse Attorneys, 1996).

The Principle of Beneficence

As nurses, our ethical framework is based on the principle of beneficence. By utilizing critical thinking skills, ethical framework, and problem-solving skills, the FNE has the ability to restore or establish in the victim a sense of self as a "real person." Beneficence in and of itself is therapeutic and sets the example for other service providers.

Cultural Implications

An important dimension of awareness in terms of intervention with battered women is an acknowledgment of the multifaceted constraints with which battered women from different cultures struggle to overcome or accommodate to domestic violence. The cultural taboos that prohibit victims from seeking help pose formidable challenges. The comprehensive knowledge base specific to the FNE may enhance his or her ability to reach out to this undiscovered population. Research and evaluation of current practices and interventions are critical to maintaining cutting-edge responses. Research, both prospective and retrospective, is an essential component. Developing risk and danger assessment tools will benefit a greater population and enhance the accomplishment of positive outcomes, which include the further development of timely and broad interventions. Evidence-based interventions that are demonstrated by retrospective study will enhance and improve current practices.

Case Study 24-1 Follow-Up Intervention

Jane M., 50-year-old divorced mother of two children, was seen in the primary care center of a local hospital with the chief complaint of "difficulty breathing." She described "feeling tired all the time" and not being able to carry out her usual activities. The physical exam, EKG, and blood work were all within normal limits. Jane stated she lives with her 16-year-old son, and her 20-year-old daughter is away at school. She described a long history of domestic violence and had been divorced for one year. Jane was referred to the mental health department for evaluation, was diagnosed with depression, was prescribed antidepression medication, and was discharged. The FNE conducting a routine case review became suspicious regarding Jane's presentation and contacted her to arrange a follow-up appointment. This follow-up revealed that Jane had been in an abusive marriage in the past and had fled to a battered women's shelter with her children. Her ex-husband, who had been arrested and incarcerated, had recently been released and was harassing her by phone both at work and at home. The FNE was able to coordinate community resources, increase safety measures, and refer Jane to a support group for battered women. Her children were also referred for intervention regarding the effects the violence in their family had on their quality of life. The FNE was also instrumental in coordinating with the legal system, sanctions, and restrictions on the activities of the former spouse, prohibiting him from any further contact with Jane. Further activities established safe contact between the children and their father based on their needs and wishes.

Case Study 24-2 Suspicions of Abuse

Her husband and eight-year-old daughter escorted Mildred, a 28-year-old married woman, to her first obstetrical clinic appointment. Mildred miscarried six months ago and was four months pregnant. Her husband insisted on remaining with her throughout her visit, and Mildred agreed to this request. She appeared somewhat uneasy, avoiding eye contact with the nurse and answering questions in a hesitating manner. Mildred's daughter was told to "sit down and be quiet" by the husband (who is not the father of the child). The child appeared to be quiet and withdrawn. During the examination, the nurse noted old bruises on Mildred's chest and neck. Her husband explained that Mildred had fallen several days ago and tended to be "clumsy" at times. The clinic nurse contacted the FNE on call and informed her of her suspicions and concerns related to the findings on physical exam. The FNE reviewed Mildred's medical records and noted that a previous specialist had indicated concerns regarding Mildred's quality of life and safety at home; however, no intervention was initiated.

The FNE advised the clinic nurse to attempt to see Mildred alone, and if this was not possible to give her an appointment to return in one week for evaluation. Mildred asked to use the bathroom; the FNE escorted her and was able to screen Mildred for domestic violence and the safety of her and her daughter. Mildred hesitantly disclosed a history of violence, fear of further harm from her husband, and the desire to return home. The FNE identified resources for both Mildred and her daughter, completed safety planning, and established a realistic follow-up plan. The nurse expressed safety concerns for the child and completed an appropriate referral to the child protection agency. Permission for photographs was obtained. Mildred chose not to keep a photograph with her, because there was a risk that her husband might discover the photograph, leading to further violence.

Rights and Remedies

Historically, police and the courts have failed to treat assaults against women as seriously as they have treated other types of assaults. Moreover, history shows that throughout the nineteenth century, state laws and cultural practice condone family violence–the belief was that it was a husband's prerogative to discipline his wife. Even when the laws changed, police and prosecutors often failed to intervene in these matters. In 1991, Senator Joseph Biden introduced the Violence against Women Act. By 1994, Congress adopted this act, which established a panel to promote research on domestic violence. The federal statute also creates a civil rights remedy: It permits victims to bring federal lawsuits against the perpetrators of domestic violence. By doing this, it reinforces state and local laws without supplanting them. Finally, for the first time in history, violence against women is being condemned at the highest levels, and the resources are available locally to do something about the abuse (Minow, 1999).

The Violence against Women Act faces continual constitutional challenges in the future, as the question posed to the court is whether Congress has the power to adopt a law that regulates interstate commerce. Members of Congress feel that Congress does have the right. Congress produced findings that domestic violence impairs a woman's ability to pursue employment and to work. It also hurts businesses due to increased employee turnover, which increases healthcare expenses and affects national healthcare costs. The next question posed to the court is whether the power of Congress to enforce the 14th Amendment's guaranteed protection encompasses the act. On this question, Congress produced extensive evidence of the widespread bias against women in the court systems. The 14th Amendment was put into place after the Civil War to make sure that states did not refuse to enforce the laws to protect all people. It is also meant to ensure that the states do not refuse to enforce the laws to protect both women and men from domestic violence. In Minow's study (1999), it stated that in order for this pattern of abuse to change, a strengthening of community policing, support for health and social services, and public condemnation of violence must be a priority.

Summary

Family violence is all-inclusive; those who experience it, those who witness it, and those who perpetrate it suffer physical and psychological trauma. A consequence of domestic violence can be the eroding of the victim's sense of self-esteem, self-worth, and spirituality.

To reduce and prevent domestic violence, an all-inclusive approach based on education and coordination of efforts must be developed. It is not "victim blaming" to understand that both men and women can contribute to this most significant social problem (Cook, 1997).

The role of the forensic nurse examiner encompasses every aspect of clinical care and is not limited to traditional hospital or medical responsibilities. Expertise in a variety of areas broadens the opportunities for recovery, rehabilitation, and community networking. The FNE evaluates forensic nursing practice for safety and cost, with a multidisciplinary approach involving the victim's significant others. Domestic violence is a purposeful and instrumental behavior, often increasing in frequency and severity over time. Continued advocacy and activism are key components to a successful response to this most destructive phenomenon. It will require the efforts of all to break the cycle of abuse and make the home and the community safer for women, men, and children.

Resources

Organizations

Clearinghouse on Family Violence Information

PO Box 1182, Washington, DC 20013; Tel: 800-394-3366

National Battered Women's Law Project

National Center on Women and Family Law, 199 Broadway, Suite 402, New York, NY 10003, Tel: 212-741-9480

National Clearinghouse for the Defense of Battered Women

125 South 9th Street, Suite 302, Philadelphia, PA 19107; Tel: 215-351-0010

National Coalition against Domestic Violence

Public Policy Office, 1633 Q Street, Suite 210, Washington, DC 20009; Tel: 202-745-1211, 800-799-SAFE(7233); www.ncadv.org

Office for Victims of Crime Resource Center

Office of Justice Programs, Department of Justice, 633 Indiana Avenue, NW, Room 1386, Washington, DC 20531; Tel: 202-307-5983, 800-851-3420

References

Abbott, J. (1997). Injuries and illnesses of domestic violence. *Ann Emerg Med, 29,* 781-785.

American Association of Nurse Attorneys (AANA). (1996). Ellicott City, MD. A comprehensive guide to legal consulting. *The Nurse Expert.*

Attala, J. M., Bauza, K., Pratt, H., et al. (1995). Integrative review of effects on children of witnessing domestic violence. *Issues Compr Pediatr Nurs, 18,* 163-172.

Ballard, T., Saltzman, L., Gazmararian, J., et al. (1998). Violence during pregnancy: Measurement issues. *Pub Health Briefs, 88,* 274-276.

Beaupre, B. (1997, April 20). A special report: No place to run for male victims of domestic abuse: Shelters, support groups rare for men. *Detroit News,* p. 9.

Campbell, J. C., & Lewandowski, L. A. (1997, June). *Mental & physical health effects of intimate partner violence on women and children* (Vol. 20, No. 2). Nursing Clinics of North America. St. Louis: Elsevier.

Coalition against Domestic Violence Voice, & Hart, B. (1989, Winter). *National estimates and facts about domestic violence,* p. 12. National Coalition against Domestic Violence Voice. Retrieved from http://outreach.missouri.edu/cfe/poverty/newsletters/pvrtys99.htm.

Colorado Domestic Violence Coalition. (1991). *Domestic violence for health providers* (3rd ed.). Denver, CO: Author. Retrieved from www.acadv.org/facts.html.

Cook, P. (1997). *Abused men: The hidden side of domestic violence.* Westport, CT: Praeger.

Davy, D. B., & Davy, P. A. (1998). Domestic violence today: What every nursing student should know. *Imprint,* 41-44.

Eisenstat, S., & Bancroft, L. (1999). Domestic violence. *N Engl J Med, 341,* 886-892.

Elliott, B. (2000). Screening for family violence: Overcoming the barriers. *J Fam Pract, 46*(2), 137. Retrieved from www.medscape.com.

Ellis, J. M. (1999). Barriers to effective screening for domestic violence by registered nurses in the emergency department. *Crit Care Nurs Q, 22*(1), 27-41.

Erikson, E. (1963). Youth: Fidelity and diversity. In E. Erikson (Ed.), *Youth: Change and challenge* (pp. 1-24). New York: Basic Books.

Feminist Majority Foundation. (1998). Facts about domestic violence in the United States Retrieved from www.feminist.org/other/dv/dvfact.html.

Fulton, D. (2000). Recognition and documentation of domestic violence in the clinical setting. *Crit Care Nurs Q, 23*(2), 26-34.

Hayward, K., & Weber, L. (2003). A community partnership to prepare nursing students to respond to domestic violence. *Nurs Forum, 38*(3), 5-10.

Hertzberger, S. (1996). *Violence within the family.* Boulder, CO: Westview Press.

Joint Commission on Accreditation of Healthcare Organizations. (2004). Hospital Accreditation Standards. Oakbrook Terrace, IL: Author.

Kircher, J. (1996). Domestic violence: Clinical and personal perspectives. Physician Assist, 20(2), 87-90.

Lamberg, L. (2000). Domestic violence: What to ask, what to do. *JAMA, 284*(5), 554. Mc Farland, J., Parker, B., & Sodken, K. (1996). Abuse during pregnancy: Associations with maternal health and infant birth weight. *Nurs Res, 45*(1), 37-41.

McAfee, R. (2001). Domestic violence as a women's health issue. *Women's Health Issues, 11*(4), 371-376.

Metropolitan Nashville Police Department. (2000). *Symptoms of abuse: Threats, power, misuse, and control. What symptoms below fit your life?* Retrieved from www.nashville.net/~police/abuse/symptoms.html.

Minow, M. (1999). Violence against women: A challenge to the Supreme Court. *N Engl J Med, 341,* 1927-1929.

Murowski, D. (1999). Is he lethal? Retrieved from www.http://groups.msn.com/SpousalAbuseSupport/areyouabused.msnw (December 6, 2004)

Pagelow, M. (1985). *Marital violence* (p. 179). Worcester, Great Britain: Billing & Sons.

Price, J. (1994, January 31). Report is a reminder men are battered too. *Washington Times,* p. 1A. Retrieved from www.vix.com/men/battery/damnabledenial.html.

Sampselle, C. (1991). The role of nursing in preventing violence against women. *JOGNN, 20*(6) 481-487.

Schwarz, T. (1999). Primary care physicians fail to spot and act on signs of domestic violence. *Am J Nurs, 99*(10), 26.

Scope and Standards of Forensic Nursing Practice–International Association of Forensic Nurses/American Nurses Association. (1997). Silver Spring, MD: American Nurses Association.

Scott-Tilley, D. (1999). Nursing interventions for domestic violence. *Am J Nurs, 99* (Suppl.) (10), 24jj-24pp.

Stark, E., & Flitcraft, A. (1996). *Women at risk.* London: Sage.

Steinmetz, S., & Luca J. (1988). Husband Battering. In Van Hasselt, V. B., et al. (Eds.), *Handbook of family violence* (pp. 233-246). New York: Plenum Press.

Straus, M., & Gelles, R. (1986). Societal change and change in family violence from 1975-1985 as revealed by two national surveys. *J Marriage Fam, 48,* 465-479.

Chapter 25 Elder Abuse

Elizabeth McGann and Barbara A. Moynihan

The Problem

Elder abuse constitutes a significant risk to a very vulnerable population. It is the last form of family violence to be acknowledged by society. According to Pillemer and Finkelhor (1988) the phrase "elder abuse and neglect" is commonly used to describe acts of commission or omission that result in harm to the health and welfare of an elder adult. The term *mistreatment* has also been used to describe physical, emotional, or financial abuse or neglect. These actions may be intentional or unintentional. Intentional harm refers to a conscious and deliberate action to inflict harm or injury to the elder. Unintentional mistreatment occurs when an inadvertent action causes harm and is often due to ignorance, inexperience, or a lack of desire to care for the elder. Self-inflicted abuse or neglect is often unrecognized and a serious consideration for evaluation and intervention.

It is against the law to abuse, neglect, exploit, or violate the rights of the elderly. The Ohio Revised Code defines *elder abuse* as the infliction upon an adult by himself or others of injury, unreasonable confinement, intimidation, or cruel punishment with resultant physical harm or mental anguish.

As a result of a congressional hearing in 1978, elder abuse gained national attention. Soon afterward, state laws were passed requiring the reporting of suspected or actual elder abuse. Demographic, societal, and healthcare trends contribute to the problem of elder abuse. The incidence of elder abuse is increasing with the burgeoning elder population (Fulmer, 1989). A 1991 report from Congress suggests that between 1.5 million and 2 million older adults (over 60 years old) are abused annually in the US. The aging population is growing at the same time that the American birth rate is dropping and the rate of women entering or returning to the workforce is increasing. These trends result in fewer family members, mostly the daughters and daughters-in-law, being available for informal caregiving. This creates additional stress on families and can contribute to elder mistreatment. Additionally, the extended family is more mobile, which makes family members less available. The stressors of single parenthood also impinge on the ability for adult children to provide care for elderly parents. Blended families can sometimes have more parents and grandparents than adult children, with the added complication of geographic distance. Healthcare trends such as shortened hospital lengths of stay result in elder individuals returning home in fragile states of health, less able to care for themselves both physically and emotionally.

Key Point 25-1

With only about 5% of persons over age 65 and about 10% of persons over age 85 being institutionalized, elder abuse is most likely to be found among community-dwelling elders.

A special note of appreciation is due to Judy Sugarman, Ombudsman, Connecticut State Department of Protective Services for the Elderly, whose generous commitment of time and energy helped to complete this project.

Incidence

In 1986, the federal government allocated funds to establish a center for the collection of data on elder abuse. This agency was the National Aging Resource Center on Elder Abuse (NARCEA). Federal support for NARCEA ended in 1992. Subsequently, the National Center on Elder Abuse (NCEA) was created in 1993. In 1986, the NARCEA estimated that there were 140,000 reports of abuse, neglect, or exploitation. In 1996, the NCEA recorded the number of reported cases at 293,000. This is an increase of 150.4% in 10 years. Recent statistics indicate that over 2 million older adults or 1 in 20 elder adults are abused annually in the US. One half of these elders are victims of self-neglect. In 1996, the median age of elder abuse victims was 77.9 years, and for self-neglecting elders it was 77.4 years. In cases of caregiver elder abuse, the abuse is usually by a caretaker who is a relative, friend, or other individual upon whom the elderly person is dependent. Each state has legislation for the reporting of abuse; however, elder abuse is seriously underreported. Some reasons for this are ignorance, fear, or lack of concern. Phillips (1986) found that if a caregiver is perceived as doing his or her best, no matter how compromised the care, elder abuse is often not identified. It is estimated that only one out of five cases of elder abuse is reported (Bourland, 1990; Frost & Willette, 1994). It is only slightly less common than child abuse. The dynamics of elder abuse are similar to abuse of younger people, but there are subtle differences. The elder person may be reluctant to ask for help, acknowledge the maltreatment, and identify the abuser who may be a close relative or friend. These people may fear retaliation by the abuser, being institutionalized, or abandonment. In far too many instances abuse has occurred in healthcare settings, which should have been safe; thus, assessment for safety should be routine for every individual. Assessment, intervention, and referral conducted for each patient, regardless of age or presentation, will help to clear the path to safety in healthcare.

Types of Elder Abuse

Abuse to the elderly is manifested in several ways. These forms include physical, psychological, and financial abuse, and neglect by self or caregiver. Withholding of medications or treatment constitutes a more subtle form of abuse and neglect and may be less easily identifiable. Elders may fall prey to several types of abuse simultaneously.

Physical Abuse

Physical abuse accounted for 14.6% of the substantiated reports of elder abuse in 1996. Physical abuse is the infliction of physical harm or injury and can include sexual abuse. It may take the form of hitting, slapping, pushing, pinching, punching, or burning. Any unexplained injury or bruising should alert the nurse to the possibility of physical abuse. Identification of physical abuse is often complicated by normal age-related changes, which may mimic trauma. Bruising can result even with gentle handling of an elder with friable skin and capillary fragility. Bilateral bruises on the upper arms, however, often are an indicator that the elder may have been shaken, pushed, or restrained by another.

Key Point 25-2

Normal changes of the skin such as capillary fragility and friability are associated with aging, and illness may mimic trauma of abuse. Bilateral bruising on the upper arms often indicates abuse involving shaking, pushing, or restraining.

Psychological Abuse

Psychological abuse may be more difficult to assess. However, demeaning, humiliating, degrading, threatening, or intimidating verbal abuse can result in depression, withdrawal, and suicide attempts by an elder person who begins to believe that he or she is worthless, is a burden for the family or caregiver, and has no purpose in living. Erickson has identified this stage of development as "late adulthood" with the task of "ego integrity versus despair." When task accomplishment is positive, the patient identifies life as meaningful; when interference or mistreatment occurs, the outcome is a life viewed as meaningless.

Financial Abuse

Financial abuse accounted for 12.3% of substantiated cases of abuse in 1996. Financial abuse or exploitation is the misuse of an elder person's funds for someone else's benefit or assets without his or her knowledge or consent. It can take the form of withdrawal of small amounts of money from bank accounts or the overcharges by housekeepers for groceries or household items. Mismanagement of funds is more difficult to identify unless during assessment the individual indicates that he or she is unable to purchase groceries, toiletries, and such because of lack of funds, which someone else controls. It is important to be aware that lifestyle preferences and income may be incongruent in persons who may not be willing to spend their funds on necessities. However, it may also be an indicator of changes in mentation that may signal early stages of dementia; thus, the role of the forensic nurse examiner is critical in determining whether or not exploitation is occurring or has occurred.

Neglect

Neglect is the failure to fulfill a caretaking obligation to provide goods or services. It is the most common form of elder maltreatment. Some examples of neglect are abandonment, denial of food or health-related services, and lack of adequate and appropriate clothing. Again, the expertise of the forensic nurse examiner is critical in the assessment and determination of causality of the findings. It can present as caregiver neglect or self-neglect.

Caregiver Negligence

Of the neglect reports substantiated in 1996, 55% involved caregiver neglect. Neglect can result from a lack of information or resources. There can be subtle signs, such as neglected medical problems, malnutrition, or failure to thrive. More overt signs include dehydration, depression, and oversedation. These manifestations may be evident in situations in which the caregiver is physically or mentally challenged or if the caregiver is an adult child who is elderly as well. Often this type of neglect situation can be ameliorated.

Neglect can also be the malicious neglect of an elder person's needs as a result of disinterest or a desire to gain financially. In these situations it is often difficult to gain access to a dwelling or obtain an accurate history of the elder's injuries (Capezuti, Yurkow, & Goldberg, 1995). Legal protections are essential in order to gain access to the compromised elder and evaluate his or her situation.

Physical neglect, inappropriate dress for the time of year, signs of poor personal hygiene, and malnutrition are causes for concern and raise the index of suspicion that proper care and treatment is not being delivered. Delay in seeking treatment, excessively detailed accounts of injuries, or overprotectiveness on the part of relatives should also be noted as evidence of possible abuse (Lynch, 1997).

Self-Neglect

Self-neglect is the neglect of personal well-being and home environment. In some cases, particularly if the person lives alone, it may be the result of dementia and mental illness. Evidence of this type of neglect is often manifested by an extreme volume of trash or newspapers around the house with little or nothing being discarded. Hoarding or food that is improperly stored or inedible are clues to investigate. It is difficult to provide services to victims of self-neglect because they are often reclusive and suspicious and may go unidentified until the situation is acute. Establishing trust is a key intervention when access to the patient is challenged. A study conducted by the National Association of Adult Protective Services Administrators in 1990 found that 79% of cases of verified adult abuse were cases of self-neglect. Most elders who do not care for themselves do not consider themselves at risk or are unaware of the seriousness of their plight. These situations pose serious social, legal, and health problems and require extensive coordination of services.

Best Practice 25-1

The forensic nurse should assess all elderly patients for signs and symptoms of abuse, neglect, and exploitation.

Profiles

Victim Profile

The expertise and knowledge of the forensic nurse examiner is invaluable in terms of coordination, assessment, and planning to improve the quality of life for the compromised elder. The typical victim of elder abuse is a white frail female over the age of 75, with a physical or mental impairment, who is living with a relative. In 1996, 66.4% of the victims of elder abuse were white, and 18.7% were black. Hispanic elders accounted for 10%, yet less than 1% were Native Americans or Asian Americans/Pacific Islanders. The majority of elder abuse victims are female. In 1996, 67.3% of all reports of abuse involved female victims.

Perpetrator Profile

As Shakespeare wrote in the Merchant of Venice, "The quality of mercy is not strain'd, it droppeth as the gentle rain from heaven upon the place beneath: it is twice blest: it blesseth him that gives and him that takes." Sadly, the stress experienced by the caregiver often interferes with the ability to be merciful.

According to the National Center on Elder Abuse, more than two thirds of elder abuse perpetrators are family member of the victims. Adult children are the most frequent abusers of the elderly.

Other family members and spouses ranked as the next most likely abusers of elders. Abusers frequently have some form of mental illness, a substance abuse problem, poor self-image, and difficulty with self-control. They often have a history of ineffective coping when experiencing stressful events. Often abusers live with the victim and are dependent on the victim for housing or financial support. Abusers may have been mistreated as a child or spouse and may retaliate against the fragile elder. Clinicians are advised to remain alert to high-risk situations, which include alcohol, substance abuse, and a history of violence. Other factors to consider are the age of the caregiver and other caregiving responsibilities (i.e., children, spouse). The abuser may also be socially isolated and may be struggling with high levels of stress or poor health. It is incumbent on the part of the healthcare provider to request a consultation by the forensic nurse examiner whenever the suspicion of elder abuse exists. The FNE often will be involved with intervening with both the victim and the perpetrator.

Risk or Vulnerability Factors

A myriad of risk factors place the elder at risk for abuse. There is often a family history of intergenerational violence, insufficient income, poor social supports, frustration, perceived burden, and transgenerational conflict or violence (Frost & Willette, 1994). Those who care for both their own elders and young children are sometimes described as the "sandwich generation." Dependency and problem behaviors such as belligerence on the part of the elder can serve as stressors for the caregiver and can trigger abuse. The onset of new cognitive impairment is also associated with elder abuse and neglect (Coye, Reichman, & Berbig, 1993; Lachs, Williams, & O'Brien et al., 1997a). Violence on the part of persons with Alzheimer's disease on their caregivers has been associated with caregiver depression (Paveza, Cohen, & Hanrahan et al., 1992). Alcohol consumption by the caregiver has also been implicated in elder abuse (Homer & Gilleard, 1990). Lachs, Berkman, Fulmer, and Horowitz (1994) identified the risk factors of functional disability, minority status, older age, and poor social networks as being associated with investigations of elder abuse, neglect, exploitation, and abandonment. According to a nine-year study conducted by Lachs and colleagues (1997a), the following were identified as risk factors that contributed to elder abuse in a cohort of 2812 community dwelling adults: female gender, poverty, minority status, functional disability, and worsening cognitive impairment. The FNE with specialized knowledge will be in a position to key into situations that include any of these factors and can develop a more comprehensive assessment intervention and safety plan for continued monitoring and follow-up of the elderly person.

The Nurse's Role

Assessment

The nurse is often the first person to interface with a victim of abuse. The nurse may encounter abusive situations in need of assessment in the community or home care setting, emergency department, long-term care setting, or acute care unit. In suspected cases of elder abuse, it is important to interview the victim privately so that the person's account of events is not influenced or compromised by relatives. The history of the injury or presenting problem is significant. Assessing suspected cases of physical abuse requires a thorough physical examination with attention to all bruises, lacerations, pattern injuries, parallel injuries, and burns. The victim needs to be treated with utmost respect and needs to be reassured that the interview is confidential. The nurse must maintain professionalism at all times and may even reassure the patient that his or her situation has happened to others in order to reduce self-blame and promote dialogue. It is important for the nurse to assess the decision-making capacity of the elder to determine if the elder has the ability to provide informed consent for any needed interventions. A mental status examination, along with a physical and social assessment, is part of a comprehensive assessment.

> **Best Practice 25-2**
>
> The forensic nurse must perform a through assessment of the caregiver as a component of the nursing assessment of an elderly patient.

Assessment must include considerations regarding the risk of suicide in the elderly despondent patient. The FNE is in a prime position to evaluate the risk for a suicide attempt by the depressed, lonely, or abused elder. The more subtle indicators include alcohol abuse, noncompliance with medications, and lack of attention to dietary or comfort measures. Elders for whom there is a high suspicion of self-neglect should also undergo a comprehensive depression and suicide evaluation. The nurse must assess the level of function, quality of life, coping strategies, and support systems of the elder, and can broaden the evaluation to include direct questions regarding any ideas, thoughts, or plans to end one's life; such a discussion could offer some relief to the elder who feels trapped in a life without hope.

In cases of suspected financial abuse it is important to determine if anyone has been coercing the elder to sign any documents or has been taking any possessions or money from the home. Query the elder regarding the ability to meet expenses or whether there may be any financial difficulty (e.g., not enough money to purchase prescriptions or other necessities).

The following questions should be posed:

- What sort of difficulty have you experienced recently, either at home or somewhere you go every day or every week?
- Has anyone been having difficulties at home?
- Has anyone touched you in a hurtful way?
- Has that happened before? Does it happen a lot?
- Is the hurting getting worse?
- Has anyone made you do anything or sign anything when you didn't want to?
- Does anyone at home take your things or money?
- How are you eating at home?
- Who prepares your meals?
- Do you take any medications?
- Are you able to meet all your expenses?
- Do you depend on anyone to help you?
- Does that person give you the help you need?
- How can we plan to keep you safe?

The nurse will also need to assess the caregiver. It is important to determine the caregiver's perception of the problem, the issues and concerns related by the caregiver, and the degree of burden the caregiver is experiencing. Questions should elicit information about the kind and amount of care necessary, how much of the care is the responsibility of the caregiver, the available support system, and the degree of obligations outside the home that this caregiver is responsible for accomplishing. The level of awareness of the problem on the part of the family may be important if it is difficult to discern caregiver neglect versus self-neglect.

The following questions should be posed to the caregiver directly:

- What do you think is the problem here?
- What do you think is important for us to know?
- What kind of care does the elder person require?
- How much of that care is your responsibility?
- How difficult is it for you to provide this care?
- What can the elder person do for himself/herself?
- Do you have any support?
- What obligations do you have outside the home?
- Are you able to coordinate these responsibilities?
- Have you noticed (state the condition that brought the person to your attention)?
- Do you know how this occurred?
- What are the sources of the elder person's income?
- Does the elder person manage his/her own finances?

This initial assessment will direct the plan, intervention, and eventual disposition. The competent patient's right to self-determination must be respected. The adult patient is in charge of decision making until she or he delegates responsibility voluntarily to another or the court grants responsibility to another. Freedom is more important than safety; that is, the person can choose to live in harm or even self-destructively provided she/he is competent to choose, does not harm others, and commits no crimes. In the ideal case, the protection of adults seeks to achieve freedom, safety, least disruption of lifestyle, and least restrictive care alternative.

Plan

The FNE builds on the information and findings gleaned during the initial assessment. A complete physical examination, including laboratory tests, radiological studies, and a complete mental health and mental status examination, must be conducted. The person's nutritional status, as well as a complete and thorough systems review, is also critical to the comprehensive delivery of services to this most vulnerable population.

The intervention must go beyond the clinic or hospital to include the individual's living conditions, physical space, and condition of the living quarters. Is the apartment or facility comfortable, cheerful, accessible, and in a safe location? In terms of integrating the skills of the forensic nurse examiner into the nursing process, the following guidelines might be helpful:

- Is there a need for a forensic gerontological assessment?
- Should the local police department or ombudsman be contacted?
- Is it safe for the patient to return home or to the residential facility where he or she is residing?
- Is a home visit needed?
- Who is the primary caregiver?
- What clues are the patient communicating that raise your index of suspicion?

Planning by the FNE extends beyond the delivery of medical and nursing care. Is the plan realistic in terms of follow-up appointments and accessibility to resources? Does the individual need assistance of any form to return to a previous lifestyle? Can the intervention, resource identification, and support result in an improvement in the quality of life for this individual?

Interventions

The major goals of intervention are securing or restoring the safety of the elder and breaking the cycle of abuse. It is in this area that the special skills of the forensic nurse can make the difference between safety and increased risk. Legal protections for this population should be included in the planning of any intervention. Discharge planning for the elder victim of abuse involves linking and networking with appropriate home care or residential treatment facilities. If caretaker stress is a causative factor, service for the caretaker, including respite services support groups and ongoing monitoring, will be required in order to decrease the potential for further abuse. Relocation of the elderly may be necessary in order to protect her/him from further harm. The forensic nurse examiner having the education and expertise to identify these issues and needs, is a vital link to additional services. The nurse's skills, critical thinking ability, and partnerships with community services contribute to holistic care and empowerment for the individual.

Best Practice *25-3*

A multidisciplinary approach utilizing social workers, healthcare providers, lawyers, and the police, and coordinated by the forensic nurse examiner is the optimal approach to intervention in these situations.

Outcomes and Evaluation

It is often difficult, under the best of circumstances, to evaluate the effectiveness of a comprehensive assessment, intervention, and discharge planning protocol. The forensic nurse examiner, once having completed a multitude of interventions, must now develop a reliable and viable tool to periodically assess the patient and evaluate whether or not all goals and objectives were met and realistic outcomes achieved. Planning for evaluation of the outcomes of interventions begins as soon as the person presents for treatment.

Reduction and Prevention of Elder Abuse

The Older American Act (OAA) provides grants to support state elder abuse prevention activities provided by State Units on Aging (SUA). The State Elder Abuse Prevention Program created by the 1987 amendments to the OAA was consolidated into the new Vulnerable Elder Rights Protection Activities, Title VII, when the OAA last was reauthorized in 1992. Title VII provides the state's discretion in setting priorities for spending these funds. States have tended to focus elder abuse prevention activities in four major areas:

1. Professional training
2. Coordination
3. Technical assistance
4. Public education

Primary prevention activities need to be directed toward early identification of those at risk of becoming victims of elder abuse. Forensic nurse examiners are eminently qualified in methods of nonviolent conflict resolution and specialized therapeutic communications skills, which are essential in dealing with potential victims of elder abuse and their families. Measures directed toward reducing caregiver stress are also important prevention interventions. Careful attention to known risk factors and evaluation of patient and family in terms of potential abusive situations that may be evolving are additional facets of primary prevention. Is primary prevention possible in coordinating the care and treatment of the elder? It is difficult to control for the family member who may harbor the potential for abusing the dependent elder; however, with planning, coordinating, screening, and selection of staff other than family, an essential first step is taken in terms of primary prevention regarding those who care for the dependent and frail elder. Respite care, support groups, and community education regarding the unique needs of the aging population will enhance sensitivity and awareness of these issues.

Reporting Elder Abuse

Mandated reporting statistics were developed to assist and protect the elder person. However, mandatory reporting is required by only 42 states. Familiarity with these mandates will enhance protection for the patient. In 1996, 22.5% of all elder abuse reports came from healthcare providers, 15.1% came from service providers, and the remainder came from family members, friends, neighbors, police officers, and victims themselves. State legislatures in all 50 states have passed some form of legislation that authorizes the state to protect and provide services to vulnerable, incapacitated, or disabled adults. In more than three quarters of the states, the services are provided through the state social services department or adult protective services. In the remaining states, the State Units on Aging have the major responsibility. Calls are screened for potential seriousness; some states operate 24-hour hotlines. It is essential that the office with the jurisdiction over the geographical area where the elder resides is contacted whenever elder abuse or neglect is suspected, regardless of the severity. These numbers can be found in the government pages of the phone book or by calling the Eldercare Locator at 1-800-677-1116, which is sponsored by the Administration on Aging (AOA).

According to state law, the following persons must report suspected, actual, or threatened cases of elder abuse:

- Any licensed or registered health-related professional
- Employees or officers of any public or private institution that provides social, medical, or mental health services; long-term care; or adult day care
- Medical examiners or coroners
- Law enforcement agency personnel

Any person required to report within the specified time, but fails to do so, is subject to a fine. Once the immediate situation has been addressed, the adult protective services (APS) agency continues to monitor the victim's situation. The APS agency personnel are assisted by a myriad of agencies specializing in services for elders. The Administration on Aging (AOA) administers the Older Americans Act (OAA), which supports a nationwide aging network consisting of the AOA and hundreds of offices at the regional, state, and local levels, representing over 27,000 community service providers. The majority of elder abuse reports are substantiated after investigation. In 1996, 64.2% of all reports made were eventually substantiated. Of those, 31% were self-neglect cases and 25.4% were cases of abuse by others.

Ombudsman Programs

Twenty-five years ago the AOA began the Long-Term Care Ombudsman Program. Professional ombudsmen working with citizen volunteers have made a dramatic difference in the lives of nursing home residents. An ombudsman may come with preparation in the disciplines of nursing, gerontology, or social work. Ombudsmen have jurisdiction to investigate nursing home complaints relative to poor resident care or violations of a patient's rights. They provide inservice to resident advocates who serve as volunteer ombudsmen and assist resident advocate councils in long-term care facilities. In 1995, 6400 certified volunteer ombudsmen backed by 900 paid staff investigated 218,455 complaints from residents of long-term care facilities, family members, and professionals; 70% of these were fully or partially resolved. One third of these complaints were about poor resident care ranging from cold food and enforced early bedtimes to verbal abuse, medical neglect, and even wrongful death.

Funding for ombudsmen programs totaled $40.9 million in 1995: 60% came from federal funding and the remainder was obtained from state and local funds. Although this seems like a sizable sum, insufficient funding is placing a strain on ombudsmen programs throughout the country. In 1994, a National Academy of Sciences study of the Long-Term Care Ombudsman Program recommended hiring 300 additional ombudsmen nationwide to lower the current estimated ratio of one full-time professional ombudsman for every 2700 nursing home beds to one for every 2000 beds.

Some states also have community ombudsmen who investigate suspected cases of abuse, neglect, exploitation, and abandonment among community dwelling elders. They determine corrective action needed and make referrals to appropriate agencies for food, shelter, transportation, or home care. They are authorized to make emergency dispositions such as hospital admission if necessary. Often, ombudsmen facilitate legal action. Ombudsmen must be cognizant of relevant state and federal law, statutes, and regulations, and must have knowledge of the community resources and agencies that can assist the elderly and disabled. Skills needed by the ombudsman are knowledge of crisis intervention, interpersonal skills, considerable oral and written communication skills, ability to provide education related to forensic issues, and supervision to a host of ancillary personnel. A specialist in forensic nursing is uniquely qualified to serve in this role.

Standards of Practice

Elderly victims of physical abuse have substantial interactions with emergency departments and these visits frequently result in admission (Lachs, Williams, & O'Brien et al., 1997b). The Joint Commission on the Accreditation of Healthcare Organizations (JCAHO) approved the adoption of new standards in 1978 that require emergency departments to develop written protocols to deal with victims of suspected child or elder abuse and to provide continuing education to their staffs in detection and management of clinical forensic cases. The hospital's role in collection, retention, and safeguarding of specimens, photographs, and other evidence and notification is clearly defined. It provides guidance for the proper documentation in the medical record and mandates that a list be maintained that includes private and public community referral agencies (Capezutti, Yurkow, & Goldberg, 1995). Accurate unbiased documentation is critically important. Quotes should be clearly indicated and injuries accurately described using anatomical landmarks as reference points. Records can be invaluable in terms of alerting the next provider, should the patient be readmitted or return for follow-up care. Records may be subpoenaed as evidence should the legal system become involved. Photographs can provide dramatic corroboration of the history of abuse, neglect, or maltreatment. Each agency, hospital, clinic, and institution should have specific policies and guidelines in place to be utilized in these situations.

Implications for Nursing Education

Historically, nursing curricula have not included content on interpersonal violence. Limandri and Tilden (1996) found in a sample of several hundred nurses in Oregon that a majority of the participants had little or no formal course work related to child, spouse, or elder abuse. Respondents described that they felt ill prepared to credibly document suspected cases of abuse and felt more certain of their intuitions than they could substantiate legally.

Several workshops conducted at the National League for Nursing Convention in 1995 (Woodtli & Breslin, 1997) encouraged nurse educators to examine opinions and make suggestions about the societal increase in violence and its effect on nursing education. Faculty thought that students needed to have planned and focused clinical experiences in settings where victims of abuse are served. For elders, these sites might include adult day care centers, respite care programs, senior centers, home care agencies, or long-term care facilities. Contemporary nursing education must go beyond including behavioral and physical indicators of abuse and the need to report in curricula. This represents the core of forensic nursing science. They must begin to incorporate more content on family dynamics, assessment, and intervention strategies. Students need to develop beginning skills in nonviolent methods of conflict resolution, debriefing, and crisis intervention. Specialized therapeutic communication skills with victims or survivors of violence and abusive episodes should be part of the curriculum. However, there is a lack of faculty preparation and expertise in the area of violence assessment and intervention, and faculty who are teaching today are unlikely to have had extensive content in their own professional preparation.

Faculty must take an active role in updating their knowledge and skills in this area. Faculty agreed that violence-related content must be infused across the continuum of the curriculum and not be just another "add-on topic." For example, assessment for abuse and family violence should be an integral component of any introductory health assessment class. Faculty need also to be aware of the student perceptions of fear related to domestic violence and assumptions or stereotyping of victims and perpetrators. Additionally, faculty need to be able to recognize what their own students may be experiencing or be at risk for domestic violence or abuse, know how to assist them via school support services, maintain student confidentiality, and appreciate how this might affect student learning and performance. A survey conducted in Ontario nursing schools yielded a similar faculty perspective (Hoff & Ross, 1994). There are many barriers to help-seeking by victims of various forms of abuse; however, the presence of a knowledgeable professional nurse skilled in forensic nursing, assessment, and interviewing and confident in providing appropriate intervention is a key factor in addressing these issues. Nurses who are well prepared in the classroom and have had the opportunity to enhance their knowledge through clinical experience are better prepared to assist students to intervene effectively with the fragile elderly.

Suggested Protocol for Screening Caregiver Applicants

The forensic nurse examiner is in an optimal position to influence and guide the development of policies and procedures that can make a difference for the elderly person. In the role of educator and advocate, the FNE can consult and collaborate with professionals from various disciplines to review current strategies, identify areas in need of improvement, and participate in the development of instruments to better address the needs of the elderly person. The nurse with an extensive background in forensic science can be invaluable in the development of a screening tool to be utilized whenever an individual is being considered for a position that involves caring for an elder.

Guidelines for Selecting and Screening Out Candidates

The following guidelines may be helpful in the selection of candidates who are qualified and the screening out of those who may pose a potential risk to the vulnerable elderly person:

- All candidates must be cleared through the local police department. Those with a criminal record are immediately excluded from the pool of potential employees.
- Three references should be requested from people who have either worked with or supervised the candidate; no personal friends or relatives may be used as a reference.
- The candidate's reason for applying should be discussed. This information will be helpful in revealing interest and motivations. However, many times salary alone is the single motivating factor, and this situation need not exclude the candidate who may be an asset to the elder.
- Previous work history can be significant. A history of brief employment with vague or evasive reasons for leaving should be a signal that this candidate may not be the best person to hire.
- Is the candidate qualified through education or formal or informal training and experience to meet the requirements of the position? Education will determine the precise title of the candidate. As an advanced practice nurse one may be a forensic nurse practitioner or clinical nurse specialist. If their nursing specialty is also in gerontology they may be identified as a forensic gerontology nurse practitioner (FGNP) or forensic gerontology clinical nurse specialist (FGCNS). A nurse with specific education in forensic nursing science who is credentialed as a forensic nurse and provides forensic examinations is considered a forensic nurse examiner (FNE).
- Is there a written preinterview survey to determine the candidate's knowledge about the elderly in terms of stage of development, common psychological and medical conditions, and demographics that may influence the responses of the prospective caregiver to elders? "What's Your Aging IQ," an instrument devised by the National Institute of Aging to measure attitudes and knowledge about the elderly, may be useful in the screening process. It is a simple 10-question true-false format. It is in the public domain.
- Is there a written preinterview questionnaire or survey to further explore the candidate's knowledge, attitudes, motivation, and commitment to serve this population? The Kogan Attitude toward Old People Scale (KOP) and or the Oberleder Attitude Scale may be useful in screening new or current employees or candidates for positions.

The Kogan Scale (Kogan, 1961) consists of 17 matched pairs of positive and negative attitudinal statements about elders. Respondents are asked to indicate their degree of agreement with each KOP statement on a Likert scale of six response categories ranging from strongly agree to strongly disagree. The scales are made comparable for interpretation by reverse scoring of positive items. Based on this technique, lower scores indicate more favorable attitudes and higher scores reflect more negative attitudes toward elders. Lookinland and Anson (1995) utilized the scale in a study measuring attitudes among present and future healthcare personnel. They reported Spearman-Brown reliability coefficients ranging from 0.73 to 0.83 for the negative scale and 0.66 to 0.77 for the positive scale. Construct and criterion validity were established using measures of anomie, ethnic prejudice, disability scales, and personality dimensions. Higher anomie was positively correlated with increased negative attitudes toward elders. The personality trait of nurturance was found to be strongly related to positive attitudes toward elders.

The Interview Process

Not enough can be said regarding the importance of the personal interview. The potential employer may decide to interview prior to the written application, but never before the police clearance and the receipt of a reference from at least one person or supervisor with whom the candidate has worked in the recent past (within six months). A written reference is most desirable. The potential employee may furnish a reference form with key questions for the individual who is completing the reference.

The candidate's mode of dress, manner of communication, personal hygiene, and nonverbal cues must be noted carefully; any suggestion of drugs or alcohol must be addressed and may be a reason to disqualify the candidate. The verbal interview should include problem-solving case situations. This can be extremely valuable in assessing the candidate's problem-solving skills, critical thinking ability, and fund of knowledge.

A key question to explore carefully and comprehensively, along with the reason for applying for the position, is the reason for selecting the elderly individual. The responses to these questions will be extremely valuable in making a decision.

It is beyond the scope of this discussion to address the myriad of considerations involved in making the decision regarding the selection of appropriate staff for the care of the elderly. Is the candidate herself or himself from a nurturing family? Is the gender of the candidate an issue? Is the candidate from another country? Is the candidate a member of a religious, spiritual, or other group whose rules and practices could interfere with the performance of some of the responsibilities of this position? Agencies should ensure that their employee application form is a useful tool for screening individuals who will play an important role in maintaining or perhaps developing a sense of safety, well-being, and dignity in the dependent elderly. The sophistication or simplification of the tool must be consistent with the caliber of individual being interviewed.

Although The Kogan Scale, the Oberleder Attitude Scale, "What's Your Aging IQ," and the suggested application form may be useful adjuncts for screening new or current employees or candidates for positions, the intuition of the interviewer is also a key factor. That "gut feeling," which is described by Gavin DeBecker (1998), is an important aspect of the interview process. Intuition has also been described as clinical hunch. It cannot be scientifically explained with ease, and it is sometimes difficult to express. However, intuition is a way of knowing that is the result of "deep" knowledge, tacit knowledge, or personal knowledge (Benner, 1984). It is important to remember that a finely honed intuitive sense is often the hallmark of a seasoned professional whose thought processes are grounded in extensive clinical experience and sound theoretical knowledge. All these aspects, along with the assistance of a consultant who is knowledgeable about staff selection, forensic expertise, and the special needs of the elderly, should be part of a comprehensive screening.

Facility or Agency Responsibilities

Extended care facilities, rest homes, skilled nursing facilities, and other residential facilities have an enormous responsibility to provide residents with the level of care that will enhance rather than diminish the quality of their lives. All staff, including those who provide indirect services (i.e., housekeeping, maintenance, dietary, or security), must be required to participate in ongoing in-service training and education that is a continuation and upgrading of the general orientation with emphasis on basic forensic and gerontology issues. Ongoing monitoring and evaluation of staff performance is mandatory in order to assure quality care. Direct observation, unannounced rounds, and patient satisfaction surveys (when possible) must be routinely accomplished. The following recommendations will assist in achieving and maintaining standards of excellence:

- Review of DNR (do not resuscitate) policies at orientation
- Observation of a staff member assisting a resident with activities of daily living, transferring or restraints, if ordered, as well as verbal and nonverbal communication
- CPR (cardiopulmonary resuscitation) certification for all staff
- Regular consultation with the forensic nurse clinical specialist with review of policies, procedures, and forensic considerations

Every consideration, evaluation, and monitoring of staff members must include the professional staff as well as the paraprofessional and support staff. Abusers of the elderly are not limited to one population; overlooking individuals because of their status or role can increase the risk to the dependent elder.

Case Study 25-1 Elder Abuse by a Child

Mary Smith, an 83-year-old widow, is being evaluated in a geriatric assessment clinic following what her daughter describes as a deterioration in her cognitive abilities as well as a change in her ability to care for herself. The forensic nurse examiner observes that the daughter appears to be quite tense and tends to answer for her mother. How might the nurse handle this situation? Describe the assessment process for this evaluation visit. Suggest initial intervention and plans for follow-up.

Case Study 25-2 Considerations and Risk Factors

An 80-year-old retired college professor was discovered wandering about the downtown area of a large city. He was confused, disheveled, and unable to identify either himself or his place of residence, but he was wearing an identification band with the address of a local assisted living care facility. A concerned shop owner had alerted the local police. Mr. Jones was transported to the local emergency department for evaluation. After his initial examination, the FNE was called in to consult. What are the primary considerations and risk factors that the nurse would explore? What disposition would be appropriate?

Summary

Elder abuse poses a significant threat to a very vulnerable population. The expertise and knowledge of the forensic nurse examiner is invaluable in terms of coordination assessment and planning to improve the quality of life for the compromised elder. Planning by the FNE extends beyond the delivery of medical and nursing care with the specialized knowledge to develop a more comprehensive assessment, intervention, and safety plan for continued monitoring and follow-up of the elderly person. The FNE often will be involved with intervening with both the victim and the perpetrator of elder abuse. The nurse's skills, critical thinking ability, and partnerships with community services contribute to holistic care and empowerment for the individual. A multidisciplinary approach utilizing social workers, healthcare providers, lawyers, and the police and coordinated by the forensic nurse examiner is the optimal approach to intervention in these situations of elder abuse.

Resources

Organizations

Administration on Aging (AOA)

US Department. of Health and Human Services, 330 Independence Avenue SW, Washington, DC 20201; Tel: 202-619-0724; www.aoa.dhhs.gov

Clearinghouse on Abuse and Neglect of the Elderly (CANE)

University of Delaware, Department of Consumer Studies, Alison Hall West, Room 211, Newark, DE 19716, Tel: 302-831-3525

Eldercare Locator

800-677-1116; www.eldercare.gov
Nationwide toll-free assistance directory sponsored by the National Association of Area Agencies on Aging.

National Aging Information Center (NAIC)

330 Independence Avenue SW, Washington, DC 20201; Tel: 202-619-0724

National Association of Area Agencies on Aging

1730 Rhode Island NW, Suite 1200, Washington, DC 20036, Tel: 202-872-0888; www.n4a.org

National Center on Elder Abuse (NCEA)

1201 15th Street NW, Suite 350, Washington, DC 20005; Tel: 202-898-2586; www.elderabusecenter.org

National Committee for the Prevention of Elder Abuse

1612 K Street NW, Washington, DC 20006; Tel: 202-682-4140; www.preventelderabuse.org

National Council on Aging (NCOA)

300 D Street SW, Suite 801, Washington, DC 20024; Tel: 202-479-1200; www.ncoa.org

National Institute on Aging

Building 31, Room 5C27, 31 Center Drive, Bethesda, MD 20898; Tel: 800-222-2225; www.nia.nih.gov

References

Bourland, M. (1990). Elder abuse from definition to prevention. *Postgrad Med, 87*(2), 139-144.

Benner, P. (1984). *From novice to expert: Excellence and power in clinical nursing practice.* Menlo Park: Addison Wesley.

Capezuti, E., Yurkow, J., & Goldberg, E. (1995). Meeting the challenge of elder mistreatment. *Nurs Dyn,* May 4(1), pp. 5-9.

Coye, A., Reichman, W., & Berbig, L. (1993). The relationship between dementia and elder abuse. *Am J Psychiatry, 150*(4), 643-646.

DeBecker, G. (1998). *The gift of fear.* New York: Dell Publishing.

Frost, M., & Willette, K. (1994). Risk for abuse/neglect: Documentation of assessment data and diagnoses. *J Gerontol Nurs, 20*(8), 37-45.

Fulmer, T. (1989). Mistreatment of elders. *Nurs Clin North Am, 24,* 707-715.

Hoff, L., & Ross, M. (1994). Violence content in nursing curricula: Strategic issues and implementation. *J Adv Nurs, 21*(1), 137-142.

Homer, A., & Gilleard, C. (1990). Abuse of elderly people by their caregivers. *Br J Med, 301*(6765), 1359-1362.

Kogan, N. (1961). Attitudes toward old people: The development of a scale and examination of correlates. *J Abnorm Soc Psychol, 62,* 44-54.

Lachs, M., Berkman, L., Fulmer, T., et al. (1994). A prospective community-based pilot study of risk factors for the investigation of elder mistreatment. *J Am Geriatr Soc, 42*(2), 169-173.

Lachs, M., Williams, C., O'Brien, S., et al. (1997a). Risk factors for reported elder abuse and neglect: A nine year observation cohort study. *Gerontologist, 37*(4), 469-474.

Lachs, M., Williams, C., O'Brien, S., et al. (1997b). ED use by older victims of family violence. *Ann Emerg Med, 30*(4), 448-454.

Limandri, B. J., & Tilden, V. P. (1996). Nurses' reasoning in the assessment of family violence. *Image: J Nurs Scholarship, 28*(3), 247-252.

Lookinland, S., & Anson, K. (1995). Perpetuation of ageist attitudes among present and future health care personnel: Implications for elder care. *J Adv Nurs, 21,* 47-56.

Lynch, S. (1997). Elder abuse: What to look for, how to intervene. *Am J Nurs, 97,* 27-32.

Paveza, G., Cohen, D., Hanrahan, P., et al. (1992). Severe family violence and Alzheimer's disease: Prevalence and risk factors. *Gerontologist, 32*(4), 493-497.

Phillips, L. R. (1986). Theoretical explanation for elder abuse. Competing hypotheses and unresolved issues. In K. A. Phillemer & R. S. Wolf (Eds.). *Elder abuse: Confict in the family* (pp. 198-217). Dover, MA: Auburn House.

Pillemer, K., & Finkelhor, D. (1988). The prevalence of elder abuse: A random sample survey. *Gerontologist, 28,* 51-57.

Woodtli, M., & Breslin, E. (1997). Violence in the nursing curriculum: Nursing educators speak out. *Nurs Health Care Perspect, 18*(5), 252-259.

Chapter 26 Sexual Assault

Linda E. Ledray

One of the first researchers to systematically study the impact and needs of the sexual assault survivor was a nurse, Dr. Ann Burgess (Burgess & Holmstrom, 1974). She and her colleague, Linda Holmstrom, a social worker, identified a two-stage syndrome of response which they referred to as rape trauma syndrome (Burgess & Holmstrom, 1974). Considerable additional research has occurred since that time, however, and has identified specific symptoms rather than a pattern of response. As a result of this more recent research, post-traumatic stress disorder (PTSD) resulting from sexual assault has become the term used to describe the symptom response following rape (American Psychiatric Association, 1994; Faigman, Kaye, & Saks et al., 1997). PTSD was first referred to by the American Psychiatric Association (APA) in 1980.

Nurses, including Dr. Burgess, have remained active in furthering the understanding of victim response and developing services for sexual assault survivors. The efforts of these pioneering nurses have led to the development of a new role for nurses, the forensic nurse examiner (FNE). Today, forensic nurse examiners function in a variety of roles, including clinical forensic nurse, nurse coroner, forensic investigator for the medical examiner, forensic psychiatric nurse, correctional nurse, domestic violence nurse examiner, and sexual assault nurse examiner (SANE). The legal nurse consultant and nurse attorneys also function as forensic investigators of questioned documents such as medical records and other legal issues involving healthcare and the law. Both roles serve to examine cases that involve incidents and issues pertaining to victims and offenders that are often previous patients of other FNE subspecialties. They work for hospitals and in other medical facilities, correctional institutions, law enforcement departments, prosecutor's offices, private law firms, community agencies, educational institutions, and private practice.

This chapter will focus on the largest group of forensic nurse examiners, the SANE. It will look at the history and SANE role development, the impact of sexual assault, and treatment needs of sexual assault survivors, as well as how the SANE functions today to meet these needs as a member of the sexual assault response team (SART).

SANE History and Role Development

Although men are raped, too, most victims of sexual and domestic violence are women. Because women are so often victims of violence, emergency department (ED) nurses have learned that whenever women present to an ED for even minor trauma, the etiology of their trauma must be thoroughly evaluated. ED staff must be aware of the types of injuries most likely resulting from violence, and the victim must be carefully questioned about the cause of the trauma to determine if it is the result of violence (Sheridan, 1993). When violence such as rape is identified, further evaluation may be necessary, including proper evidence collection, maintaining the chain of custody. Further care, beyond medical care, is also essential when rape is identified and will be discussed.

Only recently have our healthcare facilities begun to recognize their responsibility to have trained staff available to provide this specialized service for victims of sexual assault. Treating injuries alone is not sufficient. In 2000 a New York City hospital was successfully sued by a rape victim when she came to the medical facility after a sexual assault and a sexual assault evidentiary examination was not accurately performed. She was made to wait three hours before being examined, and then potentially significant evidence, her underwear and vaginal swabs, were lost. The Department of Health investigation also found that the hospital failed to provide complete care. It did not provide her with medication to prevent pregnancy. The authorities believed that if correct evidence collection and chain of custody had occurred, the evidence obtained may have been useful to secure a conviction against the serial sex offender charged with her rape. As a result, New York passed the Sexual Assault Reform Act requiring New York state to develop specialized sexual assault (SANE) evidence collection programs in 2001 (Chivers, 2000). Since 1992 the guidelines of the Joint Commission on Accreditation of Healthcare Organizations (JCAHO) has required emergency and ambulatory care facilities to have protocols on rape, sexual molestation, and domestic abuse (Bobak, 1992). By 1997 they also required healthcare facilities to develop and train their staff to use criteria to identify possible victims of physical assault, rape, other sexual molestation, domestic abuse, and abuse or neglect of older adults and children (JCAHO, 1997).

At the 1996 International Association of Forensic Nurses (IAFN) meeting in Kansas City, Geri Marullo, Executive Director of the American Nurses' Association (ANA), predicted that within 10 years JCAHO would require every hospital to have a forensic nurse available (Marullo, 1996). Even though JCAHO still does not require a forensic nurse examiner or SANE to be available to do the evaluation, it is no longer optional for medical facilities to identify and provide appropriate and complete services to victims of rape and abuse. In addition, JCAHO survey teams have begun to ask hospitals multiple questions about sexual abuse policies and procedures and whether they have a SANE program in place to respond. This JCAHO emphasis has effectively set the stage for the further development of forensic nursing as an important new nursing specialty.

Many healthcare facilities have recognized that the implementation of the forensic nurse examiner role is an optimal way to meet this expectation of a higher level of care and that it is an effective community marketing tool for the medical facility as well. The benefits of the FNE or SANE to the victim, other ED staff, the police, and the prosecutor have been the most effective impetus to SANE role development and utilization. The availability of funding for program development has also been an important impetus.

The landmark Violence Against Women Act (VAWA) of 1994, introduced by Senator Joseph Biden of Delaware, was signed into law on September 13, 1994, as Title IV of the Violent Crime

Control and Law Enforcement Act of 1994. In addition to doubling the federal penalties for repeat offenders and requiring that date rape is treated the same as stranger rape, this act made $800 million available for training and program development over a six-year period, with $26 million appropriated for the first year. This funding has had a significant impact on changing the availability of services to rape victims today. It was initially used by the existing rape crisis centers to hire paid staff and to professionalize their organizations, and more recently it has provided funding to establish SANE programs and SARTs across the US.

Demonstrating the Need for SANE Programs

The initial impetus to develop SANE and SART programs began with the individuals who were working with rape victims in hospitals, clinics, and other settings across the country. These workers primarily included nurses, other medical professionals, counselors, and advocates. It was obvious to these individuals that services to sexual assault victims were inadequate and were not being provided at the same high standard of care being given to other medical clients (Holloway & Swan, 1993; O'Brien, 1996). When rape victims came to the ED for care they often had to wait as long as 12 hours in a busy, public area, their wounds seen as less serious than the other trauma victims, competing unsuccessfully for medical staff time with the critically ill (Holloway & Swan, 1993; Sandrick, 1996; Speck & Aiken, 1995). They were often not allowed to eat, drink, or urinate while they waited, for fear of destroying evidence (Thomas & Zachritz, 1993). The medical professionals who eventually did care for them were often not sufficiently trained to do medical-legal examinations, and many were also lacking in their ability to provide expert witness testimony (Lynch, 1993).

When staff was trained, they often did not complete a sufficient number of examinations to maintain their level of proficiency (Lenehan, 1991; Yorker; 1996; Tobias, 1990). Even when the victim's medical needs were met, his or her emotional needs all too often were overlooked (Speck & Aiken, 1995), or even worse, the survivor was not believed or was blamed for the rape by the ED staff (Kiffe, 1996). All too often, the rape survivor faced a time-consuming examination by a succession of healthcare professionals, some with only a few hours of orientation, many with little experience, and most not comfortable doing the examination or concerned that they would be called to testify in court.

Services were inconsistent and problematic. Often the only physician available to do the vaginal examination after the rape was male (Lenehan, 1991). Approximately half of rape victims in one study were unconcerned with the gender of the examiner, but for the other half this was extremely problematic. Even male victims often prefer to be examined by a woman, as they too are most often raped by a man and experience the same generalized fear and anger toward men that female victims experience (Ledray, 1996a).

More recently, a significant influx of male SANEs have been widely accepted by victims due to their empathic approach and nonjudgmental manner. The Forensic Nurse Response Team in Houston, Texas, has three men on the team, and in over 600 cases performed by the three combined, only one instance in which a patient preferred a female examiner has been reported (Rooms, 2004). After having power and control over one's body ripped away by a male, having a male restore a sense of control by gaining consent before talking, touching, or examining the patient is often cited as restoring a more positive image of men in general. This has also been cited by men in nursing who specialize in domestic violence cases. It has been noted that the ability of the examiner to convey genuine concern, empathy, and return power and control are more important characteristics than gender. Whether it is the responding law enforcement officer, paramedic, triage nurse, physician, or SANE, men should be encouraged to understand the psychodynamics of sexual assault and attempt to quash the myth that men have nothing to offer the sexual assault patient (Rooms, 2004).

There are also many reports of physicians being reluctant to do the examination. This reluctance was the result of many factors, which included an awareness of their lack of experience and training in forensic evidence collection and not wanting to do something they knew was extremely important and that they were concerned they would not do well (Bell, 1995; Lynch, 1993; Speck & Aiken, 1995).

The lengthy evidentiary examination takes the physician away from other medically urgent or critically ill patients in a busy ED (DiNitto, Martin, & Yancey et al., 1986; Frank, 1996). In addition, whenever the physician is involved in evidence collection there is always the expectation that the doctor will later be subpoenaed and be taken away from working in the ED to testify in court and be questioned by a sometimes hostile defense attorney (Thomas & Zachritz, 1993; DiNitto, Martin, & Yancey et al., 1986; Speck & Aiken, 1995; Frank, 1996). All too often, such concerns resulted in evidence collection being rushed, inadequate, or incomplete. In rare instances physicians even refused to do the examination, and the rape victim was sent home from the hospital without having an evidentiary examination completed because no physician could be found to collect the evidence (Kettelson, 1995 DiNitto, Martin, & Yancey et al., 1986). Unfortunately, many of these same problems continue today in major medical centers in the US (Chivers, 2000).

As research with this population continued it was learned how important this initial contact might be for these survivors and how important it was to provide the most comprehensive care possible during the initial ED visit (Lenehan, 1991). For as many as 75% of sexual assault victims, the initial ED contact was the only known contact they had with medical or professional support staff regarding the sexual assault (Ledray, 1992).

SANE Program Development

As a result of this identified goal to better meet the needs of this underserved population, SANE programs were established in Memphis, TN, in 1976 (Speck & Aiken, 1995), Minneapolis, MN, in 1977 (Ledray & Chaignot, 1980; Ledray, 1993), and Amarillo, TX, in 1979 (Antognoli-Toland, 1985). Unfortunately, these nurses worked in isolation, unaware of the existence of other similar programs until Gail Lenehan, editor of the *Journal of Emergency Nursing* (JEN), recognized the importance of this new role for nurses and published the first list of 20 SANE programs (ENA, 1991). This facilitated communication, collaboration, and further SANE program development.

As a result of the collaboration fostered by the *Journal of Emergency Nursing,* 72 individuals from 31 programs across the US and Canada came together for the first time in 1992 at a meeting hosted by the Sexual Assault Resource Service and the University of Minnesota School of Nursing in Minneapolis. It was at that meeting that the International Association of Forensic Nurses (IAFN) was formed (Ledray, 1996b). Membership in IAFN surpassed the 1000 mark in 1996 (Lynch, 1996). By October 2000, there were more than 1800 members and by October 2003, the number of members had grown to nearly 3000. Although the initial SANE development was slow, with only three programs operating by the end of the 1970s, development today is progressing rapidly.

After years of effort on the part of SANEs and other forensic nurses, the American Nurses' Association (ANA) officially recognized forensic nursing as a new specialty of nursing in 1995 (Lynch, 1996). SANE is the largest subspecialty of forensic nursing. At the October, 1996, IAFN annual meeting held in Kansas City, the SANE Council voted overwhelmingly to use the title SANE, sexual assault nurse examiner, to define this new forensic nursing role.

A SANE is a registered nurse (RN) who has advanced education in forensic examination of sexual assault victims. IAFN has recommended a 40-hour didactic SANE training program, with specified content, plus clinical experience for a nurse to function as a SANE (Ledray, 1999). At the 1996 annual meeting of IAFN, the SANE Council also voted and adopted the first SANE Standards of Practice. The standards include goals of sexual assault nurse examiner programs, a definition of the practice area, conceptual framework of SANE practice, evaluation, documentation, forensic examination components, and minimum SANE educational qualifications (IAFN SANE Standards, 1996). In April 2002, the first national certification examination was given to 80 nurses. Of those 80 nurses, 70 (87.5%) passed and were the first to carry the SANE-A designation after their name, for sexual assault nurse examiner–adults and adolescents. The certification is offered through IAFN.

Sexual Assault Impact and Treatment Needs

Key Point *26-1*

The physical impact of a sexual assault on the victim includes genital and nongenital trauma as well as fear of contracting a sexually transmitted infection (STI), general health risk, fear of pregnancy, substance abuse, and all too often sexual dysfunction. The psychological impact can last for years after a sexual assault and typically includes depression, anxiety, fears, post-traumatic stress disorder (PTSD) symptoms, self-blame, and shame.

Nongenital Physical Injury

Most studies indicate that significant physical injury resulting from sexual assault is rare (3% to 5% across studies, with less than 1% of victims needing hospitalization). Even minor injury usually occurs in only about one third of the reported rapes. Injuries, when they do occur, are more common in stranger rapes and rapes by someone the victim knows intimately (domestic violence) than in date rape or acquaintance rape (Kilpatrick, Edmunds, & Seymour, 1992; Ledray, 1999; Marchbanks, Lui, & Mercy, 1990; Tucker, Ledray, & Werner, 1990).

In one study, the rate of physical injury for male rape victims (40%) was found to be higher than for female victims (26%). Although 25% of the men and 38% of the women in this study of 351 rape victims sought medical care after the rape for their physical injuries, only 61% of them told the treating physician they had been raped. The women expressed a strong preference for medical treatment and counseling by a woman. The male victims were less likely to express a gender preference (Petrak & Claydon, 1995). A more recent study of 1076 sexual assault victims, of which 96% were female, found nongenital trauma more often, 67% of the time. Physical force was, however, reported during the sexual assault in 79.6% of this population (Riggs, Houry, & Long et al., 2000).

Genital Trauma

Studies indicate the likelihood of genital trauma identification without the use of a colposcope to magnify the trauma is similar to that of nongenital trauma; 1% have severe injury, and 10% to 30% have minor injury across studies. The injury was always accompanied by complaints of vaginal pain, discomfort, or bleeding (Cartwright, Moore, & Anderson et al., 1986; Tintinali & Hoelzer, 1985; Geist, 1988). Although they do not specifically indicate if a colposcope was used on examination, Riggs et al. (2000) also found genital trauma more often, in 52% of the cases reviewed. It is uncertain if this is the result of more violence resulting in injury in their population, or more careful and consistent injury evaluation by experienced examiners.

The literature also suggests that colposcopic examination is often extremely useful to visualize genital abrasions, bruises, and tears, as they are often so minute they cannot be seen with the naked eye (Frank, 1996; Slaughter & Brown, 1992). These minor injuries are likely the result of tightened pelvic muscles, and a lack of pelvic tilt or lubrication during the forced penetration. This minor injury usually heals completely within 48 to 72 hours. With colposcopic examination genital trauma has been identified in up to 87% ($N = 114$) of sexual assault cases (Slaughter & Brown, 1992). Another study comparing vaginal trauma in sexual assault survivors to women who had consenting sexual contact found 68% of 311 sexual assault victims had genital trauma, where as only 11% ($N = 8$) of the 57 women in the study who had consenting sex had genital trauma (Slaughter, Brown, & Crowley et al., 1997). Unfortunately, this study has not yet been replicated and is problematic, as women who recanted the sexual assault were included in the control group. The findings do not indicate if they did or did not have vaginal injuries.

Both the colposcope and anoscope have been shown to improve the identification of rectal trauma; however, the colposcope may be less helpful than the anoscope. In a study of 67 male rape victims, all examined by experienced forensic examiners, 53% had genital trauma identified with the naked eye alone. This number only increased slightly, 8%, when the colposcope was used, but the positive findings increased a significant 32% when an anoscope was utilized. The combination of naked eye, colposcope, and anoscope resulted in a total positive findings in 72% of the cases (Ernst, Green, & Ferguson et al., 2000).

Because rape victims often fear vaginal trauma, it is also important when they seek a medical examination that the extent of the trauma, or the lack of trauma, is explained to them after the forensic examination is completed (Ledray, 1999). When a video colposcope is available, it can be helpful to turn the screen so that the survivor can also view the genital area.

Best Practice *26-1*

The forensic nurse examiner should disclose and explain the nature of any physical trauma associated with the sexual assault. If there are no apparent injuries, the victim should be reassured about the absence of trauma.

The ability of the examiner to identify genital trauma has improved considerably with the utilization of SANEs who are better trained in trauma identification and who are more likely to utilize a colposcope or anoscope. However, the issue has now shifted.

The question today being raised by defense attorneys is how can one be certain that genital trauma is the result of a sexual assault and not "rough" consenting sexual contact. Unfortunately, sufficient scientific information does not yet exist that determines if the trauma identified is the result of consenting or nonconsenting sexual contact. There is indeed a need of additional studies that look for a pattern of injury in consenting and nonconsenting sexual contact. What is known is that genital trauma does not prove rape and the absence of trauma does not prove consent.

Key Point *26-2*

Genital trauma can result from consenting sexual contact. Trauma does not result solely from nonconsenting sexual contact or sexual assault. Both trauma and multiple sites of trauma are more likely to occur as a result of sexual assault than from consenting sexual contact.

Sexually Transmitted Infections

Although one study found 36% of the rape victims coming to the ED stated their primary reason for coming was concern about having contracted a sexually transmitted infection (STI) (Ledray, 1991), the actual risk is much lower. The Centers for Disease Control and Prevention (CDC) estimates the risks of rape victims getting gonorrhea is 6% to 12%, chlamydia infection is 4% to 17%, syphilis is 0.5% to 3%, and HIV is much less than 1% (CDC, 1993; 1998). The specific STI risk will, of course, vary from community to community, and it is important that the forensic examiner is aware of local rates so that this information can be provided to concerned sexual assault victims.

From a forensic and clinical perspective, treating prophylactically for STIs is preferable to culturing. Culturing is very expensive and time-consuming for the survivor who must return two or three times for additional testing, and unfortunately, most victims do not return (Blair & Warner, 1992). In addition, STI cultures have not proved to be useful in court in adult and adolescent cases. It is still recommended in ongoing child sexual abuse cases and can be useful evidence. As a result most clinicians and forensic examiners recommend prophylactic treatment (ACEP, 1999, CDC, 1998; Frank, 1996; Ledray, 1999).

Best Practice *26-2*

Prophylactic treatment for sexually transmitted diseases should be a component of all forensic examinations of adolescent and adult victims of sexual assault.

There can indeed be genital trauma from consenting sexual contact. Trauma does not result solely from nonconsenting sexual contact, or sexual assault. It does, however, appear that trauma is more likely and multiple sites of trauma are more likely as a result of sexual assault than from consenting sexual contact.

Since the early 1980s, HIV has been a concern for rape survivors even though the actual risk still appears to be very low. The first case in which seroconversion, from HIV negative to HIV positive, suspected to be the result of a rape occurred in 1989 (Murphy, Harris, & Forester, 1989). Claydon et al. (1991) reported four more cases in which researchers believe a rape resulted in a subsequent HIV seroconversion. Even though these numbers are extremely low considering the number of rapes that occur every year, the impact for the individual victims is, of course, extremely significant.

In a study of 412 Midwest rape victims with vaginal or rectal penetration tested for HIV in the ED at three months after rape and again at six months after rape, not one seroconverted. Because 95% of individuals who are going to seroconvert will do so by three months after exposure and 100% will do so by six months, the researchers did not recommend routine HIV testing or prophylactic care. The study also found, however, that even if the survivor did not ask about HIV in the ED, within two weeks it was a concern of theirs or their sexual partner. Based on the recommendations of the rape survivors surveyed in this study, the researchers recommend that even if the survivor does not raise the issue of HIV or AIDS in the ED, the SANE or medical professional should, in a matter-of-fact manner, provide them with information about their risk, testing, and safe sex options (Ledray, 1999).

How to best deal with the issue of HIV is complicated and controversial (Blair & Warner, 1992). If the offender is HIV-infected, the probability of a rape victim contracting HIV from a sexual assault will depend upon the type of sexual intercourse, the presence of trauma in the involved orifice, if there was exposure to ejaculate, viral load of the ejaculate, and presence of other STIs (CDC, 2002). In most instances it is impossible to determine the HIV status of the offender in a timely fashion. In the Minnesota study described earlier, two assailants told the rape victims that they were positive. However, when one was apprehended and tested for HIV, he was found to be negative (Ledray, 1999). The likely risk of an offender being HIV-infected will vary from state to state, because the general rates of HIV infection vary from state to state and community to community. The forensic examiner must, of course, know the local infection rates.

Because good data are not available on the actual risk, the CDC does not make a recommendation regarding the appropriateness of offering postexposure antiviral therapy after sexual assault, but states the decision should be based on the likelihood of the offender being HIV positive. The decision to offer prophylactic treatment at this time should be based on the risk of the rape combined with the HIV prevalence in the specific geographic area (CDC, 2002). A rape would be considered a high-risk rape if it involved rectal contact or vaginal contact with vaginal tears or existing vaginal STIs that have caused ulcerations or open sores disrupting the integrity of the vaginal mucosa. It would also be considered high risk if the victim had some reason to know or suspect that the assailant was an intravenous drug user, HIV positive, or bisexual. The risks and options, including the impact of the drug regimen, should be explained to the victim so he or she can make an educated decision (Ledray, 1999).

Pregnancy

The risk of pregnancy from a rape is the same as the risk of pregnancy from any one-time sexual encounter: estimated to be 2% to 4% (Yuzpe, Smith, & Rademaker, 1982). Most SANE programs and medical facilities offer emergency pregnancy preventive care to women at risk of becoming pregnant, if they are seen within 72 hours of the rape and have a negative pregnancy test in the ED. One SANE program operating at a Catholic hospital went as far as to get special permission from the diocese to administer Ovral (ethinyl estradiol) (Frank, 1996). The National Conference of Catholic Bishops has agreed that "A female who has been raped should be able to defend herself against a potential conception from the sexual assault. If, after appropriate testing, there is no evidence that conception has occurred already, she may be treated with medication that would prevent ovulation, or fertilization" (National Conference of College Bishops, 1995, p. 16). The importance of offering complete care to sexual assault victims, including care to prevent pregnancy when requested by the victim, was further strengthened by the successful lawsuit against the New York City hospital that did not ensure that a victim receive a full birth control prescription to prevent pregnancy (Chivers, 2000). Washington, California, Illinois, and New York states have state laws requiring all hospitals that see sexual assault victims to offer them pregnancy prevention medications. Other states, including Minnesota and Oregon, are attempting to pass similar state laws. This is a very significant change in responsibility. Hopefully, many other states will follow suit.

Sometimes referred to as "the morning-after pill," oral contraceptives such as Ovral or Lovral are used for emergency contraception. The Yuzpe regimen using a combined oral contraceptive is currently the most common emergency contraceptive (Yuzpe, Smith, & Rademaker, 1982). A newly available progestin-only contraceptive, Levonorgestrel 0.75 mg (Plan B), is quickly becoming widely utilized. Plan B is slightly, but nonsignificantly, more effective in reducing the risk of pregnancy. When started within 72 hours of unprotected intercourse 85% of pregnancies were prevented in one study, compared to 57% using the Yuzpe regimen (Task Force on Postovulatory Methods of Fertility Regulation, 1998). The effectiveness of both methods decreases as the time between the assault and the first dose increases. When given within the first 24 hours Plan B reduced the risk of pregnancy by 95%, but only by 61% when given between 48 and 72 hours after unprotected intercourse. The significant difference was in the only side effect, nausea and vomiting, which was significantly reduced with the use of Plan B to 23.1%, from 50% with the Yuzpe method (Task Force on Postovulatory Methods of Fertility Regulation, 1998). This side effect can also be reduced by using an antiemetic one hour before giving the pregnancy prevention.

In a recent study it was found that it was as effective to give two tabs of levonorgestrel (75 mg) immediately, rather than as two doses (75 mg) 12 hours apart (Hertzen, Piaggio, & Ding et al., 2002).

General Health Risk

More medical professionals today are aware of the convincing evidence that sexual assault can have a significant and chronic impact on the general health of a sexual assault survivor.

Key Point *26-3*

The stress resulting from rape appears to suppress the immune system and increase susceptibility to disease, as well as increasing the survivor's attention to subtle physical symptoms and increasing concerns about general health (Cohen & Williamson, 1991).

Sexual assault victims interpret emotional reactions to the assault as physical disease symptoms (Koss, Woodruff, & Koss, 1990), or they may employ maladaptive coping strategies, such as an increased substance use and eating disorders that have a serious negative health impact (Golding, 1994; Felitti, 1991). Increased sexual activity with multiple partners, which also sometimes follows rape, especially in a formerly inactive adolescent, may also result in increased exposure to disease (Ledray, 1994).

Rape victims often want to avoid remembering or talking about the assault and are more comfortable seeking medical care, which they see as less stigmatizing than psychological counseling (Kimerling & Calhoun, 1994). Kimerling & Calhoun (1994) found 73% of a sample of 115 sexual assault victims sought out medical services during the first year after a sexual assault, while only 19% sought out mental health services during the same time period. Poor social support was associated with higher use of medical services, and higher levels of social support were associated with better actual physical health and better health perception in this population. Koss, Woodruff, & Koss (1990) found that a statistically significant 92% of 2291 female crime victims sought medical care in the first year following the crime and 100% sought medical care during the first two years. Those who had suffered more severe crime and victims of multiple crimes were the most likely to seek medical care. They, too, suggest that the stress of victimization may reduce resistance to disease by suppressing the immune system.

It is interesting that in their sample, Kimerling and Calhoun (1994) did not find a significant difference in the health utilization of women who had sought out psychological services. Jones and Vischi (1980) even found a 20% decrease in medical service utilization in a sample of 87 rape victims who were in psychotherapy, stressing the importance of ensuring initial crisis intervention and follow-up counseling for victims of sexual assault.

Waigandt and Miller (1986) found that rape victims made 35% more visits to a medical doctor each year than nonvictims; however, the victims who continued to have psychological problems several years later made more visits and perceived their health as worse than the recovered victims. The recovered rape victims experienced only 12% of possible physical symptoms, and the victims with psychological problems experienced 28% of the symptoms, primarily female problems such as dysmenorrhea and incontinence. These victims also exhibited twice the number of maladaptive health behaviors such as smoking, excessive alcohol use, and overeating.

Walker et al. (1995) found women with chronic pelvic pain were significantly more likely than women with no pelvic pain to be victims of sexual abuse, even though only 1 out of 10 were found to have an organic condition. The chronic pain groups were also more likely to be depressed, to have substance abuse problems, phobias, and sexual dysfunction. Eleven percent of the primary care visits were related to the chronic pelvic pain, at an average cost of $1816 per patient.

Rape disclosure can have a significant and positive impact on a woman's health.

Case Study 26-1 Disclosing Abuse

A 49-year-old woman experienced intermittent severe longstanding hypertension for which no biological cause could be identified. After a routine health visit to check her blood pressure (BP) she disclosed she had been having nightmares and was beginning to recall being raped by her sister's boyfriend when she was 14 years old. Immediately after the disclosure her BP went from 240/150 mm Hg to 150/105 mm Hg. The next morning she reported a good night's sleep, no more nightmares, and her BP was recorded at a normal 120/85 mm Hg (Mann & Delo, 1995).

Felitti (1991) compared a sample of 131 medical patients who had a history of sexual abuse to a group of matched control subjects. The majority (90%) had never before disclosed the abuse. Decades later, Felitti found the sexual assault victims to be significantly more depressed (83%) and experiencing physical symptoms of depression such as despondency, chronic fatigue, sleep disturbance, and frequent crying spells. Sixty percent had gained more than 50 lbs, and 35% had gained more than 100 lbs. Chronic unexplained headaches were common in the victim group (45%), as were recurrent gastrointestinal disturbances (64%). Another study of 100 women concluded that women with a history of sexual abuse were 60% more likely to have unexplained pelvic pain, abnormal bleeding, and more gynecological surgery than women without a sexual assault history (Chapman, 1989). Chapman (1989) found that sexual abuse victims had five times the number of hysterectomies and three times the number of pelvic and gynecological surgeries than a nonvictim control group and cautions that unexplained pain in women with a history of sexual abuse may not be removed by a surgical procedure when pain alone is the criteria for the procedure.

Koss, Koss, and Woodruff (1991) found severity of victimization was a more effective predictor of total yearly visits to a physician and outpatient costs than was age, ethnicity, self-reported symptoms, or actual injury. They found that rape victims were twice as likely to seek the help of a physician than nonvictims, and visits increased 56% in victim groups compared to 2% in nonvictim groups.

In a study comparing sexual assault (N = 99) and life-threatening physical abuse victims (N = 68) on physical health status 10 years later, Leserman et al. (1997) found overall poor physical health status was directly associated with sexual assault, especially with physical injury during the assault, multiple perpetrators, and the victim's life being threatened during the assault. Golding (1994) also found women with a history of sexual assault were more likely to complain of six or more medically unexplained somatic symptoms (29% versus 16% of nonrape victims) and to have a severe chronic disease such as diabetes, arthritis, difficulty in walking, paralysis, or fainting as well as having functional limitations (27% versus 16% of the nonrape victims). The increased incidence of overall explained and unexplained somatic symptoms of rape victims in this population was 60%, compared to 36% of the nonvictims.

Sexual Dysfunction

Considering the nature of sexual assault, it is not surprising that studies have found sexual dysfunction is a common reaction and often a chronic problem following a sexual assault. The sexual dysfunction often includes loss of sexual desire, inability to become sexually aroused, slow arousal, pelvic pain associated with sexual activity, a lack of sexual enjoyment, inability to achieve orgasm, fear of sex, avoidance of sex, intrusive thoughts of the assault during sex, or abstinence. Sexual dysfunction such as avoidance, loss of interest in sex, loss of pleasure from sex, painful intercourse, and actual fear of sex are mentioned repeatedly in the literature (Abel & Rouleau, 1995; Burgess & Holmstrom, 1979; Frazier, 2000; Kimerling & Calhoun, 1994; Koss, 1993; Ledray, 1994; Ledray, 1999; Chapman, 1989; Becker, Skinner, & Abel et al., 1986). It is important to note that even though rape victims may become sexually active again within months of the assault, they may still not enjoy sex years later. Celibacy may be a coping strategy.

Substance Abuse

In the college sample of 6159 students surveyed by Koss (1987), 73% of the assailants and 55% of the victims had been using alcohol or other drugs prior to the sexual assault. On the one hand, rape victims may indeed be more vulnerable to being raped as a result of substance abuse, which leads to intoxication and an increased vulnerability (Ledray, 1999); it is also important to recognize that rape also can result in substance abuse, possibly as an attempt to dull the memory and avoid thinking about the rape (Goodman, Koss, & Russo, 1993; Koss, 1993; Ledray, 1994). In a national sample of 3006 survivors, both alcohol and drug use was significantly increased after a sexual assault, even for women with no prior substance use or abuse history (Kilpatrick, Acierno, & Resnick et al., 1997).

Psychological Impact

There is considerable agreement among researchers that rape victims experience more psychological distress than do victims of other crimes. Fear, anxiety, depression, and symptoms of post-traumatic stress disorder (PTSD) are the most frequently recognized and documented reactions to sexual assault (Burgess & Holmstrom, 1974; Calhoun, Atkeson, & Resnick; 1982; Frazier; 2000; Kilpatrick & Veronen, 1984; Ledray, 1994; Resick & Schnicke, 1990).

Anxiety

Anxiety is also frequently recognized and documented in the literature as an immediate reaction to a sexual assault (Abel & Rouleau, 1995; Burgess & Holmstrom, 1974; Calhoun, Atkeson, & Resnick, 1982; Kilpatrick & Veronen, 1984; Ledray, 1994; Resick & Schnicke, 1990).

In one study, 82% of rape victims met the *Diagnostic and Statistical Manual* (*DSM*) criteria for generalized anxiety disorder (GAD) compared to 32% of nonvictims (Frank & Anderson, 1987). Some studies of long-term anxiety have found differences between victim and nonvictim groups (Gidcyz & Koss, 1991; Gold, Milan, & Mayall et al., 1994; Gidycz, Coble, & Latham et al., 1993), and others have not (Frazier & Schauben, 1994; Riggs, Kilpatrick, & Resnick, 1992; Winfield, George, & Swartz et al., 1990). Studies also report that rape victims were more likely to meet the criteria for panic disorder several years after the rape (Burnam, Stein, & Golding et al., 1988; Winfield, George, & Swartz et al., 1990).

Fear

Fear of death is the most common fear during the assault, and continued generalized fear after the assault is a very common response to rape (Dupre, Hampton, & Morrison et al., 1993; Ledray, 1994). Fear after a rape can be specifically related to factors associated with the sexual assault or it can be widely generalized to include fear of all men (Ledray, 1994). Because fear is subjective, it is generally evaluated using self-report measures. Although evidence of the duration and type of fear varies, reports of long-term fear following rape is common, with up to 83% of victims reporting some type of fear following a sexual assault (Frazier, 2000; Nadelson, Notman, & Zackson et al., 1982). Girelli et al. (1986) found the subjective distress of fear of injury or fear of death during rape was more significant than the actual violence as a predictor of more severe postrape fear and anxiety. It is thus important to recognize that the threat of violence alone can be psychologically devastating (Goodman, Koss, & Russo, 1993).

As might be expected, rape victims are consistently found to be generally fearful and experiencing hyperalertness to potential danger during the first year following a sexual assault. During the acute stage, up to 80% of rape victims report being generally fearful, afraid of violence, or afraid of being alone. Nearly as many, 75%, report a fear of being indoors, outdoors, or in a crowd, and 70% report a fear of death (Becker, Skinner, & Abel et al., 1986). Although fear of retaliation by the assailant is a persistent and long-term result of a sexual assault, except in domestic violence rapes, retaliation by the assailant when a victim reports is fortunately an extremely rare occurrence (Ledray, 1994).

Depression

Depression is one of the symptoms most commonly identified following a sexual assault. Depression is easily, reliably, and quickly measured by standardized self-report measures, such as the Beck Depression Inventory (Abel & Rouleau, 1995; Atkeson, Calhoun, & Resick et al., 1982; Kilpatrick & Veronen, 1984; Frazier, 2000; Ledray, 1994).

Studies that evaluate the level of depression in rape victims typically find that during the first two months rape victims are mildly depressed (Gidycz, Coble, & Latham et al., 1993; Becker, Skinner, & Abel et al., 1986; Frazier & Burnett, 1994; Ledray, 1984) to moderately depressed (Cluss, Boughton, & Frank et al., 1983; Frank & Stewart, 1984; Frazier, Harlow, & Schauben et al., 1993; Ledray, 1984; Moss, Frank, & Anderson, 1990). In studies without standardized criteria, 75% to 80% of rape victims reported feeling mildly to severely depressed six months after being raped (Kimerling & Calhoun, 1994; Norris & Feldman-Summers, 1981).

When rape victims are compared to nonvictim control groups the results consistently show that the rape victims are more depressed during the first two months after a rape (Atkeson, Calhoun, & Resick et al., 1982; Kilpatrick, Veronen, & Resick, 1979; Kilpatrick, Resick, & Veronen, 1981). Rape victims are also significantly more likely to meet the DSM criteria for major depressive disorder (MDD) than nonvictims. In one study 38% of rape victims coming to a rape crisis center (RCC) met the MDD criteria at six months after the rape, compared with only 6% of a matched control group (Frank & Anderson, 1987). Another study reported similar results, with 33% of rape victims meeting the MDD criteria at six months, compared to 11% of the control group (Sorenson, Siegel, & Golding et al., 1991).

Nightmares are a common problem following sexual assault; researchers have found that nightmares are associated with greater general distress and lead to more anxiety (Krakow, Tandberg, & Barey et al., 1995).

At one year after the assault, rape victims continue to be mildly depressed (Koss, Dinero, & Seibel et al., 1988; Mackey, Sereika, & Weissfeld et al., 1992). When compared to nonvictim control groups, rape victims are also consistently more depressed than other victims (Frazier & Schauben, 1994) and than nonvictim groups (Riggs, Kilpatrick, & Resnick, 1992; Burge, 1988; Cohen & Roth, 1987; Ellis, Atkeson, & Calhoun, 1981; Gidycz & Koss, 1989; Gidycz & Koss, 1991; Santiago, McCal-Perez, & Gorcey et al., 1985).

Suicidal Ideation

Although the completed suicide rate following a rape is considered low, suicidal ideation is a significant issue. Up to 20% may attempt suicide (Kilpatrick, Veronen, & Best et al., 1985), and many more rape victims (33% to 50%) report that they considered suicide at some point after the rape (Ellis, Atkeson, & Calhoun, 1981). During the immediate postrape period, rape victims are nine times more likely than nonvictims to attempt suicide (Kilpatrick, Saunders, & Veronen et al., 1987). It is thus essential that suicide risk is considered and addressed during the initial and follow-up visits. SANEs and other professionals working with this population must be aware of signs, and protocols to deal with this problem must be in place and utilized.

Best Practice *26-3*

SANEs and other professionals working with sexual assault victims must be aware of the potential of suicide among victims. Assessments in both initial and follow-up visits should address suicidal ideation.

Self-Blame and Shame

Self-blame is a common response in rape victims (Ledray, 1994; McFarlane & Hawley, 1993). Initially, some researchers thought some self-blame may actually be beneficial to rape victims, as it would foster a sense of future controllability and project a sense of safety from another rape, but after considerable research on internal versus external blame ascribed to victims, researchers have concluded that self-blame is associated only with past controllability, not with the perception of future controllability. All types of self-blame have been found to be associated with more depression and poor adjustment after the rape (Frazier, 1990). It is also important that forensic examiners not confuse self-blame with responsibility for the assault.

Post-Traumatic Stress Disorder

Post-traumatic stress disorder (PTSD) was first recognized and defined by the American Psychiatric Association as a diagnostic criteria in the *Diagnostic and Statistical Manual III* in 1980 (American Psychiatric Association) and therefore has been considered only in studies of rape impact designed after 1980. Rape trauma syndrome (RTS), which is not a diagnosis recognized by the American Psychiatric Association, is often described as a specific type of PTSD (Frazier, 2000).

The four basic elements are included in a PTSD diagnosis:

1. Exposure to a traumatic event
2. Re-experiencing the trauma (e.g., flashbacks; intrusive memories)
3. Symptoms of avoidance and numbing (e.g., attempts to avoid thoughts or situations that remind the survivor of the traumatic event; inability to recall certain aspect of the traumatic event; feeling disconnected from others)
4. Symptoms of increased arousal (e.g., exaggerated startle response; feeling easily irritated; constant fear of danger; physiological response when exposed to similar events)

Symptoms must be present for at least one month and must cause clinically significant distress or impairment (American Psychiatric Association, 1994).

The rate of PTSD varies greatly, depending upon the criteria used to define sexual assault. When sexual assault victims who have experienced less severe forms of sexual assault are included in studies, the rate for PTSD is lower, as low as 4% (Winfield, George, & Swartz et al., 1990). Based on a more strict definition of "attacked and raped" to define sexual assault, 80% of victims met the PTSD criteria (Breslau, Davis, & Andreski et al., 1991). It can be concluded from this that more severe forms of sexual assault appear to result in more severe symptoms of distress meeting the criteria for PTSD.

Women who report a sexual assault to the police or other authorities report higher PTSD rates (Rothbaum, Foa, & Riggs et al., 1992).

In an extensive review of the literature on the impact of rape, Frazier (2000) found that 75% to 94% of rape victims met the criteria for PTSD at two weeks after rape; 60% to 73% met the PTSD criteria at one to two months; 47% to 70% met the criteria at three to six months; and approximately 50% to 60% continue to meet the criteria at 12 months and beyond (Foa & Riggs, 1995; Rothbaum, Foa, & Riggs et al., 1992; Kramer & Green, 1991; Resnick, Yehuda, & Pitman et al., 1995; Frazier, Harlow, & Schauben et al., 1993; Santello & Leitenberg, 1993). According to Freedy and colleagues (1994), the most common symptoms at six months after rape are hypervigilance (79%) and exaggerated startle response (83%). PTSD prevalence rates for sexual assault victims several years after the rape are consistently reported to be from 12% to 17% (Frazier, 2000; Resnick, Kilpatrick, & Dansky et al., 1993; Kilpatrick, Saunders, & Veronen et al., 1987; Kessler, Sonnega, & Bromet et al., 1995).

SANE-SART Program Operation

The needs and care of sexual assault survivors extend far beyond their basic medical needs. For this reason it is essential that every SANE program operate as a part of a sexual assault response team (SART). SANE programs are based upon the belief that sexual assault survivors have the right to immediate, compassionate, and comprehensive medical-legal evaluation and treatment by specially trained professionals who have the experience to anticipate their needs during this time of crisis. As professionals, the SANE and other SART members have an ethical responsibility to provide victims with complete information about choices, so victims can make informed decisions about the care they want to receive.

Sexual assault survivors also have a right to report the crime of rape to law enforcement, even though not every victim may choose to report. Victims have a right to know what their options are and what to expect if they do or do not decide to report. Those who do report also have a right to sensitive and knowledgeable support without bias during this often difficult process. Those who do not report still have a right to expert, complete healthcare. Providing a higher standard of evidence collection and care can not only, ultimately, increase the prosecution of sex offenders and hopefully reduce rape, but also speed the victim's recovery to a higher level of functioning and prevent secondary injury or illness.

The Sexual Assault Response Team

The sexual assault response team (SART) is the group of professionals who work together to facilitate the survivor's recovery and the investigation and prosecution of the assailant by providing information, support, crisis intervention, gathering evidence, and facilitating the movement of the sexual assault survivor through the legal system. The SART members also work together or individually to improve the response to victims within their own disciplines and to educate the community they serve.

At a minimum the SART should include the SANE or forensic examiner, law enforcement, rape advocate, and prosecutor. Other valuable SART members are the crime laboratory personnel who analyze the sexual assault evidence kit, police dispatcher, EMT personnel, and other agencies serving sexual assault survivors such as domestic violence workers, social services personnel, and the clergy. Enlisting the support and involvement of individuals from key community agencies before they are needed can facilitate access to care.

How a SANE-SART Program Typically Operates

In some communities the SART members meet and interview the sexual assault survivor together in the ED or clinic where the initial evidentiary examination is completed, but in many communities the members function independently and coordinate their services. Although the conventional wisdom suggests that it is better to interview the sexual assault survivor only once so there is only one account of the assault and so it is less traumatic for the victim by eliminating the need for her to retell the account of the assault multiple times, no data support this approach. In fact, desensitization and exposure therapy, which involve having the survivor confront these fears and tell her story repeatedly, may be the most effective treatment identified to date (Foa & Rothbaum, 1990; Foa, 1997; Ledray, 1994; Muran & DiGiuseppe, 1994); thus, it is possible that multiple interviews may have a positive psychological benefit and may actually facilitate recovery. Research is needed in this area.

A SANE is usually available on call, off premises, 24 hours a day, 7 days a week to evaluate all male and female victims of sexual assault or abuse. Programs vary as to the age of victims they serve. The on-call SANE is paged immediately whenever a sexual assault or abuse survivor enters the community's response system. Although most evidentiary examinations are still completed at a hospital emergency department, the trend is for SANE-SART programs to operate outside the ED, either in a clinic area located near the ED, or in a separate community-based clinic or agency. The advantage of this is that because rape victims are seldom injured to the point that they require ED care, the high activity level and the expensive overhead of the ED can be avoided. The disadvantage to the SANE is that should additional medical evaluation be necessary, it may be more difficult to arrange. A plan must also be in place for medications and laboratory work to be completed (Ledray, 1999).

If the survivor was not accompanied by law enforcement or an advocate to the facility where the evidentiary examination will be performed and the protocol indicates that step, the rape advocate and or law enforcement officer should also be called when the SANE is paged. In most communities the sexual assault advocate will automatically be paged; however, law enforcement is paged only when the survivor agrees to make a police report.

During the time it takes for the SANE to respond (usually no more than one hour), the ED or clinic staff will evaluate and treat any urgent or life-threatening injuries. If treatment is medically necessary, the ED staff will treat the client, always considering the forensic consequences of the lifesaving and stabilizing medical procedures. Complete documentation is essential. If clothes or objects are removed from the victim by the ED staff, care should be taken utilizing forensic principles for handling and storage of the physical evidence. Whenever possible the SANE or law enforcement official should take all forensic photographs. If medical necessity dictates treatment prior to the arrival of the SANE, ED staff will take the photographs following established forensic procedures.

When the medical staff determines that the victim does not require immediate medical care, the survivor should be made comfortable in a private room near the ED. This area should enhance the victim's sense of safety and security and provide comfort and quiet in a sound-proof room with comfortable furniture, preferably a sofa to lie down, a telephone, and a locked door. Family members who accompany the victim, with the victim's permission, should be allowed to stay with the victim while they wait. If there was no oral sex, the victim may be offered something to eat or drink. If the victim is upset, and a hospital chaplain or social worker is available on site, they may be called, with the survivor's permission, to wait with the person until the SANE or advocate arrives.

In community-based SART programs that operate outside a medical facility, the survivor may first call law enforcement, who will evaluate if there are injuries that might require treatment. Typically fewer than 4% of rape victims will need treatment, as rape seldom involves serious injury (Tucker, Ledray, & Werner, 1990). If there are only minor injuries or no injuries are present, they will be transported to the community-based SANE facility by law enforcement. If moderate or severe injury is suspected, the victim may be evaluated by paramedics and taken to the designated medical facility where the SANE and advocate will meet them. After the patient is stabilized medically, the SANE will collect the forensic evidence.

SANE Responsibilities

Once the SANE arrives the nurse is responsible for completing the entire sexual assault evidentiary examination, including crisis intervention, STI risk evaluation and prevention, pregnancy risk evaluation and interception, interview and the collection of forensic evidence, and referrals for additional support and care. What the SANE will do is, however, to a great extent determined by the survivor's decision about reporting, so reporting must be addressed first.

Reporting Options

When the Victim Is Uncertain about Reporting. If the survivor has not yet decided whether to report, the SANE, in conjunction with an advocate when available, will discuss any fears and concerns and provide the information necessary for making an informed decision about reporting.

If the victim does not want to report at this time, but is unsure about reporting at a future date, the SANE will make sure the victim is aware of the options and the limitations of reporting at a later date. The SANE will also offer to complete an evidentiary examination kit that can be held in a locked refrigerator, for a specified time (usually one month or according to state statutes if any exist), in case the victim chooses to report later.

Mandatory Reporting. It is essential that the SANE and all other medical professionals are familiar with the local mandated reporting laws and the statutory rape laws. In most states statutory rape, although against the law, is not a mandated report. In states with mandatory reporting laws the SANE will follow established protocol regarding reporting after explaining the process and the nurse's responsibilities to the victim or the victim's family when a child is involved and a parent is present.

When the Victim Does Not Want to Report. If the rape survivor decides not to report and an evidentiary examination is not completed, the SANE can still offer medications to prevent STIs, evaluate a woman's risk of pregnancy, and offer pregnancy prevention for at least up to 72 hours postrape. The SANE will also make referrals for follow-up medical care and counseling and provide written follow-up information.

Evidentiary Examination

When a report is made or the victim indicates she or he will likely report, a complete evidentiary examination is conducted following the SANE agency protocol (Boxes 26-1 and 26-2). In most agencies the complete examination is conducted within 72 hours of the sexual assault. After obtaining a signed consent, the SANE will conduct a complete examination.

Box 26-1 Elements of a Sexual Assault Examination

- Interview to guide the examination and document victim's statements
- Collection of evidence in a sexual assault examination kit
- Collection of clothing potentially containing evidence
- Careful documentation of the victim's statements, evidence collected, and injuries on a sexual assault examination report (see Sexual Assault Examination Report in Appendix D.)
- Pictures of injuries
- Prophylactic care for sexually transmitted infections
- Evaluation of pregnancy risk and emergency contraception
- Crisis intervention
- Referral for follow-up medical and psychological care

Box 26-2 Evidence Collection

The sexual assault evidence collection will vary depending upon local protocol and the choice of kits. It will, however, typically include the following:

- Collection of swabs from the orifices involved in the sexual assault to look for sperm, acid phosphatase, and most important, the offender's DNA
- Collection of swabs from the skin that may have body fluids of the assailant, including blood, saliva, or seminal fluid
- Buccal swabs or blood from the survivor to identify DNA (If the victim was assaulted orally, buccal swabs should not be used, as the oral cavity may be contaminated with the suspect's DNA.)
- Collection of blood or urine for possible drug screen (especially in suspected drug-facilitated sexual assault)
- Pubic hair combing to look for the assailant's pubic hair
- Collection of debris from anywhere on the victim's body or clothing

Note: Most SANE programs no longer collect pulled head hair or pubic hair, as this is seldom useful evidence, the collection is very painful, and when it is needed it can be obtained in those few cases at a later time.

Chain of Custody

To maintain proper chain of custody each piece of evidence collected must be properly labeled with the victim's full name, the date and time of collection, the SANE's full name, and the identification of the evidence. It is then sealed and either given to law enforcement or placed into a locked refrigerator or cabinet with limited access. A signature record must also be kept of everyone who has possession of the evidence from the time it is collected by the SANE until it is given to law enforcement. Research comparing evidence collected in 97 cases, 24 by SANEs and 73 by non-SANEs, showed that the SANEs maintained chain of custody 100% of the time and non-SANEs only 52% of the time (Ledray & Simmelink, 1997). Similar results were found in a study of 100 kits, 41 completed by SANEs and 59 completed by non-SANEs.

The SANEs maintained chain of custody in 100% of the cases, and non-SANEs 81% of the time (Griswold, 1999).

Medical Care

The purpose of the SANE examination of the sexual assault survivor is specifically to assess, document, and collect forensic evidence. In addition, prophylactic treatment of STIs and prevention of pregnancy are provided by the SANE following a pre-established medical protocol or with the approval of a consulting physician. Although the SANE may treat minor injuries, further evaluation and care of any major physical trauma is referred to the ED or a designated medical facility. The SANE conducts a limited medical examination, and it is important to make clear to the sexual assault survivor that routine medical care is not a part of the SANE examination. Of course, obvious pathology or suspicious findings observed are reported to the client with a suggestion for follow-up care and referral, but evaluation and diagnosis of pathology is beyond the scope of the SANE examination.

Emotional Support and Crisis Intervention. The SANE is not an advocate, and when an advocate is present, the primary role of the advocate is to provide emotional support and information about the survivor's options. The SANE, however, is also not just a technician who collects evidence. As a professional nurse the SANE's role encompasses all aspects of the bio-psycho-social needs of all patients, including the survivor of sexual assault. The SANE will always provide emotional support and crisis intervention, working as a team with the advocate and other professionals (Ledray, Faugno, & Speck, 2001). Together the SANE must also make an initial assessment of the survivor's psychological functioning sufficient to determine suicidal ideation; orientation to person, place, and time; or need of further referral for follow-up support, evaluation, or treatment. When friends or family are present the advocate may need to spend time with them during the evidentiary examination, and thus, it may be necessary for the SANE to fill this role independently.

Discharge. If the victim is alone, the SANE or advocate will talk with him or her about whom to call and where to go from the hospital. Every effort will be made to find a place where the victim will feel safe and will not be alone. When necessary, arrangements may be made for shelter placement. If the victim is intoxicated or does not want to leave until morning, arrangements may be made to sleep in a specified area of the hospital when this type of space is available. In many facilities this will be an ED holding room or crisis center. If necessary, a community referral can be made to better meet long-term housing needs. Aftercare is one important component of competent care.

Testifying in Court. The SANE's role is not complete when the victim leaves the ED or clinic. An important part of the job is to testify as a witness in court, should the case be charged and prosecuted. Fortunately, more cases are closed through a guilty plea than through trial (Ledray, 1999). Although there is no research showing a direct link between a SANE examination and a guilty plea, case reports have demonstrated that when assailants are confronted with SANE evidence, they are willing to accept a guilty plea when they had denied committing any sexual abuse prior to seeing the evidence.

When a Case Goes to Trial. The SANE may be called to testify as a factual witness or as an expert witness. When testifying as a factual witness the SANE will simply report the facts of the examination as completed. The nurse will answer questions about what evidence she or he collected and how it was collected and will likely also testify as to what the victim told him or her about the assault and the victim's response during the examination. Because the SANE is completing a medical examination, the things the victim says are admissible in court as an exception to the hearsay rule (Ledray & Barry, 1998). The SANE may also testify as an expert witness, in which case, when qualified to do so based upon experience, knowledge, and training the SANE also will be allowed to give an opinion about what was found.

When testifying in court, the SANE should observe the following guidelines:

- Be sure to contact the attorney who subpoenaed you to review the issues in the case and get a basic understanding of what will be asked.
- Review your records so you are familiar with the basic details of the case.
- Dress professionally and in a conservative manner; women should wear minimal make-up and jewelry.
- In court, look at the attorney when questions are asked and at the jury when answering the questions, looking them in the eye.
- Always tell the complete truth. When unsure about an answer, say you are unsure or that you do not recall. If necessary, ask to be allowed to refer to your records to refresh your memory. When you do know an answer, speak with confidence, and speak clearly and loudly, so you can be heard. Listen carefully to the questions and if they are unclear, ask to have the questions clarified.
- If an objection is raised by either attorney during your testimony, stop speaking immediately and wait until the judge rules. It the objection is "overruled," you may continue. If it is "sustained," wait until there is another question.
- Always remember you are an unbiased witness, not an advocate. Don't get angry, be intimidated, defensive, evasive, or try to hide facts that may be unpleasant. If you made a mistake or left something out in your evidence collection or documentation, admit it; don't try to hide it.

Education, Training, Research, and Program Evaluation

In addition to providing direct client care and testifying in court, the SANE and other SART members need to be active in training other healthcare and community agencies to provide services to sexual assault survivors. SART programs should conduct ongoing program evaluation and periodic research to evaluate program impact, treatment needs, outcomes, and services. It is only through this continual program evaluation and research that the services for survivors tomorrow will continue to be more effective and efficient than the services available today.

Key Point *26-4*

The members of the sexual assault response team must assume the responsibilities associated with courtroom testimony and engage in education, training, research, and program evaluation activities aimed at improving services of community agencies providing services to sexual assault survivors.

Summary

The global prevalence of sexual assault is difficult to ascertain due to the high rate of nondisclosure. Available statistics show an alarmingly high rate of sexual assault across the US and that it is an undeniable problem in every country in the world. The majority of assaults are perpetrated by acquaintances, and many women suffer repeated assaults at the hands of one perpetrator, most often their husband, boyfriend, or authority figure. Because the incidence of sexual coercion peaks at the college age it is imperative that references are available to guide young victims to counseling centers and health clinics. The FNE/SANE plan of care for the victim of sexual assault should include a referral for counseling; if the victim desires legal action, the SANE should assist in contacting proper authorities and set up an aftercare program to schedule a follow-up screening within 24 to 48 hours with a second follow-up examination six weeks later. Each time an aftercare appointment is met, it provides the opportunity to reevaluate the emotional status as well. Sexual assault can have devastating effects for the victim, and these effects may last for many years after the actual attack. Risk factors for sexual assault have been identified as well as patterns of behavior commonly displayed following an assault. Barriers to both disclosure by the victim and adequate assessment by the medical/forensic examiner have been well documented in the literature. Responsibility lies with the forensic nurse examiner who specializes in sexual assault examinations to ensure that all patients are adequately screened for sequelae of sexual assault. FNE/SANEs are able to develop caring therapeutic relationships with patients and provide a viable foundation for the disclosure of sexual assault. Advanced practice nurses need to educate themselves regarding the risk factors and behavioral changes commonly associated with sexual assault. The challenge for the FNE/SANE must also put all biases aside and become comfortable with the fundamental forensic assessment guidelines used in screening patients for sexual assault. This epidemic must be brought to the forefront of the public consciousness if the stigmas and shame associated with sexual assault are to be eradicated. Unfortuately crimes against persons such as sexual assault will require constant monitoring and consistent screening. These procedures by FNE/SANEs can help raise awareness and help victims identify abusive behavior.

Resources

Organizations

Clearinghouse on Family Violence Information

P.O. Box 1182, Washington, DC 20013; Tel: 800-394-3366

International Association of Forensic Nurses (IAFN)

East Holly Avenue, Box 56, Pitman, NJ 08071-0056; www.forensicnurse.org

National Coalition against Domestic Violence

Public Policy Office, 1633 Q Street, Suite 210, Washington, DC 20009; Tel: 202-745-1211, 800-799-SAFE(7233); www.ncadv.org

National Organization on Male Sexual Victimization (US)

Box 103, 5505 Connecticut Avenue NW, Washington, DC 20015-2601; Tel: 800-738-4181; www.malesurvivor.org

National Organization on Male Sexual Victimization (Canada)

c/o BCSMSSA, 1252 Burrard Street, #202, Vancouver, BC V6Z 1, Canada

National Sexual Violence Resource Center

123 North Enola Drive, Enola, PA 17025; Tel: 877-739-3895, 717-909-0710; www.nsvrc.org

Office for Victims of Crime Resource Center

Office of Justice Programs, Department of Justice, 633 Indiana Avenue NW, Room 1386, Washington, DC 20531; Tel: 202-307-5983, 800-851-3420

References

American College of Emergency Physicians. (June 1999). *Evaluation and management of the sexually assaulted or sexually abused patient.* Dallas: Author.

Abel, G., & Rouleau, J. (1995). Sexual abuses. *Psychiatr Clin North Am, 18*(1), 139-153.

American Psychiatric Association. (2000). DSM IV: 2000 text revision. In American Psychiatric Association. *Diagnostic & statistical manual of mental disorders* (4th ed.). Washington, DC: Author.

American Psychiatric Association. (1994). *Diagnostic & statistical manual of mental disorders* (4th ed.). Washington, DC: Author.

Antognoli-Toland, P. (1985). Comprehensive program for examination of sexual assault victims by nurses: A hospital-based project in Texas. *J Emerg Nurs, 11*(3), 132-136.

Atkeson, B., Calhoun, K. S., Resick, P. A., et al. (1982). Victims of rape: Repeated assessment of depressive symptoms. *J Consult Clin Psychol, 50*, 96-102.

Becker, J., Skinner, L., Abel, G., et al. (1986). Level of postassault sexual functioning in rape and incest. *Arch Sex Behav, 15*, 37-49.

Bell, K. (1995). Tulsa sexual assault nurse examiners program. *Okla Nurse, 40*(3), 16.

Blair, T., & Warner, C. (1992). Sexual assault. *Top Emerg Med, 14*(4), 58-77.

Bobak, I. M., & Jensen, M. D. (1993). Violence against women. In *Maternity & gynecologic care: The nurse and the family* (5th ed.). St. Louis: Mosby.

Breslau, N., Davis, G., Andreski, P., et al. (1991). Traumatic events and post-traumatic stress disorder in an urban population of young adults. *Arch Gen Psychiatry, 48*, 216-222.

Burge, S. (1988). PTSD in victims of rape. *J Trauma Stress, 1*(2), 193-210.

Burgess, A., & Holmstrom, L. (1974). Rape trauma syndrome. *Am J Psychiatry, 131*(9), 981-985.

Burgess, A., & Holmstrom, L. (1979). Adaptive strategies and recovery from rape. *Am J Psychiatry, 136*, 1278-1282.

Burnam, M. S., Stein, J. A., Golding, J. M., et al. (1988). Sexual assault and mental disorders in a community population. *J Consult Clin Psychol, 147*, 843-850.

Calhoun, K., Atkeson, B., & Resick, P. (1982). A longitudinal examination of fear reactions in victims of rape. *J Couns Psychol, 29*, 655-661.

Cartwright, P. S., Moore, R. A., Anderson, J. R., et al. (1986). Genital injury and implied consent to alleged rape. *J Reprod Med, 31*(11), 1043-1044.

Centers for Disease Control and Prevention. (Sept. 24, 1993). Sexually transmitted diseases treatment guidelines. *MMWR, 42*(RR-14).

Centers for Disease Control and Prevention. (1998). Sexually transmitted diseases treatment guidelines. *MMWR, 42*, 1-102.

Centers for Disease Control and Prevention (4/25/2002). Sexually transmitted diseases treatment guidelines. Retrieved from www.cdc.gov/std/treatment/8-2002TG.htm.

Chivers, C. J. (August 6, 2000). In sex crimes, evidence depends on game of chance in hospitals. *The New York Times-Metropolitan Desk,* 1-6.

Claydon, E., Murphy, S., Osborne, E., et al. (1991). Rape and HIV. *Int J STD AIDS, 2*, 200-201.

Chapman, D. (1989). A longitudinal study of sexuality and gynecologic health in abused women. *J Am Osteopath Assoc, 89*(5), 619-624.

Cluss, P., Boughton, J., Frank, L., et al. (1983). The rape victim: Psychological correlates of participation in the legal system. *Crim Justice Behav, 10*, 342-357.

Cohen, L. J., & Roth, S. (1987). The psychological aftermath of rape: Long-term effects and individual differences in recovery. *J Soc Clin Psychol, 5*, 525-534.

Cohen, S., & Williamson, G. (1991). Stress and infectious disease in humans. *Psychol Bull, 109*, 5-24.

DiNitto, D., Martin, P., Yancey, N., et al. (1986). After rape: Who should examine rape survivors? *Am J Nurs, 86*(5), 538-540.

Dupre, A., Hampton, H., Morrison, H. J., et al. (1993). Sexual assault. *Obstet Gynecol Surv, 28*(9), 640-648.

Ellis, E., Atkeson, B., & Calhoun, K. (1981). An assessment of long-term reactions to rape. *J Abnorm Psychol, 90*, 263-266.

Emergency Nurses Association (1991). Sexual assault nurse examiner resource list. *J Emerg Nurs, 17*(4), 31-35A.

Ernst, A., Green, E., Ferguson, M., et al. (2000). The utility of anoscopy and coloscopy in the evaluation of male sexual assault victims. *Ann Emerg Med, 36*(5), 432-436.

Faigman, D. L., Kaye, D. H., Saks, M. J., et al. (1997). *Modern scientific evidence: The law & science of expert testimony.* St. Paul: West Publishing Co.

Felitti, V. (1991). Long-term medical consequences of incest, rape, and molestation. *South Med J, 84*(3), 328-331.

Foa, E. (1997). Trauma and women: Course, predictors, and treatment. *J Clin Psychiatry, 58*(9), 25-28.

Foa, E., & Rothbaum, B. (1990). Rape: Can victims be helped by cognitive behavior therapy? In K. Hawton (Ed.). *Dilemmas and difficulties in the management of psychiatric patients* (pp. 197-204). New York: Oxford University Press.

Foa, E. B., & Riggs, D. S. (1995). Posttraumatic stress disorder following assault: Theoretical considerations and empirical findings. *Curr Directions, 4*, 61-65.

Frank, C. (December 1996). The new way to catch rapists. *Redbook,* 104-105, 118-120.

Frank, E., & Anderson, P. (1987). Psychiatric disorders in rape victims: Past history and current symptomatology. *Comprehensive Psychiatry, 28*, 77-82.

Frank, E., & Stewart, B. D. (1984). Depressive symptoms in rape victims: A revisit. *J Affect Dis, 7*, 77-85.

Frazier, P. (1990). Victim attributions and post-rape trauma. *J Pers Soc Psychol, 59*(2), 298-304.

Frazier, P. (2000). The scientific status of research on rape trauma syndrome. In D. L. Faigman, D. H. Kay, M. J. Sakes, & J. Sanders. (Eds.). *Modern scientific evidence: The law & science of expert testimony* (Vol. 1.). St. Paul: West Group.

Frazier, P., & Burnett, J. (1994). Immediate coping strategies among rape victims. *J Couns Dev, 72*(4), 633-639.

Frazier, P., Harlow, T., Schauben, L., et al. (August 1993). Predictors of post rape trauma. Paper presented at the 1993 meeting of the American Psychological Association, Toronto.

Frazier, P., & Schauben, L. (1994) Causal attributions and recovery from rape and other stressful life events. *J Soc Clinical Psychol, 13*, 1-14.

Freedy, J. R., Resnick, H. S., Kilpatrick, D. G., et al. (1994). The psychological adjustment of recent crime victims in the criminal justice system. *J Interpers Violence, 9*, 450-468.

Geist, R. F. (August 1988). Sexually related trauma. *Emerg Med Clin North Am, 6*(3):439-466.

Gidycz, C. A., Coble, C. N., Latham, L., et al. (1993). Relation of a sexual assault experience in adulthood to prior victimization experiences: A prospective analysis. *Psychol Women Q, 17*, 151-168.

Gidycz, C., & Koss, M. (1991). Predictors of long-term sexual assault trauma among a national sample of victimized college women. *Violence Vict, 3*, 175-190.

Gidycz, C., & Koss, M. (1989). The impact of adolescent sexual victimization: Standardized measures of anxiety, depression, and behavioral deviancy. *Violence Vict, 4*, 139-149.

Girelli, S., Resnick, P., Marhoefer-Dvorak, S., et al. (1986). Subjective distress and violence during rape: Their effects on long-term fear. *Violence Vict, 1*(1), 35-46.

Gold, S., Milan, L., Mayall, A., et al. (1994). A cross-validation study of the trauma symptom checklist. *J Interpers Violence, 9*, 12-26.

Golding, J. (1994). Sexual assault history and physical health in randomly selected Los Angeles women. *Health Psychol, 13*(2), 130-138.

Goodman, L., Koss, M., Russo, N. (1993). Violence against Women: Physical, mental and health effects. In *Applied and preventive psychology* (Chap. 2, pp. 79-89). Cambridge: Cambridge University Press.

Griswold, Camille J. (1999). *Efficacy of sexual assault nurse examiner evidence collection: A northern Michigan study.* Thesis submitted to Grand Valley State University, Kirkhof School of Nursing, Allendale, MI.

Hertzen, H., Piaggio, G., Ding, J., et al. (Dec. 7, 2002). Low dose mifepristone and two regimens of levonorgestrel for emergency contraception: A WHO multicenter randomized trial. *Lancet, 360*, 1803-1810.

Holloway, M., & Swan, A. (1993) A & E management of sexual assault. *Nurs Standard, 7*(45), 31-35.

International Association of Forensic Nurses (IAFN). (1996). *Sexual assault nurse examiner standards of practice.* Pitman, NJ: Author.

Joint Commission on Accreditation of Health Care Organizations (JCAHO). (1997). *Comprehensive accreditation manual for hospitals: The official handbook.* Oakbrook Terrace, IL: Author.

Jones, K., & Uishi, T. (1980). Impact of alcohol, drug abuse and mental health treatment on medical care utilization: A review of the literature. *Med Care, 17*(2), 1-82.

Kessler, R., Sonnega, A., Bromet, E., et al. (1995). Post-traumatic stress disorder in the national comorbidity survey. *Arch Gen Psychiatry, 52*, 1048-1060.

Kettleson, D. (June 1995). Nurses trained to take evidence. *Unit News/District News*, District of East Hawaii.

Kiffe, B. (August 1996). *Perceptions: Responsibility attributions of rape victims.* Thesis. Augsburg College MSW, Minneapolis, MN.

Kilpatrick, D., Acierno, R., Resnick, H., et al. (1997). A 2-year longitudinal analysis of the relationship between violent assault and substance use in women. *J Consul Clin Psychol, 65*(5), 834-847.

Kilpatrick, D., Resnick, R., & Veronen, L. (1981). Effects of a rape experience: A longitudinal study. *J Soc Issues, 37*, 1050-1121.

Kilpatrick, D., Saunders, B., Veronen, L., et al. (1987). Criminal victimization: Lifetime prevalence reporting to police, and psychological impact. *Crime Delinquency, 33*, 479-489.

Kilpatrick, D., & Veronen, L. (1984). *Treatment of fear and anxiety in victims of rape* (Final report, grant No. R01NG29602). Rockville, MD: National Institute of Mental Health.

Kilpatrick, D. G., Veronen, L. J., Best, C. L., et al. (1985). Factors predicting psychological distress among rape victims. In C. R. Figley (Ed.). *Trauma and its wake.* New York: Brunner/Mazel.

Kilpatrick, D. G., Veronen L. J., & Resick, R. (1979). Assessment of the aftermath of rape: Changing patterns of fear. *J Behav Assess, 1*, 133-148.

Kimerling, R., & Calhoun, S. (1994). Somatic symptoms, social support, and treatment seeking among sexual assault victims. *J Consult Clin Psychol, 62*(2), 333-340.

Koss, M. P., Koss, P., & Woodruff, W. (1991). Deleterious effects of criminal victimization on women's health and medical utilization. *Arch Intern Med, 151*, 342-357.

Koss, M. (1993). Rape. Scope, impact, interventions, and public policy. *Am Psychol, 48*(10), 1062-1069.

Koss, M., Dinero, T., Seibel, C., et al. (1988). Stranger and acquaintance rape: Are there differences in the victim's experience? *Psychol Women Q, 12*, 1-24.

Koss, M., Woodruff, W., & Koss, P. (1990). Relationship of criminal victimization to health perceptions among women medical patients. *J Consult Clin Psychol, 58*(2), 147-152.

Krakow, B., Tandberg, D., Barey, M., et al. (1995). Nightmares and sleep disturbance in sexually assaulted women. *Dreaming, 5*(3) 199-206.

Kramer, T., & Green, T. (1991). Post-traumatic stress disorder as an early response to sexual assault. *J Interpers Violence, 5*, 229-246.

Ledray, L. E. (1991). Sexual assault and sexually transmitted disease: The issues and concerns. In Burgess, A. W. *Rape and sexual assault. III: A research handbook.* New York: Garland Publishing.

Ledray, L. E. (1993). Sexual assault nurse clinician: An emerging area of nursing expertise. In Linda C. Andrist (Ed.). *Clinical issues in perinatal and women's health nursing* (Vol. 4, p. 2). Philadelphia: Lippincott.

Ledray, L. (1984). Victims of incest. *Am J Nurs,* 84(8) 1010-1014.

Ledray, L. E. (1992). The sexual assault nurse clinician: Minneapolis' 15 years experience. *J Emerg Nurs, 18*(3) 217-222.

Ledray, L. E. (1994). Recovering from rape (2nd ed.). New York: Henry Holt.

Ledray, L. E. (1996a). Sexual assault nurse clinician: Sexual assault nurse examiner (SANE) programs. *J Emerg Nurs, 22*(5), 460-464.

Ledray, L. E. (1996b). Sexual assault: Clinical issues: Date rape drug alert. *J Emerg Nurs, 22*(1), 80.

Ledray, L. E. (1999). Sexual assault: Clinical issues: Date rape drug alert. *J Emerg Nurs, 17*(1), 1-2.

Ledray, L. E., & Barry, L. (June 1998). Sexual assault: Clinical issues: SANE expert and factual testimony. *J Emerg Nurs, 24*(3), 284-287.

Ledray, L., & Chaignot, M. J. (1980). Services to sexual assault victims in Hennepin County. *Evaluation and Change, Special Issue,* 131-134.

Ledray, L., Faugno, D., & Speck, P. (2001). Sexual assault: Clinical issues. SANE: Advocate, forensic technician, nurse? *J Emerg Nurs, 27*(1), 91-93.

Lenehan, G. P. (1991). A SANE way to care for rape victims. *J Emerg Nurs, 17*(1), 1-2.

Leserman, J., Zhiming, L., Drossman, D., et al. (1997). Impact of sexual and physical abuse dimensions on health status: Development of an abuse severity schedule. *Somatic Med, 59*, 152-160.

Lynch, V. A. (1993). Forensic nursing: Diversity in education and practice. *J Psychosoc Nurs, 132*(3), 7-14.

Lynch, V. A. (November 1996). President's report: Goals of the IAFN. Fourth Annual Scientific Assembly of Forensic Nurses Conference, Kansas City.

MacFarlane, E., & Hawley, P. (June 1993) Sexual assault: Coping with crisis. *Can Nurse,* 21-24.

Mackey, T., Sereika, S., Weissfeld, L., et al. (February 1992). Factors associated with long-term depressive symptoms of sexual assault victims. *Arch Psychiatric Nurs, VI*(1), 10-25.

Mann, S., & Delon, M. (1995). Improved hypertension control after disclosure of decades old trauma. *Psychosom Med. 57*, 501-505.

Marchbanks, P., Lui, K. J., & Mercy, J. (1990). Risk of injury from resisting rape. *Am J Epidemiol, 132*(3), 540-549.

Marullo, Geri. (1996). *The future and the forensic nurse: New dimensions for the 21st century.* Fourth Annual Scientific Assembly of Forensic Nurses Conference, Kansas City.

Moss, M., Frank, E., & Anderson, B. (1990). Victims of Incest. *Am J Orthopsychiatry, 69*(3), 379-391.

Muran, E., & DiGiuseppe, R. (1994). Rape. In Dattilio & Freeman (Eds.). *Cognitive behavioral strategies in crisis intervention* (pp. 161-175). New York: Guilford Press.

Murphy, S., Harris, V., & Forester, S. (1989). Rape and subsequent seroconversion to HIV. *BMJ, 299*, 718.

Nadelson, C., Notman, M., Zackson, H., et al. (1982) A follow-up study of rape victims. *Am J Psychiatry, 139*, 1266-1270.

National Conference of Catholic Bishops. (1995). Pamphlet on ethical & religious directives for Catholic health care services (pp. 14-17).

Norris, J., & Feldman-Summers, S. (1981). Factors related to the psychological impact of rape on the victim. *J Abnorm Psychol, 139*, 1266-1270.

O'Brien, Coleen. (1996). Sexual assault nurse examiner (SANE) program coordinator. *J Emerg Nurs, 23*(5), 532-533.

Petrak, J., Skinner C. J., & Claydon, E. J. (1995). The prevalence of sexual assault in a genitourinary medicine clinic: Service implications. *Genitourin Med, 71*(2), 98-102.

Resick, P., & Schnicke, M. (1990). Treating symptoms in adult victims of sexual assault. *J Interpers Violence, 5*(4), 488-506.

Resnick, H., Kilpatrick, D., Dansky, B., et al. (1993). Prevalence of civilian trauma and PTSD in a representative national sample of women. *J Consult Clin Psychol, 61*(6), 984-991.

Resnick, H., Yehuda, R., Pitman, R., et al. (1995). Effect of previous trauma on acute plasma cortisol level following rape. *Am J Psychiatry, 152*, 1675-1677.

Riggs, N., Houry, D., Long, G., et al. (April 2000). Analysis of 1,076 cases of sexual assault. *Ann Emerg Med, 35*(4), 358-362.

Riggs, D., Kilpatrick, D., & Resnick, H. (1992). Long-term psychological distress associated with marital rape and aggravated assault: A comparison to other crime victims. *J Fam Violence, 7*, 283-296.

Rooms, R. R. (2004). Personal letter to Virginia Lynch. (April 2004).

Rothbaum, B., Foa, E., Riggs, D., et al. (1992). A prospective study of PTSD in rape victims. *J Trauma Stress, 5*(3), 455-475.

Sandrick, K. J. (1996). Tightening the chain of evidence. *Acta Hosp Health Networks, 26*, 199-201.

Santello, M., & Leitenberg, H. (1993). Sexual aggression by an acquaintance: Methods of coping and later psychological adjustment. *Violence Vict, 8*(2), 91-104.

Santiago, J., McCal-Perez, F., Gorcey, M., et al. (1985). Long-term psychological effects of rape in 35 rape victims. *Am J Psychiatry, 142*, 1338-1340.

Sheridan, Daniel J. (1993). The role of the battered woman specialist. *J Psychosoc Nurs, 31*, 11.

Slaughter, L., & Brown, C. R. (January 1992). Colposcopy to establish physical findings in rape victims. *Am J Obstet Gynecol, 176*(3), 83-86.

Slaughter, L., Brown, C. R., Crowley, S., et al. (1997). Patterns of genital injury in female sexual assault victims. *Am J Obstet Gynecol, 176*(3), 609-616.

Sorenson, S., Siegel, J., Golding, J., et al. (1991). Repeated sexual victimization. *Violence Vict, 6*(4), 299-308.

Speck, P., & Aiken, M. (1995). 20 years of community nursing service. *Tenn Nurse, 58*(2), 5-18.

Task Force on Postovulatory Methods of Fertility Regulation. (1998). Randomized controlled trial levonorgestrel versus the Yuzpe regimen of combined oral contraceptives for emergency contraception. *Lancet, 53*, 4228-4333.

Thomas, M., & Zachritz, H. (1993). Tulsa sexual assault nurse examiners (SANE) program. *J Okla State Med Assoc, 86*(6), 284-686.

Tintinalli, J., & Hoelzer, M. (1985). Clinical findings and legal resolution in sexual assault. *Ann Emerg Med, 14*(5), 447-453.

Tobias, G. (1990). Rape examinations by GPs. *Practitioner, 2*, 34.

Tucker, S., Ledray, L. E., & Stehle Werner, J. (July 1990). Sexual assault evidence collection. *Wisconsin Med J*, (7), 3-5

Waigandt, C., & Miller, D. (1986). Maladaptive responses during the reorganization phase of rape trauma syndrome. *Response, 1*(2), 6-7.

Walker, E., Katon, W., Hansom, J., et al. (1995). Psychiatric diagnoses and sexual victimization in women with chronic pelvic pain. *Psychosomatics, 326*(6), 531-540

Winfield, I., George, L. K., Swartz, M., et al. (1990). Sexual assault and psychiatric disorders among a community sample of women. *Am J Psychiatry, 147*, 335-341.

Yorker, B. C. (1996). Nurses in Georgia care for survivors of sexual assault. *Georgia Nurs, 56*(1), 5-6.

Yuzpe, A., Smith, R., & Rademaker, A. W. (1982). A multicenter clinical investigation employing ethinyl estradiol combined with dl-norgestrel as a postcoital contraceptive agent. *Fertil Steril,* 37(4), 508-513.

Chapter 27 Sequelae of Sexual Violence

Pamela J. Dole

This chapter discusses the physical, emotional, and sexual consequences of sexual abuse. Consequences of sexual abuse include post-traumatic stress disorder (PTSD). PTSD also arises from all forms of violence and chronic abuse. Chronic abuse often escalates to physical violence that includes sexual violence. Other forms of intimate abuse include emotional abuse, economic abuse, destruction of pets or property, threats, and stalking.

Sexual violence affects the community on a variety of levels and spans across all socioeconomic and ethnocultural groups. These acts are committed more frequently against women than men, and laws related to prosecuting sexual violence reflect community culture and views regarding women. All aggression creates an economic burden for the community.

The forensic nurse examiner (FNE) who specializes in sexual assault intervention can have an impact on patients at all levels of healing and by knowing the possible consequences of sexual violence can better direct nursing care. In addition much can be done at various levels by professional and nonprofessional groups from government agencies, advocacy groups, peer support groups, law enforcement, healthcare professionals, and attorneys.

Key Point 27-1

Creating a community social consciousness that does not tolerate sexual crimes is an important role of the sexual assault nurse examiner/sexual assault forensic examiner/forensic nurse examiner (SANE/SAFE/FNE).

Social Impact of Sexual Violence

Most victims of sexual assault and childhood sexual abuse suffer lifelong effects from these acts of violence. Trauma is associated with medical, psychological, social, spiritual, and sexual health consequences and related costs. Public health concerns about trauma and its effects in the US are reflected in the *Healthy People 2010* objectives that include decreasing interpersonal violence injuries and increasing violence prevention in an effort to reduce trauma-associated morbidity (US DHHS, 2000). "The 1992 JCAHO guidelines (and sequentially thereafter) call for identification, documentation, treatment and referral procedures as well as for training of appropriate staff in ambulatory and emergency department settings" (AWHONN, 1999, p. 3). The Violence against Women Act of 1994 expresses the need for research addressing interpersonal violence. This is the first national act that addresses restructuring the philosophy, assessment, and prosecution of perpetrators while providing some privacy to the victim's lives.

The well-known acceptance of violence in America also pervades issues of violence against women (Sigler, 1995). Reform, which began in the 1980s, was originally prompted by the feminist movement. How sexual violence is defined will affect how victims view themselves, how others view them, how the crime is reported, and what types of statistics are kept. The term *rape* is considered too narrow to adequately reflect the spectrum of acts of violence surrounding nonconsensual sexual aggression because *rape* refers to actual penile penetration of the vagina and can include oral or anal penetration. Currently sexual aggression can be prosecuted *within* the context of marriage in many states, whereas it was excluded in the past.

The terms used in laws since approximately 1994 include sexual assault, sexual battery, and sexual abuse (Epstein and Langenbahn, 1994). These terms reflect the three common reforms as summarized by the National Research Council (Crowell & Burgess, 1996):

- Broadening the definition to sexual penetration of any type, including vaginal, anal, or oral penetration of any type, whether by penis, fingers, or objects
- Focusing on the offender's behavior rather than the victim's resistance
- Restricting the use of the victim's prior sexual conduct as evidence

The concepts in this reformed language are more supportive to victims and emphasize the violence of the act itself by the perpetrator. Prior to 1994, because the meaning of the term *rape* was limited, perpetrators could often beat the charges by using a condom, admitting to impotence, or confining their aggression to everything short of nonconsensual coitus. It is important when reading research and reports to distinguish whether the language describing rape is prior to 1994 or after. The more recent terminology reflects an expanded concept of nonconsensual sexual aggression, thus reducing the gap in justice for these criminal acts. Some federal branches continue to use narrow definitions such as those found in the *Uniform Crime Reports* by the Federal Bureau of Investigation (FBI) (1993). Narrow definitions and underreporting of violence against women in partner violence, sexual assault, and stalking contribute to the paucity of research in these areas.

FBI and police agencies categorize crime by the most violent act only, often missing important facts such as sexual assault. For example, an individual who is the victim of a sexual homicide is listed as homicide. Individuals who are not legally married but living together or dating are often not adequately represented in statistics. Therefore, the accuracy of crimes involving interpersonal abuse within committed but not married relationships are often lost in statistics. This is true in cases of battered women and same-sex relationships. The FBI (1993) reported that more than 75% of violent crimes against women are committed by someone known to the victim. It is further stated that an intimate partner commits approximately 29% of those crimes and that these statistics may be underreported as a result of terminology and the categories of reporting used.

Terminology often reflects current social philosophy. Research, funding, and a comprehensive understanding of the nature of interpersonal violence against women are just beginning. Data gaps exist in areas including women of color, patterns of multiple forms of victimization, and rates of perpetration (Crowell & Burgess, 1996). Few data exist about men who have been sexually assaulted, yet they also experience consequences from sexual aggression. Until this widened knowledge base is generated, proactive prevention strategies are limited. Statistics on the prevalence of this social problem remain skewed and underestimated, especially in light of the fact that the majority of women do not report sexual assaults or seek healthcare at the time of the crime. Limited statistics are confounded by the lack of adequate screening for domestic abuse or sexual assault. Funding for research and development of interventions is inconsistent, although it appears to be gaining importance in the national agenda.

Global Issues

In post-apartheid South Africa sexual assault occurs every six minutes to infants, children, and adults. Anger from poor economic stability and the lack of role definitions have pushed black men to retaliate against women of all ages and races.

A European myth from the middle-ages that having sex with a virgin would cure syphilis has a new deadly spin in the twenty-first century. In developing countries, prepubescent girls are being raped because of beliefs that this will cure AIDS or prevent the rapist from contracting HIV infection (Jewkes, Martin, & Penn-Kekana, 2002; Lema, 1997; Meel, 2003; Pitcher & Bowley, 2002). In 2001, virgin rape had become so pervasive infants as young as 6-9 months were victimized in South Africa. In some third world countries, it is not uncommon for an eight-year-old girl to have already experienced multiple rapes and to have contracted numerous sexually transmitted infections (STIs) including HIV and human papillomavirus (HPV).

Child Prostitution

Child sexual abuse in the form of child prostitution is a global concern arising from poor economic situations, gender bias, and lack of education. It is estimated that from 1 million to 10 million children are coerced or sold into the sex industry (Willis & Levy, 2002). These children have the highest rate of HIV infection (78% in China), hepatitis, tuberculosis, and STIs and generally have not received immunizations (Willis & Levy, 2002). Child prostitutes also experience malnutrition, violence, pregnancy, substance abuse, and mental illness, with suicide and PTSD rates as high as 67% (Willis & Levy, 2002).

Rape in War

For thousands of years wars have been won without ever firing a gun. Raping the women in villages, a common war strategy, erodes families and disintegrates communities. Documentaries on the war on Yugoslavia have depicted the effects of rape by conquering soldiers. Women and families speak about the decay caused by this particular war strategy on the communities and families, especially in Bosnia, Rwanda, and Kurdistan (*AIDS Weekly Plus*, 1996). Refugees and internal displacement movements also place women and children at increased risk of sexual abuse that exceeds 60% (Amowitz, Russ, Lyons, et al., 2002; Gardner & Blackburn, 1996; Kerimova, Posner, Brown, et al., 2003). The World Health Organization (WHO), the United Nations, and advocate groups (e.g., Human Rights Watch, Amnesty International) are examples of international organizations that offer investigative assistance and emotional support to communities following the devastation of war.

Until women are viewed as equals and partners, they will remain victims of sexual assault. Social risk factors restricting a woman's autonomy contribute to sexual violence against women. Community empowerments with interventions that improve a woman's self-efficacy are needed to change current social attitudes (Gollub, 1999).

Male Victims

Men are also victims of sexual assault and molestation. Statistically men are sexually assaulted significantly less than women; however, many of similar issues, concerns, and consequences exist. Men often report increased humiliation from not being able to defend themselves against the perpetrator (McEvoy, Rollo, & Brookings, 1999; Scarce, 1997). Boys sexually abused by clergy describe rage and spiritual distress pervading their life (Fater and Mullaney, 2000). Male victims of childhood sexual assault identifying as homosexual or heterosexual orientation tend to identify with abusers, and abandon their feelings as a victim (Clarke & Pearson, 2000). One study of men having sex with men who had been sexually abused by their partners experienced a 5.7% HIV seroconversion rate as a result (Relf, 2001). Male victims may be confused by traditional roles and fail to engage in self-care because of poor coping strategies. Adequate screening, research, and statistics are needed in this area.

Poverty-Related Sexual Assault

Individuals living in poverty are much more likely to be sexually assaulted. Persons with incomes of less than $15,000 are three times more likely to be raped, be sexually assaulted, or sustain violent injuries as compared to households with annual incomes greater than $15,000 (Von, Kilpatrick, Burgess, & Hartman, 1998; Grisso et al., 1999). Vulnerable populations have fewer resources to cope with the consequences of sexual abuse.

Economic Impact of Interpersonal Violence

The cost of interpersonal violence is difficult to estimate. Many individuals do not report acts of violence and their effects are thus categorized in unrelated areas. The World Health Organization (WHO) and the World Bank define disability as the "incidence, duration, and severity of the morbidity and complications associated with specific conditions" (Wolfgang & Zahn, 1983). "In 1990 the assaultive violence was estimated to account for 17.5 million DALYs worldwide" (Rosen, Mercy, & Annest, 1998, p. 1226). DALYs is the measure of disability-adjusted life years lost. Intrafamilial homicide costs were calculated to be $1.7 billion annually (Straus & Gelles, 1986). The number of victims of interpersonal violence was nine times higher in households with incomes of $19,999 or less when compared to women with household incomes of $20,000 to $49,999 (CDC, 1998). Alcohol use by male partners was strongly correlated to the risk of injuries in a controlled study of domestic violence and confirmed by 67% of the female victims (Kyriacou, Anglin, & Taliaferro et al., 1999). Characteristics of assaultive partners are strongly related to the use of cocaine and past history of arrests suggesting a pattern of violence in another study (Grisso, Schwarz, & Hirschinger, et al., 1999).

Sexual assault and battering also contribute to emergency department and related expenses. One study revealed 22% of 911 (emergency telephone line) calls were related to victims of battering (Baker, Burgess, & Brickman, et al., 1989). Injuries related to battering account for 12% to 35% of emergency room visits by women (Meyers, 1992). One third of battered women are also sexually assaulted by their partners. Healthcare costs for each individual from intimate partner violence is $1775 greater per year and costs healthcare plans 92% more than a random sample of general female enrollees (Wisner, Gilmer, Saltzman, et al., 1999). The cost of domestic violence to employers for healthcare, high turnover, and lost productivity is estimated to be $3 billion to $5 billion dollars (American Bar Association Commission on Domestic Violence, 1996; Bureau of National Affairs, 1990). Meyer (1992) calculated these same losses to be $5 billion to $10 billion per year.

Sexual assault costs are higher than for other violent crimes, costing victims $127 billion per year and $86,464 per individual (Miller, Cohen, & Weirsema, 1996). There are no statistics available on short-term disability losses or healthcare-related costs sought outside the emergency department. Nonmonetary costs to victims include fear, suffering, pain, and lost quality of life. In a controlled study, victims of sexual assault were found to increase physician visits 56% over a two-year period following their attack when compared to the nonassaulted group (Koss, Koss, & Woodruff, 1991).

Psychological, Physical, and Sexual Health Effects

Statistics represent numbers pertaining to the consequences of sexual assault and do not convey the devastation experienced by victims and the profound effects on their lives (Box 27-1). The "lived experience" of each individual varies and is experienced differently. "Understanding the meaning of violence in women's lives requires an awareness of both their life stories and the social context of the violence they have encountered" (Draucker & Madsen, 1999, p. 331). The most important aspect in opening the door to healing the effects of violence is to ask the questions of our friends, family, patients, and community. Patients presenting with discordant symptomatology are often waving a red flag and asking to be heard. Women have fewer post-traumatic problems when they posses stronger coherence and higher self-esteem (Nyamathi, 1991).

Key Point 27-2

Trauma has an impact on the entire person. The possible consequences to sexual violence are exhibited as symptoms within the context of individual experiences. Symptoms are guideposts for intervention to reduce human suffering and to restore well-being for the individual.

Post-Traumatic Stress Disorder

Post-traumatic stress disorder (PTSD) is a psychological condition often suffered by victims of violence, including sexual assault and childhood sexual abuse. This diagnosis does not capture all the symptoms experienced by victims. PTSD is defined in the *Diagnostic and Statistical Manual of Mental Disorders* (APA, 1994) and must meet the following summarized criteria:

- A1. (Criterion) Witnessed a life-threatening event or serious injury
- A2. (Criterion) Exposed to an unusual traumatic event that has produced intense fear, terror, horror, or helplessness

Associated symptoms that must last for at least one month include the following:

- Trauma that is re-experienced in ongoing dreams, thoughts, or perceptions (intrusive thoughts).
- Avoidance of related traumatic stimuli (physical and psychological avoidance), with a numbing of general responsiveness.
- Persistent hypervigilance, exaggerated startle response, increased arousal, sleep disturbances, irritability, outbreaks of anger, and cognitive and memory disturbances (Korn, 2001).

It has been postulated that PTSD may represent a severe expression of post-trauma disturbances, and anxiety and depression represent milder manifestations of the same continuum (Fullilove, Lown, & Fullilove, 1992). It should be noted that there is disagreement among psychiatrists about whether post-traumatic stress related to sexual assault actually meets the criteria for PTSD.

The Panel on Research on Violence against Women stated that PTSD did not adequately conceptualize the experiences by victims of violence. The following four categories were listed as areas not adequately represented in the preceding definition (Crowell & Burgess, 1996, pp. 83-84):

It doesn't account for many of the symptoms manifested by victims of violence. For example, thoughts of suicide attempts, substance abuse, and sexual problems are not among the PTSD criteria.

The diagnosis better captures the psychiatric consequences of a single victimization than the consequences of chronic abusive conditions.

The description of traumatic events as outside usual human experience is not accurate in describing women's experiences with intimate violence.

The diagnosis fails to acknowledge the cognitive effects of this kind of violence. People who have been untouched often maintain beliefs (or schemas) about personal invulnerability, safety, trust, and intimacy, which are incompatible with experience of violence.

Not all victims of sexual abuse or assault develop PTSD. Contributing risk factors include gender, age, race, culture, intelligence, psychological vulnerability, and proximity to trauma (Brunnello, Davidson, & Deahl, et al., 2001; Feeny, Zoellner, & Foa, 2002; Fullilove, Lown, & Fullilove, 1992; Kenny & McEachern, 2000; Korn, 2001; Seedat & Stein, 2000). Psychological treatment is most effective when it is begun as soon after the sexual assault as possible. However, the majority of sexual assault victims never report the trauma or seek treatment, and children seldom disclose to parents (secretly feeling they themselves were bad or were to blame for the abuse). The silence provides the basis for PTSD.

When evaluating the magnitude of PTSD it is important to keep in mind that economics, geography, and social support play an important part in the perception of trauma and subsequent recovery. Community rates of lifetime exposure to trauma range from 40% to 80%, while lifetime prevalence of PTSD is approximately 7% to 9% (Seedat & Stein, 2000). A study of middle class Americans reported that only 1% reported experiencing trauma from any source (Kulka, Fairbank, Jordan, & Weiss, 1990). In a study of poor blacks in Harlem (New York City) nearly all persons

Box 27-1 Possible Sequelae to Sexual Violence

PHYSICAL

Gastrointestinal

- Irritable bowel syndrome
- Severe constipation
- Vomiting and diarrhea
- Dyspepsia

Neurological

- Headaches/migraines
- Postconcussion syndrome
- Hearing loss
- Detached retina
- Stroke from strangulation

Musculoskeletal

- Arthralgia
- Chronic pain
- Osteoarthritis
- Fibromyalgia

Constitutional

- Fatigue
- Bulimia/anorexia nervosa
- Morbid obesity
- Sleep disturbances
- Decreased concentration
- Paresis

Gynecological/Obstetrical

- Chronic pelvic pain (often nonpathological)
- Dyspareunia
- STIs including HIV infection
- Vaginal infections
- Premenstrual syndrome
- Cystitis
- Unplanned pregnancy, especially in teens
- Bleeding during pregnancy
- Miscarriage
- Preterm labor and low-birth-weight infant
- Fetal injury and death

SEXUAL

- Dysfunction
- Decreased libido
- Decreased vaginal lubrication during intercourse
- Fear of coercion
- Decreased intimacy
- Increased casual sex

PSYCHOLOGICAL

- Post-traumatic stress disorder
- Decreased self esteem
- Decreased self-care, including adherence to medical appointment and regimens
- Depression
- Flattened affect
- Substance abuse, including alcoholism and prescription drugs
- Increased risk-taking behavior
- Phobias
- Panic disorders
- Hypochondria
- Dissociation and multiple personality disorders
- Poor bonding with offspring
- Poor boundary setting
- Suicide

LIFESTYLE

- Unemployment
- Homelessness
- Increased risk taking
- Incarceration
- Disturbances in children

Data from Dole, P. (1996). Centering: Reducing rape trauma syndrome anxiety during a gynecologic examination. *J Psychosoc Nurs, 34*(10), 32-37; Association of Women's Health, Obstetrics and Neonatal Nurses (AWHONN). (1999). Partner & abuse violence screen. In *Universal Screening for Domestic Violence.* Washington, DC: Author.

reported one distressing traumatic event after another (Fullilove, Fullilove, & Smith, et al., 1993). It appears that in communities experiencing high volumes of traumatic events, individuals may experience higher morbidity for risk-taking behavior, take poorer care of themselves, and suffer PTSD. This same group proposes separating violent trauma (physical or sexual assault, mugging, witnessed murder) from all other nonviolent trauma when studying PTSD.

It should also be noted that males and females respond or define acts of trauma differently, except for natural disasters or terrorism attacks from which 100% of the community may experience some form of PTSD. Residents of New York City have varying symptoms of PTSD following the 9/11 terrorism attacks of the World Trade Center that may increase over time (Ater, 2003). One study five to six weeks after 9/11 revealed that residents had a 9.7% increase in depression symptoms, and a 7.5% increase in PTSD (Viahov & Galea, 2002). Men frequently have PTSD after witnessing or being a victim of a violent crime similar to that experienced in combat (both military and on the streets). Women, however, additionally express homelessness and the loss of their children as traumatic events. It should be noted that much of the PTSD research to date has been done on men in the military or community disasters.

Impact during Childhood

Most victims of childhood sexual abuse experience some degree of PTSD. Multiple victimizations are a major contributing factor to PTSD in childhood sexual abuse (Jasinski et al., 2000; Polusny & Follette, 1995). PTSD is intensified when it is combined with increasing exposure to trauma, including adult sexual assault.

It is well documented that the cycle of violence generally begins in the home. Parents suffering from childhood victimization often victimize their children directly or indirectly (fail to provide a safe environment) (Hall, Sachs, & Rayens, 1998). One prospective study showed that 12% of male children sexually abused as children became pedophiles as adults (Salter, McMillian, & Richards et al., 2003). Adult abusers versus those who did not go on to abuse were more likely to have been abused by females (38% versus 17%), to witness physical abuse (81% versus 58%), to have lacked age-appropriate supervision (67% versus 40%), and to have demonstrated cruelty to animals (29% versus 5%) (Salter et al., 2003). Another study of men with increased risky behavior revealed that 25% had unwanted sexual activity before age 13 (Dilorio, Hartwell, & Hansen, 2002).

Previous childhood sexual trauma may interrupt the development of self-representation, contribute to the loss of self or fragmentation of self, increase concerns regarding control issues, disrupt identity issues, disrupt body-image evolution, and lower self-esteem (Hanna, 1996; Putnam, 1989). Sexual trauma is compounded if the individual is a member of a stigmatized group and is further subjected to acts of discrimination or oppression. "Stigma trauma," coined by Fullilove (1992), is often experienced by women of color in the form of gender oppression and ethnicity. Similarly, gay males may experience stigma trauma in the form of sexual orientation prejudices and bias hate crimes.

Burgess and Holmstrom (1974) coined the expression *rape trauma syndrome* (RTS) when describing the acute and long-term problems related to sexual attacks in a group of 146 victims studied four to six years later. RTS is considered a specific type of PTSD pertaining solely to consequences of trauma related to sexual assault or childhood sexual abuse and is not gender-specific. RTS is broken into the acute phase or disorganization phase, which is characterized by expressive or guarded interviews following the sexual assault. Problems experienced by victims are categorized into physical, emotional, social, or sexual reactions impacting both the acute and long-term process of reorganization.

The term "rape trauma syndrome" is a nursing diagnosis for implementing recovery strategies and is not used as a diagnostic category. RTS, however, more appropriately addresses the sequel related to sexual assault especially as experienced by women. It separates PTSD trauma experienced as a result of war or natural disaster that often happens to groups or communities and rarely involves nonconsensual invasion of the body by another individual. A wealth of research related to PTSD in nonsexual violence populations exists, but a paucity of material exists on RTS.

Recovery from sexual violence and RTS varies from person to person. One 1992 study found 94% of victims during the first week following the sexual assault had PTSD (Ledray, 1994). A 1993 study found 50% of women met the criteria for PTSD one year following sexual assault (Ledray, 1994). The 1992 National Victim Center report *Rape in America: A Report to the Nation* estimated that 1.3 million women are experiencing PTSD two years after the sexual assault and that more than twice that number of women experienced PTSD at some time following the sexual assault.

Not all individuals will suffer long-term RTS. Support systems and the social environment are key factors in recovery. How the sexual assault is perceived by the individual's support system is also critical. If the sexual assault is viewed as an act of violence rather than a sexual act, recovery appears to be predictable with fewer long-term effects, provided that the individual possesses adequate coping mechanisms. Individuals who are exposed to stigma or ongoing environmental trauma appear to have increased long-term effects represented by RTS. Draucker and Madsen (1999) found that sexually abused children experienced not only the sexual assault but may have been further traumatized by feelings of being "banished, alienated, or exiled." Sexually abused children also experienced deep-seated shame and the fear of feeling emotions producing guilt and anxiety (Zupancic & Kreidler, 1998). Individual coping mechanisms are dependent upon the resolution of developmental issues and stages. Children who are victims of sexual abuse (either incest or molestation) appear to have more compromised coping mechanism than adults of sexual abuse.

Women have twice the rates of PTSD as compared to men, especially if they were sexually abused as children (Brunnello et al., 2001; Katon, 2001; Wise, Zierler, & Krieger et al., 2001). A direct correlation between the severities of violence, the multiplicity of sexual abuse, and RTS also seems to exist (Koss, Koss & Woodruff, 1991; Ledray, 1990; Jasinski, 2000). Individuals with PTSD are 26 to 37 times more likely to develop affective illness, generalized anxiety disorder, or panic disorder (Katon, 2001).

Fear penetrates each of the categories in the acute phase and closely parallels the attack. Disturbances in sleep and eating patterns are two common occurrences caused by fear. The emotional reactions are seated in fear and phobic reactions and affect the ability to work, leave home, and relate to friends, family, and partners. Gratitude over surviving the attack is often clouded by the fear of being attacked again and possibly killed or mutilated (Hazelwood & Burgess, 1995; Koss et al., 1991). Similar to physical symptoms, emotional scars often go undetected because of poor history taking or the healthcare provider's inability or inexperience in managing or responding to acts of violence.

RTS is expressed in a complex, entangled lifestyle when an individual lacks adequate coping skills or social or medical support, or is subject to ongoing trauma in his or her environment. As time goes on the physical, emotional, social, and sexual categories impacted by the sexual attack become less segregated and more intertwined, making the exact nature of a particular problem less obvious. Comorbidities of RTS include chemical dependence (including injecting drug use and alcoholism) in 75% of veterans with PTSD (Kulka et al., 1990) and 43% of individuals with a diagnosis of PTSD (Breslau, Davis, Andreski, et al., 1991). Substance abuse, especially with alcohol, cigarettes, and cocaine, is common when victims desire to numb or cope with the pain of sexual trauma. Among various drug treatment programs, 46.4% of patients had a history of sexual assault as adults and 38.2% in childhood (El-Bassel, Gilbert, & Frye et al., 2004; North, 1996). In addition, 30.7% of women in a methadone maintenance treatment program (MMTP) had been sexually abused by a partner in the past six months, and cocaine use increased this violence (El-Bassel, 2004). Another study found that 59% of substance abusers had symptoms consistent with PTSD, yet they were undiagnosed and at the time they were admitted for detoxification had not received any treatment (Fullilove et al., 1993). In this same study 97% of women with PTSD reported one or more violent traumas compared to 73% of women without PTSD.

Women share a common history stating they were often re-victimized in subsequent rapes or domestic violence scenarios (Coid, Petruckevitch, & Feder, et al., 2001; El-Bassel, et al., 2004; Fullilove, et al., 1992; Johnson, Cunnington-Williams, & Cotter, 2003; Schafer, Caetano, & Cunradi, 2004; Teets, 1997; Wise, Zierler, & Krieger et al., 2001;). Women with a history of childhood sexual abuse may utilize substance abuse as one of the maladaptive coping mechanisms (Blume, 1998). Subsequent substance abuse following sexual assault or incest is more common in women than in men.

Key Point 27-3

Rape trauma syndrome is associated with risk-taking behavior, increased substance abuse, lowered self-esteem, depression and anxiety, and a wide range of physical and sexual dysfunctions.

Risk-Taking Behavior

Heightened risk-taking behavior is well documented among substance-abusing populations, placing women at an increased risk for HIV infection and other sexually transmitted infections (STIs). Other STIs that are commonly transmitted include hepatitis, human papillomavirus (HPV), chlamydia infection, gonorrhea, and herpes. One study of African American women showed that having a history of an STI, including HIV, placed them at an increased risk for drug use, depression, and interpersonal violence (Johnson, et al., 2003). Bitterness toward past life experiences often pushes individuals with a history of sexual abuse toward risk-taking scenarios, including multiple partners, exchanging sex for money, unsafe sexual practices, unwanted pregnancies, and revicitimization by intimates (Champion, Shain, Piper, et al., 2001; Coid, Petruckevitch, & Feder et al., 2001; El-Bassel, et al., 2004; Fergusen, Horwood, & Lynskey, 1997; Gonzales, Washienko, & Krone et al., 1999; Johnson, et al., 2003; Manfrin-Ledet & Porche, 2003; Pitzner, McGarry-Long, & Drummond, 2000; Resnick, Acierno, & Kilpatrick, 1997; Sowell, Phillips, & Seals, et al., 2002; Springs & Fredrich, 1992; Wise et al., 2001; Zierler, Feingold, & Laufer et al., 1991).

Risky sexual behavior places individuals at increased risk for acquiring HIV infection. Although risk-taking behavior is composed of many variables, the one common thread through numerous studies was a history of childhood sexual abuse in both men and women. In populations infected with HIV, between 30% and 87% of individuals had a history of childhood sexual abuse as compared to similar populations not infected with HIV (El-Bassel et al., 2001; Brady, Gallagher, Berger et al., 2002; Bedimo et al., 1997; Dilorio, et al., 2002; Fullilove, 1993; Gruskin, Gange, Celentano, et al., 2002; Johnson, et al., 2003; Miller, 1999; Mullings, Marquart, & Brewer, 2000; NIMH multisite HIV prevention trial, 2001; O'Leary, Purcell, Remien, et al., 2003; Stevens, Zierler, & Cram et al., 1995; Thompson et al., 1997; Wingood & DiClemente, 1997; Zierler et al., 1991; Wyatt, Myers, & Williams, et al., 2002). One contributing factor may be the increased rates of substance abuse, placing women at risk for continued poverty, incarceration, poor employment skills, and marginalization. This constellation often leaves men and women to depend on exchanging sex for money, to submit to continued partner abuse, and to neglect using condoms.

One study examining predictors of partner violence compared both male-to-female and female-to-male scenarios among African American, Hispanic, and white couples. While there were cultural differences in both groups, physical abuse in childhood by parents, impulsivity, and alcohol abuse remained the most constant predictors for intimate partner violence (Schafer, Caetano, & Cunradi, 2004).

Increased Substance Abuse

Men and women with a history of sexual violence have a higher incidence of substance abuse compared to populations that do not share that history (Morrill, Kasten, & Urato, et al., 2001; Wingood & DiClemente, 1997). In a study of injecting drug users, 68% of the women and 19% of the men reported histories of sexual violence (Braitstein, Li, & Tyndall, et al., 2003). Women were 4.25 times more likely to abuse substances if they had a history of sexual abuse compared with women who did not have a history of sexual abuse (Cohen, Deamont, & Barkan, et al., 2000). Chaotic and marginalized minority communities may serve as persistent external oppression, providing risky sexual behavior symbolic value (Wallace, Fullilove, & Flisher, 1996). Wallace (1996) suggests harm reduction community models that can build community networks and reduce sexual and substance abuse.

Lowered Self-Esteem

Leenerts (1999) describes how abusive relationships influence women's self-care practices in low-income white women infected with HIV. Sexual abuse confuses self-images, damages a woman's self-image, and breaks the spirit. In this study of the abused women, 58% used drugs. Disconnecting from self-care or health-promoting behavior was the emerging theme among women with a history of sexual abuse. Other studies have also found an association between poor self-esteem and competence among women who experienced violence including verbal abuse (Sowell, Seals, & Moneyham et al., 1999). Using the model that evolved from Leenerts' study (2003), forensic nurse examiners can build partnerships with victims to encourage self-care practices and build connections to self-care.

History of sexual abuse is even higher among incarcerated women, ranging from 55% to 73% (Browne et al., 1999; Dole, 1999; Harris, Sharps, & Allen et al., 2003; Leenerts, 2003; Stevens, Zierler, & Cram et al., 1995). In these samples childhood sexual abuse was reported in 30% to 59% of inmate cases. This rate reflects a significant difference from community-based studies of childhood sexual abuse reported at 18% (Finkelhor, 1994). Ethnicity and lower socioeconomic states may reflect some of the differences between incarcerated and community populations. Browne (1999) reported that childhood physical or sexual victimization prior to age 18 appeared to predispose women to significantly more physical violence by intimates in adulthood. In this same sample, women who were molested prior to the age of 18 were twice as likely to report sexual assaults by non-intimates in their adult lives. From this study the impact of interpersonal violence over time and generations is understood, as 82% of the women in this study had experienced "severe parental violence and/or childhood sexual abuse before reaching adulthood." Browne postulates that the long-term effects of violence are the primary reasons contributing to incarceration with associations to other risk-taking behaviors, such as substance abuse and being in precarious situations.

The adoption of mandatory drug sentencing in 1987 by the US Sentencing Commission was strengthened in 1996 and has resulted in increased rates of incarceration for women from 4% to 6%. Incarceration is a common consequence of substance abuse, accounting for 66% of women in federal penitentiaries and 33% of women in state prisons according to the Bureau of Justice Statistics in January 1998. This situation is further discussed in Chapter 50.

The majority of women feel betrayed, often sparking rage, as the majority are sexually violated by someone known to them. This anger can be turned inward as well as outward. Many women on death row are there because they murdered their assailant in partner violence cases (Bureau of Justice, 2001; Greenfield et al.,

1998; Justice Works, 2003). Tom Mason and Dave Mercer described two repeating themes of female psychopaths: lifetime of abuse beginning in early childhood, and revictimization by various institutions. PTSD with substantial Axis I and Axis II comorbidities has been documented in other works described in this chapter (Fischbach & Herbert, 1997; Heim, Newport, & Heir et al., 2000; Katon, 2001; Wise et al., 2001). Conversely, many more women return to abusive partners in the hope that their partner will change (Goss & DeJoseph, 1997).

Depression and Anxiety

Increased rates of depression and anxiety are frequently associated with sexual abuse. One study reported that 78% of women who had been physically or sexually abused had a mental illness (Leenerts, 2003). This illness can be expressed in substance abuse, as previously discussed, and in suicide and physical cutting. Childhood abuse (including sexual abuse) and household dysfunction have been highly correlated with suicide (Dube, Anda, & Felitti et al., 2001). In another study of triethnic adolescents, histories of sexual abuse, physical abuse, and environmental stresses were among five of the strong risk factors for suicide (Rew, Thomas, & Horner et al., 2001). Self-mutilation and self-injury are often cries for help from persons who have been sexually abused (Steighner, 2003).

Women sexually violated by strangers describe the devastating shifts in their relationships. Partners often feel helpless and at a loss to know what to do to support their partners. Two exceptional ABC broadcasts ("Partners of Rape," *Nightline,* March 27, 2000; "Domestic Violence," *The Oprah Winfrey Show,* September 25, 2002) presented couples searching for answers regarding sexual assault, trying to comprehend the process of violence and begin healing. Few of these marriages could survive the ordeal, and the majority of the couples interviewed were divorced.

Physiological Expression of Rape Trauma Syndrome

Physical symptoms often parallel sites of bodily injury. Physical force and general body trauma is found in as many as 80% of sexual assault cases (Riggs et al., 2000; Slaughter & Brown, 1992; Slaughter, Brown, Crowley, et al., 1997). Genital injuries occur in 16% to 87% of women and in 36% of males (Biggs, Sternac, & Divinsky, 1998; Bowyer & Dalton, 1997; Dumont & Parnis, 2003; Cartwright, 1987; Riggs et al., 2000; Slaughter & Brown, 1992; Slaughter et al., 1997). Gynecological manifestations (e.g., chronic vaginal problems, changes in the menstrual cycle) may also present. Premenstrual syndrome is common in women with a history of sexual abuse (Golding, Taylor, Menard, et al., 2000). These symptoms may occur for years following the original trauma and often go undetected because history taking does not illicit questions regarding sexual trauma. RTS becomes so enmeshed in the patients over time that it is difficult to adequately assess the full impact of trauma on the human body. Only a few longitudinal studies provide answers, and few studies included control groups.

Golding, Wilsnack, and Learman (1998) found sexual assault histories to be 20% to 28% in a randomized study of the general population from two regions of the US ($n = 3131$) and one national sample ($n = 963$). Symptoms of dysmenorrhea, menorrhagia, and sexual dysfunction were common risk indicators for sexual assault with an increased probability for risk correlating with increasing numbers of symptoms. Symptoms were not well correlated to women over the age of 44, especially perimenopausal women. Only 4% to 5% of the study population had all three symptoms *and* a history of sexual assault. Few women had disclosed their sexual assault history to physicians or received mental health interventions.

During the 154th Annual Meeting of the American Psychiatric Association in May 2001 several studies suggested that estrogen may alter the biochemical effects of stress in women (Brady, 2001). PTSD can alter the stress-related neurotransmitter, neurohormonal, and immune functions. Continued trauma alters the normal burst response of the hypothalamic-adrenal-pituitary (HPA) glands that secrete cortisol during a stressful encounter. Increased stress or severity of the situation produces higher levels of cortisol. A person with PTSD dysregulates this response by lowering the cortisol levels. The HPA glands also appear to be influenced by the hormonal levels of the menstrual cycle. A decrease in the stress response occurs during the follicular phase. Overall, women have lower cortisol levels when compared to men irrespective of PTSD in either gender. There are no PTSD-related differences in cytokine levels between genders. Another study also found a strong association with decreased estrogen levels and increased follicle-stimulating hormone (FSH) levels putting women into earlier menopause (Allworth, Zierler, Krieger, et al., 2001).

Another study of women with a history of childhood sexual abuse found a sixfold increase in adrenocorticotropic hormone (ACTH) response when the individual also had a major depression diagnosis (Heim et al., 2000). The findings suggest that a hyperactivity of the HPA glands and autonomic nervous system exists in women with a history of childhood sexual abuse, possibly contributing to adulthood psychopathological conditions.

Neurological impairments are common in men and women with chronic PTSD. These impairments are increased when there is a history of childhood or adult sexual abuse, and are often missed. Soft neurological signs were found in 82% of persons with a history of PTSD (Gurvits et al., 2000). Soft signs include subtle abnormalities in language and motor coordination such as motor hyperactivity, attention deficit, learning problems, or enuresis. Childhood physical abuse is associated with higher rates of migraines in adulthood (Goodwin, Hoven, & Murison et al., 2003).

Chronic abdominal pelvic pain is a common complaint of women who have a history of sexual assault and sexual abuse (Schei & Bakketeig, 1989; Carlson, Miller, & Fowler , 1994; Golding et al., 1998; Harrop-Griffiths et al., 1988; Laws, 1993; Mathias et al., 1996; Rapkin et al., 1990; Reiter, Shakerin, Gambone, et al., 1991; Walling et al., 1994; Wurtele et al., 1990). Women with a history of childhood sexual abuse were more likely to utilize more healthcare services and to report more chronic pain symptoms (Finestone et al., 2000). For healthcare providers, evaluating this symptom is frustrating because documenting the etiology is difficult. Often a history of sexual violence is not elicited.

Studies have found that women with a history of sexual assault avoid gynecological care because the pelvic examination triggers memories of fear, loss of control, and vulnerability (Dole, 1998; Golding et al., 1998; Robohm & Buttenheim, 1996). Women with a history of sexual abuse are less likely to have routine screening such as Papanicolaou (pap) smears, placing women at increased risk for undetected cervical disease (Harsanyi, Mott, & Kendell, 2003; Golding et al., 1998), and suggesting that a history of no pap smear may represent undiagnosed PTSD. Failure to screen for sexual abuse prior to a pelvic examination may actually be conceptualized as revictimization (King, 1999). Patients relive the sexual assault and often dissociate during the examination.

Professional colleagues have witnessed such extreme dissociation and anxiety that patients have leaped off the examination table while the speculum is still in place within the vagina. Labor and delivery rooms are another source of dissociation that actually potentiates the experience of being out of control and increases pain sensitivity (Heritage, 1998).

Rape Trauma Syndrome and Sexual Health

Dyspareunia and urinary tract infections are common sequelae in women with sexual trauma and may represent current intimacy problems. PTSD flashbacks, decreased sexual desire, or fears of forced intercourse with a coercive intimate partner decrease vaginal lubrication, contributing to dyspareunia and urinary tract infections. In the absence of pathological findings, current sexual coercion or RTS should be considered the primary diagnosis in dyspareunia. This "cry for help" may also represent a form of testing the professionals' ability to support her should she decide to disclose.

As previously mentioned, self-care is decreased in persons with a history of childhood sexual abuse and sexual assault. Past sexual abuse is a high predictor of not using condoms, increasing the risk of STIs previously discussed (Witte et al., 2000). It also increases the risk for unwanted pregnancy.

Thirty percent to 40% of victims reported that their sexual functioning had not returned to normal for up to six years later (Burgess & Holmstrom, 1979; Peter & Whitehall; 1998). Pattern styles of women with a history of child sexual abuse is categorized as anger, passive, reenacting, or chaotic (Perez, Kennedy, & Fullilove, 1995). These pattern styles may shape the individuals' sexual interaction affecting choice of safe partners, adoption of safer sexual practices, and whether they promptly recognize STIs. An example of the passive style is characterized by this response: "I just lay there and you do what you got to do." (Perez, et al., 1995, p. 88) The reenactment style seems to test fate and danger repeatedly in relationships, often bringing women to a new crisis or trauma. The chaotic style is particularly destructive and possibly addictive to women with a history of childhood sexual abuse. It is propelled by the need for continual crisis or trauma. The angry-styled individual is always hostile and fighting. Fragmented sense of self pervades these pattern styles, preventing healthy sexual or intimate relationships, and involves the characteristics listed in Box 27-2.

Nursing Implications

Healthcare professionals feel that they are too busy and state that histories of sexual assault or abuse are not a priority. Unfortunately, this omission often represents a missed opportunity to assist patients in beginning the healing process by telling their story. Often it simply takes "planting the seed."

Box 27-2 Barriers to Healthy Sexual Functioning

- Inability to problem solve
- Increased risk-taking behavior
- Poor boundaries
- Increased teenage pregnancy
- Continuum extremes from promiscuity to lack of sexual desire
- Decreased intimacy
- Dyspareunia
- Chronic pelvic pain

Case Study 27-1 The Patient and Healthcare Provider Relationship

A survivor of childhood incest and domestic violence shared the importance of "planting the seed" by healthcare providers in order to change the situation and heal oneself. At the time she relayed this event, she had 10 years of sobriety free from drug and alcohol use and was employed with a publishing company. Now 34 years old, this black woman described her experience on welfare and involvement in a series of abusive relationships.

She had connected with an obstetrician in one of the clinics who had seen her on several occasions. Each time the healthcare provider had examined her there were multiple bruises on her body, in various stages of healing. Each time, the obstetrician would comment on the bruises and ask if she was in a safe environment. There was never a lengthy discussion or a perceived judgmental attitude on behalf of the healthcare provider. During the fifth visit, a postpartum check up, the obstetrician observed several bruises on the patient's legs and stated, "You know, you don't have to live this way."

Several weeks later, following another battering incident, the woman remembered those words. She stated she was able to pick up her baby and go to a shelter for help. She now states that "it was the scariest yet best thing I ever did, having no money, no skills, and no support." The option to leave may not have occurred to her had the obstetrician not planted that seed. This woman added that healthcare providers don't have to "fix the situation," just raise the conscious awareness of the patient, show compassion without judgment, and support her during the process. The responsibility for reshaping her life rests with the individual.

This scenario discussed in Case Study 27-1 expresses the trust and compassion between patient and healthcare provider. The importance of such a relationship has been extensively reported in literature describing elements of adherence or harm reduction. Although few data exist evaluating follow-up programs for victims of sexual assault, perhaps drawing upon related women's health literature regarding cervical disease follow-up can provide insight. Several studies identified that personal contact by their healthcare provider was the most important variable to future appointment adherence (Abercrombie, 2000; Segnan, Senore, Giordano, et al., 1998). A tracking system is helpful to remind patients of a forthcoming appointment and to document missed appointments (Marcus, Kaplan, Crane, et al., 1998; Paskett, Phillips, & Miller, 1995). Developing a protocol that includes phone calls and letters from the sexual assault nurse examiner/forensic nurse examiner (SANE/SAFE/FNE) may be beneficial in decreasing ongoing missed appointments (Miller, Siejak, & Schroeder et al., 1997). Consideration must be given to patients' desire to be contacted, especially with minors and individuals at risk for domestic violence. Three controlled studies found that an educational brochure available in the clinic or sent to nonadherent patients significantly reduced missed appointments (Paskett, Phillips, & Miller, 1995; Paskett, Carter, & Chu et al., 1990; Stewart, Bucheggar, & Lickrish et al., 1994). Failure by healthcare professionals to communicate the possible consequences (of sexual assault) has also been found to be a primary factor in missed appointments (Lerman, Miller, & Scarborough et al., 1991).

Mental illness and childhood abuse are primary reasons for missed clinic appointments among indigent adults (Curry & Bristol, 2003; Leenerts, 2003; Pieper & DiNardo, 1998). Socioeconomic disparities in access to healthcare may contribute to undiagnosed PTSD among the poor. Mental health counseling is less available to individuals with lower income or those on Medicaid. Young low-income mothers with or without histories of sexual abuse are generally more depressed, irrespective of race and cultural backgrounds, when compared to women with higher levels of income (Salsberry, Nickel, & Polivka et al., 1999). Given the fact that lower income women are at increased risk for sexual assault and depression, strategies to increase adherence to follow up appointments is a challenge for forensic nurses working with this population.

Researchers have reported that healthcare professionals fail to elicit a history of incest, molestation, or sexual abuse. One study found that older nurses were more apt to screen for abuse (Boutcher & Gallop, 1996). For this reason, patients are reluctant to make this disclosure at their first encounter with healthcare professionals (Dole, 1999; Fellitti, 1991; Golding et al., 1998). When sexual abuse was disclosed to physicians, victims stated their physician was generally not helpful. Women who failed to disclose often harbored the impression that they caused or were somehow responsible for the sexual abuse having occurred, thus perpetuating the secrecy surrounding the "social taboo."

Victims of sexual violence have an increased utilization of medical care, especially in the emergency department (ED) and specialty areas (Koss et al., 1991; Felitti, 1991; Peter & Whitehall; 1998; Sigler, 1995). Given the underutilization of ED services by victims at the time of the traumatic event, screening for sexual violence may be the only method to unveil prior injuries and victimization. Most certainly, professionals in all areas of women's healthcare (both gynecology and obstetrics), adolescent health, and psychiatry could be trained to recognize the signs and symptoms of current and past sexual abuse. Proactive screening for sexual abuse is key to promoting healing and breaking the cycle of violence. However, curricula for medical school and extended care providers (such as physician assistants and nurse practitioners) often lack any information about the signs and symptoms of violence (Koss, 1991; Flitcraft, 1995). Graduates from these programs are not able to realize their potential to initiate services for women. Clinical medicine and psychiatric assessments fail to explore sexual histories and abuse histories regarding physical and sexual violence. It must be noted that violence is the major cause of injury to women between the ages of 15 and 44 years.

Education and Prevention

A study by Moore, Zaccaro, and Parsons (1998) found that 66% of nurses had received some education about domestic violence. Most still believed that abuse was not a problem in their population and therefore did not screen for abuse. Nurses and healthcare providers often avoid using screening tools for fear that a patient will admit to being a victim of abuse, which may cause the healthcare professionals to feel inadequate to deal with it (Nieves-Khouw, 1997). Nurses who themselves were victims of abuse and violence and had not healed their own trauma were unable to fully engage in the screening questions. Unresolved abuse and trauma impacts on the physical, emotional, sexual, and spiritual well-being of the patients and the nurse. Education is the key to empowering nurses and victims. Once verbalization begins, the FNE can begin assisting patients in creating a safer and more balanced life (Draucker & Stern, 2000).

Increasing knowledge at all levels is the best form of prevention. Utilizing the nursing process will guide nursing interventions in the hospital, community, and classroom. Curricula should include education about the myths and realities related to gender bias and unequal gender rights.

Proactive programs in secondary schools, colleges, and the workplace can facilitate decreasing the causes of interpersonal violence. Many men and women do not understand boundaries or the definitions of sexual violence (Parrot, Cummings, & Marchell, 1994; Simon & Golden, 1996; Simon & Harris, 1993a). In a longitudinal study of adolescents and college women, 88% reported at least one incident of physical or sexual victimization (Smith, White, & Holland, 2003). In this same study, 66% of the women suffered more severe forms of sexual or physical violence (Smith et al., 2003). Special attention is given to athletic departments and to providing education about acquaintance rape (Benedict, 1998). The following statements reflect this lack of knowledge:

- 15% to 25% of male college students have engaged in sexual aggression (Benedict, 1998; Malmutgh et al., 1991; Parrot et al., 1994).
- 27% of sexually assaulted college women did not consider themselves victims (Simon & Harris, 1993b).
- 84% of sexual assaults on campus are acquaintance rapes, and 84% of the campus men did not feel that what they did was rape (Koss, Gidycz, & Wisniewski, 1987; Simon & Harris, 1993b).

Providing clarity regarding definitions of sexual violence and acceptable sexual interactions are important components of a prevention program. Defining sexual objectification to both men and women with examples of escalation of aggression would be included. For example, understanding that telling sexist jokes or not intervening when listening to a sexist joke is a form of sexual violence progression. A myth such as submission is consent, combined with rape fantasies, can escalate to sexual violence. Forced sex was found to be a risk factor for victims of femicide. Forced sexual aggression (including during pregnancy) was found in 57% of women killed by their partners, compared to 14.9% of women who were in abusive relationships but not victims of homicide (Campbell, Webster, Koziol-McLean, et al., 2003). Program components include discussions of sexual harassment, threats, and stalking. Behavior characteristic of sexual abuse includes catcalls, peeping toms, voyeurism, obscene phone calls, sexual harassment, and exhibitionism with flashing to minors.

Sexual assault awareness on campuses would include a task force as well as a prevention program. Brown University (as did many other universities) began a sexual assault peer education (SAPE) program in response to escalating sexual assaults. Policies and procedures regarding sexual assault must be in place and require the support of all departments on a college campus.

Guiding children to reduced encounters of violence has to become a national agenda. The national broadcasting network and the movie industry recently agreed to tighten regulations with respect to the degree of violence shown to child audiences. Revised rating systems will reflect this new philosophy with more stringent guidelines. Parents will have a better sense of the content material being viewed and can better guide their children. Parental involvement is crucial in shaping gender roles and how violence is viewed. Forensic nurses could participate in the movement to decrease violence for our children by writing reviews of movies, television programs, CDs, books, video games, and so forth for the local newspaper. Sharing the results of usage reviews on child injuries or SANE/SAFE programs can increase community involvement through increased knowledge and understanding.

Screening and Risk-Reduction Strategies

More sexual assaults are unreported (71%) when compared with the 16% to 32% of reported cases (Ciancone, Wilson, Colette, et al., 2000; Kilpatrick & Resnick, 1994). Women who are poor, are in their twenties, have PTSD, and have a prior history of sexual assault or sexual abuse are at increased risk for revictimization, especially when combined with alcohol or cocaine abuse. The 10% of women at risk for sexual assault who have a history of childhood sexual abuse, liberal sexual attitudes, higher than average alcohol use, and a larger number of sexual partners had a risk factor twofold higher than women without this profile (Crowell & Burgess, 1996). Another study found that the use of alcohol or drugs was reported in 20% of sexual assault victims (Brechlin & Ullman, 2002).

Best Practice 27-1

It is imperative that all levels of healthcare providers identify and screen for past sexual abuse or sexual assault.

In a gynecological clinic for HIV-infected individuals, the majority of women stated that they had never been asked about past sexual victimization (Dole, 1998). It should be noted that many women were asked over several visits before they were comfortable revealing the past trauma. The time needed to assess the healthcare professional and develop a trusting rapport before disclosure may also contribute to underreporting. It is important to include sexual abuse screening with each healthcare encounter. Many healthcare professionals fail to seek the truth and remain neutral during their interviews, history taking, and assessment of patients. One study revealed that 83% of sexually abused women had never disclosed the abuse to a healthcare provider (Golding et al., 2000). Doing a gynecological examination and not asking about previous trauma or assaults can revictimize patients. Unhealed trauma fueled with environmental triggers (i.e., vaginal speculum examinations) can potentially prompt flashbacks that result in dissociation from the examination. At this point, it becomes difficult to interact with patients to complete an examination. Indeed, it is often impossible to complete required procedures. Dole (1996) provides suggestions to reduce PTSD anxiety during a gynecological examination.

Secondary revictimization by healthcare providers, SANE/SAFE/FNE, or legal or police personnel is common. Stressful situations that lack privacy and respect or blame the victim make the individual feel stigmatized or devalued. Situations that revictimize the individual include ignoring the vulnerability of the victim, discounting the trauma, patronizing the victim, and making negative or judgmental comments to the victim (Valente, 2000). Failure to assess for sexual abuse upon admission to clinics or hospitals may also inadvertently create opportunities for secondary revictimization (Garber, Grindel, & Mitchell, 1997).

As already stated, many healthcare professionals feel inadequate to handle responses related to histories of sexual assault and abuse. Many times, however, simply acknowledging the assault can open dialogue and create opportunities for healing. When the patient is ready, she/he can be referred for psychotherapy. If the patient is disclosing after years of silence, several sessions to stabilize such feelings may be needed with the FNE or health provider with whom the patient has an established relationship. Otherwise, the patient may be resistant to being referred. It is essential to reassure persons that they are not alone and that the nurse will continue to support them. The PLISSIT model (Box 27-3) can offer structure for anxious healthcare providers during initial interventions with individuals who may disclose sexual abuse (Annon, 1974).

Healthcare professionals in all disciplines need education included in their respective curricula to promote assessment and identification of sexual assault and sexual abuse (Box 27-4). The PLISSIT model adapted from the psychological discipline can be used by similar disciplines to provide specific guidelines and to decrease inadequate feelings regarding asking the questions listed in Box 27-4.

Box 27-3 Examples for Using the PLISSIT Model

P = permission
LI = limited information
SS = specific suggestion
IT = intensive therapy

Examples for using the elements of the PLISSIT model include the following:

P = Asking the question regarding sexual assault and abuse gives the person *permission* to disclose and share associated concerns.

LI = Choose the associated concern that you feel most prepared to address and make a professional statement about it. For instance, providing reassurance that many individuals experience difficult intimate relations or feel blame for the sexual assault generates a sense that they may share similar experiences with others. Patients at this point are generally feeling like they are the only ones with this concern or difficulty. Providing *information* specific to the concern can assist the individual in feeling less alone in the process and relieve guilt or shame. Perhaps the patient is experiencing dyspareunia related to psychological effects of sexual trauma (pathological etiologies have been eliminated), and you suggest that fear may be decreasing a woman's ability to lubricate sufficiently for sexual intercourse. Providing *limited information* conveys reassurance to enter into open dialogue. Those who doubt the healthcare professional's willingness to engage in the process of sorting out the consequences of the sexual assault may be relieved by this interaction.

SS = Providing a *specific suggestion* or task to complete before returning assures the patient that you are concerned about his or her well-being and return to health. Often asking if the patient is ready to forgive the perpetrator to promote the patient's own health provides the health professional insight as to where the patient is in the healing process and what coping mechanisms he or she may have. Asking patients to think about what they would like to accomplish and what trauma-related concerns may be holding them back will provide information about what to specifically suggest. With respect to the dyspareunia, suggesting the use of K-Y Jelly or Astroglide prior to penetration during sex provides individuals with a possible solution to problematic situations with their partner. Ask the patient to report back on the suggestion's effectiveness. This type of dialogue can be ongoing, contributing to the patient-provider relationship.

IT = *Intensive therapy* generally involves a referral to a therapist, support group, pastoral care, or whatever seems appropriate for the individual.

Box 27-4 Sexual Assault Screening Questions

- Have you been hit, slapped, kicked, or otherwise hurt by someone in the last year? If so, by whom?
- In your lifetime have you ever been forced to have sex when you didn't want to?
- In your lifetime have you ever had your private areas touched when you didn't want them touched?
- Is there a partner from a previous relationship who is making you feel unsafe now?
- Are you safe in your present relationship?
- Has a partner ever embarrassed, humiliated, or insulted you?
- Do you fear for your safety or the safety of your children from a past or present partner?
- Has a partner ever withheld money from you or your children?
- Did you seek professional assistance for this/these incidence(s) or report to the police?
- How can I assist you with these concerns?

Data from Association of Women's Health, Obstetrics and Neonatal Nurses (AWHONN). (1999). Partner & abuse violence screen. In *Universal screening for domestic violence* (p. 12). Washington, DC: Author; Campbell, J. C. (1995). *Assessing dangerousness: Violence by sexual offenders, batterers, and child abusers* (p. 84). Thousand Oaks, CA: Sage Publications; Straus, M. A. (1979). Measuring family conflict and violence. The conflict tactics scale. *J Marriage Fam, 41*, 75-88; Straus, M. A. (1990). Measuring intrafamily conflict and violence: The conflict tactics scales. In M. A. Straus & R. J. Gelose (Eds.), *Physical violence in American families: Risk factors and adaptations to violence in 8,145 families* (pp. 29-47). New Brunswick, NJ: Transaction Publishers.

Forensic nurse examiners can facilitate ease for nurses and healthcare providers using these questions by providing continuing education courses. Providing knowledge and a safe environment to practice new skills will increase the likelihood that patients are routinely asked the difficult questions about their safety and unresolved trauma. Levels of consciousness and awareness can be elevated during such classes. The success of SANE programs has shifted patients' care primarily to the FNE. EDs reported that 10% or less of the sexual assault cases seen require additional examination by physicians (Ciancone et al., 2000). There is an understood, basic concept that the forensic examination is performed by a nurse with forensic education. The forensic process during an examination for child sexual abuse, sexual assault, domestic violence, or elder abuse is essentially the same, requiring the foundations of nursing and forensic science.

Follow-Up Care

The follow-up rate of sexual assault victims is low across the US and in other countries and is rarely reported above 25% (Ciancone et al., 2000; Holmes, Resnick, & Frampton, 1998; Rambow, Atkinson, & Frost, 1992). Ciancone and colleagues (2000) found that 73% of sexual assault programs could not provide information on the follow-up of their victims. This may be the result of various factors. Many victims want to forget the experience and fail to follow up appointments in an attempt to do so. Others may fear retribution from perpetrators (known or unknown) including partner violence. This is often the onset of a cascade of consequences that has already been described in this chapter. Statistics reveal that only 8% of sexual violence victims who present for treatment and evaluation to an ED receive immediate follow-up care. Early intervention has been shown to decrease the consequences of trauma, especially when coupled with social supports.

Best Practice *27-2*

The forensic nurse examiner should ensure that healthcare systems have a strong program in place to increase adherence with follow-up appointments related to sexual assault. Strict monitoring and specific remediations should be an integral component of such programs.

Other factors that may contribute to low follow-up rates include a range of possibilities. The ED is often the first contact for victims of violence. Yet the ED is not designed to do follow-up appointments. Often, there are no clear guidelines directing responsibility for missed appointments between interdepartmental referrals. Some victims refuse further contact from the healthcare facility. Outcome measures of SANE/SAFE/FNE protocols and forensic nurse performance need to include detailed methods of follow-up and referrals. SANE/SAFE/FNE programs that exist separate from the ED have the potential to excel in the area of patient follow-up. Evaluation methods must keep the victimized patient anonymous during use reviews to ensure integrity to the judicial process.

Many sexual assault programs operate through EDs. Appointments are given to return either to providers in the clinic or outside the ED. Victims are reluctant to see providers unknown to them at a time they are feeling vulnerable. The ED is often not conducive to follow-up appointments with the same provider. SANE/SAFE/FNE programs may not have strong community networks for referral and follow-up. Personnel with forensic knowledge for bridging the care between the ED and the community may not exist. This is a weakness in the many of SANE/SAFE/FNE programs.

Nurses must evaluate all patients in the same manner, regardless of whether they are medicolegal patients or not (want to prosecute or not). At trial, prosecutors may reinforce this format, as it is easier for the case when there is no additional contact with the person who collected the sexual assault evidence kit. The defense attorney may try to complicate the case with advocacy issues when there is further contact from the healthcare provider. Forensic nurse examiners often need to educate attorneys. Nurses are more than technicians who merely document evidence and collect kits. The FNE will be challenged to listen and to assess each person to develop appropriate care with patients.

Standard of care includes follow-up for any traumatized individual irrespective of the nature of trauma. Many brochures and publications have one sentence or one paragraph referring to follow-up and referral for the treatment of infectious diseases or injuries. Neither of these national guidelines provides proactive strategies to decrease the short- and long-term sequelae of sexual assault beyond infectious diseases or injuries. If healthcare providers including forensic nurses are to diagnosis, assess, treat, and refer to maximize well-being, how is this being actualized? It may be time to reexamine the guidelines and mechanisms for follow-up in all SANE/SAFE/FNE programs.

Forensic nurse examiners prepared in critical incident stress debriefing (CISD) can provide a valuable service to both patients and healthcare providers in evaluating stress related to traumatic events. It is conceivable that adding this component to SANE/SAFE/FNE curriculum would enable nurses to mobilize victims sooner and access healthcare, including keeping follow-up appointments.

Forensic nurses need to examine how they cope with stress and difficult cases in order to prevent burnout. Local chapters of the International Association of Forensic Nurses (IAFN) can provide education as well as support to nurses dealing with the devastation related to forensic cases. It is imperative for nurses to identify and outline a plan for coping with the ongoing stress related to forensic nursing.

Creating a Healing Environment

Creating a healing environment for both our patients and ourselves is essential to the promotion of wellness and to decrease burnout (Duquette, Kerouac, & Sandhu et al., 1994). Using holistic and nursing frameworks such as Martha Rogers' science-based nursing practice can guide nurses' worldview of their place within the total environment. Patients, too, are inclusive within the total environment. Traumatized patients bring disorganized energy patterns to this environmental field that affect the nurse as well as others in the periphery of this field. The SANE/SAFE/FNE who has just had an argument with another person and is entering the room to care for the patient brings disorganized energy patterns to the environment. However, the nurse who is "centered," well rested, and has an optimistic outlook on life brings a calm, caring, organized energy pattern to the environment. This harmonious energy pattern has the potential to defuse the traumatized disorganized field of the patient.

Best Practice *27-3*

A healing environment should be created for caregivers as well as victims of sexual assault.

Centering provides the nurse access to inner peace and tranquility. It also provides the nurse with a shield from the violent energy patterns of the victimized patient. Continued exposure to chaotic and violent energy can be detrimental to nurses and other healthcare providers and may contribute to burnout over time (Duquette, Kerouac, & Sandhu et al., 1994; McKivergin, Wimberly, & Loversidge et al., 1996). Centering allows the individual to access the inner self where tranquility prevails and suffering does not exist. Teaching patients to center can provide them with a tool to help heal and manage the current trauma. Asking patients what method they utilize to access calm and quiet, then assisting the patient to reach such a state, may help to empower patients during a difficult situation. Nurses who center during the forensic examination are less likely to be traumatized by the event and can potentiate a healing environment. (For more information regarding centering see Krieger, 2002; Krieger, 1997; Laurie & Tucker, 1993; and Macrae, 2001.)

Reducing the external chaotic energy of a busy ED will be beneficial to promoting calm. Earth tone colors and classical music that is wordless and grounded but not airy can also promote a sense of calm. However, all the external finishing will not replace the power of the internal tranquility of the centered nurse. Sometimes the nurse will develop adverse associations to the colors, music, or situations that parallel those of the forensic examination room. This may be an indication that the nurse was not centered and could place the nurse at risk for burnout and PTSD (Box 27-5).

Box 27-5 Signs and Symptoms of Burnout

PHYSICAL

Insomnia and fatigue
Stiff neck or shoulders
Upper back pain
Chest or abdominal pain
Palpitations
Clammy hands
Dry mouth
Diarrhea
Anorexia or unusual hunger

EMOTIONAL

Frustration
Isolation from friends and peers
Grief, numbed to suffering of patients and loved ones
Depression
Sense of powerlessness
Fear
Anxiety
Inflexibility
Rage
Criticizing others
Self-righteousness
Hopelessness
Sense of worthlessness
Behavioral problems
Short attention span
Overactivity
Irritability
Grinding teeth
Short temper
Control or power trips
Crying easily
Blaming
Procrastination
Negative attitude
Chattering endlessly
Changes in libido
Taking risks
Driving recklessly

AT WORK

Distancing from patients
Negative self-evaluations

Many resources are available to meet the psychosocial needs of sexual violence victims. Nurses should not overlook even the simplest and most obvious options during follow-up appointments. At all stages of recovery it is important to take every opportunity to empower patients. Offering patients choices as often as possible creates a mutual participatory process that is freeing and allows the individual to transform (Barrett, 1990).

Summary

Forensic nurse examiners can identify the needs of their community and state in caring for victims of interpersonal and sexual

Power Enhancement

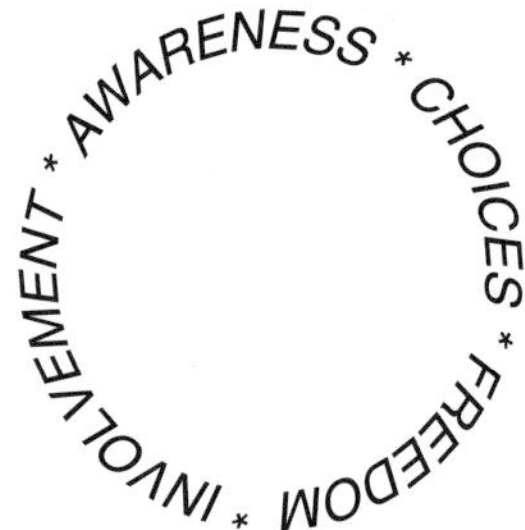

Fig. 27-1 Model showing elements of power enhancement. (From Barrett, E. A. (1998). Power Enhancement. *Nurs Sci Q, 11,* 94-96.)

violence. The more diverse a forensic program can be within a community, the more choices are available both to the community and the victim. With choices, knowledge, and participation communities and individuals feel free and empowered. Communities and victims can reduce the effects of trauma and associated PTSD when they perceive that they have power (Fig. 27-1).

Forensic nurse examiners can pave the way by developing community friendly SANE/SAFE/FNE programs, raising the awareness of communities regarding the problems and morbidity related to sexual abuse, and developing a community initiative in all areas of the government agencies, private businesses, schools, and hospitals. Lobbying for adequate healthcare coverage and economic foundation for such programs is also crucial. Some of the current challenges for forensic nurses include enacting laws, securing sufficient funding for forensic programs, keeping the state board of nurse examiners informed, educating communities, standardizing SANE/SAFE/FNE programs and education, developing standards of care that now include certification, and conducting research while caring for victims of violence.

Nurses have caring practices that are artful, knowledgeable, and lifesaving (Benner, 2000). Morse and Penrod (1999) describe the pathways of hope as a process of emerging from the trauma to a resultant state of transcendence. Victims who endure sexual assault are often uncertain of the outcome. Suffering is a level of knowing that acknowledges the assault. Forensic nurse examiners can facilitate hope or acceptance of the sexual assault and provide an opportunity to victims to dream about the future again. Drawing from a holistic foundation, based on sound judgment and filled with experiential wisdom, the art of nursing is a dynamic profession able to provide creative and compassionate forensic models to care for victims of sexual abuse immediately following the assault and in the months and years following the traumatic event.

Resources

Organizations

International Association of Forensic Nurses (IAFN)

East Holly Avenue, Box 56, Pitman, NJ 08071-0056; www.forensicnurse.org

National Organization on Male Sexual Victimization (US)

Box 103, 5505 Connecticut Avenue NW, Washington, DC 20015-2601; Tel: 800-738-4181

National Organization on Male Sexual Victimization (Canada)

c/o BCSMSSA, 1252 Burrard Street, #202, Vancouver, BC V6Z 1, Canada

National Sexual Violence Resource Center

123 North Enola Drive, Enola, PA 17025; Tel: 877-739-3895, 717-909-0710; www.nsvrc.org

Nurse Healers–Professional Associates International

4550 West Oakey Boulevard, Suite 111-R, Las Vegas, NV 89102; Tel: 702-870-5507; www.therapeutic-touch.org

Office for Victims of Crime Resource Center

Office of Justice Programs, Department of Justice, 633 Indiana Avenue NW, Room 1386, Washington, DC 20531; Tel: 202-307-5983, 800-851-3420

References

Abercrombie, P. R. (2000). Improving adherence to abnormal pap smear follow-up. *J Obstet Gynecol Nurs, 30*(1), 80-88.

AIDS Weekly Plus. (1996). Violence against women in war: Rape, AIDS, sex slavery (1996). *AIDS Weekly Plus*, Nov. 25-Dec. 2, 13-14.

Allworth, J. E., Zierler, S., Krieger, N., et al. (2001). Ovarian failure in late reproductive years in relation to lifetime experiences. *Epidemiology, 12*(6), 676-681.

American Bar Association Commission on Domestic Violence. (1996). *The impact of domestic violence on your legal practice.* Washington, DC: American Bar Association.

American Psychiatric Association (APA). (1994). *Diagnostic and statistical manual of mental disorders* (DSM-IV-TR). Washington: Author.

Amowitz, L. L., Russ, C., Lyons, K. H., et al. (2002). Prevalence of war-related sexual assault, violence, and other human rights abuses among internally displaced persons in Sierra Leone. *JAMA, 287*(4), 513-521.

Annon, J. S. (1974). *The behavioral treatment of sexual problems.* Honolulu: Enabling Systems.

Ater, R. W. (2003). Post-traumatic stress disorder. *On the Edge: The Official Publication of the International Associaton of Forensic Nurses, 9*(3), 4-7.

Association of Women's Health, Obstetrics and Neonatal Nurses (AWHONN). (1999). Partner & abuse violence screen. In *Universal screening for domestic violence.* Washington, DC: AWHONN.

Baker, T. C., Burgess, A. W., Brickman, E., et al. (1989). *Report on District of Columbia police response to domestic violence.* Joint project of the D.C. Coalition Against Domestic Violence and the Women's Law Center. Washington, DC: D.C. Coalition Against Domestic Violence.

Barrett, E. A. M. (1990). Rogers' science-based nursing practice. In E. A. M. Barrett (Ed.), *Visions of Rogers' science-based nursing* (pp. 31-44). New York: National League for Nursing.

Bedimo, A. L., Kissinger, P., & Bessinger, R. (1997). History of sexual abuse among HIV-infected women. *Int J STD AIDS, 8,* 332-335.

Benedict, J. R. (1998). *Athletes and acquaintance rape.* Thousand Oaks: Sage Publications.

Benner, P. (2000). The wisdom of our practice. *AJN, 100*(10), 99-105.

Biggs, M., Sternac, L. E., & Divinsky, M. (1998). Genital injuries following sexual assault of women with and without prior sexual intercourse experience. *Can Med Assoc, 159*(1), 33-37.

Blume, S. B. (1998). Addictive disorders in women. In R. J. Frances & S. I. Miller (Eds.), *Clinical textbook of addictive disorders* (2nd ed). New York: Guilford Press.

Boutcher, F., & Gallop, R. (1996). Psychiatric nurses' attitudes toward sexuality, sexual assault/rape, and incest. *Arch Psychiatric Nurs, 10*(3), 184-191.

Bowyer, L., & Dalton, M. E. (1979). Female victims of rape and their genital injuries. *Br J Obstet Gynaecol, 104*(5), 17-20.

Brady, K. (2001). Gender differences in PTSD. Retrieved on 1/6/02 from www.medscape.com/medscape/cno/2001/APACME/Story.cfm?story_id=2257.

Brady, S., Gallagher, D., Berger, J., et al. (2002). Physical and sexual abuse in the lives of HIV-positive women enrolled in a primary medicine health maintenance organization. *AIDS Patient Care STDs, 16*(3), 121-125.

Braitstein, P., Li, K., Tyndall, M., et al. (2003). Sexual violence among a cohort of injecting drug users. *Soc Sci Med, 57*(3), 561-569.

Brechlin, L. R., & Ullman, S. E. (2002). The roles of victim and offenders alcohol use in sexual assaults: Results from the National Violence Against Women Survey. *J Stud Alcohol, 63*(1), 57-63.

Breslau, N., Davis, G. C., Andreski, P., et al. (1991). Traumatic events and post-traumatic stress disorder in an urban population of young adults. *Arch Gen Psychiatry, 48*, 216-222.

Browne, A., Miller, B., & Maguin, E. (1999). Prevalence and severity of lifetime physical and sexual victimization among incarcerated women. *Int J Law Psychiatry, 22*(3-4), 301-322.

Brunnello, N., Davidson, J. R., Deahl, M., et al. (2001). Posttraumatic stress disorder: Diagnosis and epidemiology, comorbidity and social consequences, biology and treatment. *Neuropsychobiology, 43*(3), 150-162.

Bureau of Justice. (1998). *Statistics: Substance abuse among offenders.* Washington, DC: Author.

Bureau of Justice. (2001). *Crime characteristics: Violent crime-victim/offender relationship.* Washington, DC: Author. Retrieved from www.ojp.gov/bjs/cvict_c.

Bureau of National Affairs. (1990). *Violence and stress: The work/family connection.* Special report #32. Washington, DC: Author.

Burgess, A. W., Fehder, W. P., & Hartman, C. R. (1995). Delayed reporting of the rape victim. *J Psychosoc Nurs, 34*(10), 21-29.

Burgess, A. W., & Holmstrom, L. L. (1974). Rape trauma syndrome. *Am J Psychiatry, 131*(9), 981-986.

Burgess, A. W., & Holmstrom, L. L. (1979). Rape: Sexual disruption and recovery. *Am J Orthopsychiatry, 49*, 648-657.

Campbell, J. C., Webster. D., Koziol-McLean, J., et al. (2003). Risk factors for femicide in abusive relationships: Results from a multisite case control study. *Am J Public Health, 93*(7), 1089-1097.

Carlson, K. J., Miller, B. A., & Fowler, F. J. (1994). The Maine women's health study: II. Outcomes of nonsurgical management of leiomyomas, abnormal bleeding, and chronic pelvic pain. *Obstet Gynecol, 83*(4), 566-572.

Cartwright, P. S. (1987). Factors that correlate with injury sustained by survivors of sexual assault. *Obstet Gynecol, 70*(1), 44-46.

CDC. (1998). Lifetime and annual incidence of intimate partner violence and resulting injuries–Georgia, 1995. *MMWR, 47*(40), 849-853.

Champion, J. D., Shain, R. N., Piper, J., et al. (2001). Sexual abuse and sexual risk behaviors of minority women with sexually transmitted diseases. *West J Res, 23*(3), 241-254.

Ciancone, A. C., Wilson, C., Collette, R., et al. (2000). Sexual assault nurse practitioner programs in the United States. *Ann Emerg Med, 35*(4), 353-357.

Clarke, S., & Pearson, C. (2000). Personal constructs of male survivors of childhood sexual abuse receiving cognitive analytic therapy. *Br J Med Psychol, 73*(2), 169-177.

Coid, J., Petruckevitch, A., Feder, G., et al. (2001). Relationship between childhood sexual and physical revictimisation in women: A cross-sectional survey. *Lancet, 358*(9280), 450-454.

Cohen, M., Deamant, C., Barkan, S., et al. (2000). Domestic violence and childhood sexual abuse in HIV-infected women and women at risk for HIV. *Am J Public Health (AJPH), 90*(4), 560-565.

Crowell, N. A., & Burgess, A. W. (Eds). (1996). *Understanding violence against women.* Washington, DC: National Academy Press.

Curry, M., & Bristol, J. (2003). The effects of childhood abuse on adherence and health. *Focus, 18*(5), 5-6.

Dilorio, C., Hartwell, T., & Hansen, N. (2002). Childhood sexual abuse and risk behavior among men at high risk for HIV infection. *Am J Public Health, 92*(2), 214-219.

Dole, P. (1996). Centering: Reducing rape trauma syndrome anxiety during a gynecologic examination. *J Psychosoc Nurs, 34*(10), 32-37.

Dole, P. (1998). Examining sexually traumatized incarcerated women. *HEPP News (HIV Education Prison Project), 2*(6), 5.

Dole, P. J. (May 15-29, 1999). The impact of PTSS on GYN clinic adherence of paroled women with HIV disease in a New York City hospital based program. (Abstract). American Academy of Nurse Practitioner's Annual Meeting, Atlanta, GA.

Draucker, C. B., & Madsen, C. (1999). Women dwelling with violence. *Image: J Nurs Scholarship, 31*(4), 327-332.

Draucker, C. B., & Stern, P. N. (2000). Women's responses to sexual violence by male intimates. *West J Nurs Res, 22*(4), 385-306.

Dube, S. R., Anda, R. F., Felitti, V. J., et al. (2001). Childhood abuse, household dysfunction, and the risk of attempted suicide. *J Am Medical Assoc, 286*(24), 3089-3095.

Dumont, J., & Parnis, D. (2003). Forensic nursing in the context of sexual assault: Comparing the opinions and practices of nurse examiners and nurses. *Appl Nurs Res, 16*(3), 173-183.

Duquette, A, Kerouac, S., Sandhu, B. K., et al. (1994). Factors related to nursing burnout: A review of empirical knowledge. *Iss Ment Health Nurs, 15*, 337-358.

El-Bassel, N., Gilbert, L., Frye, V., et al. (2004). Physical and sexual intimate partner violence among women in methadone maintenance treatment. *Psychology of Addictive Behavior, 18*(2), 180-183.

El-Bassel, N., Witte, S. S., Wada, T., et al. (2001). Correlates of partner violence among female street-based sex workers: Substance abuse, history of childhood abuse, and HIV risks. *AIDS Patient Care STDs, 15*(1), 41-51.

Epstein, J., & Langenbahn, S. (1994). The criminal justice and community response to rape. In *Issues and practices in criminal justice.* Washington, DC: National Institute of Justice, US Department of Justice.

Fater, K., & Mullaney, J. A. (2000). The lived experience of adult male survivors who allege childhood sexual abuse by clergy. *Iss Ment Health Nurs, 21*(3), 281-295.

Federal Bureau of Investigation (FBI). (1993). *Uniform crime reports.* Washington, DC: US Department of Justice.

Feeny, N. C., Zoellner, L. A., & Foa, E. B. (2002). Treatment outcomes for chronic PTSD among female assault victims with borderline personality characteristics: A preliminary examination. *J Personal Disord, 16*(1), 30-40.

Felitti, V. J. (1991). Long-term medical consequences of incest, rape, and molestation. *South Med J, 84*(3), 328-331.

Fergusen, D. M., Horwood, L. J., & Lynskey, M. T. (1997). Childhood sexual abuse, adolescent sexual behaviors and sexual revictimization. *Child Abuse Neglect, 21*(8), 789-803.

Finestone, H. M., Stenn, P., Davies, F., et al. (2000). Chronic pain and health utilization in women with a history of childhood sexual abuse. *Child Abuse Neglect, 24*(4), 547-556.

Finkelhor, D. (1994). The international epidemiology of child sexual abuse. *Child Abuse Neglect, 18*, 409-417.

Fischbach, R. L., & Herbert, B. (1997). Domestic violence and mental health: Correlates and conundrums within and across cultures. *Soc Sci Med, 45*(8), 1161-1176.

Flitcraft, A. (1995). From public health to personal health: Violence against women across the lifespan. *Ann Intern Med, 123*, 800-801.

Fullilove, M. T., Fullilove, R. E., Smith, M., et al. (1993). Violence, trauma, and post-traumatic stress disorder among women drug users. *J Trauma Stress, 6*(4), 533-543.

Fullilove, M. T., Lown, E. A., & Fullilove, R. E. (1992). Crack "hos and skeezers": Traumatic experiences of women crack users. *J Sex Res, 29*(2), 275-287.

Garber, A., Grindel, C., & Mitchell, D. (1997). Assessing for sexual abuse. *J Psychosoc Nurs, 35*(3), 26-30.

Gardner, R., & Blackburn, R. (1996). People who move: New reproductive health focus. *Pop Rep, 24*(3; Series J, #45), 1-13.

Golding, J. M., Wilsnack, S. C., & Learman, L. A. (1998). Prevalence of sexual assault history among women with common gynecologic symptoms. *Am J Obstet Gynecol, 179*(4), 1013-1019.

Golding, J. M., Taylor, D. L., Menard, L., et al. (2000). Prevalence of sexual abuse history in a sample of women seeking treatment for premenstrual syndrome. *J Psychosom Obstet Gynecol, 21*(2), 69-80.

Gollub, E. L. (1999). Human rights is a US problem, too: The case of women and HIV. *Am J Public Health, 89*(10), 1479-1482.

Gonzales, V., Washienko, K. M., Krone, M. R., et al. (1999). Sexual and drug-use risk factors for HIV and STDs: A comparison of women with and without bisexual experiences. *Am J Public Health, 89*(12), 1841-1846.

Goodwin, R. D., Hoven, C. W., Murison, R., et al. (2003). Association between childhood physical abuse and gastrointestinal disorders and migraine in adulthood. *Am J Public Health, 93*(7), 1065-1066.

Goss, G. L., & DeJoseph, J. (1997). Women who return to abusive relationships: A frustration for the critical care nurse. *Crit Care Nurs Clin North Am, 9*(2), 159-165.

Greenfield, L. A., Rand, M. R., & Craven, D. (1998). *Violence by intimates: Analysis of data on crimes by current or former spouses, boyfriends, and girlfriends.* Washington, DC: US Dept. of Justice.

Grisso, J. A., Schwarz, D. F., Hirschinger, N., et al. (1999). Violent injuries among women in an urban area. *N Engl J Med (NEJM), 241*(25), 1899-1905.

Gruskin, L., Gange, S. J., Celentano, D., et al. (2002). Incidence of violence against HIV-infected and uninfected women: findings from the HIV Epidemiology Research (HER) study. *J Urban Health, 79*(4), 512-524.

Gurvits, T. V., Gilbertson, M. W., Lasko, N. B., et al. (2000). Neurological soft signs in chronic posttraumatic stress disorder. *Arch Psychiatry, 57*, 181-186.

Hall, L. A., Sachs, B., & Rayens, M. K. (1998). Mothers' potential for child abuse: The roles of childhood abuse and social resources. *Nurs Res, 47*(2), 87-95.

Hanna, B. (1996). Sexuality, body image, and self-esteem: The future after trauma. *J Trauma Nurs, 3*(1), 13-20.

Harris, R. M., Sharps, P. W., Allen, K., et al. (2003). The interrelationship between violence, HIV/AIDS, and drug use in incarcerated women. *J Assoc Nurses AIDS Care, 14*(1), 27-40.

Harrop-Griffiths, J., Katon, W., Walker, E., et al. (1988). The association between chronic pelvic pain, psychiatric diagnoses, and childhood sexual abuse. *Obstet Gynecol, 71*(4), 589-594.

Harsanyi, A., Mott, S., & Kendell, S. (2003). The impact of a history of child sexual assault on a woman's decisions and experiences of cervical screening. *Aust Fam Physician, 32*(9), 761-762.

Hazelwood, R. R., & Burgess, A. W. (1995). *Practical aspects of rape investigation: A multidisciplinary approach* (2nd ed.). Boca Raton, FL: CRC Press.

Heim, C., Newport, D. J., Heit, S., et al. (2000). Pituitary-adrenal and autonomic response to stress in women after sexual and physical abuse in childhood. *JAMA, 8*, 2321-2322.

Heritage, C. (1998). Working with childhood sexual abuse survivors during pregnancy, labor, and birth. *J Obstet Gynecol Nurs, 27*(6),671-677.

Holmes, M. M., Resnick, H. S., & Frampton, D. (1998). Follow up of sexual assault victims. *Am J Obstet Gynecol, 179*(2), 336-342.

Jasinski, J. L., Williams, L. M., & Siegel, J. (2000). Childhood physical and sexual abuse as risk factors for heavy drinking among African-American women: A prospective study. *Child Abuse Neglect, 24*(8), 1061-1071.

Jewkes, R., Martin, L., & Penn-Kekana, L. (2002). The virgin cleansing myth: Cases of child rape are not exotic. *Lancet, 359*(9307), 711.

Johnson, S. D., Cunnington-Williams, R. M. & Cotter, L. B. (2003). A tripartite of HIV-risk for African American women: the intersection of drug use, violence, and depression. *Drug and Alcohol Dependence*, 70, 169-175.

Justice Works. (2003). Mothers in prison national facts. Retrieved on 6/8/03 from www.justiceworks.org/factsheets/mip.

Katon, W. (2001). Complex posttraumatic stress disorder. Retrieved from www.medscape.com/Medscape/CNO/Story.cfm?story_id=2260.

Kenny, M. C., & McEachern, A. G. (2000). Racial, ethnic, and cultural factors of a childhood sexual abuse: a selected review of the literature. *Clin Psychol Rev, 20*(7), 905-922.

Kerimova, J., Posner, S. F., Brown, Y. T., et al. (2003). High prevalence of self-reported forced sexual intercourse among internally displaced women in Azerbaijan. *Am J Public Health, 93*(7), 1067-1070.

Kilpatrick, D. G., & Resnick, H. S. (March 1994). Rape, other violence against women, and post-traumatic stress disorder: Critical issues in assessing the adversity-stress-psychopathology relationship. 84th Annual Meeting of the American Psychopathological Association, New York, NY.

King, P. (March 7, 1999). Personal communication.

Korn, M. (2001). Emerging trends in understanding post-traumatic stress disorder. Retrieved from www.medscape.com/medscape/cno/2001/APACME/Story.cfm?story_id=2258.

Koss, M. P., Gidycz, C. A., & Wisniewski, N. (1987). The scope of rape: Incidence and prevalence of sexual aggression and victimization in a National Sample of Higher Education Students. *J Consult Clin Psychol, 55* (2), 162-170.

Koss, M. P., Koss, P. G., & Woodruff, W. J. (1991). Deleterious effects of criminal victimization on women's health and medical utilization. *Arch Intern Med, 151*,342-347.

Krieger, D. (2002). *Therapeutic touch as transpersonal healing.* New York: Lantern Books.

Krieger, D. (1997). *Therapeutic Touch.* Santa Fe: Bear & Company.

Kulka, R. A., Fairbank, J. A., Jordan, B. K., et al. (1990). *Trauma and the Vietnam war generation.* NY: Brunner/Mazel.

Kyriacou, D. N., Anglin, D., Taliaferro, E., et al. (1999). Risk factors for injury to women from domestic violence. *N Engl J Med, 341*(25), 1892-1898.

Laurie, S. G., & Tucker, M. J. (1993). *Centering: A guide to inner growth* (2nd ed.). Rochester, VT: Destiny Books.

Laws, A. (August 1993). Sexual abuse history and women's medical problems. *J Gen Intern Med, 8*, 441-443.

Ledray, L. E. (1994). *Recovering from rape.* New York: Henry Holt.

Ledray, L. E. (1990). Counseling rape victims: The nursing challenge. *Perspect Psychiatr Care, 26*(2), 21-27.

Leenerts, M. H. (1999). The disconnected self: Consequences of abuse in a cohort of low-income white women living with HIV/AIDS. *Health Care Women Int, 20*, 381-400.

Leenerts, M. H. (2003). From neglect to care: A theory to guide HIV-positive incarcerated women in self-care. *J Assoc Nurses AIDS Care, 14*(5), 25-38.

Lema, V. M. (1997). Sexual abuse of minors: Emerging medical and social problem in Malawi. *East Afr Med J, 74*(11), 743-746.

Lerman, C., Miller, S. M., Scarborough, R., et al. (1991). Adverse psychological consequences of positive cytological cervical screening. *Am J Obstet Gynecol, 165*, 658-662.

Macrae, J. A. (2001). Nursing as a spiritual practice: A contemporary application of Florence Nightingale's views. New York: Springer Publishing Company.

Mathias, S. D., Kuppermann, M., Liberman, R. F., et al. (1996). Chronic pelvic pain: Prevalence, health related quality of life, and economic correlates. *Obstet Gynecol, 87*(3), 321-327.

Malmutgh, N. M., Sockloskie, R. J., Koss, M. P., et al. (1991). Characteristics of aggressors against women: Testing a model using a national sample of college students. *J Consult Clin Psychol, 59*, 670-681.

Manfrin-Ledet, L., & Porche, D. J. (2003). The state of science: violence and HIV infection in women. *J of the Ass Nurses in AIDS Care, 14*(6), 56-68.

Marcus, A., Kaplan, C., Crane, L., et al. (1998). Reducing loss-to-follow-up among women with abnormal pap smears. *Med Care, 36*, 397-410.

McEvoy, A., Rollo, D., & Brookings, J. (1999). *If he is raped: A guide for parents, partners, spouses, and friends.* Holmes Beach, FL: Learning Publications.

McKivergin, M., Wimberly, T., Loversidge, J. M., & Fortman, R. H. (1996). Creating a work environment that supports self-care. *Holistic Nurs Pract, 10*(2), 78-88.

Meel, B. L. (2003). The myth of child rape as cure for HIV/AIDS in Transkei: A case report. *Med Sci Law, 43*(1), 85-88.

Meyers, H. (January 6, 1992). The billion-dollar epidemic. *Am Med News*. American Medical Association.

Miller, T. M., Cohen, M. A., & Weirsema, B. (1996). *Victim costs and consequences: A new look*. Research Report NCJ 155282. Washington, DC: US Department of Justice, Office of Justice Programs, and US Department of Health and Human Services, Maternal and Child Health Bureau.

Miller, M. (1999). A model to explain the relationship between sexual abuse and HIV risk among women. *AIDS Care, 11*(1), 3-20.

Miller, S., Siejak, K., Schroeder, C., et al. (1997). Enhancing adherence following abnormal pap smears among low-income minority women: A preventive telephone counseling strategy. *J Natl Cancer Inst, 89*, 703-708.

Moore, D. B. (2000). Make them laugh: Therapeutic humor for patients with grief-related stress or anxiety. *Adv Nurse Practitioners, 8*(8), 34-37.

Moore, M. L., Zaccaro, D., & Parsons, L. H. (1998). Attitudes and practices of registered nurses toward women who have experienced abuse/domestic violence. *J Obstet Gynecol Neonat Nurs, 27*(2), 175-182.

Morrill, A. C., Kasten, L., Urato, M., et al. (2001). Abuse, addiction, and depression as pathways to sexual risk in women and men with a history of substance abuse. *J Substance Abuse, 13*(1-2), 169-184.

Morse, J. M., & Penrod, J. (1999). Linking concepts of enduring, uncertainty, suffering, and hope. *Image: J Nurs Scholarship, 31*(2), 145-150.

Nieves-Khouw, F. C. (1997). Recognizing victims of physical and sexual abuse. *Crit Care Nurs Clin North Am, 9*(2), 141-148.

Nightingale, F. (1959). *Notes on nursing: What it is and what it is not.* New York: Dover Publications (original work published in 1860).

NIMH multisite HIV prevention trial. (2001). A test of factors mediating the relationship between unwanted sexual activity during childhood and risky sexual practices among women enrolled in the NIMH multisite HIV prevention trial. *Women Health, 33*(1-2), 163-180.

North, C. S. (1996). Alcoholism in women: More common–and serious–than you think. *Postgrad Med, 100*(4), 221-224, 230, 232-233.

Nyamathi, A. M. (1991). Relationship of resources to emotional, somatic complaints, and high-risk behaviors in drug recovery and homeless minority women. *Res Nurs Health, 14*, 269-277.

Nyamathi, A. (1991). Relationship of resources to emotional distress, somatic complaints and high-risk behaviors in drug recover and homeless minority women. *Res Nurs Health, 14*, 269-277.

O'Leary, A., Purcell, D., Remien, R. H., & Gomez, C. (2003). Childhood sexual abuse and sexual transmission risk behaviour among HIV-positive men who have sex with men. *J Assoc Nurses AIDS Care, 15*(1), 17-26.

Parrot, A., Cummings, N., & Marchell, T. (1994). *Rape 101: Sexual assault prevention for college athletes*. Holmes Beach, FL: Learning Publications.

Paskett, E. D., Carter, W. B., Chu, J., et al. (1990). Compliance behavior in women with abnormal pap smears, developing and testing a decision model. *Med Care, 28*, 643-656.

Paskett, E. D., Phillips, K., & Miller, M. (1995). Improving compliance among women with abnormal Papanicolaou smears. *Obstet Gynecol, 86*, 353-359.

Peter, L. M., & Whitehall, D. L. (1998). Management of female sexual assault. *Am Fam Physician, 58*(4), 920-926.

Perez, B., Kennedy, G., & Fullilove, M. T. (1995). Childhood sexual abuse and AIDS. In A. O'Leary & L. S. Jemmott (Eds.), *Women at risk: Issues in the primary prevention of AIDS*. New York: Plenum Press.

Pitcher, G. J., & Bowley, D. M. (2002). Infant rape in So. Africa. *Lancet, 359*(9303), 274-275.

Pieper, B., & DiNardo, E. (1998). Reasons for missing appointments in an outpatient clinic for indigent adults. *J Am Acad Nurse Pract, 10*(8), 359-364.

Pitzner, J. K., McGarry-Long, J., & Drummond, P. D. (2000). A history of abuse and negative life events in patients with a sexually transmitted disease and in a community sample. *Child Abuse Neglect, 24*(5), 715-731.

Polusny, M. A., & Follette, V. M. (1995). Long-term correlates of child sexual abuse: Theory and review of the empirical literature. *Appl Prev Psychol, 4*, 143-166.

Putnam, F. W. (1989). *Diagnosis and treatment of multiple personality disorders*. New York: Guilford Press.

Rambow, B., Atkinson, C., Frost, T. H., et al. (1992). Female sexual assault medical and legal implications. *Ann Emerg Med, 21*, 727-731.

Rapkin, A., Kames, L., Darke, L., et al. (1990). History of physical and sexual abuse in women with chronic pain. Obstet Gynecol, *76*, 92-95.

Reiter, R. C., Shakerin, L. R., Gambone, J. C., et al. (1991). Correlation between sexual abuse and somatization in women with somatic and nonsomatic chronic pelvic pain. *Am J Obstet Gynecol, 165*(1), 104-109.

Relf, M. (2001). Battering and HIV in men who have sex with men: A critique and synthesis of literature. *J Assoc Nurses AIDS Care, 12*(3), 41-48.

Resnick, H. S., Acierno, R., & Kilpatrick, D. G. (1997). Health impact of interpersonal violence 2: Medical and mental health outcomes. *Behavior Med, 23*(summer), 65-78.

Rew, L., Thomas, N., Horner, S. D., et al. (2001). Correlates of recent suicide attempts in a triethnic group of adolescents. *J Nurs Scholarship, 33*(4), 361-367.

Riggs, N., Houray, D., Long, G., et al. (2000). Analysis of 1,076 cases of sexual assault. *Ann Emerg Med, 35*(4), 358-362.

Robohm, J. S., & Buttenheim, M. (1996). The gynecological care experience of adult survivors of childhood sexual abuse: A preliminary investigation. *Women Health, 24*(3), 59-75.

Rosen, M. L., Mercy, J. A., & Annest, J. L. (1998). The problems of violence in the United States and globally. In R. B. Wallace (Ed.), *Maxcy-Rosenau-Last: Public health & preventive medicine* (14th ed). Stamford, CT: Appleton & Lange.

Salsberry, P. J., Nickel, J. T., Polivka, B. J., et al. (1999). Self-reported health status of low-income mothers. *Image: J Nurs Scholarship, 31*(4), 375-380.

Salter, D., McMillian, D., Richards, M., et al. (2003). Development of sexually abusive behavior in sexually victimed males: A longitudinal study. *Lancet, 361*, 471-476.

Scarce, M. (1997). *Male on male rape: The hidden toll of stigma and shame.* New York: Insight Books–Plenum Press.

Schafer, J., Caetano, R., & Cunradi, C. (2004). A path model of risk factors for intimate partner violence among couples in the United States. *Journal of Interpersonal Violence, 19*(2), 127-142.

Schei, B., & Bakketeig, L. S. (1989). Gynaecological impact of sexual and physical abuse by spouse: A study of a random sample of Norwegian women. *Br J Obstet Gynaecol, 96*, 1379-1383.

Seedat, S., & Stein, D. J. (2000). Trauma and post-traumatic stress disorder in women: A review. *Int Clin Psychopharmacol, 15*(suppl 3), S25-33.

Segnan, N., Senore, C., Giordano, L., et al. (1998). Promoting participation in a population screening program for breast and cervical cancer: A randomized trial of different invitation strategies. *Tumori, 84*, 348-353.

Sigler, R. T. (1995). The cost of tolerance for violence. *J Health Care Poor Underserved, 6*(2), 124-134.

Simon, T., & Golden, B. (1996). *Dating: Peer education for reducing sexual harrassment and violence among secondary students.* Holmes Beach, FL: Learning Publications.

Simon, T. B., & Harris, C. A. (1993a). *Sex without consent: Peer education training for secondary schools* (Vol. 1). Holmes Beach, FL: Learning Publications.

Simon, T. B., & Harris, C. A. (1993b). *Peer education training for colleges and universities* (Vol. 2). Holmes Beach, FL: Learning Publications.

Slaughter, L., & Brown, C. R. (1992). Colposcopy to establish physical findings in rape victims. *Am J Obstet Gynecol, 166*, 83-86.

Slaughter, L., & Brown, C. R., Crowley, S., & Peck, R. (1997). Patterns of genital injury in female sexual assault victims. *Am J Obstet Gynecol, 176*(3), 609-616.

Smith, P. H., White, J. W., & Holland, L. J. (2003). A longitudinal perspective on dating violence among adolescent and college-age women. *Am J Public Health, 98*(7), 1104-1109.

Sowell, R. L., Phillips, K. D., Seals, B., et al. (2002). Incidence and correlates of physical violence among HIV-infected women at risk for pregnancy in the southeastern United States. *J of the Assoc of Nurses in AIDS Care, 13*(2), 30-42.

Sowell, R., Seals, B., Moneyham, L., et al. (1999). Experiences of violence in HIV seropositive women in the South-eastern United States of America. *J Adv Nurs, 30*(3), 606-615.

Springs, F. E., & Friedrich, W. N. (1992). Health risk behaviors and medical sequelae of childhood sexual abuse. *Mayo Clinic Proc, 57*, 527-532.

Steighner, K. (2003). Breaking the cycle of pain. *On the Edge: The Official Publication of the International Associaton of Forensic Nurses, 9*(3), 4-7.

Stevens, J., Zierler, S., Cram, V., et al. (1995). Risks for HIV infection in incarcerated women. *J Women's Health, 4*(5), 569-577.

Stewart, D. E., Bucheggar, P. M., Lickrish, G. M., & Sierra, S. (1994). The effect of educational brochures on follow-up compliance in women with abnormal Papanicolaou smears. *Obstet Gynecol, 81*, 280-282.

Straus, M. A., & Gelles, R. J. (1986). Societal change in family violence from 1975 to 1985 as revealed in two national surveys. *J Marriage Fam, 48*, 465-479.

Teets, J. M. (1997). The incidence and experience of rape among chemically dependent women. *J Psychoactive Drugs, 29*, 331-336.

Thompson, N. J., Potter, J. S., Sanderson, C. A., & Maibach, E. W. (1997). The relationship of sexual abuse and HIV risk behavior among heterosexual adult female STD patients. *Child Abuse Neglect, 21*(2), 149-156.

US Dept. of Health & Human Services (USDHHS). (2000). *Healthy People 2010* (Vols. 1 and 2). Washington, DC: Author.

Valente, S. M. (2000). Evaluating and managing intimate partner violence. *Nurse Pract, 25*(5), 18-35.

Viahov, D., & Galea, S. (2002). N.Y. study shows increase in PTSD and depression after Sept. 11. *Mental Health Weekly, 12*(13), 1.

Von, J. M., Kilpatrick, D. G., Burgess, A. W., et al. (1998). Rape and sexual assault. In R. B. Wallace (Ed), *Maxcy-Rosenau-Last: Public Health & Preventive Medicine* (14th ed). Stamford, CT: Appleton & Lange.

Wallace, R., Fullilove, M. T., & Flisher, A. J. (1996). AIDS, violence and behavioral coding: Information theory, risk behavior and dynamic process on core-group sociogeographic networks. *Soc Sci Med, 43*(3), 339-352.

Walling, M., O'Hara, M. W., Reiter, R., et al. (1994). Abuse history and chronic pain in women. II. A multivariate analysis of abuse and psychological morbidity. *Obstet Gynecol, 84*, 200-206.

Willis, B. M., & Levy, B. S. (2002). Child prostitution: Global health burden, research needs, and interventions. *Lancet, 359*(20), 1417-1422.

Wingood, G. M., & DiClemente, R. J. (1997). Childhood sexual abuse, HIV sexual risk, and gender relations of African-American women. *Am J Prevent Med, 13*(5), 22-24.

Wise, L. A., Zierler, S., Krieger, N., et al. (2001). Adult onset of major depressive disorder in relation to early life violent victimization: A case-control study. *Lancet, 358*(9285), 881-887.

Wisner, C. L., Gilmer, T. P., Saltzman, L. E., et al. (1999). Intimate partner violence against women: Do victims cost health care plans more? *J Fam Pract, 48*(6), 439-443.

Witte, S. S., Wada, T., El-Bassel, N., et al. (2000). Predictors of female condom use among women exchanging street sex in New York City. *Sex Transm Dis, 27*(2), 93-100.

Wolfgang, M. E., & Zahn, M. A. (1983). Criminal homicide, In S. H. Kadish (Ed.), *Encyclopedia of crime and justice*. New York: Free Press.

Wurtele, S. K., Kaplan, G. M., & Keairnes, M. (1990). Childhood sexual abuse among chronic pain patients. *Clin J Pain, 6*(2), 110-113.

Wyatt, G. E., Myers, H. F., Williams, J. K., et al. (2002). Does a history of trauma contribute to HIV risk of women of color? Implications for prevention and policy. *Am J Public Health, 92*(4), 660-665.

Zierler, S., Feingold, L., Laufer, D., et al. (1991). Adult survivors of childhood sexual abuse and subsequent risk of HIV infection. *Am J Public Health, 81*, 572-575.

Zupancic, M. K., & Kreidler, M. C. (1998). Shame and the fear of feeling. *Perspect Psychiatric Care, 34*(3), 29-34.

Chapter 28 Bereavement and Sudden Traumatic Death

Paul T. Clements, Joseph T. DeRanieri, and Gloria C. Henry

A sudden traumatic death is typically violent in nature and often the result of interpersonal violence or crime (Vigil & Clements, 2003). This form of death can be uniquely painful for the survivors, otherwise known as co-victims or victims by extension (the family members and friends who are experiencing the associated loss) (Henry-Jenkins, 1993; Spungen, 1997). A review of the bereavement literature suggests that when death occurs from sudden and unexpected circumstances, the reactions are more severe, exaggerated, and complicated. Subsequently, coping and adaptation can be overwhelmed by ongoing symptomatology related to intrapsychic and emotional trauma, grief, and bereavement, and a potential derailing of everyday functioning (Clements, Benasutti, & Henry, 2001; Clements & Weisser, 2003; Doka, 1996; Rando, 1993).

Although the cause of death varies across a vast continuum, all deaths are ultimately assigned to one of five standard manners of death: natural, accidental, homicide, suicide, and undetermined (DiMaio & DiMaio, 1993). Intuitively, it would seem that sudden traumatic deaths would include those in the categories of accidents, homicide, and suicide.

Key Point *28-1*

Natural deaths and those for which a manner of death is undetermined can also be sudden and traumatic in nature, and they may evoke a significant and complicated traumatic bereavement response in co-victims.

Death is a subject that is still spoken about in whispers and often with great trepidation, a concept society finds difficult to grasp or come to terms with (Clements, Vigil, & Manno et al., 2003; DeSpelder & Strickland, 1996). The death of a loved one is, in and of itself, a difficult situation for most. Additionally, the ensuing grieving process is a complicated and often lonely trek for those left in death's chaotic wake, and the bereaved mourner's path may be guided by ethnic and cultural traditions (Clements & Henry, 2002; Clements, Vigil, & Manno et al., 2003).

Compounding this grief process is the potential eruption and upheaval of emotions that occur in response to deaths that are sudden and traumatic. Deaths of this type are often thought of as "untimely" and "unfair," contributing to disbelief, shock, and anger from the onset. In addition, sudden traumatic death triggers a medicolegal investigation. Even though the victim can no longer speak for him- or herself, examination of the body, the surrounding environment, and related circumstances can, via the physical or trace evidence it yields, often speak for the victim. (Clements, Reid, & DeRanieri, 2003). Although the cause and manner of death may ultimately be determined, bringing an end to the medicolegal investigation, for the surviving family members and friends, the pain and suffering are just beginning.

This chapter will describe the various types of sudden traumatic death, explore the impact on survivors, describe complicated grief and bereavement after sudden traumatic death, and suggest interventions for the forensic nurse examiner (FNE) or nurse coroner (NC) who may encounter this client population.

Case Study 28-1 The Shocking Reality

Mr. and Mrs. Hatcher arrived at the medical examiner's office at 11:00 A.M. in June 1988. The combination of apprehension, confusion, and disbelief were evident on their faces as they walked through the door. After inquiring with the pleasant receptionist in the lobby, they were instructed to take a seat in the waiting area, and told that the investigator would be with them shortly. Ten minutes later, which seemed like hours, a young man approached the Hatchers. "Are you the Hatcher family?" asked the man. "Yes." replied Mrs. Hatcher, "I'm Celeste Hatcher, and this is my husband Anthony." The man replied, "I am Michael, one of the medical examiner's investigators, and I need to confirm the identity of a person who I unfortunately believe to be your daughter, Amanda." As their anxiety rapidly reached a panic level, Mr. Hatcher said "Obviously there has been some kind of mistake. Our daughter can't be dead. She is a good girl and never gets into any kind of trouble. She is in college and is getting all good grades."

The investigator, seemingly oblivious to the details of Amanda's long list of good qualities, asked the Hatchers to accompany him to the identification room, where the Hatcher's worst fears were confirmed. There lay the body of their 21-year-old daughter, Amanda. She had been badly beaten and had a single gunshot wound to her forehead. In the midst of their gasps of disbelief and tears, the investigator informed them that Amanda was beaten and brutally raped at gunpoint, and then shot in the head by the perpetrator, resulting in immediate death. Her body was found by a man walking his dog in an alley behind one of the local nightclubs. For Amanda, the pain and suffering had ended when she died at the hands of her perpetrator, but for her parents, the conflict and grief from the sudden and traumatic death of their daughter was just beginning. Mr. Hatcher commented that when he woke up that morning and put on his shoes to start the day, he never, in his wildest thoughts, imagined claiming the body of his murdered daughter at the city morgue, the result of a sudden traumatic death.

The Impact

It is impossible to accurately define or describe the impact that sudden traumatic death has on co-victims; grief and pain are very personal feelings, individually based, and potentially guided by ethnic and cultural norms (Clements & Henry, 2002; Clements, Vigil,

& Manno et al., 2003). However, grief, bereavement, and trauma are all issues that cause an unpleasant response in most humans, and these responses, relative to sudden and traumatic deaths, can be potentially disruptive and derailing to the functional tasks of everyday life. There are several pivotal points along the continuum of grief related to sudden traumatic death: death notification, the police investigation, the experience of the medical examiner's office, the media, the judicial system, the healthcare system, and reentry into the community. Each of these facets can lead to complicated bereavement and delay successful integration of the loss (Clements, 2001; Doka, 1996; Henry-Jenkins, 1993; Vigil & Clements, 2003).

Death Notification

Death notification typically heralds the beginning of traumatic bereavement for the family and friends of the victim. The police often have the unfortunate responsibility of ringing the doorbell and announcing to an unsuspecting family that their loved one is dead. Most police officers dislike this facet of their job and are often the unfortunate target of the family's denial and anger. It is important to remember that grief and bereavement intervention is not a part of the police academy's preparation for certification as a police officer. They, too, often feel overwhelmed and unprepared when making a notification of death.

Mr. Karch, whose daughter was killed by a drunk driver, recalls the police visit to his front door:

> *They asked me if I had a daughter named Annie. I knew what was coming next but I couldn't seem to hear the words coming out of the officer's mouth. It was so weird . . . I saw his mouth moving but it was like nothing was coming out! Then I was so angry at him. How dare he come to my home this late at night and tell me my daughter was dead and already down at the morgue! Poor fella . . . I look back now and feel sorry for the things I must have said to him, half of which I don't even remember. Having thought about it over and over again, I have decided that there just isn't a good way to tell someone that somebody they love is dead. There is no way to sugar-coat it and make it nicey-nice. When they are dead, it's a terrible truth. Although I still get mad when I think about the officer's words that night, I have to admit that I am still glad that he was honest with me about Annie and the way she died. Lying to somebody to save their feelings doesn't change the harsh cold reality they have to face as they wake up every morning for the rest of their lives.*

When the death is sudden and traumatic, it is difficult to grasp the concept immediately and integrate into the neural circuits of reality. When there is significant injury, dismemberment, or predeath violence or torture, there is an immediate sense of impossible rescue that can consume the surviving family members (Clements, Faulkner, & Manno, 2003). There is often an overwhelming need to think about how the loved one's death might have been made less traumatic and less painful. This intense need quickly and repeatedly collides with the ever-resurfacing reality that the loved one is already dead, and that there is nothing that can be done to save them. Even worse is the repetitive realization that it is impossible to bring them back. The permanence and irreversibility of death is a uniquely painful experience.

Although shock, numbness, and disbelief prevail, there is little time to integrate the reality of the loss before dealing with the multifaceted preparations for the funeral, the questions of family and friends, and the quest for answers that may never be found (Clements & Burgess, 2002; DeRanieri, Clements, & Henry, 2002). Many of these questions are answered with yet more questions if there is a police investigation.

Best Practice *28-1*

The forensic nurse examiner should anticipate a wide range of emotional responses from family members who have just received notification about the sudden traumatic death of a loved one. Their reaction may include anxiety, anger, and physical displays of aggression and may vary among family members.

The Police Investigation

Because the decedent may have been the victim of a crime, occupational accident, motor vehicle accident, or suicide, the event may involve unusual circumstances requiring additional exploration and investigation. It is frequently the role of the police to initiate an investigation toward understanding and clarification of the surrounding circumstances and conditions. A subsequent police investigation can be disturbing for some family members. Some family members have expressed anger at the police for making it seem as if their loved one was somehow responsible for their own tragic death.

Mr. Austin remembers when his 17-year-old son was the victim of a homicide while walking home from school:

> *The officer kept asking me if my son had any enemies, or if he was doing drugs. . . . Bo, my son, was a straight-A student, and was a good boy. He was run over on the way home from his job at the car wash, where he worked for a few hours every day so that he could take his girlfriend to the mall or to the movies on Friday night. My son was probably killed as a result of a random accident or drunk driver. I was getting really pissed off at this cop for making it sound like my Bo was involved in his own death. I know the cop was just doing his job, but my Bo was a good boy, and he hadn't been dead more than three hours, run over like a dog, and here some cop, who didn't even know my Bo, was making it sound like he did something to deserve it.*

The other dynamic that can enrage families is being questioned about the death but not being able to get any answers. As family members search for reasons in the midst of such a shocking event, desperately seeking an explanation that might somehow reduce the emotional pain and loss with which they are grappling, any person in a real, or perceived, position of authority will often be asked for answers. Unfortunately, many of the official personnel who are initially encountered are in search of answers themselves. This frustrating situation may lead to the family getting more questions instead of answers, creating a conundrum of chaos, confusion, and pain. The first person who may offer some definitive answers to the questions surrounding the death is the medical examiner, the forensic pathologist, or the nurse coroner. However, this portion of the grief process holds its own unique dynamics and burdens.

The Medical Examiner's Office

Although the work and commitment of the medical examiner's office (MEO) are of utmost importance, the MEO is unfortunately

Best Practice 28-2

Because families are often looking for answers that are not necessarily available at that time, forensic nurse examiners can enhance care by being a good listener. Taking a stance that displays care and concern can lessen the family's anxiety about not being able to get answers at that time.

tied to and intertwined with the concept of death. In fact, it is probably safe to say that no one comes through the doors of the MEO with the anticipation of a pleasant experience.

The medical examiner is responsible for determining the cause and manner of death. Frequently, this information is gleaned from the scene investigation and forensic autopsy that provides the surviving family members with the details surrounding their loved one's last minutes of life. Although painful, this knowledge forms a double-edged sword for family members, involving two types of pain that are equally unique: the pain of finally knowing the potentially gruesome facts surrounding their loved one's death, or the pain of not knowing and not reaching resolution (an "undetermined" manner of death).

For many families, the pain and confusion are further perpetuated by the need for an autopsy on the decedent. Families often struggle with what may be perceived as an additional violation and destruction of their loved one (Clements, Reid, & DeRanieri, 2003). An autopsy can be very difficult to accept in addition to the violence and pain that the victim may have already suffered prior to death. Compounding these feelings can be horrific fantasies about the autopsy in which the family may fear more pain for their loved one when the body is cut, that their loved one will be additionally mangled and disfigured.

Religious or cultural issues may also contribute to the anxiety surrounding an autopsy. Some religious practices may prohibit touching of the body by nonfamily members; religious edicts may require burial within a specific timeframe; removal of any body tissues or organs may represent loss of a portion of the dead loved one's soul (Clements, Vigil, & Manno et al., 2003). The need for additional investigation and autopsy may disrupt such practices, for the medical examiner has the legal power to delay the release of the body until all necessary specimens are collected and the autopsy is completed. This can be a complex and emotionally painful hurdle for many families. However, the autopsy may be a necessary step in the systematic medicolegal determination of cause and manner of death. Subsequently, it requires sensitivity, education, and support of families as they proceed through this segment of the aftermath of sudden traumatic death.

Key Point 28-2

The MEO plays a critical role in the aftermath of a sudden traumatic death. The findings of the MEO become the voice of the victim. Because the victim can no longer tell the facts surrounding the death, it is the role of the medical examiner to identify the circumstances surrounding the victim's death, including the cause and manner.

Best Practice 28-3

Forensic nurse examiners can promote a reduction in family anxiety levels by proactively providing education about the purpose and process of the forensic autopsy. Discuss the information in a matter-of-fact manner and reinforce the importance of the autopsy and how it may potentially result in information that increases an understanding of the details surrounding the sudden traumatic death of their loved one.

The Media

When someone dies from a sudden traumatic death, it may become news. Although most deaths are treated with confidentiality, some may become of interest to the commonwealth of the people. For example, when someone is murdered, it is usually on the news (Henry-Jenkins, 1993). Murder is a crime against the commonwealth, whose members want to know how this event will impact them and their community. Occupational deaths, which occur as the result of industrial accidents, might be brought into the media spotlight as people attempt to deconstruct how such an accident could occur (Clements, DeRanieri, & Fay-Hillier et al., 2003). Motor vehicle accidents, especially those involving drunk drivers and which have deadly results, may be reviewed on news broadcasts, describing the details of the gruesome scene, or perhaps, as in recent years, a broadcast of the accident scene itself, with bodies still strewn on the highway (Halm, 1996; Marshall & Oleson, 1996; Stayduhar & Sekhon, 1998).

Families may find themselves instantly and unexpectedly thrown into the media spotlight. They may be barraged with microphones placed in their path, being asked repeatedly: "How do you feel?"—a question they may not be able to answer. Depending on the circumstances surrounding the death, the family may find little escape from reliving the horrible details of the death if it is aired on the news in the morning, noon, dinnertime, and bedtime. The face of their loved one may be flashed repeatedly across the screen with the accompanying broadcast; an ongoing reminder of the death, which they already feel powerless to do anything about.

Just as some families cannot escape the media focus, counterintuitively, other families are outraged that their loved one's death received little to no media coverage, seeming to further diminish the importance of their life. One mother expressed her anger:

> *My son was shot by mistake as he came out of a Chinese restaurant and minding his own business. All of a sudden he was no more than a "twenty-something-year-old black male found shot in the Brookside section of the City." They didn't know my son at all! But the way they announced it on the TV screen made it seem like just another black boy who got shot because he was doing something he shouldn't have been doing!*

It is imperative to acknowledge the implications of the media to promote expression and understanding in families. Many families may be embarrassed to share this issue with nurses; however, it is a significant issue in relation to the bereavement process, which can be normalized with acknowledgment, exploration, and guidance (Clements & Burgess, 2002; DeRanieri, Clements, & Henry, 2002).

The Judicial System

Just as many families are beginning to heal from the sudden and traumatic loss of their loved one, the court proceedings may begin. If a criminal action was related to the death, such as homicide, motor vehicle accident, or occupational circumstance, families are confronted with the choice of attending the courtroom trial. Most families express feeling obligated to attend the proceedings, if only as a sign of family commitment and support in the memory of the life of their loved one.

Much to their surprise, family members quickly discover that they are mere spectators in an arena of justice that often seems unfair for the deceased victim. The basic tenets of the judicial system set forth that the defendant is indeed innocent until proved guilty. In addition, the defense attorney doing his or her job to the utmost of his or her ability will attempt to paint a picture of innocence for the defendant, or at least attempt to raise the question of reasonable doubt. At times, this may seem as though the defense attorney is proposing that the deceased was, at least in part, responsible for his or her own death.

Families are often outraged at being forbidden to come to the defense of the loved one. Already distressed by the unexpected loss, families can rapidly become very distraught and incensed when the defense attorney seemingly suggests that the defendant is innocent. Yet, they are not permitted to call out, or even speak, lest they be removed from the courtroom and barred from attending subsequent sessions.

Many families have expressed that in spite of having "won" the case, the victory is hollow. One mother stated:

> *In winning, everybody still ends up losing. Winning didn't bring my son back. Now another mother has lost her son to prison. But even then, at Christmas-time, that mother can go visit her son in prison; I get to go visit the cold hard dirt at my son's gravesite. Everybody loses.*

The Healthcare System

Many family members do not consciously make the connection between grief and the way that it can affect the body and the ability to complete daily functions of life. Fortunately, healthcare education and clinical approaches are returning to the brain and behavior correlates, which promote understanding of human response patterns to various types of traumatic situations. Grief is a strong example of the gray area between physical and psychological conditions, for it can, and almost always does, manifest itself with symptoms of both types. One father who had lost his daughter in a plane crash said:

> *Grief can make you sick! I just kept seeing her strapped in that seat as the plane was going down. I couldn't sleep or eat, I just kept thinking about it. I couldn't concentrate. I felt so guilty. I bought her that trip for her graduation. I just couldn't help but think that somehow I was partly to blame for her death. I finally got so weak that I ended up in the hospital with "exhaustion." They kept giving me pills to make me sleep. Nobody ever even really asked me why I was so "exhausted." I felt like they all knew, but that they were afraid they would upset me. Finally they sent some psychiatric nurse lady in to see me. She said she was very sorry about my daughter, and asked me how I was doing. I just busted-up into tears. I talked to her for an hour, and told her everything I had been thinking. I felt so much lighter afterward. Funny thing is, she really didn't do anything but listen and give me the time of day, but she really cared about me as a person. Her ears did a hell of a lot more for me than all those damn pills!*

Best Practice *28-4*

It is helpful for the FNE to understand that facilitating the expression of a survivor's feelings is one of the most basic and important tenets of the healing process. It is not unusual for family members to seek out healthcare intervention to alleviate the discomforting symptoms that accompany grief. These symptoms might include sleep or dietary disturbances, intrusive thoughts, depression, anxiety, and anger. Frequently, families might seek a "pill" to make these symptoms "go away." However, without appropriate diagnosis, education, and follow-up, the family member might experience concern and confusion when the "pill" is seemingly not successful. It is important to tell families that any pharmacological intervention is effective only when used in unison with concomitant grief counseling.

Reentry into the Community

After the crisis, chaos, and completion of the funeral rites, the weary truth is that many friends and relatives must return to the daily routines that prevailed prior to the death. The house, which may have been suddenly burgeoning with love, support, and numerous shoulders to cry upon, may now seem more like an empty shell, filled with haunting reminders and echoes of the person who is now dead and buried (Clements, Vigil, & Manno, 2003).

"The silence was deafening," one mother said, as she struggled with feeling overwhelmed by staying home alone in the house, and yet she found herself too weak and apathetic to go out and engage in other activities.

Key Point *28-3*

Eventually, each mourner must return to the realm of the living, and be confronted with a reentry, which can be fraught with sometimes unexpected reactions and interactions.

Returning to work, school, or church can be quite a discomforting experience. One mother shared her frustration:

> *I went back to church about a month after my husband was killed by a drunk driver. I was so hurt! Not a soul said a word about my husband. They all said how sorry they were, and that I was "in their prayers," but not one person asked me one question about the outrageous and unfair act of a drunken woman who took my husband away without warning and without respect. I wondered to myself "who are these people?" If I thought I felt lonely with the loss of my husband, it seemed like this drunk woman had killed off all of my friends, too!*

Although people are sincerely saddened by the loss of a loved one, many of them may also be unsure of what to say or how to act. They may fear that bringing up the subject will only upset the surviving family members. In light of society's ongoing struggle with the discomforting topic of death, many well-wishers may not think about asking the survivor about their thoughts and feelings related to the death, yet this can be helpful if done with guidance and permission from the survivor (Clements & Henry, 2002).

Typical Patterns of Bereavement

In providing support to those in the throes of a sudden traumatic death, it is important to understand the typical response patterns. This is no simple task, because grief is a unique and individual experience. Grief response patterns will vary, based on previous losses, past grieving issues, the relationship to the current decedent, the nature and circumstances of the death, and any specific grieving rituals (Clements & Henry, 2002; Doka, 1996; Vigil & Clements, 2003). Some basic guidelines can be applied to understanding the phases of bereavement, and giving the necessary support to assist with identification and understanding of the tasks for functional grieving.

Many survivors express feeling like they are "going crazy," when in reality they are experiencing intense but normal grief. Support, education, and genuine appreciation of their loss is the most effective conduit toward healthy grieving and integration of the loss. In the earliest phase after the death, the survivor will typically be in some state of shock and disbelief (Clements & Henry, 2002). It is difficult to understand and accept the loss.

Best Practice *28-5*

During this period, it is important to keep in mind that survivors may not remember much of what is being said to them. Repetition and reminders are critical as you proceed. Contact numbers, educational information, and other important information should be provided in both oral and written formats because the survivors may need to read it repeatedly or refer to it later when their level of concentration and comprehension begin to improve.

During this time it is important to acknowledge all the rapid events that require thought and attention. These responsibilities include arranging the funeral, notification of family and friends, the wake, the burial, and legal matters. Much of this may get accomplished with the assistance and support of surrounding family and friends during the time of the funeral. After the funeral, the grieving and mourning really begins and can be a roller coaster ride of emotions (Clements & Henry, 2002).

The following sensitive questions should be asked of people who are coping with the sudden loss of a loved one (Clements, DeRanieri, & Fay-Hillier et al., 2003, p. 2):

- What are the family's cultural traditions and rituals for coping with dying, the deceased's body, and honoring the dead?
- What are the family's beliefs about what happens after death?
- What does the family feel to be a normal expression of grief and acceptance of the loss?
- What does the family consider to be the roles for each member in coping with the death?
- Are certain types of death less acceptable (e.g., suicide), or are certain types of death especially difficult to handle for the family's culture (e.g., the death of an infant or child)?

Once the survivors are left alone to deal with the grief, their emotions may run the gamut. The survivor may experience any or all of the following:

- Denial; refusal to accept that their loved one is gone
- Intense feelings of anger
- Sensing the deceased loved one's presence (expecting the lost victim to come home at the regular time; thinking he is calling when the phone rings)
- Hearing the deceased loved one's voice or momentarily mistaking someone else for the decedent
- Mood swings; outbursts of tears or anger
- Insomnia
- Guilt (there may be thoughts and feelings that perhaps there was some way that something could have been done to prevent the death; "if only . . ."; "maybe if I would have . . .")
- Sense of abandonment, betrayal, or fear
- Tightness in the throat or heaviness in the chest
- Headaches
- Empty feeling in the stomach
- Shortness of breath
- Fatigue
- Trembling
- Nausea and vomiting
- Confusion; forgetfulness
- Recollection (the need to tell the story over and over again)

Any or all of these symptoms are a normal grief response. However, it is important to remind a grieving individual to seek medical or psychological assistance if any of these symptoms become unbearable or disabling. If this is necessary, the survivor should be reminded to tell the healthcare provider that he or she has recently lost a loved one to a sudden traumatic death (Bendersky-Sacks, Clements, & DeRanieri et al., 2000; Bendersky-Sacks, Clements, & Fay-Hillier, 2001; Clements & Henry, 2002; Jacobs, 1993).

Everyone reacts differently to sudden traumatic deaths. Some may appear calm (laughing and talking as if nothing has happened), others stoic (just staring and not really reacting to anything), and some hysterical (screaming, running around the room, fainting, vomiting), yet others may be angry, lashing out at random people, even those attempting to provide assistance or support. It is important not to personalize these reactions to grief. It may even be directed at the care provider. However, drugs, alcohol, and violence are not a normal part of the grieving process, and anyone displaying such behavior should be referred to a professional (Clements & Henry, 2002).

Best Practice *28-6*

It is critical for the forensic nurse examiner to establish a network for follow-up and evaluation for surviving family members. This intervention may include referrals for counseling and medical assessment. Bereavement exists on a continuum and will require additional assessment, intervention, and evaluation over time.

Case Study 28-2 Complicated Grief and Bereavement

A family, who had arrived at the medical examiner's office to identify the body of their loved one, consisted of the mother, father, aunt, and uncle of the decedent. When taken to the identification room, the father, aunt, and uncle all agreed on the positive identification of the decedent. The mother, on the other hand, looked at the picture of the decedent and announced very calmly, "That's not my son." Her relatives looked at her, stunned and confounded by her statement. They attempted to talk with her about the fact that it was indeed her son. She continued to calmly refute that the person whose photo was before her was her son. She insisted on obtaining dental records to "prove" that this was her son. The dental records matched without deviation. Still, the mother calmly denied that this was her son; in her mind, this was a clear case of mistaken identity. The body was eventually released and the funeral ensued. Later the following week, the mother came in to attend a support group meeting at the bidding of her family, who were concerned for the welfare of her mental health. During the group session, one family member asked her about the funeral. The mother replied: "It was nice. They said it was my son that was buried, but it wasn't really my son." This mother represents an example of a person who is in extreme denial and who is clearly in need of professional help.

Case Study 28-3 Adaptive Coping

One mother was so devastated and grief-stricken when her son was "shot down in the street and left to die" that it took several months of grief counseling before she could even acknowledge his death. She had discovered that her son's death was the result of a drug deal that "went bad." This information compounded her grief and shock because she was not aware that he was involved in drug-related activities. As she was trying to grasp the reality of her son's death, she was also trying to grasp the reality of her son's apparent "secret life." She was in disbelief about the things she was hearing about her son. She became so angry that her only way to cope was to begin a mission to help the police find her son's killer. She became so intensely involved that her family and friends feared for her safety. She would admittedly roam the streets at night, looking at passers-by, wondering, "Are you my son's killer?"

After many hours of grief counseling over the phone and in person, she began to channel her anger in a positive manner. She began to write articles to the local newspaper, describing her son's death, and the injustice that she felt. Eventually, her son's killer was arrested and prosecuted. She was beginning to gain some closure on the long process of grief. Two years after her son's death, she and her family founded an organization named in memory of her son. The organization does seminars for college students, educating them about the potentially lethal impact of drugs, not just from using drugs, but from the violence that is often associated with that climate.

The Forensic Nurse's Role

The forensic nurse, as a medicolegal investigator and counselor, may be confronted with an extensive list of problems. The nurse must be mindful that the collection of forensic information must be carefully and sensitively intertwined with concomitant grief counseling. Lynch described a set of interventions that are geared toward assisting the survivor in identifying the appropriate tasks and responses.

- Assure the survivors that their difficulty in planning and taking action is not unusual in the aftermath of a sudden traumatic death.
- Provide an environment with decreased stimuli and distraction to promote clarification of the interaction and interview as well as decreasing unanticipated sources of stress and tension.
- Avoid lengthy and abstract communications.
- Be able to tolerate silence when the survivor seems to need quiet time; conversely, be able to tolerate apparently unmotivated outbursts of anger and hostility.
- Reflect the survivor's feelings and concerns from time to time in order to avoid possible misinterpretations and to indicate that you are listening.
- Focus on the reality of the current circumstances.
- Assist the survivor in identifying the various things that must be done in the immediate future (the funeral, notification of friends and family, legal issues, etc.).
- Assist the survivor in identifying appropriate alternatives.
- Encourage the survivor to prioritize tasks that must be accomplished.
- Be alert to the possible physical effects of the survivor's psychological reactions.

Additionally, Clements & Henry (2002) identified the following goals for healing, which can be helpful to share during the initial interface between healthcare providers and grieving families:

- Set goals for yourself.
- Start accomplishing with small, short goals.
- Accept the fact that what you are feeling is real and may be painful.
- Remember that the pain of loss might manifest itself in many different ways.
- Know that you must mourn the loss and allow yourself to do just that.
- Go with your feelings and do not attempt to minimize the fact that the pain of loss exists.
- Cry if and when you feel like it.
- Do not allow yourself to go into a state of loneliness and avoid those who care about you.
- Do not allow guilt or fear to set you back. We often feel that we could have or should have done something to prevent what happened and may begin to worry about future losses.
- Experience your thoughts and feelings one day at a time.
- Each person grieves differently and at his own speed. It is important not to rush through your grief.
- Don't be too hard on yourself by thinking you should be feeling well and be "over it" in a month or two. Grief-related symptoms are typical for at least the first year with increasing thoughts and emotional triggers as the anniversary date approaches, and may be considered normal for up to two years. (However, extreme grief-related symptoms may require medical or mental health intervention.)
- Do not allow others to define the loss for you. Decide for yourself what the loss means to you.

- Allow yourself to "backslide." Just because you felt great yesterday does not mean that you may feel the same today, tomorrow, or next week. Grief is a process with peaks and valleys along the way.
- It's acceptable to feel angry, betrayed, fearful, tired, confused, or ill; these symptoms can be normal grief responses. However, if they persist, do contact your healthcare provider.
- Don't be surprised if you find yourself repeating the story of your loss over and over. This helps to make the loss real and helps you to explore what the loss really means to you.

Summary

Sudden traumatic deaths can be disruptive on many levels of everyday life. The trauma caused from this type of death begins with the death, but the path that follows is fraught with many potential complicating factors and interfaces with the many facets of the medicolegal system. It is critical for clinicians to be aware of these complicating factors. It is imperative to confront these issues in a timely and sensitive manner.

As a survivor moves forward in the grieving process, the goal is to be able to reinvest in life and to return to daily life (Attig, 2001; Clements & Henry, 2002). Often, the grieving survivor will try to forget the death and in essence try to forget the decedent. This is an impossible, unrealistic, and unhealthy goal. The goal should be to remember the decedent, and to be able to become progressively less emotionally and physically affected by the loss (Clements & Henry, 2002; Clements, 2001). To reinvest in life, grieving survivors must acknowledge and determine the impact that the death has had in their life (Attig, 2001). Without completing this task, life will be complicated and filled with anxiety and avoidance, especially surrounding any issue of the death.

It is difficult to determine when healing actually begins. One day the survivor realizes that he has more energy, he is sleeping better, the appetite is improved, life seems more organized, and decision making seems easier. The survivor is able to start thinking about the decedent without a burst of tears or wave of rage. The survivor may even begin to laugh and smile again. These are all indications that the survivor is beginning to place the death of the loved one into a healthy perspective and reinvest in life.

Resources

Books and Articles

Cox, G., Bendiksen, R., & Stevenson, R. (Eds.) (2001). *Complicated grieving and bereavement: Understanding and treating people experiencing loss.* Amityville, NY: Baywood Publishing.

Janoff-Bulman, R. (1992). *Shattered assumptions: Towards a new psychology of trauma.* New York: Free Press.

Matsakis, A. (1992). *I can't get over it: A handbook for trauma survivors.* Oakland, CA: New Harbinger.

Sunderland, R. (1995). Helping children cope with grief: A teachers guide. In *Picking up the pieces* (2nd ed.). Fort Collins, CO: Services Corporation International.

References

Attig, T. (2001). Relearning the world: Always complicated, sometimes more than others. In G. Cox, R. Bendiksen, & R. Stevenson (Eds.), *Complicated grieving and bereavement: Understanding and treating people experiencing loss.* Amityville, NY: Baywood Publishing.

Bendersky-Sacks, S., Clements, P. T., DeRanieri, J., et al. (March 2000). Calming workplace tragedy. *Nurs Spectrum, 9*(6), 6-7.

Bendersky-Sacks, S., Clements, P. T., & Fay-Hillier, T. (2001). Care after chaos: Utilization of critical incident stress debriefing after traumatic workplace events. *Perspect Psychiatric Care, 37*(4), 133-136.

Clements, P. T. (2001). Homicide bereavement: Scary tales for children. In G. Cox, R. Bendiksen, & R. Stevenson (Eds.), *Complicated grieving and bereavement: Understanding and treating people experiencing loss* (pp. 41-52). Amityville, NY: Baywood Publishing.

Clements, P. T., Benasutti, K., & Henry, G. C. (2001). Drawing from experience: Utilizing drawings to facilitate communication and understanding with children exposed to sudden traumatic deaths. *J Psychosoc Nurs, 39*(12), 12-20.

Clements, P. T., & Burgess, A. W. (2002). Children's responses to family member homicide. *Family Community Health, 25*(1), 1-11.

Clements, P. T., DeRanieri, J. T., Fay-Hillier, T., et al. (2003). The benefits of community meetings for the corporate setting after the suicide of a co-worker. *J Psychosoc Nurs, 41*(4), 44-49.

Clements, P. T, Faulkner, M., & Manno, M. S. (July 2003). Family member homicide: A grave situation for children. *Medscape Online J, 3*(3). Retrieved from www.medscape.com/viewarticle/458064.

Clements, P. T. & Henry, G. C. (2002). The process of grieving. *On the Edge: The Official Newsletter of the International Association of Forensic Nurses, 7*(4), 1, 9–10.

Clements, P. T, Reid, P. C., & DeRanieri, J. T. (March 2003). Providing assistance to families of murder victims in the emergency department. Retrieved from www.forensictrak.com/member/article2.php.

Clements, P. T., Vigil, G. J., Manno, M. S., et al. (2003). Cultural considerations of loss, grief & bereavement. *J Psychosoc Nurs, 41*(7), 18-26.

Clements, P. T., & Weisser, S. (2003). Cries from the morgue: Guidance for assessment, evaluation and intervention with children exposed to homicide of a family member. *J Child Adolescent Psychiatric Nurs, 16*(4), 153-161.

DeRanieri, J. T., Clements, P. T., & Henry, G. C. (2002). When catastrophe happens: Assessment and intervention after sudden traumatic deaths. *J Psychosoc Nurs, 40*(4), 30-37.

DeSpelder, L., & Strickland, A. (1996). *The last dance: Encountering death and dying* (4th ed.). Mountain View, CA: Mayfield Publishing.

DiMaio, D., & DiMaio, V. (1993). Medicolegal investigative systems. In D. DiMaio and V. DiMaio (Eds.). *Forensic pathology* (pp. 1-19). Boca Raton, FL: CRC Press.

Doka, K. (Ed.) (1996). *Living with grief after sudden loss: Suicide, homicide, accident, heart attack and stroke.* Washington, DC: Hospice Foundation of America.

Halm, K. (1996). MADD services available to assist emergency nurses. Mothers Against Drunk Driving. *J Emerg Nurs, 22*(6), 595-596.

Henry-Jenkins, W. (1993). *Just us: Understanding homicide bereavement.* Omaha: Centering Corporation.

Jacobs, S. (1993). *Pathological grief: Maladaptation to loss.* Washington, DC: American Psychiatric Press.

Marshall, M., & Oleson, A. (1996). MADDer than hell. *Qualitative Health Res, 6*(1), 6-22.

Rando, T. (1993). *Treatment of complicated mourning.* Champaign, IL: Research Press.

Spungen, D. (1997). Homicide: The hidden victims. In *Interpersonal violence: The practice series.* Thousand Oaks, CA: Sage Publications.

Stayduhar, K., & Sekhon, L. J. (1998). Comprehensive plan to prevent adolescent injuries and violence: The role of clinicians. *Physician Assistant, 22*(3), 83, 86, 89-90.

Vigil, G. J., & Clements, P. T. (2003). Child and adolescent homicide survivors: Complicated grief and altered worldviews. *J Psychosoc Nurs, 41*(1), 30-39.

Chapter 29 Stalking Crimes

Ann Wolbert Burgess

Forensic nurse examiners (FNEs) will encounter the crime of stalking in their work with victims of sexual harassment, assault, rape, domestic violence, and death. This chapter provides information on the classification of stalkers using the format established by the Behavioral Science Unit at the FBI Academy in Quantico, Virginia (Douglas, Burgess, & Burgess et al., 1992).

Over the last two decades of the twentieth century the term "stalking" became part of the American vocabulary and a new classification of crime. The mental health and legal communities have been especially sensitized to this abnormal social behavior (Meloy, 1996) by the forensic cases of Prosenjit Poddar (*Tarasoff v. Regents*, 1976) and John Hinckley Jr. (Caplan, 1987).

Key Point 29-1

Stalking is pursuit; it is victimization of another human being by acts of following, viewing, communicating with, or moving threateningly or menacingly toward him or her.

Stalking, in contrast to an actual attack, involves pursuit of a victim (Sohn, 1994) and is the act of following, viewing, communicating with, or moving threateningly or menacingly toward another person. Stalking behavior has many dimensions that include written and verbal communications, unsolicited and unrecognized claims of romantic involvement on the part of victims, surveillance, harassment, loitering around, and following that produce intense fear and psychological distress to the victim. In addition, these behaviors can take the form of telephone calls, vandalism, unwanted appearances at a person's home or workplace, and electronic mail communication.

Stalking is an ongoing, usually long-term, crime without a traditional crime scene. The stalking will occur at the target's residence, place of employment, shopping mall, school campus, or other public place. There will be a number of aborted or obscene phone calls and/or anonymous letters addressed to the target professing love or knowledge of the target's movements. Written communications or symbolic items are often left on vehicle windows or placed in mail boxes or under doors by the stalker. The tone of communications may progress from protestations of adoration, to love, to annoyance at not being able to make personal contact, and eventually to threatening and menacing.

Although the actual number of stalking incidents has yet to be fully documented, a congressional report estimated that approximately 200,000 victims have been subjected to the terror of threatened violence in the recent past. Estimates provided by professionals suggest that 1 in every 40 individuals may be a target of a stalker (Flynn, 1993). All 50 states in the United States have passed stalking legislation in an attempt to fill the gaps left by criminal statutes prohibiting such activities as "threats of violence," "criminal trespassing," and "harassment" and to provide victims with enhanced legal remedies beyond "orders of protection" (Gerberth, 1992). In response to public fears, the states have passed antistalking laws, and the National Institute of Justice, together with the National Criminal Justice Association, published a model antistalking law (Fein, Vossekuil, & Holden, 1995).

Motivation for Stalking

Isolated research efforts have reported findings from cases involving the pursuit of public figures (Dietz, Matthews, & Martell et al., 1991) and serial homicide (Ressler, Burgess, & Douglas, 1988) or describing the personalities and motivations of a small sample of stalkers (Hazelwood & Douglas, 1980; Gerberth, 1992). Newspaper and anecdotal accounts are more prevalent than the academic literature; however, these accounts reveal little about the overall dynamics of the crime beyond the specific incident.

Stalker crimes are primarily motivated by interpersonal aggression rather than by material gain or sex. The purpose of stalking resides in the minds of stalkers who are compulsive individuals with a misperceived fixation. Stalking is the result of an underlying emotional conflict that propels the offender to stalk or harass a target.

Because of the cognitive component to the behavior, stalking can be conceptualized as occurring on a continuum from nondelusional to delusional behavior. Delusional behavior may indicate the presence of a major mental disorder such as a schizophrenia, psychosis, or delusional disorder (American Psychiatric Association, 2000). Nondelusional behavior, while reflecting a gross disturbance in a particular relationship and a personality style or disorder, does not necessarily indicate a detachment from reality. This distinction is significant because of the potential legal implications (e.g., pleas of insanity). What most readily distinguishes the behavior on this spectrum is the nature of the relationship an offender has had with his target and the content of the communication.

Although the research on menacing, harassing, and stalking behaviors in persons who have or had a prior relationship is relatively new (Walker, 1979), the psychiatric literature has been building a classification scheme on a subgroup of stalkers diagnosed with erotomania in whom the relationship exists only in fantasy and delusion. Doust and Christie (1978) and Ellis and Mellsop (1985) noted that erotomania has long been known to be associated with stalking behaviors of both men and women and to have the potential to lead to overt aggression, and they provide a historical perspective on both the forensic aspects of stalking and the psychodynamic components. The early writings of an erotic delusion syndrome, named after the physician De Clerambault in his book *Les Psychoses Passionelles*, outlines the features of the syndrome. De Clerambault (1942) observed that erotomania began with love and hope but then disintegrated into resentment and anger. The patients, usually female, were described as holding the delusional belief that a man, usually older and of an elevated social rank, was passionately in love with them. This love becomes the purpose of the patients' existence and they may send letters and telephone the person both at home and at work.

Raskin and Sullivan (1974) observed that the patients may be dangerous and may threaten the life of their victim or his family, especially when the patient reaches the stage of resentment or hatred, which replaces love. Meloy (1989) has suggested the dynamics of blurring of unrequited love and the wish to kill.

Rekindling an interest in the forensic aspects of erotomania has been credited to Goldstein (1978) and Taylor, Mahendra, and Gunn (1983). Zona and colleagues (1993) analyzed police files and classified persons as either erotomanic, love obsessional, or simple obsessional. Stalkers have been classified from a mental health intervention standpoint using short-term crisis intervention to assist survivors (Roberts & Dziengielewski, 1996) and a law enforcement perspective (Wright et al, 1996) based on the nature of the relationship (nondomestic or domestic), the content of communication (nondelusional or delusional), level of aggression (low, medium, or high), level of victim risk, motive of stalker, and outcome. Forensic studies of obsessional harassment and erotomania have occurred in criminal court populations (Harmon, Rosner, & Owens, 1995; Meloy & Gothard, 1995). Meloy and Gothard (1995) have suggested the term "obsessional follower" for someone who engages in an abnormal or long-term pattern of threat or harassment directed toward a specific individual. In cases of stalking in domestic relationships, the escalation of aggression can be associated with violence and death. Consequently, stalking patterns in domestic violence are now seen as dangerous and the forensic aspect is being tested (Perez, 1993). Erotomania in and of itself is insufficient for explaining stalking behavior. When focusing on relationships involving romantic attachment and domestic activities, empirical investigation demonstrates different characteristics associated with stalking behaviors than those found in erotomania (Meloy, 1996).

Key Point *29-2*

The erotomania stalker often has a long-term relationship with a victim through written and telephonic communications, surveillance, and attempts to approach; with the passage of time, preoccupation and stalking activities become more intense and may lead to injury or death.

As with other classifications of stalking, the activity of the erotomania stalker is often long-term with written and telephonic communications, surveillance, attempts to approach the target, etc. With the passage of time, the activity becomes more intense. Or the preoccupation with the victim becomes all-consuming and may ultimately lead to the death or injury of another party. John Hinkley Jr., both an attempted political assassin and a celebrity stalker, is one such example. His erotomanic obsession with Jodie Foster was never destined to be consummated in a realistic relationship. According to Fischoff (1998), Hinckley is an identity-seeking celebrity stalker. Such stalkers seek a self-identity through actions or fantasies, often (but not exclusively) electronic relationships with targets. All actions are ultimately designed to fill the bottomless personality void, designed to bring media attention to someone with serious personality and social defects. Research shows that even if the stalkers are successful in their pursuit of a celebrity, they have no meaningful agenda at the ready. The chase, according to Fischoff (1998), is all, and it is the process, not the outcome, that drives the engine and gives the stalker's anemic sense of self some momentary transfusion. Such stalkers, like Hinckley, are likely to transfer targets of obsession. Indeed, Hinckley first staked out Jimmy Carter and only settled on Ronald Reagan when access to Carter eluded him. He injured both target and surrounding victims. In Hinckley's 1998 release petition hearing, a state witness, Commander Jeanette Wick, testified to the effect that Hinckley was stalking her–he had gathered information about her personal schedule, recorded love songs for her, and when ordered not to contact her, disobeyed by sending her a package. A state mental health expert testified that Hinckley's psychotic disorders were in remission but that Hinckley was still dangerous. The expert based his opinion on Hinckley's "relationship" with the commander, stating it was strikingly similar to the "relationship" he had with Jodie Foster (Caplan, 1987).

On the extreme delusional end of this spectrum there is usually no actual relationship; rather, such a relationship exits only in the mind of the offender. On the nondelusional end of the spectrum there is usually a historical relationship between the offender and the victim. These tend to be multidimensional relationships such as marriage or common-law relationships replete with a history of close interpersonal involvement. In between these two poles are relationships of varied dimensions and stalkers who exhibit a mix of behavior. The offender may have dated his target once, twice, or not at all. The target may only have smiled and said hello in passing or may in some way be socially or vocationally acquainted. For the purpose of classification, this spectrum of stalking behavior is divided into three general types: domestic (nondelusional), nuisance (a mix of nondelusional and delusional behavior), and erotomania (delusional).

For purposes of this chapter the terms *target* and *victim* are not necessarily interchangeable. Target is used to describe the primary recipient of the stalker's attention. However, in many cases those people around a stalker's target become victims of the stalker's behavior.

Domestic Stalker

Domestic stalking occurs when a former boyfriend, girlfriend, family member, or other household member threatens or harasses another member of the household. This definition includes common-law relationships as well as long-term acquaintance relationships. The domestic stalker is initially motivated by a desire to continue or reestablish a relationship and can evolve into an attitude of "If I can't have her, no one can."

A study by Burgess and colleagues (1997) examined data from 120 male and female batterers of varied age and marital, educational, and economic status, who attended group treatment for batterers or who were charged with domestic violence in a district court setting. One third of the sample admitted to stalking and the behavior indicated there can be a continuance of violent acts even though separation with the partner has occurred. There is both open and clandestine stalking. At this point, it is not clear if this represents a particular pattern. Part of stalkers' openness includes their feeling that they have a right to do what they do. It also suggests bragging and control. It seems that the triggering event is less predicated on behavior of the victim and resides more in the fantasy life of the stalker. The provocation of the nonstalker may be a displacement (e.g., being humiliated or disappointed in other areas of life and coming home and beating the wife).

Factor analysis of batterers who stalk compared to nonstalking batterers found three stalking patterns of pursuit. First, stalkers are open in their attempts to contact their ex-partner; when this fails they begin to contact others and discredit the partner. The second factor is the conversion of positive emotion of love to the negative of hate. They essentially go underground with the clandestine behavior, being nonrevealing and including anonymous or hang-up phone calls and entering the residence without permission. Just before they go public again, there is a phase of ambivalence, indicating the splitting of love and hate, when they send gifts and flowers. When they move from the mix of public and secret behavior to a public display of stalking and targeting behavior, they suddenly explode and, in this sample, entered the victim's residence and were very violent.

Victimology

The target knows the stalker as an acquaintance or may have a familial or common-law relationship which the target has attempted to terminate. The target is aware of the stalking and may have requested a restraining order or assistance from law enforcement on prior occasions. In addition, there is a history of prior abuse or conflict with the stalker. The target may report a sense of being "smothered" in the prior relationship.

Crime Scene Indicators

The domestic stalking case often culminates in a violent attack directed at the target. Usually the scene of this attack involves only one crime scene and it is commonly the target or stalker's residence or place of employment. The crime scene reflects disorder and the impetuous nature of the stalker. A weapon will usually be brought to the scene. There could be signs of little or no forced entry and no sign of theft. The crime scene may also reflect an escalation of violence, (e.g., the confrontation starts as an argument, intensifies into hitting or throwing things, and could culminate in the target's death and would then be classified as domestic homicide). Others such as family members and boyfriends/girlfriends may be involved in an assault. If the target has taken steps to keep the stalker away (changed phone number, changed residence, restraining order, etc.), the only access the stalker may have is at the target's place of employment. In such cases, coworkers, security personnel, and customers may become victims. In some instances, the stalker will abduct the target in an attempt to convince her to stay with him.

Best Practice *29-1*

The forensic nurse examiner should consider all reports of domestic stalking very seriously and take appropriate actions because these cases often culminate in violence or hostage-taking at the victim's residence or place of employment.

The stalker may be at the scene when law enforcement or emergency medical personnel arrive or may commit suicide. The stalker may make incriminating statements.

Common Forensic Findings

Alcohol and drugs may be involved. There usually are forensic findings consistent with a personal type of assault. Depersonalization, evidenced by facial battery, and a focused area of injury indicative of anger are examples of a personal assault.

Investigative Considerations

If the crime occurs in the target's residence, domestic stalking should be considered. When other family members are contacted, they often describe a history of domestic violence involving the target and stalker. This claim is often supported by police reports. A history of conflict due to external stressors (e.g., financial, vocational, alcohol) is a common element of domestic stalking. The stalker may have demonstrated personalized aggression in the past as well as a change in attitude after the triggering event.

Search Warrant Suggestions

Although most of the evidence will be left at the crime scene, the nurse may request diaries as well as financial and medical records to verify any premeditation of the crime.

Best Practice *29-2*

The forensic nurse examiner should consider all documentation that might assist in substantiating premeditation of a crime; these evidentiary materials may include medical records, journals, telephone records, computer files, letters, photographs, reading materials, credit card records, ticket stubs, and travel receipts.

Nuisance Stalker

The nuisance stalker is one who targets an individual and interacts with that target through hang-up, obscene, or harassing telephone calls; unsigned letters; and other anonymous communications or continuous physical appearance at the target's residence, the target's place of employment, shopping mall, or school campus. The stalker is often unknown to the target. It is unlikely the target will become aware of being stalked until the stalker's activity is well under way. Only after the stalker has chosen to make personal or written contact will the target realize the problem.

Victimology

The target, usually a female, has often crossed paths with the stalker, most likely without noticing him or her.. The target, therefore, will have no knowledge of the stalker's identity. The relationship between the stalker and the target is one way. The target will eventually become aware of the physically present nuisance stalker.

Other potential victims are spouses, boyfriends or girlfriends, or any others who are viewed as an obstacle between the stalker and his target.

Crime Scene Indicators

Stalking is an ongoing, usually long-term, crime without a traditional crime scene. The stalking will occur at the target's residence, place of employment, shopping mall, school campus, or other public place. There will be a number of aborted or obscene phone calls or anonymous letters addressed to the target professing love or knowledge of the target's movements. Written communications are often left on vehicle windows or placed in mail boxes or under doors by the stalker. The tone of communications may progress from professing adoration, to declaring love, to expressing annoyance at not being able to make personal contact, and eventually may become threatening and menacing.

The stalker may place himself or herself in a position to make casual contact with the target, at which time verbal communication may occur. A description of this contact may be used in a later communication to terrorize or impress upon the target that the stalker is capable of carrying out any threats.

Investigative Considerations

Trace telephone calls and perform threat analysis of the written or phone communications. Careful analysis of early communications may provide leads for identifying the stalker. Observe target's places of employment, residence, mall, or campus for stalker. Because communications are often left on or in a target's vehicle, observation of vehicles can often lead to the identity of the stalker. The target should be interviewed about any suspicious "accidental" contacts she may have had in the recent past, such as being bumped into while shopping, door-to-door salesmen, telephone solicitations, a stranger asking to use the telephone or asking for directions, and so on.

Search Warrant Suggestions

The primary items to search for are photographs, literature (newspaper articles, books, magazine articles), and recordings concerning the target. Diaries, journals, calendars, or surveillance logs detailing the stalker's preoccupation or fantasy life with the target may also be found. Recordings of telephone calls to targets are often made and retained.

Other items to look for are evidence of contact or attempted contact with the target: telephone records or returned letters. Credit card records, ticket stubs, and hotel receipts are often kept as souvenirs and may be helpful in documenting travel in pursuit of a target. Computer equipment should not be overlooked as a repository for information.

Case Study 29-1 Nuisance Stalker

A man who stalked a woman was arrested outside her house carrying weapons, a stocking mask, and other items. The woman told police she recently found her bathing suit taped to the windshield of her car. On one other occasion she found some of her undergarments draped on the car's mirror. One week prior, the victim found cartridge casings from a handgun taped to the car's window.

On the night of the arrest of the stalker, the victim saw a man outside her apartment and called the police. Minutes later the police arrested the stalker, who months prior to this incident had been acquitted of burglarizing the woman's home.

The stalker was found sitting in his vehicle less than 100 yards from the victim's apartment. Officers searched the stalker and found a knife and a key to the victim's residence.

In his vehicle they found a .22-caliber pistol and ammunition, a stun gun, Mace, a camera and film, two sets of binoculars, two tape recorders, two flashlights, pictures of the victim's residence and car, rubber gloves, cotton gloves, a stocking mask, a large nylon bag and a bag with a change of clothes, several condoms, a book of nude pictures, a gun cleaning kit, and a cooler filled with ice and beer.

Erotomania Stalker

Erotomania-related stalking is motivated by an offender-target relationship that is based on the stalker's fixation. This fantasy is commonly expressed in such forms as fusion (the stalker blends his personality into his target's) or erotomania (a fantasy-based idealized romantic love or spiritual union of a person, rather than sexual attraction). The stalker can also be motivated by religious fantasies or voices directing him to target a particular individual. This preoccupation with the target becomes consuming and ultimately could lead to the target's death. The drive to stalk arises from a variety of motives, ranging from rebuffed advances to internal conflicts stemming from the stalker's fusion of identity with the target. In addition to a person with high media visibility, other victims include superiors at work or even complete strangers. The target almost always is perceived by the stalker as someone of higher status. Targets often include political figures, entertainers, and high media visibility individuals but do not have to be public figures. Sometimes the victim becomes someone who is perceived by the stalker as an obstruction.

When erotomania is involved and the target is a highly visible media personality (usually someone unattainable to the stalker) the target becomes the imagined lover of the stalker through hidden messages known only to the stalker. The stalker builds an elaborate fantasy revolving around this imagined love. Male erotomaniacs tend to act out this fantasy with greater force than do female.

Victimology

The target is aware of the stalker through many prior encounters or communications (letters or phone calls). The target often has high media visibility. Many times the initial contact with a public figure will be in the form of "fan mail."

Crime Scene Indicators

As with other classifications of stalking, the activity of the erotomania stalker often involves long-term written and telephonic communications, surveillance, and attempts to approach the target. With the passage of time, the activity becomes more intense with the stalker's attitude shifting to the familiar "If I can't have her, no one can."

The majority of erotomania-motivated attacks are close range and confrontational. The stalker may even remain at the scene. These close-range encounters tend to be more spontaneous, as reflected by a more haphazard approach to the target: evidence is left, and there are likely to be witnesses. This does not mean the stalker did not fantasize, premeditate, and plan the stalking; all of these elements characterize this crime. Rather, the actual act is usually an opportunistic one. The stalker takes advantage of opportunity to interact with the target as it is presented to him.

Common Forensic Findings

Firearms are the most common weapon carried by stalkers, especially with a distance stalking. Occasionally, they will use a sharp-edged weapon, such as a knife. The sophistication and type of weapon will help establish the degree of stalker sophistication. If the target of the stalker is killed, the vital organs, especially the head and chest, are most frequently targeted.

Investigative Considerations

The stalker almost always surveys or stalks the target preceding the encounter with the target. Therefore, the availability of the target's itinerary and who may have access to it is one investigative consideration. There is a likelihood of preoffense attempts by the stalker to contact the target through telephone calls, letters, gifts, and visits to the target's home or place of employment. There may even be an incident involving law enforcement or security officers having to remove the stalker from the target's residence or workplace.

The stalker's conversation often will reflect this preoccupation or fantasy life with the target. When those associated with the stalker are interviewed they will most likely recall that much of the stalker's conversation focused on the target. He or she may have claimed to have had a relationship with the target and may have invented stories to support this encounter.

Assistance should be requested from FBI's Investigative Support Unit or mental health professionals experienced with these complicated cases.

Search Warrant Suggestions

The primary items to search for are photographs, literature (newspaper articles, books, magazine articles), maps, letters from a celebrity target to a stalker, surveillance photos of the target, and recordings concerning the target. Diaries and journals detailing the stalker's preoccupation or fantasy life with the target may also be found.

Other items to look for are evidence of contact or attempted contacts with the target: telephone records, returned letters or gifts, motel receipts, gas bills, rental agreements, or airline/bus/train tickets implying travel to locations the target has been. Credit card records also may be helpful in this regard.

Case Study 29-2 Erotomania Stalker

On the morning of March 15, 1982, Arthur Richard Jackson, 47, was waiting near Theresa Saldana's West Hollywood apartment house. As Saldana, 27, rushed out to a music class at Los Angeles City College, Jackson approached. When Saldana paused to unlock her car, Jackson asked "Excuse me, are you Theresa Saldana?" Saldana replied, "Yes."

Saldana's identity confirmed, Jackson began stabbing Saldana with a hunting knife. He stabbed and slashed her so hard, and so often that the knife bent. Hearing Saldana's screams, a delivery man rushed to her aid and wrested the weapon away from Jackson.

The intervention of the delivery man, heart-lung surgery, and 26 pints of blood saved Saldana's life. Jackson, convicted of attempted murder and inflicting great bodily injury, was given the maximum sentence of 12 years in prison.

Arthur Jackson was born in Aberdeen, Scotland, in 1935 to an alcoholic father and a mother whom investigators believe may have been schizophrenic. He was an odd and fanatical child who often became lost in fantasy. In an 89-page autobiographical letter addressed to Saldana, written in 1982 shortly after his arrest, Jackson wrote that when he was 10 years old, he became fixated on a neighbor girl called Fiona. At 13 he described a sexual encounter with an older boy.

It was also in this letter to Saldana that he expressed his "torturous love sickness in my soul to you combined with a desperate desire to escape into a beautiful world I have always dreamed of (the palaces of gardens of sweet paradise), whereby the plan was for you, Theresa, to go ahead first, then I would join you in a few months. . . . I swear on the ashes of my dead mother and on the scars of Theresa Saldana that neither God nor I will rest in peace until this special request and my solemn petition has been granted."

At 17, he suffered his first nervous breakdown. It took a full year before Jackson was released from the Scottish psychiatric hospital where he sought treatment. After his release, he began a trip across two continents; working in London as a kitchen porter, in Toronto as a zoo helper, and in New York as a jack-of-all-menial-trades.

In 1955 he joined the US Army. While in the army he fell in love with a fellow soldier and suffered another nervous breakdown. He was sent to Walter Reed Hospital in Washington, D.C., for psychiatric treatment. While in the hospital he was given a weekend pass in honor of his twenty-first birthday in 1956. Jackson celebrated his birthday by going to New York. While in New York he attempted suicide with an overdose of sleeping pills.

Discharged from the Army, he continued to wander the US. In 1961, the US Secret Service arrested Jackson for threatening President John F. Kennedy. Later that year he was deported to Scotland, where he occasionally lived with his widowed mother. During this time he was a vagrant on the dole and seldom stayed in one place for more than a few months.

In 1966, Jackson reentered the US through Miami and was given a six-month visitor's visa. He was again deported when he overstayed the six months.

He first became aware of Saldana in 1979, when he sat in an Aberdeen theater and watched "I Want to Hold Your Hand," a film about Beatlemania. Movies were Jackson's only reality. Jackson conceived mad passions for women in movies whom he thought of as stars.

Two years later he saw Saldana in "Defiance," a movie in which she plays a girl trying to make a life for herself in a crime-ridden slum. When costar Jan-Michael Vincent was attacked in the movie by a street gang, the scene provoked vivid memories of his 1956 suicide attempt. Focusing his macabre excitement on Theresa, Jackson convinced himself he could win the actress by "sending her into eternity."

He began stalking Saldana in early 1982, the year he illegally returned to the US. Jackson would make several cross-country bus trips in this single-minded quest.

He initially went to New York City, where he tried to contact Saldana's relatives and business associates, pretending to be an agent with a hot script. He was unable to locate Saldana. A trip to Los Angeles also yielded nothing. Only after he had returned to New York from California did he manage to trick one of Saldana's relatives into telling him the actress lived in Hollywood.

While he stalked Saldana, he tried to purchase a gun in many different states but was prevented by state laws requiring a minimum of a driver's license for identification. The only weapon available to Jackson was a hunting knife.

After returning to Hollywood, he hired a private detective, who provided Saldana's address. During questioning by the police he was asked why he had tried to kill Saldana. Jackson replied, "Read my diary. It's all in there." Jackson had kept a diary of his quest in his knapsack.

While in custody Jackson confessed to the murder of two people during a robbery of a London bank in 1962.

Jackson continues to write to Saldana as well as reporters about his quest for Saldana. Jackson became eligible for parole in 1991.

Summary

In summary, the nuisance stalker may know the target through social contact (business, school, etc.) or from a random meeting in a public place (store, mall, sporting event, etc.). Targets of the nuisance and erotomania stalkers are selected by the stalker based on love, hate, religion, or voices heard by the stalker. The selection process may be known only to the stalker. These targets are unaware of the initial reason for their selection.

The domestic stalker is known to the target and had a close personal relationship with the target. These cases are the most likely to end in a violent confrontation.

The erotomania stalker's target is typically a public figure. Television appears to be the most probable source because it provides visual and auditory material for the fantasy being developed by the stalker.

The stalker is usually unable to develop meaningful relationships with others and is classed as a loner. Stalkers often have prior involvement with law enforcement (arrests, trespass complaints, etc.) and with psychiatric facilities. They may have attempted suicide in the past. The stalker may have engaged in similar activity on prior occasions. The education and investigative skills of the forensic nurse examiner will become an important issue when treating or investigating the circumstances surrounding victims of interpersonal and sexual violence as well as understanding and reporting stalking crimes. The FNE who specializes in forensic mental health and the behavior of the mentally disordered offender will be able to better identify the symptomology associated with the perpetrator and potential risk of violence.

Resources

Organizations

National Center for Victims of Crime

2000 M Street NW, Suite 480, Washington, DC 20036; Tel: 202-467-8700; www.ncvc.org

National Criminal Justice Reference Service

P.O. Box 6000, Rockville, MD 20849-6000; Tel: 313-519-5000, 800-851-3420; www.ncjrs.org

National Domestic Violence Hotline

P.O. Box 161810, Austin, TX 78716; Tel: 800-799-7233; www.ndvh.org

National Organization for Victim Assistance (NOVA)

1757 Park Road NW, Washington, DC 20010; Tel: 800-879-6682, 202-232-6682; www.trynova.org

Survivors of Stalking (SOS)

P.O. Box 173655, Tampa, FL 33672; www.soshelp.org

Web Sites

National Victim Center: help guide for stalking victims
www.ojp.usdoj.gov/ovc/assist/nvaa/ch21-2st.htm

Privacy Rights Clearing House
www.privacyrights.org

Stateside Iowa Domestic Abuse Hotline Stalking FAQ
www.state.ia.us/government/ag/stalker.htm

Stalking Behavior
www.stalkingbehavior.com

Government Reports

Cyberstalking: A New Challenge for Law Enforcement and Industry: A Report from the Attorney General to the Vice President
www.usdoj.gov/criminal/cybercrime/cyberstalking.htm

DOJ First Annual Stalking Report to Congress (1996)
http://ncjrs.org/txtfiles/stlkbook.txt

References

American Psychiatric Association (APA). (2000). *Diagnostic and statistical manual of mental disorders* (4th ed.). Washington, DC: Author.

Burgess, A. W., Baker, T., Greening, D., et al. (1997). Stalking behaviors within domestic violence. *J Family Violence, 12*, 389-403.

Caplan, L. (1987). *The insanity defense and the trial of John W. Hinckley, Jr.* New York: Dell.

De Clerambault, C. G. (1942). Les psychoses passionelles. In *Oeuvres psychiatriques* (pp. 315-322). Paris: Presses Universitaires de France.

Dietz, P. E., Matthews, D. B., Martell, D. A., et al. (1991). Threatening and otherwise inappropriate letters to members of the United States Congress. *J Forensic Sci, 36*, 1445-1468.

Douglas, J. E., Burgess, A. W., Burgess, A. G., et al. (1992). *Crime classification manual: A standard system for investigating and classifying violent crimes.* New York: Lexington Books/Macmillan.

Doust, J. W., & Christie, H. (1978). The pathology of love: Some clinical variants of de Clerambault's syndrome. *Soc Sci Med, 12*(2A), 99-106.

Ellis, P., & Mellsop, G. (1985). De Clerambault's syndrome: A nosological entity? *Br J Psychiatry, 30*, 619-621.

Fein, R. A., Vossekuil, B., & Holden, G. A. (1995). *Threat assessment: An approach to prevent targeted violence. NIJ research in action.* Washington, DC: US Department of Justice.

Fischoff, S. (1998). Stalker ever after. *Forensic Echo, 2*, 10.

Flynn, C. P. (1993). New Jersey antistalking law: Putting an end to a "fatal attraction." *Seton Hall Legislative J, 19*, 297.

Gerberth, V. J. (1992). Stalkers. *Law Order, 40*(10), 138-143.

Goldstein, R. L. (1978). De Clerambault in court: A forensic romance. *Bull Am Acad Psychiatry Law, 6*, 36-40.

Hall, D. M. (1997). Stalking often linked to sexual assaults. *Sexual Assault Rep, 1*(1), 6.

Harmon, R. B., Rosner, R., & Owens, H. (1995). Obsessional harassment and erotomania in a criminal court population. *J Forensic Sci, 40*(2), 188-196.

Hazelwood, R. R., & Douglas, J. E. (1980). The lust murderer. *FBI Law Enforcement Bull, 49*, 18-22.

Lindesmith, A. R., & Dunham, H. W. (1941). Some principles of criminal typology. *Soc Forces, 19*, 307-314.

Meloy, J. R. (1989). Unrequited love and the wish to kill. *Bull Menninger Clin, 53*, 477-492.

Meloy, J. R. (1996). Stalking (obsessional following): A review of some preliminary studies. *Aggression Violent Behav, 1*, 147-162.

Meloy, J. R., & Gothard, S. (1995). Demographic and clinical comparison of obsessional followers and offenders with mental disorders. *Am J Psychiatry, 152*(2), 258-263.

Perez, C. (1993). Stalking: When does obsession become a crime? *Am J Crim Law, 20*, 264-290.

Raskin, D. E., & Sullivan, K. E. (1974). Erotomania. *Am J Psychiatry, 131*, 1033-1035.

Ressler, R. K., Burgess, A. W., & Douglas, J. E. (1988). *Sexual homicide: Patterns and motives.* New York: Free Press.

Roberts, A. R., & Dziegielewski, S. F. (1996). Assessment typology and intervention with the survivors of stalking. *Aggression Violent Behav, 1*, 359-368.

Sohn, E. F. (1994). Anti-stalking statutes: Do they really protect victims? *Crim Law Bull, 30*, 203-241 (NCJ 148872).

Taylor, P., Mahendra, B., & Gunn, J. (1983). Erotomania in males. *Psychol Med, 13*, 645-650.

Tarasoff v. Regents of the University of California, 17 Cal. 3d 425 (1976).

Walker, L. E. (1970). *Battered woman.* New York: Harper & Row.

Wirtz, P., & Harrell, A. V. (1987). Police and victims of physical assault. *J Crim Justice Behav, 14*, 81-92.

Wright, J. A., Burgess, A. G., Burgess, A. W., et al. (1996). A typology of interpersonal stalking. *J Interpersonal Violence, 11*, 487-502.

Zona, M. A., Kaushal, K. S., & Lane, J. (1993). A comparative study of erotomania and obsessional subjects in a forensic sample. *J Forensic Sci, 38*, 894-903.

Chapter 30 Child and Adolescent Sex Rings and Pornography

Ann Wolbert Burgess

The number of reported cases of child sexual abuse is increasing. This prompts questions as to whether this increase is due to better reporting by victims, to a more responsive criminal justice system, or to increased sexual deviance. For forensic nurse examiners (FNE), however, the fact remains that skills are needed for assessment, diagnosis, treatment, and expert testimony. This chapter will outline the phenomena of child and adolescent sex rings and the use of pornography.

Child Sexual Abuse

The study of the sexual victimization of children has primarily focused on incest or family member (intrafamilial) abuse of female children. As reports have indicated a growing number of abusers who are outside the family (extrafamilial) and who abuse both males and females, attention has expanded to include this type of sexual deviancy. There is a need for health professionals and law enforcement to increase their efforts concerning sex ring cases involving multiple victims of the same offender.

Key Point *30-1*

Child sexual abuse includes incest, interfamilial abuse, and multiple types of exploitation emerging from pornography and child sex rings. Healthcare professionals, baby-sitters, day-care workers, teachers, coaches, parents, siblings, and law enforcement officers must maintain ongoing vigilance to identify victims.

Sex ring crime is a term describing sexual victimization in which there are one or more adult offenders and several children who are aware of each other's participation. There are three different types of child sex rings. The solo sex ring involves one or two adult perpetrators and multiple children. There is no exchange of photographs, nor are there sexual activities with other adults. By contrast, a syndicated sex ring involves multiple adults, multiple child victims, and a wide range of exchange of items including child pornography and sexual activities (Douglas, Burgess, & Burgess et al., 1992).

At a level between these two types of rings is the transition sex ring, in which the children and pornography are exchanged between adults, and often money changes hands. These three types of rings are further described in this chapter with case studies.

Child pornography can be defined as any visual or print medium depicting sexually explicit conduct involving a child. More simply stated, child pornography is photographs or films of children being sexually molested. Sexually explicit conduct includes sexual intercourse, bestiality, masturbation, sadomasochistic abuse, and lewd exhibition of the genitals or pubic area. The child or children visually represented in child pornography have not reached the age of consent.

Solo Child Sex Rings

Solo child sex rings are characterized by the involvement of multiple children in sexual activities with one adult, usually male, who recruits the victims into his illicit behavior by legitimate means (Douglas, Burgess, & Burgess et al., 1992). This offender can be assessed by his methods for access to and sexual entrapment of the children, control of the children, maintaining the isolation and secrecy of the sexual activity, and by the particulars of ring activities. The events surrounding disclosure of the ring and the victims' physical and psychological symptoms are also important elements of the ring. Victims can be both male and female, and their ages can range from infancy to adolescence. The distinguishing factor is the age preference of the offender. Victims are found in nursery schools, baby-sitting and day-care services, youth groups, and camps.

Crime Scene Indicators

The crime scene is usually the offender's residence, vehicle, or group meeting hall. There can be many locations. The pornographic material is usually hidden in the residence of the offender. The most recent crime scene will usually have the camera and equipment needed to create the pornography as well as props, collateral material, and goods used to bribe the victims.

Forensic Findings

The victimization is usually reported by a third party and little, if any, forensic evidence is immediately available. To obtain forensic evidence detailed medical and psychiatric examinations of the victims are required. Medical evidence could include anal or vaginal scarring, bruises, and other marks.

Investigative Considerations

Obtain a search warrant for the offender's residence. Check telephone and financial records for purchases of materials needed to create the pornography. Be sensitive to props and collateral used to bribe the targeted age group. Interviews with the victims should be conducted carefully by an investigator specially trained for interviewing children.

Aspects of a Solo Sex Ring

In brief, sexual encounters between adults and children usually fall into a predictable pattern: access to and sexual entrapment of the child by the adult; isolation and secrecy of the sexual activities; and disclosure of the victimization, which includes short- and long-term outcomes and impact for the child and his family. In outlining these phases with the case under consideration, one notes the consistency in the patterns and phases.

Key Point 30-2

Sexual abuse of a child is a consciously planned, premeditated behavior. The adult is usually someone known to both the child and parent and who has ready access to the child.

Access and Entrapment

The sexual abuse of a child is a consciously planned, premeditated behavior. The adult is usually someone known to both the child and parent and who has ready access to the child. The offender stands in a relationship of dominance to the child. Ambivalence as a component of the decision-making process is a characteristic of the young person's emotional life, and the offender trades on this. The desire for domination by the adult is aimed at breaking the internal resistance of the subordinate. After gaining access to the child, the adult engages the child into the illicit activity through the power and authority that adulthood conveys to the child as well as misrepresenting moral standards.

In one case, the adult was an authority figure vis-à-vis his position as a sports director with the YMCA. The families were supportive of their sons being involved in activities at the local YMCA because of its program for assisting in the positive development of young males. While in the role as sports directors, both the sports director and his associate became acquainted with the young boys and almost immediately began paying special attention to specific boys both at the YMCA during the activities at summer day camp and when the boys would be invited to their home.

Isolation and Secrecy

When an offender is successful in abusing his victim, he must try to conceal the deviant behavior from others. More often than not, he will try to pledge the victim to secrecy in several ways. Secrecy strengthens the adult's power and control over the child and perpetuates the sexual activity. It is important to understand that the child usually keeps the secret; some children never tell anyone. There are many reasons why the abuse is kept secret. The child may fear people will not believe such behavior, fear people will blame the child for the activity, fear there will be punishment for disclosure, or fear the adult will carry out the threats, and the child may want to protect the abuser.

In this case, the sports directors programmed the boys to believe that they needed to be educated about sex and that this kind of activity was practiced between men and their students. Pornographic magazines depicting heterosexual acts were shown to normalize the activity. The boys did not tell because of loyalty to their coach and a belief that they were very special to the adult. The boys were unaware of each other's involvement with the adult.

Sexual Activities

A wide range of sexual behaviors may occur between the adult and child in combination with psychological pressure or physical force. There may be a slow progression of advancing sexual acts perpetrated with the characteristics of sexual seduction, or the acts may be forceful and sudden to the child.

In this case, youths described sexual acts including fondling, mutual masturbation, kissing, and escalating over time to oral and anal sex. Nude photographs and videos were taken of the youths without their knowledge. The boys were also shown pornographic videos.

Key Point 30-3

During sexual abuse scenarios, children are confused about power and authority associated with being trapped and participating in sexual activity in isolation and secrecy.

Encapsulation Phase

As part of the isolation stage, the child is trapped in the sexual activity, having to participate, yet having to be silent. Much of the psychological injury derived from the exploitation can be linked back to the manner of entrapment, the length of time of encapsulation, and nature of the sexual activity. Children are confused over the use of power and authority, and abuse has a disorganizing impact on their thinking. As the abuse continues, their belief about sex between adults and children shifts from wrong to right. Some think they can intervene and stop. The child often tries to protest the activity and begins to reenact and repeat the abuse, first to himself and then to others. The resistance is normal and always there if one carefully looks for it. However, there is also the component of arousal disharmony and because of the trauma learning the behavior is usually reenacted.

In this case the overt protest behaviors were noted in various boys in that some had minimal contact with the adults and others had extended contact. With disclosure the boys' behavior begin to deteriorate.

Disclosure

Child sexual abuse is usually discovered and disclosed in two ways: accidentally and purposefully. In accidental disclosure, a third party may observe the abuse, or symptoms may be noted in the child. In purposeful disclosure, a child consciously decides to tell an outsider or parent about the abuse. When there is disclosure, then the social meaning of the abuse becomes known; that is, the child must deal with the reactions of people (i.e., parents, friends, authority) to the knowledge of the abuse. It becomes important that people believe the child, understand the confusion and fear that permeates the experience, and take protective action on behalf of the child.

Best Practice 30-1

The forensic nurse should ensure that specific actions are taken to support the child after disclosure because the child will be confused and frightened and may require protection.

In this case, after disclosure occurred, parents were notified by the police. Some of the boys continued to deny their involvement with the offenders until photographs and videotapes surfaced.

Psychological Injury

The impact of child sexual abuse will be discussed in terms of critical issues in general, specific injury, insult, and psychological damage.

The repetitive secret nature of the sexual abuse requires the victim to psychologically compartmentalize (encapsulate) the event; that is, the victim keeps it separate from the rest of his or her life. It is through this process that the coping mechanism of dissociation is derived ("I thought of other things while he was doing

[it]"). Inherent in the dissociation is cognitive confusion. At some level the child knows it is wrong because it has to be kept secret. Thus, he does not let the outside world know. There is a break with social ties. Commitment and social ties to values lose their color and dominance.

Further along in the dissociation is the mechanism of splitting. In this particular case, the real disruption is evidenced in the splitting of parental relationships. There is a strong lack of trust in people and the attachment or bonding nonsexually to people is missing. To attach in a social way requires some trust and faith, and this component has been shattered and destroyed for the youths. Rather than developing a normal trusting social bond with others, the bonding was to the deviant sexual activities. The boys were trapped.

The youths were inhibited from exerting any action to protect themselves and to prevent or stop the exploitation. Self-protection was inhibited and adult protection nonexistent. Because this inhibition cut the boys off from self-assertive behaviors, the aggressive drive was compromised and displaced in its direction. Thus, anger and aggression were noted in symbolic and inappropriate behaviors. Several of the youths showed anger and aggression, which derived from the fact that they could not protect themselves.

Impact on Victim

The evaluation of the impact that sexual abuse has on an adolescent's life may be noted in several ways:

- Reviewing the details and circumstances of the sexual abuse and noting any unusual or out-of-the ordinary features
- Listing the symptoms that reflect the post-trauma features
- Citing the dynamics of the abuser's behavior

In the first method, the details and circumstances of the sexual abuse and exploitation help to evaluate the major impact the abuse has had on the youths' lives.

The betrayal of a trusted relationship was critical in this case. In the case of the YMCA sports directors, the boys were programmed to become overly attached to them. The youths were at a critical developmental period and vulnerable for attention from an adult male. The coach gave what appeared to the boys to be love and attention, meeting the narcissistic wish of a child to be the center of attention. The exchange for being taught about sex and to be special was secrecy about the sex. The youths' rage stemmed from the betrayal of this special status and the humiliation of the knowledge that many other boys were so treated.

The second way to evaluate the post-trauma effects is to document symptoms that a boy develops as a result of the abuse. Symptoms, which include the intrusive thoughts and phobic/avoidance behavior, evidence the major impact the abuse had and continues to have, on the youths' lives.

In addition, the youths became unusually quiet, confused, less active, and less energetic. Behavior was of depression, moodiness, preoccupation. Other symptoms included difficulty sleeping (trouble falling asleep, sleeping restlessly, sleeping more, bad dreams, nightmares) and an exaggerated startle reflex.

After disclosure, the youths had difficulty in listening: they did not hear people as clearly and had trouble concentrating and paying attention. Of major concern was the amount of aggression and violence displayed by the youths.

Symptoms noted for youths under the age of 15 were primarily conduct behaviors: skipping school, running away, starting fights, forcing others to have sex, hurting an animal on purpose, hurting other people (other than in a fight), deliberately damaging things not their own, setting fires, lying, and stealing or robbing (Burgess, 1984).

Best Practice *30-2*

When children have been victimized by pornography and sex rings, the forensic nurse must plan support systems for them that permit attachment to an experienced therapist with expertise in child and adolescent trauma.

Treatment Issues

Some of the general treatment issues for the youths included the following:

- Attachment to a caring, therapeutic figure who is experienced in child and adolescent trauma. This attachment is critical to reduce the potential of the youth acting out in a self-directed or other-directed manner.
- Attention and assessment of the youth's thought processes are important in the early sessions. It is critical to find out what is on the youth's mind. For example, how entitled versus disregarded did he feel in his family? Does he believe his family is uncaring; these are the premises laid down by the offender. He has been supported in transgressions by the offender. Are these thought still operant?
- The sexually abusive experience needs to be first linked with current symptoms. People can have a conscious awareness of upsetting events but may be totally incapable of connecting it to ongoing symptomatic behavior. The anger and rage exist because of the violation, the exploitation, and the compromising. The defense of anger is easier to manage than to deal with the loss of innocence and the loss of the trusted coach who lied that they were special.
- The youths remain at a crossroad. They need to attach to a therapist in order to begin to trust and reduce anxiety. Then there can be work on the issues evolving from the traumatic experience. If the alienation from people continues, they will be at risk for acting on their aggressive and suicidal thoughts.

Transitional Child Sex Rings

The transitional child sex ring involves multiple offenders as well as multiple victims. The offenders are known to each other and collect and share victims (Douglas, Burgess, & Burgess et al., 1992).

Victimology

In the transition sex ring, multiple adults are involved sexually with children, and the victims are usually pubescent. The children are tested for their role as prostitutes and thus are high risks for advancing to the syndicated level of the ring, although the organizational aspects of the syndicated ring are absent in transition rings. It is speculated that children enter these transition rings by several routes: (1) they may be children initiated into solo sex rings by pedophiles who lose sexual interest in the child as he or she approaches puberty and who may try, through an underground network, to move the vulnerable child into sexual activity with pederasts (those with sexual preferences for pubescent youths); (2) they may be incest victims who have run away from home and who need a peer group for identity and economic support; (3) they may be abused children who come from disorganized families in which parental bonding has been absent and multiple neglect and abuse are present; (4) they may be missing children who have been abducted or kidnapped and forced into prostitution.

It is difficult to identify clearly this type of ring because its boundaries are blurred and because the child may be propelled quite quickly into prostitution. Typically the adults in these transition rings do not sexually interact with each other, but instead have parallel sexual interests and involvements with the adolescents who exchange sex with adults for money as well as for attention or material goods.

Crime Scene Indicators

The crime scene can be the offenders' residence, a vehicle, group meeting hall, or hotel/motel. There are usually many locations. The pornographic material is usually hidden in the residences of the offenders. The most recent crime scene will usually have the camera and other materials needed to create the pornography as well as props, collateral material, and goods used to bribe the victims.

Forensic Findings

The victimization is usually reported by a third party and little, if any, forensic evidence is immediately available. To obtain forensic evidence detailed medical and psychiatric examinations of the victims are required. In addition to the general forensic findings described earlier, there could be anal or vaginal scarring, bruises, and other injuries.

Investigative Considerations

Obtain a search warrant for the offenders' residences. Check telephone and financial records for purchases of materials needed to create the pornography. Be sensitive to props and collateral used to bribe the targeted age group. Interviews with the victims should be carefully done by an investigator specially trained for interviewing children.

Case Study 30-1 Transitional Child Sex Ring

A classic case example of a transitional child sex ring is more than 20 years old. From December 1977 to December 1978, described by one gay Boston newspaper as the year of the witch hunt, Boston was in the spotlight regarding a male youth prostitution ring. Earlier that year, the investigation of a solo child sex ring had led an assistant district attorney and police to uncover a second generation of rings. In the apartment of a man who had an extensive history of convictions for child molesting, investigators found numerous photos of naked youths as well as pornographic films. Sixty-three of the depicted youths were located and interviewed, and 13 agreed to testify before a grand jury. From this testimony, additional men (many with professional and business credentials) were indicted on counts of rape and abuse of a child, indecent assault, sodomy, and unnatural acts.

By December 1978 the trial of the first defendant, a physician, began. Testimony from four prosecution witnesses revealed the link between the two types of rings. According to news reports, the first witness, a man who was serving a 15- to 25-year term after pleading guilty to charges derived from the child solo ring, admitted to having sexual relations with boys as young as 10 during the 13 years he had rented the apartment. He testified that he could be considered a "master male pimp" and that he became involved in the sex-for-hire operation after meeting one of the other defendants. He said that initially no money was involved, but after a few months expenses increased, so the men were charged and the boys were given $5 to $10 for sexual services.

Newspapers reported that another prosecution witness, an assistant headmaster at a private boys' school, admitted visiting the apartment more than 40 to 50 times over a five-year period. He denied being a partner in a scheme to provide boys for hire but admitted to taking friends to the apartment with him and paying to have sex with the boys.

A prosecution witness, a 17-year-old, testified to being introduced into homosexual acts by the first witness, who had told the boys they could make all the money they wanted. "All we had to do was lay there and let them do what they wanted to us," he said.

Another victim testified that at age 12 he had met the third witness through friends. He received gifts of clothes and money for going to the man's apartment. While there, he would drink beer and smoke pot, and watch stag movies. He brought his younger brother to the apartment and they both had sex with the man. At age 14 he was "turning tricks" and charging $10 for oral sex and $20 for anal sex. At that point he met the defendant.

The defendant, a pediatrician and psychiatrist, claimed in his defense that he went to the apartment as part of a research study, which was submitted to a journal after his indictment and subsequently published in a sex research journal.

The jury, sequestered for the 19-day trial, deliberated two and a half days before reaching a verdict of guilty. The judge sentenced the physician to five years' probation on the condition that he undergo psychiatric treatment. More than a year later the state board of medicine revoked his license. The other defendants in the ring plea-bargained their charges, and there were no further trials.

Syndicated Child Sex Rings

A syndicated child sex ring uses a well-structured organization that involves the recruitment of children, the production of pornography, the delivery of sexual services, and the establishment of an extensive network of customers (Douglas, Burgess, & Burgess et al., 1992).

Victimology

The syndicated ring involves multiple offenders as well as multiple victims. The syndicated child prostitution ring is a well-established commercial enterprise.

Crime Scene Indicators

There can be many locations. There are many levels of material created. Information and details about locations can be obtained from the pornography itself. The most recent location will have all the equipment necessary to create the material.

Forensic Findings

The victimization is usually reported by a third party and little, if any, forensic evidence is immediately available. To obtain forensic evidence detailed medical and psychiatric examinations of the victims are required.

Investigative Considerations

Investigation requires an understanding of typical operation of a syndicated ring. The organizational components of the syndicated ring include the items of trade, the circulation mechanisms, the supplier of the items, the self-regulating mechanism, the system of trades, and the profit aspect.

Items of Trade

Items of trade include the children, photographs, films, and tapes. The degree of sexual explicitness and activity may vary. For example, photographs range from so-called innocent poses of children in brief attire taken at public parks, swimming pools, arcades, or similar places where children congregate to carefully directed movies portraying child subjects in graphic sexual activities. In the films, the child is often following cues provided by someone standing off-camera. Also, in audiotapes the children may be heard conversing with age-appropriate laughter and noises as well as using language that is highly sexual and suggestive of explicit behaviors.

Circulation Mechanisms

Various mechanisms for circulation include the mail (photographs, coded letters), tape cassettes, CB radio, telephone, and beepers. The mail is a major facilitator for circulation of child pornography. Often, a laundering process may be used. For example, buyers send their responses to another country; the mail, received by the overseas forwarding agent, is opened and cash or checks are placed in a foreign bank account; the order is remailed under a different cover back to the US. This procedure ensures that the subscriber does not know where the operation originates and that law enforcement has difficulty tracing the operation.

Suppliers

Suppliers of child pornography include pedophiles, professional distributors, and parental figures. Pedophiles with economic resources and community status may organize their own group to have access to children and to cover their illegal intentions, or they may work within the framework of existing youth organizations. The professional distributors include the pornographer, that has access to an illegal photographer, who in turn generally owns a clandestine photo laboratory and film processor. These photo laboratories can provide services to many illegal operations; thus, they also present some problems to the professional pornographers, that may find their photographs or films in magazines or adult bookstores without their knowledge and prior to their own distribution. The professional procurers who supply children also provide photographs and films through wholesale distributors and adult bookstores. Another source of professional distribution is photographic processing facilities. A photographic development laboratory often has a storefront business that handles photographic orders such as holiday pictures, while its mail-order business is advertised in magazines. One such facility had a mail-order division that promised, through its advertisements in "adult" magazines, confidential photo finishing. These advertisements were also found in periodicals catering to clientele with special sexual interests. Parental figures who supply children for pornographic and prostitution purposes include natural parents, foster parents, and group home workers. The supplier may operate a foster home, as in the case of a self-proclaimed clergyman, who by his own estimates sold approximately 200,000 photos per year, with an income from this operation in excess of $60,000. The technique used by the man was to have older boys engage younger boys in sex acts. If a youth did not submit, he was beaten and abused by an older youth. After the youth submitted, he was photographed in the sexual acts and the man would then use the boys for his own sexual purposes. In order to ensure secrecy, a pornographer often keeps a blackmail file on each boy.

Self-Regulating Mechanism

Syndicated child pornography operations do not have recourse to law enforcement or civil process for settling disputes that arise in matters of theft, unauthorized duplication of photographs, or resources of supply. Thus, a self-regulating mechanism develops for the elimination of members guilty of actions deemed unfair. Violators are eventually identified by evidence such as the grade of paper, characteristic of typewriter keys, number of letters, as well as the sincerity and insistence of the correspondence. Letters are kept as a security measure. Recriminations between the offender and guilty party become extremely bitter, and support by fellow members in chastising the guilty party is solicited through immediate correspondence. Members of the syndicates are alert to law enforcement efforts against the group in general or with respect to their syndicate in particular.

System of Trade

One rule for trading is that members of the syndicate may assist each other in finding items of interest to other collectors. Through a system of trades, photographs held by syndicate members are traded, and those pictures chosen to be retained are kept by the receiving member.

Profit

The financial profit of child pornography appears to be an individual matter. Some collectors trade items for their personal use, and others trade items for personal as well as commercial purposes. The financial lure of pornography is seen in the actual cost of production and verified in the correspondence of the pornographers. Frequently collectors who sell photographs actually are selling duplicate copies of items in their collection, thereby having income to purchase additional photographs from other sources. Identification of additional victims can be made from the pornography obtained with a search warrant.

Case Study 30-2 Syndicated Child Sex Ring

A child sex ring involved 10 boys and one girl. In October, information regarding the offender (Paul) was brought to the attention of a West Coast FBI office. The children involved ranged in ages from 8 to 16. Paul befriended a family with two boys and one girl; both parents worked. The parents grew to trust Paul and invited him to live in their house, renting out a bedroom to him. He drove a Cadillac equipped with a telephone, and he handed out business cards advertising a 24-hour limousine service that he provided with his Cadillac. At one point Paul made his child prostitutes wear beepers so that he could call the child he thought would best suit his customer's desires. Paul was constantly trying to recruit more children, and he would pick up runaways and use the children to recruit others.

Paul never gave any of his child prostitutes money, as he felt this would ruin them. Instead, he provided food and clothing, bought them various toys, and took them to amusement parks, sporting events, movie shows, and roller rinks.

The offender kept an apartment in a complex with a swimming pool and tennis courts. He used this apartment as a "crash pad" for many of his child prostitutes, and they used the pool and tennis courts. The older boys were told by Paul to keep the younger ones in line. Paul was sexually involved with several of his child prostitutes and provided Quaaludes to all the children. He also had a sizable collection of child pornography.

Because it was determined that no federal laws applied to Paul's activities, the case was turned over to local police. In November, Paul was convicted on seven felony counts (19 felony counts were dismissed), and in May he was sentenced to 13 years' imprisonment and was declared a mentally disturbed sex offender.

Internet Child Pornography

Computer technology has provided another means for access of the pedophile with a child target. Investigating and prosecuting Internet cases is a subspecialty called cyberstalking cases (Douglas, Burgess, & Burgess et al., 1992). Although cyberstalking can involve adults, many pedophiles are also exploiting this technology. The use of a computer in child pornography offenses requires an above-average intelligence and economic means, both common features of pedophiles (Armagh, 1999).

In *US v. Reinhart (1997)* the court granted the government's motion for pretrial detention. The defendant was charged with producing and distributing child pornography. On government's motion for pretrial detention under the Bail Reform Act, the district court held that (1) defendant's case involved crime of violence; (2) there were no conditions of release, which could reasonably assure safety of community and appearance of defendant; and (3) defendant also posed risk of flight.

This case is critically important for its illustration of the use of the Internet as a tool for pedophiles and child pornographers. This case clearly links a pedophile's use of technology to access children for sexual purposes, to gain control over the child and his family, to recruit new victims, and to communicate with other pedophiles. The amount of detail, care, and compulsiveness that is demonstrated in the profile of a career pedophile is exemplified in this case.

Pedophiles' social networks are other pedophiles. They socialize, telephone, write letters, Email, network, and share strategies for continuing their deviant relationships with children, even when in prison. In Florida, one convicted child pornographer used his prison post office box number to expand his distribution of child pornography until he was discovered.

Pedophiles can move from an isolated position of solo operator into a network of perpetrators (e.g., Reinhardt had a codefendant). It is no wonder, now that elaborate and organized networking is well under way on the Internet both nationally and internationally. This case emphasizes the Internet pedophile as an entrepreneur having a product line on his own home page. Reinhardt provides advice to a "chat room" correspondent on how to build a long-term relationship with a young boy, how to manipulate parents so that they do not "cause problems," and teaches his victims on how to answer questions about the ongoing sexual relationship. Reinhardt videotaped instructing his victim in how to type in responses to sexually oriented questions being sent from a chat room. His home page contained images of nude children and his victims as well as an image of his own penis wherein he had a minor assist in the scanning of his genitalia, an act serving as a permanent document of his sexual entrapment of the boy.

Pedophiles are totally preoccupied with their sexual interest in children. In this case, the probation office identified nine jobs Reinhardt held between 1986 and 1997 in four states. His obsession with the Internet was noted in his owning several computers while living in a trailer. The reason for his job instability seemed to depend upon whether the job was in the service of sexual deviation or whether his compulsion for children interfered with his work productivity.

This case reveals the inner workings of pedophiles and child pornographers. The general public can now access all dimensions of child sexual exploitation through the Internet. They can call up a pedophile's home page or talk with him in a "chat room." Although Internet pedophile activities will lose their clandestine nature, it means the pedophile can be more discriminating in selecting and testing his victims by remaining anonymous.

Internet pedophiles are sophisticated in the investigative aspects and have developed ways to bypass the restrictions (e.g., the growing use of encryption). Investigators report that such coded messages are sometimes impossible to intercept.

A critical question concerns whether or not children can be protected from the Internet pedophile. In March 1997 Senate hearings examined the risks of victimization to children in cyberspace. The result was the March 1998 establishment of the cybertipline (www.missingkids.com/cybertip). The tipline has been created at the National Center for Missing and Exploited Children for parents to report suspicious or illegal Internet activity online. The intent is to ensure that the Internet not be allowed to become a sanctuary for pedophiles, child pornographers, and others who prey upon children.

A more recent phenomenon is the solicitation of sex over the Internet. A survey conducted by Crimes Against Children Research Center at the University of New Hampshire found that one in five youths who regularly use the Internet received a sexual solicitation or approach by a stranger who wanted "cybersex" within the past year (Finkelhor, Mitchell, & Wolak, 2000). One in four were exposed to unwanted sexual material, with 6% of the regular Internet users reporting an exposure to unwanted sexual pictures that distressed them in the last year.

In conclusion, child pornography is a central part of most sex rings, in which an individual or group of offenders sexually abuses one or more children. Child pornography produced in sex rings is used for the collection of the offenders in the ring and often for sale, publication, or exchange. Child victims, in these rings, are usually forced to perform sexual acts, participate in the production of pornography, or recruit other children.

Summary

Child sexual abuse is increasing, at least in part to increasing sexual deviance. Today's forms of mass communication and media have facilitated the escalation of child pornography and sex rings, contributing to deviant sexual behaviors involving children and adolescents. The forensic nurse examiner needs to be skilled in assessment, diagnosis, and treatment, as well as prepared to offer courtroom testimony as a fact or expert witness. This role involves an understanding of crime scene indicators, forensic findings, and investigative considerations. The victim impact of pornography and sex rings is far-reaching, and in order to plan appropriate interventions, the nurse must appreciate the impact of specific injuries, insults, and psychological damage that are associated with these phenomena.

The dynamics of child sex rings have been described as a pipeline in which offenders control the victims through bonding, competition, and peer pressure. Children are recruited, seduced, molested, and discarded. Offenders use blackmail if a child tries to leave the ring because they have the pornography that depicts the forced sexual acts and thus are able to silence the child.

Child pornography may also play a different role in different types of sex rings. In a solo ring, the offender usually uses the pornography for his own personal use. In rings involving more than one offender sexually involved with several children, the offender may exchange or sell the child pornography they produce. Child victims may also be pressured and recruited to participate in more structured rings consisting of sexual offenders and numerous sexually abused children. Large amounts of child pornography may be sold or exchanged within the rings.

The Internet has greatly expanded the access pedophiles and child molesters have to children. One national response is the National Center for Missing and Exploited Children's cybertipline (www.cybertipline.com). The NCMEC maintains a 24-hour child pornography tipline to assist in the investigation of child sexual exploitation of children.

Resources

Organizations

Child Exploitation and Obscenity Section

Criminal Division, US Department of Justice, 1400 New York Avenue NW, Suite 600, Washington DC 20005; Tel: 202-514-5780

Federal Bureau of Investigation (FBI)

Innocent Images Initiative: www.fbi.gov/hq/cid/cac/innocent.htm
Locate your local FBI field office: www.fbi.gov/contact/fo/fo.htm

Human Rights Watch

1630 Connecticut Avenue NW, Suite 500, Washington, DC 20009; Tel: 202-612-4321; www.hrw.org

International Child Pornography Investigation and Coordination Center

US Customs Service, 45365 Vintage Park Road, Suite 250, Sterling, VA 20166; Tel: 703-709-9700, ext. 353

National Center for Missing and Exploited Children

Charles B. Wang International Children's Building, 699 Prince Street, Alexandria, VA 22314-3175; Tel: 703-235-3900, 800-THE-LOST; www.missingkids.com

The UN Convention on the Rights of the Child

www.unicef.org/crc

Publications

Children and Prostitution: How Can We Measure and Monitor the Commercial Sexual Exploitation of Children?

www.childwatch.uio.no/cwi/projects/indicators/prostitution/index.html
Literature review and annotated bibliography. A collaboration between UNICEF Headquarters, New York, Centre for Family Research, University of Cambridge, and Childwatch International.

The Commercial Sexual Exploitation of Children in the US, Canada, and Mexico

http://caster.ssw.upenn.edu/~restes/CSEC.htm
Results of a two-year study conducted by the University of Pennsylvania regarding child sexual exploitation in the Americas; links to full report, abstracts, appendices and tables. Download full text of report in PDF format: www.hri.ca/children/CSE/Estes_Weiner_19sept01.pdf

References

Armagh, D. S., Battaglia, N. L., & Lanning, K. V. (1999). *Use of computers in the sexual exploitation of children.* Washington, DC: Office of Juvenile Justice and Delinquency Prevention, Portable Guides in Investigating Child Abuse (US Department of Justice).

Burgess, A. W., Hartman, C. R., & McCausland, M. (1984). Response patterns in children and adolescents exploited through sex rings and pornography. *Am J Psychiatry, 141*(5), 656.

Douglas, J. E., Burgess, A. W., Burgess, A. G., et al. (1992). *Crime classification manual.* San Francisco: Jossey-Bass.

Finkelhor, D., Mitchell, K. J., & Wolak, J. (2000). *Online victimization: A report on the nation's youth.* Alexandria, VA: National Center for Missing and Exploited Children.

United States v. Reinhart, 975 F, Supp. 834 (W.D, La, 1997).

Chapter 31 Male Victims of Interpersonal Violence

Cris Finn and Paul T. Clements

The issues surrounding male interpersonal violence have received increased attention in the past decade. In many industrialized countries, male sexual assault is a reportable and prosecutable crime (Criminal Justice and Public Order Act, 1994; National Center for Victims of Crime [NCVC], 2004). Precedent convictions for sexual assaults against males have occurred (NCVC, 2004; Rogers, 1995; 1997); however, this attention has not resulted in significant clinical breakthroughs relative to increased reporting or with which to help male survivors overcome the impact of sexual assault (Coxell & King, 1996; Frazier, 1993). Little is known about prevalence, mode, and manner of assault; physical and psychosocial consequences faced by male survivors; or effective therapeutic options. The limited amount of clinical or scientific evidence suggests that male survivors develop post-traumatic stress disorder (PTSD) or post-traumatic rape syndrome (PTRS) following the assault. Although the development of PTSD in female rape survivors is now fairly well documented, few systematic studies have enhanced the understanding of PTSD in male survivors of interpersonal violence or sexual assault. This chapter will examine the extant literature to identify the current state of knowledge regarding male interpersonal violence, specifically sexual assault; provide suggestions for enhanced and sensitive assessment, intervention, and planning by forensic nurse examiners (FNE); and identify implications for future research and policy development regarding this vulnerable population of victims.

Background and Significance

Male sexual assault is not a new phenomenon, having occurred for centuries. In ancient times, defeated male enemies were often raped by their victors as an expression of dominance and superiority. As a result, men who were sexually penetrated by force were believed to have lost their manhood and were no longer considered warriors or rulers, thereby adding to postassault shame and stigma. The gang rape of a male was used as punishment by the Romans for adultery and by the Persians and Iranians for violation of a harem (Donaldson, 1990).

In spite of centuries of existence, sexual assault, in general, remains a significantly underreported crime. This is particularly true when the victim is male (NCVC, 2004; Scarce, 1997). In part, this is due to stigma or public attitudes about male sexual assault. For example, myths persist that men are strong enough to prevent sexual assault, that sexual assault against males is very rare, that male sexual assault victims are, as a result, homosexual, and that manhood is lost after sexual assault (Coxell & King, 1996; NCVC, 2004; Scarce, 1997). Adding to the confusion created by these myths, most men are potentially more ashamed or humiliated to report sexual assault if they consequently obtained an erection or ejaculated during the violation. These physiological responses which are typical during such stimulation (Plaud & Bigwood, 1997) are often misinterpreted and misunderstood as some form of consent or enjoyment. In fact, some offenders may purposefully try to stimulate their victims to erection or orgasm to reinforce the fantasy of complete and total control and support any existing thinking errors about the victims' enjoyment of the assault. Additionally, some offenders feel if the victim ejaculates, he will be much less likely to report the crime (Brochman, 1991; Groth & Burgess, 1980; NCVC, 2004).

The available clinical research suggests that male rape victims experience significant physical and psychological trauma from the assault (Coxell & King, 1996; Goyer & Eddleman, 1984; NCVC, 2004), and limited empirical research suggests that, like their female counterparts, male sexual assault victims are held somewhat responsible for being assaulted (Whatley & Rigio, 1993). Societal stereotypes continue to perpetuate the myth that all sexual assault victims are at least somewhat responsible for the event (Dietz & Byrnes, 1981; Kanekar & Kolsawalla, 1980; Muehlenhard & Cook, 1988; NCVC, 2004; Scarce, 1997). Although most of these stereotypes are still applied to female victims, an often overlooked and underestimated sexually aggressive behavior is that of male-on-male or female-on-male sexual assault. This type of sexual assault has been recognized as a widespread occurrence in prisons (Ben-David & Silfen 1993; Sagarin, 1976; Scacco, 1982), and in recent years there have been a growing number of clinical reports on male sexual assault among non-incarcerated adults (Goyer & Eddleman, 1984; Groth & Burgess, 1980; Hickson, Davies, & Hunt et al., 1994; Scarce, 1997). However, there remains a significant paucity of related empirical research related to male sexual assault (Whatley & Riggio, 1993).

Key Point 31-1

Male sexual assault is an underreported crime, in part, because of stigma or public attitudes. This impairs the collection of realistic epidemiological data and thwarts comprehensive investigative studies.

Scope of the Problem

An accurate picture of the frequency of male sexual assault in the general population is difficult to determine. Surveys of college students have indicated that a significant proportion of college males have been pressured or forced into sex by both males and females (Struckman-Johnson, 1988; Struckman-Johnson & Struckman-Johnson, 1994). A recent survey of sexual assault among homosexual men in England found that approximately 25% of the sample had been subjected to non-consensual sex at some point in their lives (Hickson, Davies, & Hunt et al., 1994). However, such surveys reflect a broad range of sexually harassing and sexually aggressive behaviors other than male sexual assault. Adding to the lack of accurate statistics, the Federal Bureau of Investigations (FBI) Uniform Crime Reports (UCR) does not compile figures for male rape because the agency definition lists rape as a sexual assault involving a female victim (Allison & Wrightsman, 1993, Federal Bureau of Investigations, 2000). Therefore, available crime statistics provide only a crude estimate of the true incidence of male sexual assault.

According to 1995 crime estimates, approximately 19,390 males above the age of 12 were the victims of rape or attempted rape (US Department of Justice, 1997). Ultimately, the vast majority of male sexual assaults are thought to go unreported (Calderwood, 1987; NCVC, 2004; Scarce, 1997). Given the poor monitoring mechanisms and poor reporting due to ongoing associated social stigma, it is likely that male sexual assault is even more underreported than those involving female victims.

Typically, male sexual assault is perceived to be what happens to young boys by homosexual men or what happens between men in prison. Although these are the most commonly reported forms of male sexual assault, there are also male sexual assaults perpetrated by females. Some would argue that it is not sexual assault if a female takes advantage of a man while he is sleeping and has an erection. Some purport that it is not sexual assault because the female does not invade the body cavity of a man; specifically, she does not penetrate a male as a male would penetrate a female. If held as the benchmark, then only vaginal penetration would be a violation. Sexual assault is not simply about intercourse; it is about an act of violence, power, and control. Therefore, if a female takes advantage of a situation, which may or may not result in penetration, these actions constitute acting-out in a violent manner and exerting non-consensual power and control over another individual.

Some initial preliminary studies in the US have provided early insight into the prevalence of male sexual assault. Kaufman and colleagues (1980) reported an alarming increase in the number of male victims of rape presenting at a medical center in New Mexico. Sorenson and colleagues (1987) found that a survey of the general population revealed that 1480 men who were interviewed about past sexual experience represented 7.2% having experienced at least one episode of forced sexual contact. However, a significant and ongoing problem is that statistics from rape counseling facilities vary across the US. For example, in 1990, the San Francisco Rape Treatment Center reported that of 528 victims, 9.8% were men. A similar report from Boston's Beth Israel Hospital indicates that 10% of patients were men. Other reports estimate that between 5% to 10% of all rapes in the US involve male victims. In a study done at a New York emergency department, 27 male sexual assaults were documented during a four-year period. This accounted for 12% of all sexual assaults seen at this emergency department (Centers for Disease Control, 1996). According to the Bureau of Justice Statistics (1994), there were approximately 60,000 sexual assaults of males over the age of 12 in the US in 1992. The 1985 report "The Crime of Rape," also from the Bureau, indicated that over 123,000 men were sexually assaulted over a ten-year period. Again, because of issues related to underreporting, it is probable that these numbers do not accurately reflect the actual number of male sexual assaults.

In *Sexual Assault of Men: College-Age Victims*, Isely (1998) looks into many studies of sexual assault of college-aged men. Like authors of other studies and articles, he concludes that this is an underreported crime with few statistics and only a small body of empirical evidence. In a recent survey of sexual assault treatment centers, results indicated 130 sexual assaults at various campuses from 1972 to 1991. This number appears small but when placed in perspective, noting the years of the study and the reluctance to report sexual assault by the male population in general, it highlights the ongoing poor support for studies with this victimized group.

Dynamics of Male Sexual Assault

Clinical research on male sexual assault has a gradually increasing appearance in the scholarly literature, but tends to examine a relatively small number of patients presenting to forensic nurse examiners in emergency rooms or seeking psychological treatment or support (Goyer & Eddelman, 1984; Kaufman, DiVasto, & Jackson et al., 1980; Myers, 1989). These limited studies do not support the stereotypical dynamic of homosexual assailants against heterosexual victims as the primary motivating factor. In contrast, both homosexual and heterosexual assailants assault men of either sexual orientation (Hickson, Davies, & Hunt et al., 1994). Typically, male sexual assault victims are sodomized or forced to perform fellatio on their attacker(s) and are often physically assaulted as well. In addition, male victims are more likely than female victims to be gang-raped (Mitchell & Hirshman, 1999). Although the stereotype that men are not as significantly affected by such an event, particularly within the commonly held belief that men are "supposedly" tougher emotionally and better able to cope, there is a notable similarity in the post-assault responses among male sexual assault victims and the diagnostic criteria for rape trauma syndrome observed in female victims (Calderwood, 1987; Coxell & King, 1996; Mezey & King, 1989; Scarce, 1994).

Key Point *31-2*

Post–sexual assault response patterns are unique in comparison to other forms of assault, particularly since victims of other interpersonal crimes are not typically viewed with such suspicion and doubt regarding their own involvement and responsibility.

If heterosexual men have strong fears about reporting their assault, it is conceivable that their fears and shame-related avoidance may be due to anticipation of negative and stereotypical responses from healthcare providers, police officers, and family and friends. Supporting this supposition, Mezey and King (1990) noted that many homosexual victims did not report being sexually assaulted based on a belief that police would be unsympathetic and perceive them as "asking for it" (Mezey & King, 1990).

The prevalence and dynamic underpinnings of male sexual assault continue to be unclear, underreported, and further hampered by minimal scientific studies and poor epidemiological statistical data. These factors may perpetuate the ongoing misunderstanding about sexual victimization occurring in males as well as females. Although it is likely that male sexual assault occurs far less frequently than female sexual assault, this lower incidence may be a reinforcing factor leading to a reduced level of care for the male victim. An ongoing lack of reporting and comprehensive care is likely due in part to a poor understanding of the plight of the male sexual assault victim, which in turn contributes to insufficient training and protocol development in healthcare settings.

Global Implications of Male Sexual Assault

Male sexual assault is gradually becoming an increasingly noticed public health problem worldwide. For example, the narrow definition of rape did not change in the United Kingdom until 1994 with the passage of the Sexual Offences Act, which changed the inadequacies in the law (Criminal Justice and Public Order Act, 1994; King & Woollet, 1997). This law was changed to state that vaginal *or* anal penetration of a person, male *or* female is now legally considered rape. *Survivors*, an English counseling organization, established in the late 1980s to counsel male victims of sexual assault, conducted a study from January 1993 to December 1994 using a standardized format. In this study some interesting facts were provided to increase the data bank on specific details of surrounding male victims. Of the 115 men in the study, 87% reported assaults by other men, 7% were assaulted by women, and 6% reported that assailants were both sexes. More remarkable is the fact that 61% of the study participants were younger than 16 years old at the time of the assault. It is also reported that 75% of study participants sought no help after the assault. Similar to female victims, it was noted that male victims often had some knowledge of their assailants (King & Woolett, 1997).

Although there appears to be no reported data available on male rape in Western Europe, in the US between 5% to 10% of total rapes are reported against men. Up to 10% of victims reporting to treatment centers are also men (King & Woolett, 1997).

Ongoing underreporting, cultural conditioning, and archaic laws worldwide need to be addressed by healthcare workers and lawmakers alike. Many of the victims, years later, become sexual predators themselves as they enter the cycle of trauma learning. This trauma learning may lead to the survivor committing the same forms of violent acts against others in dysfunctional attempts at mastery of the original trauma (Burgess, Hartman, & Clements, 1995). Such dysfunctional attempts often occur within a framework of inadequate coping skills and little or no treatment for the victim. This compulsion to repeat the original trauma of the sexual assault contributes to an increase in sexual assaults throughout the world.

Another commonality among male and female sexual assault victims is that they frequently know their assailant. Most sexual assaults are not committed by strangers, but rather by someone known to the victim, which supports the tenet that sexual assault of both sexes is perpetrated not solely for sexual gratification but for reasons of anger and power. After exposure to such power and control, both genders can experience significant disruption of psychological functioning that can manifest itself in a variety of behaviors, including sexual difficulties, mood disturbances, and somatic problems. These sequelae can create lifelong emotional and developmental disturbances for the victim, and result in a diagnosis of PTSD.

Laws regarding sexual assault vary from state to state and country to country. There are still some international laws that dictate only vaginal penetration can be considered rape or sexual assault. This reinforces societal beliefs that men cannot be victims of sexual violence as women are. In some countries, however, other laws and legal terms address the sexual violation of male victims but do not carry the weight of implications associated with rape.

Community rape crisis centers across the US are becoming more aware of the male victim of sexual assault and his related needs. This awareness has been significantly expanded and highlighted with the increase in sexual assault nurse examiners (SANEs). More and more programs are teaching SANE examination techniques unique to postassault assessment of males. SANE and advanced practice nurses who specialize in forensic nursing have a responsibility to inform the public at large about the prevalence of sexual assault of males and the services available to all victims of sexual assault, both male and female. Forensic nurse examiners help educate the world community by being aware of, examining, and educating regarding the realities surrounding male interpersonal violence and sexual assault. This approach includes examining new modes of assault, including, for example, the use of date rape drugs such as Rohypnol and GHB. Males can be "date raped" just as women can.

Best Practice *31-1*

The forensic nurse examiner must consider the fact that certain physical indicators of male sexual assault are transient or difficult to detect. The absence of apparent injury should not be construed to mean that physical trauma was not incurred.

Collection of Evidence

The most common type of sexual assault on men is sodomy (STAR, 2002). Although this is typically the only sexual activity that occurs in the assault, oral penetration is not uncommon. Physical evidence is most often difficult to detect due to a delay in or lack of seeking treatment, rapid healing of wounds, or lack of physical signs of injury. When physical injuries do occur, they most commonly include perianal erythema, scarring or swelling, anal fissures, bite marks, and bruising of the foreskin or scrotum. Immediate signs of anal penetration include laxity and decreased anal sphincter tone. This will resolve quickly, so timely reporting is essential. Reporting and early assessment and intervention by the FNE can be significant in promoting good health and adaptive coping in the male sexual assault victim.

The Forensic Nurse's Role

Public awareness regarding the scope and practice of the forensic nurse examiner can play an important role. By recognizing the injuries seen in trauma centers or emergency departments and by acknowledging the occurrence of male interpersonal violence, forensic nurses can begin the assessment process. Most victims are searching for compassion, understanding, and validation of the traumatic experience they have endured. FNEs are perfectly suited for this role. An environment of acceptance and a nonjudgmental stance must be demonstrated to promote trust so that men feel safe disclosing their trauma.

Key Point *31-3*

Forensic nurse examiners can assist in dispelling myths about male sexual assault by conducting scientifically based research, reporting their findings, and developing community awareness programs to assists all victims.

For the few male victims who seek medical attention, the intervention of a forensically trained practitioner is essential. SANEs are subspecialty trained forensic nurse examiners. The SANE provides targeted and enhanced services in sexual assault investigation. The protocol of the SANE (Crowley, 1999) (see Chapter 26) includes a forensic examination and treatment; collection, preservation, and documentation of evidence; providing emotional stabilization, treatment, and referral; and court testimony. Treatment includes a complete forensic examination, assessment of the patient's injuries and psychological state, and documentation of the patient's affect and demeanor during the examination. Following the forensic examination, the patient is offered prophylactic treatment for the prevention of sexually transmitted infections.

Best Practice *31-2*

The SANE will conduct and document a thorough sexual assault evidentiary examination for male sexual assault victims, based on local regulations governing evidence collection and preservation as well as the regulations governing testifying in the legal system.

The SANE will collect numerous samples, which most commonly include semen, saliva, urine, hair, involved area swabs, and blood samples. Of note, the gender of the SANE seems to be of minimal concern to the victims interviewed. The key is the concern, passion, and respect for the patient. (See Appendix E for the guidelines for a male sexual assault examination.)

Traumatic Effects of Male Sexual Assault

Post-Traumatic Stress Disorder

Post-traumatic stress disorder (PTSD) was included in the *Diagnostic and Statistical Manual of Mental Disorders* as a diagnosis in 1980 (American Psychiatric Association, 1980); however, the effects of trauma have been long recognized, with "traumatic neurosis" (Kardiner, 1941) and "shell shock" (Southard, 1919) being two earlier attempts at describing specific post-traumatic symptoms. The current diagnosis of PTSD using DSM-IV-TR (American Psychiatric Association, 2000) is assigned when a person who is exposed to an extreme trauma later develops three persistent clusters of symptoms: reexperiencing the trauma, avoidance of trauma-related stimuli, and symptoms of increased arousal. The symptoms must be present for more than one month and cause significant impairment of function. To date, the relationship between trauma and PTSD has been researched across a number of different traumatized populations (Helzer, Robins, & McEvoy, 1987). One such population has been the victims of sexual crime, although male sexual assault has received significantly less study than female sexual assault. Possible reasons for this lack of study may be that male sexual assault survivors are less likely to seek help after the assault (Calderwood, 1987; Kaufman, DiVasto, & Jackson et al., 1980). Furthermore, male survivors appear to develop a loss of masculinity, with confusion about sexual orientation (Myers, 1989). Some men believe that the assault occurred because they were not "man enough" to avoid or escape the situation. They may keep reviewing the incident for years, trying to resolve what they should have done to prevent it (Groth & Burgess, 1980).

Owing to the lack of males seeking help following their assault, it is difficult to determine the true severity and impact of male sexual assault. However, other areas of study support the link between the development of PTSD and male sexual assault. Rowan & Foy (1993) reviewed the relationship between PTSD in both male and female survivors of child sexual abuse. They concluded that there is clearly sufficient evidence to support continued empirical research in this area. There is also some evidence that suggests that most male survivors who present to forensic services suffer from PTSD. Huckle (1995) reported on 22 male rape survivors who had been referred to a forensic psychiatric service over a six-month period (representing 12.5% of male referrals): of these 22 subjects, 9 (41%) had a diagnosis of PTSD.

Studies on the impact of sexual assault on females are more readily available in the literature, with the relationship between female rape and PTSD being more clearly documented. For example, Rothbaum and associates (1992) found that 94% of female study participants had PTSD shortly after their rape, and 47% continued to have PTSD three months later; Kilpatrick and coworkers (1987) found that 16.5% of women had PTSD, on average, 17 years after the assault. These studies clearly demonstrate a significant relationship between sexual assault and PTSD in females, and although not empirically supported at this time, it is reasonable to expect a similar response in males.

Post-Traumatic Symptoms

Post-traumatic symptoms among male sexual assault survivors may be similar but will vary depending on the circumstances surrounding the assault and aftermath. An increase in reporting and analysis of PTSD responses is needed for clinicians to ascertain whether specific outcomes are common among male sexual assault survivors. As previously mentioned, Huckle (1995) described the long-term emotional effects of 22 male sexual assault survivors who were referred to a forensic psychiatric service. Commonly noted problems included embarrassment and shock, rape-related phobias, increased anger, irritability, conflicting sexual orientation, and sexual dysfunction. Davison and coworkers (1994) reported the case of a man with mild learning disabilities who was sexually assaulted while in prison. A clear description of the impact included flashbacks, intrusive thoughts, fear of being alone in his room, sleep difficulties, and avoidance of triggers that reminded him of prison; the patient was also depressed and had attempted self-harm and suicide. All the response patterns described in these study findings are congruent with a diagnosis of PTSD.

PTSD includes a bewildering array of mental and emotional symptoms that are experienced after exposure to a life-threatening trauma or related horror and helplessness. In some cases a single terrifying event can trigger PTSD. In others it develops after exposure to an ongoing trauma, such as typically experienced by children who are abused. "In PTSD our fight-or-flight system, the one that prepares us for coping with danger, seems to chronically malfunction," says Dr. Matthew Friedman, Executive Director of the National Center for PTSD at the Department of Veterans Affairs. "People see the world as threatening and continue to respond to it that way until recovery takes place" (Wartik, 1998).

A national survey conducted by researchers at the University of California at Los Angeles (Butler, 1997) suggests that nearly three quarters of Americans will face a traumatic stressful event at least once in their lives. These events may include sexual assault, motor vehicle accidents, drive-by shootings, muggings, fire, domestic violence, earthquake, or other natural disasters. In the days and weeks that follow, at least 25% will suffer, if only briefly, from the symptoms of PTSD. It is possible for the symptoms of PTSD to fade in a week, a month, or a year. However, for some, the related symptoms become hard-wired, intractable, and unresponsive to therapy.

First officially diagnosed in veterans of the Vietnam War, PTSD is now known to strike millions of survivors of civilian disasters, such as the Oklahoma City bombing or the September 11 World Trade Center attack. In the nineteenth century, doctors encountered similar behaviors with Civil War veterans and survivors of train wrecks, and subsequently nicknamed it "soldier's heart" and "railroad spine." The psychologists of the twentieth century's two World Wars called it "shell shock," "traumatic neurosis," and "battle fatigue." Recently, in victims of sexual assault, the diagnostic criteria have been modified to include "rape trauma syndrome."

Rape Trauma Syndrome

Rape trauma syndrome (RTS) was first coined by Holmstrom and Burgess (1978) to describe the physical, emotional, cognitive, behavioral, and interpersonal traumas experienced by rape victims in the aftermath of rape (Luo, 2000). Previous research indicated that most victims experience a strong acute reaction, such as anxiety, fear, and depression, during the immediate aftermath following the sexual assault. Although noted that some sexual assault victims experience significant symptom reduction by the third month following the attack, others continue to experience chronic problems for an indefinite period of time. These persistent problems fall under the categories of fear and anxiety (Resick 1993; Ruch, Arnedeo, & Leon et al., 1991), self-blame and guilt (Katz & Burt, 1988; Ruch, Arnedeo, & Leon et al., 1991), disturbed social adjustment (McCann & Pearlman, 1990; Ruch, Arnedeo, & Leon et al., 1991), sexual dysfunction (Becker Skinner, & Abel et al., 1984), and PTSD (Holmstrom & Burgess, 1978; Foa, Rothbaum, & Riggs et al., 1991).

Treatment Issues

Due to the high comorbidity in PTSD and RTS, treatment is not always straightforward. King (1995) suggests that when PTSD develops following male sexual assault, cognitive-behavioral therapies that use imaging and real-life exposure may be helpful. The benefit of exposure with female sexual assault survivors has been clearly demonstrated by Foa and coworkers (1991). In a study of 45 female sexual assault survivors with PTSD they found prolonged exposure to be superior to other therapies at follow-up on all PTSD symptoms (Foa, Rothbaum, & Riggs et al., 1991); however, treatment may not always be this selective. Experience with male survivors with PTSD/RTS suggests that a range of treatments may sometimes be needed. Usually the most common treatment priority is managing the risk to self and others. Some clients attempt suicide and many are depressed at the time of treatment. Many victims have significant problems with anger control. Davidson and Foa (1991) provide a review of comorbidity issues. Common problems reported are somatization disorder, schizophrenia, panic disorder, social phobia, obsessive-compulsive disorder, general anxiety, and depression.

Key Point *31-4*

The main focus of initial treatment for male sexual assault victims involves reducing depression and suicide risk by medication and cognitive-behavioral therapy.

Stress inoculation training for anger control problems can also be very useful in helping to reduce the risk to others. Helping the client manage immediate risks often helps engagement, and targeting the most immediate problem areas allows the patient to gain some mastery over his problems before working on treatment specifically related to the sexual assault.

As a foundational approach toward treatment, a general awareness of the various ways a male can be sexually assaulted is needed. An FNE who shows surprise at the victim's account of the assault will only reinforce any previous negative reactions that the victim may have received or feared. Although it is impossible for FNEs to be aware of every possibility, a general awareness of some of the issues (e.g., that men can sometimes involuntarily ejaculate when sexually assaulted) will diminish the likelihood of a surprised response. It is sometimes useful to raise the issue of the gender of the FNE during the assessment. Some male clients may prefer a female nurse, citing they are less intimidated and find the female examiner more nurturing. However, as in female victims, the gender of the examiner is less important than the character and attitude of the nurse or physician. Forensic nurse examiners are best able to evaluate the situation and respond immediately to the patient's needs.

Some men may find it helpful to hear about the biobehavioral functions of the body as a method of understanding the way they are feeling. For example, up to the mid-1980s, the study of emotions and the study of the nervous system were separate fields; most psychiatrists assumed that PTSD was a purely emotional reaction to events that had shattered lifelong assumptions. Few considered whether it had any basis in the neurochemistry of the brain. But since that time a new breed of scientists, trained in both psychiatry and neurobiology, have established otherwise. These clinical neuroscientists have discovered that moments of overwhelming horror appear to alter the chemistry, perhaps even the structure, of the brain. It does not seem to matter whether the trigger was a year of combat in Vietnam, nightly sexual assaults in a childhood bedroom, or a brief crisis such as experiencing a hurricane, assault, or car crash. Any uncontrollable stress can have the same biological impact. The transformation is believed to begin at the moment of the life-threatening danger. The nervous systems "kick" into survival mode, releasing a cascade of adrenaline and other neurochemicals that prepare the body for fight, flight, or prolonged struggle. Anyone who has ever felt the senses quicken and the mind clear knows the benefits of an adrenaline rush. If the threat is prolonged, the body releases other hormones, including cortisol and brain opioids, to suppress inflammation and numb what would otherwise be excruciating pain. These are the biological forces that can stanch potentially fatal bleeding or allow an injured mountaineer to hobble out of the wilderness on a broken foot. But a response that saves lives in the short run can have long-term impact on the brain. Moderate levels of adrenaline may stimulate our hearts and help us outrun or fight off an assault, but excessive amounts can induce confusion and impair learning and memory. In laboratory animals high levels of adrenaline can cause amnesia (Butler, 1997). Psychiatrist Bessel van der Kolk, a leading trauma researcher at Boston University School of Medicine and Clinical Director of the HRI Trauma Center in Brookline, Massachusetts, states the system gets overtaxed and starts flailing (Butler, 1997). It is a breakdown of the normal stress response.

Providing male victims with this type of information can erode many commonly held fears and myths and plant seeds for recovery and reinvestment in life.

Neurobiological Implications for Treatment

Decades after their service in Vietnam, some veterans remain on biochemical alert. A 1987 study at Yale University found abnormally high daily levels of adrenaline in the urine of traumatized veterans, more than 20 years after their tours of duty (Butler, 1997). High adrenaline levels were also found in a recent National Institutes of Health study tracking 80 sexually abused girls ages 7 to 14 (Butler, 1997). Researchers now believe these high levels of fight-or-flight hormones trigger the emotional reactivity of PTSD. Dr. John Krystal, a psychiatrist and researcher at Yale University Medical School, states these people become jumpy, more sensitive, more guarded, and have the feeling that something bad is about to happen. Some researchers thought flashbacks were just psychological, with no basis in the physiology of the brain; however, now it is obvious there is more physical involvement (Butler, 1997). Trauma may somehow damage tiny brain receptors that normally slow and calibrate the body's release of adrenaline. These "alpha-2 receptors" within brain cells act as dimmer switches, sensing levels of adrenaline and reducing them when they get too high. One Yale study (Butler, 1997) found that PTSD patients have 40% fewer alpha-2 receptors than people without PTSD. When enough alpha-2 receptors are not there to do their job, adrenaline levels rise, increasing the startle response and resulting in increased flashbacks and intrusive thoughts.

Recent research suggests that trauma may also damage the hippocampus, a seahorse-shaped structure deep in the brain that is crucial for learning and memory. In two studies, Yale neuroscientists, J. Douglas Bremner and Dennis Charney, found that the hippocampi in 38 male and female survivors of combat or severe childhood abuse were 8% to 12% smaller than in a group of people without PTSD (Butler, 1997). Similar results were presented in a study at the University of San Diego that examined brain scans of 43 clients of a women's health clinic, half of whom had traumatic sexual assault histories (Butler, 1997). It is not known if individuals with a small hippocampus are simply more prone to develop chronic PTSD or whether stress-related hormones actually harm the brain. If there is damage, Bremner believes it may be caused by prolonged exposure to high levels of cortisol, which have been linked to injured brain cells and shrunken hippocampus in stressed laboratory animals. Other researchers, however, have found abnormally low levels of cortisol in trauma survivors. Whether the brain changes associated with PTSD are permanent, or can be reversed through therapy, is controversial. Neurochemist Rachel Yehada, a trauma researcher at the Bronx Veterans Affairs Medical Center, believes the science is far too preliminary to warrant pessimism. "It's irresponsible to lead trauma survivors to think they're walking around with permanent brain changes as a result of their experience. Therefore, we created the diagnosis of PTSD to validate the idea that traumas can have long-lasting effects, not to turn survivors into permanent victims" (Butler, 1997).

Psychosocial Implications for Treatment

Research suggests that trauma survivors can head off long-lasting symptoms by identifying and utilizing a social network and anchor for safety (Burgess, Hartman, & Clements, 1995). Sharing thoughts and feelings with family and friends and confronting traumatic memories early with professional guidance can potentially mitigate the frequency and severity of the trauma-related symptoms. Although there are limited data on the effects of therapies related to sexual assault, activists set up rape counseling hotlines in the 1970s on the intuition that immediate counseling might reduce rape victims' initial and perhaps even long-term pain. Pioneering PTSD researcher Edna Foa, a cognitive-behavioral psychologist, provided further confirmation in 1995 when she showed that early rape counseling can be of significant benefit in the recovery trajectory. In a study at the Allegheny University of the Health Sciences, Foa recruited 20 Philadelphia women who had been raped or otherwise assaulted. Ten received four weekly sessions of cognitive-behavioral therapy, beginning within three weeks of the rape. The other 10 women received no treatment. In therapy the women were educated about common reactions to rape, encouraged to repeatedly talk about and relive their attacks emotionally, and gently but logically challenged when they expressed the notion that their rapes or assaults indicated they were helpless, incompetent, or somehow to blame (Butler, 1997). Two months after the rape, seven of the untreated victims still reported the flashbacks and agitation of PTSD. Only one of the 10 women who received therapy reported such symptoms. None of the women who received therapy were even moderately depressed five months after the attack; half of those in the untreated group were depressed (Butler, 1997). Foa et al. (1991) advised trauma victims to talk to a lot of other people to prevent their social withdrawal.

Legal Issues

Until recently, male sexual assault did not exist under the law as a prosecutable offense. Historically, sexual assault referred to the penile penetration of the vagina and excluded anal sex. Therefore, sexual assaults against men could not be legally prosecuted. Forced anal penetration of a man was considered to be nonconsensual buggery and carried a lesser penalty. However, evolving and expanding clinical anecdotes and scientific inquiries have contributed to reconsideration of legal interpretations and statutes. For example, Groth and Burgess (1980) found that of the 14 male rape victims they treated, one victim was anally penetrated with an object, five victims were forced to perform fellatio on their assailant, and in two cases the victim was forced to perform various sex acts on another victim. In another case the victim had to masturbate the offender. Additional studies describe the violational behaviors of perpetrators (Goyer & Eddleman, 1984; Groth & Burgess, 1980; Johnson & Shrier, 1987; Myers, 1989). To date, only minimal evidence supports the legal view that the "act" of the assault is "exclusively" through anal intercourse; clinical research, although limited, suggests that the most likely characteristic of forced sexual assault is that the victim has to perform a sex act on another person, with oral sex being the most common.

Implications of Sexual Assault in Special Populations

Prison Environment

The majority of reported male sexual assaults occur in the prison environment. This is not a cultural or environmental issue limited to the US but rather a worldwide concern. According to Mallory (1999), each year more than 300,000 prisoners in the US are sexually abused. Sexual assault in prison, like sexual assault outside the locked gates, reflects the same underlying dynamics of a violent act committed within the context of power and control and not primarily one of sexual desire. Sexual assault in prison is often used as a form of punishment or ownership among inmates. In prison there exists a caste system in which those at the top are the perpetrators; those at the bottom are the victims (Mallory, 1999). Once a man has been raped by anal or oral penetration it is said, among prisoners, that he has had his "manhood" taken away. He becomes the slave of another prisoner and is relegated to the bottom ranks of the caste system. This reinforces the theory of sexual assault as a method of exerting power and control in all settings.

Military Environment

Male sexual assaults occur in many military organizations worldwide at an alarming rate as well as in the civilian communities in which they reside. One report indicated an incidence in 1994 of a sexual assault on a sleeping male soldier by five members of his platoon in the Canadian military. He reported waking to find urine, semen, and saliva on his body. He reported this to his superior officers and the five men were all charged with a variety of low level offenses. The victim lost his trust in his comrades and shortly thereafter left the service. His self-reported postassault symptoms were similar to those encountered by sexually assaulted females.

In May and September of 1996, while investigating other cases, the Ontario Provincial Police discovered another abuse case involving two male members of the armed services. It was only by chance that this incident was discovered and investigated. At the time of discovery the matter was in the process of being covered. The fear of reprisal was so strong on the base that service members were afraid to come forward with such allegations (O'Hara, 1998).

These situations should not be tolerated. Development of an independent agency to oversee investigations into such matters, with official reporting to the appropriate command level, could ensure appropriate prompt justice with treatment for the perpetrator(s), as well as appropriate prompt counseling and treatment for the victims. It is believed that even in the military, predators are victimizing these males and are using the fear of "outing" or press coverage to intimidate them from reporting the crimes. One should also consider that the perpetrators are not homosexuals, as sexual assault, against men or women, is not primarily based on sexual orientation but rather on the foundations of violently exerting the dynamics of power and control.

Domestic Violence

For many, the initial reaction upon hearing about the topic of battered men is one of incredulity or humor. Battered husbands are often a topic for jokes, such as the cartoon image of a woman chasing her husband with a rolling pin, or being called "henpecked" or "whipped." One researcher noted that wives were the perpetrators in 73% of the depictions of domestic violence in newspaper comics (Saenger, 1963). One reason researchers and clinicians may have minimally investigated incidents of male partner battering is because it was thought to be a fairly rare occurrence. Police reports seem to support this thinking, as Steinmetz (1977) noted 12 to 14.5 female victims to every male victim. However, this study is reasonably dated and may not reflect accurate occurrences in contemporary society. Additionally perpetuating this gender-specific stereotype may be that women are more vulnerable to attack than men, and that men are also viewed as more sturdy and self-reliant. Therefore, the study of abused husbands seems to historically have had relatively little importance in research or clinical anecdotes.

Although family violence persists as an extremely serious concern, in the majority of families men and women do not engage in physically abusive behavior. When physical abuse does occur, however, men and boys are as likely to be victims as women and girls, according to research done on family systems (Biller, 1995). Systemic sociological research reported by Murray Strauss and colleagues (1986) indicates that, on average, despite men being more aggressive outside domestic relationships, women are at least as likely to initiate physically abusive acts within the household. Researchers find that in approximately 50% of abusive families, male and female adults are acting in a reciprocally aggressive fashion. Of the remaining households, about 25% reflect what is misleadingly portrayed as the model situation, with men abusing relatively passive women. The other 25% involve women being the consistently aggressive protagonists toward their male partners (Biller, 1995). Compared to men, women are usually more at risk for serious physical injury; however, even in the case of spousal murder, approximately 35% to 40% of victims are men killed by their female partners (Biller, 1995). Although in some families, women who severely injure or even kill men may be acting in self-defense, it is misleading to assume that females behave violently toward males only when protecting themselves or their children.

Recent study highlights find that mothers more often physically abuse children than do fathers. Moreover, males are more frequently the victims of severe maternal physical abuse than females. Certainly there is increasing evidence of both men and women maltreating children, but mothers more often batter, or even kill, their children, than do fathers (NIS-3 US Dept. HHS, 1997). Much domestic violence involves men whose relationship to women and children is rather transitory. A large proportion of violent households are those in which the man and the woman are not married or one adult, typically the male, has not shared in the child-rearing responsibilities. Compared to those living with their own families, men who move in with women and children are more at risk to become physically abusive. Boys and girls are as apt to witness domestic abuse initiated by mothers as by fathers; they are as likely to see their mothers mistreat males as they are to see their fathers mistreat females. Both men and women must be held accountable and concentrate more on increasing constructive male-female relationships inside and outside the family unit. In *When She Was Bad: Violent Women and the Myth of Innocence* (1997), Patricia Pearson makes the case that women perpetrate the vast majority of newborn murders and a large number of spousal abuse and sibling violence.

The male with a bruised lip or a cut on his face may be especially reluctant to seek medical aid if he thinks medical personnel may find out he was hit by his wife. More women than men seem to seek medical care for minor injuries such as a swollen lip or a superficial cut. Studies that have examined specific injuries rather than decision making related to seeking medical assistance usually yield a smaller gap between male and female victims of domestic violence. In the book *The Violent Couple* by Hanson Shupe, Lonnie Hazelwood, and William Stacey (1994), based on case studies from the Family Violence Diversion Network in Austin, Texas, the overall "injury index" (combined score of the percentages who have sustained a given type of injury) is 158 for men and 335 for women. In particular, 4% of men and 17% of women sustained broken teeth or bones (about four times as many women as men); 10% of men and 38% of women had a split lip; 4% of men and 21% of women had a black eye; and 10% of men and 47% of women had multiple bruises. Cuts were sustained by 22% of men and 31% of women; the same percentage of women and men (4%) had cuts requiring stitches. More men than women (53% compared to 49%) had scratches. Overall, the differences, although minor, still justify attention and further study.

There may be many reasons an abused male is silent. He may repress the memories of the experience, he may believe there is no help available for him, and he may feel ashamed. When the abused man is asked to recall his experience he may (1) deny the event or (2) relive the event via post-traumatic symptoms. If he denies the event, he is likely to say that he was not abused or at least to minimize the attacks. If he relives the experience, he may become affectively charged. Society at present provides minimal shelter for the abused man. Reporting remains very difficult for these men, as many have experienced law enforcement personnel who "laugh at" a male caller and doubt the validity of the report. Adding to this barrier to care, most hotlines are not trained or equipped to handle male victims and the legal system has little experience in helping these men.

Violence against women is clearly a problem of national importance. However, little empirical data or clinical anecdotal information is available regarding the prevalence of women who commit acts of violence against men. Although the very idea of men being beaten by their wives runs contrary to many of society's deeply ingrained beliefs about men and women, female violence against men is a documented phenomenon almost completely ignored by both the media and society. For example, a December 12, 1990, police report detailing the beating of Stanley G. by his wife stated, "... she started pawing and ripping at him with her fingers, scratching his back and face ..." The hospital emergency department record of the same incident described his injuries as "multiple bruises, abrasions and lacerations ... chest wall contusion ... psychological trauma" (McNealy and Mann, 1990).

Violence takes various forms. However, according to Professors R. L. McNealy and Coramae Richey Mann (1990), "The average man's size and strength are neutralized by guns and knives, boiling water, bricks, fireplace pokers and baseball bats" (Menweb, 2004). In fact, a 1984 study of 6200 cases of reported domestic assault found that 86% of female-on-male assaults involved weapons, but only 25% of male-on-female violence did (McNealy & Mann, 1990).

According to many women's rights advocates, female violence against men is purely a self-defense response to male violence. Several studies, however, indicate that women initiate about one quarter of all domestic assaults, men initiate another quarter, and the remaining half are classified as "mutual." Other researchers claim that because women are physically weaker and do less damage, only "severe assaults" should be compared. The results of that analysis show men are only slightly more likely (35% by men, 30% by women) to initiate the violence. Overall, Dr. Strauss and associates (1986) found that whether the analysis is based on all assaults or is focused exclusively on dangerous assaults, "about as many women as men attack a spouse who has not hit them during a one year period." (Strauss, 1986)

If female-on-male domestic violence is occurring, it raises the question about minimal reporting and related treatment. According to the 1990 Department of Justice Survey of Criminal Victimization, men report all types of violent victimization 32% less frequently than women. This may be due to intergenerational foundations for the socialization of boys and men, especially regarding male role expectations. For example, men may fear society's traditional reaction to reporting. In eighteenth and nineteenth century France, a husband who had been pushed around by his wife would be forced by the community to wear women's clothing and to ride through the village, sitting backward on a donkey, holding its tail. If he tried to avoid the punishment, the crowd would instead punish the man's closest neighbor, for having allowed such a travesty to occur so close to his own home. This humiliating practice, called the *charivari*, was also common in other parts of Europe. In Brittany, villagers strapped wife-beaten husbands to carts and "paraded them ignominiously through a booing populace" (Steinmetz & Lucca, 1988).

Modern versions of the charivari persist today. Consider Skip W., who participated in a program on domestic violence aired on the short-lived Jesse Jackson show in 1991. Skip related how his wife repeatedly hit him and attacked him with knives and scissors. The audience's reaction was exactly what male victims fear most: laughter and constant, derisive snickering. Even when they are severely injured, men may go to great lengths to avoid telling anyone what they have been through. Dr. Ronn Berrol, an emergency room physician at Mercy Hospital in San Diego, sees a lot of men with hot-water burns on the face, deep cuts on the hands, and other injuries consistent with being on the receiving end of domestic violence. But when Berrol asks how they were injured, most of these victims are evasive and claim they somehow did it themselves or that their kids accidentally dropped something on them (Menweb, 2004). A few men are willing to demonstrate the courage necessary to call the police when they have been abused by their wives. Although police officers are very careful to claim that "domestic violence calls are all handled the same way, regardless of the gender of the victim," many male victims tell a very different story.

Case Study 31-1 Battered Husband

Tracy T., a 36-year-old professional man, was regularly attacked by his wife and, just as regularly, called the police. "But every time they'd show up, they'd just laugh it off and tell me not to take it so seriously." One evening, after his wife had hit him with a shoe and thrown a phone at him, Tracy says he finally decided enough was enough. When she came at him again, he slapped her. "She immediately stopped hitting me and called the police." When they arrived a few minutes later, Tracy tried to explain what had happened. "There I was, cuts and bruises all over my arms, but when I told the cops I'd only slapped her in self-defense, they told me I was under arrest for beating my wife."

Many healthcare providers seem uninterested in confronting their own stereotypes about domestic violence. One abused man, Dan Z., had an experience that demonstrates the significant gaps in comprehensive mental healthcare for male victims. Dan and his then-girlfriend went to see a therapist to discuss, among other things, her violence toward him. During one session, Dan told the therapist about an occasion when he had fallen asleep on the couch while watching TV. About 2 a.m., he was awakened by his girlfriend, pounding on the front door. After Dan opened the door to tell her to go home, she suddenly clobbered him over the head with a glass seltzer bottle. After hearing the incident, the therapist looked at Dan and asked: "Do you often fall asleep in front of the TV?"

When it comes to domestic violence, society seems to have one set of rules for men and another for women. Perhaps it is related to gender-specific socialization, which is more accepting of women's violence than men's violence. A 1989 study published in the *Journal of Interpersonal Violence* found that "both men and women evaluated female violence less negatively than male violence" (Saunders, 1995). When it came to domestic violence, the researchers found that ". . . physical violence of any kind was perceived less negatively when the female in the arguing couple was the aggressor" (Saunders, 1995). The double standard for violence apparently extends as far as murder. A survey (Szabo, 1998) of 60,000 people over 18 years of age, conducted by the Department of Justice, found that people believed a husband's stabbing his wife to death 40% worse than a wife's stabbing her husband to death.

There are several very serious effects from society's reluctance to acknowledge the female potential for violence. First, women are subtly encouraged to be more violent. Dr. Strauss (1986) found that "a large number of girls have been told by their mothers, 'If he gets fresh, slap him.' " Images of women kicking, punching, and slapping men with complete impunity are not only wide-spread in movies, TV, and books, but the viewer's reaction is usually "good for her." Second, although it is possible to argue that a slap is unlikely to do any severe damage, not recognizing that a slap is still violence sets a rather dangerous precedent. Arresting a man who slaps a woman, while dismissing a woman who slaps a man as "nothing to worry about," both condones violence and reinforces a double standard that historically has been used to oppress women in the name of "protection."

Male victimization is a fact. Nevertheless, a few questions remain: First, if men are so much bigger and stronger, why don't they protect themselves? Often, little girls are being taught that it's acceptable to slap, while little boys are being told to "never hit a girl." Then, when these little boys grow up, they are told that any man who hits a woman is a bully. But if a woman hits him, he is supposed to "take it like a man." James B., for example, is a battered husband who was repeatedly told by his therapists that his wife's violence was something he'd "just have to put up with." Second, according to Professor Suzanne Steinmetz, director of Family Research Institute at Indiana University-Purdue University at Indianapolis (IUPUI), men recognize the severe damage they are capable of doing and therefore consciously try to limit it. Some men are simply unable to offer any resistance to their partner's violence. One man who was blind was regularly abused by his girlfriend. "She'd just turn the TV up real loud," he said, so he "could never tell when she was coming" at him.

Not fighting back is one thing, but why would any person stay in an abusive relationship? It may surprise some people to learn that men's reasons differ little from women's: economics and concern for the children. Although the average male victim of domestic abuse has more financial resources available than his average female counterpart, this appears to be changing fast as more and more women enter the workforce. Additionally, more men than women lost their jobs in the recent recession, leaving them completely dependent on their wives' income and unable to support themselves alone. Many abused women fear that if they leave their husbands, the violence they have experienced may be directed against the children. Abused men, too, are just as concerned for their children's safety.

For a man, the decision to leave an abusive relationship is only half the battle. The other half is, "Where do I go?" For women, shelters and support groups exist, although still scarce and pathetically underfunded. But where are the facilities for men? The views of society are often that "men's victimization is statistically irrelevant," and "any violence women may do is purely the result of living in a violent patriarchy." The only shelter for battered men in the entire state of California is run by Community United Against Violence (CUAV) in San Francisco, an organization dealing exclusively with gay men. Even straight men who are brave enough to risk the stigma of admitting victimization are unlikely to turn to a group of gay men for support. In some other states, attempts are being made to help abused men. In St. Paul, Minnesota, George Gilliland, Sr., the director of the Domestic Right Coalition, has been trying to set up a shelter for battered men. Gilliland's wife hit him in the head with a board with a nail in it, missing his eye by a fraction of an inch. He attributes part of the delay to efforts by battered women's groups and other women's organizations to block the project. In San Luis Obispo, California, David Gross is organizing the Allen Wells Memorial Fund for Battered Husbands. Mr. Wells was a battered man who could find no help and finally committed suicide after losing his children to his violent wife in a custody battle. While battered men find few facilities or support, there are a variety of programs to help abusive men deal more effectively with their violence. However, for violent women no comparable treatment programs exist. This fact further illustrates a serious problem: society is simply unwilling, or unable, to acknowledge and deal with violent women. Dr. Suzanne Steinmetz (1988) states there are plenty of women who have been violent to their husbands or who are feeling out of control and are afraid they will hurt someone. But these women have no place to turn. When they call women's shelters or support groups, they are often told that they "can't do any real damage anyway," and that "their violent feelings are nothing to worry about."

Despite all the evidence about female-on-male violence, many groups actively try to suppress coverage of the issue. McNealy, PhD, a professor at the School of Social Welfare at the University of Wisconsin-Milwaukee, and Gloria Robinson-Simpson, EdD, published "The Truth about Domestic Violence: A Falsely Framed Issue" (1987). The article examined various studies on domestic violence and concluded that society must recognize that men may be victims "or we will be addressing only a part of the phenomenon." In the rare instances when female-against-male violence is publicly acknowledged, the woman's responsibility is frequently mitigated. In the CBS movie "Men Don't Tell" (1993) (which told the story of a physically abused man), for example, the abusive woman was clearly mentally ill, a fact that made her more pathetic to the viewers.

The victims and the perpetrators of domestic violence, women and men alike, have been suffering for too long. As the sharp distinctions between traditional men's and women's roles continue to blur, women are more frequently behaving in ways once erroneously thought to be the exclusive province of men. Many experts believe that the problem of female-initiated violence must be exposed, "legitimized," and addressed by the media, the forensic practitioner, the mental health and law enforcement communities, and the legislature. Resources and facilities to combat domestic violence are in short supply as a result of cutbacks in almost all social services. Acknowledging men's victimization in no way involves denying that women are victims. Women's groups that help battered women could also help battered men, and men's groups that counsel abusive men could make their expertise available to violent women as well.

Continuing to portray spousal violence solely as a women's issue is not only wrong, it is counterproductive. Encouraging such unnecessary fragmentation and divisiveness will ultimately do more harm than good to society. No one has a monopoly on pain and suffering. Until society as a whole confronts its deeply ingrained stereotypes and recognizes all the victims of domestic violence, the problem will not be solved. Domestic violence is neither a male nor a female issue. It is simply a human issue.

"Husband abuse should not be viewed as merely the opposite side of the coin to wife abuse. Both are of the same problem, which should be described as one person abusing another person. The problem must be faced and dealt with not in terms of sex but in terms of humanity" (Langley & Levy, 1977).

Summary

Sexual assault is a costly societal health issue. Historically, rape has been defined in such a way that little credibility was given to the victim's experience or the long-term health consequences. The cost of assault is a burden to victims of crime, society, the criminal justice system, and healthcare and financial providers. Furthermore, the scientific literature is deficient regarding the implications for forensic nursing research in the area of preventive intervention following sexual assault.

PTSD has benefited from increasing research over recent years, but there are many areas that have been largely ignored. Male sexual assault is one such area, and although it is important to study the similarities and connections between traumatic groups, there is also a need to examine the differences, if recognition and treatment are going to improve. The efficacy of exposure-based therapies has been demonstrated when treating different populations, but there is a tremendous need to replicate such work regarding victims of male interpersonal violence. Forensic nurses should lead the way in these endeavors.

Resources

Organizations

International Association of Forensic Nurses

East Holly Avenue, Box 56, Pitman, NJ 08071-0056; Tel: 856-256-2425; www.forensicnurse.org

MaleSurvivor

Box 103, 5505 Connecticut Avenue NW, Washington, DC 20015-2601; Tel: 800-738-4181; www.malesurvivor.org

References

Allison, J. A., & Wrightsman, L. S. (1993). *Rape: The misunderstood crime.* Newbury Park, CA: Sage.

American Psychiatric Association (APA). (1980). *Diagnostic and statistical manual of mental disorders* (3rd ed.). Washington, DC: Author.

American Psychiatric Association (APA). (2000). *Diagnostic and statistical manual of mental disorders* (4th ed.). Washington, DC: Author.

Becker, J. V., Skinner, L. J., Abel, G. G., et al. (1984). The effects of sexual assault on rape and attempted rape victims. *Victimology, 7,* 106-113.

Ben-David, S., & Silfen, P. (1993). Rape, death and resurrection: Male reaction after disclosure of the secret of being a rape victim. *Med Law, 12,* 181-189.

Biller, H. B. (March 1995). The battered spouse may be male. *Brown Univ Child Adolescent Behav Lett, 3,* 1-3.

Brochman, S. (1991). Silent victims: Bringing male rape out of the closet. *The Advocate, 582,* 38-43.

Bureau of Justice Statistics. (1994). *Criminal victimization in the United States, 1992.* Washington, DC: Author.

Burgess, A. W., Hartman, C. R., & Clements, P. T. (1995). The biology of memory in childhood trauma victims. *J Psychosoc Nurs, 33*(3), 16-26.

Burgess, A. W., & Holmstrom, L. (1979). Adaptive strategies and recovery from rape. *Am J Psychiatry, 136,* 1278-1282.

Butler, K. (1997). After shock. *Health, 7,* 104-109.

Calderwood, D. (1987). The male rape victim. *Medical aspects of human sexuality. 21*(5), 53-55, 181-189.

Centers for Disease Control. (1996). *Hospital ambulatory medical care survey: 1994 emergency department advance data* (p. 275). Atlanta: Author.

Criminal Justice and Public Order Act (1994). *Part XI, Sexual offences, rape.* Retrieved from http://www.hmso.gov.uk/acts/acts1994/Ukpga_19940033_en_15.htm.

Crowley, S. R. (1999). *Sexual assault: The medical-legal examination.* Stamford, CT: Appleton & Lange.

Coxell, A. W., & King, M. B. (1996). Male victims of rape and sexual abuse: Sexual and marital therapy. *J Assoc Sex Marital Therapists, 11*(3):297.

Davidson, J. R., & Foa, E. B. (1991). Diagnostic issues in posttraumatic stress disorder: Considerations for the DSM-IV. *J Abnorm Psychol, 100,* 346-355.

Davison, F. M., Clare, I. C. H., Georgiades, S., et al. (1994). Treatment of a man with mild learning disability who was sexually assaulted whilst in prison. *Med Sci Law, 34,* 346-353.

Dietz, S. R., & Byrnes, L. E. (1981). Attribution of responsibility for sexual assault: The influence of observer empathy and defendant occupation and attractiveness. *J Psychol, 108,* 17-29.

Donaldson, S. (1990). Rape of males. In Dynes W. R. (Ed.), *Encyclopedia of homosexuality.* New York: Garland Press.

Federal Bureau of Investigation. (2000). *Crime in the United States. Uniform crime reports.* Retrieved March 16, 2004 from www.fbi.gov/ucr/cius_00/00crime2_4.pdf.

Foa, E. B., Rothbaum, B. O., Riggs, D. S., et al. (1991). Treatment of posttraumatic stress disorder in rape victims: A comparison between cognitive-behavioral procedures and counseling. *J Consult Clin Psychol, 59,* 715-723.

Frazier, A. (1993). A comparative study of male and female rape victims seen at a hospital-based rape crisis program. *J Interpersonal Violence, 8*(1), 65-76.

Goyer, P. F., & Eddleman, H. C. (1984). Same sex rape of nonincarcerated men. *Am J Psychiatry, 141,* 576-579.

Groth, A. N. & Burgess, A. W. (1980). Male rape: Offenders and victims. *Am J Psychiatry, 137,* 806-810.

Helzer, J. E., Robins, L., & McEvoy, L. (1987). Post-traumatic stress disorder in the general population. *N Engl J Med, 317,* 1630-1634.

Hickson, F. C., Davies, P. M., Hunt, A. J., et al. (1994). Gay men as victims of nonconsensual sex. *Arch Sex Behav, 23,* 281-291.

Holmstrom, L. L., & Burgess, A. W. (1978). *The victim of rape. Institutional reactions.* New York: Wiley.

Huckle, P. L. (1995). Male rape victims referred to a forensic psychiatric service. *Med Sci Law, 35,* 187-192.

Isley, P. J. (1998). Sexual assault of men: College-age victims. *NASPA J, 35,* 305-317.

Johnson, R. L., & Shrier, D. (1987). Past sexual victimization by females of male patients in an adolescent medicine clinic population. *Am J Psychiatry, 144,* 650-652.

Kanekar, S., & Kolsawalla, M. B. (1980). Responsibility of a rape victim in relation to her respectability, attractiveness, and provocativeness. *J Soc Psychol, 112,* 153-154.

Kardiner, A. (1941). *The traumatic neurosis of war.* New York: Hoeber.

Katz, B. L., & Butt, M. R. (1988). Self-blame in recovery from rape: Help or hindrance? In A. W. Burgess (Ed.), *Rape and sexual assault* (Vol. II, pp. 191-212). New York: Garland.

Kaufman, A., DiVasto, P., Jackson, R., et al. Male rape victims: Noninstitutionalized assault. *Am J Psychiatry, 137,* 221-223.

Kilpatrick, D. G., Saunders, B. E., Veronen, L. J., et al. Criminal victimization: Lifetime prevalence, reporting to police and psychological impact. *Crime Delinquency, 33*, 479-489.

King, M. (1995). Sexual assaults on men: Assessment & management. *Br J Hosp Med, 53*, 245-246.

King, M., & Woollet, E. (1997). Sexually assaulted males: 115 men consulting a counseling service. *Arch Sex Behav, 26*, 579-589.

Langley, R., & Levy, R. C. (1977). *Wife beating: The silent crisis.* New York: Pocket Books.

Luo, T. Y. (2000). Marrying my rapist?! The cultural trauma among Chinese rape survivors. *Gender Soc, 4*, 581-608.

Mallory, J. (Nov/Dec 1999). The sexual assault in prison: The numbers are far from funny. *Touchstone I*, 5.

McCann, L., & Pearlman, L. A. (1990). *Psychological trauma and adult survivor: Theory, therapy, and transformation.* New York: Brunner Mazel.

McNealy, R. L., & Mann, C. R. (1990). Domestic violence is a human issue. *J Interpersonal Violence, 5*, 129-132.

McNealy, R. L., & Robinson-Simpson, G. (1987). The truth about domestic violence: A falsely framed issue. *Social Word, 32*, 485-490.

Menweb. (2004). Husband battering. Men's issues page. Retrieved from www.menweb.org/throop/battery/commentary/brott-hidden.html

Mezey, G., & King, M. (1989). The effects of sexual assault on men: A survey of 22 victims. *Psychol Med, 19*, 205-209.

Mitchell, D., & Hirschman, R. (1999). Attributions of victim responsibility, pleasures, and traumas in male rape. *J Sex Res, 4*, 369-373.

Muehlenhard, C. L., & Cook, S. W. (1988). Men's self reports of unwanted sexual activity. *J Sex Res, 24*, 58-72.

Myers, M. F. (1989). Men sexually assaulted as adults and sexually abused as boys. *Arch Sex Behav, 18*, 203-215.

National Center for Victims of Crime (NCVC). (2004). Information for victims. Retrieved from www.ncvc.org/ncvc.

Nisonoff, L., & Bitman, I. (1979). Spouse abuse: Incidence and relationship to selected demographic variables. *Victimology, 4*, 131-140.

O'Hara, J. (May 19, 1998). When the victims are men. *MacLean's Magazine, 111*, 22.

Pearson, P. (1997). *When she was bad: Violent women and the myth of innocence.* New York: Viking Press.

Porter, E. (1986). *Treating the young male victim of sexual assault.* Brandon, VT: Safer Society Press.

Plaud, J. J., & Bigwood, S. J. (1997). A multivariate analysis of the sexual fantasy themes of college men. *J Sex Marital Ther, 23*, 221-231.

Resick, P. A. (1993). The psychological impact of rape. *J Interpersonal Violence, 8*(2), 223-255.

Rogers, P. (1995). Male rape: The impact of a legal definition on the clinical areas. *Med Sci Law, 35*, 4.

Rogers, P. (1997). Post-traumatic stress disorder following male rape. *J Mental Health, 6*, 5-10.

Rothbaum, B. O., Foa, E. B., Riggs, D. S., et al. (1992). A prospective examination of post-traumatic stress disorder in rape victims. *J Traumatic Stress, 5*, 455-475.

Rowan, A. B., & Foy, D. W. (1993). Post-traumatic stress disorder in child sexual abuse survivors: A literature review. *J Traumatic Stress, 6*, 3-20.

Ruch, L. O., Arnedeo, S. R., Leon, J. J., et al. (1991). Repeated sexual victimization and trauma change during the acute phase of the sexual assault trauma syndrome. *Women Health, 17*, 1-19.

Saenger, G. (1963). Male and female relations in the American comic strips. In M. White & R. H. Abel (Eds.), *In the funnies: An American idiom* (pp. 219-223). Glencoe, IL: The Free Press.

Sagarin, E. (1976). Prison homosexuality and its effect on post-prison sexual behavior. *Psychiatry, 39*, 245-257.

Saunders, D. G. (1995). The tendency to arrest victims of domestic violence: A preliminary analysis of officer characteristics. *J Interpersonal Violence, 10*, 147-158.

Scacco, A. (1982). *Male rape.* New York: AMS Press.

Scarce, M. (1997). *Male on male rape: The hidden toll of stigma and shame.* New York: Insight Books.

Shupe, H., Hazelwood, L., & William, S. (1994). *The violent couple.* Westport, CT: Praeger.

Sorenson, S. B., Stein, J. A., Siegel, J. M., et al. (1987). The prevalence of adult sexual assault: The Los Angeles epidemiologic catchment area project. *Am J Epidemiol, 126*, 1154-1164.

Southard, E. E. Shell shock and neuropsychiatric problems. Boston, Leonard. 1919.

Standing Together Against Rape (STAR). (2002). Sexual assault topics: Male victim of sexual assault. Retrieved from www.star.ak.org/Library/files/mv.htm.

Steinmetz, S. K. (1997-1978). The battered husband syndrome. *Victimology 2*, 499.

Steinmetz, S. K., & Lucca, J. S. (1998). Husband battering. In V. B. Van Hasselt, Morrison, R. L., Bellack, A. S., and Hersen, M. (Eds.), *Handbook of family violence* (pp. 233-246). New York: Plenum Press.

Strauss, M. A., Gelles, R. J., & Steinmetz, S. K. (1986). *Behind closed doors: Violence in American families.* New York: Doubleday.

Struckman-Johnson, C. (1988). Forced sex on dates: It happens to men, too. *J Sex Res, 24*, 234-241.

Struckman-Johnson, C., & Struckman-Johnson, D. (1994). Men pressured and forced into sexual experience. *Arch Sex Behav, 23*, 93-114.

Szabo, P. (1998). Violence against men. In *Tragic tolerance of domestic violence.* (Chapter 3, pp. 24-34). Retrieved from www.fact.on.ca/tragic_t/tragic_t.htm.

US Department of Health and Human Services. (1997). *Third national incidence study of child abuse and neglect* (NIS-3). Washington, DC: Author.

US Department of Justice, Bureau of Justice Statistics. (1997). *Sourcebook of criminal justice statistics–1995.* Washington, DC: US Government Printing Office.

Wartik, N. (1998). Survivor syndrome. *Harper's Bazaar, 3436*, 250-252.

Whatley, M. A., & Riggio, R. E. (1993). Gender differences in attributions of blame for male rape victims. *J Interpersonal Violence, 8*, 502-511.

Chapter 32 Approach for Emergency Medical Personnel

Russell R. Rooms and Paul D. Shapiro

First Response

Skilled personnel who respond to medical emergencies outside the hospital setting have various titles: emergency medical technicians (EMTs), paramedics, rescue squad members, and search-and-rescue teams are only a few. Whether these personnel work as volunteers or are paid, function otherwise as firefighters, are hospital employees, or work for private emergency medical service companies, these first responders constitute a vital link in both the patient's survival and in the management of any forensic evidence associated with the event. The multiple levels of medical training and experience should not interfere with the education and concepts required to think forensically and preserve evidence.

Forensic evidence is most frequently lost during the interval between the victim's initial injury and death, generally as a result of medical intervention or movement of the body. Preserving forensic evidence is less complicated when a person dies at a residence or in a contained crime scene, rather than in a transportation accident, industrial explosion, or mass disaster. In a more confined accident or death scene, barricade tape can be placed to afford security for medical examiners, detectives, and forensic investigators. Here, in this "controlled" environment, an investigative team can take the time necessary to conduct a thorough crime scene search, ensuring that vital evidence is not overlooked, lost, or altered and that it is collected using proper procedures.

When a person is subjected to life-threatening trauma, forensic evidence moves or becomes unstable in relationship to the victim's body. The crime scene often has only a few bystanders or witnesses initially, but may quickly become crowded when news of the event is heard. Within minutes, police officers, firefighters, and emergency medical personnel arrive. Due to the number of people interfacing with elements within the crime scene, evidence that could aid in the determination of circumstances before, during, and after the injury or death is frequently lost, destroyed, or simply disappears.

Cases of life-threatening injury are not the only situations at risk for loss of critical evidence. Loss of evidence can also occur when patients with minor physical injury, such as sexual assault victims, are transported to an emergency department or other specialized location designated for examination. Highly perishable and fragile evidence used to identify and prosecute a sexual offender successfully requires special handling. Prehospital personnel and others who are among the first to come into contact with these cases must be educated in the recognition, preservation, collection, and transmission of biological evidence (Ryan, 2000).

Many seminars on crime scene preservation focus on the passive role of the first responder. The standard warning in crime scenes, "don't touch anything," is not an option for first responders. However, EMTs and paramedics are often called to crime scenes immediately after the incident occurs. Medical protocols demand that they accomplish physical assessments, control hemorrhage, intubate, defibrillate, perform cardiopulmonary resuscitation, immobilize, and transport patients to the hospital as necessary. To "not touch anything" is impossible. Prehospital personnel focus first on the attempt to save life; recognition and preservation of perishable forensic evidence become secondary. However, these objectives are not mutually exclusive when prehospital personnel are educated and trained in medicolegal protocol and procedures. Rather, basic forensic evidence collection tends to become automatically integrated into practice without creating delays in medical care.

> **Key Point 32-1**
>
> Evidence is often fragile or perishable and can be altered or lost during medical procedures. Once evidence is recognized, it should be documented, collected, and preserved in accordance with established forensic procedures.

> **Key Point 32-2**
>
> Lifesaving medical care is the top priority for medical personnel and should not be delayed in order to document, collect, or preserve on-scene evidence.

Principles discussed in this chapter are useful not only for EMTs and firefighters, but also for emergency nurses who are first responders in the clinical environment or flight nurses at a crime scene. Aeromedical transport has a great impact on criminal investigations. Frequently, patients are injured in a rural setting and must be transported to a trauma center (or other comprehensive care facility) in a distant section of the state or in another state entirely. When a crime is committed in one locale and the patient is transported by ground or air to an institution in a different county or state and subsequently dies, the coroner or medical examiner for the jurisdiction where the death was pronounced will be responsible for the investigation. Such investigators will no longer have access to forensic evidence left at the scene of the traumatic event or crime.

The clinical forensic principles and techniques for first responders that are outlined in this chapter pertain to all scenes, emphasizing the recognition, preservation, collection, and transmission of evidence. The chapter is divided into three sections. The first section discusses death scenes, in which medical intervention is not required; the second section addresses crime scenes in which it is required. The final section presents practical issues (e.g., preservation strategies, chain-of-custody concerns, documentation, and legal testimony).

Forensic Evidence

Courts of law recognize three types of evidence: direct, circumstantial, and real. Direct evidence is an eyewitness account of what happened or statements from witnesses who possess firsthand knowledge of the event in question. Circumstantial evidence is physical evidence or statements that establish circumstances from which one can infer other facts. Real evidence is a physical, tangible object that may prove or disprove a statement in question; such evidence may be direct or circumstantial. Everything from trace physical evidence to eyewitness statements can be considered either direct or circumstantial (indirect) evidence. The difference between direct and circumstantial evidence may best be described in the following example:

Someone looks outside the window and sees that water is falling from the sky and collecting in puddles on the ground. This is good direct evidence that it is raining. Therefore, this person could provide eyewitness testimony that it had rained. Conversely, if someone went outside to find the car covered in beaded droplets and pooling of accumulated water, there is good circumstantial evidence that it had rained. The definition of circumstantial evidence is "indirect evidence by which principal facts may be inferred." This evidence does not result from actual observation or knowledge of the facts in question, but from other facts which can lead to deductions that indirectly confirm the facts being sought (Nash, 1992).

The evidence collected by first responders can be either direct or circumstantial. According to Locard's principle of exchange theory, when a criminal comes into contact with an object or person, a cross-transfer of evidence occurs (Saferstein, 2003). Therefore, if one can link the offender to the scene and the victim to the scene, a conclusion can be drawn that the offender and the victim are linked.

Nonmedical Intervention

Death at Home

State law regulates the delineation of authority in regard to the declaration of death. Most states allow first responders to declare death when conclusive signs are present. Furthermore, advanced prehospital care providers, such as paramedics, may often declare death when faced with an advanced directive or inability to regain a perfusing rhythm after a set number of interventions. The patient is then classified as dead on arrival (DOA). Often, when first responders reach the scene, they have had advanced information that indicates they should not expect to find a viable patient. The initial 911 call information, scene dynamics, and direct statements from bystanders will provide these clues. In these cases, prehospital teams should approach the body with minimal equipment and supplies and then do a rapid immediate assessment to confirm death while disturbing the scene as little as possible. Personnel and bystanders should enter and leave the death scene by the same route to minimize risks of altering environmental elements at the scene. The first responder team must document all information surrounding the encounter for law enforcement officials and the medical examiner. This documentation should include the times from dispatch, the time the pronouncement of death was made, scene entrance and exit routes, and any disturbances made to the scene by personnel involved in intervention. Physical assessment procedures or other medical care should be noted, including information about any areas of the body that were touched in the process. Disposable equipment used on the patient (e.g., defibrillator pads) should be left in place for the medical examiner. Gloves or other expendable items used by the care team should be placed in a paper bag, labeled, and left at the scene as well.

Death Outside the Home

Pronouncement of death outside a domestic dwelling produces a different set of challenges for the first responder. Many of these deaths are on major roadways where there may be an increased number of people interacting with the scene of the crime or death. Additionally, wildlife can invade the scene and remove elements that may potentially be considered evidentiary. Because the area is open to the public, the first priority is to isolate the scene. The principles of patient care and scene management are identical to those for "at home" deaths. As soon as death has been confirmed, the immediate area should be sealed with crime scene barrier tape while awaiting law enforcement officers and crime laboratory personnel who will further document and search the scene for evidence. For detailed directions pertaining to large crime scene preservation see Chapter 10.

Interventions: Life-Threatening Trauma

Firearm Injuries

Injuries caused by firearms have altered dramatically in the last decade, not only in the number of incidents of gun-related violence but also in the increasingly variable population of those using guns and falling victim to gunfire (Perkins, 2003). Without the education of all personnel involved, from first responders through surgeons, evidence needed to properly evaluate and prosecute cases will be lost (Evans & Stagner, 2003).

For example, when the first responder comes into contact with a shooting victim, the responder will normally expose the affected area identified by the loss of continuity of the clothing surface, or by the obvious location of hemorrhage. It may seem natural to take trauma shears and cut up to and through the hole in the clothing, or even to use the bullet hole as a starting point in the exposure process. This must not be done, however, because cutting through bullet holes creates the first breach in preserving vital forensic evidence.

When a bullet is fired from a weapon, heated gases emerge, as well as burning and unburned gunpowder. This gunpowder comes to rest on the first surface with which it comes into contact, frequently the victim's clothing. Investigators can use this clothing in several ways. First, the gunpowder itself can be examined and may give an indication about the type of ammunition used. Second, the investigators can take the suspected weapon, along with the suspected ammunition and test fire it to determine the distance (range of fire) between the perpetrator and the victim when the gun was discharged. Last, the test fire is matched to the victim's shirt. These procedures make it imperative *not* to cut through the hole caused by the bullet or gases.

Clothing collection is also vital to forensic investigation. Garments should be placed in paper bags, not thrown onto the floor, tossed into a stairwell, left in the ambulance, or crammed into a biohazard bag. If time does not permit proper packaging, clothing should be preserved by hanging it (or placing it) over paper (or on a clean white sheet) to facilitate air drying. Any clothing that is still wet should be noted as such, packaged and immediately turned over to law enforcement personnel so that the technical investigative services can complete the drying process. New (nonrecycled) paper bags should be readily available on the ambulance and in the emergency department. Do not place clothing into a plastic biohazard bag. When enclosed in plastic, biological specimens will undergo chemical changes, degrading their value as forensic specimens. Biological evidence *must* be preserved in a receptacle that permits airflow in and out of the container. However, if clothing is sufficiently saturated with blood or bodily fluids that it cannot be contained in double or triple layered paper bags, place the entire paper packaged and sealed garment in a plastic biohazard bag, leaving it open to air.

Best Practice *32-1*

Do not discard clothing. Do not cut through bullet holes or other defects mechanically inflicted in clothing. Place articles of clothing in a paper bag to permit air-drying.

Next, in cases involving firearm shootings, first responders should observe and document the characteristics of wounds. Rather than classifying the wound as an entrance or exit wound, describe in detail the characteristics that would support such a classification. Most important, documentation should consist of location (including measurement from obvious landmarks), the presence or absence of an abrasion ring, the direction of the weighted border of the abrasion ring, and the presence of stippling or soot (Fig. 32-1). Unless absolutely necessary, do not clean the wound or disturb the patient's or victim's hands. Sophisticated tests may be required to determine whether or not gunshot residue (GSR) is present on the victim's or patient's hands. Paper bags should be placed over the hands and taped at the wrist to prevent any loss of the substance.

Arguments have been made that the hands may be needed for vascular access. However, current standards in trauma care call for large-bore peripheral intravenous lines (IVs) to be placed in the antecubital fossa. Experience demonstrates that the only chance for vascular access may be in the hand or wrist. In these cases, cleansing beyond the venipuncture site should be avoided.

Best Practice *32-2*

Gunshot victims with or without visible or suspected gunpowder residue on their hands should have a paper bag placed over the hands and taped at the wrist to prevent loss of residue. Bullets or bullet fragments must be transferred with gloves or rubber-tipped forceps and placed into a suitable specimen container. Deceased victims of sexual assault should also have paper bags placed over the hands to protect trace evidence.

After arriving at the emergency department, bandages covering any wounds should be removed by hospital staff and preserved for examination for the presence of gunshot residue. Any bullets or bullet fragments should be preserved by picking them up with either a gloved hand or rubber-tipped (shod) forceps and placing them in a small envelope or padded specimen container for transfer to the proper law enforcement authorities (Evans & Stagner, 2003).

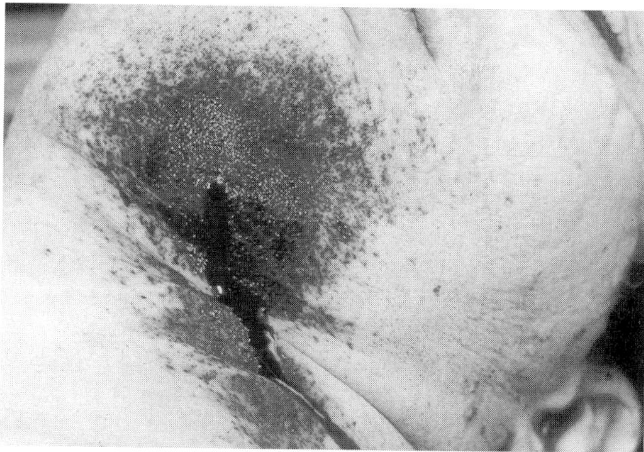

Fig. 32-1 Gunshot wound with stippling.

Sharp Force Trauma

First responders encounter several different types of sharp force trauma from which two distinctive categories emerge: incised wounds, including cuts and slashes, or punctures such as stab wounds.

All sharp force trauma produces smooth edges without bridging of tissue. Abraded or contused margins are also usually absent, except when the instrument used is particularly dull or serrated. Incised wounds are classified as such because their length exceeds their depth. Conversely, stab or puncture wounds have a depth that exceeds their surface length. Incised wounds usually give little information about the offending object itself. However, the observation of tailing, which is created when the angle at which the sharp object loses contact with the tissue becomes increasingly shallow, demonstrates the direction of the offending forces (Fig. 32-2). The main objective in preserving evidence of sharp force trauma is accurate documentation of the characteristics of the wounds, as well as their locations on the victim's body.

Blunt Force Trauma

There are four primary types of blunt force trauma: abrasions, lacerations, contusions, and fractures. Frequently, a determination can be made from these injuries as to the circumstances that surrounded and caused the injury.

Abrasions

These injuries occur when the epidermal layer of the skin is removed secondary to friction against a rough surface. They are

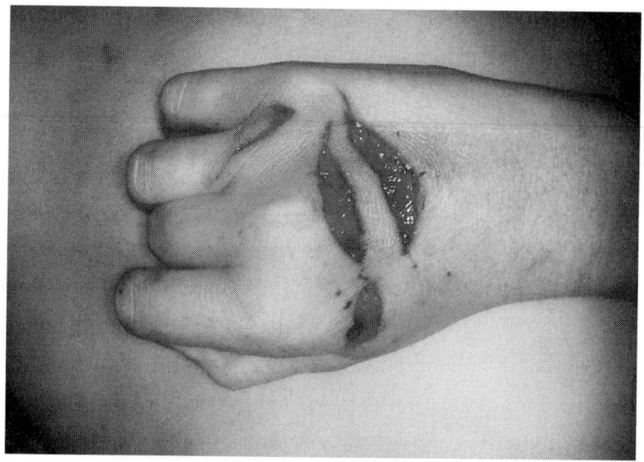

Fig. 32-2 Tailing injury suggesting the direction of force.

subclassified into four categories. First, the scratch abrasion is known for its thin linear formation that resembles that of a cat scratch, whereas graze abrasions are more commonly referred to as "road rash." The third type (impact abrasions) results when the offending object stamps the skin, thus removing the epidermal layer. Finally, linear pressure with movement, often seen in cases involving hanging, creates friction abrasions.

Evidence related to abrasion injuries is used to assist investigators in determining the direction of the forces applied to the patient, manifested by linear markings within the wound as well as skin tags seen on the leading edges of the wound. Debris from the offending object or frictional surface can be transferred to the wound. In the prehospital setting wounds may have been covered or dressed before the first responders have arrived to the scene. If the wound is rebandaged, the original dressings should be saved as evidence. Hospital personnel in the emergency department must also understand the importance of saving all prehospital dressings, which may contain evidence. Trace elements of the offending object or surface may be imbedded in the dressings. Place these items into a paper bag and notify law enforcement of their existence.

Best Practice *32-3*

The characteristics and appearance of wounds should be noted prior to any cleaning. Wound dressings applied in the field to treat gunshot wounds or blunt force injuries should be collected as forensic evidence.

The appearance of the wound must be documented and forensic evidence collected before cleaning, debridement, or suturing. Failure to do so will result in scrubbing away trace evidence, losing the direction of skin tags, and altering the wound's characteristics.

Lacerations

Lacerations are the results of blunt injury. They are commonly misclassified by healthcare personnel. They are characterized by their irregular edges, bridging tissue, localized swelling, and contused margins. They differ greatly from sharp injuries (e.g., slashes and punctures). Although a type of laceration referred to as a split may mimic a sharp injury due to the smoother edges of the wound, bridging of tissue inside the wound will be present.

Contusions or Bruises

These injuries are produced when blood extravasates from the circulating vasculature into the interstitial space. Contrary to popular belief, age determinations cannot be made based on the appearance or colorations of contusions. Contusions with varied color patterns do, however, suggest that the injuries occurred at different times. Of utmost importance to first responders is the presence of a pattern injury that can lead to the identification of the offending object. Whether these are bruises, caused by a hand during manual strangulation, or an extension cord impression on the body of a child, all pattern injuries require extensive documentation. Photographic documentation at the emergency department should be conducted at the earliest possibility before healing diminishes the quality of the evidence. Furthermore, follow-up photographs should be taken within 24 hours if the patient is admitted to the hospital.

Fractures

Fracture, the remaining form of blunt force trauma, results in the loss of continuity of the bone and can be direct or indirect (DiMaio & DiMaio, 2001). Direct fractures include focal, crushing, and penetrating types. Focal fractures, such as transverse fractures, result from a force applied to a small area, and may be associated with little or no soft tissue damage overlying the fracture site. In contrast, a crush-type fracture occurs when a large amount of force is applied over a larger body surface area, resulting in comminuted fractures and greater soft tissue damage. Penetrating fractures, the third type of direct fracture, are produced when a large amount of force is applied to a small body surface area. Usually only seen in association with firearm injury, these wounds, while often bone shattering, present with little overlying soft tissue damage.

Indirect fractures caused by forces remote to the fracture site include traction, angulation, rotational, and vertical compression fractures, or combinations thereof. Athletic activity commonly leads to indirect fractures when activities such as jumping, running, and quick turning create linear traction, angular, rotational, or compression forces on the bone. Rotational injury may manifest as spiral fractures in the physical abuse of children. The standard guidelines for fracture management in the prehospital setting work well to preserve fracture characteristics that are vital for forensic investigation regarding the mechanical forces of injury. Short of creating a new fracture or causing a closed fracture to reopen, the fracture evidence should not deteriorate because use of rigid and traction splints preserves the fractures well.

Motor Vehicle Collisions

Motor vehicle collisions (MVCs) are among the most common events that require responses from the prehospital care provider. With these collisions comes a host of different circumstances that call for the recognition, preservation, and collection of forensic evidence. The kinematics associated with even low-velocity collisions can still lead to both blunt and sharp injuries. In many instances, the keen first responder can look at the damage of a vehicle and deduce possible injuries sustained by the patients involved.

Some questions regarding patient position before the collision arise when investigating motor vehicle collisions. Occasionally, however, when a death results from the collision, people still alive at the scene profess to be passengers and not the driver, even when found behind the wheel of the damaged vehicle. Sometimes everyone associated with the vehicle is ejected and unable to explain the positions of the passengers in the car.

Fortunately, clues exist that will give a consistent indication about the position of the occupants when the accident happened. Windshield glass is laminate and composed of two sheets of glass with a plasticized film sandwiched in between. When this type of windshield breaks, it shatters into long slivers of glass that will cause longitudinal sharp injuries on the faces of those sitting in the front seat. In contrast, the side window glass is composed of tempered glass, which shatters into many angular pieces when it breaks (Fig. 32-3), which will cause angular sharp injuries to the victim on the same side as the window. Therefore, a passenger in the front seat will traditionally have linear cuts down the front of the face, and angular cuts–or what forensically are known as dicing injuries–to the right side of the face or even to the shoulder (Fig. 32-4).

Drivers, following the same line of reasoning, would be expected to have dicing injuries on their left sides. Other injuries that suggest

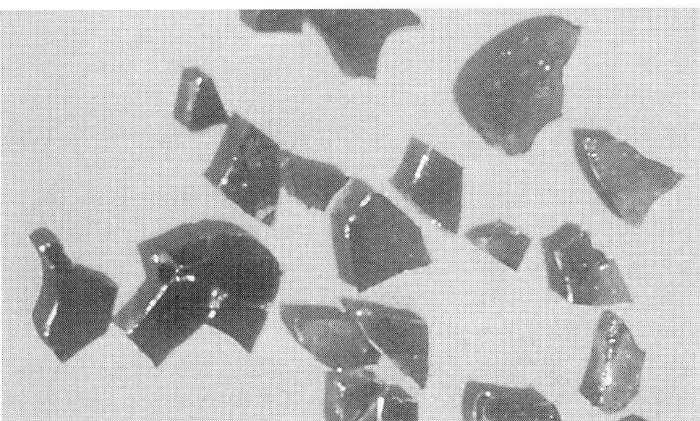

Fig. 32-3 Tempered glass pieces revealing characteristic shards in broken automobile windows.

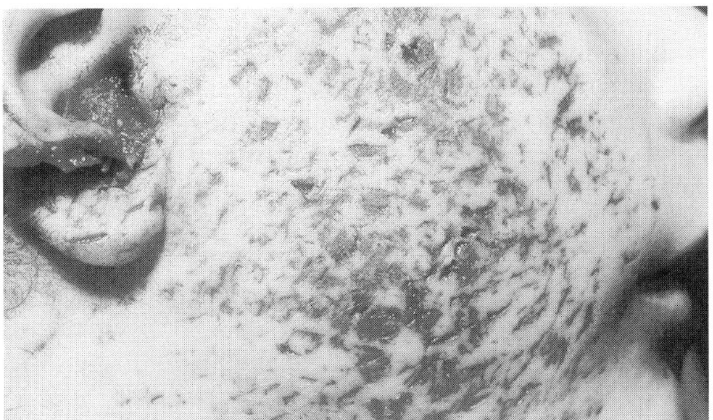

Fig. 32-4 Dicing injury incurred from head impact with tempered automobile glass.

the patient's place in the vehicle include pattern contusions or impact abrasions caused by the steering wheel or automobile company logos that are frequently found on the dashboard (Fig. 32-5). In the absence of obvious sharp injuries, look for glass fragments that may be caught in the clothing of suspected automobile occupants. Any such glass fragments or shards should be collected and placed in a solid container and preserved as evidence, along with any other debris, such as paint chips, plastic, metal pieces, plant, or grass material.

Clothing should be preserved. Clothing may contain the previously listed forensic evidence, as well as trace evidence from contacts made with the car, street surface, and other objects. Additionally, clothing evidence may also provide key blood spatter evidence that will allow investigators to determine the direction of force and injury. A frequently overlooked and underappreciated piece of forensic evidence is the footwear of people involved in serious motor vehicle collisions. Shoes may be used to determine the occupant's position in the vehicle or even the manner of death, as in the case of suspected vehicular suicide. Impressions on soles from desperate braking attempts, for example, may validate the driver of the car.

Investigations of the scenes of motor vehicle collisions usually occur long after emergency medical providers have transported the last victim from the area. When occupants are thrown from the vehicle and subsequently transported, the investigating officers frequently lack vital information pertaining to where the patient's body landed, as well as its initial position. If photographic documentation is not available, the conscientious first responder would see to it that detailed references to patient's location and position

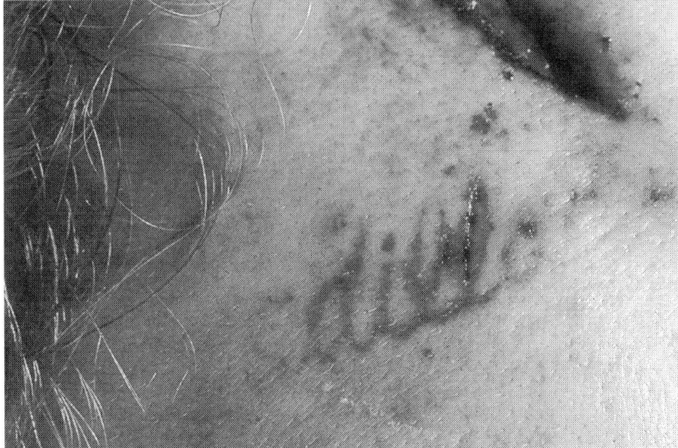

Fig. 32-5 Dashboard impression revealing impact with steering wheel.

are made available to investigators. This can be done with tape, chalk, or other method indicating the patient's position. The same method is used when investigating auto-pedestrian injuries.

Best Practice *32-4*

When managing victims of vehicular collisions, on-scene personnel should document the details regarding the state of the crashed vehicles, the location or apparent position of the occupants at the time of impact, and any other physical factors that could be helpful in predicting the forces of injury.

Overdose or Poisoning

When first responders encountered a patient who may have "overdosed" or may have been a victim of intentional poisoning , care should be taken to recover suspected substances within the immediate environment. Investigators will eventually need to determine whether an elderly person who is admitted to the emergency department was confused, was suicidal and intentionally ingested an overdose of medication, or whether the medication was administered to the patient by another individual with the intent to do harm. Bottles, pill containers, and syringes should be handled carefully in order to preserve fingerprints or other artifacts that might be important for the forensic investigating team. Gloves should be worn, and a tool such as a hemostat should be used to move containers or to transfer them to a clear plastic or paper bag. When dealing with cases involving suspected poisoning or overdose by injection, especially if they should become lethal, it is often confusing for the medical examiner to determine which punctures are therapeutic (e.g., missed IV sticks or lab draws) and which were caused by dosing of the illicit substance. To assist these future investigators, forensic first responders can circle the therapeutic puncture sites they created, using ink, to allow investigators to differentiate the two types. Although this method is generally considered acceptable, it should first be cleared with the local medical examiner or coroner. Finally, in preserving evidence of overdose and poisoning, all emesis should be retained and preserved as evidence. If vomiting is going to be induced, first responders should take saline moistened sterile swabs and swab the inside of each nostril and preserve the swab as evidence to prevent destruction of any toxic substances that may have been inhaled. The swabs must then be air-dried before packaging in an envelope in order to prevent cross-contamination.

Best Practice *32-5*

The containers or delivery device for any toxic substance should be transported with the patient to the hospital along with any emesis produced.

Asphyxia

One area in the prehospital setting that has a great impact on criminal investigations is the generic category of asphyxia. Asphyxia is also one topic in which first responders traditionally receive minimal formal education. Without outward signs of trauma, asphyxia can be unidentifiable at autopsy, making well-documented information from the accident or crime scene vital in assuring the proper medicolegal outcome.

First responders should be able to distinguish between the three broad categories of asphyxia–suffocation, strangulation, and chemical asphyxiation–each of which also comprises several subdivisions. Awareness of these classifications provides a knowledgeable first responder with a better conception of the pertinent information needed to adequately document the circumstances surrounding a particular incident.

Suffocation

Suffocation is asphyxiation in which oxygen fails to reach the bloodstream. Inadequate oxygen supply leads to entrapment or environmental asphyxias. Smothering results from obstruction or occlusion of the external airways (e.g., placing a pillow or plastic bag over the victim's face). Choking can occur when air is blocked from entering the airway passages within the throat (choking on an object), whereas external pressure placed on the thorax or trachea is referred to as mechanical asphyxia or strangulation, respectively. One must be clear when documenting choking or stragulation. Choking is generally accidental in nature whereas strangulation may be either accidental or intentional. Finally, suffocating gases can displace oxygen from the atmospheric air (e.g., carbon dioxide and methane). Combinations of events can occur, such as mechanical asphyxia coupled with smothering, often seen in children sleeping in the same bed as an adult (lying-over deaths). Although mechanisms of suffocation differ, they all involve the failure of oxygen to reach the bloodstream.

Strangulation

This cause of death includes hangings, ligature or manual strangulation, and autoerotic asphyxiation. Hangings are characterized by the use of a noose or constricting band, with asphyxia resulting from compression of the neck vessels by the body's weight. Ligature strangulation also involves the use of a constricting band, although tightened by a force other than the victim's body weight. Use of the hand, forearm, or other limb to compress the neck vessels defines manual strangulation. Autoerotic asphyxia is caused by intentionally inducing hypoxia for intensifying sexual gratification.

Chemical Asphyxia

This type of asphyxia is caused by inhaled substances that prevent oxygen from reaching the cells. Some examples of these potentially lethal chemicals include carbon monoxide, cyanide, and hydrogen sulfide.

Physical findings most common to the asphyxias, in general, are petechial hemorrhages, found in the eyes and on the face, and Tardieu spots (Fig. 32-6), found in the dependent extremities, both of which findings are secondary to vascular congestion. Another important point in documentation is the presence (or absence) of a furrow and its characteristics, because the continuity and track of a furrow may differentiate between homicidal and suicidal asphyxiation. Most cases of hanging involve patients with a furrow that goes around the neck and ends with the point of suspension in an angular position at some point in the track (Fig. 32-7). Ligature strangulation usually produces a furrow that travels circumferentially around the neck. Victims who struggle may create breaks in the continuity of the furrow by placing their fingers between the neck and the constricting implement. With accurate descriptions and documentation of these physical findings, law enforcement officials may access information vital to an investigation that could easily be lost during resuscitative efforts.

Other Prehospital Scenarios

Rape and Sexual Assault

Most sexual assaults that occur in the US are not physically life-threatening to the victims, which makes psychological trauma the

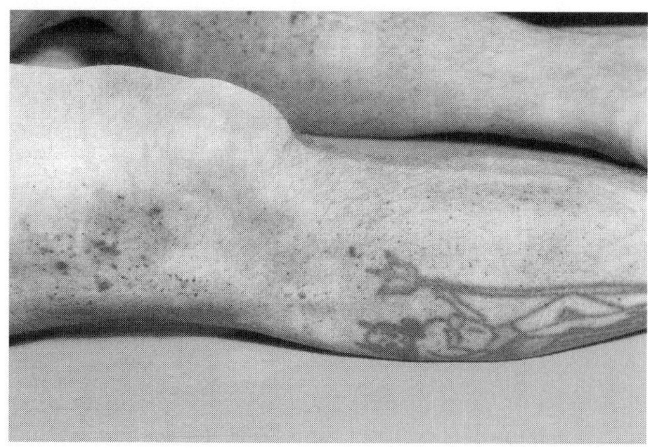

Fig. 32-6 Tardieu spots created from vascular congestion in asphyxia.

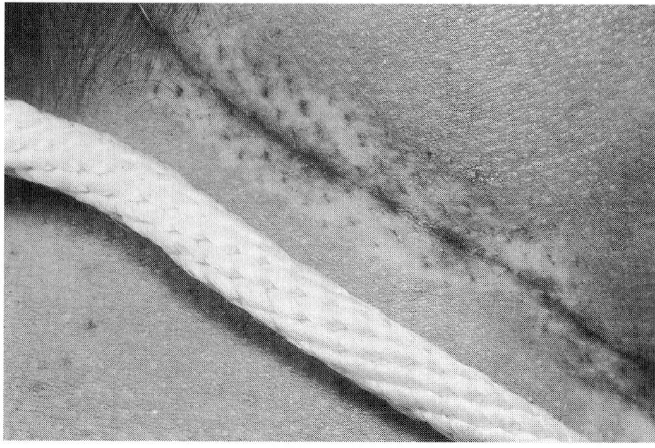

Fig. 32-7 Hanging furrow created by neck ligature.

primary concern when assisting most patients who have been sexually assaulted or abused. Police or family members usually transport victims of sexual assault to the hospital. Although ambulances may also sometimes transport sexual assault victims, lifesaving prehospital care is rarely required. Several things regarding prehospital care for victims of rape or sexual assault must be mentioned. Foremost, all patients need to be treated with dignity and respect. Whenever possible, allow patients to make decisions about what is going to happen to them. Some controversy exists over the necessity of having female caregivers provide care to female victims of sexual assault. The role of an empathetic male caregiver who returns power to the patient can be very helpful to the female patient and her recovery. It is also important to provide privacy and shelter from public scrutiny or media attention.

For medical treatment and assessment, it is imperative that the first responders touch *only* those areas of the victim's body necessary for stabilization and assessment. Unless absolutely necessary, avoid the patient's perineal area. If the victim is at home and has the opportunity to get clean clothing, it is permissible to bring the clothing to the hospital or examination facility. Explain that the clothing worn during the assault may need to be taken as evidence.

First responders must diligently document any information surrounding the assault volunteered by the victim. Their statements should be placed in quotes and in their exact words. These statements may later be used in court as an excited utterance. It is not, however, warranted to interrogate the patient or investigate details of the actual assault other than information absolutely necessary or openly offered. This consideration will be appreciated by the victim, if not immediately, then later, after they have been asked to repeat the details of the attack several times.

Finally, after transferring care of the victim to the hospital or examination facility, provide the medical staff with the linens from the ambulance stretcher, because dirt, hair, and fibers that may have fallen off the patient during the transport to the hospital would otherwise be lost. The linens should be packaged in a *paper* bag after being folded inward to prevent loss of contents. Ensure that there is a chain-of-custody form and if possible, turn this evidence over to law enforcement immediately.

Child Abuse

News stories depict the tragedy of child maltreatment that occurs daily across North America and throughout the world. Many children who die at the hands of an abuser have made hospital or clinic visits before the fatal attack. First responders must always be observant for the possibility of child abuse and neglect.

The primary advantage that first responder personnel have in the investigation of child maltreatment and abuse is the ability to observe a child in his or her natural environment. The conditions of the dwelling in which the patient lives can often provide signs of abuse or neglect. First responder's documentation should include objective statements regarding the living conditions and the way the child interacts with the caregiver.

When the least amount of suspicion arises, first responders should attempt to separate caregivers before ascertaining the circumstances surrounding the injury and document their responses accurately and in quotes. Later, their versions may change or become more consistent when they have had the chance (and time) to create an improved story. Parents should be questioned about feeding difficulties and inconsolable crying of infants in a nonthreatening manner, because these are often triggers for abusers with poor self-control. Challenges with toilet training are also a common trigger for abuse.

In addition to the inconsistency of the history, often the appearance of the injury is not consistent with the physical surroundings present. Again, detailed descriptions of suspicious injuries and the possible causative factors are required. First responders occupy a unique position that the physicians and nurses in the hospital rarely do. If parents report the child brushed up against a hot radiator, first responders have the ability to see whether the radiator is actually hot. Are the other radiators on in the house, or was this radiator turned on for some "special" reason? Does the child have pattern marks on his or her skin? Is there anything obvious that could have caused those marks? Only first responders have the opportunity to see the scene immediately after the report of the abuse or injury occurred. Therefore, it is essential to document anything that could be used later to either confirm or refute the reported mechanism of injury. Remember that the victim and siblings may be potential sources of important and reliable information, too.

Most states have child welfare laws that require notification to the police or other specified authority if child abuse or maltreatment is suspected. Be familiar with local jurisdiction's requirements and reporting procedures.

Domestic Abuse or Intimate Partner Violence

As with cases of sexual assault and child maltreatment, first responders can either aid or destroy the patient's ability to escape domestic abuse or intimate partner violence. The first responsibility, of course, is to ensure the safety and protection of the patient by removing them from the situation, either to an ambulance, police car, or neighbor's residence. After the patient is in a safer environment, assessment and treatment of injuries and psychological intervention can begin.

First responders usually enter the scene during the explosion phase during which fear for one's life or the concern of a family member or neighbor has initiated an emergency response. In the emergency department, abuse becomes even more complicated because many victims of intimate partner violence present with complaints other than battery. In either case, when taking a history, compassionate but straightforward questions will usually prompt the patient to engage in factual conversations regarding his or her abuse (Ellis, 1999). Whether the patient elects to press legal or criminal charges, the best aid for these patients is to document their history and physical injuries and provide resources quickly if and when they choose to leave the violent situation. Documentation may also be used later if additional attacks prompt legal action. The forensic first responder must also be aware that with currently developing legislation, cases of domestic violence may require mandated prosecution in some jurisdictions. The first responder should always encourage patients to accept transport to a medical facility, not only for the evaluation and treatment of current injuries, but also for a more extensive examination and consultation with specialized personnel who are skilled in providing support and assistance to the patients of intimate partner violence.

Forensic Responsibilities

Prehospital Evidence Preservation

Methods used for forensic evidence preservation follow some general rules; all specific local and state protocols and their approved guidelines, as well as laboratory specific qualifications, must also be consistently observed. Therefore, it is of paramount importance that before collecting any evidence the local collection methods must be procured and used as a basis for the forensic protocols. From documentation of victim's statements to types of laboratory procedures, all evidence must be preserved with the intention that it will end up in court. All local guidelines and protocols must be followed to ensure admissibility.

First responders have a large supply of equipment that is strategically placed on response vehicles; however, three important items should be added to the equipment list to ensure the proper preservation of forensic evidence:

- Paper bags of various sizes should become standard issue equipment. Contact the local law enforcement agency for a supply of their recommended collection bags because the evidence ultimately will be used for their investigations.
- A small camera with a built-in flash unit should also be added and include the "one-step" or disposable cameras. Although it is not appropriate for first responders to delay or compromise patient care to photograph evidence, when feasible, it may be beneficial to photograph motor vehicle collisions, atypical injury situations, and other unusual occurrences. Photography is recognized as the ultimate method of documentation.
- Finally, chain-of-custody forms for evidence should always be among the first responder's basic supplies in order to document evidentiary items and to serve as a record for transfers.

Chain of Custody

Chain-of-custody forms are available through commercial vendors and law enforcement agencies or can be produced by the individual service. Forms should contain the patient's name, other identifying information such as social security number, date of birth, the emergency medical service (or run) number, and a description of the specimen or suspected evidence being preserved. A list of the people who have had control of the evidence at any point of security and transmission should also be included, complete with the date and times of each transfer. The chain of custody starts with the person who initially collected the evidence and continues through the police, the forensic investigators, the laboratory technicians, and anyone else who may have reason to handle or examine the evidence. First responders who gather evidence in the field should also note on their ambulance call report (or other agency form) that evidence of a particular type was preserved and should list the first transfer that was made. An appropriate notation, for example, would be "white T-shirt with suspected bullet hole was preserved in a paper bag and custody was transferred to Officer Smith at the scene."

Eliminating unnecessary transfers helps to preserve the continuity of the chain of custody. Handing evidence to the officer or technical investigator responsible would take the emergency department staff out of that chain, leading to fewer points of attack for attorneys trying to dispute the integrity of the evidence. Finally, when responsible for the evidence, be certain that it can be accounted for at all times. If the evidence must be left in the back of the ambulance while going into the hospital with the patient, note where the vehicle was located at a specific time. Preferably, store the evidence in a double-locked cabinet within the locked vehicle itself.

Prehospital Blood Specimens

As previously mentioned, the medical examiner or coroner is ultimately responsible for determining the cause and manner of death. Manner of death may include homicide, suicide, accidental, natural, and undetermined. Forensic laboratories must frequently examine blood specimens that have been diluted by IV fluids, medications, and blood products administered by field responders and emergency department staff. Although these agents are essential in resuscitation efforts they may complicate accurate forensic analysis. In many jurisdictions, advanced life support personnel are authorized to draw blood samples for in-hospital testing when they initially establish IVs, which are far more representative of the patient's condition just before (or after) death has occurred. Although some hospital emergency departments have policies against using blood samples not drawn by their staff, first responders should not allow their samples to be discarded. The medical examiner/coroner's office may be interested in having access to them at a later date.

It is imperative that first responders abide by all local protocols regarding the drawing of blood samples. Although in the course of time a nationwide forensic protocol standard will be developed to ensure proper use of prehospital blood samples, guidelines of individual agencies, county protocols, and statewide regulations must be followed.

Documentation

The best way to protect oneself and the rights of patients is to perfect documentation skills, because the emergency response record is at times the only way to preserve forensic evidence. For example, the first responder is often the only one to hear a patient's dying declaration that could implicate a perpetrator of crime. Primarily, however, meticulous documentation provides a legal record that will contain information to reconstruct the circumstances surrounding an emergency response, the condition in which the patient was found, and the treatment provided throughout the encounter. Documentation must be accurate, complete, objective, and legible (Dernocoeur, 1990).

Accuracy involves providing details to prevent uncertainty about what occurred, when, where, and to whom it occurred, and what injuries resulted. When documenting injury, record measurements in relationship to well-known landmarks or from the top of the head and from the sagittal plane separating the right and left halves of the body. Accuracy also requires use of the correct terminology when describing wounds. Labeling a wound caused by the edge of a well-sharpened kitchen knife as a laceration is not only inaccurate but also could have the report and its associated eyewitness testimony disallowed in court. This would be embarrassing as well as tragic if such testimony would reveal that the patient's last words were "Johnny did it."

Further, avoid inaccuracies created by making assumptions, such as classifying gunshot wounds by caliber or as entrance or exit wounds. A 22-caliber gun found at the scene is not necessarily the gun that caused the injury, and entrance and exit wounds should be labeled only after technical investigation and surgical exploration or autopsy. Instead, describe the injury by its shape, and length, presence or absence of an abrasion ring, stippling, or powder residue. With sharp injury, the presence of tailing or a hilt or guard abrasion should be noted.

Patient and bystander statements should be verbatim, and assessment data should be precise. The first responder should avoid documentation of "within normal limits (WNL)" as assessment data. For example, capillary refill should be "< 2 seconds," and bowel sounds should be "hyperactive," "hypoactive," or "active." Document specific patient behavior and statements as opposed to general statements about the patient's behavior such as "out of control" or "depressed."

The record must be legible, because accurate, complete, and objective documentation proves worthless if the investigators are unable to decipher it. In addition, a defense attorney may enlarge a run report to poster size, point out spelling and grammatical errors, and ask the author to read unintelligible scribble, all of which produces a poor perception of the first responder's education, undermines his or her professionalism, and may lead to the discrediting of testimony.

Photodocumentation

Injury can require more than a thousand words to describe it accurately. Therefore, photodocumentation provides a great tool to supplement written documentation. Many first response vehicles are carrying the "one-step" type cameras to bring the kinematics of a motor vehicle collision to the emergency department physician, and to document injury before dressing the wound(s) or surgical intervention. After an initial orientation shot that includes the patient's face in proximity to the wounds for identification purposes, each injury should be photographed twice from the same distance and angle, once with some type of scale, ruler, or standard such as a coin or pencil, and the other without the scale. Without an orientation shot, the wound photograph may not be admissible in court, particularly if it does indicate who the victim was. The patient's name, date, time, and the photographer's name should be placed on the photograph. A policy should be developed to address the disposition of the photographs. Sealing them in an envelope and transferring to the investigating officer with a chain of custody would be ideal. Again, do not delay or compromise patient care to photograph injuries. Bystanders and other first response personnel are perfect choices for photographers and can be of great assistance when the emergency care providers are busy. For detailed information on photodocumentation see Chapter 18.

Legal Testimony

Testifying in court can be a nerve-wracking experience for many first responders. Although experience remains the best way to overcome the apprehension and uneasiness, a courtroom rookie should always consider the following guidelines.

The reputation of one's agency, one's profession, and the criminal justice system are at risk in the courtroom. Dress conservatively and exhibit exemplary professional behavior. Unless otherwise advised by the attorney, do not wear uniforms. Both men and women should wear dark or gray business suits. Jeans, sweatshirts, jogging suits, shorts, sneakers, and similar casual attire are not appropriate in the courtroom.

On receiving notice of a pending court appearance, contact one's supervisor and local attorney immediately. Request a copy of the prehospital report. Testify only on what is specifically remembered about the case and what is included in one's report. Do not speculate. When on the witness stand, listen to the questions carefully, and if unsure, ask for clarification. Be calm. Stay calm. Speak slowly and confidently. Above all else, be prepared. Knowing in advance the summoning attorney's questions will help alleviate the apprehension associated with appearing in court. If possible, review questions and facts of the case with the attorneys before taking the stand. If testifying as an expert witness, be aware of the state's scientific testimony standards and be prepared with the appropriate materials to support your opinions and testimony.

Summary

The nation has focused on improved responses to victims of trauma and violent crime in the new millennium, and prehospital personnel may ensure the first vital link in preservation of key forensic evidence. First responders must remember that any accident or death scene can be the subject of future legal action. It is imperative to recognize, preserve, collect, and transmit forensic evidence, using proper procedures and techniques. Although medical treatment is always the primary goal of prehospital personnel, it does not preclude secondary and concurrent attention to forensic details on the scene or in the emergency department.

Case Study 32-1 Removing Evidence

Forensic pathologist Milton Helpern (1967) relates a story in his book *Where Death Delights*, regarding an interesting case that provides a great example of how first responders can make the pathologist's job difficult.

One morning Dr. Helpern was performing an autopsy and he could not determine how the woman had died. After pondering it all morning he decided to go to lunch. The autopsy laboratory was housed in the basement of the old Bellevue Hospital in New York City, and as he was walking down the hall a nurse stopped him.

"What did you find out about that suicide?" she asked.

"What suicide?" he replied.

"The one you've been working on all morning."

"What makes you think that it was a suicide?" he asked.

"Well, because of the plastic bag around her head at the scene that was removed for resuscitation."

Although the information was obviously known to the first responder and passed on to the emergency department nurse, it was not placed in the official documentation provided by either one.

Data from Helpern, M. (1967). *Where Death Delights*. New York: Coward-McCann Inc.

Resources

Organizations

National Registry of Emergency Medical Technicians

Rocco V. Morando Building, 6610 Busch Boulevard, P.O. Box 29233, Columbus, OH 43229; Tel: 614-888-4484; www.nremt.org

US Department of Transportation

National Standard Curriculum Emergency Medical Technician Paramedic (EMT-P), NHTSA; www.nhtsa.dot.gov

References

Dernocoeur, K. B. (1990). *Streetsense: Communication, safety, and control* (2nd ed.). Englewood Cliffs, NJ: Prentice Hall.

DiMaio, D. J., & DiMaio, V. J. (2001). *Forensic pathology* (2nd ed.). Boca Raton, FL: CRC Press.

Ellis, J. M. (1999). Barriers to effective screening for domestic violence by registered nurses in the emergency department. *Crit Care Nurs Q, 22*(1), 27-41.

Evans, M. M., & Stagner P. A. (2003). Handling forensic evidence in the operating room. *AORN J, 78*, 4.

Helpern, M. (1967). *Where death delights.*New York: Coward-McCann.

Nash, J. R. (1992). *Dictionary of crime*. New York: Paragon House.

Perkins, C. (2003). Weapon use in violence crime. *National Crime Victimization Survey 1993-2001*. Washington, DC: National Center for Victims of Crime.

Ryan, M. T. (2000). Clinical forensic medicine. *Ann Emerg Med, 36*(3), 271-273.

Saferstein, R. E. (2003). *Criminalistics: An introduction to forensic science* (8th ed.). Englewood Cliffs, NJ: Prentice-Hall.

UNIT SIX

Death Investigation

Chapter 33 The Forensic Investigation of Death

Virginia A. Lynch

Health and Justice

Society's need to understand the disease mechanisms and biomechanical factors associated with death is essential to systems of public health and the administration of justice. These processes, which help to determine the precise precipitating factors and causes of death, not only benefit medical science but also serve the public's general welfare by ensuring that natural, accidental, and crime-related fatalities are systematically identified and investigated in regard to cause, manner, and mechanism of death.

Regardless of the circumstances of death, there are usually acute emotional reactions of significant others as well as inherent legal consequences. For example, the precise way individuals die and the events that surround the dying process can determine the execution of last wills and testaments, life insurance distributions, rights of survivorship, and more. Death cannot be viewed apart from the consideration of civil and criminal laws and collective justice principles that govern human existence from a social, moral, and religious perspective.

In a typical social structure, the loss of a loved one is a disruptive and often devastating experience. Many questions exist about why the death occurred and if it somehow could have been prevented. In addition, if death comes suddenly or unexpectedly or involves a violent act, it now becomes a forensic case, demanding a systematic legal inquiry. Police, medical examiners, coroners, and other representatives of the court are interjected into a poignant event, compounding the many emotions and stressors that are present when someone dies.

Historically, nurses have been among the key individuals to care for both the dying patient and the bereaved in that delicate period before and after death. They often participate in lifesaving intervention or resuscitation efforts and perhaps later prepare the deceased for postmortem procedures or release to a funeral home. Nursing roles and responsibilities in death investigation have been predicated on the natural extension of nursing interventions that emerge from a respect for human life and social responsiveness. Furthermore, contemporary nursing practice mandates forensic accountability as a priority in sudden, unexpected, and questioned deaths, a duty deemed second only to lifesaving interventions or resuscitation efforts. With these factors in mind, one can readily appreciate the appeal of death investigation as a forensic nursing career choice.

Historical Perspective of Forensic Death

Death is defined as the permanent cessation of all vital bodily functions: the end of life (Dorland's, 2000). The causal factors of death establish the principal foundation of medical science: sustaining and improving the quality of life. Without knowledge regarding *why* people die, it would be virtually impossible to establish preventive healthcare practices. From the beginning of civilization, death roused the interest and curiosity of the public to determine what separated the living from the dead. As a result of human deaths, medical science and the law initiated a search that has lasted from antiquity until the present. The question of why people die has unfolded criteria for both natural and unnatural death, yet even now there remains a requisite mystery surrounding unexplained deaths. The need for absolute accuracy is compelling. Forensic medicine becomes the "application of clinical and scientific knowledge that provides answers to questions of law and/or patient treatment involving court related issues" (American Academy of Forensic Science [AAFS], 2002).

In the US, *forensic pathology* is a subspecialty of anatomical pathology and forensic medicine charged with the responsibility of determining the cause and manner of questioned deaths. The manner of death will determine whether or not a crime has been committed. As a social and cultural issue, the interface between investigators of death, the decedent's family, and the public at large has been recognized as a framework in need of reform. This is an important area where the forensic nurse examiner (FNE) can bring clinical management skills and expertise to the grieving and bereaved.

A Multidisciplinary Task

Justice Blackmun referred to the circumstances of death investigation as the *unavoidable intersection* between law and medicine that requires cooperation and understanding, rather than distance and isolation between investigating agencies (*Law & Politics Book Review,* 1998). This essential cooperation has expanded to include nurses in the facilitation of social justice for patients who have been injured or die as a result of intentional or nonintentional trauma. Accordingly, nurses must be aware of the circumstances of death and the legal statutes that unite them with law enforcement agencies in the role of a clinical investigator. Whether the patient has committed a crime or is the victim of a criminal act, the nurse has explicit legal responsibilities that cannot be compromised. The universal application of nursing accountability includes the scientific investigation of death.

The historical development of forensic pathology, questioning why people die, has been recorded as long as literature has existed. The earliest application of forensic medicine dealt with suicide, generally regarded as a crime against public interest since classical times (Baden, 1989). The criminality of suicide and the penalty involved included condemnation of the offender by the Roman Catholic Church. For the violation of canon law by suicide to be confirmed, the investigation of death evolved from the need to determine the accurate cause of suicidal deaths (Spitz & Fisher, 1993). During these times, the investigation relied solely on the circumstances of death without a specific examination of the body.

Not until the thirteenth century did the autopsy become a standard of practice in the postmortem evaluation of death. China is the first country known to have developed extensive, detailed instructions on necropsy pathology and the autopsy. The Chinese handbook *Hsi Yuan Lu* specified precise protocols addressing the types of wounds inflicted by sharp versus blunt instruments, death by drowning versus submersion in water after death, and death by fire versus burning after death (*Hsi Yuan Lu* in Camps, Robinson, & Lucas, 1976).

Since these earliest beginnings, there has been an intense and ever-expanding interest in death investigation, specifically as it relates to solving crimes. New technologies have emerged to complement the examination and dissection of the body. Contemporary death investigation incorporates the application of infrared videography, ultraviolet lights, lasers, spectrographs, neutron activation analysis, computer software, scanning electron microscopes, and DNA analysis. However, the contribution of the autopsy remains basically unchanged and irreplaceable.

Death Investigation and the Law

Every death has actual or potential legal implications. Death investigation procedures are designed to determine the precise factors surrounding death, which will aid medical science and, in some cases, foster the administration of justice. Health or disability insurance payments, survivor benefits, transfer of estates, anatomical tissue or organ donations, and criminal charges are dependent on information emerging from autopsy findings. Data that suggest suicide, evidence of torture, presence of toxicological residue, or the discovery of an unknown pregnancy can significantly impact subsequent judicial proceedings, as well as determining the corpus delicti in criminal liability. *Corpus delicti* refers to the substantial and fundamental *fact* necessary to prove the commission of a crime (Dorland's, 2000). This term is often used erroneously to designate the physical body of the homicide. For example, the corpus delicti of homicide is the fact that a person died from unlawful violence (Adelson, 1974). This legal term literally refers to the body of the crime or offense, *not* the corpse of the decedent, and must be determined for successful prosecution of a criminal death.

Key Point *33-1*

The *cause of death* is the factor that initiated the sequence of events that culminated in death, such as cancer or multiple injuries from a vehicle incident.

The *manner of death* refers to the circumstances from which the cause of death emerged—that is, natural, accidental, homicidal, suicidal, or undetermined.

Fundamentals of Death Investigation

Death investigation is a process that involves the collection and analysis of data, physical evidence, and circumstances of the event from which conclusions are derived or hypothesized. These data will direct further investigation as appropriate to establish the identification of the decedent, approximate interval of time since death, and the cause, manner, and mechanism of death.

The investigation process is systematic and ongoing. This involves both subjective and objective data and an assessment of those data from which a plan of investigation is derived. The actual conduction of an investigation, evaluation of data obtained during the investigation, and the reinvestigation and reevaluation of data as necessary stem from the medical investigation of death. The process is consistent with established guidelines for the individual manner of death being investigated. The findings and conclusions derived are validated by the data obtained. The cause of death is certified and supported by the findings of the investigation.

Death is the actual state of nonbeing. To declare a person dead is a legal issue that should mandate medical knowledge. The sequence of physiological events that relate specifically to the process of dying is a medical issue. This responsibility demands knowledge of the presumptive signs of death as well as laws governing determination of death. Although most legal rights are suspended at death, certain laws pertain to an inquiry into the circumstances of death, security of personal property, and disposition of the body, as well as individual human rights, which remain in death. The rights of the decedents and their families become legal issues once the processes of death are complete.

After life is concluded, the body becomes a nonentity without conscious needs. Attention then turns to the family's needs, once the body becomes the property of the law in cases of traumatic or unexpected deaths, or where the cause of death is unknown. These cases require the body to be identified, categorized, labeled, and transported to the forensic facility where questions pertaining to *who, what, when, where, why, and how* death occurred will be answered or remain undetermined.

The medical investigation of forensic deaths include evaluations to determine a cause and manner of death. Classic questions are asked:

- *Who* is/was the person? (confirm the identity beyond any doubt)
- *What* happened? (stabbing, beating, fall, collision, or exsanguination)
- *When* did the person die? (the best estimate of the time of death)
- *Where* did it happen? Where did the person die? (e.g., in the street and then in the hospital)
- *Why* did it happen? (argument, lost consciousness, defective product)
- *How* did it happen? (a car spun on ice, rotated, glanced off a building, then struck a pedestrian)

Beyond the initial issues of *who* the decedent may be, one must determine *what* vectors and forces caused the death. *When* the death occurred is often essential information to help determine the circumstances and manner of death. *Where* represents the location the body was found. Did the death occur here, or was the person killed elsewhere? Did the person walk to her or his death, or was the body transported to this particular place? *Why* refers to the series of sequential circumstances pertaining to events prior to death, at the time of death, and immediately afterward. *How* refers to a descriptive account of the circumstances of *why* in an investigator's report.

Answers to these questions will help establish the cause of death. The answers are often determined at the time of autopsy but may remain undetermined if no cause can be identified. Although *what* is often the most controversial issue in the investigative process and courtroom debate, each aspect of the investigation must interface with the others in order to provide a precise conclusion. Determining what occurred depends on the quality of scene investigation, recovery and preservation of evidence, the autopsy, and toxicology evaluation.

The final diagnoses are based on the answers to these issues. The issue of *what* occurred is of paramount importance in determining whether or not a crime has been committed. The need for absolute accuracy is paramount in establishing the cause of death (Besant-Matthews, personal communication, April 2004). These questions and their answers will guide the investigator through a plan of action and provide an evaluation of outcomes.

Causes of Death

There are two major categories of the *cause* of a medical death: disease and trauma. Most medical deaths occur when pathology or injuries impact the vital functions of the central nervous system or heart and lungs. The *manner of death* may be natural or unnatural. A medical death is deemed *natural* if it stems from congenital anomalies or disease that interferes or disables vital organ functions. Natural deaths may involve degenerative infections of metabolic or neoplastic origins.

Unnatural deaths involve intentional acts such as homicide or suicide as well as nonintentional traumatic antecedents. When deaths result from violence or acts of war, poisonings, fire, abuse, neglect, or environmental toxins, they are termed unnatural.

Basic knowledge regarding the scientific investigation of death involves the following:

- Identification of trauma, natural disease processes, self-inflicted wounds versus those inflicted by another, pharmacology, toxicology, entomology, anthropology, anatomy and physiology, risk factors, statistics, and human behavior.
- Recognition of wound characteristics related to injuries resulting from weapons used to inflict death range from the subtle, innocuous signs of abuse or neglect to catastrophic fatal injuries or mutilation of bodies before and after death.
- Recovery and documentation of evidence, collection and preservation of highly perishable and fragile specimens, and the security of such material are primary responsibilities of the death scene investigator.
- Notification of next of kin in a personal, timely, compassionate, and sensitive approach.

At the scene of death, the responding investigator assesses the circumstances of death, observing for indicators of violence, poisoning, homicide, suicide, or accident. The investigator interviews the decedent's family or significant others at the scene to determine if the person has a notable medical history, obtains the name of the attending physician, and documents any medications or other clues at the scene that might reveal an associated medical condition. At this time, the investigator may request the family to contact a mortuary or inform them that the body will be sent to a morgue for further assessment. In the latter case, the investigator is responsible for arranging legally secure transportation of the body to the medical examiner or coroner's facility. Emergency medical personnel on the scene will rarely assume this role since they must be immediately available to respond to calls involving living persons. If the death is deemed to be a natural death and if the decedent's physician has agreed to sign the death certificate, the medical examiner or coroner may permit the body to be taken to the funeral home while awaiting certification.

The body should not be embalmed prior to a postmortem examination. It is vital to ensure that the death is not a forensic case prior to any mortuary procedures because embalming may introduce artifacts or destroy evidence, especially in cases of poisoning.

Best Practice *33-1*

Forensic autopsy should precede embalming procedures, because body alterations and use of embalming fluids affect the appearance and characteristics of body surfaces, organs, and tissues and the blood.

Although embalming temporarily preserves the condition of the body and significantly reduces the risk of infection from the corpse, it is essential to accomplish any investigative procedures first. When the body is released for burial the mortician will obtain permission according to the wishes of the family to proceed with embalming techniques (Adelson, 1974).

Forensic Pathologist/Coroner at the Scene

Generally, the elected coroner or appointed medical examiner is not mandated to go to a death scene. Often, depending on the law within their jurisdiction, the forensic examiner may decide to respond to the scene or send a designee to oversee the medical investigation. The presence of a forensic medical professional enhances an understanding of the case. Although it would be ideal, the shortage of forensic pathologists limits the time and opportunity to respond to the scene with few exceptions. However, most scenes require the attendance of a forensic pathologist or medical investigator, coroner or deputy coroner. Other cases may require neither. Because the majority of all reported deaths consist of natural deaths, many cases can be confirmed by a telephone interview with the attending physician. In most jurisdictions, the coroner's deputy, or the medical examiner's investigator can authorize the removal of the body by preexisting arrangements or after consulting with the police and the removal service.

When the presence of a forensic medical professional is required at a scene, the professional is notified by the responding law enforcement agency once it has been determined a death has occurred. In a coroner's system, the coroner or coroner's deputy will respond to the scene. The chief medical examiner, independently or through an appointed forensic medical investigator, will respond to a scene within jurisdictional boundaries. The medical examiner (ME), coroner, or his or her investigator has the authority to conduct an inquiry and an investigation to certify the death of those who die under the legislative mandate of their jurisdiction.

The medical examiner, coroner or designee appointed to conduct a medicolegal death investigation has the authority to take custody and control of the body, respond to and investigate the scene, take possession of evidence, and review medical records. Only the ME or coroner, however, is authorized to certify the cause and manner of death under independent authority, unfettered by political or other influences.

The forensic nurse as the medical investigator or deputy coroner responsible for representing the medical examiner or coroner collects information that may be used to confirm the identification of the decedent and establish an approximate date and time of death. These data will assist the forensic pathologist at the time of autopsy and contribute to the determination of cause, manner, and mechanism of death.

Consent to the removal of the body from a scene of suspicious death must come from an authority of either system. The body and the scene should be photodocumented in a sequential and detailed series for presentation to the forensic pathologist at the time of autopsy. These photographs should represent the scene and position of the body, as well as any medical evidence pertaining to the cause of death on or around the body, to provide a virtual assessment of the circumstances of death in the absence of the pathologists at the scene.

Law enforcement has absolute jurisdiction over the scene of crime. The officiator of death has unconditional jurisdiction over the body. After law enforcement officials have completed their scene investigation, the body should be removed with as little disturbance as possible. The clothing, weapons, dressings, or other paraphernalia should remain intact and later viewed in detail within a laboratory environment. Here, the clothing should be delicately removed to prevent the loss of any trace or physical evidence. Photographs should be taken of the body while clothed and after clothing is removed, prior to dissection.

Death Investigation Systems

Systems structured for the investigation of death are organized to conduct a professional practice within the framework of standards developed and approved by the discipline's governing body and within the parameters of legislative authorities. A medicolegal death investigation system may operate under the direction of an appointed chief medical examiner (forensic pathologist certified by the American Board of Forensic Pathology) or an elected coroner as authorized by state law.

Governing statutes, administrative rules, and professional performance standards define the duties and responsibilities of those who are appointed to conduct a forensic death investigation. Medical examiner or coroner systems are responsible for determining the cause and manner of questioned deaths. Forensic cases require the investigation of all violent, sudden, or unexpected deaths as well as any other identified by legal statutes that may include the following:

- Any death which may be due entirely or in part to any factor other than natural disease
- Natural deaths (approximately 65% of investigations in small jurisdictions and 31% in urban areas) in which the decedent does not have a personal physician familiar with the patient's medical history, social or environmental situation, or the circumstances of the terminal event
- Deaths from violence, accidents, or acts of suicide or homicide
- Suspicious deaths (unusual, unexpected, unexplained with no history of significant heart disease or other condition associated with sudden death)
- Deaths suspected to be a result of sudden infant death syndrome (SIDS)
- Deaths that occur during or in association with, or as a consequence of, a diagnostic, therapeutic, or anesthetic procedure (during trauma treatment, under general anesthesia, or from complications of diagnostic or therapeutic procedures)
- Any death in which a fracture of a major bone has occurred within the past six months.
- Deaths in which a person died while an inmate of a public institution or in the custody of law enforcement personnel

Death investigation jurisdictions in the US operate in various systems within the different states. The objectives, however, remain the same. The office of the chief medical examiner (OCME) or office of the chief medical investigator (OCMI) system (unique to New Mexico), coroner (medically qualified or lay-coroner), or a combination of mixed systems (such as sheriff-coroner/public administrator system, or a medical examiner system) comprises the primary death investigation systems in the US. A new system becoming recognized is the nurse-coroner system. The coroner is an elected official who appoints deputies; qualifications are set by each state, and coroners are not required to be physicians in many states. According to Marion Cumming, "The coroner is a public official who is primarily charged with the duty of determining how and why people under the coroner's jurisdiction die" (Cumming, 1995).

Where the law provides for a system of death investigation under the jurisdiction of the medical examiner, coroner, or mixed system, the death will become a point of legal inquiry from both a medical and a legal perspective. The law states that certain categories of deaths are to be reported to the county or state death authority for its participation in the investigation. All trauma deaths are categorized as forensic cases and require investigation until any suspicious circumstances have been confirmed or ruled out. Because trauma providers work in an area most likely to come in contact with forensic cases, they should be aware of death investigation protocols as well as the legal statutes pertaining to traumatic deaths. This includes suspicious or questioned deaths, unattended deaths, anesthesia-related deaths or deaths related to medical treatment, and a number of others specific to medical-forensic mandates.

Key Point *33-2*

All trauma deaths are categorized as forensic cases and require investigation.

Medical examiners are generally physicians, predominantly forensic pathologists who are appointed officials who in turn appoint deputy medical examiners. These may be forensic pathologists, medical investigators (lay-persons with a variety of nonmedical backgrounds) or forensic nurses. Due to the lack of board-certified forensic pathologists in North America, an appointed physician may not have forensic education and training, but will receive competency and experience through on-the-job training. There are fewer than 400 board-certified forensic pathologists in the US and Canada; the distribution is uneven, and smaller states may have far fewer than needed to cover the number of deaths in their jurisdiction. Jurisdictions may be defined by the state or county depending on state law. Medical examiner agencies function either as an independent governmental unit or as a division of some other unit. Medical forensic investigators are appointed to represent the authority of the chief medical examiner at the scene of death.

Forensic nurse examiners serve as elected coroners and assistants to forensic pathologists or coroners at the crime scene, residence or the hospital, as well as during postmortem examinations, autopsies, exhumations, and in disaster site recovery. Efficient, well-equipped, well-trained investigators contribute significantly to a successful investigation and removal of remains in catastrophic, unexpected, or unattended natural deaths. Smooth functioning and close cooperation between the first responders, police agencies, fire department officials, emergency services, mortuary personnel, and death scene investigators demonstrate a high level of continued confidence in medicolegal matters to the community.

Intuitively, it appears to be a better choice to have someone with a healthcare background and clinical expertise to fill this important role. Nurses are particularly prepared to recognize signs and symptoms of natural disease processes, to interact with physicians or other healthcare professionals, and to interact with grieving families. The nurse investigator or nurse coroner must also collaborate with scientific and legal personnel, law enforcement agents, and other investigative agencies involved in the medicolegal investigative process.

Jurisdiction of Death

Legislative statutes of the state, province, or country of residence establish jurisdiction and authority for the medical examiner, medical investigator, and coroner systems in forensic deaths. Legal statutes defining jurisdiction differ according to the local, state, federal, or provincial levels, and vary in different countries; however, the categories of death generally remain the same or similar in nature.

State or provincial statutes define jurisdiction over the body of any person who dies as a result of trauma, violence, accident, suicide, or homicide, or whose death is unattended or involves any suspicion of foul play. The medical examiner or coroner may also be notified depending on the circumstances of death of persons who have no known pertinent medical history. This category of death is intended to include those about whom nothing medical can be found–for instance, a traveler passing through the state who dies at the bus station. It does not include a person who is found dead under nonsuspicious circumstances whose regular attending physician or other clinical physician is unwilling to certify death simply because the physician was not present to observe the death. Certification of death is based on the physician's ability to determine the cause of death based on reasonable medical certainty. The medical examiner or coroner has no authority to assume jurisdiction over the body of a person who has died of an obvious natural disease in nonsuspicious circumstances or to be summoned into the case merely because the decedent's private physician is temporarily unavailable or unwilling to sign. Some jurisdictions do not include nursing home deaths, as all patients have attending physicians, unless suspicious circumstances are reported or suspected.

Key Point *33-3*

Certification of death is based on the physician's ability to determine the cause of death based on reasonable medical certainty.

Furthermore, it is necessary to eliminate natural deaths from being sent to the medical examiner when possible. This is an important consideration where forensic nurse investigators or nurse coroners can examine and evaluate the death from a medical perspective, releasing the body directly to the funeral facilities. The ability to divert the natural deaths from the forensic facility helps in three important categories:

1. Reduction of cost to county government
2. Reduction of unnecessary workload on the forensic pathologist
3. Reduction of emotional trauma to the family

Death Defined

The diagnosis of death is traditionally made using the *Triad of Bichat,* which states that death is "the failure of the body as an integrated system associated with the irreversible loss of circulation, respiration and innervation." This is also known as somatic death or clinical death (University of Dundee, 2003). The American College of Legal Medicine defines death in the following manner: "For legal purposes, a human body with irreversible cessation of total brain functions, according to usual and customary standards of medical practice, shall be considered dead" (Liang & Snyder, 2004).

Brain Death

Brain death is a state in which that organ is incapable of sustaining spontaneous respiration and circulation as a result of severe and irreversible injury (American Bar Association and the National Conference of Commissioners of Uniform State Laws 1968, cited in Spitz & Fisher, 1993). Brain death is further defined by the Iowa Statewide Organ Procurement Organization as the irreversible loss of all functions of the brain. It can be determined in several ways. One criterion is that no electrical activity is occurring within the brain as demonstrated by EEG. Another criterion for brain death is that no blood is flowing to the brain. Finally, when there is absence of functioning in all parts of the brain as determined by clinical assessment (no movement, no response to stimulation, no breathing, no brain reflexes), the conditions for brain death are met.

There are several ways in which a person can become brain dead. These include anoxia, ischemia, intracranial hematoma, gunshot wound to the head, intracranial aneurysm, or tumor mass. When any of these occurs, they cause swelling of the brain. Because the brain is enclosed in the skull, it does not have room to swell, thus intracranial pressure increases. This can stop blood flow to the brain, kill brain cells, and cause herniation of the brain. When brain cells die, they do not regenerate; thus, any damage caused is permanent and irreversible (Emory, 2003).

Key Point *33-4*

A person who is declared brain dead is legally dead.

Criteria for brain death must be present for 30 minutes at least six hours after onset of coma and apnea. All appropriate diagnostic therapeutic procedures must be performed. A confirmatory test of cerebral blood flow is necessary if any standard is doubtful or not tested. These include the presence of coma or cerebral unresponsiveness, apnea, dilated pupils, absent brain stem reflexes and electrical silence of vital brain tissue.

In spite of some differences in legal definitions of brain death in various states, physicians can meet the requirements of all by using commonly accepted criteria of brain death or by having two physicians, one of whom is a neurologist, make the determination. To avoid any appearance of impropriety when the death of an organ or tissue donor is being certified, physicians should not be members of the recipient's transplant team. Brain death must be declared prior to disconnection of artificial ventilation and before removing any organs or tubes (Spitz & Fisher, 1993). Cessation of brain function can be confirmed by a flat EEG for five minutes and the absence of physical movements and sensations.

Molecular Death

Molecular or cellular death is a definitive sign of death. It is the death of individual organs and tissues of the body consequent upon the circulation. Different tissues die at different rates depending on their oxygen requirements. Thus, within four minutes of the blood supply to the brain ceasing, the central nervous system is irreversibly damaged (University of Dundee, 2003).

Signs of Death

Postmortem Body Changes

Nurses are familiar with early signs of death that include changes in the eyes and skin as well as a general cooling of the body. Upon death, the pupils dilate and there is no reaction to light. Corneal reflexes are absent and the cornea gradually becomes cloudy. A thin film of cornea cloudiness may be observed within two to three hours if eyes remain open; if eyes remain closed, it may take up to 24 hours. In the postmortem period in a dry environment, there is a blackish brown discoloration on the exposed area of the eyes between the eyelids called *taches noires* (Fig. 33-1). Other changes include a loss of pressure in eyeballs and the *railroad or boxcar phenomenon.* This common phenomenon induced by the settling of red blood cells in a boxcar pattern within the fundi of the eyes is an immediate sign of death. The absence of respiration and electrical and mechanical heart action for five minutes or more also constitute death.

Early Signs of Death

Cooling of the Body

Soon after death, the body loses heat through conduction, convection, and radiation. These combined processes, sometimes augmented by small amounts of evaporative cooling, reduce the core temperature until it reaches ambient temperature. This process is usually complete in 16 to 20 hours. In usual environmental conditions surrounding death, the rate of cooling may be either accelerated or retarded.

Changes in the Skin and Muscle

Livor Mortis. The skin becomes a pale ashy white and loses tone and translucency. *Livor mortis* (Fig. 33-2) (also termed postmortem lividity) is a purplish blue discoloration noted on dependent areas of the body due to gravitational pooling of blood after circulation ceases. This process typically starts in one to three hours post-death and begins as mottled patches of color, but over the next three to six hours it gradually spreads, affecting larger areas. Livor mortis reflects the postmortem interval (i.e., the time between death and discovery of the body). There are certain situations that impact livor mortis development including body position or position changes and even poisoning.

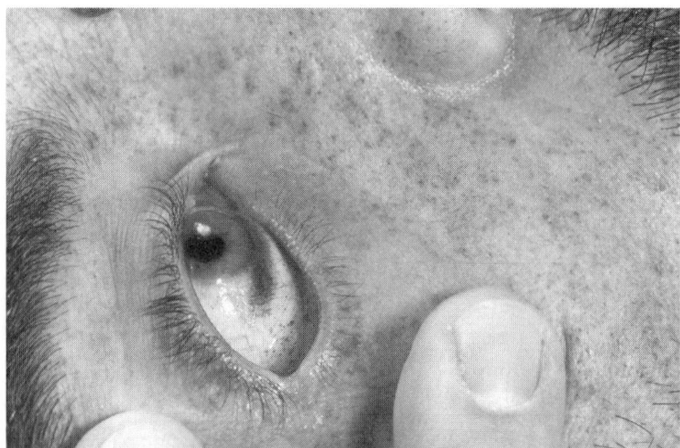

Fig. 33-1 In the postmortem period in a dry environment, blackish-brown discoloration of the exposed eyeball, termed *taches noires*, occurs.

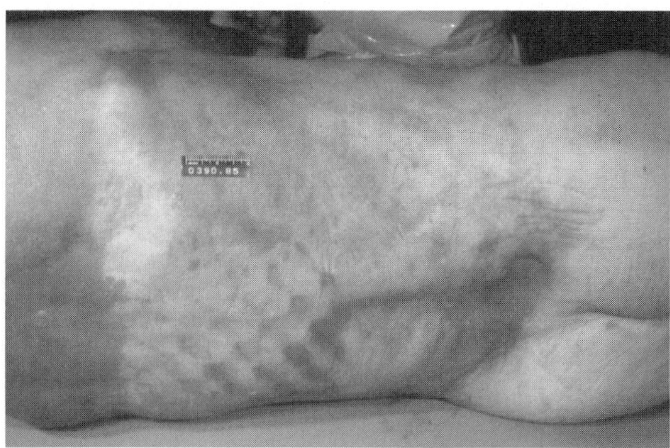

Fig. 33-2 *Livor mortis* (also termed postmortem lividity) is the purplish blue discoloration noted on these dependent areas of the body due to gravitational pooling of blood after circulation ceases.

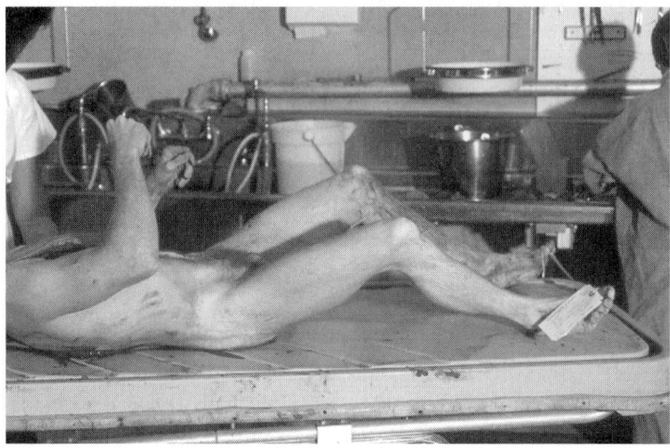

Fig. 33-3 This individual displays the characteristics of postmortem *rigor mortis.*

Rigor Mortis. Muscles become flaccid soon after death, but within 30 minutes or more and in average temperate conditions, they become increasing more rigid resulting in a condition termed *rigor mortis* (Fig. 33-3). This condition is induced by a stiffening and shortening of muscles after death due to loss of adenosine triphosphate (ATP). Actin and myosin form a stiff gel in both involuntary and voluntary muscles and affect the body from head to toe. The process of rigor mortis starts within half an hour to two to three hours depending on environment and temperature. It is usually complete in 12 hours and gradually subsides within the next 12 to 24 hours. The period of rigor mortis is affected by many external and internal factors such as climate and extreme physical exertion immediately prior to death, but may last up to 36 hours. Along with livor mortis, its presence helps to define the postmortem interval for estimating the time of death. If rigor mortis is dramatically accelerated or retarded, it may suggest poisoning by strychnine or unusual environmental conditions, respectively.

Late Signs of Death

Decomposition

Later signs of death include changes in color and composition of body tissues. The presence of sulfmethemoglobin creates a greenish discoloration over the sacrum, flanks, abdomen, genitalia, and other body parts.

Putrefaction

Putrefaction results from tissue autolysis that is induced by microorganisms and other environmental factors. Putrefaction is accompanied by discoloration and a foul smell caused by accumulating gases. Ammonia, hydrogen sulfide, carbon dioxide, methane, phosphorated hydrogen, indole, skatole, and mercaptan are among these foul-smelling substances. At this point, the body surfaces appear taut and the face, abdomen, and genitalia are bloated due to escalating gas pressures in body tissue and cavities. Certain skin surfaces may develop blisters and appear denuded. There may be an evacuation of dark body fluids of decomposition through the nose and mouth as a result of increased pressures within the body. This phenomenon is termed *purging* (Fig. 33-4). Maggots may also be evident at this stage. The climate and ambient tissue as well as the predeath health status of the individual often influence the rate and amount of putrefaction. The earliest external manifestations of decomposition (24 to 48 hours) affect the lower abdominal wall, which presents as a greenish discoloration over the bowels. Internal manifestation of early decomposition includes the stomach, intestine, spleen, liver, omentum, mesentery, larynx, trachea, and brain. Later decomposition, which occurs over a two- to three-day period, affects the heart, lungs, kidneys, urinary bladder, esophagus, pancreas, diaphragm, blood vessels, testes, prostate, and uterus. Several other changes also occur, each helping to identify the postmortem interval. Teeth are loosened in three to seven days, skeletonization occurs in one to three months, and bones are usually totally destroyed in 25 years. In the postmortem period, three weeks to one year, under conditions of high temperature and diminished airflow, a waxy substance called *adipocere* may form. Adipocere creates a waxy appearance of fatty tissue in the face, extremities, buttocks, and female breasts. In some rare instances of high environmental temperature, low humidity, and good ventilation, mummification rather than adipocere will result

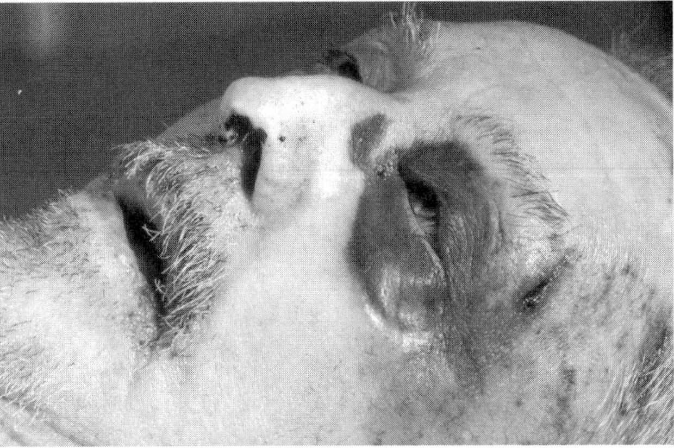

Fig. 33-4 Note the dark drainage from the nostril induced by increased gaseous pressures within the body during decomposition. This is referred to as *purging*.

Postmortem Interval Determination

Estimation of the time of death is based on a determination of the postmortem interval, that period of time between death and the time the body was found. Clues of value to the death investigator are the presence of biochemical changes as well as circumstantial evidence (clothes and belongings, extent of digested food, urine and fecal matter, crime scene) (Gorea, 2004).

Certification of Death

Death certification is the accurate determination of the cause, manner, and mechanism of death. Certification is essential to differentiate the homicidal death from deaths resulting from suicide, accident, or natural causes. Appropriate assessment and investigative analysis are based on data collected, evidence recovered, and physical findings obtained during the investigation and autopsy examination.

In spite of scientific advances in forensic pathology and the investigation of death, some things remain unchanged. Lester Adelson, MD, one of the pioneering *greats* in the annals of forensic pathology, emphasizes the importance of both the medical and legal aspects of evidence of the cause and manner of death. The cause and mechanism of death are derived from the assessment data obtained during research and exploration of the death. These data are supported by investigative findings and are validated by the examination of the remains and review of appropriate medical and other documents. The manner of death is consistent with the cause of death and is corroborated by investigative findings.

The most significant concern in validating the death certificate is the accuracy of terms used. A clear understanding of following terms is essential: The *cause* is defined as that which initiates the series of events ending in death. The *manner* is defined by those circumstances in which the cause arose. The five manners of death include *natural, accidental, homicide, suicide,* or *undetermined* (NAHSU). The mechanism (or mode) refers to the physiological or biochemical disturbance as a result of the cause. This terminology is essential knowledge to the individual responsible for the investigation as well as certification of death (Adelson, 1974).

Terminology of Injury

Accurate medical terminology is essential in documentation of injury and death, whether in legal proceedings or in public health. The certification of death becomes the foundation for the many national statistics used in the prevention of crime, violence, communicable diseases, and death by unnatural causes. The National Center for Health Statistics (NCHS) compiles data from death certificates. In contrast, the FBI Uniform Crime Reports are based on police reports (National Committee for Injury Prevention and Control, 1989).

The accurate terminology of wound characteristics is critical to the education of medicolegal investigators of death. Considering the importance of correct terminology to describe wounds associated with the cause of death and evidence of patterned injury that may describe the weapon used to inflict them, familiarity with blunt and sharp trauma is essential knowledge.

Special Aspects of Certification of Death

An important aspect of certification of death is related to the disposal of the body by cremation. Various laws, forms, signatures,

The cause of death means the disease, abnormality, injury, or poisoning that caused the death, not the mode of dying, such as cardiac or respiratory arrest, shock, or heart failure.

In Part 1, the immediate cause of death is reported in line (a). Antecedent conditions, if any, which gave rise to the cause are reported on lines (b), (c), and (d). The underlying cause should be reported on the last line used in Part 1. No entry is necessary on lines (b), (c), and (d) if the immediate cause of death on line (a) describes completely the train of events. ONLY ONE CAUSE SHOULD BE ENTERED ON A LINE. Additional lines may be added if necessary. Provide the best estimate of the interval between the onset of each condition and death. Do not leave the interval blank, if unknown, so specify.

In Part 2 enter other important diseases or conditions that may have contributed to death but did not result in the underlying cause of death given in Part 1.

See examples below.

CAUSE OF DEATH

35. PART 1 ENTER THE DISEASES, INJURIES OR COMPLICATIONS THAT CAUSED THE DEATH. DO NOT ENTER THE MODE OF DYING SUCH AS CARDIAC OR RESPIRATORY ARREST, SHOCK, OR HEART FAILURE. LIST ONLY ONE CAUSE ON EACH LINE.

			Approximate Interval Between Onset and Death
IMMEDIATE CAUSE (Final disease or condition resulting in death) →	a.	Rupture of Myocardium	Mins.
Sequentially list conditions, If any, leading to immediate cause. Enter UNDERLYING CAUSE *(disease or injury that initiated events resulting in death)* LAST	b.	Acute Myocardial Infarction	6 days
	c.	Chronic Ischemic Heart Disease	5 years
	d.		

PART 2 OTHER SIGNIFICANT CONDITIONS CONTRIBUTING TO DEATH BUT NOT RESULTING IN THE UNDERLYING CAUSE GIVEN IN PART 1 (i.e., substance abuse, diabetes, smoking, etc.)

Diabetes, Chronic Obstructive Pulmonary Disease, Smoking

36a. AUTOPSY? ☒ YES ☐ NO

36b. AUTOPSY FINDINGS AVAILABLE PRIOR TO COMPLETION OF CAUSE OF DEATH? ☒ YES ☐ NO

37. DID TOBACCO USE CONTRIBUTE TO DEATH: ☒ YES ☐ PROBABLY ☐ NO ☐ UNKNOWN

38. DID ALCOHOL USE CONTRIBUTE TO DEATH: ☐ YES ☐ PROBABLY ☒ NO ☐ UNKNOWN

39. WAS DECEDENT PREGNANT
AT TIME OF DEATH ☐ YES ☒ NO ☐ UNK
WITHIN LAST 12 MO ☐ YES ☒ NO ☐ UNK

EXAMPLE

CAUSE OF DEATH

35. PART 1 ENTER THE DISEASES, INJURIES OR COMPLICATIONS THAT CAUSED THE DEATH. DO NOT ENTER THE MODE OF DYING SUCH AS CARDIAC OR RESPIRATORY ARREST, SHOCK, OR HEART FAILURE. LIST ONLY ONE CAUSE ON EACH LINE.

			Approximate Interval Between Onset and Death
IMMEDIATE CAUSE (Final disease or condition resulting in death) →	a.	Cerebral Laceration	10 mins.
Sequentially list conditions, If any, leading to immediate cause. Enter UNDERLYING CAUSE *(disease or injury that initiated events resulting in death)* LAST	b.	Open Skull Fracture	10 mins.
	c.	Automobile Accident	10 mins.
	d.		

PART 2 OTHER SIGNIFICANT CONDITIONS CONTRIBUTING TO DEATH BUT NOT RESULTING IN THE UNDERLYING CAUSE GIVEN IN PART 1 (i.e., substance abuse, diabetes, smoking, etc.)

36a. AUTOPSY? ☒ YES ☐ NO

36b. AUTOPSY FINDINGS AVAILABLE PRIOR TO COMPLETION OF CAUSE OF DEATH? ☒ YES ☐ NO

37. DID TOBACCO USE CONTRIBUTE TO DEATH: ☐ YES ☐ PROBABLY ☒ NO ☐ UNKNOWN

38. DID ALCOHOL USE CONTRIBUTE TO DEATH: ☐ YES ☒ PROBABLY ☐ NO ☐ UNKNOWN

39. WAS DECEDENT PREGNANT
AT TIME OF DEATH ☐ YES ☒ NO ☐ UNK
WITHIN LAST 12 MO ☐ YES ☒ NO ☐ UNK

Fig. 33-5 Death certificate.

and authorities are involved in the cremation of human remains. This extensive procedure may vary in different states or countries, but it generally requires the application by relatives for cremation and the signature of the registered medical practitioner in attendance at the time of death who has also signed a death certificate. Finally, the authority to cremate is issued by the medical referee, medical examiner, or coroner. A record of the cremation and disposition of the remains is noted (Gresham & Turner, 1979).

Death Certificate

The death certificate provides legal proof that an individual is deceased: prima facie evidence of the fact of death. Accurate certification of death is one of our most important vital statistics (Fig. 33-5).

Implications for the persons immediately concerned and for society as a whole are addressed on the official death certificate. Viewing the perceived value of this document and the inferred outcomes of death reflected in this document, one would assume that all medical personnel authorized to certify death would be required by law to demonstrate a command of knowledge pertaining to the cause, manner, and mechanism of death. This is not the case. Failure to correctly identify the cause of death in the death certification process has been and remains a constant problem for the Department of Vital Statistics and law enforcement agencies. Nonforensic physicians and nonmedical coroners alike have historically been at fault in determining the precise cause of death and entering it correctly on the death certification document.

The death certificate is written and certified utilizing standard nomenclature for classification of diseases and injuries and conforms to established guidelines in the country of death. The certification document in countries subscribing to the World Health Organization's universal definition of death includes language on the death certificate specifically stating *"do not enter the mode (mechanism) of death such as cardiac arrest, cardio-respiratory arrest, shock, or heart failure below*" referring to the circumstances under which the death occurred, the cause of death. Yet it continues to happen. Unfortunately, this results in misinterpretation of statistical data on which public health budgets are based as well as research that indicates persons and conditions of high risk for death. In rare instances, one may include a mechanism of death and or the immediate cause of death in part 1 of the death certificate where clinical clarification is needed. However, an etiologically specific cause of death must also be included as the underlying cause.

Pronouncement of Death

Pronouncing death is a confirmation of the death of an individual who has met the criteria of death. The time and day of death is documented on the death certificate along with the signature of the physician who pronounced death. Although nurse pronouncement laws have been enacted in the US, nurses in this country do not sign the death certificate. In South Africa, however, the death certificate identifies the *professional nurse* as one who is authorized to sign for the certification of death. With advanced practice, forensic nurse examiners are certifying natural deaths in certain jurisdictions as independent practitioners who are licensed healthcare professionals. Although US law varies from state to state, the elected coroner (nurse or otherwise) may certify death.

Time of Death

Determining the exact time of death is an inexact science. Accurate and precise methods have not been discovered due to external factors; consequently, the determination of *time of death* presents a challenge to those who investigate death. Precise techniques for determining time of death are highly desirable but have not yet been achieved despite extensive research (Evans, 1996). The basis for estimation of time of death and the variables that make these estimation techniques unpredictable involve physical evidence, biochemical changes, environmental influences, and crime scene evidence.

Careful attention to the physical changes that occur after death such as livor mortis, rigor mortis, degree of decomposition, body temperature, and stomach contents is used to help determine the time of death. Without witnessing the event of death, it is all but impossible to indicate the precise time death occurred. Each of these variables can be hastened or slowed by a number of factors, such as ambient temperature, physique, exercise, alcohol, and drugs.

Where deaths are witnessed, the *time of death* is the time that resuscitation efforts were stopped and the pronouncement of death is recorded. Generally, the principle of sequential postmortem changes following death can be utilized in the estimation of time of death and the related destructive and or artifactual changes that may simulate premortem injury or modify toxicological findings (Spitz & Fisher, 1993).

These criteria may be used to evaluate time of death:

1. Scene findings.
2. Physiochemical changes evident in direct examination of the body.
   - Changes in body temperature.
   - Development of livor mortis and rigor mortis.
   - Extent of decomposition.

   (Note: none of these postmortem parameters are independently reliable.)
3. Evaluation of physiological processes establishing progress rate and cessation at death (e.g., presence of gastric contents affected by time of digestion and the gastric emptying time).
4. Changes in chemical composition of body fluids or tissues (e.g., postmortem potassium concentration of vitreous fluid).
5. Postmortem residual reactivity of muscles to electrical or chemical stimuli (e.g., electrical stimulation of the masseter muscle and reaction of the iris to chemicals); may be limited to European practices and is uncommon in the US.
6. Survival time after injuries, particularly when time of infliction is known. The nature, extent, and severity of injury and quantitative association of complications are often considered in determining time of death (e.g., amount of bleeding, early tissue reaction to injury).

The nature, extent, and severity of injury and quantitative association of complications are often used in determining time of death. The established criteria for determining the rate of temperature as it falls after death are approximately one degree per hour. Considering that the musculature and ambient temperature may significantly affect the rate of change, the following formula is widely used for estimating the time of death:

Normal temperature (37.0° C, 98.6° F)	–	Rectal temperature	=	Approximate number of hours since death

It must be emphasized that none of these considerations is consistently accurate and only by evaluating all possible factors can a likely time of death be established.

Entomology and Time of Death

Although time of death remains an inexact science, the study of entomology or insect activity at the scene or on the body can provide important information, narrowing the window between the time death occurred and the discovery of the body. Forensic entomology is the analysis of insects and their offspring that inhabit decomposing remains. Any flying, crawling, and burrowing insects need to be collected. Some insects burrow themselves under a corpse. If the postmortem period is greater than three weeks, several samples of soil need to be removed from beneath the corpse.

Fleas, body lice, and all insects found on the body need to be collected during the autopsy. Maggots and other insects such as blowflies and beetles that are on the body are important in determining an approximate time of death. This can be determined by studying the stages of insect growth. It is important for investigators to recognize the differences between the adult and the larvae stages of each insect. These insects become important evidence when the forensic entomologist analyzes them by coordinating the growth stages from the egg to the adult. These stages help to establish a time frame of the human death within the period of growth, death, and the next generation of insects.

Cycles of Growth

Ova	18-36 hours
Maggots	24 hours
Pupa	4-5 days
Adults	4-5 days

Detailed descriptions of the techniques of proper collection, preservation, and rearing entomological specimens are available through the forensic science literature on forensic entomology. Problems arise when relying solely on these criteria, and major problems result due to the variation in the environmental and individual factors on the magnitude and kinetics of postmortem phenomena (Knight, 1996; Rodriguez & Lord, 1997; Spitz & Fisher, 1993).

Cause of Death

The cause of death is the injury, disease, or the combination of the two responsible for initiating the train of physiological disturbances, brief or prolonged that produce the fatal termination. When trauma results in immediate death, the injury is both the proximate and the immediate cause of death. If the sequence of events leading to death is sufficiently prolonged to develop pneumonia, peritonitis, or a massive pulmonary embolism, these sequelae would become the immediate cause of death (complications of underlying cause). The original injury would become the proximate (initiating event) or underlying cause of death. Thus, the cause of death must be etiologically specific.

One primary objective of the postmortem evaluation is to determine the *cause of death*: natural or unnatural (violent). The second is the *manner of death*. If it is known or determined to be a *natural death*, the pathology of disease must be documented and health authorities notified of any threat to public health and safety. If the death is known or determined to be an *unnatural death*, the pathology of trauma or homicide must be documented and reported to local law enforcement agencies.

In addition to inquiring into sudden and unexpected deaths, the determination of *jurisdiction* must be considered due to the possibility of delayed effects of injury. There is no statute of limitations for fatal injuries in certifying the cause of death (Adelson, 1974; Gorea, 2004). For example, if an individual is hospitalized for smoke inhalation due to an accidental fire, later develops pneumonia, and dies six months or a year later, then the cause of death is smoke inhalation (rather than pneumonia, which would be a natural death) and the manner is accidental.

Asphyxia

Mechanical (Traumatic)

Asphyxia encompasses a variety of conditions that result in interference with the uptake or utilization of oxygen with failure to eliminate carbon dioxide. Subnormal oxygen in the blood supply to the brain causes rapid unconsciousness. Microscopic evidence of central nervous system damage occurs as early as 30 to 40 seconds after oxygen deprivation. One category, mechanical or compression asphyxia, results from external compression of the chest or neck. Ventilation is prevented by weight of an object (Spitz & Fisher, 1993).

Drowning

Cause of death in drowning is a complex combination of asphyxia (10% to 12%) and inhalation of large amounts of water. However, drowning is a complicated diagnosis that requires extensive evaluation of the scene and the drowning medium, whether fresh water, brackish water, or sea (salt) water. Recovery of a corpse from water raises two critical questions (Adelson, 1974; Spitz & Fisher, 1993):

1. Was death a result of drowning or from some other cause, natural or unnatural?
2. If death was caused by drowning, was it accidental, suicidal, or homicidal?

Gunshot Injury

Gunshot Wound to the Head

Guns are involved in approximately two-thirds of all homicides in the US. Handguns, automatic pistols, and revolvers are most common. Rifles and shotguns are less common. Gunshot wounds of the brain will frequently show signs of intracranial pressure where the vital centers were not injured, but pressure causing deformation toward the foramen magnum still occurs. Pressure secondary to the deformation may be the fatal mechanism in these cases (DiMaio, 1985). For a detailed explanation of injury associated with firearms, see Chapter 20.

Manner of Death

Manner of death refers to the circumstances in which the cause of death occurred: *homicide, suicide, accident,* or *natural.* If the manner of death cannot be determined, it will be designated *undetermined* on the death certificate. The manner of death should be given when there is a preponderance of evidence based on all available knowledge of the case. The manner of death is an opinion that can change with the presentation of substantive additional information. The manner of dying will direct the civil or criminal investigation. Prosecutors of *crimes against persons* find it difficult, although not always impossible, to successfully prosecute a case where the medical cause or manner of death is not determined. However, it may be possible to determine the manner of death without determination of the medical cause of death based on the circumstances of the event. The manner of death influences the legal ramifications of the investigation, charges that may be filed, or lack of evidence to determine the cause or manner of death.

In his book *Pathology of Homicide*, Adelson wrote:

> *Until the pathologist has demonstrated that death was produced directly or indirectly by some kind of violence or culpable negligence, there is no homicide to investigate . . . if he misdiagnoses a nonexistent homicide, he may place an innocent person in jeopardy. . . . Conversely, if he fails to give adequate weight to the part played by violence and concludes that the death resulted entirely from natural causes, a murderer goes free and a crime goes unpunished. (1974, p. 15)*

Various typologies of deaths are defined in five specific categories denoted as *manner of death*:

1. Homicide
2. Suicide
3. Accident
4. Natural
5. Undetermined

Homicide

Literally the killing of a human being, homicide is legally defined as the destruction of human life by the act, agency, procurement, or culpable omission of another person or persons.

Criminal Homicide

Criminal homicide includes violent deaths that are legally classified as murder, generally in the first or second degree or as manslaughter.

Child Homicide

The violent deaths of children constitute a specific category of death investigation known as child homicide.

Noncriminal Homicide

Justifiable or excusable homicides constitute the noncriminal category. These homicides are carried out by law enforcement officers legally performing their duties when acting under competent authority or non-law-enforcement persons resisting attempts at murder or serious harm to themselves and others or in defending their homes or property.

Excusable Homicide

Accidents or mishaps resulting in the unanticipated and unintended death of another, or those that have occurred as a result of a lawful act carried out in a lawful way with lawful means (such as state-ordered executions) are recognized as excusable homicides.

Sexual Homicide

In sexual homicide, the sexual element provides a basis for the sequence of acts leading to murder. Performance and significance of this sexual element vary with the offender. The act may range from rape (either before or after death) to a symbolic sexual assault. This category is divided into organized sexual homicide, disorganized sexual homicide, mixed sexual homicide, and sadistic murder (Olshaker, Jackson, & Smock, 2001).

Suicide

Intentional death inflicted by one's self. As proof of suicide, it must be demonstrated that the individual could have carried out the act alone. Methods of suicide vary. Shooting, hanging, and drug overdoses are among the most common causes of suicidal deaths. Self-stabbing is rare and self-inflicted wrist cutting or throat-cutting rarely lead to death.

Accident

Determination of accidental death is essential to rule out intent by self or others or natural causes. An unintentional death resulting from a chance event or carelessness not due to any fault or misconduct by the individual but from the consequences of such entity or circumstance is categorized as accidental.

Natural

The majority of reported deaths in medical examiner or coroner's jurisdictions are natural deaths. Death due to the natural circumstances of life involving disease and degenerative aging processes involves the forensic system when the death is unattended by a physician, or if physician will not sign the death certificate for a variety of reasons. Unexpected deaths from natural causes usually involve a medical history that can be readily verified. However, each death must be approached with an index of suspicion until any suggestion of foul play, however slight, has been ruled out and the cause of death has been clearly determined.

Undetermined

The cause of death is designated as undetermined if (1) there are insufficient physical findings at autopsy, (2) toxicology and microscopic examinations yield nonspecific or insignificant results, (3) massive injuries or decomposition prevent identification of a specific cause, or (4) a final case review concludes that circumstances surrounding the death are elusive or impossible to confirm with a degree of certainty. Undetermined cases may result from trauma or violence, or from natural causes.

Mechanism of Death

The *mechanism of death* is defined as the physiologic derangement or biochemical disturbance incompatible with life, which is initiated by the cause of death. It may also be referred to as the mode of death as often seen on the death certificate. Mechanisms of death (not causes) include hemorrhagic (hypovolemic) shock, metabolic disturbances (acidosis and alkalosis), cardiac asystole and ventricular fibrillation, respiratory depression and paralysis, cardiac tamponade, sepsis with profound bacterial toxemia, and so on (Adelson, 1974). The mechanism of death is distinct from the cause, which initiates the mechanistic sequence of factors incompatible with life. For example, a stab wound (cause) may lead to blood loss and collapse of lung, resulting in hemorrhagic shock (mechanism).

A mechanism may be included in Part 1 of the Death Certificate where clinical clarification of a specific etiology is appropriate, provided both the mechanism and the underlying etiology are listed.

Clinical Autopsy versus Forensic Autopsy

There are significant differences between the clinical (hospital) autopsy and the forensic autopsy:

- The clinician is mainly concerned with the inside of the body and with the processes of nature, as well as the location/presence/absence of natural disease.
- The forensic autopsy is mainly concerned with the exterior of the body, vectors, forces, directions, body positions, physical capabilities, cause and manner of death.

Deaths that occur during hospitalization of a patient and are referred to the clinical/anatomical pathologist are of natural causes. The attending physician can, and generally does, sign the death certificate. Clinical (hospital) autopsies are generally performed at the request of the physician or the family to determine the origin or extent of a disease process or the effectiveness of treatment regimes. This procedure requires the permission of the family and is a primary resource for medical research. Any death other than natural falls within the medical examiner/coroner jurisdiction.

Best Practice *33-2*

Autopsies should be performed only by physicians solidly grounded in gross and microscopic anatomy and pathology to avoid errors in procedures or analyses of derived findings. (Adelson, 1974)

Postmortem Evaluations

External Examination versus Forensic Autopsy

An external (*view*) examination refers to a postmortem examination limited to external findings and a review of medical records and investigative information to arrive at the cause and manner of death without internal organ examination and evisceration. The term *autopsy*, which is a type of postmortem examination, indicates that in addition to an external examination, the body is opened and organs and structures are examined. The purpose of a forensic autopsy is to determine the cause, manner, mechanism of death, identification of the body, time and place of death, and reconstruction of the fatal episode.

The forensic autopsy is specific to the investigation of suspected criminal cases or where the cause of death is unknown. These autopsies are required by law and do not require the permission of the family. Forensic autopsies focus on the external body and are a primary resource to public health and law enforcement agencies.

Necropsy Pathology: The Autopsy

The examination of the body after death is most often referred to as the autopsy (Greek: *autopisa,* to see for one's self; *opsesthai,* with one's own eyes). A more technically correct term for the evisceration and dissection is *necropsy,* or looking at the dead. The objective of the autopsy is to establish the identification of the body and the medical cause of death (Wright, 2003). The terms *autopsy, necropsy,* and *postmortem procedures* are generally synonymous. *Autopsy* is the term most commonly used in the US, the term *morbid anatomy* is a British term, and *necropsy* is most commonly used in Latin America and European countries.

The autopsy provides valuable information through postmortem analysis such as cause of death, mechanism of injury, multi-organ system failure, and communicable diseases, etc. Since the forensic examination is directed mainly toward the cause and manner of death, it is a mistake to assume that all bodies handled in a coroner or medical examiner setting will be opened and fully examined. In fact, a significant proportion will be examined externally only.

Prerequisites to Autopsy

The forensic pathologist will depend on an incisive report of circumstances of death and documentation of the scene of death as observed by the medical investigator, coroner or deputy coroner, the police, or other first responders prior to initiating postmortem procedures. An insightful investigator will collect reports from other agents at the scene; compile a photographic documentary of the body, the scene, and the evidence; recover and review medical records from the hospital; interview with the family physician; and review statements from witnesses in order to compile a complete and comprehensive evaluation of information pertaining to cause and manner of death.

Police reports may contain valuable information regarding the criminal investigation of death, yet they may be unrelated to the medical cause of death. In the same sense, shared information related to the medical investigation of death may be invaluable to the criminal investigator to confirm or rule out whether or not a crime has been committed.

Autopsy Procedure

A detailed visual inspection of the clothing prior to removal must precede the examination of injury or condition of the body. Photographic and written or dictated inspection of forensically significant evidence on the clothing before it is removed is a priority. Clothing should not be disturbed or removed at the scene. The entire clothed body should be wrapped in a clean sheet to protect any trace, physical, or biological evidence on the garments.

The dissection of the human body generally entails the removal of the internal organs through incisions of the chest, abdomen, and head. The most prevalent technique used in the US has been the *inframammary incision,* or Y-shaped incision, to initiate the autopsy dissection. This procedure begins at each shoulder and extends downward, to the midline of the body in the lower chest, then extending to the top of the pubic bone, resulting in a Y-shaped incision. The T incision has been adopted for facilitation of the examination of the tongue and neck (Wright, 2003). Examination of the brain requires an incision from behind one ear to the other, reflecting the scalp backward and sawing the skull in a circular cut followed by the removal of the skullcap.

After the removal of organs, each is weighed and dissected to determine disease or injury. Information derived from the medical history, witness statements, scene examination, and the autopsy determine further dissection or analysis of tissue that may be performed following the routine procedures just described (Wright, 2003).

Documentation of each step of the scene of death and autopsy procedures is essential to ensure relevant and ultimately admissible evidence in court. The forensic nurse examiner must remain aware that any involvement in death investigation–from the scene, the hospital, the residence, interviews, evaluation or examination of injuries, and so on–may or may not result in legal testimony. All forensic professionals consider testifying as a requisite of their position and must be prepared to explain actions or opinions to the court.

Autopsy examination may determine what type of weapon caused injury and death, determine whether injuries are antemortem or postmortem in nature, and determine if a single or multiple injuries are responsible for death. Determination of the postmortem interval, the lapse of time between death and discovery of the body, and the probable duration between injuries or incapacitation or death is essential in understanding the circumstances of death.

Special Cases

When infant or maternal deaths occur, documenting evidence of trauma and history of abuse is essential. These deaths are categorized as forensic cases and will necessitate an adaptation of routine autopsy procedures. Special procedures are required in newborn or stillborn infant deaths. Investigation of these cases requires certain aspects of information surrounding the birth and death, as well as history of prenatal care if it exists.

Generally, autopsy procedures are similar to that of the adult, with a few notable exceptions. Modifications may be required in the removal of specific organs such as the heart and brain. It is often important to discover the actual age of the fetus in relation to the duration of the pregnancy. Fetal age is generally determined by the weight and measurements of the body, specifically the circumference of the head. The centers of bone growth also indicate the state of maturation at the end stage of a normal pregnancy.

The presence of *lanugo,* a fine delicate hair over the shoulders of a fetus, indicates immaturity, as does the lack of fingernail growth. Any postmortem examination of a stillborn infant is incomplete without examination of the placenta, which should be sent with the baby from the hospital. Placental abnormality is frequently a cause of fetal death, and without it, a diagnosis is often impossible (Gresham & Turner, 2003). Epidemiological data suggest that one in every two American women will be a partner in a violent relationship. Approximately one third of all emergency department visits by women are related to domestic violence. Of these visits, only 5% are recorded as battering or maltreatment on the hospital record. In addition, 37% of pregnant women have a history of physical abuse, which is considered to be the leading cause of infant mortality and birth defects. Yet America is not alone. Battering by an intimate partner may be the single most common cause of injury to women worldwide and the cause of traumatic death in pregnancy.

Findings from various studies indicate the incidence of abuse occurs in 10% to 26% of all pregnancies. Despite the fact that battered women are frequently seen in the emergency department setting, the diagnosis of abuse is often missed. Historically, healthcare professionals have not been trained to recognize, identify, or intervene for the battered woman. The number of women who have experienced domestic violence has not been routinely detected or reported by emergency department physicians and nurses. Before help can be offered to women, they must first be identified in the healthcare setting.

The US Joint Commission on the Accreditation of Healthcare Organizations (JCAHO) has established guidelines requiring routine assessments for abuse in emergency and ambulatory settings, as well as education for healthcare providers who come into contact with such victims. Because many women seek medical assistance in acute care settings, and only a small percentage of domestic violence cases are detected, it has become a mandate that all women presenting to an emergency department or prenatal clinics undergo routine screening for interpersonal violence. Forensic nurse examiners assigned to urgent care and mother-baby units have proved to be beneficial in reducing and preventing the number of deaths of mothers and the unborn. This futuristic approach to case management of the forensic patient is being developed in contemporary healthcare institutions worldwide (Lynch, 2003).

Key Point 33-5

Trauma is noted to be the leading cause of maternal death during pregnancy.

Anatomy and Physiology of the Autopsy

Understanding the anatomy and physiology of the body is fundamental in relation to the autopsy dissection and determination of cause of death. This includes the classification of the organs that comprise the systems and well as the precise terminology. The relationship between cause, manner, and mechanism of death requires in-depth inductive and deductive reasoning to assure an accurate investigation of why people die. An astute understanding of these processes begins with the three major systems of the body: nervous system, cardiovascular system, and respiratory system. Other body systems include gastrointestinal, genitourinary, endocrine, musculoskeletal, integumentary, and lymphoreticular.

Momentary interruption of any one of these three main systems may commence an irreversible potentially fatal process (e.g., interruption of circulation for four minutes causes irreversible brain damage). The only other mechanism that leads to irreversible damage quickly is hemorrhage. Such rapid hemorrhage would involve blood loss through a breach of artery.

No External Findings

In sudden and unexpected deaths with no external or obvious cause of death, which may result in classifying the cause as undetermined, one should consider the following conditions:

- Disease or injury of heart or brain
- Asphyxia chemical or mechanical (carbon monoxide or smothering)
- Alcohol or drugs
- Hyperthermia or hypothermia
- Dehydration
- Electrocution (45% of low-voltage cases have no marks)
- Abusive head trauma in children with no external findings

Rapid Death versus Delayed Death

When death takes place rapidly, it is generally a result of severe multiple traumas. When death takes time to occur, such as when death occurs as the result of burns, the patient may die later of complications such as infection. Law enforcement officers may perceive terminal diseases as homicides due to the presence of blood, such as cirrhosis of the liver or bleeding gastric ulcers. Blunt injuries resulting from collapse may be misinterpreted as an assault.

Identification of the Body

Methods and Means

Upon arrival at the scene, identification of the body is a priority. The investigator's first question should be to ask if the body has been identified. If the identity of the body is unknown, every effort must be taken to establish who the individual was. If complete identification is not possible, noting the height, weight, age, sex, tattoos, and scars should contribute to the process of identification. Factors such as dental status, race, religion, and other characteristics may also assist in verification of identity (Fierro, 1993).

Visual

Identification of the decedent by a close family member or companion is the most readily available method of ensuring the particulars of a known person. Yet even the most intimate and significant other may not recognize the body due to the emotionally traumatic effect of the death or the condition of the body. Visual identification is often unreliable and frequently leads to misidentification (e.g., for a fire victim, the hair may be gray due to smoke or singed a brassy color and skin wrinkles may flatten due to heat; or bodies in water for long periods will turn black). If visual identification must be made in the direct presence of the body (e.g. without a glass partition), the friend or family member should be advised not to touch the decedent. This provides protection for the chain of evidence if there is any suspicion of homicide as well as to maintain legal security of the body.

Fingerprints

The first book on fingerprints as a method of identification was published as early as 1892. When the body is unclaimed and no known relation or other individual is present to identify the decedent, the method most readily available and least expensive is fingerprints. No two individuals have the same fingerprints; even identical twins have different ridge patterns. Fingerprints fall into three basic types: latent, visible, and molded (or plastic). The latent print is the most common and the most durable; it can last for centuries when left on a hard, protected surface. Assuredly, many citizens remain outside the list of millions of fingerprints, but chances are significant that the likelihood of fingerprint identification is worthwhile (Evans, 1996). Other than fingerprints, scientists have found footprints and lip prints to be suitable for identification as well. Footprints of children under age 14 have become routine in identification comparisons. One forensic task that may be considered for the forensic nurse consultant is fingerprinting. One California police department inquired if forensic nurses could be trained to take fingerprints, stating they had an overwhelming workload and were considering contracting this job to civilians.

Forensic Odontology

Forensic odontology is the application of the arts and sciences of dentistry to the legal system (Glass, 2003) and refers to the specialized science of dental identification. No part of the human body outlasts the teeth after death, so they provide an ideal means of identification. Often the teeth may be the only means of identification, specifically in severely burned or decomposed bodies. If no fingerprints are available and no visual identification can be made, dental identification is generally the second step. Teeth are also useful in determining age after death. However, dental comparison cannot be used if the identity of the body is unknown. It is imperative to have both ante- and postmortem dental records; without known dental record, there is nothing to compare. Forensic odontologists can also confirm a crime suspect's identification through the interpretation of human bite marks. Human dentition provides irrefutable evidence when compared to the bite mark on tissue, based on individual class characteristics of the accused (Evans, 1996).

DNA

Deoxyribonucleic acid (DNA) forms the building blocks of life. DNA provides powerful, compelling evidence. For the past century, science has been trying to identify what makes each living thing unique. Each individual has the potential to be identified by his or her biological fluids or trace evidence. As in dental identification, however, if there is no one known or suspected to be the decedent, a confirmation of identification remains unknown. DNA evaluation is time consuming and expensive, generally out of the reach of most budgets in routine death investigations. In a criminal investigation, the specimens are generally blood, hair, blood-stained clothing, semen, saliva, or any cell of human tissue. The estimate that two individuals would have the same DNA is on the order of one in the billions. There is nothing to suggest at this time that DNA is anything other than the most significant forensic breakthrough since the discovery of the forensic application of fingerprints (Evans, 1996).

Computer or Video Identification

The use of computer-enhanced imagery is a rapidly growing method of identification. This is a revolutionary computer program that simulates aging. When criminals or victims have been missing for a number of years, this program can simulate the appearance of the individual based on a psycho/social profile of lifestyle and project a likely current appearance. Such features as sags, wrinkles, or receding hairline help to produce the suspected appearance concurrently with the number of years the individual has been missing. Equipment designed to manipulate photo images to remove blemishes has been used to create a likeness of how a battered corpse had looked when alive. Video superimposition is another method of identification in which a photograph is placed over an image of a skull to determine whether the two are the same person. Using a high-resolution video camera and known photographs of the individual in question can result in an exact match. Follow-up with fingerprints or DNA for further confirmation is used with both computer-enhanced imagery and video superimposition (Evans, 1996).

Facial Reconstruction

The art of reconstructing a face from a skull is not a recent development. As early as 1895, anatomists began creating human likenesses for the purpose of identification. Modern practitioners of facial reconstruction, known as forensic sculpture, have continued to work with various art forms that have proved to be remarkably similar to the subject in question. Initial evaluation of unidentified skulls begins with establishing skin thickness at strategic points over bone. Modeling clay is then applied in accordance with carefully delineated measurements of the mouth and cheeks. However, because cartilage decomposes quickly after death, the nose poses one of the most difficult aspects of reconstruction. Prosthetic eyes and the appropriate color of wigs (where hair may have been found with the body) produce amazing results and often provide accurate identification of the unknown dead (Evans, 1996).

Death Scene Control and Processing

Body at the Scene

The crime scene and associated criminal evidence remains within the jurisdiction of the police in the criminal investigation of death. The body and associated medical evidence pertaining to the cause of death is within the jurisdiction of the medical examiner or coroner. The forensic investigation of a crime scene involves interagency cooperation, scene examination, and preservation as well as photography and field notes. Law enforcement is present to accomplish an investigation; however, the coroner or medical investigator achieves a separate and concurrent investigation. The two entities must function as a team. Both may perform interviews of witnesses and next of kin. The objectives of each agency are different, as are the responsibilities.

Best Practice *33-3*

Essential steps in managing a body at a scene include identification, photography, creation of a scene diagram, documentation of the condition of the body and clothing, preservation of trace evidence, and bagging of the hands and the body of the deceased.

Natural Deaths

Because 60% to 75% of reportable deaths occur without an attendant physician, it is reasonable to expect death to transpire in a residence or elsewhere in the community. When the decedent has not been admitted to the hospital prior to death, a significant amount of time may lapse before the body is discovered when the individual lives alone. Without prior arrangements with legal and medical authorities, such as hospice cases, the investigators must proceed to the residence to pronounce and examine the scene of death.

When death occurs in the community, prompt removal of the body from the scene or from public view may be in the best interest of the family, bystanders, or traffic. However, a thorough investigation is time consuming, and related legal statutes are specific regarding the protection of the body and scene. Statutes that govern the investigation of forensic deaths define guidelines for the removal of a body from the scene of death. Generally, it is a violation of law for the body to be moved or any items removed from the body prior to the completion of the scene investigation. There are a few exceptions, however; for example, if the body is in an unsafe location or is blocking traffic, it may be removed to a site near the place of death until the investigation is complete.

Investigators who wish to perform their duties without interference or annoyance from people observing the situation at the location of death should consider which forensic functions may be completed after removal.

Until a search of the scene is completed by law enforcement, failure to comply will often result in a conflict with the criminal investigators. After an initial observation and evaluation of the body, an extensive medical examination should only be conducted within the confines of the autopsy laboratory or mortuary.

Exhumation

Circumstances in an investigation may come to light after the burial of an individual that requires an exhumation of the body for further evaluation to clarify the cause and manner of death. An autopsy on an exhumed body is rare. The legal removal of a body from the site of burial requires permission of the family or the law. An exhumation involves disinterment of the body to investigate a suspected homicide, to establish doubtful identity, or to answer claims for compensation or charges of malpractice. The body is in the jurisdiction of the medical examiner or coroner once disinterred and remains so until buried again. The pathologist must be present at the scene of exhumation and document every step of the procedure with photography (Knight, 1997). Special courses on the identification of clandestine gravesites and the exhumation of human remains are taught at the Joseph H. Davis Forensic Center in Dade County, Miami, Florida. The classes are for forensic pathologists, coroners, forensic nurse investigators, non-nurse forensic investigators, and police investigators.

Recovery of Skeletal Remains

Quite often, all that remains of a body are bones, generally dry, brown, fragile, and sometimes they may clearly be ancient. These bones are often accidentally discovered and reported to law enforcement agencies that are responsible for notifying the medical examiner or coroner. Prior to any removal, determination of human or animal origin is preferred. It is not uncommon for officials or investigators not skilled in the forensic sciences to request an investigation and postmortem examination of remains later determined to be that of an animal.

Precise guidelines for the removal of skeletal remains must be outlined before entering the scene of death. Homicide detectives lead the investigation at the scene with an initial evaluation of the location. Measurements must first be taken of the distances involved from the central mass of the body to each item of evidence, and next, to three stationary objects for scene reconstruction purposes. Each item of evidence must be located, staked with an identifying flag, photographed, and measured before any removal of the remains can occur. The removal procedures are strictly the responsibility of the medical examiner or coroner's office. It is not exceptional for a rural scene investigation to take two to three days before actual recovery of skeletal remains is transported to the autopsy laboratory. Disaster scenes such as the World Trade Tower bombing or passenger plane crashes may involve weeks or months. This type of scene investigation requires intensive cooperation and coordination of the investigative team between law enforcement and the medical investigators.

Forensic Anthropology

Forensic anthropology can be defined as a broad application of the theory and methods of anthropology to legal issues. This subspecialty of physical anthropology, the study of human biological functions and variations, refers specifically to skeletal biology (Sorg, 2003).

Several basic questions arise with the discovery of any skeletal remains. Forensic anthropologists are trained to evaluate the conditions and circumstances of how a person lived and died through an incisive examination of the structure of the human body. The age at the time of death, sex, race, and height of the person remain the most forensically significant observations when determining the identification of the decedent or the cause of death. Whether the remains are of the ancient or recently dead, whether they are those of servicemen killed in military action or the passengers of airline disasters, skeletal remains can unfold the history of debilitating diseases, healed fractures, right- or left-handedness, and even possibly the occupation of the person in life. This information may be invaluable to the evaluation of the quality and quantity of forensic evidence made available through forensic anthropology.

Case Study 33-1 Death Investigation

A 62-year-old white male is reported dead at his residence by the spouse. Law enforcement officers arrive and notify the forensic nurse examiner on duty. The decedent is identified as L.B.D. by his wife. Death is pronounced at 0900 hours. There are no weapons or obvious signs of breaking and entering, and there is no evidence of struggle. The doors were locked from the inside when the wife returned home. Evidence at the scene includes copious amounts of blood on the floor, ceiling, walls, and furniture. Bloody footprints from the central area of the house to the location of the body are observed. Blood is pooled underneath the decedent's head. The body is observed on the floor in the bedroom in a supine position; it is cold to touch and in full rigor, and early stages of decomposition are noted. The decedent is wearing black, knee-length shorts only. The body presents with a pale yellow discoloration, consistent throughout, with numerous irregular patches of bruising. Blood is exuding from the nose and mouth. No open wounds are observed. Severe distention of the abdomen is present. Aspirin and cigarettes are located on the bedside table. A large bottle of vodka on the bed is noted. Police suspect foul play. This case is being investigated as a homicide until proved otherwise (Figs. 33-6, 33-7, and 33-8).

Medical history: The decedent is known to have been under the care of a family physician for several years. His wife states that the decedent has not been compliant with medication or medical appointments for the past year until he was recently treated for alcohol withdrawal. Complaints include hallucinations, flapping tremors, abdominal pain (acute pancreatitis), and shortness of breath (postural asphyxia).

Diagnosis: End-stage cirrhosis of the liver

Cause of death: Exsanguinating hemorrhage from ruptured esophageal varices

- due to cirrhosis of the liver
- due to chronic alcoholism

Signs and symptoms: Jaundice, ecchymosis, acites, projectile vomiting of blood

Summary

Death investigation is a vital part of the forensic sciences because every death has actual or potential legal implications. Detailed

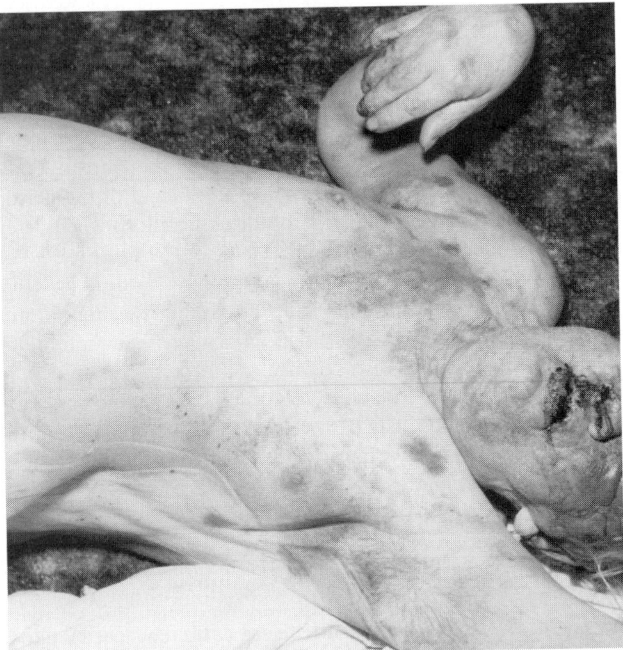

Fig. 33-6 Initial observations at death scene suggest a violent death.

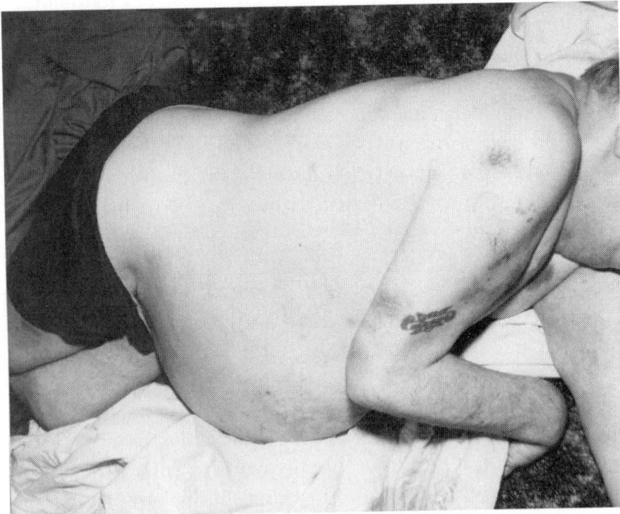

Fig. 33-7 Further examination reveals multiple old bruises and a large, distended abdomen.

procedures are required to determine the cause, aid medical science, and contribute to the administration of justice. The forensic autopsy is a vital part of the death investigation process, which is systematic and ongoing. It involves the collection and analysis of data and physical evidence from which certain assumptions and conclusions are derived. These data serve as a basis for further investigations to establish the identification of the decedent, the approximate interval of time since death, and the cause, manner, and mechanism of death.

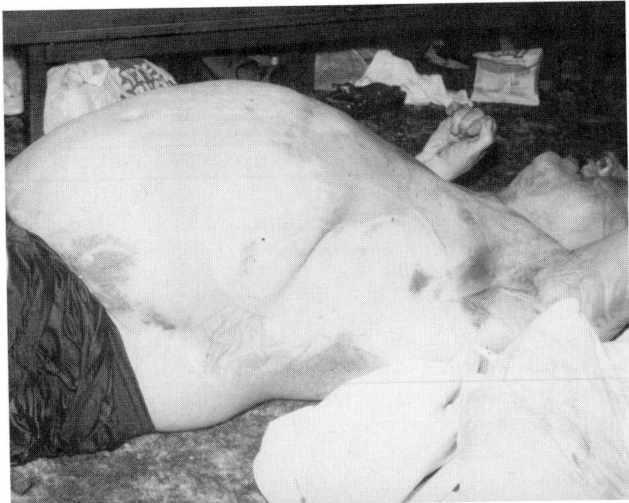

Fig. 33-8 Side profile confirms the presence of ascites and other skin changes consistent with cirrhosis.

Resources

Books

DiMaio, V. J., & DiMaio, D. J. (2001). *Forensic pathology* (2nd ed.). Boca Raton, FL: CRC Press.

Dix, J. (1999). *Color atlas of forensic pathology.* Boca Raton, FL: CRC Press.

Haglund, W. H., & Sorg, M. H. (Eds.). (1997). *Forensic taphonomy: The postmortem fate of human remains.* Boca Raton, FL: CRC Press.

Spitz, W. U. (Ed.). (1993). *Medicolegal investigation of death* (3rd ed.). Springfield, IL: Charles C Thomas.

Journals

American Journal of Forensic Medicine and Pathology

Lippincott Williams & Wilkins, Philadelphia, PA; www.amjforensicmedicine.com

Journal of Forensic Sciences

American Academy of Forensic Sciences, ASTM International, 100 Bar Harbor Drive, PO Box C700, West Conshohocken, PA 19428; Tel: 610-832-9585

Web Sites

Armed Forces Institute of Pathology

www.afip.org

National Association of Medical Examiners, Writing Cause of Death Statements

www.thename.org/CauseDeath/COD_main_page.htm

References

Adelson, L. (1974). *Pathology of homicide.* Springfield, IL: Charles C Thomas.

American Academy of Forensic Sciences. (2002). Informational brochure. Colorado Springs, CO: Author.

Baden, M. (1989). *Unnatural deaths: Confession of a medical examiner.* New York: Random House.

Cumming, M. F. (1995). The vision of a nurse-coroner: A "protector of the living through the investigation of death." *J Psychosoc Nurs Ment Health Serv 31*(11), 7-14.

DiMaio, V. (1985). *Gunshot wounds.* New York: Elsevier.
Dorland's illustrated medical dictionary (29th ed.). (2000). Philadelphia: W.B. Sanders.
Emory, S. (2003, December). *What is brain death?* Iowa Statewide Organ Procurement Organization. Retrieved from www.transweb.org.
Evans, C. (1996). *Forensic detection.* New York: John Wiley and Sons.
Fierro, M. (1993). Identification of human remains. In W. Spitz & R. Fisher (Eds.), *Medicolegal investigation of death* (3rd ed., pp. 71-117). Springfield, IL: Charles C Thomas.
Glass, T. (2003). Forensic odontology. In S. James & J. Nordby, *Forensic Science* (pp. 61-62). Boca Raton, FL: CRC Press.
Gorea, R. (2004). Adapted from Course Outline, Signs of Death. Government Medical College Patiala, Punjab, India.
Gresham, G., & Turner, A. (1979). *Post-mortem procedures.* (An illustrated textbook). Chicago: Year Book Medical.
Hsi Yuan Lu. (1976). Instructions to coroners, as cited in F. Camps, A. Robinson, & B. Lucas (Eds.), *Gradwohl's legal medicine* (3rd ed., p. 7). Chicago: Year Book Medical.
Knight, B. (1996). *Simpson's forensic medicine* (11th ed., chap. 3). Bedfordshire, UK: Arnold.
Law & politics book review. (1998, December). American Political Science Foundation. University of Maryland, *8*(2), 447-449.
Liang, J. W., & Snyder J. W. (2004). Legal medicine (6th ed.). American College of Legal Medicine. St. Louis, MO: Mosby.
Lynch, V. (2003, September 6). *Domestic violence in pregnancy.* Paper presented at 6th World Congress on Perinatal Medicine, Osaka, Japan.
National Committee for Injury Prevention and Control. (1989). *Injury prevention: Meeting the challenge.* New York: Oxford University Press.
Olshaker, J., Jackson, M. C., & Smock, W. (2001). *Emergency forensic medicine.* Philadelphia: Lippincott.
Rodriguez, W. C., & Lord, W. D. (1997). *Other means of estimating time of death* (11th ed., p. 25). Oxford: Oxford University Press.
Sorg, M. (2003). Forensic anthropology. In S. James & J. Nordby. *Forensic science.* Boca Raton, FL: CRC Press.
Spitz, W., & Fisher, R. (Eds.). (1993). *Medicolegal investigation of death* (3rd ed.). Springfield, IL: Charles C Thomas.
University of Dundee. (2003). *Brain stem death and organ transplantation (molecular death defined).* Retrieved from www.dundee.ac.uk/forensicmedicine/llb/brstem.htm.
Wright, R. (2003). Role of the forensic pathologist. In S. James & J. Nordby, *Forensic Science* (pp. 19, 20). Boca Raton, FL: CRC Press.

Chapter 34 The Forensic Nurse Examiner in Death Investigation

Virginia A. Lynch

Death as a Phenomenon

Death is considered one of the great rites of passage of human existence. Death involves more than the physical medical sciences that require attention to postmortem procedures and burial practices. Death is one factor that defines each culture and the theological concepts surrounding the bioanthropology of its people. Regardless of any given society's belief–that life continues beyond death, or that it ends at that moment of death, or that existence after death is unknown–death is a shared phenomenon of the human experience. As nurse scientists, skilled in the forensic investigation of death, each of these phenomena are to be considered as one ventures into the realm of questioned deaths. It is the forensic nurse examiner's duty, then, to tread cautiously as interpretations are made, taking particular care to avoid judgmental reactions toward attitudes of death that may differ from one's own. The scientific and social phenomenon of death represents the two primary aspects of death investigation on which the practice and philosophy of forensic nursing science is founded. These principles will guide the forensic nurse examiner (FNE) toward the expected outcomes of holistic forensic care, which includes body, mind, spirit, and the law.

The medicolegal aspects of death investigation are defined by forensic thanatology (*thanatos* meaning "death" and *logos* meaning "science," or simply the study of death). It is a known phenomenon that death occurs in two stages: (1) somatic, systemic, or clinical death and (2) cellular or molecular death. The term *death* as commonly employed refers to somatic death, which is due to complete and irreversible cessation of vital functions of the brain, followed by the heart and lungs. Previously, cessation of the beating heart and respirations were used as the criteria for death. Now, with the advent of cardiac transplantation, the emphasis has shifted to irreversible cessation of brain function (Parikh, 1999).

Among death's phenomena, perhaps the most difficult for families to understand is the beating-heart cadaver. What emotional trauma could be greater than having to make the ultimate decision to remove someone from a perceived life source: artificial ventilation. It is often confusing to the family and to the nursing staff to accept that death exists while oxygen still infuses the lungs, the blood still circulates, and the body is soft and warm. These phenomena reflect centuries of confusion over how, exactly, to define death, that precise moment when the intangible life force ceases to exist. Before brain activity could be measured, the absence of a beating heart had long been considered the defining moment. Yet the brain survives for 6 to 10 minutes after the heart has failed. Considerable fears surround the family while contemplating these issues: *Could there be hope? What if we make the wrong decision? How can we live with the anxiety and doubt once the decision is made?*

When emotional support is needed at times such as this, who is up to the task? Who can explain brain death with clarity, but nonetheless in a way that a person in denial can understand? What of the need for compassion, for empathy? Or what if the bereaved is a suspect in the death of the patient? Of all the issues involved, this circumstance presents the most difficult professional responsibility while, at the same time, providing the necessary psychosocial intervention in case the suspicion is invalid. Experience in forensic nursing and guidelines in death investigation help provide the *ways of knowing* and *critical thinking* that determine the basis on which accurate case management of questioned deaths can be provided.

The Science of Death Investigation

Death has become a respectable field of inquiry, particularly in the social and behavioral sciences, as well as an acceptable topic of study in the curricula of institutions of higher learning. The science of death investigation joins with nursing science to address the physiological, psychological, and legal aspects of death and dying. Certainly, the most refreshing change is the emphasis on a human caring. This approach to the scientific investigation of death seems to parallel trends in other sectors of society, which are attuned to the advancement of humanity. Previously the emphasis on mechanism of injury, cause, and manner of death and knowledge of the law stood alone within the forensic arena of death investigation.

Death brings with it innocent, living victims by extension, those who survive the loss of lives they cherished. According to those who work with individuals, families, and communities that suffer from the catastrophic impact of tragic death, the forensic response alone is not enough. Grief psychologist Jerry Harris in Fort Worth, Texas, stated, "In a science which stresses the careful collection and accurate documentation of evidence, it is interesting that the psychological impact of traumatic death on survivors receives little attention in actual practice" (Harris, 1989). Recognition of this concept reflects the distinction between normal and pathological mourning, unresolved grief, and mental illness, and calls for a complete reexamination of the premise on which views of death and dying are traditionally based. There is definitely a place in nursing and other health sciences for the recognition and application of a more empathic discipline pertaining to questioned death than has existed in the past. Intervention in grief must be seen and supported as a means toward adaptation and health (Lynch, 1993).

The Aftermath of Terrorism

Should one question the validity of this approach, consider the grief that remains unresolved in the tragic aftermath of September 11, 2001. Unresolved grief, anger, rage, fear, and depression continue to haunt the nation at large, as well as the nations of the world. One can consider the individual families or the entirety of the victim's families as one, and recognize the dramatic and tragic toll under which those who survived and those left behind continue to suffer.

Although many people were touched by the devastation of this criminal act, none were as damaged as the immediate survivors and the decedent's next of kin. The destruction and wreckage of lives inflicted on the living in the wake of such loss and a continuing fear of the unknown represents the despair of human tragedy.

Violent death is not an uncommon event in the world's war on terrorism, at home and abroad. No single event, with the possible exception of an epidemic, brings more tension into the health and justice systems than sudden, traumatic death. Whether it is a commercial aircraft disaster or the bombing of a federal building, these dramatic events bring criminal justice agencies into the emergency department and into the lives of ordinary people, along with medical examiners, coroners, and a host of other agencies. Because homicide from mass disasters is a leading category of death worldwide, it stands to reason that public service operatives will experience these events frequently.

Innumerable public servants served with honor in response to the massive emergencies surrounding the tragedy of the World Trade Towers. Regardless of the real heroes of those times, however, many direct survivors and decedent's families have accused others of unethical, unprofessional practices and violations of individual human rights. A significant number of those most intimately involved in 9/11 have resented the manner in which some–not all–agency professionals and first responders who attended the injured and dead, at the scene and in the aftermath, performed–or failed to perform–their duties. Much of this reaction is justified. The resentment lies deep. The pain is unrelinquished. Demonstrations of resentment and psychological pain continue to be displayed privately and publicly.

What lessons can be learned from catastrophes such as these? How can health and justice professionals prepare to better address critical concerns involving human tragedies, to recognize the essentials of healing and prevent unresolved grief? In contemporary public administration, tight budgets and retrenchment, agency and institutional management oftentimes lends little credence to social service programs and ideas that cannot be exactly and efficiently countered. In the absence of designated others, the forensic nurse examiner often provides the essential crisis intervention and follow-up during ongoing death investigations.

Unique to Nursing

As health and justice systems enter the twenty-first century, forensic nursing provides the partnership that has historically existed in every medical specialty with the exception of one: forensic medicine. In 1986, Dr. John Butt, chief medical examiner in Alberta, Canada, was the first to recognize that the registered nurse represented a valuable resource to the field of death investigation. After conducting a five-year study to determine the ideal professional related to medical investigation, he concluded that it was the registered nurse who provided the qualities and professionalism essential to a scientific, social, and cultural investigation of death. In 1975, Dr. Butt established a program using nurses as medical examiner's investigators, citing the nurses' biomedical education and emphasizing their knowledge of natural disease processes, medical terminology, and pharmacology, as well as their ability to empathize as their most important qualifications. The nurse's experience in public relations is also a major priority in representing the medical examiner at the scene of death, handling confidential material and being comfortable relaying sensitive information to family members (Lynch, 1993)

Butt stressed the importance of coordination and cooperation between the criminal and biomedical investigative personnel. He expressed concern that medically untrained officers often disregarded medical evidence, maintained poor sensitivity, and were noncommunicative with grieving families. Conversely, healthcare professionals recognize the integrity of criminal evidence, the suspect interview, and the investigation of leads.

The ability to review health histories and medical records; understand medical terminology; interpret medical abbreviations; communicate with physicians and paramedical personnel; evaluate the impact of surgical or chemical interventions prescribed and performed prior to death; and relate social, financial, and interpersonal relationship factors of a psychological autopsy must also be included in the armamentarium of the investigator of forensic deaths. These skills are unique to nursing. Essential knowledge regarding the investigation of sudden and unexpected death or the clarification of suspicious or natural deaths across the life span must begin with an incisive understanding of the phenomenon of death. An elucidation of these issues may become a point of contention in a court of law.

Forensic Intervention

Medical professionals, criminalists, and police officers alike recognize the strategic benefits of the forensic nursing role. Nurses recognize this as an opportunity to expand their professional horizons and promote their professional goals. The concept of forensic nursing, which embraces a multidisciplinary approach to abuse detection and community mental health, enhances the quality of community life through effective systems coordination. The tri-care systems approach, involving healthcare, forensic science, and the law, provides an interdisciplinary team approach as the nurse death investigator works closely with the crime laboratory, law enforcement operatives, and community legal service agencies to identify possibilities of human abuse in questioned deaths. A comprehensive total health and justice program in any progressive community will provide the three major components of forensic intervention: (1) prevention of death, (2) intervention at the time of death, and (3) post-death care (post-vention) for the decedent's significant others. To recognize these essential elements of dying as a life process, with a greater shift toward human caring, is to provide an insightful contribution to nursing science and to humanity.

Related research has sought to identify behavioral responses to death, both physiological and psychological, in an attempt to categorize significant etiological factors that serve to promote or inhibit change in the public health status. Forensic nurses are in a position to make primary contributions to the long process of restoring homeostasis to the bereaved. These strategies are supported by what seems to be of paramount importance as new perspectives arise for considering the familiar phenomena of health, illness, and death in relation to human life.

Forensic Nurse Investigation

Nurses are exceptionally capable to interact with police, physicians, grieving families, and collaborate with other professionals in forensic investigations. In the initial phases of establishing a forensic nurse investigative team, however, police, prosecutors, or physicians without awareness of the accomplishments forensic nurses have attained will often express objections and fail to fully support the integration of a nurse into their investigative agenda.

Forensic nurses do not participate as criminal investigators, but rather as clinical investigators, though the interface and assistance to criminal investigation is extensive. It has been noted, however, that the interface between clinical nurses and law enforcement officers has often been rife with strife and resentment. This is not limited to nurses and police in the emergency department setting, but between forensic nurses and criminal investigators as well. Law enforcement officers have, at times, resented the idea of working with nurses, of having to share responsibility or to communicate with a discipline so foreign to their own. Frequently, this professional friction is based on suspicion of the unknown, untested or simply untried. Although the benefits of forensic nursing are well documented and increasingly accepted, arguments against the concept have been touted in the fields of health and justice. The significance of forensic nurse examiners in death investigation and the unique qualifications they contribute to a field often lacking in biomedical professionals is primarily based on a lack of understanding–or funding. This can create rejection or lack of acceptance.

However, according to Z. G. Standing Bear, retired federal agent and criminologist, "Forensic nursing brings together the necessarily neutral, detached and suspicious arena of the law enforcement investigator with the empathic, involved and accepting dimensions of psychosocial nursing" (Standing Bear, 1987, p. 7). He further advised:

> *Forensic nurse examiners and forensic nursing services are a revolutionary concept for utilizing nursing abilities in an arena of human services not previously explored by nurses. Nurses can make significant contributions to the area of death investigation as well as services to survivors. In a world where academic camps are alienated from and even hostile toward one another, this idea speaks to a refreshing blend of energy and cooperation. Breaking down these old barriers of competition and building up new cooperative programs cannot help but benefit humankind. The obvious benefits of this new idea contribute to the quality of community life, as well as bringing together of two historically different disciplines with a common and worthwhile purpose. (Standing Bear, 1995, p. 63)*

Other arguments oppose the use of registered nurses in death investigation because nursing education is primarily based on the common assumption that the goal of nursing is the preservation of life. This view holds that using nurse death investigators is inappropriate or even a waste; that nurses would do well to disregard the carnage and loss of human life and rather focus on the needs of the living. Countering this argument are those who assert that death and dying are as much as part of the life cycle as birth and that those who die leave the living in need of care as a result of their deaths (Lynch, 1993).

Until now, a limited number of job opportunities posed the greatest argument in preparing nurses for professional roles in this field. Because of the existing medical-legal systems, there is little demand or opportunity for nurses to become involved in the death investigation field. Although interest in the field remains high, without hope of employment, there is limited motivation to pursue advanced practice for those not already in the system. There are, however, numerous archaic death investigation systems in the US and abroad that are, albeit slowly, converting toward biomedical professional models. As this occurs, the potential for the employment of nurses in greater numbers appears promising. As this is a pioneering arena for nurses, salaries are typically low in contrast to clinical nursing. Conversely, with the emerging emphasis placed on higher standards in death investigation, forensic nurse examiners in enlightened jurisdictions are receiving competitive salaries, commensurate with advanced education and clinical forensic experience.

Previously, forensic investigative staff generally consisted of nonbiomedical personnel, often retired law enforcement officers or morticians. Upon being interviewed, one forensic pathologist, when asked why policemen without education in the physical and psychosocial sciences were used to investigate traumatic death and interface with grief-afflicted families stated that "retired homicide detectives were more economically budgeted because they receive a retirement salary and can subsist on the low-salary position created for nonmedical personnel." As forensic nurses pursue advanced education in the forensic and nursing sciences, attaining postgraduate degrees in the forensic investigation of death and specializing in a variety of related fields such as forensic anthropology, bioterrorism, and disaster management, government agencies and scientific institutions are investing in these professionals to enhance the medicolegal management of death investigation.

One of the most significant contributions to nurses in death investigation was initiated in Canada as early as 1975. At the insistence of John Butt, who initiated the first formal position for forensic nurse death investigators, the salary and benefits were established equivalent to that of clinical nurses with equal education and experience. These pioneering nurses were also required to maintain their nursing licensure and national nursing association membership. These requirements should be incorporated into any forensic nurse investigator or nurse coroner program. Failing to do so was the single greatest mistake by those employing nurses in medicolegal investigation as this concept moved from Canada into the US. Although many clinical nurses have chosen to work in this field, they were unable to without sufficient financial compensation. This alone would have moved forensic nurse examiners forward into the realm of forensic pathology and the investigation of death decades ago.

Caring for the Dead

Although nurses have traditionally been recognized as the primary caretaker of the living, it must be recognized that nurses throughout history have also been the caretakers of the dead. In addition, as a component of the caregiver role, nurses comfort or console those who survive, including other members of the healthcare team who share in the grief and mourning process. Hospice nurses become experts in death and dying. Oncology nurses are prepared to provide terminal patients and their families with insightful perspectives on the stages of death and essential emotional support during those last moments of life. Neonatal nurses are exceedingly familiar with loss of life in the neonatal intensive care unit and the impact of grief that undermines the traditional joy accompanying birth. No department in the hospital faces the trauma of death and dying more frequently than the emergency department, as those who are admitted suddenly and unexpectedly due to random violence, catastrophic mass disasters, and natural or unknown causes often fail to survive.

To identify and recover microscopic bomb fragments while debriding a wound and to relate them to a detonator associated with known criminals, to relate wound characteristics to distinctive weaponry from crimes of this century and the last (such as the Unabomber, Oklahoma City Federal Building, the World Trade Tower, and others), is to acknowledge healthcare's accountability in combating crime. The US has displayed great national sensitivity in the recovery, identification, and memorial of the public, private, national dead. So, too, have other nations where civility and respect for death has brought together governments and families in mourning. The forensic sciences are responsible for the primary identification and repatriation of the war dead. Military nurses have launched initiatives in forensic nursing and Veterans Administration hospitals have established specific procedures to guide the clinical investigations of suspicious deaths among their patient populations. The presence of the military FNE would limit the physical and psychological abuse resulting from unethical interrogation, torture, and degrading humiliation of prisoners of war. This role would further reduce and prevent questioned deaths within these secured environs.

William Gladstone, a nineteenth-century British prime minister, spoke of the value of caring for the dead as a reflection of the morals and ethics of a society when he wrote one of his most famous statements, one that has memorialized the dead of wars over the centuries: "Show me the manner in which a Nation cares for its dead and I will measure with mathematical exactness, the tender mercies of its people" (Jalland, 1996). Cited at the momentous dedication of the Vietnam Veterans Memorial in Washington, D.C., in 1986, this statement has specific meaning for those who have lost loved ones in war or in peace.

Gladstone addressed death from a diverse perspective, as both good and bad. He stated that "death is an inevitable experience for us all, but the manner of dying varies greatly, as do individual and family responses to death and their mourning rituals" (Jalland, 1996). The French historian Michel Vovellehas observed that death "in the human adventure stands as an ideal and essential constant" (Jalland, 1996). Though it remains a constant in the reality of death, it is relative in relationship to the times of the social and religious perspectives of death. As times of social change continue to evolve, so does the manner in which people die. This concept was further emphasized by Pierre Chaunu in that every society gauges and assesses itself in some way by its system of death. In the same manner, the study of death and bereavement in the past has helped people to understand the present, the study of medicolegal death investigation, historical or in the recent past, helps people to evaluate and improve a systems approach to the scientific investigation of death.

Attitudes, customs, and beliefs relating to death impact the behavior of people from all levels of society in the management of the dying as well as the care of the dead. Cumulative experience with death and dying and social interaction derived from helping grief-stricken survivors, combine to shape the beliefs and behaviors that the forensic nurse death investigator (FNDI) brings into practice. It should not be surprising that the registered nurse has been found to be an ideal clinician to fulfill the requirements of the death investigator role.

Death investigation is an essential part of the healthcare and the judicial systems. However, clinical physicians are typically ill prepared to assume the responsibility inherent to the medicolegal management of questioned death cases. In North America, few medical schools provide curricula that include forensic medicine; even fewer address the psychosocial interventions associated with death. These two topics are essential aspects of developing a socially appropriate death investigation system. Furthermore, many physicians are not attracted by the prospect of becoming a public governmental employee with fixed income, continuing public scrutiny, and bureaucratic constraints. This has led to a dearth of qualified forensic medicine practitioners to work within the death investigation systems at a point in history when the need for this role is expanding exponentially. These circumstances have resulted in an increased opportunity for nurses to fulfill forensic roles in death investigation and clinical forensic practice. Forensic nurse examiners are stepping forward to assume these responsibilities in hospitals, clinics, and the community at large.

Forensic Nurse Examiner

Nurses are serving as the officiator of death in numerous areas throughout the US. The forensic nurse examiner specializing in death investigation as an elected coroner (an independent authority) or medical investigator (under the direction of a forensic pathologist) has brought a higher standard of administration and case management to questioned deaths than has existed in the past. Titles vary from one jurisdiction to another depending on the role and preference designated by the chief medical examiner or coroner. These titles evolve as existing roles are filled by nurses or as new roles are developed for nurses in the forensic investigation of death.

As an elected or appointed official, the title of coroner or deputy coroner is used in South Carolina, Wisconsin, Georgia, Colorado, and California, among others. In some states, for example in North Carolina, the forensic nurse has replaced the nonforensic physician. This nurse holds the title of district medical examiner and serves under the authority of the state medical examiner. In certain settings, such as the military or international death investigation systems, titles such as special investigator or chief forensic nursing officer may be appropriate. Among other titles assumed by nurse investigators in medical examiner systems are field investigator, field agent, forensic investigator, forensic nurse investigator, medical investigator, medicolegal investigator, medicolegal death investigator and forensic nurse death investigator (FNDI). Where nurses fill a supervisory role, titles may include chief investigator, senior investigator, or coordinator of the investigative team. Regardless of the title, authority and jurisdiction over the body at the scene of death remains the same. Forensic nurse examiners present the requisite skills and knowledge acquired as a natural extension of their nursing assessment proficiency and healthcare education. Nurses are valued components of the medicolegal death investigation team in jurisdictions of both coroners and medical examiners (Allert & Becker, 2002).

The title forensic nurse examiner (FNE) is appropriate to adapt to any one of the subspecialties of forensic nursing science where forensic examinations are performed on either living or deceased individuals. The FNE conducts an investigation of trauma or death, provides a forensic examination of physical, psychological, or sexual assault trauma, and examines the questioned analysis of medical records or court-ordered evaluation of mental status, provided the educational and experiential requirements and qualifications of a forensic nurse are met.

Nurse Coroner

Where the law does not require the coroner to be a physician, this position remains open to anyone who has reached the minimum age of 18 years, can provide proof of county residency for the past one or two years, and obtains the majority of votes. Although the statutes regulating this position vary from state to state, it remains accessible to the unskilled, untrained, nonmedically oriented and politically driven elected official known as a lay-coroner. However, according to Cumming, "This person must possess medical knowledge in order to be able to make critical judgments based on symptoms, medical history, postmortem appearance, toxicology and other diagnostic studies, combined with evidence revealed by other aspects of the investigation" (Cumming, 1995, 29-33).

Contemporary communities recognize that the expectations and qualifications for an officiator or investigator of questioned deaths must incorporate medical, psychological, and environmental acumen in a scientific and accurate determination of cause and manner of death. These communities elect and employ forensically skilled nurses who are well qualified to differentiate between postmortem changes and signs of victimization, understand interpretative toxicology, correlate mechanism of injury to cause of death, associate psychosocial histories with manner of death, comfort survivors, and provide appropriate referrals and support (Cumming, 1995).

A Nurse Coroner's Perspective

Charles E. Kiessling Jr., RN, BSN, CEN, who serves as the Lycoming County Coroner in Westport, Pennsylvania, is one example of an FNE who exemplifies quality death investigation. According to Kiessling, nurses are well qualified to fill the role of an officiator of death. Kiessling describes his role and experiences as typical of those who serve as the elected official in a growing number of US jurisdictions (Kiessling, no date):

> *Nurse Coroners have a thorough understanding of the pathophysiology necessary in determining the cause of death. In most counties across Pennsylvania the Coroner is called to the scene to investigate the cause and manner of death. Registered Nurses, through their nursing education and clinical experience, make excellent medical legal death investigators. Nurses also have significant experience in dealing with death and dying, frequently helping patients and families during some of the most difficult times of their lives. Who better to serve as an advocate for injury and death prevention than nurses who have experienced firsthand the catastrophic loss of life in their communities?*
>
> *The Nurse Coroner has the ability to monitor causes of death in the community and effect changes through such organizations as: SAFE KIDS, Child Fatality Review Teams, DUI Advisory Boards, Emergency Medical Services and Driver Safety Task Force. Nurse Coroners are also well versed on community resources to not only deal with the investigation of the death scene, but also to assist families deal with the aftermath of sudden deaths including such services as grief counselors and support groups as necessary. As elected officials, Nurse Coroners are generally well positioned with political contacts to recommend legislative changes when necessary.*
>
> *Law enforcement personnel in Lycoming County generally perceive most nurses as fellow professionals. As long as nurses recognize their limited knowledge regarding processing of crime scenes and legal procedures and remain willing to work cooperatively with law enforcement personnel, they will work well as Nurse Coroners. Conversely, law enforcement personnel will generally look to the nurse coroner for their expertise in medical pathophysiology, pharmacology, toxicology and mechanisms of injury in traumatic deaths.*

Kiessling is presently working to change hospital policy and procedures regarding the retention of critically ill and or injured patients that may eventually end up as coroner's investigations. Presently the local hospitals hold blood and urine specimens for three days and then discard these specimens unless directed to do otherwise. In 2003, a drug delivery case resulting in death was nearly lost because of the loss of these initial specimens. Fortunately autopsy findings were consistent with a methadone overdose, witnesses identified the suspect, and he then confessed. In the future these specimens will be retained until the patient is discharged or dies and the coroner clears these specimens for disposition. This change will assure that specimens are available to develop the prosecution's case against drug dealers who deliver drugs that result in deaths.

Implications for Forensic Nursing

Most laws have relegated medical-forensic tasks strictly to physicians within clinical and community environs. Exceptions were made, however, to include paramedical personnel, law enforcement officers, and elected officials in order to activate death investigation procedures. Currently in the US, many physicians and nonphysician professionals who hold these positions are not required to have forensic expertise. This role is often filled with laypersons (nonmedical and nonforensic personnel) who wish to run for public office. Their responsibility is to determine the cause and circumstances of death, provide a comprehensive scene investigation, request a postmortem evaluation as required, and notify the next of kin. This requires a systematic and methodical approach to confirm or rule out events disclosed prior to, during, and immediately after death occurs. A miscarriage of justice often results where specific knowledge related to the medical, legal, and social aspects of death investigation does not exist.

Until recent times, neither clinical nor community agencies nor institutions extended nurses the authority to pronounce death. Exception was extended to the nurse as an elected or appointed official in the county's medicolegal jurisdiction–not because the person was a nurse, but because she or he was an official or forensic investigator. Excluding clinical nurses appears to be an oversight that is incongruent with the education, experience, and professionalism of nurses when compared with that of paramedics and police or the local lay-coroner. Within the past two decades, however, nurse pronouncement laws have changed significantly. Where these laws exist, they provide nurses with the authority to pronounce death. Families no longer have to await the arrival of a physician to pronounce a terminal patient dead and can proceed with rites of passage and funeral arrangements without the anxiety of unnecessary delay.

In these jurisdictions, the attending physician no longer has to come to the hospital or nursing home to pronounce an expected death in order to release the body to mortuary services. Law enforcement officers at the scene of death or at the hospital appreciate the timeliness of nurse pronouncements and reduction of time required to remain with the body. Physicians find that this is an appropriate responsibility assumed by nurses that also helps to reduce the unnecessary pressure of being on call.

Laws continue to be updated and some nurses can pronounce death; however, only a physician may sign a death certificate in the US. One exception is the nonphysician coroner who may be authorized to certify death in certain states. This exception, however, can present a series of problems where the nonmedical coroner may fail to require an autopsy or recognize the accurate cause of death. Other common problems include the hesitation to release transplantable organs, inaccurate documentation, or the lack of important information regarding the circumstances of death.

As in any field of practice, all coroners cannot be judged by the same failures to practice satisfactory death investigation. In many jurisdictions, the elected coroner may be a general medical practitioner, a nurse, a paramedical professional, or a veterinarian.

Others may be lawyers, muffler repairmen, tow-truck operators, or sheriffs–without medical or nursing proficiency. Some 500 counties in the US employ morticians as coroners in spite of the fact that this is considered to be a conflict of interest in certain states. The California attorney general's opinion–which is next to law–considers this conflict of interest to be unethical where there is more than one mortician practice in a single jurisdiction. In Washington State, morticians are prohibited from seeking the elected position of coroner. However, one cannot judge the qualifications of an official by the title; in some states, the coroner may be a board-certified forensic pathologist. The law determines the title of the officiator of death as well as the term limits.

The Forensic Science Foundation in Colorado Springs, Colorado, estimates that where lay-coroners rule in questioned deaths, 10% to 50% of felonious deaths go unrecognized and unreported. These statistics also estimate that lay-coroners rule 40 percent more heart attacks than medically oriented officiators do due to the lack of glaring evidence of foul play (such as gunshot or stab wounds) (Fields, 2004). For example, in Texas, the lay-coroner is known as justice of the peace, an antiquated system practiced over a century (since 1869) that still prevails. Qualifications for justice of the peace require the candidate to be at least 18 years old and to have resided in the county for 12 months, yet justices of the peace have the authority to certify death, to initiate murder charges, and to influence life insurance claims, malpractice suits, and other important proceedings.

Critics state that homicides go undetected, accidental deaths are mistakenly ruled natural, life-threatening occupational and environmental hazards are missed, and child abuse deaths and suicides are underreported. Because the nonmedical, non-nursing coroner (or justice of the peace) does not have the necessary training to determine the exact cause of death, such as fatal infectious diseases, communities may be at peril when such cases go unrecognized and unreported. The lay-coroner may fail to recognize the subtle signs and symptoms of natural disease processes that generate concern when one considers that 60% to 65% of reportable deaths in the US are natural deaths, such as the complications of a diabetic coma, a gastrointestinal bleed, end-stage cirrhosis of the liver, or status epilepticus. These are frequent causes of deaths of individuals who die alone or unattended (Lynch, 1993). US Census 2002 estimated that 2,537,000 deaths occurred. Of that number, 20% were certified by US coroners and medical examiners. The remaining 80% were certified by attending physicians. Thus, over half a million people, approximately 507,400, constitute the number of medical examiner/coroner cases each year requiring an investigation of death.

Traditionally, individuals hired as death investigators have had an extensive background in law enforcement, although advances in forensic and nursing science indicate the need for investigators with a stronger background in anatomy and physiology, psychology, pharmacology, medical terminology, and a comprehensive knowledge of communicable and natural diseases (Lynch, 1986). Medical examiners and coroner systems that employ forensic nurse investigators find that the nurse who is cross-trained in forensic science and legal issues provides a collaborative practice approach, which is beneficial to forensic science professionals. A forensic specialist in nursing represents an innovative concept in an area of human services not previously explored by nurses but that is ideally suited for the forensic nurse examiner.

Forensic analysis provides data to develop trauma care systems and clinical practice standards. Thus, a hospital trauma care system's program for quality assessment helps to identify preventable deaths in order to modify care protocols and outcomes in subsequent cases. Clinical and community health nurses should also include clinical history and documentation of evidence. These components are critical elements in the administration of justice.

Forensic Nursing Services

Death Investigation and the Nursing Process

The unexpected death is most often responsible for arousing suspicion. The presence of the FNE initiates an investigation based on the Scope and Standards of Forensic Nursing Practice approved by the American Nurses Association Congress of Nursing Practice and the International Association of Forensic Nurses. The application of the nursing process forms the basis for the investigation of injury, illness, disease, disorder, or death in all human health conditions. Whether the individual at the center of the investigation is a patient in the hospital or dies at a scene of crime, in a residence or in police custody, the evaluation of circumstances surrounding the death requires a systematic, scientific approach, which is applicable through the nursing process.

The duties of a nurse death investigator are carried out in accordance with the performance standards and procedures established under the medical examiner or coroner's system of death investigation and the jurisdictional regulations. The standards established by the National Association of Medical Examiners, the Coroners Association, the International Association of Forensic Nurses, and the American Nurses Association conform to legislation and professional policies and procedures, administrative rules, and standards for professional practice. Coping with death-related grief is a manifest problem. Grief is seen as a social role, not only a "condition," and treatment plans are designed to alleviate this problem.

In approaching death investigation from a nursing process standpoint, collaterally, death investigations are not unlike traditional bedside nursing. Each investigation involves the following processes:

Assessment. Careful observation of the scene and circumstances of death are noted; discussions are held with the law enforcement officer at the scene, the family and or witnesses are debriefed, the attending or personal physician is interviewed regarding past medical history and recent hospital or clinic visits, and medications and injuries or illnesses are noted.

Planning. Decisions concerning each situation are made, further investigation into circumstances is developed, and appointments with pertinent persons are scheduled.

Interventions. The body and scene are documented with photography, evidence on or around the body pertaining to cause of death is recovered, notification of death is carried out and survivor needs are assessed, and referral for counseling sessions are planned as necessary. Referrals to appropriate professional agencies are made as needed. At programmed intervals, personal property is secured.

Evaluations. Evaluations are conducted concerning the investigation, interpretations of laboratory tests are reviewed, and medical records are compared as the autopsy report is examined. Further discussion with detectives and the family are reconsidered and implemented as appropriate. Peer review is routine and case notes are assessed.

Nurses employed or appointed to perform the duties of a forensic death investigator are skilled in forensic and nursing science. They are expected to meet or exceed established criteria for qualifications in education and research. Governing statutes, administrative rules, and professional performance standards define the duties and professional responsibilities of those appointed to conduct a forensic death investigation.

The nurse investigator works as one member of the multidisciplinary team in the scene investigation process requiring an in-depth evaluation of cases such as homicides, suicides, accidents, and cases of unknown or unrecognized trauma. In jurisdictions where the majority of the medical examiner's caseload is composed of natural deaths, which do not require a high investigative profile involving law enforcement officials, the forensic nurse assumes legal custody of the body until mortuary services arrive. This prevents police officers from being unnecessarily detained with a natural death and allows them to devote more time to criminal investigation. Forensic nurses do not compete with, replace, or supplant other practitioners–rather, they fill voids by accomplishing selected forensic tasks concurrently with law enforcement agencies.

Although both law enforcement agents and the forensic nurse investigator (FNI) are present at the scene of death, two distinct jurisdictions prevail. In most medical examiner/coroner jurisdictions, the crime scene belongs to the police, and the body belongs to the medical investigator. Each must recognize boundaries and coordinate specific aspects of the investigation, clearly designating individual and mutual responsibility. Failure to clarify roles and authority can result in unnecessary friction, territoriality, and even liability when matters go wrong (Lynch & Weaver, 1998).

Best Practice *34-1*

Respect Boundaries: The law enforcement agent's jurisdiction is the crime scene; the agent's objective is to determine if a crime has been committed and who committed the crime. The medical examiner/coroner's jurisdiction is the body, and the objective is to determine the cause and manner of death (i.e., why and how death occurred).

Death in the Clinical Environs

The priority to save lives is obvious to emergency department nurses in catastrophic near-death treatment. Yet the importance of properly identifying, securing, and preserving items that can later be considered as evidence may be forgotten as the patient dies. The medical examiner and the crime laboratory rely on the attending staff to provide an accurate and detailed description of wounds, to collect and preserve admission or postmortem blood and body fluids, and to recognize and recover trace evidence. The forensic nurse examiner on duty will be responsible for gathering essential documents, contacting appropriate authorities and agencies, ensuring notification of death, and intervening with the decedent's family.

The *dead on arrival* (DOA)–or those who die during trauma treatment, in the operating room, delivery room, or any other area of the hospital–require specific considerations when certifying the place of death. The pronouncement of death will determine the place of death, even if the initial trauma or end stage of the disease process responsible for death occurred elsewhere. If the decedent's body is removed from the site of death or dies during transport and pronounced DOA, the hospital becomes the place of death and is documented as such on the death certificate. Thus, the trauma room, for example, becomes a scene of death and should be protected as a crime scene until the body is removed and final evidence collection and documentation are completed.

When identification of the decedent is not in doubt, as with most individuals who die in the hospital, the investigation is simplified to a certain extent. When the *cause of death* is not in doubt and is not a traumatic or suspicious death but is required to be reported by law, the attending physician generally signs the certificate of death and the medical examiner's jurisdiction is waived. The body is released to the funeral home and the investigation is completed. Yet each death must be considered on the merits of the individual case. Under known or unknown circumstances, it is beneficial to have a death investigator with a biomedical background and who has the ability to review medical records and to interpret medical abbreviations and nurses' notes, natural disease processes, and surgical interventions. The death investigator should also be familiar with pharmacology in order to eliminate or confirm medication errors. Clinical nurses must recognize the ME/C jurisdiction of the case and maintain chain of custody over the body, scene, and evidence while awaiting the arrival of the death investigator. The FNI will interview clinical personnel, family or friends, and police at the hospital; collect evidence; document the condition of the decedent; and assume chain of custody before transferring the body to the forensic pathology laboratory.

Generally, information not readily available at the scene of death is available on the admission note or medical records. Medical history, diagnosis, time of death, and names of the next of kin and attending physician are available upon request to the death investigator. Laws in the US provide for access to this information involving forensic cases of death. The medical examiner or coroner has no jurisdiction over living persons but has ultimate authority over all questioned deaths within his or her jurisdiction. The exception would be in states where the coroner has jurisdiction over mental health-related issues.

Nurses who hesitate to divulge information related to a patient's death can be considered to be *obstructing justice* when failing to cooperate with the medical examiner or coroner. Medical investigators generally carry documents that provide the authority to access medical records. If the healthcare professional refuses to comply, a special warrant is required to obtain the documents (primarily due to complications in health privacy laws). When a person dies in the hospital and there are no relatives, generally, the health authority is lawfully in charge of the body.

Under a medical examiner or coroner system, the body is transferred to the investigative facility for a reasonable length of time so that the relatives can be located. After approximately 48 hours, if no relation can be traced, the health authority can authorize an autopsy. The health authority is equally responsible for the disposal of the body by burial or cremation. The health authority must bear the cost of the disposal of the body (Box 34-1).

Box 34-1 Body at the Hospital

- Clothing: Recover, dry, and pack in paper container (not plastic)
- Hair: Recover and package
- Treatment records: Obtain necessary copies and information
- Hardware: Do not remove; rather tie off or clamp
- Bag hands: Any patient that died of sexual assault or gunshot injuries
- Preserve evidence in general

Clinical nurses are continuously required to contact the ME/C's office to report deaths that occur in hospitals and nursing homes. Frequently, nurses are unaware of the specifics of death-reporting procedures or the laws that govern which deaths must be reported to the medicolegal system. Failure to report a forensic death and insufficient or erroneous information may cause investigation procedures to be hampered, and interagency relations may be jeopardized.

Key Point *34-1*

Nurses and other medical professionals, law enforcement agencies, forensic scientists, and public health authorities must engage in interagency cooperation for optimum death investigation processes to succeed.

Death-Reporting Initiatives

The clinical forensic nurse educator on the hospital staff should incorporate the following information in a death-reporting orientation for emergency services personnel and other departments. Ideally, nurses should know the law prior to facing legal issues in sudden and unexpected death. Nurses should keep a laminated copy of the law and of the information required for reporting to the ME/C in the desk or ambulance for ready reference and create a death information checklist. Nurses should also know what to report (anything other than natural death or a natural death that falls within the parameters of the law), what number to call (ME/C), who to ask for (medical investigator or deputy coroner), and what information that person will request. The forensic nurse should not release personal property to the next of kin without the permission of the police, the coroner, or the medical examiner. Patient's personal belongings often constitute forensically significant evidence. This includes clothing, valuables, or other property. Once the property has been released, the chain of custody has been severed and it is no longer admissible in court.

Proper Body Handling

When a person dies in the hospital, nurses are typically instructed to follow the clinical protocol for preparing the body, which is generally outlined in the nursing procedure manual. If the decedent is to be sent to the ME/C office, routine postmortem care is no longer appropriate. Although contrary to general procedure, the wrists and ankles should not be tied together. Binding limbs with gauze or other material will leave marks that can be confused with ligature or handcuff marks or may destroy any such impressions that preexist. Although limbs have traditionally been tied in order to assist those who are handling the body after death, it is preferable to wrap the body in a clean white sheet, tying each end together to protect the body and extremities.

Suspicious Deaths

When a traumatic death is pronounced on arrival or shortly after being admitted, or when any suspicion of circumstances has been reported to the police or ME/C, routine postmortem care is no longer appropriate. Do not remove clothing or treatment paraphernalia, and do not wash the body. The FNE should distinguish those features caused from injury from those caused by life-saving intervention or medical treatment. Document these features on the patient's chart or use a skin marker on the body with ME/C approval. This should be cleared by contacting the local medical examiner or coroner for preferences in procedures and be written into the hospital's forensic protocol.

Case Study 34-1 Attempted Killing of Patients by Muscle Relaxants

A nurse was accused of killing and attempting to kill 30 patients by injecting them with nondepolarizing muscle relaxants (gallamine triethiodide or pancuronium) leading to respiratory muscle paralysis and transient or permanent respiratory arrest. These scenarios occurred over the period of June 1996 to April 1997 in the neurosurgical department intensive care unit at the Faculty of Medicine Hospital, Alexandria, Egypt. Only one quadriplegic victim was exhumed and autopsied, four days after burial. The body was severely putrefied and blood was positive for Flaxidil (gallamine triethiodide). However, medical files indicated that the patient suffered from hypostatic pneumonia before death and was taking approximately 12 drugs that could give false positive results during the chemical analysis.

Reviewing files of 30 suspected victims revealed several signs and symptoms not consistent with muscle relaxants, such as convulsions, bradycardia, and severe hypertension. "Apnea" was observed in the majority of cases after surgical intervention. Medication was absorbed through brain tissue near the brain stem or through the ventricles. A confession was taken from the accused nurse a few hours after she fell from the second floor of police headquarters (attempted suicide) during confession. She was suffering from multiple pelvic fractures, was bleeding internally and externally, and had taken several drugs prior to interview that affect memory and concentration.

The purpose of this case study is to direct attention of medicolegal authorities to establish an internationally approved medicolegal system in the fields of medical and nursing responsibilities in an attempt to protect them against false accusation during their professional practice, particularly in criminal courts, and to urge the International Association of Forensic Sciences to establish a hotline information center approved by the ministries of justice around the world, specifically in developing countries. Such centers would assist investigators in identifying criminal behavior in healthcare facilities and also in reducing and preventing further deaths of this nature.

Data from El Shennawy, I. (1999). *Mass killings and attempted killings of 30 patients by muscle relaxants.* Proceedings of the International Association of Forensic Sciences, Los Angeles.

Notification of Death

The consequences of violence and other unnatural causes of death take a tremendous toll on individuals, families, and communities. These consequences are not only legal issues but also add difficulty to times of great personal crisis. The immediate aftermath of a sudden, unexpected, and unexplained death requires direct and intimate communication. Notification of death is one of the most traumatic moments in the lives of individuals closely related or intimately involved with someone who has died suddenly or unexpectedly, whether a result of catastrophic events or casualties common to community lives. A family's immediate response to the news of a death is often unpredictable. Death is a difficult topic to discuss, both personally and professionally. With the death of a child or parent, or the anticipatory grief of family elders for those closest to them, for that moment, the living experience a distortion of reality.

Key Point *34-2*

Violent deaths are more stigmatizing and traumatic. Violent deaths trigger feelings of guilt, hatred, perplexity, resentment, panic, confusion, and rage.

The office of the medical examiner or coroner is ultimately responsible for the notification of deaths within their jurisdiction. Because nurse coroners generally employ nurses as deputy coroners, the staff is well prepared to intervene with the unknown and unexpected emotional reactions to death notification.

The use of forensic nurse death investigators is growing in the US and becoming preferred in many medical examiners' jurisdictions. Forensic pathologists who employ nurse investigators stress the importance of teamwork between criminal and biomedical investigative personnel. They have expressed concern that medically untrained officers often disregard medical evidence, maintain poor sensitivity, and are not communicative with bereaved families (Butt, 1993). Forensic nurse examiners who fill the role of death investigator or coroner contribute holistically by bringing together clinical expertise, forensic technique, and empathy.

Vernon McCarty, the coroner for Washoe County, Nevada, has employed nurses in his office for longer than two decades and is an advocate for using nurses in death investigations. He states:

> *The medical investigator will often play a key role in notification of the next of kin, advisement as to death related events, and grief counseling. The investigator should never overlook this opportunity to provide social support. The investigator should be acquainted with grief related responses. In doing so it is realized that not only will the investigative function be much simplified and that an important human need will be fulfilled. Medical examiner's investigators are required to make judgments and solve problems on their own initiative and in liaison with other disciplines. The consequences of error are great, with effects that could lead to aggravation of grief or litigation. (Handbook for Death Reporting, no date)*

When a sudden and unexpected death occurs, the first responders are generally the police, emergency services, and the death investigator or coroner. They usually share in the responsibility of interviewing the survivor and documenting the evidence. The task of communicating with the decedent's survivors requires tact and human caring. When the shock of the loved one's death is compounded by violence, the death notification is frequently an overwhelming scenario of grief, despair, and anguish. Whether the interface with the next of kin or significant other is at the scene of death or in the emergency department, the alleviation of human suffering remains the objective of the empathetic health and justice professional.

Social scientists have begun to study the survivors left behind in the wake of traumatic grief. These individuals display signs and symptoms of post-traumatic stress disorder resulting from not only the death trauma, but from "secondary wounds" due to the circumstances surrounding the aftermath (Herzog, 1979). This begins with the notification of death.

How can the FNDI help the survivors of catastrophic death trauma? The relatives and friends of the victim are recognized as *victims by extension*, often requiring crisis intervention and grief therapy. Shneidman (1984) indicated that "post-vention" (i.e., appropriate and helpful acts after the tragedy) will render immediate and on-the-scene crisis intervention. Post-vention reduces the aftereffects of a traumatic event for the victim-survivors.

Defense Mechanisms

As healthcare professionals, FNEs have a responsibility to the family to understand the verbal and nonverbal clues and to determine how to help them. The most common defense mechanisms often present are one's reactions to the notification of a sudden death and include shock, panic, guilt, confusion, rage, and resentment.

As an immediate source of support, the death investigator making the notification provides the opportunity for the bereaved to vent their feelings. The FNE cannot prevent the primary injury and emotional trauma caused to the victim-survivors by death. However, the FNE's responsibility is to prevent the secondary wounds from an insensitive or inappropriate notification of death.

Best Practice *34-2*

Forensic nursing must apply the practices of human caring to the study and practice of the biological and social sciences in the scientific investigation of death.

Death notification is a sensitive and delicate message that needs to be delivered in person and as soon as possible. The investigator responsible for making the notification should have developed a flexible system of notification, interviewing, and questioning before approaching the family. Because emotional defense mechanisms are unique to each individual, one must understand that any reaction from the next of kin is their way of coping under stress. Often the bearer of sad news is the first to receive the brunt of an emotional outburst of anger, rage, or grief. This should not be taken personally, but rather the FNE should adjust to the reactions of the adult or child in a way that offers assistance in this difficult time.

Key Point *34-3*

An important part of the coroner or medical examiner's work is to serve as a liaison with the next of kin. This facilitates the grieving process, assists families in expressing emotion, and decreases guilt by ensuring families that grief is a natural reaction.

A historic lack of comprehensive training for investigators or officiators with criminal investigative backgrounds has resulted in definitive problems related to notification of death. Police have been cited as lacking sensitivity and the ability to display empathy. Families state they perceive this interaction with law enforcement officers to be cold, callous, and indifferent. This lack of emotion most often negatively affects the mental health of grieving relations (Lynch, 1995). It is difficult for a staff without appropriate education to understand the basic needs of the bereaved as well as provide the necessary cooperation from the standpoint of interagency and interpersonal communication. The educational preparation of a death investigator must include psychosocial skills in order to reduce and prevent further emotional trauma or the negative issues often associated with law enforcement investigators in notification of death procedures.

Human consolation is not the objective of criminal investigation. Officers often state that they find it necessary to operate according to *unstated rules* in order to remain objective and maintain control. These unstated rules include the following:

- Don't get too close.
- Don't ask unnecessary questions.
- Don't focus on feelings of the survivors.
- Don't get personally involved.

This is without criticism of law enforcement officers. In regard to criminal investigation, they are trained to display traits necessary to gain their objectives. In the same sense that professionals in any field cannot be judged alike, all law enforcement agents cannot be judged by the negative behavior of some. Empathy is a learned behavior as well as a personality trait. Many officers are sincerely concerned with the impact of sudden death on parents, children, or significant others and provide a sensitive and perceptive approach when addressing those who are victims by extension.

Conversely, a chief complaint often accorded to nurses addresses their failure to be objective, suspicious, or remain alert to potential indicators of criminality when families express sentiments of emotion and shock. The forensic nurse, however, is taught to maintain a strong sense of suspicion in behavioral evaluation, while at the same time providing a perceptive and observant assessment. Based on their cross training in criminal justice and forensic science technique, forensic nurses are cautioned to approach each death as if it were a homicide until proved otherwise. In the same manner, clinical FNEs are taught to consider unrecognized or unidentified injuries as abuse until confirmed or ruled out.

Current nursing theories and practices emphasize a caring response to the complex and sensitive issues surrounding death and dying. Emotional trauma resulting from abnormal grief or inappropriate adaptation to stress directly affects health and disease orientation. Intervention in grief must be seen and supported as a means toward adaptation and health. Forensic nursing is a part of an essential shift in human consciousness that represents a much needed and long overdue concern for survivors. For further information on responses to grief and management of the bereaved, see Chapter 28.

Proper Notification Technique

The National Organization for Victims Assistance Bulletin 110 (NOVA, no date) advises the following notification procedures:

- *Never* make a notification by telephone. This can generally be avoided by contacting a local chaplain that works with the police department or other agency skilled in the notification of death in a different city or country and request personal notification.
- Arrange a personal contact.
- Project warmth and compassion.
- Convey the information simply and directly.
- Be aware of the survivors' medical history.
- Use concise terms, such as *dead, died,* or *was killed.* Avoid ambiguous terms such as *passed on, expired, is gone.* These terms are easily misunderstood and create false hope.
- Never refer to the decedent as "the body"; instead use the decedent's name or familial status.
- Don't fear emotional involvement; don't be afraid to join the survivors in their grief.
- Be empathic and let the survivors know you care about them and their loss.
- Encourage them to cry freely, expressing their grief in whatever way they wish and for as long as they wish.

Forensic nurse death investigators are often the first to come in contact with the next of kin in the immediate post-death period. A sensitive approach should include the application of psychosocial interventions among those listed here:

- Consoling the survivors
- Listening
- Talking about the decedent
- Evaluating the emotional status of the survivors
- Offering referral information
- Sharing strength and concern through touch
- Not being in a rush to leave
- Never leaving them alone
- Encouraging them to express other emotions; anger and guilt need to be ventilated/shared
- Reassuring them that the death was not their fault
- Maintaining a policy of availability to relatives who often have no place to turn with their questions about the most delicate circumstances of the death
- Giving them as much information as possible
- Supporting their need to repeat questions
- Encouraging them to seek additional support
- Never saying, "I understand," "It was God's will," or "At least you have other children"

Psychosocial Intervention

Post-vention is described as appropriate and helpful acts after a tragedy and provides immediate and on-scene crisis intervention. It also helps to reduce the aftereffects of a traumatic event in the lives of the survivors. Three psychological stages of post-ventive care include the following:

1. Resuscitation: Working with the initial shock and grief in the first 24 hours
2. Rehabilitation: Consultations with family members from the first to the sixth month
3. Renewal: Healthy tapering off of mourning process from the sixth month on (Shneidman, 1984)

Caution: Although the nurse investigator must not let emotions interfere with professionalism, the family's loss must always be recognized. This requires a balance of objectivity and empathy, never becoming so insensitive that their loss cannot be felt. The nurse investigator should always say, "I'm sorry," and let the next of kin know he or she is sincere.

Guidelines for Approaching the Family

- Do not make death notifications from the doorstep!
- Identify yourself and ask to come inside. Tell them your position. Ask for their names.
- Make eye contact. Eye contact and a quiet voice convey caring and establish some rapport.
- Offer to find a place where everyone can be seated. Never stand when a victim-survivor is seated.
- It is appropriate to "anchor" them with a touch–hold a hand, touch a shoulder. Brief physical contact conveys compassion.

- Start with, "I have very difficult news to bring you" or "It's about your son, it is very serious," then "Your son was killed today."
- Never draw out the point of the notification–the longer the news is drawn out, the greater the stress.
- Never give them too much information at one time. Wait until they ask the next question before continuing with the information. Hesitate between each sentence, giving them the time to react and absorb what they are being told.
- Speak slowly. Slowing down helps the family to gradually grasp the news. They will be in shock and will not want to believe what they are hearing. They will have an immediate onset of physical symptoms from the rush of adrenaline. Their hands will be cold, respirations rapid, and heartbeats fast.
- Explain what the next sequence of events will be. Leave written information. They may not remember later what was said: the instructions regarding the investigation, the coroner, the autopsy, the mortician, and so on.
- Activate at least one source of support. Contact a family member, clergy, neighbor, or victim advocate. It is not appropriate to leave someone in acute grief alone. They are vulnerable, in shock, and fragile. Newly bereaved individuals are often at risk for serious accidents.
- Follow up with a phone call, letter, or visit (some ME/coroner offices have specially prepared letters). The FNE will be remembered with gratitude and respect and will not be forgotten. The FNE will become part of their healing process (adapted from Monroe, 2003).

Viewing of the Body

Whenever possible, allow the family or significant other to see their loved one. With rare exception, it is essential that they be allowed to view the body if they have requested to do so. Prepare them for what they may see. Explain the condition of the body and give them the opportunity to change their minds. If they are confident this is what they wish, give them a moment to organize their thoughts while the body is arranged for viewing.

In a forensic case, any treatment paraphernalia from the body should not be removed and the face should not be washed. Cover any injured body parts and drape the body with a clean white sheet. If the head is injured, wrap a clean white towel around the hair and lower the room lights. Be prepared to support them both emotionally and physically as the situation demands. However, they should *never* be alone with the body. Explain that they cannot touch the body. This is a precaution for the security of evidence in a forensic case. The FNE has custody of the chain of evidence initiated with the body. It is not uncommon for the spouse, parent, or others close to the decedent to be the primary suspect. The nurse investigator or coroner should supervise the entire viewing process as well as protect the body and evidence from any disturbance throughout.

This supervision should be of particular consideration in child deaths. Children are most frequently killed by their parents or primary caretakers. Until the autopsy has been completed and suspicion of abuse or murder has been eliminated, no one should be allowed to touch, to hold, or to be alone with the body. Within the nursery (neonatal or infant class of deaths), significant concern has been expressed by nurses who are requested by the ME or coroner *not* to allow the parents to hold the baby's body before releasing it for autopsy. Although the hospital's intention is to allow the parents to initiate some extent of closure, one must also consider the risk that a suspected sudden infant death syndrome case might actually be a homicide. If the body is to be autopsied, no one should come in contact with the body or evidence. The nurse investigator should explain that the death is now an ME/C case, and contact is not allowed. The reason for this precaution is to prevent loss or cross-contamination of evidence. The explanation should be kept simple, brief, and firm (it is not necessary to explain that the parent may be considered a suspect). Generally parents are considerate of this request. If the death is not an ME/C case and is of natural causes, parents should always be allowed the opportunity to hold, touch, and share last moments with the infant or child.

Attempts to lessen traumatic shock when viewing the body or making visual identification during the initial post-death period is an important responsibility of the forensic nurse. Medical examiners and coroners recognize this need and often provide special viewing rooms for privacy and security of the body. A small, quiet, comfortable room with a plate-glass window or closed-circuit television visualization to observe the body is beneficial to the one making identification. This helps to distance the impact of trauma, eliminates smells, and provides for security of the body. Some facilities have a chapel that also serves as a viewing room. Polaroid photographs have proved to be a significant visual identification method in mass disasters, eliminating the need for an actual viewing of the body. This helps to reduce the time management and emotional trauma of families when dealing with mass disasters. These bodies are removed directly from the scene to the forensic pathology facilities for identification and autopsy, and they are often stored in refrigerated transportation units. The next of kin, in these cases, would likely prefer to make identification from the photographs. However, it is the special presence of the forensic nurse that provides the physical and psychological support that often helps to stabilize the family members in this difficult experience. How they are treated is significant postvention care–something they will remember always.

As a clinical nurse cares for the dying and counsels their families during the hospital stay, the forensic nurse death investigator is able to continue in the role of a nurse. In a very real way, the planning is continued as originated in the clinical setting. The nurse sees to the needs of those left behind and is a visible part of the community care system. The position description of the forensic nurse examiner in death investigation falls within the parameters of the standards of nursing care and meets the criteria of the nursing process. There is ongoing evaluation of the position description as FNEs work with other members of the profession.

The Question

It is not uncommon to be asked why a nurse would want to perform the duties of an investigator of death. Generally, peer professionals in the clinical setting (even some nurse educators) or in the public eye cannot imagine why anyone would choose this role. They cannot conceive of the scenarios faced by the nurse investigator and the risk of vicarious trauma that can, and may, affect the psychological well-being of those most often to first come in contact with the family, to bear the brunt of sudden shock and grief. It must be remembered that the decedents, regardless of the circumstances of death or the condition of the body, are the same individuals often treated in the emergency department, only they are no longer breathing.

Each person is our patient. Whether someone dies on the trauma table or on an interstate highway, of a natural death or violent causes, FNEs have a responsibility to treat the individual as if the victim were a member of his or her own family. Who wants to think that when the time of death comes that anyone should be afraid or repulsed to tend to our last needs? There was a time when each family was responsible for the care of the dead, their own dead. Although it must have been difficult, it was surely done with love and tenderness. That no one would want to do this job–with care–is a reflection on our lack of humanness. It should be considered an honor to become the deceased's last friend, to represent the deceased as one would the disabled, to speak for the dead, with the deceased's family or in a court of law.

The ultimate goal of death investigation, to determine why one dies, is to save lives of a similar nature in the future. To make recommendations for public health and safety is one vital aspect of health and justice objectives. Death investigation is intellectually stimulating; each case is a challenge, an anticipation of the unknown. One must consider the contribution to society–the reduction and prevention of injury, illness, and death. To know you have performed a job that few others would want, to diminish human suffering in some small way, and to care when others do not–these acts bring their own reward.

Cultural Competency

In many countries, as well as in some cultures within the US, the family remains the primary caretaker of the dead. It is important to consider the ethnic, religious, burial, and grieving practices of each family and accept each with respect. Cultural competency in death-related cases, from a forensic nursing perspective, includes three interacting viewpoints: objective, subjective, and the cross-cultural encounter (Lipson, 1996). The objective component focuses on the decedent, family, and cultural and social characteristics including communication and worldview. Subjective perspectives reflect the FNE's personal and cultural characteristics involving self-awareness, values, beliefs, and communication style. Communication barriers based on ethnocentric or bias toward a particular ethnic group, religion, or political group can interfere with effective interviewing during an investigation. Interpersonal sensitivity is essential regarding diversity in death rituals, preparation of the body, and funerary requirements, or cultural beliefs when interfacing with immigrants and refugees or those whose sociocultural background is different from one's own. Except for the American Indian, immigrants from all parts of the world populated the US throughout different eras (Lipson, 1996). These issues cannot be addressed appropriately in making notification of death by telephone, which should not even be considered. There is rarely a situation that cannot be managed by personal notification. If this exceptional situation should occur, one must rely on nursing's *ways of knowing and critical thinking skills* with consideration for the next of kin's ability to communicate and understand, as well as the person's age and health, and the presence of a companion.

Diversity is part of the fabric of social life, not only in the US, but also in most countries due to our transient society. Some specific considerations include the family's language skills, tone of voice, nonverbal communication, privacy, personal space, eye contact, touch, and time orientation, socioeconomic status and social class, sexual orientation, disability, and death rituals.

Although consent to autopsy is not a choice in ME/C cases, consideration of other cultural and religious beliefs will provide sensitivity and enhance the investigative relationship during the immediate post-death period. Although a nurse coroner or nurse investigator is one of the first to meet the survivors and discuss the death, being able to offer support to the grieving family is a rewarding part of a difficult job.

The professional philosophy of the forensic nurse examiner, which parallels nursing philosophy in general, is *prevention*. This philosophy is embodied in an earnest attempt to accomplish a reduction in human destructiveness between individuals or as a result of self-annihilation, from communicable disease or the manufacture of unsafe products, from interpersonal violence or terrorism, in time of war or at peace. This reflects the belief that people who experience human kindness in the midst of trauma will recover faster, and those who give caring and respect human dignity to others find the greatest satisfaction in personal fulfillment and professional reward.

The Future

Forensic nursing science has contributed significantly to both the forensic sciences and to traditional nursing practice. The forensic nurse continues to be of assistance in the evolution of a health and justice-oriented system of care based on society's values and needs. This continuing evolution will require varying degrees of assistance in stabilizing and advancing forensic nursing as a discipline and as a science. Society demands a specific kind of help from persons specially qualified to care for the situations and circumstances often called for in human death.

Consider, now, another turning point in the ever-expanding role of the forensic nurse. Forensic nurse examiners and the future of death science are clearly interrelated. Scientifically, nurses are prepared to participate in and to assist with all aspects of the investigation of death, from the scene of death to the autopsy laboratory, from the hospital and the community setting to a court of law. The forensic nurse examiner serves as a liaison between the medical examiner/coroner's office and the police, news media, governmental agencies, families, and other individuals. For families, the forensic nurse examiner extends a more sensitive approach to death investigation. For the pathologist, the forensic nurse is the natural protégé.

Advancing the Scope of Forensic Science

After the implementation of the first graduate program to prepare nurses as medicolegal investigators at the University of Texas at Arlington, the question was "Where will we go?" In 1988, Dr. Charles Petty, chief medical examiner in Dallas County, Texas, when queried regarding the status of nurses in death investigation, replied in a personal letter to Lynch:

> *The basic premise is that death investigation is better carried out by individuals with medical training. This was recognized over 100 years ago, first in Massachusetts when the first medical examiner system was established. Gradually since then, more and more death investigation systems have incorporated physicians as medical examiners, supplanting the old lay-coroner system. In many large metropolitan areas, the physician medical examiner does not have the time to conduct the basic death investigation in person. Individuals who are trained by the medical examiner to visit scenes and to carry out telephonic investigations do this. Until recently, nurses were not engaged in this type of investigation. However, in this office, we have now, and have had in the past, registered nurses*

who proved to be excellent death investigators because of the past medical training possessed by them. (Petty, 1988)

As forensic pathology became the preferred method of death investigation and was considered the standard by which all questioned deaths were to be evaluated, a significant limitation was recognized due to the shortage of those qualified to practice as medical examiners. Forensic medicine remains the second smallest specialty in the practice of US medicine. Inevitably, this leaves a serious deficit of specialists to manage the multitude of forensic cases reported in North America.

One solution to this shortage is to utilize forensic nurse examiners. This approach utilizes a preexisting resource, one who is educated and skilled as forensic professional for the role of coroner, deputy coroner, or forensic nurse death investigator in adjunct to a forensic pathologist. Where the law does not require this position to be filled by a physician, the forensic nurse examiner provides an ideal solution to existing problems within the system of death investigation.

Petty further stated, "This is a new field for nurses and I believe will become one that will be most acceptable to both nurses and medical examiners. I can foresee the time when in metropolitan areas nurses will be involved as death investigators, possibly supplanting others." Petty explained the rationale for a preference to nurses or lay-investigators, as opposed to the use of police officers as field agents in medical investigation. He stated that it was more advantageous to take an individual with a medical background and train him or her in investigative technique than it was to teach a criminal investigator about medical knowledge and technique.

This has become the principle on which nurse coroners and nurse death investigators have been recognized as uniquely qualified to serve as officiators of death and to represent the forensic pathologists at the scene. This principle, originating with John Butt in 1975, has been embraced by many US jurisdictions and has reached into the distant areas of Africa and Asia. Butt believes that forensic nurses fill a multifaceted role beyond scene investigation, expanding their nursing skills to touch the lives of the grieving and bereaved in a manner that has brought a new respect to the field of death investigation.

From the history of nurses and death investigation, the following information is excerpted from an interview at a nursing conference in Alberta, Canada, on June 3, 1996:

As a result of the Canadian trend toward nurse death investigation, Dr. Nizam Peerwani, Chief Medical Examiner, Tarrant and Parker County Medical Examiner District in Ft. Worth, Texas, appointed Virginia Lynch to the position of Medical Investigator in his jurisdiction. Lynch became the first registered nurse, the first female, and the first death investigator for Parker County in 1984, serving an area of 960 square miles. In charge of investigating all reported deaths in rural Parker County with 65,000 residents, she was frequently on duty 24-7 for the next six years. As a result of these early experiences in death investigation, Lynch recognized the intrinsic value of forensic science to clinical nursing in criminal and liability-related trauma. This concept and its application to nursing practice would eventually be recognized as an important element of public health and safety. Peerwani served as a mentor to Lynch and later became a faculty member in the first Forensic Nursing Master's degree program at the University of Texas at Arlington, which she designed and initiated. The end results became the evolution of a new era of nursing practice: Forensic Nursing Science.

Figures 34-1 through 34-3 show the initial investigation at an apparent homicide scene.

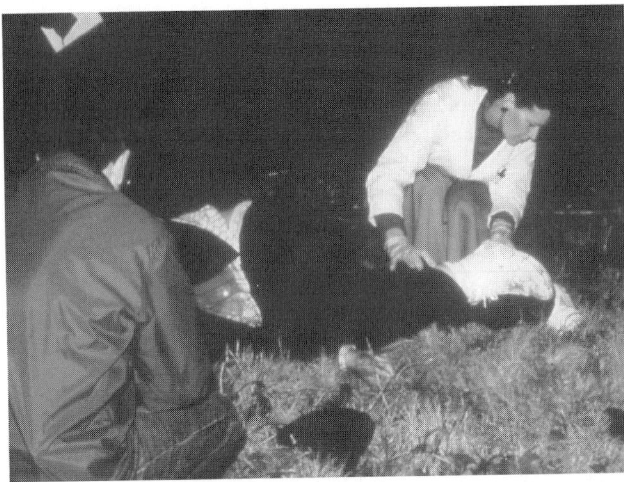

Fig. 34-1 A forensic nurse examiner makes an initial assessment while investigating an apparent homicide scene in conjunction with law enforcement officers.

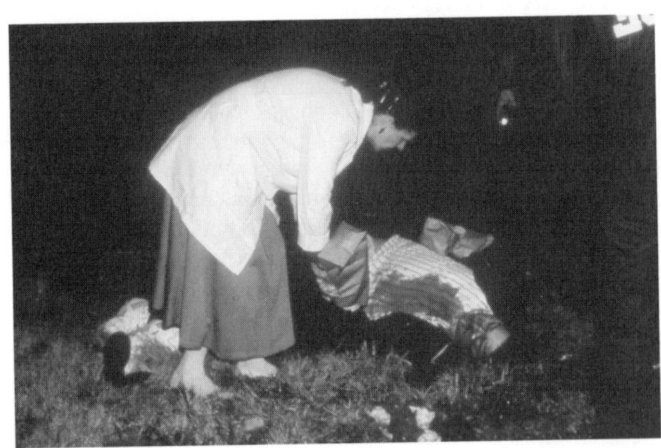

Fig. 34-2 Bags have been placed over victim's hands to preserve trace evidence.

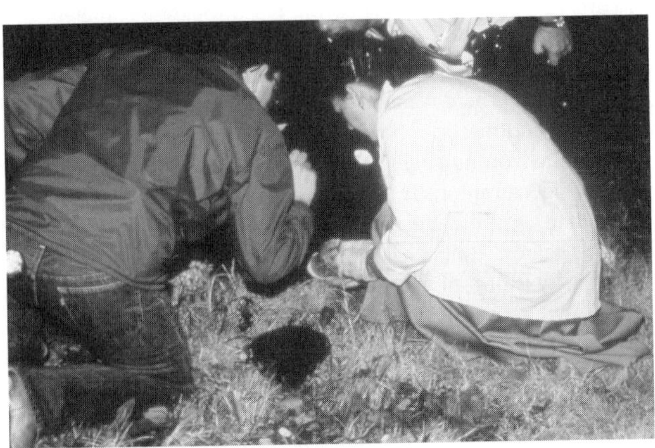

Fig. 34-3 Law enforcement officer and FNE scrutinize another potential evidentiary item at scene.

Advanced Practice in Death Investigation

Forensic nursing has come of age. A viable conceptual system has been established, one that provides comprehensive, relevant guidelines for theory building and research. No longer are FNEs overly concerned with status as forensic nurse scientists, but instead they are concerned with the phenomena of life and death as equal counterparts in human care. FNEs are beginning to realize their potential for discovering a particular kind of knowledge that is relevant to other disciplines and essential to nursing. The problem of the past has been the dearth of forensic nursing knowledge. The problem of the future will be the acceleration of that knowledge into every aspect of each nursing specialty, for there is no nursing specialty that cannot benefit equally from the application of this knowledge. There is no nursing specialty that does not come in contact with the realities of human violence as a public health concern.

Although our charge was clear more than 100 years ago, Florence Nightingale envisioned a better world for humankind through nursing. Nurses have always cared for victims of crime—and for the dead. Yet because of the direction nurses have taken in search of nursing knowledge, only recently have they begun to discover that truth and justice also lie within the nucleus of nursing care. Nursing is on the threshold of an exciting venture into new domains of knowledge, science, and the law. Its application to traditional nursing practice will be enhanced by forensic nursing as a tool for preventing human abuse, premature deaths, and social injustice. Forensic nursing is at a new juncture of development and has led this emerging discipline toward a new image and profile. At the same time, it has lent a new level of sophistication and prestige to forensic medicine through the acceptance of highly skilled and competent counterparts in forensic nursing. This collegial relationship and association represents a value that is seen as both necessary and desirable in reinforcing a degree of security within both professions as FNEs work together to conduct mutual research and outcomes nonexistent in the past.

To join with other health professionals in expanding concepts that cross the barriers of tradition for tradition's sake is invigorating. Nursing has long recognized the need to focus on topics such as the right to die, children and death, youthful suicide, grief and bereavement, sudden death trauma, and defining death. Perspectives on death emphasize quality of life issues that cannot be quantified in psychosocial and scientific research. Theories and practices share caring responses to the complex and sensitive issues surrounding death and dying. The social services available to those facing death, dying, and grief are reported in a complex intermingling of disciplines that include nursing, medicine, law, genetics, philosophy, psychology, religion, sociology, anthropology, political science, economics, and education. Such complexity affects the role of every professional concerned with the quality of life for humankind. Considering the increasing effects of the life span of humankind, the greater number of elderly will have a significant impact on healthcare and on death investigation where prevention of exploitation, abuse, and quality of life interface with health, peace, and quantification of years.

The education and experience of the forensic clinical nurse specialist or the forensic nurse practitioner provides a distinctive knowledge base and clinical skills appropriate for an advanced role in death investigation and other forensic services. Although registered nurses with a specialized education in death investigation have proved exceptional investigators or coroners, advances in the forensic and medical sciences are persuading a greater number of nurses than ever before to attain advanced degrees. Progressive academic institutions are currently providing the opportunity for innovative programs of study for nurses who wish to attain a master's degree or PhD in forensic nursing science. As in any other career, the trend to maintain quality continuing education and formal credentials impacts the professional benefits of the forensic nurse as well. These futuristic insights into the advanced realm of forensic nursing practice will provide unlimited potential and an exciting career path in role development yet to be imagined and fulfilled.

The continual evolution of forensic nursing practice is being considered for more advanced roles as associates in forensic pathology, in scientific research, and in clinical trials with goal-directed outcomes, involving education, publications, supervisory positions in large institutional facilities, and as direct service providers in medical examiner and coroner systems. Advanced specialists in forensic nursing will provide an enhanced image to the complex field of death investigation, a field once viewed with disdain by clinical professionals, families of the dead, and the public at large. Considering that the major status of the forensic nurse is, foremost, nursing, it is the nursing process and nursing ingenuity that guides the investigative actions of the forensic nurse. As nursing becomes more independent, the nurse investigator's level of practice will be subjected to greater scrutiny requiring more sophisticated education, qualifications, and skills.

In the US and increasingly in other countries, governments, and nongovernment organizations (NGOs) are turning to forensic nurse examiners with expectations to fill a void where a deficient number of forensically skilled physicians have resulted in inadequate prosecutions, loss of evidence, long delays in response time, and the loss of human lives. Forensic nursing services can assist law enforcement and emergency physicians in meeting the expectations of victims and their families through accessible and cost-effective programs. The expectations are as follows:

1. Utilize nursing principles and skills in communication, interviewing, and physical assessment through appropriate nursing interventions with the decedent, the decedent's family, and other relevant persons in the community.
2. Synthesize and apply skills of physical assessment and knowledge of biomedical investigation to assess, plan, provide, and evaluate nursing interventions, with and on behalf of the deceased, the family, and the community.
3. Participate effectively on the multidisciplinary medical examiner/coroner team to plan and provide direct and supportive nursing care; to assess needs for and make referral to other healthcare services and to counsel individuals and families through periods of stress.
4. Participate in investigations under the direction of the medical examiner/coroner to determine circumstances surrounding sudden death. This includes, but is not necessarily limited to, the following:
   - Visiting the scene of death and working with the police
   - Independently identifying and developing health details and collecting medical evidence related to the cause of death in both criminal and noncriminal cases
   - Interpreting the patient's health history and circumstances prior to death
   - Researching health records and preparing case history summaries to facilitate death investigation
   - Interviewing physicians and other healthcare providers to help establish cause and manner of death
   - Providing direction in handling the body and personal effects of the deceased

  - Arranging transportation of the body when necessary
  - Conducting interviews with persons reporting deaths and with other persons as appropriate
  - Conducting follow-up interviews with the family members and assessing for unresolved grief and stress-related diseases with referral to appropriate agencies
5. Plan and implement forensic educational programs for nurses, other healthcare providers, and the community, such as in child abuse, child safety, grief counseling, and health maintenance, promotion, and prevention programs for people at risk for major health problems
6. Assume accountability as a forensic nurse examiner by accepting responsibility as a nurse clinician, recognizing one's own abilities and limitations, and consistently seeking guidance, counseling, direction, and learning experiences that promote professional and personal development.
7. Demonstrate a leadership role in forensic nursing–including innovation, consultation, advocacy, accountability, and responsibility–to improve services to the family, the community and as appropriate, the criminal justice system in cases of sudden death.

One of the most recent advances in the development of forensic nurse death investigators is in Houston, Texas. The Harris County medical examiner's office has acquired a cadre of forensic nurse investigators and is projecting the employment of more in the near future. The following letter reflects the evolution of nurses in death investigation that was predicted by Charles Petty in 1988, as addressed earlier. Dr. Luis Sanchez, chief medical examiner of Harris County, has committed human and fiscal resources to the development of a system of forensic investigators: exclusively nurses. In an effort to recruit the quality of nurses for positions in the Harris County program, Sanchez addressed the need, the purpose, and the goal of this system of nurse death investigators in a letter in 2003 (Fig. 34-4).

It is interesting to note that over the past two decades, FNEs have stayed the course. From the Canadian model to the worldview of forensic nursing, the foundation of practice has been maintained with clarity. Forensic nurse Laynese Guay, a pioneer in death investigation, addressed the essence of forensic nursing from the twofold perspective: physical intervention in death and psychological intervention in society. In introducing the role of the nurse in death investigation to the Canadian Nurses Association in 1985, Guay noted that medicolegal investigation is a relatively new role for nurses, but it is neither a shadowy occupation nor a morbid experience. Rather it is a role that can make considerable contributions to important aspects of social justice, public service, and community mental health. Indeed, helping to establish the exact cause of sudden death can, in itself, provide for adjudication of criminal cases, instill confidence in public administration and be a way of helping survivors work through their grief. The future progress of the profession of nursing displays many facets in an increasingly demanding society. The opportunity to be a part of the development of a new specialization is an exciting challenge: We have expanded our role in the last century, and we continue to break new ground as nurses. The role of the caregiver continues.

Summary

The need for a new generation of medical investigators blending biomedical training with the investigation of death indicates a new trend in the forensic sciences. Recent advances in medical and forensic science indicate a need for individuals with a background in anatomy, physiology, and pharmacology, along with an emphasis on grief and crisis intervention. Forensic pathologists and criminalists alike recognize forensic nurses as professionals who can make diverse contributions to the scientific investigation of death (Lynch 1986).

The forensic nurse examiner is well prepared to meet the scientific demands of death investigation by assisting law enforcement officers in the recovery of medical evidence while meeting the needs of grieving and bereaved families. The forensic nurse can provide an immediate support system and play a key role in the tragic and traumatic environment of sudden and unexpected death. The opportunity to provide adequate social support should never be overlooked, although the investigator's primary mandate remains (Lynch, 1995).

The education of the forensic nurse is exceptionally extensive, ranging from on-the-scene management of the decedent and medical evidence, incorporating legal authority and jurisdiction, to a wide range of concepts and procedures pertaining to death and dying. The ability to maintain an index of suspicion while providing a sensitive yet probing interview with family members takes tact and skill. Such an incisive education also prepares the forensic nurse to identify aspects of academic research involving the epidemiology of death, to apply deductive reasoning in evaluating potential prevention analysis, and to make concluding assessments of the agents and forces that result in the loss of human life. "Whether those vectors be physical, environmental, chemical, microbiological or unknown, the knowledge between survivable injury and death is simply a matter of degree–the pattern of injury is the same" (Anderson & Gay, 1996). Clinical knowledge and nursing experience remain the basis for expertise in the medical investigation of death, separating the forensic nurse examiner from the lay-investigator and from the criminal investigation of death.

Marion Cumming, a Wisconsin nurse coroner for 17 years, has advised that the "utilization of the nursing process defines the foundation for evaluation in forensic nursing practice that includes immeasurable skills in caring and empathy." When she began her practice as coroner, Cumming was advised by the Wisconsin State Board of Nursing that "any role that relies on one's nursing education and nursing skills is by definition a nursing role." By using the knowledge acquired in the school of nursing, experience attained in more traditional nursing roles, familiarity with death investigation, and now suggestions for a more holistic approach, the forensic nurse investigator will assist the living (Cumming, 1995).

The essence of forensic nursing, the philosophy called upon whether in the clinical environs or at the scene of death, is summarized here:

> *The forensic nurse examiner has a unique presence. It is taught, learned, and perhaps inherent in those called healers. Presence is a delicate yet powerful sense referred to as empathy. For the survivors of loss, the forensic nurse not only looks, but also sees, being alert to a subtle gesture. The forensic nurse carries the history and spiritual tradition of true contact and intimacy that has long been the core value of nursing. It is a quiet sense, a feeling deeply heartfelt and honored. It is a privilege to care and a duty to prevent further suffering. (Hirtz, 2001, p. 1)*

By empowering the forensic nurse examiner as a coroner or death investigator, the holistic collaboration of person, public prosecution, and prevention emerge as one.

Luis A. Sanchez, M.D.
Chief Medical Examiner

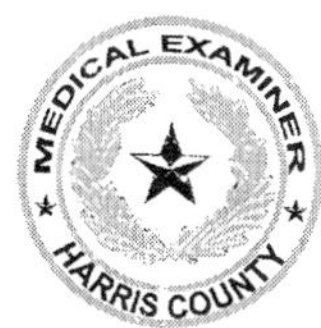

(713) 796-9292
FAX : (713) 796-6844

JOSEPH A. JACHIMCZYK FORENSIC CENTER

October 23, 2003

Virginia A. Lynch, MSN, RN, FAAFS, FAAN
Forensic Nursing and Forensic Health Science
Beth El College of Nursing and Health Sciences
University of Colorado, Colorado Springs
1420 Austin Bluffs Parkway
Colorado Springs, CO 80933-7150

Dear Ms. Lynch,

I take great pride in sharing with you the latest innovation at the Harris County Medical Examiner's Office (HCMEO), that being the addition of Forensic Nurse Investigators to our Investigative Division. The first Master's prepared registered nurse joined the office last year and is now the program coordinator/supervisor. This year, we created 12 additional positions, two of which have been filled, one by a nurse with a Master's Degree in Forensic Nursing, and the second by a nurse who is completing her Master's in a Nursing program.

Our new team of nurses will ensure that the HCMEO has forensic nursing coverage 24 hours a day! We are, therefore, eagerly seeking well trained and highly motivated nurses to fill our recently created positions. Although a Bachelor's Degree in Nursing is required, our ideal candidates will have experience in Forensic Nursing and will have attended forensic degree programs.

Forensic nurses bring a unique perspective to forensic medicine and pathology, fusing the principles of the forensic disciplines with the nursing knowledge base. Our nurses work with assigned pathologists, conduct external examinations, obtain follow-up information, perform scene investigation, review medical records, interact with family members and facilitate communications between law enforcement personnel and the District Attorney's offices. Because the nurses are present during autopsies, they are able to view the examinations, discuss the findings with the pathologist and, in the doctor's absence, address family inquiries in a timely manner.

Our nurses contribute enormously to our office by both evaluating the content of medical records to help determine whether an autopsy or external examination is performed, and by conducting external examinations under the direct supervision of the attending pathologists. In light of the National Association of Medical Examiners' position statement endorsing the role of pathology assistants in the forensic autopsy (allowing non-physicians to conduct examinations with supervision), we are taking full advantage of our nurses' documentation and assessment skills to enhance the quality and output of the Medical Examiner's Office.

1885 Old Spanish Trail, Houston, Texas 77054
www.co.harris.tx.us/me

Fig. 34-4 Letter from Dr. Luis A. Sanchez. *(Continued)*

Virginia Lynch, MSN, RN, FAAFS, FAAN
October 23, 2003
Page 2

In addition, forensic nurses may also be called upon to conduct scene investigations, even in cases where children die in a hospital. According to the 2000-2001 Houston/Harris County Child Fatality Review Team Report, seventy-one percent (71%) of child deaths reported, including deaths from SIDS, were due to natural causes. The nurses are able to respond directly to these death scenes and conduct thorough investigations, including physical assessments.

Where a child dies in a hospital, the nurse may conduct a dual investigation with the homicide investigator. The nurse and the homicide investigator meet at the home or site where the child was found and conduct a home assessment, photograph the scene and discuss medical/social history. This protocol facilitates communication between the law enforcement agencies and the pathologist conducting the examination.

Finally, our forensic nursing staff maintains a working relationship with the clinical forensic program at the Memorial Hermann Health System (MHHS), the largest clinical forensic nurse program in the Houston area. The MHHS clinical program evaluates patients who are victims or perpetrators of violence or traumatic accidents. Our nurses play an integral role in the MHHS clinical program by conducting trainings and collaborating on cases that progress from the local hospital to the Medical Examiner's Office.

I know you appreciate the satisfaction I feel in helping to create a highly functioning team of forensic nurses (the largest in Texas), who are conducting death investigations and may be on their way to making a little bit of history. Thank you so much for your contributions to our program. Stacey Mitchell (nee, Lasseter), Stacey Drake and Teresa Royer, all of whom you recommended, are forensic nurses of exceptional quality and highly valued members of our team. We look forward to your continued insights and support as we move forward to expand our program.

Sincerely,

Luis A. Sanchez, M.D.
Chief Medical Examiner

LAS/jlr

1885 Old Spanish Trail, Houston, Texas 77054
www.co.harris.tx.us/me

Fig. 34-4 Letter from Dr. Luis A. Sanchez.—Continued.

Where criminal or civil issues are involved in the death assessment of traumatic injuries or the subtle indications of abuse and neglect, nurses have a professional and ethical responsibility to address the decedent's legal rights through the recovery and proper documentation of evidence. Through the implementation of healthcare policies that address forensic issues, the biomedical investigation of a vast number of cases of child abuse and crimes against women and the elderly will aid law enforcement agencies in meeting the objectives of criminal investigation. Nurses who provide a forensic assessment share common interests and role behaviors with social and justice advocates in the medicolegal management of the dead, the dying, and their families. This includes the assessment, case management, intervention, and evaluation of death scene investigation, as well as a forensic holistic concern for *body, mind, spirit, and the law.*

Resources

Organizations

Harris County Medical Examiner Office

1885 Old Spanish Trail, Houston, TX 77054; Tel: 713-796-9292; www.co.harris.tx.us/me

American Board of Medicolegal Death Investigators

c/o Division of Forensic Pathology, St. Louis University School of Medicine, 1402 South Grand Boulevard, St. Louis, MO 63104-1028; Tel: 314-977-5970; www.slu.edu/organizations/abmdi

Forensic Medical Death Investigation Course

Dr. Mary Dudley, Chief Medical Examiner, Sedgwick County Kansas; www.forensicmi.com/Course%20Description.htm

Investigation of Injury and Death, Forensic Nursing and Forensic Health Sciences

Beth El College of Nursing, University of Colorado, Colorado Springs, CO; Undergraduate, Graduate, and Certificate Programs; http://web.uccs.edu/bethel

Training Programs

Introduction to Medicolegal Death Investigation: A Nursing Internship; for more information on this program contact South Charleston coroner Susan Chewing at susan@charleston.net.

Injuries and Death Investigation through the Eyes of the Forensic Nurse; Metropolitan Dade County, Medical Examiner Department, One Bob Hope Road, Miami, FL 33136-1133

References

Allert, L., & Becker, M. (2002). Death investigation. In *The Forensic Nurse*, premiere issue, pp. 16-18.

Anderson, W., & Gay, R. (1996, February). The Forensic Sciences in Clinical Medicine, workshop presented at the American Academy of Forensic Sciences, Nashville, TN.

Butt, J. (1993). Forensic nursing: Diversity in education and practice. Cited in V. Lynch, *J Psychosoc Nurs Ment Health Serv, 31*(11), 7-14.

Cumming, M. F. (1995). The vision of a nurse-coroner: A "protector of the living through the investigation of death." *J Psychosoc Nurs Ment Health Serv, 33*(5), 29-33.

Fields, K. (2004). *Cause of death uncertain.* Historical Archives, American Academy of Forensic Sciences. Colorado Springs, CO.

Handbook for Death Reporting, Office of the Coroner, Washoe County, Reno, NV (n.d.)

Harris, J. (1989, February 11). Personal communication.

Herzog, W. (1979). Prevention, intervention and post-vention of suicide. *Ann Intern Med,* 453-458.

Hirtz, S. (2001). *The forensic nurse coroner.* Unpublished manuscript.

Jalland, P. (1996). *Death in the Victorian family.* Oxford: Oxford University Press.

Kiessling, C. (no date). *A nurse coroner's perspective.* Unpublished manuscript.

Lipson, J., et al. (1996). *Culture and nursing care.* San Francisco: University of California at San Francisco Nursing Press.

Lynch, V. (1993). Forensic nursing: Diversity in education and practice. *J Psychosoc Nurs Ment Health Serv, 31*(11), 7-14.

Lynch, V. (1995, November). Forensic nursing: Management of crime victims from trauma to trial. *Crit Care Nurs Clin North Am,* 497-501

Lynch, V. (1986, February). *The registered nurse functioning as an investigator of death: A new field for the profession.* Paper presented at the American Academy of Forensic Sciences. New Orleans, LA.

Lynch, V., & Weaver, J. (1998). Forensic nursing: Unique contributions to international law. *J Nurs Law, 5*(4), 23-34.

Monroe, A. (2003). How to deliver tragic news. Workshop brochure.

National Organization for Victims Assistance (NOVA). (no date). Network information bulletin 110 (2-3), Washington, DC: Author.

Parikh, C. (1999). *Textbook of medical jurisprudence, forensic medicine and toxicology.* Edition 6. Section 3, p.1. Ministry of Law, Justice and Company Affairs, Government of India, CBS Publishers and Distributors, New Delhi.

Petty, C. (1988, January 27). Personal communication. Dallas, TX.

Shneidman, E. (1984). *Death: Current perspectives.* Palo Alto, CA: Mayfield.

Standing Bear, Z. G. (1987, April). Interview in the *Valdosta Daily Times,* Valdosta, GA.

Standing Bear, Z. G. (1995). Forensic nursing and death investigation: Will the vision be co-opted? *J Psychosoc Nurs Ment Health Serv, 33*(5), 59-64.

Chapter 35 Profiling Homicides

Robert K. Ressler

Since the 1970s, investigative profilers at the FBI's National Center for the Analysis of Violent Crime have been assisting local, state, and federal agencies in narrowing an investigation by providing criminal profiles. Profiling does *not* provide the specific identity of the offender. Rather, it indicates the kind of person most likely to have committed a crime by focusing on certain behavioral and personality characteristics.

Key Point 35-1

Profiling does *not* provide the specific identity of the offender. Rather, it indicates the kind of person most likely to have committed a crime by focusing on certain behavioral and personality characteristics.

Criminal Profiling from Crime Scene Analysis

The ability to solve a crime by describing the perpetrator is a skill of the expert investigative profiler. Evidence speaks its own language of patterns and sequences that can reveal the offender's behavioral characteristics. Special agents at the FBI Academy have demonstrated expertise in crime scene analysis of various violent crimes, particularly those involving sexual homicide.

Profiling techniques have been used in various settings, such as hostage taking (Reiser, 1982). Law enforcement officers need to learn as much as possible about the hostage taker in order to protect the hostages. In such cases, police are aided by limited verbal contact with the offender and possibly by access to the offender's family and friends. The police must be able to assess the subjects in terms of what courses of action they are likely to take, and what their reactions to various stimuli might be.

Profiling has also been used in identifying anonymous letter writers (Casey-Owens, 1984) and persons who make written or spoken threats of violence (Miron & Douglas, 1979). In cases of the latter, psycholinguistic techniques have been used to compose a *threat dictionary*, whereby every word in a message is assigned, by computer, to a specific category. Words used in the threat message are then compared with those used in ordinary speech or writings. The vocabulary usage in the message may yield *signature words* unique to the offender. In this way, police may be able not only to determine that several letters were written by the same individual, but also to learn about the offender's background and psychological state.

Rapists and arsonists also lend themselves to profiling. Through careful interview of the rape victim about the rapist's behavior, law enforcement personnel build a profile of the offender (Hazelwood, 1983). The rationale is that behavior reflects personality; and by examining behavior the investigator may be able to determine what type of person is responsible for the offense. For example, common characteristics of arsonists have been derived from an analysis of the *Uniform Crime Reports* (Rider, 1980). Knowledge of these characteristics can aid the investigator in identifying suspects and in developing strategies for interviewing these suspects. However, studies in this area have focused on specific categories of offenders such as serial rapists, mass murderers, or terrorists.

Criminal Profiling in Serial Sexual Homicides

Criminal profiling has been found to be of particular usefulness in investigating the crime of serial sexual homicide. These crimes create a great deal of fear because of their apparently random and motiveless nature, and they are also given significant publicity. Consequently, law enforcement personnel are under great public pressure to apprehend the perpetrator as quickly as possible. At the same time, these crimes may be the most difficult to solve precisely because of their apparent randomness. There has been a considerable upswing in these types of murders. In the 1990s, the rate of serial sexual homicide climbed to an almost epidemic proportion. Estimates of these types of criminals indicate that from 35 to 40 individuals are at large roaming the US, according to US Department of Justice officials. Some of the more noted cases have had victims numbering from 33 in the case of John Wayne Gacy in Chicago, to as many as 165 in the case of Henry Lee Lucas in Texas and his friend Ottis Elwood Toole in Florida.

While it is not completely accurate to say that these crimes are motiveless, the motive may all too often be one understood by only the perpetrator, and thus unknown to the investigating officers. Lunde (1976) demonstrated this issue in terms of the victims chosen by a particular offender. As Lunde has pointed out, although the serial murderer may not know the victims, their selection is not random. Rather, it is based on the murderer's perception of certain characteristics of those victims that are of symbolic significance to the perpetrator. An analysis of the similarities and differences among victims of a particular serial murderer provides important information concerning the "motive" in an apparently motiveless crime. This, in turn, may yield information about the perpetrator. For example, the murder may be the result of a sadistic fantasy in the mind of the murderer and a particular victim may be targeted because of a symbolic aspect of the fantasy (Ressler, Burgess, & Douglas et al., 1985).

In such cases, the investigating officer faces a completely different situation from a case in which a murder occurs as the result of jealousy, a family quarrel or during the commission of another felony. In those cases, a readily identifiable motive may provide vital clues about the identity of a perpetrator. In the case of the apparently motiveless crime, the investigative profilers must look to other methods, as well as to conventional investigative techniques, in their effort to identify the perpetrator. In this context, criminal profiling has been productive, particularly in those crimes where the offender has demonstrated repeated patterns at the crime scenes.

Acknowledgment goes to John E. Douglas, Ann W. Burgess, and Carol Hartman for contributions to concepts discussed in this chapter.

The Profiling of Murderers

Traditionally, two very different disciplines have used the technique of profiling murderers: (1) mental health clinicians who seek to explain the personality and actions of a criminal through psychiatric concepts and (2) law enforcement agents whose task is to determine the behavioral patterns of a suspect through investigative concepts. Forensic nurse examiners (FNEs) who work with victims and perpetrators of sexual assault are being utilized by forensic pathologists to provide rape homicide examinations in many jurisdictions across the US. Because FNEs also works with homicide detectives during an investigation and are often requested to accompany law enforcement officers to the scene, it is important for this group of professionals to be knowledgeable of the actions and behaviors of the lust murderer and any evidence that may be indicative of the criminal.

Psychological Profiling

In 1957, the identity of George Metesky, the arsonist in New York City's Mad Bomber case (which spanned 16 years), was aided by psychiatrist-criminologist James A. Brussel's staccato-style profile: "Look for a heavy man, middle-aged, foreign born, Roman Catholic, single, lives with a brother or sister; when you find him, chances are he'll be wearing a double-breasted suit, buttoned." Indeed, the portrait was extraordinary in that the only variation was that Metesky lived with two single sisters. Brussel, in discussion about the psychiatrist acting as Sherlock Holmes, explained that a psychiatrist usually studies a person and makes some reasonable predictions about how that person may react to a specific situation and about what he or she may do in the future. Profiling, according to Brussel, reverses this process. By studying an individual's deeds, one deduces what kind of person the individual might be (Brussel, 1968).

The idea of constructing a verbal picture of a murderer using psychological terms is not new. In 1960, Palmer published results of a three-year study of 51 murderers who were serving sentences in New England. Palmer's "typical murderer" was 23 years old when he committed murder. Using a gun, this typical killer murdered a male stranger during an argument. He came from a low social class and achieved little in terms of education or occupation. He had a well-meaning but maladjusted mother, and he experienced physical abuse and psychological frustration during his childhood.

Similarly, Rizzo (1981) studied 31 accused murderers during the course of routine referrals for psychiatric examination at a court clinic. His profile of the average murderer listed the offender as a 26-year-old male who most likely knew his victim, with monetary gain the most probable motivation for the crime.

Criminal Profiling

Techniques used by law enforcement today seek to do more than describe the typical murderer, if in fact there ever was such a person. Investigative profilers gather their information from the crime scene in order to analyze what it may reveal about the type of person who committed the crime.

Law enforcement has had some outstanding investigators; however, the skills, knowledge, and thought processes of these investigators have rarely been captured in the professional literature. These people were truly the experts of the law enforcement field, and their skills have been so admired that many fictional characters (Wilkie Collins, Sherlock Holmes, Hercule Poirot, Mike Hammer, Charlie Chan) have been modeled on these experts. Although Lunde (1976) believes that the murders of fiction bear no resemblance to the murders of reality, a connection between fictional detective techniques and modern criminal profiling methods may indeed exist. For example, it is attention to detail that is the hallmark of famous fictional detectives; the smallest item at a crime scene does not escape their attention. This trait is seen in Sergeant Cuff, a character in Wilkie Collins's *The Moonstone*, widely acknowledged as the first full-length detective study. At one end of the inquiry there was a murder, and at the other end there was a spot of ink on a tablecloth that nobody could account for. "In all my experience . . . I have never met with such a thing as a trifle yet." However, unlike detective fiction, real cases are not solved by one tiny clue but the analysis of all clue and crime patterns.

Criminal profiling has been described as a collection of leads; as an educated attempt to provide specific information about a certain type of suspect (Geberth, 1981); and as a biographical sketch of behavior patterns, trends, and tendencies (Vorpagel, 1981). Geberth (1981) has also described the profiling process as particularly useful when the criminal has demonstrated some form of psychopathology. As used by the FBI profilers, the criminal profile–generating process is defined as a technique for identifying the major personality and behavioral characteristics of an individual based on an analysis of the crimes he or she has committed. The profiler's skill is in recognizing the crime scene dynamics that link various criminal personality types who commit similar crimes.

The task of an investigative profiler in developing a criminal profile is quite similar to the process used by forensic clinicians to make a diagnosis and treatment plan: data are collected and assessed, the situation reconstructed, hypotheses are formulated, a profile is developed and tested, and the results are reported. Investigators traditionally have learned profiling through brainstorming, intuition, and educated guesswork. Their expertise is the result of years of accumulated wisdom, extensive experience in the field, and familiarity with a large number of cases.

An investigative profiler brings to the crime scene the ability to make hypothetical formulations based on his or her previous experience. A formulation is defined here as a concept that organizes, explains, or makes investigative sense out of information and that influences profile hypotheses. These formulations are based on clusters of information emerging from the crime scene information and from the investigator's experience in understanding criminal actions. A basic premise of criminal profiling is that the way a person thinks (e.g., his or her patterns of thinking) directs that individual's personal behavior.

Best Practice *35-1*

Forensic investigators should gather detailed information from the crime scene to assist profilers in determining the type of person who committed the crime.

Generating a Criminal Profile

Investigative profilers at the FBI's National Center for the Analysis of Violent Crimes (NCAVC) have been analyzing crime scenes and generating criminal profiles since the 1970s. Their description of the construction of profiles represents the offsite procedure as it is conducted at the NCAVC, as contrasted with on-site procedure (Ressler, Burgess, & Douglas et al., 1985). The criminal profile–generating process is described as five stages with the sixth, the outcome, being the apprehension of a suspect (Fig. 35-1).

The criminal profile-generating process has produced hundreds of profiles. A series of overlapping steps lead to the final goal of apprehension. These steps include the following:

1. Profiling inputs
2. Decision-process models
3. Crime assessment
4. The criminal profile
5. Investigation
6. Apprehension

There are two key feedback filters: (1) achieving congruence with the evidence, decision models, and investigation recommendations and (2) adding new evidence.

Profiling Inputs

The profiling input stage begins the criminal profile–generating process. Information recorded by local law enforcement officers at the site or location of the crime is gathered and detailed. A thorough inspection of the specific crime scene yields information about physical evidence, patterns of evidence, body positions, and presence of weapons and other pertinent information.

The focus then moves to factors pertaining to the victim. An in-depth examination of the background and activities of the victim(s) provides information on the victim's background, habits, family structure, and occupation, as well as when the victim was last seen. At this time, a decision is made about whether or not the victim was of low or high risk. If low risk is the determination, questions about why the victim was targeted by the subject are formulated. More information on determining risk is discussed later in the chapter.

Forensic information is compiled about cause and type of death, pre- and postmortem wounds, and sexual acts committed

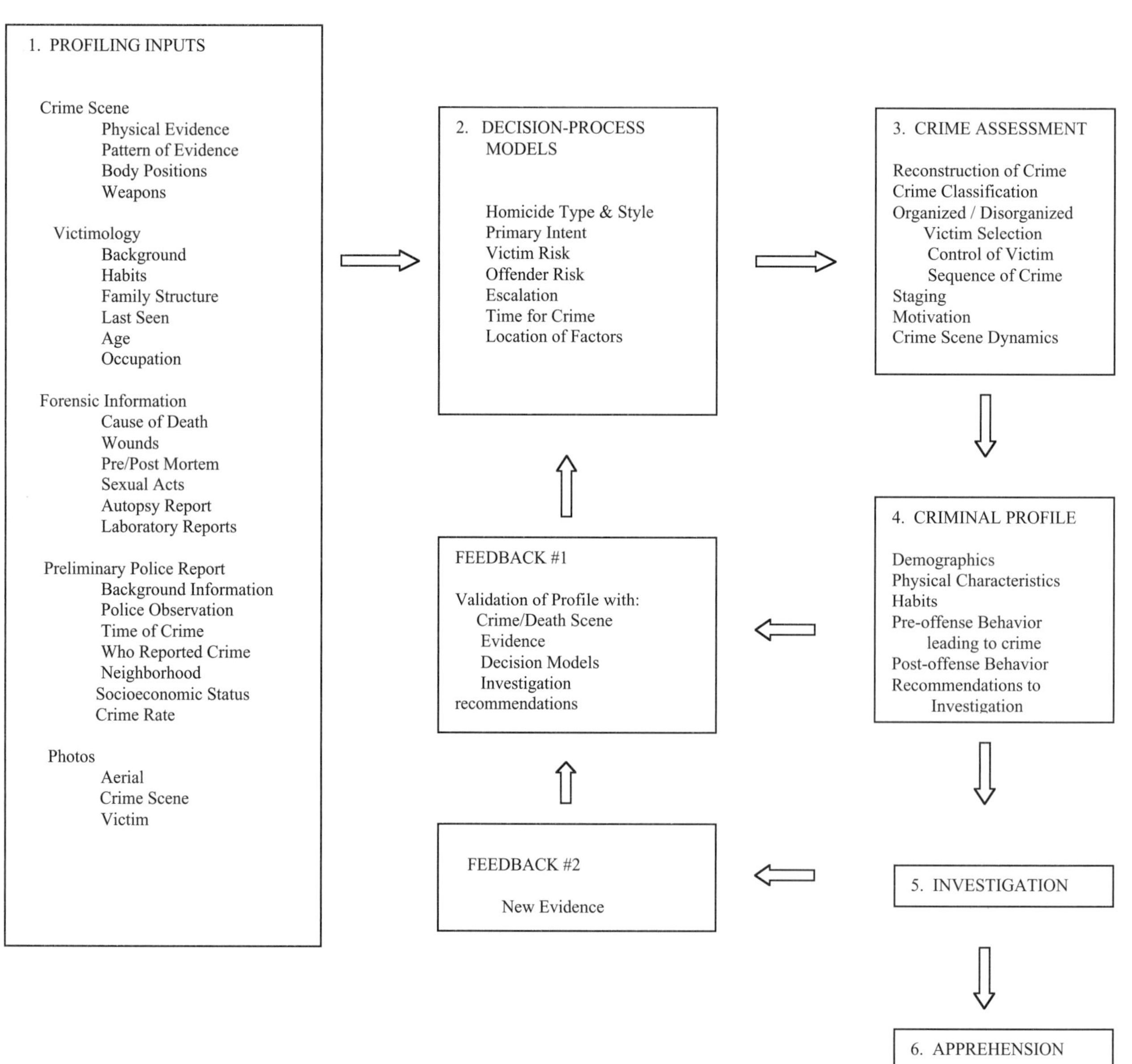

Fig. 35-1 Criminal profile generating process.

with the victim. Laboratory and autopsy reports provide a clear picture of the extent of the wounds, which allows the investigator to determine the amount (or lack) of control the offender exhibited during the crime. For example, stabbings randomly made to the body (as contrasted with stabbings in one part of the body) suggest the offender had difficulty controlling the victim. Crime photographs may be used for such purposes as identifying the offender's emotional state (such as anger, in the case of overkill).

Preliminary police reports and investigative documents that include background information, police observations, time of crime, who reported the crime, socioeconomic status and crime rate of the neighborhood, and photos (aerial, crime scene, and victim) are sent for evaluation. The personal observations of the officers called to that scene as well as the circumstances under which they were called are all important. These reports do not include suspect information from local law enforcement.

Best Practice *35-2*

The forensic examiner should use written and photodocumentation to precisely preserve details about the homicide victim's wounds and sexual acts, as such information is essential for homicide profiling.

Decision-Process Models

The decision process begins the organizing and arranging of the inputs into meaningful patterns. Seven key decision points, or models, differentiate and organize the information from Step 1 and form an underlying decisional structure for profiling.

Homicide: Type and Style

As noted in Table 35-1, type and style classify homicides. A single homicide is one victim, one homicidal event; a double homicide is two victims, one event and in one location; and a triple homicide has three victims in one location during one event. Anything beyond three victims is classified as a mass murder–that is, four or more victims in one location and within one event.

Classic Mass Murderer. There are two types of mass murderers: classic and family. A classic mass murderer involves one person operating in one location at one period of time. That period of time could be minutes or hours and might even be days. Classic mass murderers are usually described as mentally disordered individuals whose problems have increased to the point that they act against groups of people unrelated to these problems. The murderer unleashes this hostility through shootings or stabbings. One classic mass murderer was Charles Whitman, a man who armed himself with boxes of ammunition, weapons, ropes, radio, and food; barricaded himself in a rooftop tower in Austin, Texas; and opened fire for 90 minutes, killing 16 people and wounding more than 30 others. He was stopped only when he was killed on the roof. James Huberty was another classic mass murderer. With a machine gun, he entered a fast-food restaurant and killed and wounded many people. Responding police also killed him at the site. Pennsylvania mass murderess Sylvia Seegrist (nicknamed Ms. Rambo for her military style clothing) was sentenced to life imprisonment for opening fire with a rifle aimed at shoppers in a mall in October 1985, killing three persons and wounding seven. In a Littleton, Colorado, high school, anger had been building in students Eric Harris and Dylan Klebold. On the 110th anniversary of Adolf Hitler's birth, they swept through the corridors in a rampage leaving 13 dead, 25 injured, and a community in shock.

Family Member Mass Murderer. A second type of mass murderer is one who kills several family members. If more than three family members are killed and the perpetrator commits suicide, it is classified as a mass murder/suicide. Without the suicide and with four or more victims, the murder is called a family killing. One example of such killings involves William Bradford Bishop from Bethesda, Maryland, who beat to death his wife, mother, and three children in the family residence in March 1976. He then transported them to North Carolina in the family station wagon where their bodies, along with the family dog, were buried in a shallow grave. Bishop was under psychiatric care and had been prescribed antidepressant medication. No motive was determined. Bishop was a promising midlevel diplomat who had served in many overseas jobs and was scheduled for higher-level office in the US State Department. Bishop is a federal fugitive and has never been captured. There is strong indication his crimes were carefully planned and he had made provisions for leaving the country.

John List, an accountant and employed as an insurance salesman, killed his entire family. In a front room, the bodies of List's wife and three children (ages 16, 15, and 13) were discovered lying side by side facing up. Each was meticulously covered with a white sheet and their arms were folded across their bodies. Each had been shot once behind the left ear except for one son who had been shot 16 times. A further search of the residence revealed the body of List's mother, also shot once behind the left ear. Furthermore, she also had been neatly laid out and covered with a white sheet. He disappeared after the crime and is a federal fugitive. It is uncertain whether or not Bishop and List have committed suicide.

Spree and Serial Murderers. Two additional types of multiple murderers are spree and serial murderers. A spree murder has killings at two or more locations and no emotional cooling-off period. During the 1940s, New Jersey spree murderer Howard Unruh took a loaded German Luger with ammunition and randomly fired his handgun at people, while walking through his neighborhood. Many people were killed. This is not classified as a mass murder because the killer moved to different locations.

Serial murderers are involved in three or more separate incidents with an emotional cooling-off period between homicides.

Table 35-1 Homicide Classification by Style and Type

STYLE	SINGLE	DOUBLE	TRIPLE	MASS	SPREE	SERIAL
Number of victims	1	2	3	4+	2+	3+
Number of events	1	1	1	1	1	3+
Number of locations	1	1	1	1	2+	3+
Cooling-off period	Yes	Yes	Yes	Yes	No	Yes

This killer usually premeditates homicide. The serial murderer plans and fantasizes, and when the time is right and the killer has cooled off from the first homicide, the next victim is selected. The cool-off period can be days, weeks, or months and is the main element that separates the serial killer from the other multiple killers.

However, there are other differences. The mass murderer and the spree murderer are not concerned with who their victims are; they will kill anyone that comes in contact with them. In contrast, a serial murderer selects victims. These murderers think they will never be caught. A serial murderer controls the events, whereas in a spree murder the events control the killer. The spree murderer can barely control what will happen next. The serial killer is planning, picking, and choosing, and sometimes stopping the act of murder.

A serial murderer may commit spree homicides. In 1984, Christopher Wilder, an Australian racecar driver, went on a murder spree, starting in Florida and traveling across the US for a period of several months. Wilder would target victims at shopping malls or would abduct them after meeting them through a beauty contest setting or dating service. While a fugitive as a serial murderer, Wilder was investigated, identified, and tracked by the FBI and almost every police department in the country. Wilder's classification changed form serial to spree murderer because of the multiple murders and the lack of a cooling-off period. The tension due to his fugitive status and to the high visibility of his crime gave Wilder (and other noted spree murderers) a sense of desperation. Their acts are open and public, and this usually means no cooling-off period. They know they will be caught, and the coming confrontation with police becomes an element in their crimes. Their goal appears to be that they will be killed on sight.

Key Point *35-2*

The mass murderer and the spree murderer are not concerned with who their victims are; they will kill anyone that comes in contact with them.

Classifying Homicides

It is important to classify homicides correctly. For example, a single homicide is committed in a city; a week later, a second single homicide is committed; and the third week, a third single homicide. Three seemingly unrelated homicides are reported, but by the time there is a fourth, there is a tie-in, both through forensic evidence and an analysis of the crime scene. These four single homicides now point to one serial offender. It is not mass murder because of multiple locations and a cooling-off period, thus being a serial homicide. The correct classification assists in profiling and properly directs the investigation. Similarly, profiling of a single murder may suggest a repeat, either in the past or in the future.

Primary Intent of the Murderer

Murder may have both primary and secondary intentions. Classification of a murder in terms of the killer's primary intent is outlined in Table 35-2. A killer may be acting either on his or her own or as part of a group. The primary intent may involve criminal enterprise. Criminal enterprise includes people who are involved in the business of crime. Their livelihood is through criminal business and sometimes murder becomes part of it, even though there is no personal malice. For example, food may be poisoned during an extortion attempt of a business (i.e., extortion notes are written to a company demanding money and threatening the poisoning of products). The primary motive is financial. In the 1950s, a young man placed a bomb in his mother's suitcase, which was loaded aboard a commercial aircraft. The aircraft exploded; his motive was collecting on a life insurance policy he purchased for her flight. Criminal enterprise murders involve a group (e.g., contract murders, gang murders, competition murders, political murders).

When the primary intent of the murderer involves emotional, selfish, or cause-specific reasons, individuals may kill for self-defense and compassion (e.g., mercy killings where life-support systems are disconnected). Family disputes/violence may lie behind infanticide, matricide, patricide, and spouse and sibling killings. Paranoid reactions may also result in murder as in the previously described Whitman case. Mentally disordered murderers may commit a symbolic crime or have a psychotic outburst. Assassinations, such as those committed by John Hinkley and Mark Chapman, also fall into the emotional intent category. Murders in this category involving groups are committed for a variety of reasons: religious (Jim Jones and the Jonestown, Ghana, case), cult (Charles Manson), and fanatical organizations such as the Ku Klux Klan and the Black Panthers Party of the 1970s.

Finally, the murderer may have sexual reasons for killing. Individuals may kill as a result of or to engage in sexual activity, dismemberment, mutilation, evisceration, or other activities that have sexual meaning only for the offender. Occasionally two or more murderers commit these homicides together, such as in the 1980s California case of Lake and Ng.

Victim Risk

The concept of the victim's risk is involved at several stages of the profiling process and provides information about the suspect in

Table 35-2 Primary Intent of Murderers

NUMBER OF MURDERED	CRIMINAL/ENTERPRISE	EMOTIONAL/SELFISH CAUSE SPECIFIC	SEXUAL
One	Insurance collection Contract killing	Self-defense Compassion (i.e., mercy killings) Family violence Paranoid reaction Emotional disorder Assassination	Rape and other sexual activity Mutilation Dismemberment Evisceration
Two or more	Gang Competition Political	Religious Cult Fanatical	Same as above

terms of how he or she operates. Risk is determined using such factors as age, occupation, lifestyle, and physical stature of the victim and is classified as high, moderate, or low. High-risk victims are those targeted by the murderers who know where they can find victims. Killers seek high-risk victims at locations where victims may be vulnerable, such as bus depots or isolated areas. The young and the elderly may be high-risk victims due to their lack of resistance ability. Students may be classified as moderate-risk, as it is known that predators may target college campuses. Low-risk types include those whose occupation and daily lifestyle do not lend themselves to easy targeting. The information on victim risk helps to generate an image of the type of perpetrator being sought.

Offender Risk

Data on victim risk integrate with information on offender risk, or the risk the offender was taking to commit the crime. For example, abducting a victim at noon from a busy street is high-risk. Thus, a low-risk victim snatched under high-risk circumstances generates ideas about such offenders, such as personal stresses they are operating under, their beliefs that they will not be apprehended, or the excitement they seek in the commission of the crime.

Escalation

Information about escalation is derived from an analysis of facts and patterns from the prior decision-process models. Investigative profilers are able to deduce the sequence of acts committed during the crime. From this deduction, they make determinations about the potential of the criminal, not only to escalate the crimes (for example, from peeping to fondling, to assault, to rape, to murder) but also to repeat the crimes in serial fashion. One case example is David Berkowitz, the Son of Sam killer, who started his criminal career with the nonfatal stabbing of a teenage girl. His killing escalated to the subsequent .44-caliber killings.

Time Factors

There are several time factors that need consideration in generating a criminal profile. These factors include the length of time required (1) to kill the victim, (2) to commit additional acts with the body, and (3) to dispose of the body. The time of day or night that the crime was committed is also important, as it provides information on the lifestyle and occupation of the suspect (and also relates to the offender risk factor). For example, the longer an offender spends with a victim, the more likely it is that the killer will be apprehended at the crime scene. In the case of New York murder victim Kitty Genovese, the killer carried on his murderous assault to the point where many people heard or witnessed the crime, leading to his eventual prosecution. A killer who intends to spend time with his victim therefore must select a location to preclude observation.

Location Factors

Information about location–where the victim was first approached, where the crimes occurred, and if the crime and death scenes differ–provides yet additional data about the offender. For example, such information provides details about whether the murderer used a vehicle to transport the victim from the death scene or if the victim died at the point of abduction.

Crime Assessment

The crime assessment step in generating a criminal profile involves the reconstruction of the sequence of events and the behavior of both the offender and victim. Based on the various decisions of the previous steps, this reconstruction of how things happened, how people behaved, and how they planned and organized the encounter provides information about specific characteristics that help to generate the criminal profile. Assessments are made about the classification of the crime, its organized/disorganized aspects, the offender's selection of a victim, strategies used to control the victim, the sequence of crime, the staging (or not) of the crime, the offender's motivation for the crime, and crime scene dynamics.

The classification of the crime is determined through the decision process outlined in the first decision-process model. The classification of a crime as organized or disorganized includes factors such as victim selection, strategies to control the victim, and the sequence of crime. An organized murderer is one who appears to plan the murders, to target victims, to display control at the crime scene, and to act out a sexually violent fantasy against the victim. For example, Ted Bundy's planning was noted through his successful abduction of young women from highly visible areas (i.e., beaches, campuses, ski lodge). He selected victims who were young, attractive, and similar in appearance. He controlled the victims through physical force. These dynamics were important in the development of a desired fantasy victim.

In contrast, the disorganized murderer is less apt to plan the crime in detail, obtains victims by chance, and behaves haphazardly during the crime. For example, Herbert Mullin, who killed 14 people of varying types (e.g., an elderly man, a young girl, a priest) over a four-month period, did not display any specific planning or targeting of victims; rather, the victims were people who happened to cross his path, and their murders were based on impulse as well as on fantasy.

The question of whether or not the crime was staged (i.e., was the subject truly careless or disorganized or did the offender make the crime appear that way to distract or mislead the police) helps direct the investigative profiler to the killer's motivation. In one case, a 16-year-old high school junior, living in a small town, failed to return home from school. Police, responding to the father's report of his missing daughter, began their investigation and located the victim's scattered clothing in a remote area outside the town. A crude map was also found at the scene, which seemingly implied a premeditated plan of kidnapping. The police followed the map to a location, which indicated a body might have been disposed in a nearby river. Written and telephoned extortion demands were sent to the father, a bank executive, for the sum of $80,000. The demands warned police in detail not to use electronic monitoring devices.

Was this crime staged? The question was answered in two ways. The details in one aspect of the crime (scattered clothing and tire tracks) indicated the subject was purposely staging a crime while the details in the other (extortion) led the profilers to speculate who the subject was: specifically that he had a law enforcement background and therefore had knowledge of police procedures concerning crimes of kidnap and extortion. Thus, the crime was determined to be a staged extortion, hiding the primary intent. With this information, the investigative profiler hypothesizes that the behavior would escalate and the subject become bolder. Instructions were transmitted to the suspect to look for the extortion envelope in a specific location with the result that the suspect was apprehended at the location. It was then ascertained that the primary intent of the crime was rape.

Motivation is a difficult factor to judge because it requires dealing with the inner thoughts and behavior of the offender. Motivation is more easily determined in the organized offender, whose premeditation, planning, and ability to carry out a plan of action is logical and complete. On the other hand, the disorganized offender carries out crimes by motivations that frequently are derived from mental illnesses and accompanying distorted perceptions (resulting from delusions and hallucinations). Drugs and alcohol as well as panic and stress resulting from disrupted plans in carrying out the crime are additional criteria that must be accounted for in the overall assessment of the crime scene.

Crime Scene Dynamics

Crime scene dynamics are the numerous circumstances common to every crime scene, which can be misunderstood or misinterpreted by investigating officers. Examples include location of the crime scene, cause of death, method of killing, positioning of body, excessive trauma, and location of wounds or lack of mutilation.

Investigative profilers read the dynamics of a crime scene and interpret them based on their viewing of similar crimes. They can thereby relate these crime scene dynamics to similar cases where outcomes of such crime are known and available. Extensive research by the behavioral science unit at the FBI Academy and in-depth interviews with incarcerated felons who have committed such crimes have provided a vast body of knowledge of common threads that link crime scene dynamics to specific criminal personality patterns. For example, a common error of some police investigators is to assess a particularly brutal lust-mutilation murder as the work of a sex fiend and to direct their investigation toward known sex offenders when such crimes are commonly perpetrated by youthful unsophisticated teenagers with no criminal record.

Crime Profile

The fourth step in generating a criminal profile deals with the type of person who committed the crime and that individual's behavioral orientation with relation to the crime. Once this description is generated, the strategy of investigation can be formulated, as this strategy requires a basic understanding of how an individual will respond to a variety of investigative efforts.

Included in the criminal profile are background information (demographics), physical characteristics, habits, beliefs and values, pre-offense behavior leading to the crime, and post-offense behavior. It may also include investigative recommendations for interrogating or interviewing, identifying, and apprehending the offender.

This fourth stage has an important means of validating the criminal profile; this is called Means Feedback 1. The profile must fit with the earlier reconstruction of the crime, the evidence, and the key decision-process models. In addition, the investigative procedure developed from the recommendations must make sense in terms of the expected response patterns of the offender. If there is lack of congruence, then profiling investigators must review all available data.

Once the congruence of the criminal profile is determined, a written report is provided to the requesting agency and added to its ongoing investigation efforts. The investigative recommendations generated in Stage 4 are applied, and suspects matching the profile are evaluated. If identification, apprehension, and a confession result, the goal of the profile effort has been met. If new evidence is generated (e.g., by another murder or crime) or a suspect is not identified, then reevaluation occurs via Feedback 2. The information is reexamined and the profile revalidated.

Apprehension

Once a suspect is apprehended, the agreement between the outcome and the various stages in the profile generating–process are examined. When an apprehended suspect admits guilt, it is important to conduct a detailed interview and to affirm the total profiling process for validity and quality. This process is similar to the nursing process and scientific process with the requisite feedback loops.

Case Study 35-1 Crime Scene Evidence

A young woman's nude body was discovered at 3:00 p.m. on the roof landing of the apartment building where she lived. She had been badly beaten about the face and strangled with the strap of her purse. Her nipples had been cut off after death and placed on her chest, and scrawled in ink on the inside of her thigh was: "You can't stop me." The words "Fuck you" were scrawled on her abdomen. A pendant in the form of a Jewish sign (Chai), which she usually wore as a good luck piece around her neck, was missing and presumed taken by the murderer. Her underpants had been pulled over her face; her nylons were removed and very loosely tied around her wrists and ankles near a railing. The murderer had placed symmetrically on either side of the victim's head the pierced earrings she had been wearing. An umbrella and ink pen had been forced into the vagina, and a hair comb was placed in her pubic hair. The woman's jaw and nose had been broken and her molars loosened. She suffered multiple face fractures caused by a blunt force. Cause of death was asphyxia by ligature (pocketbook strap) strangulation. There were postmortem bite marks on the victim's thighs, as well as contusions, hemorrhages, and lacerations to the body. The killer also defecated on the roof landing and covered it with the victim's clothing.

Elements of Case Analyses

Profiling Inputs

In terms of *crime scene evidence* in the case study, everything the offender used at the crime scene belonged to the victim. Even the comb and the felt-tip pen used to write on her body came from her purse. The offender apparently did not plan this crime; he had no gun, ropes, or tape for the victim's mouth. He probably did not even plan to encounter her that morning at that location. The crime scene indicated a spontaneous event; in other words, the killer did not stalk or wait for the victim. The crime scene differs from the death scene. The initial abduction was on the stairwell; then the victim was taken to a more remote area.

Investigation of the *victim* revealed that the 26-year-old, 90-pound, 4′11″ white female awoke around 6:30 a.m. She dressed, had a breakfast of coffee and juice, and left her apartment for work at a nearby day-care center, where she was employed as a group teacher for handicapped children. She resided with her mother and father. When she would leave for work in the morning, she would either take the elevator or walk down the stairs, depending on her mood. She was a quiet young woman who had a slight curvature of the spine (scoliosis).

The *forensic information* in the medical examiner's report was important in determining the extent of the wounds, as well as how the victim was assaulted and whether evidence of sexual assault was present. No semen was noted in the vagina, but semen was found on the body. It appeared that the murderer stood directly over the victim and masturbated. There were visible bite marks on the victim's thighs and knee area. He cut off her nipples with a knife after she was dead and wrote on the body. Cause of death was ligature strangulation, first manual, then with the strap of her purse. The fact that the murderer used the strap from the victim's pocketbook indicates that he did not prepare to commit this crime as he used a weapon of opportunity. He probably used his fist to render her unconscious, which may be the reason no one heard any screams. There were no deep stab wounds and the knife used to mutilate the victim's breasts apparently was not big, probably a penknife that the offender normally carried. The killer used the victim's belts to tie her right arm and right leg, but he apparently untied them in order to position the body before he left.

The *preliminary* police report revealed that another resident of the apartment building, a white male, age 15, discovered the victim's wallet in a stairwell between the third and fourth floors at approximately 8:20 a.m. He retained the wallet until he returned home from school for lunch that afternoon. At that time he gave the wallet to his father, a white male age 40. The father went to the victim's apartment at 2:50 p.m. and gave the wallet to the victim's mother.

When the mother called the day-care center to inform her daughter about the wallet, she learned that her daughter had not appeared for work that morning. The mother, the victim's sister, and a neighbor began a search of the building and discovered the body. The neighbor called the police. Police at the scene found no witnesses who saw the victim after she left her apartment that morning.

Decision-Process Models

This crime's *style* is a single homicide with the murderer's primary intent making it a sexually motivated *type* of crime. There was a degree of *planning* indicated by the organization and sophistication of the crime scene. The idea of murder had probably occupied the killer for a long time. The sexual fantasies may have started through the use of pornography.

Victim risk assessment revealed that the victim was known to be very self-conscious about her physical handicap and size and she was a plain-looking young woman who did not date. She led a reclusive life and she was not the type of victim that would or could fight an assailant or scream and yell. She would be easily dominated and controlled, particularly in view of her small stature.

Based on the information on occupation and lifestyle, this was a low-risk victim living in an area that was at low risk for violent crimes. The apartment building was part of a 23-building public housing project in which the racial mixture of residents was 50% black, 40% white, and 10% Hispanic. It was located in the confines of a major police precinct. There had been no other known crimes reported in the victim's or nearby complexes.

The crime was considered very *high-risk* for the offender. He committed the crime in broad daylight, and there was a possibility that people who were up early might see him. There was no set pattern for the victim taking the stairway or the elevator. It appeared that the victim happened to cross the path of the offender.

There was no *escalation* factor present in this crime scene.

The *time* for the crime was considerable. All his activities with the victim–removing her earrings, cutting off her nipples, masturbating over her–would have taken a substantial amount of time. The extended amount of time the murderer spent with his victim increased his risk of being apprehended.

The *location* of the crime suggested that the offender felt comfortable in the area. He had been there before, and he felt that no one would interrupt the murder.

Crime Assessment

The crime scene indicated that murder was one event, not one of a series of events. It also appeared to be a first-time killing, and the subject was not a typical organized offender. There were elements of both disorganization and organization; the offender might fall into a mixed category.

A reconstruction of the crime/death scene provides an overall picture of the crime. To begin with, the victim was not necessarily stalked but instead was confronted. What was her reaction? Did she recognize her assailant, fight him off, or try to get away? The subject had to kill her to carry out his sexually violent fantasies. The murderer was on known territory and thus had a reason to be there at 6:30 in the morning: either he resided there or he was employed at this particular complex. He felt comfortable at the crime location.

The killer's control of the victim was through the use of blunt force trauma, with the blow to her face the first indication of his intention. Because she didn't fight, run, or scream, it appears that she did not perceive her abductor as a threat. Either she knew him or he looked nonthreatening (i.e., he was dressed as a janitor, a postal worker, a police officer, or a businessman).

In the sequence of the crimes, the killer first rendered the victim unconscious and possibly dead; he could easily pick her up because of her small size. He took her up to the roof landing and had time to manipulate her body while she was unconscious. He positioned her body, undressed the victim, and acted out certain fantasies, which led to masturbation. The killer took his time at the scene, and he probably knew that no one would come to the roof and disturb him in the early morning. The crime scene was not staged. Sadistic ritualistic fantasy generated the sexual motivation for murder. The murderer displayed total domination of the victim. In addition, he placed the victim in a degrading posture, which reflected his lack of remorse about the killing.

The crime scene dynamics of the covering of the killer's feces and his positioning of the body is incongruent and needs to be interpreted. First, as previously described, the crime was opportunistic. The crime scene portrayed the intricacies of a long-standing murderous fantasy. Once the killer had a victim, he had a set plan about killing and abusing the body. However, within the context of the crime, the profilers noted a paradox–the covered feces. Defecation was not part of the ritual fantasy and thus it was covered. The presence of the feces also supports the length of time taken for the crime, the control the murderer had over the victim (her unconscious state) and the knowledge that he would not be interrupted.

The positioning of the victim suggested the offender was acting out something he had seen before, perhaps in a sadomasochistic pornographic magazine. Because the victim was unconscious, the killer did not need to tie her hands. Yet he continued to tie her neck and strangle her. He positioned her earrings in a ritualistic manner; he wrote on her body. This reflects some sort of imagery that he probably had repeated over and over in his mind. He took her necklace as a souvenir, perhaps to carry around in his pocket. The investigative profilers noted that the body was positioned in the form of the woman's missing Jewish symbol.

Crime Profile

Based on the information derived during the previous stages, a criminal profile of the murderer was generated. First, a physical description of the suspect stated that he would be a white male, of the same general age as the victim, and of average appearance. The murderer would not look out of context in the area. He would be of average intelligence and would be a school or college dropout. He would not have a military history and may be unemployed.

The degree of lack of sophistication in how the crime was carried out relates to the age factor. The presence or absence of control of the victim would also be due to the suspect's age. However, because of the organization at the crime scene, the killer would not be a teenager. Rather, his age would be between 25 and 35.

The murderer knocked his victim unconscious in order to deal with her. He would be sexually inexperienced, sexually inadequate, and never married. He would have a pornography collection. The fact that he did ejaculate indicated that he would be not sexually dysfunctional. The subject would have sadistic tendencies; the umbrella and the masturbation act are clearly acts of sexual substitution. The sexual acts showed controlled aggression, not unleashed rage. Rage or hatred of women was not observed. The murder was not a reaction to rejection from women as much as to morbid curiosity.

In addressing the habits of the murderer, the profile revealed there would be a reason for the killer to be at the crime scene at 6:30 in the morning. He could be employed in the apartment complex, be in the complex on business, or reside in the complex.

The killer's occupation would be blue collar or skilled. In carrying out his crimes, he demonstrated a degree of sophistication. Alcohol or drugs did not assume a major role as the crime occurred in the early morning.

Although the offender might have preferred his victim conscious, he had to render her unconscious because he did not want to be caught. He did not want the woman screaming for help.

The murderer's infliction of sexual, sadistic acts on an inanimate body suggests that he was disorganized. He was not a psychopathic personality, a sexual sadist, or sexual psychopath. He probably would be a very confused person, possibly with previous mental problems. If he had carried out such acts on a living victim, he would have a different type of personality. The fact that he inflicted acts on a dead or unconscious person indicated his inability to function with a live person.

The killer would have difficulty maintaining any kind of personal relationships with women. If he dated he would date women younger than himself, as he would have to be able to dominate and control in relationships.

The crime scene reflected that the killer felt justified in his actions and that he felt no remorse. He was not subtle. He left the victim in a provocative, humiliating position, exactly the way he wanted her to be found. He challenged the police in his message written on the victim; the messages also indicated the subject might well kill again.

Investigation

The crime received intense coverage by the local media because it was such an extraordinary homicide. The local police responded to a radio call of a homicide. They in turn notified the detective bureau, which notified the forensic crime scene unit, medical examiner's office, and the county district attorney's office. A task force was immediately assembled of approximately 25 detectives and supervisors.

An intensive investigation resulted, which included speaking to, and interviewing, more than 2000 people. Record checks of known sex offenders in the area proved fruitless. Handwriting samples were taken of possible suspects to compare with the writing on the body. Mental hospitals in the area were checked for people who might fit the profile of this type of killer.

The FBI's behavioral science unit was contacted to compile a profile. In the profile, the investigation recommendation included that the offender knew that the police sooner or later would contact him because he either worked or lived in the building. The killer would somehow inject himself into the investigation, and although he might appear cooperative to the extreme, he would really be seeking information. In addition, he might try to contact the victim's family.

Apprehension

The outcome of the investigation was apprehension of a suspect 13 months following the discovery of the victim's body. After receiving the criminal profile, police reviewed their files of the 22 suspects they had interviewed. One man stood out. This suspect's father lived down the hall in the same apartment building as the victim. Police originally had interviewed his father, who told them his son was a patient at the local psychiatric hospital. Police learned later that the son had been absent without permission from the hospital the day and evening prior to the murder.

They also learned he was an unemployed actor who lived alone; his mother had died of a stroke when he was 19 years old (11 years previous). He had had academic problems of repeating a grade and dropped out of school. He was a white 30-year-old, never-married male who was an only child. His father was a blue-collar worker who also was an ex–prize fighter. The suspect reportedly had his arm in a cast at the time of the crime. A search of his room revealed a pornography collection. He had never been in the military, had no girlfriends, and was described as being insecure with women. The man suffered from depression and was receiving psychiatric treatment and hospitalization. He had a history of repeated suicidal attempts (hanging/asphyxiation) both before and after the offense.

The suspect was tried, found guilty, and is serving a sentence of 25 years to life for this mutilation murder. He denies committing the murder and states he did not know the victim. Police proved that security was lax at the psychiatric hospital in which the suspect was confined and that he could literally come and go as he pleased. However, the most conclusive evidence against him at his trial were his teeth impressions. Three separate forensic dentists, prominent in their field, conducted independent tests and all agreed that the suspect's teeth impressions matched the bite marks found on the victim's body.

Sexual Homicide

Sexual homicide results from one person killing another in the context of power, control, sexuality, and aggressive brutality. The psychiatric diagnosis of sexual sadism, sometimes applied to the victimizer, states that the essential feature of this deviant behavior (i.e., paraphilia) is the infliction of physical or psychological suffering on another person in order to achieve sexual excitement. It is difficult to gather dependable statistics on the number of sexual homicide victims for several reasons: (1) the victim is officially reported as a homicide statistic and not as a rape assault; (2) there is a failure to recognize any underlying sexual dynamics in a seemingly "ordinary" murder; (3) those agencies that investigate, apprehend, and assess the murderer often fail to share their findings, curtailing the collective pool of knowledge on the subject; and (4) conventional evidence of the crime's sexual nature may be absent. When law enforcement officials cannot readily determine a motive for murder, they examine its behavioral aspects. In developing techniques for profiling murderers, FBI agents have found that they need to understand the thought patterns of murderers to make sense of crime scene evidence and victim information. Characteristics of evidence and victims can reveal much about the murderer's intensity of planning, preparation, and follow-through. From these observations, the agents begin to uncover the murderer's motivation, recognizing how dependent motivation is to the killer's dominant thinking patterns. In many instances, a hidden, sexual motive emerges, a motive that has its origins in fantasy. The role of fantasy in the motive and behavior of suspects is an important factor in violent crimes, especially sexual murders. Since the 1970s, the role of sadistic fantasy has been explored in several studies (Brittain, 1970; Reinhardt, 1957; Revitch, 1980; West, Roay, & Nicholas, 1978), with MacCulloch and colleagues (1983) suggesting that sadistic acts and fantasy are linked and that fantasy drives the sadistic behavior (Figs. 35-2, 35-3, and 35-4).

Standard data collection forms should be utilized. The forms not only provide guidelines for interviewing subjects but also establish a system of recording and coding relevant data to permit computer analysis and retrieval. Information is requested about the offender and the offender's background, the offense, the victim, and the crime scene. Subjects are asked questions about childhood, adolescent, and adult behaviors or experience that might be related to violence. This provides quantitative analysis of background data and qualitative analysis of interview data from murderers.

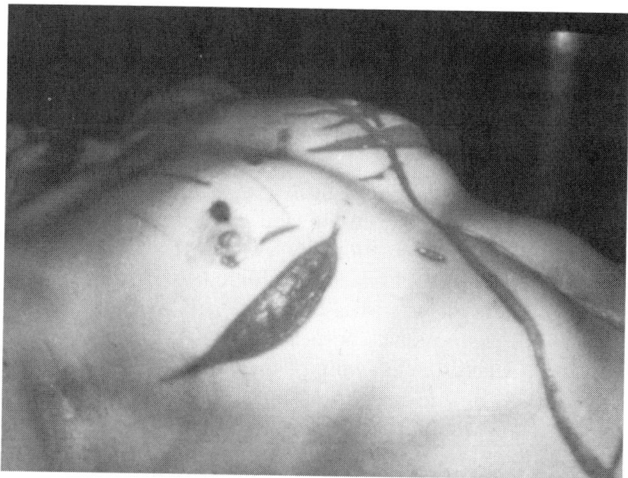

Fig. 35-2 Mutilation of the breasts of a sexual homicide victim.

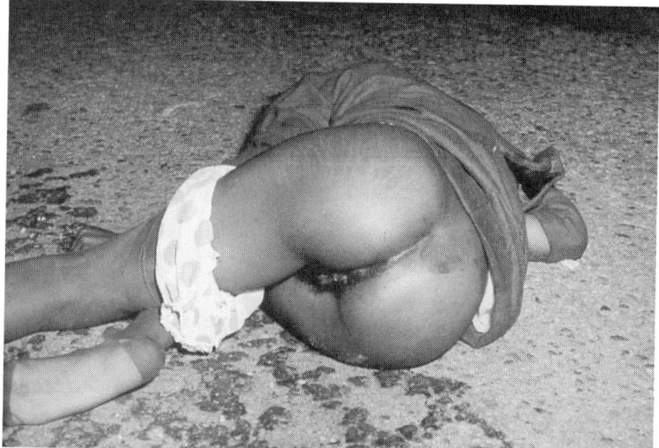

Fig. 35-3 Sexual homicide victim was killed with Phillips screwdriver.

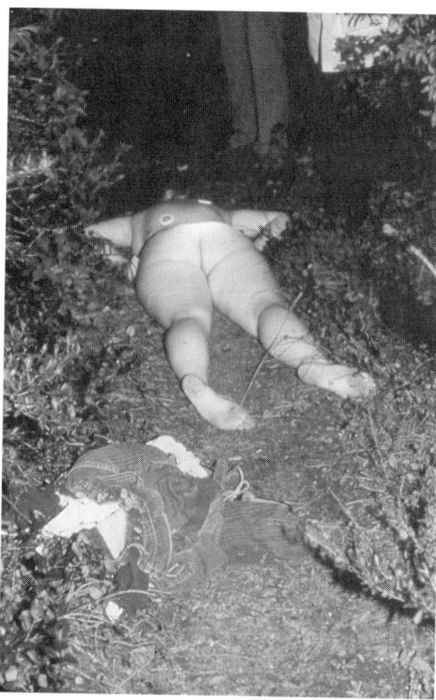

Fig. 35-4 Crime scene will provide investigator valuable clues for profiler of serial sexual homicide.

Implications

Statistics from the FBI Uniform Crime Reports clearly indicate that violent crimes represent a serious national problem. Some Americans feel society is increasingly violent and have support for that belief through mortality statistics. Public pressure is great on law enforcement officials when a community member is victimized by a violent, senseless, "motiveless" crime. In the case of a homicide, a community is generally shocked over the crime and demands swift and positive action from law enforcement in investigating and identifying the suspect. Once a suspect has been arrested and charged, the public then looks to the forensic behavioral sciences for an explanation of the murder's mental state and motivations.

The advancement of law enforcement techniques requires a knowledge base of the criminal personality. However, there are major hurdles inherent in the study of criminal personality. First, it is difficult to gather sufficient numbers of cases in an unbiased manner. More frequently, single cases are reported often by healthcare clinicians not trained in the forensic sciences. Second, although murder can be classified as an interactional situation involving at least two parties, the literature contains more reports on the murderer than on the victim. Third, prior to trial as well as after conviction, offenders rarely cooperate in an interview because the material may incriminate them as they continue the appeal process. Fourth, there is a paucity of data from staff managing offenders in their daily institutional routine that could lend significant understanding to an offender's state of mind. And fifth, the various disciplines whose work brings them into contact with offenders focus on only one small part of the total picture. They concentrate only on the problem from their specialty perspective.

Interagency cooperation through sharing of information and collaborating on cases is not practiced to any high degree. Mental health staff members are not knowledgeable about the details of the crime or how the suspect acted during initial arrest or interrogation. Clinicians see the suspect when the individual's frame of mind is different because the clinical environment is unlike the crime scene, the police station, or prison. Similarly, investigators do not see the offender in the structure of a prison or hospital to note adaptive or maladaptive behavior. All of these factors require a systematic multidisciplinary perspective to the investigation.

The psychological assessment is an important factor in the process. As the violent crime rate continues to spiral and as criminals become increasingly sophisticated with their crimes, so must the investigative tools of law enforcement be sharpened. Over past years, one tool being developed at the Behavioral Science Unit of the FBI Academy is criminal profiling–the psychological assessment of a crime.

Psychological profiling is defined as the process of identifying the gross psychological characteristics of an individual based on an analysis of the crimes he or she committed and providing a general description of the person utilizing those traits. This process normally involves five steps: (1) a comprehensive study of the nature of the criminal act and the type of persons who have committed these offenses, (2) a thorough inspection of the specific crime scene involved in the case, (3) an in-depth examination of the background and activities of the victim(s) and any known suspects, (4) a formulation of the probable motivating factors of all parties involved, and (5) the development of a description of the perpetrator based on the overt characteristics associated with his or her probable psychological makeup.

It is not known who first used this particular process to identify criminals; however, the general technique was used in the 1870s by Dr. Hans Gross, an examining judge in the Upper Styria Region of Austria, and according to some, the first practical criminologist. More recently Dr. James Brussel, a New York psychiatrist, who provided valuable information in such famous cases as the Mad Bomber, the Boston Strangler, and the Coppolino murders, popularized a similar approach to criminal investigation.

The FBI, to assist local police in finding the perpetrator of a homicide, first used the procedure in 1971. Though the profiling was done on an informal basis in connection with classroom instruction, the analysis proved to be accurate and the offender was apprehended. In the following years, profiles were informally prepared on a number of cases with a reasonable degree of success, and as a result, requests for the procedure by local authorities increased steadily. The requests for profiling, provided by the Behavioral Science Unit, Training Division, have continued to increase since that time and today represent a significant commitment of agency power.

In 1981, the Institutional Research and Development Unit of the FBI Training Division was asked to initiate a cost-benefit study to determine the extent to which the service had been of value to the users. Specifically, the analysis was undertaken to examine two questions: (1) what was the nature and extent of any assistance provided by psychological profiling, and (2) what were the actual results of utilization of a psychological profile in terms of offender identification or savings in investigative agent days.

A review of the material submitted by the various field divisions for analysis revealed that requests had originated within the jurisdictional areas of 59 field offices located within the US and two FBI Liaison Representatives assigned to American embassies abroad. While the majority of these submissions were from city police (52%), requests came from all levels of law enforcement including county police or sheriff, FBI, state police, state investigators, and state highway patrol. As might be suspected, most of the requests for psychological profiling were submitted in an effort to identify the individual(s) responsible for one or more murders (65%). The second highest offense requested was for rape (35%) with other offenses including kidnapping, extortion, threat/obscene communication, child molestation, hostage situation, accidental death, and suicide. Most of the cases submitted involved a single victim (61%), although 10% involved at least two, and 17 contained six or more victims. Based on the total requests (n = 192), the suspect(s) were identified in a total of 88 or 46% of the cases. In these cases, responding agencies indicated that psychological profiling was useful in the following ways:

- It focused the investigation properly.
- It helped locate possible suspects.
- It identified suspects.
- It assisted in the prosecution of suspect(s).

Only in 15 cases was the profiling stated to be of no assistance. In attempting to document the cost-benefit aspect, the study suggested that the use of psychological profiling resulted in a total saving of 594 investigative agent-days. That number is considered a substantial figure when such matters as salaries, support costs, and availability of personnel for other assignments are considered. Variables that have been found at levels of significance can now be tested against cases that have been profiled by the Behavioral Science Unit agents.

Summary

The refinement of these investigative tools means faster suspect identification and apprehension and prevention of additional victims. Further, research efforts by law enforcement agencies are important to their development of additional skill in reading the seemingly inert characteristics of crime scene evidence. Understanding the motivational and behavioral matrix of the offender increases law enforcement's use of the connection between patterns of thinking and behaviors. Law enforcement agencies that employ forensic nurse examiners will benefit from the advent of forensic nursing science and the multidisciplinary cooperation needed to bring clinical and criminal investigation together.

Resources

Organizations

U.S. Department of Justice

950 Pennsylvania Avenue NW, Washington, DC 20530-0001; www.doj.gov

U.S. Federal Bureau of Investigation: Behavioral Science Unit

J. Edgar Hoover Building, 935 Pennsylvania Avenue NW, Washington, DC 20535-0001; www.fbi.gov/hq/td/academy/bsu/bsu.htm

Genetest Corporation: Forensic DNA Criminal Profiling

2316 Delaware Avenue, Buffalo, NY 14216; 877-404-4363 or 877-964-2436; www.genetestlabs.com/forensic/forensicscriminalprofiling.htm

National Association of Medical Examiners

1402 South Grand Boulevard, St. Louis, MO 63104; Tel: 314-577-8298; http://expertpages.com/org/name.htm

Websites

John Douglas, Criminal Profiler
www.johndouglasmindhunter.com

References

Brittain, R. P. (1970). The sadistic murderer. *Med Sci Law, 10,* 198-207.

Brussel, J. A. (1968). *Casebook of a crime psychiatrist.* New York, Grove Press. Excerpts retrieved January 8, 2005, from: www.crimelibrary.com/terrorists_spies/terrorists/metesky/10.html?sect=22

Casey-Owens, M. (1984). The anonymous letter-writer–psychological profile? *J Forensic Sci, 29,* 816-819.

Gerberth, V. J. (1981). Psychological profiling. *Law and Order,* 46-49.

Hazelwood, R. R. (1983). The behavior-oriented interview of rape victims: The key to profiling. *FBI Law Enforcement Bull,* 1-8.

Lunde, D. T. (1976). *Murder and madness.* San Francisco: San Francisco Book Company.

MacCulloch, M. G., Snowden, P. R., Wood, P. J., et al. (1983). Sadistic fantasy, sadistic behavior and offending. *Br J Psychiatry, 143,* 20-29.

Miron, M. S., & Douglas, J. E. (1979). Threat analysis: The psycholinguistic profile. *FBI Law Enforcement Bull, 48*(9), 5-9.

Palmer, S. (1960). *A study of murder.* New York: Thomas Crowell.

Reinhardt, J. M. (1957). *Sex perversions and sex crimes: A psychocultural examination of the causes, nature and criminal manifestations of sex perversions. Police science series.* Springfield, IL: Charles C. Thomas.

Reiser, M. (1982). Crime-specific psychological consultation. *The Police Chief,* 53-56.

Ressler, R. K., Burgess, A. W., Douglas, J. E., et al. (1985). Criminal profiling research on homicide. In A. W. Burgess (Ed.), *Rape and sexual assault: A research handbook.* (pp. 343-349). New York: Garland.

Revitch, F. (1980). Genocide and unprovoked attacks on women. Correctional and Social Psychiatry, 26, 6-11.

Rider, A. O. (1980). The firesetter: A psychological profile, part 1. *FBI Law Enforcement Bull, 49*(6), 6-13

Rizzo, N. D. (1981). Murder in Boston: Killers and their victims. *Int J Offender Ther Comp Criminol, 26*(1),36-42.

Vorpagel, R. E. (1981). *Painting psychological profiles: Charlatanism, charisma, or a new science?* Paper presented at the FBI behavioral sciences class.

West, D. J., Roy, C., & Nicholas, F. L. (1978). *Understanding sexual attacks.* London: Heinemann.

Chapter 36 Autoerotic Fatalities

Ann Wolbert Burgess

This chapter concerns deaths occurring in the course of autoerotic activities in which a potentially injurious agent was used to heighten sexual arousal. Autoerotic fatalities are deaths that occur as the result of or in association with masturbation or other self-stimulating activity. Such seemingly obscure deaths, estimated to be between 500 to 1000 reported each year, affect not only the victims but also their survivors and those whose professional roles demand knowledge of these matters (Hazelwood, Dietz, & Burgess, 1997).

There are important forensic nursing considerations. The majority of autoerotic fatalities involving injurious agents are accidental, but their features sometimes lead to mistaken impressions of suicide or homicide. The fact that many autoerotic fatalities share common characteristics with suicide, such as a finding that the victim was alone in a locked room or that he died by hanging, sometimes leads to initially classifying an autoerotic death as a suicide. Other features, such as the presence of a blindfold, a gag, or physical restraints, have led to mistaken suspicions of homicide. Thus, understanding the important features of the autoerotic death scene, the classification of such fatalities, and the family response to the untimely death of the victim provides the forensic nurse with knowledge for advanced practice.

Best Practice *36-1*

The forensic nurse investigator should carefully analyze all circumstances in order to differentiate autoerotic death scenes from those of suicide.

Human Sexuality

Sexual arousal is that internal state in which the probability of orgasm is increased. Major studies of the past 50 years have measured the circumstances under which such arousal occurs for men (Kinsey et al., 1948) and women (Kinsey et al., 1953) in the general population and the anatomic and physiological bases of arousal and orgasm (Masters & Johnson, 1966). The former studies show the who, what, where, and when of human sexuality; the latter show the how of orgasm. Between these two charted territories, however, lies an area where measurement is even more difficult: the processes in the brain through which sensory stimulation and fantasy combine to heighten arousal and carry it forward to the point at which orgasm is inevitable (Hazelwood, Dietz, & Burgess, 1997). Each of the major theories of human behavior can be invoked, with greater or lesser success, in an attempt to understand the evasive linkage.

Regardless of the theoretical vantage point, sexual arousal has both universal and individual features. Direct tactile stimulation of significant sexual parts of the body is a universal feature of sexual arousal, though the most effective forms of tactile stimulation and the specific area of the body that hold sexual significance vary among individuals.

Available evidence is consistent with the widely shared view that individual variations in the effectiveness of and preference for specific types of sensory stimulation and fantasy originate in the life histories of individuals. This view, however, does not help one in understanding sexual arousal, for individual life-history experiences range from the prenatal environment (Money & Ehrhardt, 1972), through early childhood experiences, to learning that continues through adolescence and adulthood by the repeated pairing of stimulation and fantasy with pleasure and orgasm. Researchers and clinicians are at an even greater loss when attempting to understand unconventional forms of stimulation and fantasy that produce sexual arousal for only a relatively small segment of the population such as the erotic risk-taking group.

Key Point *36-1*

Fantasy—the mental representation of sights, feelings, and other sensations—is a universal component of sexual arousal, though the specific mental imagery that is most effective varies widely among individuals.

Erotic Risk Taking

Among the activities that some individuals find arousing are procedures that carry an inherent risk to life. In the broadest sense, no human activity is without risk, but here the activity has an inherent greater risk of death than that associated with such everyday activities as crossing a busy street or driving in heavy traffic.

The recognized forms of erotic risk taking that result in death are discussed in this chapter but may represent only a small fraction of the total number of fatalities resulting from erotic risk taking. Based on what is known of the recognized forms, it is suspected that there may be many individuals who engage in risk-taking behavior at least in part because it arouses sexual feelings. Such individuals do not necessarily suffer any form of psychosexual disorder. The brain centers involved in sexual behavior are closely linked with those involved in aggressive behavior, and this proximity may underlie part of the association between sexuality and aggression. The biochemical and hormonal linkages between sexual arousal, risk taking, and aggression are only now being investigated. Studies showing the production of an amphetamine-like substance in the body during parachute jumps (Paulos & Tessel,

Key Point *36-2*

The individuality of sexual preferences is such that activities abhorrent to most people are sexually arousing to some.

1982) and elevations of a hormone involved in male sexuality among men behaving violently when they died (Mendelson et al., 1982), to cite just two examples, are fertile sources for speculation about these as-yet-uncharted linkages.

Of all the recognized forms of erotic risk taking, none results in death more frequently than asphyxia. The term *asphyxia* has a variety of meanings, but in this chapter is used synonymously with hypoxia, a decrease in the availability of oxygen to the tissues of the body, particularly the brain. A mild degree of asphyxia results in the familiar feeling of being out of breath, causing an increase in the frequency and depth of respiration in an unconsciously controlled effort to restore the normal levels of oxygen and carbon dioxide in the blood. Greater degrees of asphyxia produce cyanosis, loss of consciousness, convulsions, brain damage, and death. Relief from asphyxia and prompt intervention may interrupt this process at any stage prior to death and may be lifesaving.

Autoerotic Fatalities Study

In the spring of 1978, the Federal Bureau of Investigation (FBI) issued a mandate that original in-depth research be conducted on matters relevant to the law enforcement community. In response to this mandate, Supervisory Special Agent Robert Hazelwood requested that students at the FBI Academy submit cases for the study. One-hundred and fifty-seven suspected cases were submitted to the Behavioral Science Unit over a three-year period.

The materials submitted varied somewhat between cases. In all instances, investigative reports were submitted along with either a description or photographs of the scene of death. Additional information was obtained related to interviews with the person who found the body and statements made by relatives. Writings, drawings, photographs, or notes that had been made by the victim were submitted in a number of cases. Although this collection of cases cannot be said to be a probability sample, it appears to be the largest collection of thoroughly investigated reported cases.

Sample Characteristics

The 157 cases were classified into four types of autoerotic death: asphyxial, atypical, partner-involved, and suicide.

Asphyxial Autoerotic Death

Asphyxial autoerotic activity was the most common form of death, accounting for 132 deaths or 84% of the sample. The asphyxial techniques most commonly recognized are compression of the neck through hanging or strangulation, exclusion of oxygen with a plastic bag or other material covering the head, obstruction of the airway through suffocation or choking, compression of the chest preventing respiratory movements, and replacement of oxygen with anesthetic agents.

It is important to note the distinction between autoerotic or sexual asphyxia on the one hand and asphyxia as a cause of death on the other. Autoerotic or sexual asphyxia refers to the use of asphyxia to heighten sexual arousal, more often than not with a nonfatal outcome. Although not necessarily fatal, sexual asphyxial practices are clearly dangerous. The autoerotic-asphyxia practitioner who dies while engaged in autoerotic asphyxiation most often dies from an unexpected overdose of asphyxiation when, for one reason or another, the person becomes unable to terminate this means of enjoyment. From time to time, however, someone engaged in autoerotic asphyxia may die a nonasphyxial death (for example, from a heart attack, stroke, or exposure) during this activity. Conversely, it is theoretically possible that someone engaged in nonasphyxial autoerotic activities might die an asphyxial death (for example, carbon monoxide poisoning from a faulty heater or automobile exhaust system).

The overwhelming majority of victims in this sample were male and white. Of 132 persons who died by asphyxiation, 5 were female. There were four black males, one black female, one Native American male, one Hispanic male, and one Hispanic female. The mean age of decedents was 26.5 years. Four victims were preadolescent, 37 were teenagers, 46 were in their twenties, 28 in their thirties, 8 in their forties, 6 in their fifties, 2 in their sixties, and 1 in his seventies. Although 76 (67.9%) of the 112 decedents for whom marital data was known were single, 41 of the 132 decedents were under age 20. Available data on social class suggest that the decedents were more often middle class than upper, working, or lower class. This is an unusual observation for cases coming to the attention of medical examiners and law enforcement agencies, for members of the lowest social strata usually are disproportionately represented among traumatic deaths.

Atypical Autoerotic Fatalities

There are forms of dangerous autoerotic activity that do not involve the purposeful use of asphyxia. These activities involve a wide variety of potentially dangerous activities, such as the use of nonasphyxial sexual bondage, infibulation, electricity, insertion of foreign bodies in the urethra, vagina, or rectum, and life-threatening games.

Although it cannot be said with certainty whether these nonasphyxial dangerous practices are more widely practiced than sexual asphyxia, with the exception of electricity they seem less likely to result in death. Deaths from such activities are less prevalent than deaths during autoerotic asphyxia, and they are therefore referred to as atypical autoerotic fatalities.

Nonasphyxial autoerotic practices can result in a variety of causes of death. There were 16 such cases submitted, including death by electrocution (6), heart attack (4), poisoning (4), exposure (1), and undetermined (1). In two other atypical cases, autoerotic asphyxia resulted indirectly in an asphyxial death due to aspiration of vomitus. These 18 decedents are made up of 16 white males and 2 black females.

Sexual Asphyxial Fatalities Including a Partner

Sexual asphyxial deaths also occur in the presence of a partner. Most often, these are homicides in which a male assailant strangles, smothers, or otherwise asphyxiates a rape victim (male or female). Cases in which it was obvious that this is what occurred were not requested for this study, and none was submitted. A less common occurrence is the death by asphyxia of an individual who apparently consented to engage in sexual activity. In such instances, it is likely that there will be considerable difficulty in determining willful murder from negligent manslaughter. In addition, under certain circumstances, there may be difficulty in determining whether a sexual partner was present at the time of death.

It is also possible that a person engaged in autoerotic activity may incidentally become a homicide victim. The autoerotic activity may have nothing to do with the homicide. For example, an individual may be engaged in autoerotic activity when a burglar enters his home and kills him. The autoerotic activity may have some bearing on the homicide. In one case (not from the study sample), a wife shot and killed her husband in his bed, believing him to be her husband's lover. What she did not know at the time of the shooting was that her husband was a transvestite and had fallen asleep dressed in his female clothing after engaging in autoerotic activity.

A remote possibility that must always be borne in mind is that of a homicide scene staged to appear to be accidental autoerotic death. In one unusual case from the study, the decedent's wife, who had previously observed him engaging in autoerotic asphyxia, altered the death scene to make it appear like a homicide. Her effort was singularly unsuccessful, for she left the noose within sight and inflicted a minor stab wound that was readily shown to have been inflicted after death by asphyxia.

Autoerotic Suicides

True autoerotic suicides are rare. Over the years, many autoerotic fatalities have been mistaken for suicide, largely because the investigators were unaware of the phenomenon of autoerotic asphyxia. Thus, cases described as a suicide by unusual methods or a bizarre form of suicide are scattered throughout the literature.

In addition, some cases are factitious suicides in which family members or others have removed evidence of sexual activity in order to make the manner of death appear to be suicide. In one study case, for example, the decedent's wife removed the female clothing he had been wearing at death and dressed his body in a suit before calling the police.

Two study cases were autoerotic suicides that could be documented as such on the basis of antemortem behavioral indicators, such as a suicide note. There is no possible means by which to determine with certainty how often other cases may have involved clear suicidal intent. It is certainly feasible that an individual fond of dangerous autoerotic activity will include that behavior in a purposeful suicide. It is conceivable that a suicidal individual, having heard of sexual asphyxia, might choose an asphyxial method of suicide over other options in order to lessen discomfort, but this possibility remains highly speculative. Also, an individual who repetitively engages in dangerous autoerotic practices might decide to end his or her life, although there is no proof of this ever having occurred. More likely, individuals fond of sexual risk taking might escalate the risk to their lives purposefully with full knowledge that death might ensue, but without formulating a conscious intent to die on one particular occasion. Courts deciding whether to award accidental-death benefits in asphyxial autoerotic fatalities have presumed the intent of the decedent, ruling that the fact of the insured's having engaged in an obviously life-threatening act is sufficient evidence of the intent to bring about "the natural and probable consequences of the act," quite apart from whether any particular consequence was consciously intended in a given instance.

The Autoerotic-Death Scene

As in all death investigations, the autoerotic-death scene should be preserved through photographs and sketches to complement the written record. The possibility of a victim's parent or spouse legally challenging the cause or manner of death listed on the death certificate should be anticipated. There have been cases where parents have litigated cases believing their child was murdered or pressuring a local coroner to change a ruling from accident during autoerotic acts to accident due to physical exertion. And the decedent's insurance company may also contest the manner of death when accidental-death benefits are at stake. Thus, a careful investigation and documentation of the death scene is of utmost concern.

Location

Sexual fantasies precede and accompany an autoerotic act. Thus, the individual preparing to act out his fantasies typically selects a secluded or isolated location. The locations involved in the study sample included locked rooms; isolated areas of the victim's residence such as attics, basements, garages, or workshops; motel rooms; places of employment during nonbusiness hours; summer residences; and wooded areas. The victim's desire for privacy is paramount in the selection of location. Such acts require concentration on the fantasy scenario and, depending on the use of props, may require considerable preparation time. Thus, the individual takes precautions to avoid disruption. The location itself may play a role in the victim's fantasy (Figs. 36-1 and 36-2).

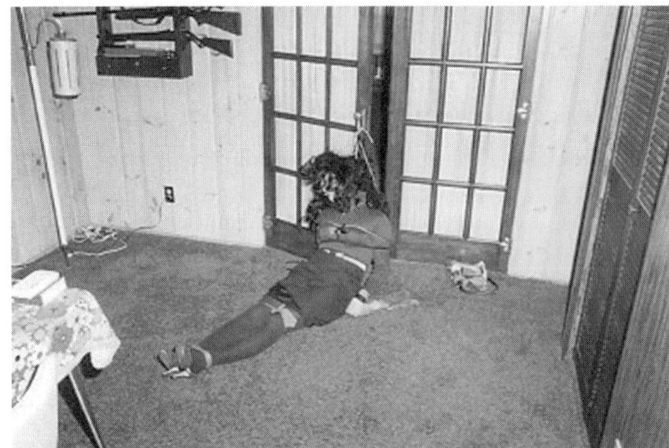

Fig. 36-1 Autoerotic-death scene with female victim hanging in secluded place. Note the breast binding and bound ankles.

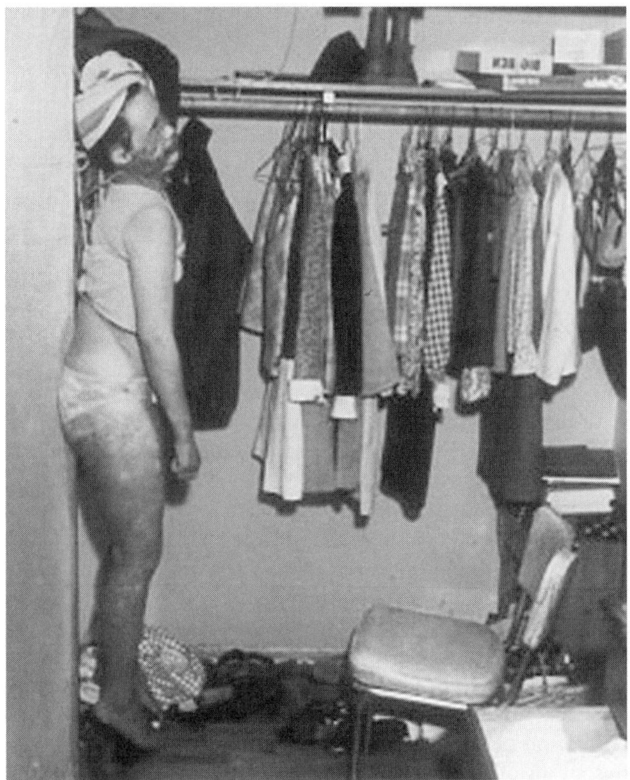

Fig. 36-2 Male cross-dressed victim who suffered autoerotic asphyxial death.

Case Study 36-1 Location of the Body

A 28-year-old repairman was discovered dead by coworkers when he failed to return to the office. His repair truck was located on a rural road approximately two miles from his last service call. The body was located in a heavily wooded area 250 feet from the roadway. The victim was lying facedown with the upper portion of his body resting on his forearms. Around his neck was a 3/8-inch hemp rope secured by a slipknot. The rope extended from his neck to a tree limb approximately six feet overhead. To the left front of the victim were four magazines depicting nude females. The victim's pants were undone, and his underwear had been lowered sufficiently to expose the penis and scrotum. Medical authorities recorded the cause of death as asphyxiation due to constricted carotid arteries.

Victim Position

Most commonly, the victim's body is partially supported by the ground, floor, or other surface. Occasionally, the victim is totally suspended. The most common position noted in the study was one in which the deceased was suspended upright with only the feet touching the surface. In most such cases, some type of ligature was around the neck and affixed to a suspension point within the reach of the victim. Accidental-death victims have been found sitting, kneeling, lying face upward or downward, or suspended by their hands.

Key Point *36-3*

The forensic specialist should not be unduly influenced in deciding whether a death is accidental or homicidal by the fact that the body position seemingly indicates the involvement of a second party.

The Injurious Agent

The forensic nurse death investigator at the death scene is charged with the responsibility of gathering information that will allow determination of any action or lack thereof that contributed to the victim's death. That includes that the injurious agent be studied in great detail, including a careful search for and analysis of possible malfunctioning.

In the study, the most common injurious agent was a ligature of some sort that compressed the neck. Other injurious agents included devices for passing electrical current through the body; restrictive containers; obstruction of the breathing passages with gags; and the inhalation of toxic gases or chemicals through masks, hoses, and plastic bags.

In the construction or use of these devices, the individual risks miscalculation. Depending on the mechanism used, the individual may misjudge the amount of time, substance, pressure, or current.

The Self-Rescue Mechanism

The self-rescue mechanism is any provision that the victim has made to reduce or remove the effects of the injurious agent. The self-rescue mechanism may be nothing more than the victim's ability to stand up straight, thereby lessening the pressure about his neck, or it may be as involved as an interconnection between ligatures on the extremities and a ligature around the neck, thereby allowing the victim to control pressure on his neck by moving his body in a particular way or pulling on a key point. Any of a wide variety of items or potential actions that the practitioner had available may have been intended as a self-rescue mechanism. If the injurious agent is a ligature, a slipknot or knife may be

Case Study 36-2 Injurious Agent: Ligature

A 32-year-old fully clothed man was found lying on his stomach on his floor. A handkerchief was over his mouth and tied behind his head. A length of rope wound around his neck and was tied with a slipknot. The rope ran down his back and was attached to a brown leather belt, which held his ankles together. His feet were pulled toward his head by the rope connecting his neck and feet. Blood had trickled from his nose and ears. The responding officers initially thought the death to be a homicide. An examination of the decedent's head revealed no blunt-force trauma, and the ear and nose bleeding was properly attributed to asphyxiation. They also noted the victim's arms were free: had he not lost consciousness, he could have released the ligature by the slipknot at his neck or by cutting the rope with the serrated steak knife found on the floor nearby. On a table beside the body were two similar pieces of rope that had been tied with slipknots. He had probably practiced with those two pieces of rope before engaging in the lethal act.

Case Study 36-3 Injurious Agent: Chloroform

A 23-year-old single white male college student was found dead clad in a pair of shorts in his apartment that he shared with another male. His hands were secured in a pillory that rested across his shoulders. This restraining device consisted of two pieces of wood secured at one extreme by a spring-loaded hinge. Two holes, lined with gray rubber, held his wrists, and a 6-inch hole had been cut to fit the neck. Situated between the neck and one wrist aperture was a padlock. Approximately 2 1/2 feet from the victim's body was a set of keys, one of which fit the padlock securing the pillory. He was wearing a full-face gas mask with a hose leading from the mask to a metal canister, which contained 13 cotton balls saturated with chloroform, a wadded washcloth, two sheets of toilet paper, and a small bottle containing chloroform. He apparently dropped the keys, was unable to retrieve them, and lost consciousness. He died from chloroform inhalation.

Case Study 36-4 Self-Rescue: Slipknot

A 23-year-old white female died as a result of ligature strangulation. The woman had used an extension cord to interconnect her ankles with her neck. She had used a slipknot as a self-rescue mechanism. Examination of the slipknot revealed that in tying it, her hair had become entangled in the knot, thereby preventing her from disengaging it.

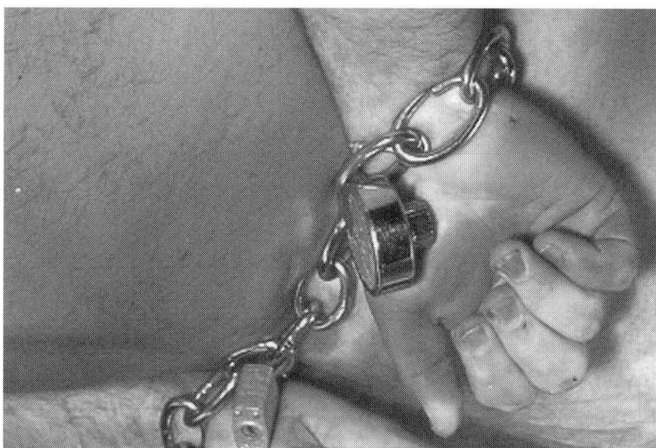
Fig. 36-3 Evidence of bondage using locked wrist restraints.

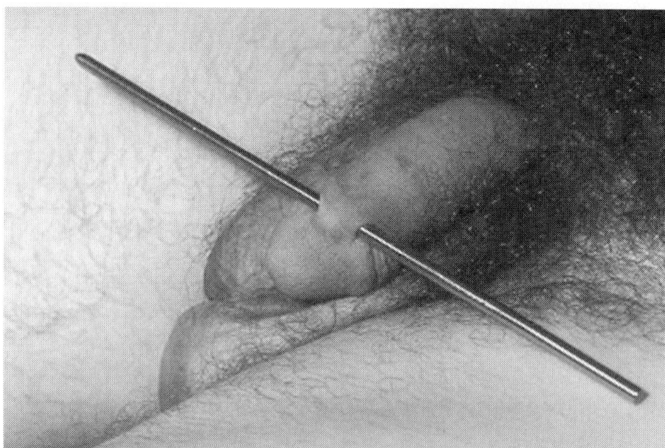
Fig. 36-4 Infibulation of penis using steel pin.

involved; if locks are involved, a key may be present; if chains are involved, a pair of pliers may be nearby. As with the injurious agent itself, the possibility of a malfunction of the self-rescue mechanism must be carefully considered.

Bondage

The terms *bondage* and *domination* are used to describe a range of sexual behaviors closely related to the features commonly associated with autoerotic deaths. Bondage refers to the physical restraining materials or devices that have sexual significance for the user. This factor is important, for its involvement is most often responsible for the misinterpretation of these deaths as homicidal rather than accidental (Fig. 36-3). In one case, a man covered himself entirely with mud prior to placing a ligature around his neck. As the mud dried, it caked and constricted the skin. Examples of restrictions on the organs of sensation and expression identified in this study include hoods, blindfolds, and gags. In addition, belts, decorative chains, and other features have been observed that were presumed to be elements of symbolic bondage for the victim, as they often are for individuals who engage in other forms of sexual bondage behavior.

Physical restraints in the study included ropes, chains, handcuffs, and other similar devices that restricted the victim's movement. Even in obvious cases, the death investigator needs to prove it was physically possible for the victim to have placed the restraints as they were discovered. It may be necessary to duplicate bindings or knots, and for that reason, the knots should not be cut or undone prior to scrutiny.

Case Study 36-5 Constriction and Restriction

A 40-year-old man was discovered dead by his wife in the basement of their home. He was totally suspended by a rope that had been wrapped several times around an overhead beam. Around his neck was a hangman's noose that had been meticulously prepared. The body was dressed in a white T-shirt, a white panty girdle with nylons, and a pair of women's open-toed shoes. His hands were bound in handcuff fashion with the wrists approximately 10 inches apart. Over his head was another girdle, and his ankles were bound with a brown leather belt. On discovering the body, the wife assumed her husband had been murdered.

The investigators correctly assessed the death as accidental and attributed the bound wrists, ankles, and covered head to sexual bondage. They recognized that the girdle covering his head was a bondage-related feature. Bodily restraint through bondage includes not only restrictions in the movement of the body but also constriction of the body and restriction of the organs of sensation and expression. Constrictive materials identified in this study included elastic garments (for example, girdles, support hose, and tight underwear) and other materials such as ace bandages.

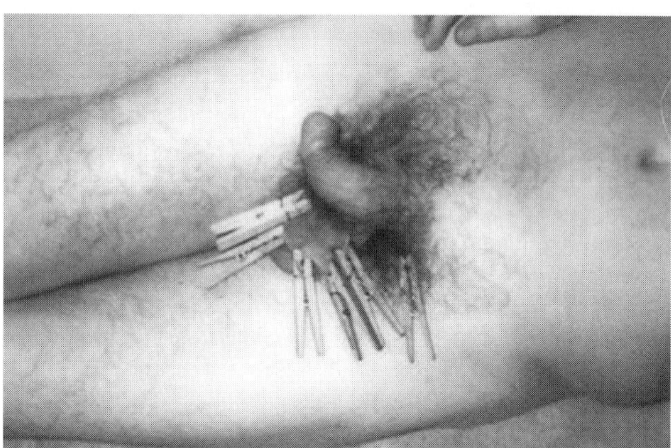
Fig. 36-5 Clothespins and other devices attached to testicles used for autoeroticism.

Sexually Masochistic Behavior

It will sometimes be observed that the decedent had inflicted pain upon his genitals, nipples, or other areas of the body. In addition to whatever pain may be associated with bondage restraints or constrictive materials, pain may have been induced mechanically, electrically, or through self-induced burns, piercing, or frank mutilation. Cases in the study have included a belt tightened around the scrotum, clothespins affixed to the nipples, electrical wire inserted into the penis or anus, an electrified brassiere, and cigarette burns to the scrotum. The term infibulation is used to describe the passing of needles or pins through the body, most often through the scrotum, penis, or nipples, but sometimes through an earlobe or the nose (Figs. 36-4 and 36-5). In one case, pins had been passed through each of the decedent's nipples. The self-mutilation may be more extreme, as in the following case.

Case Study 36-6 Masochistic Behavior

A 31-year-old white male was found suspended from a beam by a hangman's noose around his neck. His feet were touching the floor. He was nude except for a black leather belt around his waist. Handcuffs secured his wrists in front, and a key to the handcuffs was found in his right hand. Examination of his penis revealed a surgery-like incision around the circumference of the shaft. Inserted and tightened into the incision was a metal washer. The outer edge of the washer was flush with the penis shaft.

Attire

Sometimes the victim is attired in one or more articles of female clothing, especially undergarments. Nylon, lace, leather, rubber, or other materials that hold sexual significance for the victim are commonly part of his attire. The investigator needs to be aware that the attire may have been adjusted, altered, or completely changed by family members prior to the arrival of the investigative team. In the instances where this had been done, family members said they attributed their alterations to shame, embarrassment, or impulse.

Case Study 36-7 Attire

A 16-year-old white male was discovered dead in his room by his father. When the police arrived, they found the victim lying on his back and wearing blue jeans, a T-shirt, jockey shorts, and wool socks. A belt looped on one end was near his head, as were his glasses. His father informed the officers that when originally found, his son was wearing only his T-shirt and socks. The victim's underwear and pants were on the floor at the end of the bed. The father said that he did not know why his son had been undressed when first found and that he had dressed his son without thinking.

Had the adjustment in attire not been discovered, the death might have been ruled a suicide. Close examination of the body and its lividity may reveal that attire or restraints have been adjusted, altered, or completely changed, or that the body has been moved since death.

Protective Padding

Frequently, the victim will be found with soft material between a ligature and the adjacent body surface. The purpose of this protective padding is to prevent abrasions or discoloration that might prompt inquiries from family or friends. In the previous case study, the parents had no idea their son was involved in such dangerous activities. His mother, however, recalled that some months prior to her son's death she had noted burn marks on both sides of his neck. When she inquired as to their cause, he had explained the marks as having occurred when he had been grabbed by his jersey while playing football. When he was discovered dead, there was no protective padding in place (Fig. 36-6).

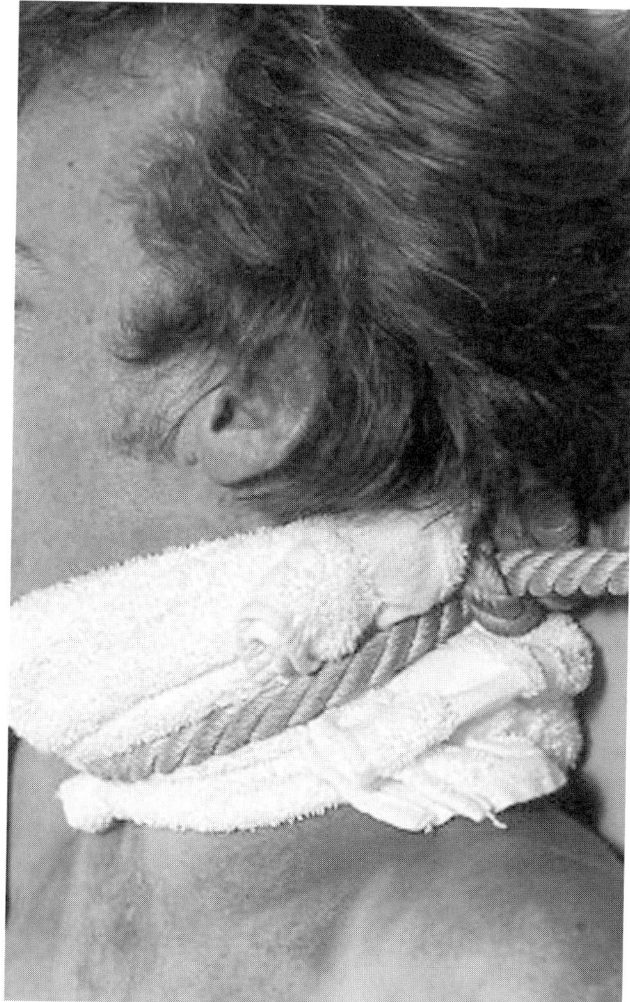

Fig. 36-6 Padded ligature mechanism used by victim in autoerotic sexual acts.

Sexual Paraphernalia

Sexual paraphernalia was found on or near the victim in many cases in the study sample. These paraphernalia included vibrators, dildos, and fetish items such as female garments, leather, and rubber items. Often materials that are present are not recognized as having a sexual meaning for the victim because they do not appeal sexually to the investigator and are dismissed as inconsequential. All items at the scene and their proximity to the body should be noted and photographed in their original positions for later interpretation. In the case of a 51-year-old single male victim, discovered fully dressed with the exception of wearing two leather jackets, and suspended by a rope around his neck and attached to a tree limb, a search of his residence revealed the following: more than 50 leather coats; ropes; chains; handcuffs; leg irons; a penis vice; scrotum weights; electrical shock devices; discipline masks; traffic cones with fecal material on them; 107 pairs of leather gloves of which 29 were determined to have seminal stains inside; a mace with chain and spiked ball; canes; whips; and assorted padlocks.

Props

Items found at the death scene may have been used as fantasy props. Items so identified in this study included mirrors, commercial erotica, photographs, films, and fetish items. One wife volunteered that the bondage magazine found by her husband's body was open to his favorite bondage picture. She said he would replicate to exact detail every knot and tie in the picture. Magazines about women's fashions and hairstyles were also found in the possession of some cross-dressers. In one case, a movie projector threaded with a pornographic film was found, indicating the victim had been watching the film prior to or during his final autoerotic act. One man found bound and hanging, with mirrors arranged such that he could view himself, had been watching an explicitly sexual movie on cable television.

Masturbatory Activity

The victim may or may not have been engaged in manual masturbation during the fatal autoerotic activity. The presence of seminal discharge is not a useful clue in determining whether a death is due to sexual misadventure. Seminal discharge frequently occurs at death, irrespective of the cause or manner of death. To be sure, the existence of seminal stains on the victim or nearby surfaces should be noted, photographed, and collected for possible blood-type determination and comparison to the victim, but the mere presence of seminal staining is not evidence of sexual activity.

Manual masturbation may be suggested by finding the victim's hand on or near the genitals, but it is to be remembered that the extremities may twitch or move in the final movement of life. Other indicators of sexual activity include such findings as a dildo or vibrator in or near the body, the penis wrapped in cloth to prevent staining of garments, or exposure of the genitals of a victim who is otherwise dressed. Individuals committing suicide by hanging avoid nudity (except for prisoners). Complete nudity in death is presumptive evidence of an autoerotic death.

Frequently no direct evidence of manual masturbation exists. Indeed, some living practitioners of autoerotic asphyxia have reported that they did not manually masturbate while asphyxiating themselves but rather used asphyxiation to arouse themselves sexually, after which they would manually masturbate.

Evidence of Previous Experience

Five types of information were found in the study that are useful in judging the extent of the victim's prior experience: information from relatives and associates, permanently affixed protective padding, suspension-point abrasions, complexity of the injurious agent, and collected materials.

Information from Relatives and Associates

Although family members, sexual partners, and friends sometimes have no awareness of the victim's dangerous autoerotic practices, they may nonetheless have observed behavior that gains meaning in retrospect. One father noted that his son was always tying knots. Another father knew that his son occasionally put a belt around his neck and tightened it until becoming weak.

Permanently Affixed Protective Padding

One factor indicative of prior practice is the permanent affixing of protective padding to ligatures or devices used in the activity. This suggests that the victim has engaged in similar acts in the past and intended to do so in the future. The padding indicates the victim's intent to prevent leaving marks on the body.

Suspension Point Abrasions

If the victim's death involved the use of ligatures over or around suspension points, the forensic specialist should examine those areas and others like them for abrasions or grooves caused by similar use in the past. A young white male died while suspended from a braided leather whip that went around his neck and over the top of a closet door. The whip was secured to a wheel and tire on the opposite side of the door. His hands were free, but his ankles were loosely bound with leather thongs. The door top revealed several grooves and abrasions from previous use.

Complexity of the Injurious Agent

When the injurious agent is highly complex, it is likely that the apparatus became complex through repetitive experience and elaboration over time. One 26-year-old victim was discovered dead wearing a commercially produced discipline mask and had a bit in his mouth. A length of rope was attached to each end of the bit and ran over his shoulders, going through an eyelet at the back of a specially designed belt he was wearing. The pieces of rope ran to eyelets on both sides of his body and were connected to wooden dowels that extended the length of his legs. The ropes were attached to two plastic water bottles, one on each ankle. The bottles were filled with water and each weighed 7 pounds. The victim's ankles had leather restraints about them. A clothespin was affixed to each of the victim's nipples. The victim's belt had a leather device that ran between his buttocks and was attached to the rear and front of the belt. This belt device included a dildo that was inserted into his anus and an aperture through which his penis protruded. His penis was encased in a piece of pantyhose and a toilet-paper cylinder. A small red ribbon was tied in a bow at the base of his penis.

Collected Materials

The type, quantity, complexity, and cost of sexual materials collected by the victim provide indirect evidence of the duration of these activities. While in most instances the victim will be found in close proximity to this collection of sexual materials, the forensic specialist should assess other areas that are known to be under the control of the victim for additional materials.

Family Response

Although the forensic and law enforcement literature describes the investigative and medical components of autoerotic deaths, little exists in the behavioral or social science literature that describes this type of fatality or the response of family members and others. This absence may be attributed largely to (1) misdiagnosis of suicide or homicide rather than accident, and thus an underreporting of this manner of death, (2) a general acceptance and encouragement of all types of consenting sexual activity and a concomitant reluctance to acknowledge or emphasize the dangerous component in certain sexual activities (e.g., sexual bondage), and (3) social stigma surrounding sexually motivated death.

Clearly there is a need to alert forensic nurses and mental health professionals about young people who engage in this type of activity in order that they and their families can be counseled. This need has been heightened through the study by learning of parents of young victims who had been shocked at the sudden death of their children and who had known nothing about the manner of these deaths. If parents who have lost children to this type of death believe it is timely to talk about the subject, not only to investigators but to the news media, then forensic nurses whose work may bring them into contact with families need accurate information also.

Traumatic News

There is no news that has so great a psychological effect on survivors as the death of a family member or close associate.

Although many factors influence the severity of a stress reaction to a traumatic grief event, the emotional response is particularly devastating when the discovery of the body is made by a family member on friend, when the death is untimely, when the decedent is young, and when the death is sexual in nature. These are the factors generally present in autoerotic fatalities.

The discovery of the body can occur in several ways. In the majority of cases in this sample, the victim was found dead by a family member or friend. Of the 34 cases with data from the teenage group, 25 parents discovered their son dead. Of the 17 cases with data on married victims, 11 were found dead by their wives. In the unmarried group, out of 59 cases with data, 10 parents and 9 relatives found the decedent. More frequently in this group, the victim was found dead by friends, roommates, landlords, janitors, maids, employers, colleagues, police, or search parties.

Upon learning of the victim's death, friends and family were invariably stunned and shocked. The victim was usually described as having been in good spirits and physical health, as active, and having a future orientation. There was rarely any suspicion of suicidal ideation.

A sexual death resulting from the use of an injurious agent during a masturbatory ritual is considered an unusual type of death because many people, professionals included, have never heard of it. Although many people are familiar with autoerotic practices using manual stimulation, it appears that a significantly smaller number of people are aware of techniques for reducing oxygen to the brain to achieve an altered state of consciousness and to enhance erotic sensations and fantasy. The sexually associated features of this type of death puzzle and confuse family members.

Family members often helped investigators to determine if the victim had prior experience with autoerotic asphyxia. Some associates or relatives reported no prior awareness of the victim's activity. In other cases, relatives made pertinent observations but, lacking the knowledge of dangerous autoerotic activity, failed to attach significance to the victim's preoccupation with tying knots, signs of red marks on his neck, bloodshot eyes, or confused behavior for short time periods.

The families' reactions to the manner of death depended on how, when, and what they were told. There were cases in which the manner of death was quickly determined to be accidental and reported to the family. In others, the death was initially labeled a suicide or homicide and later reversed to accidental. Thus, the family may have to deal with change in its conception of the manner of death or with uncertainty for a time.

Families were noted to respond in several ways to the manner of death. In some cases, the families accepted the victim's death because they had strong feelings about alternative manners of death, with one mother commenting this type of death was "just a shade below suicide." There are some families who accepted that the victim had died accidentally but would not accept the nature of the death as sexual. Parents of a 21-year-old college student were successful in having the cause of death changed on the death certificate. And there were a few cases in which the family would not accept the determination that the death was accidental. Most often these families believed the death was a homicide and became angry with investigating officers for closing the case prematurely. Some families were upset and angry with the victim and refused to believe anything. One family refused to bury a son after learning that his death was sex related.

Forensic Issues

The most frequent question that arises in the death investigation of sexual fatalities is whether an individual who was alone committed suicide or died accidentally. Less often, the question posed is whether another person had been present and, if so, whether the death was intended or not. These questions involve complex issues of fact, behavior, and intent and are not always answerable. Opinions should not be rendered in such cases without detailed information about both the death scene and the victim's history.

Case Study 36-8 Accident or Suicide?

A 30-year-old married man had stayed home alone for three hours while his wife, who was eight months pregnant, and their two children went to a church-related activity. Upon her return, she discovered him dead in an upstairs bedroom that he was converting to a nursery. The victim was suspended from a rope that encompassed his neck and was attached to a pulley. A second rope passed over the pulley and ended in his left hand. The pulley was hooked to a metal bar, which extended between two beams in the roof. His feet were touching the floor, his pants were around his ankles, his underwear was semen-stained in front, and his shirt had been rolled up to expose his chest. The cause of death, as determined by the medical examiner, was asphyxiation due to hanging.

This case was submitted for opinion by the attorney for the executrix of the decedent's estate. His widow was involved in litigation with her husband's insurance company concerning the accidental-death-benefits clause of his life insurance policy.

The evidence in this case is consistent with accidental death. The victim used a pulley apparatus with two ropes. One rope went over the pulley and attached to his neck with a hangman's noose; the second rope served a control or braking function. By maintaining pressure on a braking rope, he could prevent the pulley from turning. This, in turn, would allow the noose to compress his neck and alter the flow of blood to his brain, producing a transient hypoxia, the extent of which he could control, at least while conscious. He could then loosen the ligature by allowing the control rope to slip or, should he lose consciousness, the control rope would slip from his grasp, automatically slackening the rope attached to his neck: a dead man's release. On this occasion, one rope had slipped off the track and jammed the pulley, preventing its rotation and resulting in his body weight being suspended from the rope, thereby causing his death.

The victim hid this sexual activity from his family and friends. At the time he died, his family had been at church, and he had removed the telephone from its cradle to prevent calls from interrupting his autoerotic activity.

The hangman's noose used for the ligature had symbolic value to the victim, who probably had an execution fantasy. His history also suggested a fascination with bondage activities in that he collected handcuffs, ropes, and locks and was very knowledgeable about the various types of knots.

The complexity of the apparatus he used strongly suggests prior practice. Rather than simply hanging himself, he used a sophisticated pulley system as part of his autoerotic ritual. On prior occasions, he was apparently able to engage in this activity without serious consequences.

The victim was described as being in excellent spirits, oriented toward the future, enjoying good physical health, and being interested in his work and family. His recent weight reduction was said to have improved his self-image. There were no precipitating stresses identified and no history of psychiatric disorder. His wife reported their life together as being at its highest point, with good prospects both financially and personally. If he had intended suicide, he would not have required an elaborate pulley system to achieve this aim.

Summary

There are problems for the person engaging in autoerotic activity because the stigma and secrecy surrounding the behavior prevent him or her from disclosing. There are problems for families in dealing with this type of sexual activity because they may not know about it or how to look for signs or what to do if they do discover their child with sexually oriented equipment. There are problems for therapists because there is no specific psychiatric diagnosis or appropriate discussion of this behavior.

Attention has been called to autoerotic activity because of the awareness of the sizable number of deaths resulting from it, such that mental health clinicians cannot ignore it. Forensic nurse specialists can educate about the type of activity and warn of its lethality. The study emphasized that families want basic information about the manner in which they have lost their loved ones, as well as emotional support through the grieving process.

Resources

Organizations

American Academy of Forensic Sciences

410 North 21st Street, Colorado Springs, CO 80904-2798; Tel: 719-636-1100; www.aafs.org

American Foundation for Suicide Prevention

120 Wall Street, 22nd Floor, New York, New York 10005; Tel: 212-363-3500 or 888-333-AFSP; www.afsp.org

National Association of Medical Examiners

430 Pryor Street SW, Atlanta, GA 30312; Tel: 404-730-4781; www.thename.org

Web Sites

Law-Forensic.com

www.law-forensic.com/autoerotic_2.htm
Literature review of autoerotic asphyxia and fatalities.

Silent Victims

www.silentvictims.org

References

Hazelwood, R. R., Dietz, P. E., & Burgess, A. W. (1997). *Autoerotic fatalities.* West Newton, MA: Awab.

Kinsey, A. C., Pomeroy, W. B., Martin, C. E., et al. (1948). *Sexual behavior in the human male.* Philadelphia: W. B. Saunders.

Kinsey, A. C., Pomeroy, W. B., Martin, C. E., et al. (1953). *Sexual behavior in the human female.* Philadelphia: W. B. Saunders.

Masters, W. H., & Johnson, V. E. (1966). *Human sexual response.* Boston: Little, Brown.

Mendelson, J. H., Dietz, P. E., & Ellingboe, J. (1982). Postmortem plasma luteinizing hormone levels and antemortem violence. *Pharmacol Biochem Behav, 17,* 171-173.

Money, J., & Ehrhardt, A. A. (1972). *Man & woman, boy & girl: The differentiation and dimorphism of gender identity from conception to maturity.* Baltimore: Johns Hopkins University Press.

Paulos, M. A., & Tessel, R. E. (1982). Excretion of B-phenethylamine is elevated in humans after profound stress. *Science, 215,* 1127-1129.

Chapter 37 Postmortem Examination of Sexual Assault Victims

Virginia A. Lynch and Jamie J. Ferrell

"Sex-related homicides have been thought uncommon and more often a stranger-to-stranger crime. Because of this, many sex-related homicides may have been and continue to be unrecognized. When investigating a sex-related homicide, it is important to realize that one is not generally dealing with a killer who has raped, but with a rapist who has killed," according to Tara Henry, coordinator of the Sexual Assault Response Team in Anchorage, Alaska. As a forensic nurse examiner (FNE), Henry has provided postmortem sexual assault examinations for the forensic pathologists at the Alaska state medical examiner's office in Anchorage since 1999 (Henry, 2003).

A stranger may often commit a sex-related homicide, but they are more likely to be committed by an acquaintance, family member, or current or former intimate partner. The FBI's Uniform Crime Report 2000 reported that 44.3% of all murder victims knew their offender and that 33% of female murder victims were killed by their husbands or boyfriends. It is essential to keep in mind the prevalence of sexual assaults in domestic violence relationships when investigating a domestic homicide. The autopsy on a female victim of a domestic homicide should include a postmortem evaluation and evidence collection for a sexual assault. It is not unusual for the clinical and criminal investigators to find they are dealing with not only a domestic homicide, but also a sex-related homicide (Henry, 2003).

Historical Perspective

From the annals of medical and legal history, perversion of the sexual instinct has confounded those who have studied the psychopathology of the sexual sadist, investigated the crime scenes, examined the bodies of the dead, and attempted to explain the association of lust and murder. Such are the cases of sadistic sexual homicide and sex-related murder. During the most intense emotion in which serious injury, wounds, or death are inflicted on the victim, lust and cruelty become unbounded in a psychopathic individual (Von Krafft-Ebbing, 1892). The perverse sexual acts resulting from psychopathology of the offender are of the greatest importance clinically, socially, and forensically. Therefore, they must receive careful consideration regarding the active cruelty combined with violence and lust (Box 37-1).

It is interesting to note that sex-related homicides are not unique to this century but have been documented throughout the annals of forensic and psychiatric medicine. The same *modus operandi*, victimology, and traumatology present at scenes of sex-related homicides over a hundred years ago continue to impact those who practice contemporary forensic science, including the FNE.

"Sexually sadistic offenders commit well-planned and carefully concealed crimes. Their crimes are repetitive, serious, and shocking; and offenders take special steps to prevent detection. The harm that these men wreak is so devastating and their techniques so sophisticated that those who attempt to apprehend and convict them must be armed with uncommon insight, extensive knowledge, and sophisticated investigative resources." (Hazelwood, Dietz, & Warren, pp. 474-475).

Box 37-1

The Whitechapel murderer, who still eludes the vigilance of the police and medical science today, probably belongs in the category of psychosexual monsters. The absence of uterus, ovaries, and labia in the victims of this modern Bluebeard allows the presumption that he seeks and finds still further satisfaction in anthropopathy.

In other cases of lust-murder, for physical and mental reasons (vide supra) violation is omitted, and the sadistic crime alone becomes the equivalent of coitus. Yet in other groups, following the perversions of the sexual instinct (which arise from hyperaesthesia and paraestheisa sexualis with retained virility) comes naturally the necrophiles and mutilation of corpses.

Adapted from Von Krafft-Ebing, R. (1892). *Psychopathia sexualis: Contrary sexual instinct: a medico-legal study*. New York: Arcade.

Equally, however, it is essential for the forensic nurse examiner (FNE), whether serving as a forensic nurse death investigator (FNDI) or sexual assault nurse examiner (SANE), to understand that there is often a difference between the pattern of behavior of the sexual sadist and the sexual torture of victims sanctioned by governments for purposes of intimidation and interrogation. This is a common human rights violation in countries worldwide.

Because of these critical components in the criminal investigation of sex-related homicides, it would stand to reason that the clinical investigator would be of significant value in the collection, preservation, and photodocumentation of evidence on the body of the crime. The partnership between homicide investigators and FNEs provides the strongest link among the apprehension, prosecution, and incarceration of the sexual predator.

General Principles

The FNE's role is one of collaboration with a multidisciplinary team of investigators. FNEs bring years of study and experience with living sexual assault victims into a sex-related homicide investigation. The ability to mobilize via a sexual assault response team (SART) enhances the contribution to investigative efforts. Technology used to augment the postmortem genital examinations includes colposcopic 35-mm photography, toluidine blue dye, and ultraviolet light (Wood's lamp). Reflective light imaging via alternate light source can also be incorporated.

The nature and pattern of postmortem genital findings are described in a manner consistent with conventional forensic designation (i.e., sharp versus blunt force trauma). The model developed for evaluation of bite marks by forensic odontologists is also ideal for description of nongenital injuries in the sexual homicide victim. The sexual homicide database provides a conceptual framework in which to collect data and evidence and categorize both normal and abnormal physical findings. The database will facilitate the study of salient postmortem characteristics and allow eventual comparison of the genital findings in sexual homicide victims to a control group of individuals who died of unrelated causes.

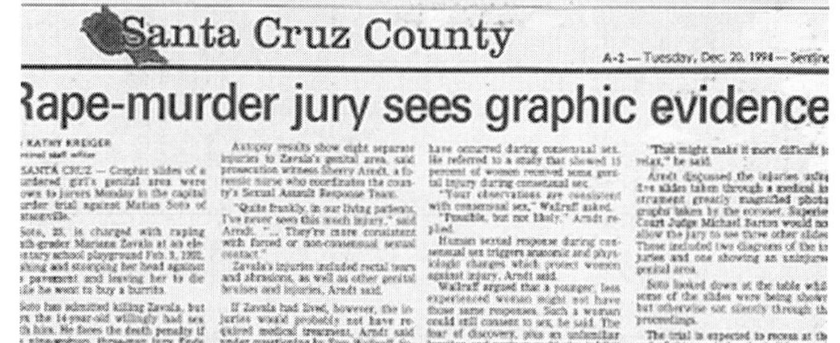
Santa Cruz County

A-2 — Tuesday, Dec. 20, 1994 —

ape-murder jury sees graphic evidence

Fig. 37-1 The headlines proclaim that nurse testimony and photograph documentation helped federal jury decide outcome in rape/homicide case.

Acumen of the Forensic Nurse Examiner

The FNE specializes in the identification, collection, and documentation of evidence of individuals who have been sexually assaulted, abused, neglected, or intentionally injured or killed. Their objectivity, scientific, and clinical expertise makes them ideally suited to perform examinations of either the victim or perpetrator of this category of criminal act.

The FNE is exceptionally skilled in the nuances of the sexual assault evidentiary examination and can serve as a valuable consultant to attorneys, government agencies, forensic pathologists, coroners, healthcare institutions, and police departments. Typically, FNEs are qualified without difficulty as expert witnesses, based on their specialized education and experience with such cases, for courtroom testimony in cases of sexual assault and human abuse.

Homicide detectives and district attorneys in many areas of the US have originated the initial request to the medical examiner/coroner to involve the FNE in these complicated cases. Having become familiar with the expertise of the FNE in cases of living victims, detectives and attorneys recognize the necessity of applying current standards and state-of-the-art equipment that often makes a critical difference in the success of prosecutions.

FNE Preparation and Certification

FNEs are generally skilled in either or both pediatric and adult sexual assault examinations. Education, experience, and training of the FNE are important considerations to the supervising forensic pathologist who will be relying on the nurse's testimony regarding the evaluation and documentation of trauma for courtroom presentation. In one such case in a federal court, the forensic pathologist testified regarding the autopsy and the FNE testified to injury specific to the sexual assault. When interviewed after the trial, the jury stated that it was the nurse's testimony and the photo-documentation that assisted them in clearly understanding the crucial circumstances of the rape/homicide case (Fig. 37-1). Credentialing has become an important aspect of qualifying as expert status in court testimony. However, few states had made provisions for credentialing sexual assault examiners who practice within their own jurisdiction. Recognizing the need for national certification, the International Association of Forensic Nurses launched a certification examination for sexual assault nurse examiners, which is anticipated to be a globally accepted credential for those who specialize in this field.

With the advent of the FNE as a specialist in sexual assault examinations, the US FBI CODIS Project recognized this registered nurse, qualified as an FNE skilled in the identification and documentation of sexual trauma, as the ideal clinician to provide the medical/forensic examination, collection of biological evidence and testify in court.

Best Practice *37-1*

The FNE, a registered nurse qualified in the identification and documentation of sexual trauma, should be selected to provide the medical/forensic examination and collect biological evidence in postmortem sex-related cases.

Postmortem Examination of Sexual Assault Victims

The criminal investigation of sexual homicide requires collaboration of several specialists to ensure a detailed analysis of the crime scene environs and the victim's body with emphasis on identification of the perpetrator. It is vital to link the clinical and criminal investigators at the onset of the investigation in order to maximize the effectiveness of their unique skills. Productive investigations are more likely to result when the clinical sexual assault investigator and criminal sexual assault detective work as a unit from the time the investigation is launched until the legal proceedings are finalized.

The ability to perform medical/legal examinations as soon as possible is paramount to successful outcomes. Autopsies may be conducted in various mortuaries instead of a central morgue; thus, the ideal system is a mobile unit, yet comprehensive enough to include all necessary adjunctive equipment required for the optimal examination. Along with recognition of the need for research in sexual homicide in particular and postmortem genital exams in general was the realization that successful study required a method that would bring equipment to where the body was located.

Although the FNE works in conjunction with the forensic pathologist when called to perform a postmortem examination for sexual assault, the FNE should be knowledgeable in the identification and interpretation of postmortem changes that occur in the body after death. This prevents misinterpreting a normal postmortem change for injury on the genitalia and anus of a sex-related homicide victim. Postmortem anal dilation is a common "normal" finding at autopsy but may be alarming to clinicians accustomed to examining live patients. FNEs must also remain aware of other conditions commonly confused with genital trauma by unskilled personnel (Henry, 2003).

The FNE should be fully informed regarding the circumstances surrounding the death as early as possible prior to the postmortem examination. This can be accomplished by talking with the investigating law enforcement agency, the medical death investigators, and the forensic pathologist. The identification of significant evidentiary injury and diagnosis of sexual abuse at autopsy may have serious implications for the criminal justice system, victim's families, and suspected offenders.

Henry indicates that postmortem examination for sexual assault is similar in both the living and the deceased. The following procedural details are essential to successful prosecutions. Begin the examination with the careful inspection of any clothing present on the body; inspect for defects in the garments and determine if those defects correspond to any wounds on the body (e.g., stabbing, gunshot wounds, strangulation). Photograph all clothing and visible trace evidence. Document and collect trace evidence from the clothing such as hairs, fibers, and debris *prior* to removal of the clothing from the body. Examine for additional trace evidence on the body after the clothing has been removed. As in a sexual assault examination of a living victim, the routine sexual assault evidence collection protocol should be followed:

- Collection of combed and pulled head and pubic hair samples
- Scraping and swabbing of the fingernails
- Use of an ultraviolet light source to identify fluorescence of possible body fluids
- Collection of oral swabs (including the lips)
- Flossing the teeth of the victim if feasible (this may increase the chance of collecting semen that may be present in the oral cavity)
- Swabbing of the breasts and any suspected bite marks
- Examination of the genitalia and anus using instrumentation (e.g., speculum, anoscope, colposcope)

Moving the trunk of the body to the end of the autopsy table will allow for better visualization of the genitalia and anus, thus making it easier to perform the speculum and anoscope examinations. Assistance is often required to hold the legs in a position so the colposcopic examination can be accomplished. Rigor mortis may need to be broken at the joints in order to complete the exam. With rigor mortis, the introitus and vaginal walls may not be as pliable, which occasionally makes speculum examinations difficult.

Henry has advised if the genital tissue is not displaying signs of decomposition or is in the early stages of decomposition, the FNE will be able to manipulate the genital and anal tissue as one would with a living victim without causing injury. The tissue is pale without the circulating blood. Genital and anal injuries such as redness and swelling that may be present in live victims are not apparent in the deceased. Lividity appears pink to red in the tissue and could be misinterpreted as bruising by an inexperienced examiner. Areas that are thought to be bruising can be incised to confirm extravasation of blood into the tissue. The anus is often gaping in both children and adults postmortem and should not be misinterpreted for sexual abuse or assault (Henry, 2002).

Adjunct Techniques for Evidentiary Examinations

Staining Procedures: Toluidine Blue

The use of toluidine blue dye can enhance the ability of FNEs to identify injury related to forced genital contact in both living and deceased victims. According to McCauley and colleagues (1987), the use of toluidine blue dye in adult women reporting sexual assault increased the incidence of positive findings of genital injury from 24% to 40% in one study (Lauber & Souma, 1982). In adolescents reporting sexual assault, positive findings increased from 4% to 28%, and in pediatric victims reporting sexual abuse the increase in positive findings was 16.5% to 33%. At autopsy, it is a preferred method to aid in the detection of genital and anal injuries due to child sexual abuse.

The application of TB dye should occur after the collection of external forensic evidence to avoid interference with laboratory evaluations for the presence of semen. It should only be utilized when the postmortem examination is done within a few hours after death and the victim's skin is relatively intact (Bays & Lewman, 1992). The following method of TB dye use has been employed to document genital and perineal lacerations following suspected sexual assault (Box 37-2).

Forensic nurses performing postmortem sexual assault examinations with the aid of toluidine blue must understand the following:

- A negative finding is indicated by no uptake or light, diffusely stippled uptake of dye
- A positive result is indicated by deep staining in skin defects (Bays & Lewman, 1992)

A 0.25% acetic acid solution works well to remove the toluidine blue dye in postmortem exams (Bays & Lewman, 1992). Reexamination of the tissue should be done after the speculum and anoscope removal to document tearing or sloughing of the

Box 37-2 Toluidine Blue (TB) Dye Application in the Sexual Assault Forensic Examination

PURPOSE

To aid in the detection and visualization of minor injury to the genital area that is not readily identified on inspection. This is a procedure for external use only. TB dye does not stain the surface layers of the skin but will dye nucleated squamous cells in the deeper layers of epidermis exposed by even superficial lacerations.

SUPPLIES

Toluidine blue dye 1% aqueous solution
Squirt bottle containing 1% acetic acid
Lubricating jelly
Cotton swabs
4 X 4 gauze

PROCEDURE

1. Collect all external genital specimens as indicated by history or examination prior to TB dye application and consider photodocumentation.
2. Prior to speculum examination or instrumentation to area, apply TB dye by using a sterile cotton swab to genital area in question (avoid inserting dye into vaginal vault).
3. Dye application may be used on the labia majora, labia minora, posterior fourchette, hymen, perineal body, and perianal area.
4. Allow to dry for approximately 1 minute.
5. Using spray bottle, gently, with broad spray, flood the area until excess TB dye is flushed away.
6. Gently blot the area with 4 X 4s. *Do not* rub the area.
7. Consider photodocumentation of area following TB dye application.

PATIENT TEACHING

Advise the living patient that small traces of TB dye may shed in the clothing over the next two days.

tissue, if present, that occurred during the speculum and anoscope exam. Vaginal, anal, and rectal swabs can be collected prior to, or at time of, the speculum and anoscope exam.

When analyzing and interpreting data derived from postmortem sexual assault examinations, limitations of the technique should be appreciated. Staining by toluidine blue merely indicates that the skin has been broken. Other causes of dye uptake may include, diaper dermatitis or vulvovaginal disease. The examiner must consider that certain injuries may have occurred before or during autopsy, and they are unrelated to sexual abuse. These may include fissures due to constipation, perirectal abscess, surgical procedures, maceration, insect damage, or accidental injury (Devine & Debich, 1990).

Augmented Visualization: Foley Catheter

The Foley catheter balloon technique is a primary method associated with the expansion of medical/forensic examination protocol in the living menarche and older patient and can have an important impact on the postmortem evaluation of female infants and adolescents. The sole purpose of this technique is to assist with the visualization of the estrogenized hymen in sexual assault/abuse victims. This technique was first introduced in menarche and older adolescent healthcare and was adapted to the evaluation of deceased victims by Ferrell (1995). This nurse examiner has been actively engaged in teaching physicians and nurses in the US, Canada, El Salvador, Honduras, South Africa, Zimbabwe, and Kosovo about the benefits of the Foley evaluation in sexual assault survivors and rape/homicides. When instructing forensic examiners, she has emphasized that as in the living, the Foley technique helps to ensure accuracy of examination findings which has a crucial impact on the judicial system (Bays & Jenny, 1990).

In a full-scale FNE program that evaluates patients of all ages for sexual assault, the examinations of children and adolescents are particularly challenging. For young girls and adolescents, the determination of whether there has been vaginal penetration invariably focuses on the hymen, which is not always easily or consistently addressed. The use of a little-known but effective technique used with adolescent patients helps FNEs to meet this challenge (Box 37-3) (Hazelwood & Burgess, 2001). For the purpose of this chapter, the term adolescent means any female patient who has begun her menses. At this level of development, patients are appropriate candidates for the Foley catheter balloon technique. Chronological age does not accurately reflect the developmental changes seen in the female external genitalia. Most of these changes are influenced by various levels of estrogen found in the female at different times of her infancy, childhood, and adolescence. Estrogen is present at birth in the female infant due to maternal estrogen effects and can continue to be present in the genital tissue up to two to four years old. This is demonstrated most often by small amounts of mucus and bloods being secreted vaginally into the diaper as maternal estrogen dissipates. Estrogen then returns at puberty and is demonstrated with the onset of menses. The effect of estrogen to the female genitalia has tremendous impact in the evaluation of sexual assault. With estrogen present, tissue is more elastic and not sensitive to touch. However, estrogen contributes to a hymenal enlargement that makes visualization quite difficult, thus making evaluation of the hymen at this stage more challenging than in the unestrogenized hymen. The sole benefit of the Foley catheter balloon technique is to evaluate the estrogenized hymen in the menarche and older female for the presence or absence of injury in the patient reporting sexual assault. This technique can provide an invaluable part of the genital examination in sexual assault evaluations. Variations of this technique are based on the visibility of acute injury and will differ within the living patient population and postmortem victim evaluation.

In the living patient population, the Foley catheter technique is reserved for the menarche age and older. It is *not* used in the living infant. The stage of menarche fluctuates by age and is further influenced by a range of variables. The onset of menses can begin at age 10 or earlier. In this patient population, the Foley catheter technique can prove to be beneficial for injury evaluation. Answers to the question "Is there injury present, and if so to what extent?" are best derived by use of the Foley catheter technique.

As with any sexual assault examination, all forensic specimens and culture specimens should be collected before the Foley technique is used. Numerous FNE programs have used this simple technique for adolescents, as well as other patients at different stages of maturity. It has become an invaluable diagnostic tool and has made other techniques of evaluating hymenal trauma in adolescents obsolete.

The comfort level of the clinician is accomplished by practicing this skill in her or his particular patient population to acquire competency with the technique itself as well as variations in the technique. Once competency is acquired, the Foley catheter balloon technique is a valuable examination tool and provides great precision in the medical/forensic sexual assault evaluation.

Box 37-3 Method of Examination

1. Select an indwelling Foley catheter, size 18F or larger with a 5-ml capacity balloon.
2. Collect a 60-ml syringe that will attach to the balloon pigtail.
3. Fill the syringe with 50 ml of air and test the integrity of the balloon before the examination.
4. Insert the Foley catheter into the vaginal vault to the point where the balloon is estimated to be midway in the vagina.
5. Inflate the balloon with 40 to 50 ml of air (not water, because water is so heavy it decreases the buoyancy of the balloon and thus decreases the visualization of the posterior hymen) or an amount that is comfortable for both the patient and examiner.
6. Insert the index finger and carefully guide the balloon to the hymen edge while tugging gently and carefully on the Foley catheter with the other hand. The hymen will be expanded to its full capacity and the edge of the hymen will be readily visualized for the presence or absence of signs of trauma.

From Hazelwood, R., & Burgess, A. W. (2001). *Practical aspects of rape investigation: A multidisciplinary approach* (3rd ed.). Boca Raton: CRC Press.

Fatal Child Abuse

The investigation of fatal child abuse requires the skills of a multidisciplinary team involving clinical experts in pediatric medicine, FNEs as clinical investigators, police department child protection units, sex crimes detectives, coroners and forensic pathologists who may also be members of the state and local child death review team. The use of toluidine blue dye, colposcope magnification, and alternate light source at autopsy indicates the mutual responsibility and benefit of collaboration between forensic nursing, forensic pathology, and criminal investigation.

A possible oversight by forensic pathologists can involve the definitive diagnosis of sexual assault in cases of fatal child abuse. Often, the prosecuting attorney is dependent on the autopsy report to provide the determination of sexual assault in order to ensure that appropriate charges are filed and to instill confidence in the jury and public that justice has been served. However, the forensic pathologist is often unable to confirm or rule out the presence of sexual assault without the utility of advanced techniques and scientific technology that is brought to the armamentarium of FNEs through highly specialized training, peer reviews, certification, and continuing education activities.

The statistical analysis of child sexual homicides perpetrated worldwide and investigated by FNEs and child protection agents in special law enforcement units will provide a greater understanding of the crime of child sexual/homicide, the victims, perpetrators, families, and commonalties among cases.

Key Point *37-1*

The infant victim is likely to have a history of physical abuse, exhibit colic-like behavior, and other symptoms of neglect. The caretaker-perpetrator in these types of cases is most likely the biological father or the substitute father figure.

Case Study 37-1 Postmortem Sodomy of a Four-Year-Old

A four-year-old male examined three days postmortem presented with ligature marks around the neck and left ankle and with feces smeared around the anus, perineum, and inside of right thigh. His anus was gaping open, and two small lacerations were visible at the anal verge. No mucosal tears or bleeding were present. After dissecting out the anus and lower rectum, colposcope examination identified three lacerations at the anal verge. With the application of toluidine blue dye, more than 15 lacerations became visible. The presence of multiple injuries at the anal verge without mucosal hemorrhage indicated that sodomy had occurred postmortem, which was later confirmed by the subsequent confession of the perpetrator.

Case Study 37-2 Sexual Assault and Suffocation

A three-month-old female infant was examined in the ED as a suspected SIDS case. The staff became suspicious after they noticed blood and apparent injuries around the anus. Roentgenograms of the body revealed a healing fracture of the left tibia, and birth records revealed positive urinary toxicologic findings for cocaine and methamphetamines. Several tears noted around the anus where toluidine blue was utilized indicated deep staining at regular intervals. The dye also identified a previously undetected tear of the anterior frenulum of the labia minora and a stippled pattern of staining at the posterior fourchette and midline of the perineal body. Forensic specimens showed no evidence of semen; rather the injuries were determined to be by sexual penetration with a foreign object. The cause of death was suspected to be suffocation.

Clinical Research in Sex-Related Homicides

Research in postmortem examination and genital anatomy, presented at the 2001 Meeting of the American Academy of Forensic Sciences by Sharon Crowley, a forensic clinical nurse specialist in Santa Cruz, California, represents one of the leading research projects in the field. Often, one of the most complicated decisions for forensic pathologists is to determine whether or not the decedent has been sexually assaulted (prior to or after death). The fact alone that sexual assault occurred will contribute to the charges filed against the suspect. This information is critical to the district attorney as well as to the public or private defense attorney. Because the question at hand is critical to the outcome of the trial, absolute accuracy is essential. However, for many years, the US FBI did not keep separate statistics that differentiated between rape and rape homicide. During early periods of research in the behavioral sciences, all homicides were simply categorized as homicides, with no differentiation as to specifics of sexual motivation. As knowledge related to patterns and motives of sexual homicide developed, the awareness of the necessity of identifying the psychological profile of the sexual sadist and other sexually motivated deaths became indispensable data to the FBI. Furthermore, it is known among those who specialize in sexual assault evaluations that it is often difficult to document physical finding regardless of the extent of sexual contact. Therefore, prosecutors, specifically, must be confident in the data they present in order to provide equal justice. The FBI statistics indicate that 37% of those accused of rape are exonerated by DNA evidence. With this in mind, FNEs, as experts in sexual assault examination, are charged with accountability for the evidence and documentation they provide.

Crowley's research, initiated in 1995, described the salient findings accumulated during the clinical adaptation of sexual homicide. The purpose of this initial research was to study the nature and pattern of genital trauma in sexual homicide victims. The successful finding in this study has led to further research in other important areas adjunct to the postmortem genital examination. This includes the study of a system of mobile technology that augments the exam in multiple settings, such as central morgues and independent mortuaries. The value of colposcopy and colposcopic photography as an integral component of the postmortem genital examination cannot be undervalued. The development of a sequential methodology for the genital examination of the sexual homicide victim is essential in the collection of evidence and photodocumentation. The salient tenets of published clinical research on genital trauma in living sexual assault victims allows for the comparison and contrast findings with a control group of women who engaged in consensual sexual activity. They include both genders and all age-groups.

Previous research described the patterns of genital trauma in living female sexual assault victims that were examined with colposcope (Slaughter, Brown, & Carl et al., 1997). During the autopsy, gross visualization alone may preclude the detection of the more subtle characteristic injuries usually found in sexual assault victims–namely, tears/lacerations, ecchymosis, microabrasions, redness, and swelling (TEARS acronym). This may explain the paucity of physical findings traditionally found on genital examinations of deceased victims. The magnification and photographic capability of the colposcope not only enhances visualization, but also provides a mechanism of photodocumentation of the evidentiary examination and provides important material for peer review.

By 2002, the value of Crowley's research had been well recognized by the multidisciplinary team of investigators, forensic pathologists, and prosecutors who rely on current developments and data applicable to sexual homicide. Collaboration of an FNE with a criminal investigative analyst illustrates the complementary nature of the two disciplines during the investigation of sexual homicides (Devine & Debich, 1990).

A sequential methodology for the examination of sexual homicide victims (Ferrell, personal communication, 2002) was developed to respond to the need for a systematic approach to the genital examination of deceased sexual homicide victims (Micromedex, 1998). Crowley's protocol, which incorporated colposcopic magnification, was refined and other aspects were expanded. These included the collaborative role of the FNE and the forensic pathologist and the use of reflective and fluorescent imaging, integrating the sexual homicide database (Ferrell, 2002).

According to Crowley, the use of the colposcope in examining the living sexual assault victim is well established. Patterns of injury have been described and compared to a control group of women who engaged in consensual sex (Crowley, 1999). Prior to the incorporation of the colposcope in the evaluation of living sexual assault victims, traditional methods of exam yielded a paucity of physical findings (10% to 30%). Similarly, during the autopsy, gross visualization alone may not allow detection of the more subtle findings that usually constitute genital trauma during sexual assault. The colposcope affords both magnification and photographic capability. This enhances visualization, provides photodocumentation, and makes peer review possible. Higher magnification makes it feasible to study the effects of the postmortem interval and other factors on the anogenital tissue.

Key Point *37-2*

During autopsy, gross visualization alone may not allow detection of the more subtle findings that usually constitute genital trauma during sexual assault; colposcopic augmentation affords improved visualization, magnification, and photographic capability.

Research Methodology Used by Crowley

Crowley's research involved a study of 18 deceased patients (15 female, 3 male). These subjects were evaluated using a protocol involving the colposcope. Causes of death included suicide, accidental, and natural. All cases were examined using the mobile system of technology described by Crowley et al. (2000). Examinations were done in collaboration with Brian Peterson of the Forensic Medical Group, Inc., of Fairfield, California. Photographs were available for review on 10 cases, all female, in this group; the ages ranged from 6 years to 72 years old with a mean of 48.8 years. The postmortem interval varied from less than 24 hours to several days with active decay. All but one of the cases were examined with the colposcope, using a fixed magnification of either 7.5X or 15X. In most cases, photographs were also obtained using a 35-mm SLR camera, for comparison with colposcopic images. Two cases were documented only with macrophotography. The cases were assigned an identification number and entered into a modified version of the Sexual Homicide Database (Crowley & Prodan, 1996). Data included the age, ethnicity, race, date of exam, postmortem interval, cause of death, major medical conditions, reproductive status, known gynecological history, gross nongenital trauma, and exam technique. Eleven anatomical sites were included for review. These included the labia majora, labia minora, periurethral area, posterior fourchette, fossa navicularis, hymen, vagina, cervix, perineum, anus, and rectum. The nature and pattern of postmortem genital findings are described in a manner consistent with conventional design (i.e., sharp versus blunt force). The database provides a conceptual framework in which to analyze and categorize postmortem findings. This will eventually facilitate comparisons to the anogenital physical characteristics in sexual homicide victims.

Best Practice *37-2*

Postmortem sexual assault examinations should be performed with the benefit of binocular microscopy and sequenced photography to document the presence or absence of genital or other injuries.

FNE Protocol Requested by Coroner

Suspected rape/homicide examinations are being referred to FNEs with increasing frequency as forensic pathologists and coroners are becoming aware of this option. Because many forensic nurses have not yet participated in postmortem sexual assault examinations, their initial reaction and response may be one of concern. These concerns are valid, and one should be prepared for such an event in order to provide the quality of injury identification and recovery of evidence expected to confirm or rule out criminality in a court of law.

Recognition of the FNE's Role

Paul Jones, assistant coroner for Richland County, Ohio, contacted FNE Roe on a Sunday afternoon regarding the investigation of the death of a 26-year-old female. The history given by others present indicated that in the early morning hours of a party, the patient or victim became unresponsive and began shaking. Three men had offered to take her into a room and take care of her–alone. At approximately 11 a.m. Saturday morning, party members noticed that she was having trouble breathing and placed a call to 911. She was admitted to the emergency department (ED) and promptly intubated and cared for, but no toxicology evidence was collected at that time. She was pronounced dead later that evening from a subdural hematoma. Coroner Paul Jones was called in at the time of her death. Upon a review of the history, and as a great supporter of sexual assault nurse examiners, he contacted the prosecuting attorney for Richland County and requested to have a sexual assault examination with evidence collection performed. (See Box 37-4.)

Box 37-4 Perspectives of a Forensic Nurse Examiner: Teresa Roe

Having never participated in the examination of a rape/homicide case, I was initially overwhelmed, challenged, and then honored when Coroner Paul Jones requested the forensic services of our sexual assault nurse examiner team. I had never given thought to examining a deceased patient. I didn't know if there were legal ramifications to consider since the decedent was in the hospital morgue. I didn't know if there was any special education needed to examine a deceased patient. I contacted the ED nurse manager who gave me full support and advised me to contact the director of nursing (DON). The DON was also encouraging as I related my concerns. She provided her full support and praised our team for the opportunity. As I thought about the exam, I knew the SANE exam should not deviate from the International Association of Forensic Nursing SANE standards for a living patient, but that I would obviously proceed with special considerations.

Outcome Analysis

The body was taken to the forensic pathologist the next day for autopsy. The pathologist was impressed at the extent of the examination, the use of TB dye, and colposcopic photography. The pathologist further stated that if the routine procedure done at autopsy were used, the extent of the sexual assault exam and evidence collection would have only consisted of vaginal swabs after gross visualization. Coroner Paul Jones expressed confidence in his decision to include the sexual assault nurse examiner team during his investigation. Jones believed the specifics of this examination "helped to tell the story that the victim couldn't tell."

Rape-Homicide Investigations and the FNE

The sexual assault nurse examiner who works with living patients may have some reservations about assuming a role that extends to the deceased. However, the evidence gathered in these latter cases is no less important to law enforcement or the judicial system. Sexual assault nurse examiners who routinely perform postmortem evidentiary examinations offer some helpful tips for working with the deceased victim.

Procedural Tips for Beginning Postmortem Examiners

- Initially it may be difficult to touch and move the body. It can be surprising how coldness and rigor mortis impact the procedure.
- A full body scan should be performed with a Wood's lamp. Carefully examine the hair for fibers.
- If areas of hair are clumped together, carefully cut the locks of hair containing the unidentified substance. It could be electrode paste or semen deposits.
- A tongue ring often has a considerable amount of debris lodged underneath. First swab around it carefully, remove the tongue ring (with assistance) by prying the mouth open just enough to remove the jewelry.
- Check to see if the posterior body surface displays postmortem lividity. Note and distinguish between bruising acquired prior to the incident and bruises noted from IV attempts. Follow strict forensic documentation, noting the exact location, size, and description of each bruise, laceration, or cut. The forensic pathologist will determine the age of the injury.
- The examination of the genitalia includes detailed assessment, external swabbings, toluidine blue (TB) dye, and an internal speculum examination. Positioning of the body for colposcope/genital examination is often a challenge. The labia majora can be discolored due to postmortem changes.
- If a laceration (tear) is observed during inspection with the colposcope, obtain swabs and apply TB dye.
- The TB dye should be applied prior to insertion of the speculum to ensure no injury was caused during the examination due to the loss of skin pliability. Because of the loss of skin elasticity, the Foley catheter technique may not be used.
- If unable to position the patient at the foot of the table, insert the speculum upside down in the vaginal vault, as this eliminates the difficulty of the handle resting on the table.
- Cervical changes are apparent at the postmortem examination. The cervix changes from a full, thick, pink appearance to bluish and creased from the loss of circulating blood.
- Insert 3 cc distilled water into the vaginal vault; collect evidence using a pipette.
- The inner thighs should be inspected again after completion of the exam to ensure that no tissue damage occurred as a result of the abduction of the legs.

Collaboration with Forensic Pathologists

In response to a query regarding the use of FNEs to provide the documentation of injury and collection of evidence in rape/homicide cases, Dr. M. G. F. Gilliland, a regional forensic pathologist of the North Carolina state medical examiner system, stated:

> *As a forensic pathologist I would be very pleased to have additional competent individuals involved in the gathering of time-critical evidence. Persons with specialized training in such evidence collection in the living could be of great assistance to the investigators, pathologists, litigators, and triers-of-fact.*
>
> *As long as we are all working together to gather information, establish the truth, convey it clearly and neutrally, we should be able to do some good for victims and for suspects. (Lynch, personal communication, 2000)*

Future of Postmortem Forensic Analysis

Problems relating to sexual assault are multiple and diverse. As society has sought to strike a balance between the rights of the accused and the rights of the victims, the role of the FNE is becoming important to the police, prosecutors, public and private defenders, victim assistance programs, the victim, and the accused. The effectiveness of the FNE is reflected in their research and practice involving complex sexual crimes, which can enhance the outcome of sexual offense investigations involving the health and justice systems. The FNE can be a powerful tool in the multidisciplinary team approach to reducing and preventing sexual crimes against persons. Increased integration and support of these programs by the law enforcement community are the keys to progressive intervention and continued success of investigations. Although legal and social reforms have been slow in coming, the disciplines of forensic science, nursing science, and criminal justice have made a global commitment to combine their skills and efforts in a mutual responsibility to this cause.

The goals of forensic nursing specialists involved in sexual assault care and the scientific investigation of death are as follows:

- To provide a comprehensive overview of knowledge involving sexual assault in the living and the deceased subject
- To educate the forensic healthcare community regarding the incidence and prevalence of traumatic victimization in the pediatric and adult population by sexual homicides

A combination of both areas of expertise is interdependent on the research, technique, method of documentation, and the skills of the specific examiner/investigator and the clinical and criminal analyst. Working in unison will provide a greater response from the criminal justice and healthcare system involving the crime characteristics of the offenders, victims, and the scene of crime. Past attention to the social/sexual crimes of the twentieth century identified an existing gap in continuity of care between the healthcare institution, the police, and the medical examiner/coroner's systems. Significant to the resources are the forensic nursing researcher, educator, clinician, and policymaker who commit their knowledge of forensic skills in the living to assist the deceased victim through a scientific approach to the reduction of sexual violence.

Summary

Among the primary principles and philosophies of forensic medicine is the concept that the investigation of death is for the benefit of the living: the public's right to know, the family's right to know, and the administration of justice. Prevention is the underlying motivation of those who investigate death. This *prevention philosophy* has also been adopted by the science of forensic nursing. As in any clinical evaluation, one must first know and understand the normal in order to identify the abnormal. In the same sense, one must know and understand the anatomy of the living in order to apply the principles and standards of clinical evaluation to the decedent. This is especially applicable in the examination, evaluation, and documentation of sexual assault crimes. When the patient cannot speak for himself or herself, whether nonverbal infants or deceased victims, the skill and expertise of the forensic nurse examiner will speak for the victim.

Case Study 37-3 The Foley Catheter in Use

In the deceased patient, the Foley catheter balloon technique also serves as a valuable tool to assess the hymen of the infant and young child where estrogen is present (a residual of maternal estrogen) prior to autopsy.

History

A three-month-old female patient presented with no pulse or respirations. Full resuscitation efforts were in progress by the paramedics. No history was presented other than that the infant was found lifeless in its crib. Upon arrival to the emergency department, the infant was pronounced dead. One of several concerns upon examination was the ecchymotic labia minora. After consultation with the medical examiner's office, a sexual assault evaluation was requested prior to autopsy.

Examination

During the postmortem evaluation, after specimen collection, the Foley catheter balloon technique is demonstrated on this three-month-old infant (Fig. 37-2a).

In a nonesterogenized deceased infant or child, this technique is not necessary due to the absence of estrogen and the tissue tension that occurs with application of the traction technique. Under these conditions, a clear view of the hymenal edge is readily observed.

Once again, the steps of evaluation begin with inspection of external female genitalia, progressing to separation of the labia majora, then separation of the labia minora (Fig. 37-2b).

Oftentimes, the examination would end at this point due to the "closed or intact" appearance of the hymen as perceived by the inexperienced or ineffectual practitioner. The examination should continue with the *traction technique* in order to evaluate the edge of the hymen or rim of the hymen tissue. In the evaluation of a child, *traction* is accomplished by gently tunneling the tissue of the labia majora outward toward the clinician. As Figure 37-2 shows, the rim of the hymen has very pronounced projections with an obvious opening (Fig. 37-2c).

Due to the postmortem state of the infant, this provides the opportunity to use the Foley catheter balloon technique to clearly answer the question "Is there presence of well-healed tears?" or "Due to estrogen, is this a hymen with prominent projections whose appearance will smooth out with stretching?"

A 12 French Foley catheter is then inserted just past the hymen and inflated with 30 cc of air. Visualized in Figure 37-2d, the projections smooth out, and the examiners unquestionably conclude that the projections were not caused by injury. The hymen viewed has no injury present.

Resources

Books

American College of Emergency Physicians. (1999). *Handbook on evaluation and management of sexually assaulted or sexually abused patients.* Dallas: Author.

Burgess, A. W. (1984). *Child pornography and sex rings.* Lanham, MD: Lexington Books.

Davies, M. (1996). *Women and violence.* Atlantic Highlands, NJ: Zed Books.

Hazelwood, R., & Burgess, A. W. (2001). *Practical aspects of rape investigation: A multidisciplinary approach* (3rd ed.). Boca Raton, FL: CRC Press.

Girardin, B., Faugno, D., Seneski, P., et al. (1997). *Color atlas of sexual assault.* St. Louis, MO: Mosby.

Articles

Dietz., P. E., Hazelwood, R. R., & Warren, J. J. (1990). The sexually sadistic criminal and his offenses. *Bull Am Acad Psych Law, 18*(2), 163-178.

Organizations

International Society for Prevention of Child Abuse and Neglect

245 West Roosevelt Road, Building 6, Suite 39, Chicago, IL 60601; Tel: 630-876-6913; www.ispcan.org

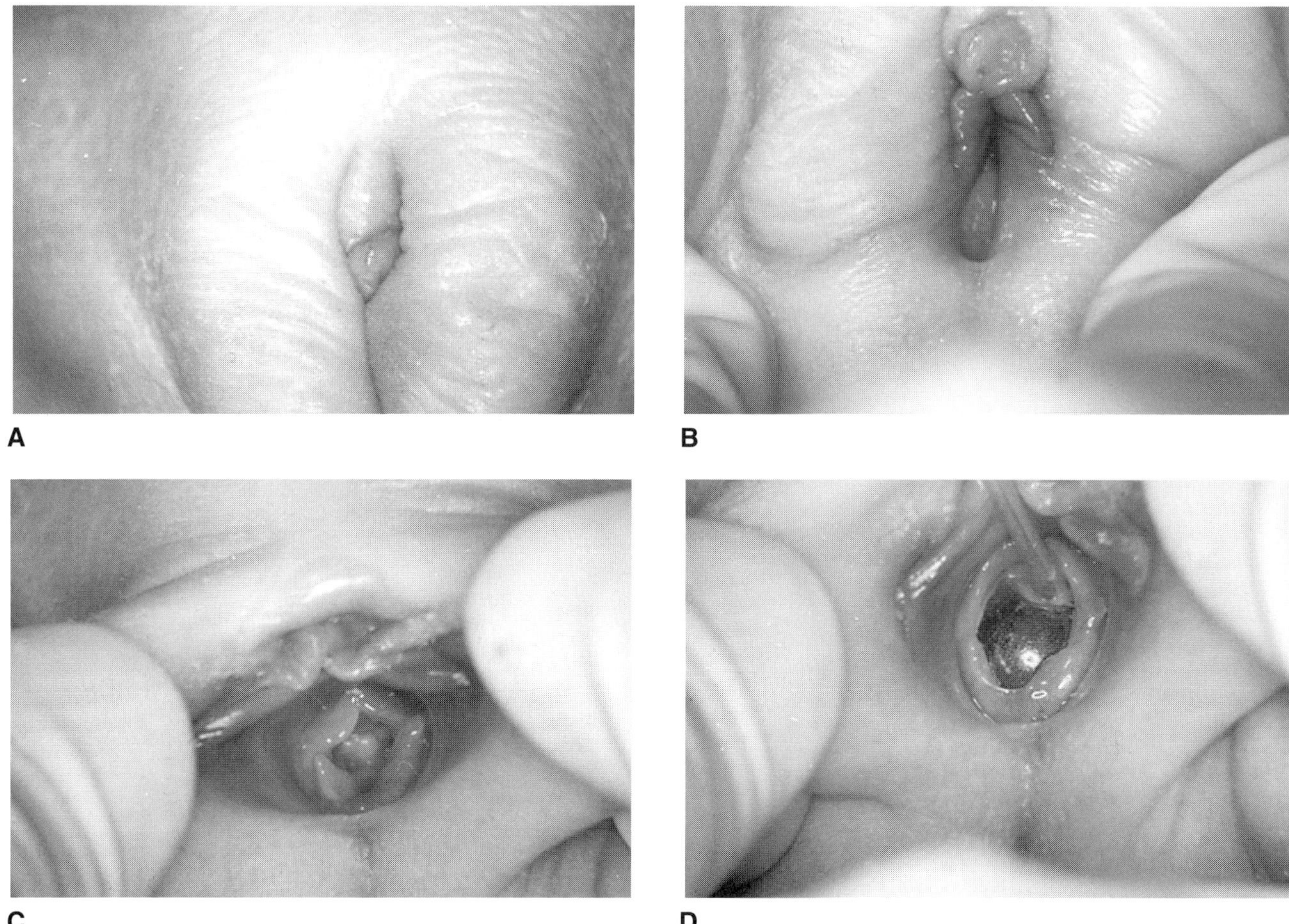

Fig. 37-2 *A,* 3-month-old postmortem infant evaluation; inspection of external female genitalia. *B,* 3-month-old postmortem infant evaluation; separation of the *labia majora* and *minora* providing visualization of the hymen tissue. *C,* 3-month-old postmortem infant evaluation demonstrating use of the traction technique by gently tunneling the *labia majora* tissue in order to provide evaluation of the rim of the hymen tissue. As visualized, the rim of the hymen has very pronounced projections with an obvious opening. *D,* 3-month-old postmortem infant evaluation. An uninflated 12 French Foley catheter inserted past the hymen and inflated with 30 cc of air. As visualized here, the projections smooth out and the hymen has no injury present. The Foley technique is only to be used in the living child after menarche age.

National Center for Missing and Exploited Children

Charles B. Wang International Children's Building, 669 Prince Street, Alexandria, VA 22314; Tel: 703-274-3900, 800-THE-LOST; www.missingkids.com

Web Sites

American Academy of Forensic Sciences (AAFS)

www.aafs.org

American Academy of Pediatrics

www.aap.org

American Professional Society on the Abuse of Children

www.apsac.org

International Association of Forensic Nurses

www.forensicnurse.org

National Center for Victims of Crime

www.ncvc.org

References

Bays, J., & Jenny, C. (1990). Genital and anal conditions confused with child sexual abuse trauma. *Am J Dis Child, 144,* 1319-1322.

Bays, J., & Lewman, L. (1992). Toluidine blue in the detection at autopsy of perineal and anal lacerations in victims of sexual abuse. *Archives Pathol Lab Med, 116,* 620-621.

Crowley, S., Barsley, R., Peterson, B., et al. (2000, February 21-26). Proceedings of the American Academy of Forensic Sciences, Reno, NV.

Crowley, S. (1999). *Sexual assault: the medical-legal examination.* Stamford, CT: Appleton & Lange.

Devine, W. A., & Debich, D. E. (1990). Damage to the head and neck of infants at autopsy. *Pediatr Pathol, 10,* 475-478.

Ferrell, J. J. (1995) Foley catheter balloon technique for visualizing the hymen in female adolescent sexual abuse victims. *J Emerg Nurs, 2,* 585-586.

Ferrell, J. J. Personal communication, April 2002.

Hazelwood, R., Dietz, P., & Warren, J. (2001). The Criminal Sexual Sadist. In Hazelwood, R., & Burgess, A.W. (2001) *Practical aspects of rape investigation: A multidisciplinary approach* (3rd ed.). Boca Raton, FL: CRC Press.

Hazelwood, R., & Burgess, A. W. (2001). *Practical aspects of rape investigation: A multidisciplinary approach* (3rd ed.). Boca Raton, FL: CRC Press.

Lauber A., & Souma G. (1982). Use of toluidine blue for documentation of traumatic intercourse. *Obstet Gynecol, 60,* 644-648.

McCauley, J., Guzinski, G., Welch, R., et al. (1987). Toluidine blue in the corroboration of rape in the adult victim. *Am J Emerg Med, 5*(2), 105-108.

Micromedex, Inc. (1998). *Volume 95: Tolonium-toxicologic managements.* Engelwood, CO: Author.

Slaughter, L., & Brown, C. (1992). Colposcopy to establish physical findings in rape victims. *Am J Obstet Gynecol, 166*(1), 83-86.

Slaughter, L., Brown, C., Crowley, S., et al. (1997). Patterns of genital injury in female sexual assault victims. *Am J Obstet Gynecol, 176*(3), 609-616.

Von Krafft-Ebing, R. (1892, 1998). *Psychopathia sexualis.* New York: Arcade.

Chapter 38 Taphonomy and NecroSearch

John R. McPhail

Science of Taphonomy

Taphonomy is the study of the fate of human remains after death (Haglund and Sorg, 1997). A vivid imagination is required to entertain all of the physical, environmental, and circumstantial possibilities that might alter a body that has been hastily abandoned in the woods or buried in a shallow grave as opposed to one that received a contemporary burial when the body is carefully prepared, perhaps embalmed, protected in a sealed casket and vault, and placed into the ground or mausoleum crypt. Without today's funerary expertise, some ancient cultures had developed techniques to mummify and preserve human remains. When Egypt's King Tutankhamen's tomb was opened in 1923, scientists were amazed at the excellent state of his body, which had been encrypted since 1343 B.C. Another example is the "Ice Man" found in the Alps in 1991. The body, its clothing, and its associated artifacts have provided a fascinating glimpse into the Neolithic period, 5300 years ago (Spindler, 1994). These landmark cases and others emphasize the many factors that determine the fate of human remains and how the burial site itself interacts with the body. As Haglund notes, at clandestine grave sites, the body influences the surroundings as much as the surroundings influence what happens to the body (James & Nordby, 2005). This dynamic interaction can assist medical death investigators in determining when the body was deposited at a given location and whether or not it has been moved, be it by criminal design or by the acts of nature, animal scavengers, or other natural forces.

Taphonomy in the Forensic Context

Taphonomy was developed within the disciplines of paleontology, archaeology, and paleoanthropology (Haglund & Sorg, 1997). Forensic taphonomy focuses on reconstructing events at and following death. This is done through collection and analysis of data, distinguishing peri- and postmortem alteration of remains, estimating how long the remains have been at the site, and estimating time of death. In this way, forensics differs from and extends the reach of taphonomy (Box 38-1).

Consulting Scientists in Death Investigation

Several types of scientists may be enlisted to assist the forensic medical examiner in determining the cause and manner of death when the death has been recent and the identity of the individual is known. However, when a partially decomposed body or skeletal remains are discovered in a remote area or at a clandestine grave site, new questions arise that mandate the use of additional experts, including forensic anthropologists, archaeologists, botanists, naturalists, and climatologists. Anthropologists can be very helpful in answering certain questions, such as:

- Are the bones from an animal or a human?
- If human, what is the approximate age, race, gender, and stature of the individual?
- Have scavenging animals disarticulated the body or damaged bones?
- If there are defects in the body assemblage, were they caused by premortem or postmortem events?
- What effects have plants, animals, weather, and climate had on the body over time?

In some instances, archaeologists will be involved in distinguishing contemporary burials from ancient ones. When the geological period of the burial site is in question, paleontologists are consulted. Botanists, naturalists, climatologists, and geologists can also help to answer many questions for forensic death investigators.

Taphonomy Research

The practice domain of those interested in taphonomy is diverse. Understandably, laws, ethics, social customs, emotions, taboos, and legislation largely prohibit the inquiry into how a human body deteriorates or responds to the elements in a given physical area after death. Scientists cannot merely deposit human remains in various locations or subject such human remains to a specified set of conditions to learn more about these factors. A majority of what has been learned thus far has been gleaned from research work accomplished at Indian burial sites, battlegrounds, and other mass grave areas in the US. These studies have resulted in valuable insights into pre-, peri-, and postmortem conditions of those individuals and in some instances were able to identify the victim and provide clues regarding the biomechanical injury forces or disease factors contributing to the death. Recently, the trend to limit studies on ancient Indian burial grounds and to repatriate the remains of these Native Americans has curtailed the work of some researchers working at such sites.

Known Grave Sites

When burial grounds and cemeteries are relocated to make way for construction or contemporary land uses, scientists gain a fair appreciation of the impact of time and other factors on the traditionally buried body, embalmed and unembalmed. It is well known that the type of casket and vault containment alters the rate and degree of decomposition as well as how water, weather, and long-term climate conditions affect body tissue preservation, breakdown, and dispersal (Box 38-2). Although this information is of interest to those who exhume bodies for forensic purposes, it has limited value for taphonomists who tend to concentrate on clandestine burial locations. However, when forensic personnel encounter bodies of unknown origin, certain known characteristics can be used to distinguish cemetery findings that may have been "unearthed" by accident or vandalism from other remains. Remnants of caskets, clothing, artifacts, and embalmed tissue are useful markers to corroborate that the body originated from a cemetery (Berryman, 1997).

Box 38-1 Forensics and Taphonomy

Forensic work extends the reach of taphonomy in several key ways:

- The forensic investigator concentrates on the process immediately surrounding death and the postmortem timeline, which can be days to years. Death investigation concentrates on estimating time of death and whether events happened before, during, or after death. This timeline is different from those used by paleontologists and archaeologists.
- Forensics focuses on the closest period of corpse transformation. In addition, greater emphasis is placed on soft-tissue changes as part of decomposition.
- Forensic concerns are at the individual level, where the taphonomist may focus on populations of organisms.
- Forensic investigation has multijurisdictional concerns and potential medicolegal consequences with matters such as chain of custody and testimony.

Data from Haglund, W. D., & Sorg, M. H. (1997). Method and theory of forensic taphonomy and research. In W. D. Haglund and M. H. Sorg, *Forensic taphonomy: The postmortem fate of human remains* (p. 14). Boca Raton, FL: CRC Press.

Box 38-2 Order of Tissue Decomposition

1. Intestines, stomach, accessory organs of digestion, heart, blood and circulation, heart muscle
2. Air passages and lungs
3. Kidneys and bladder
4. Brain and nervous tissue
5. Skeletal muscles
6. Connective tissues and integument

Data from Gill-King, H. (1997). Chemical and ultrastructural aspects of decomposition. In W. D. Haglund and M. H. Sorg, *Forensic taphonomy: The postmortem fate of human remains* (Pp. 97-98). Boca Raton, FL: CRC Press.

Other Body Sources

Human remains are periodically discovered in remote locations such as in fields, forests, and deserts and in or near bodies of water. Each of these sites is likely to produce important information regarding the length of time since death and how body decomposition and dispersal has been affected by the unique environmental characteristics of each locale. Water is a prime example of a variable that provides vital information to the forensic team. Is the body in question one that was deposited at the site of its finding, or was it transported over great distance to the site by a flowing body of water or tidal washing onto a beach? Could the body have been washed ashore after a legitimate, recorded burial at sea, or did an individual attempt to illegally deposit the human remains in a large body of water, trusting that it would never be seen again (Box 38-3)? Is trauma on the body the result of premortem impacts, or did the remains strike rocks and other objects while beingswept downstream, creating soft-tissue and skeletal defects? Have the remains been scavenged by marine life such as sharks, or are arms and legs missing as a result of premortem events? There is considerable and well-researched information regarding the effects of water sources on human remains. Among these are observations that contribute to the taphonomist's understanding of findings. Transport time and distance can vary widely, by days and months and hundreds of miles, based on whether the body is submerged or partially floating at times. Bodies disarticulate with marine scavenging and mechanical impacts; therefore, body parts may be discovered in separate and distinct locations, often great distances from one another. The biochemical contents of water, the presence of silt or sediment, and the general river-bottom morphology affect water flow currents and thus the transport of human remains over areas and distances. Even the size and density of the body can influence how easily it surfaces and how much resistance is imposed in transit (Nawrocki, Pless, & Dawley et al., 1997).

Box 38-3 Factors That May Indicate a Bona Fide Burial at Sea

- Remains in a canvas body bag and chain mesh (as recommended by the Environmental Protection Agency)
- Evidence of an autopsy (e.g., Y-shaped incision, removal of internal organs)
- Applications of mortuary techniques (e.g., eye caps, wiring of the jaws, formalin)
- Unexpected combination of postmortem changes in the remains (e.g., bones that are eroded but have no tooth marks or crushing features, suggesting the remains were tumbling or dragging on the ocean floor)
- Presence of an urn

Data from Haglund, W.D., & Sorg, M. H. Method and theory of forensic taphonomy and research. In W. D. Haglund and M. H. Sorg, *Forensic taphonomy: The postmortem fate of human remains* (Pp.620-621). Boca Raton, FL: CRC Press.

Mountains, glaciers, deserts, rain forests, and farm fields are other places human remains may be encountered, and it is imperative to answer questions about what happened to the body prior to death, at the time of death, and after the remains ultimately reached a final resting place. The taphonomist, working with other forensic investigators, is better able to answer these questions after having studied similar scenarios where known characteristics can be matched. However, it must be appreciated that some of these case findings are so unique that little or no prior information is known about the normal processes of decomposition and disarticulation in that given location. The increasing importance of such knowledge was the stimulus for the origination of the NecroSearch project, formed to find such answers through scientific inquiry using swine models.

NecroSearch

NecroSearch International, Inc., is a nonprofit, volunteer organization dedicated to research, education, and investigation in the location of clandestine graves, the recovery of the remains, and the investigation of associated evidence in and around the graves (France, Griffin, & Swanburg et al., 1997). Volunteers consist of individuals from law enforcement, investigations, serology and chemistry, forensic nursing, forensic anthropology, archaeology, entomology, geology, pedology, geophysics, geochemistry, petrology, photography and aerial photography, thermal imagery, meteorology, botany, wildlife biology, and criminal psychology. Naturalists and computer data analysts are other valuable personnel associated with the project. Scent-detecting dogs and their handlers, as well as other outside resources, may be obtained as needed in certain phases of the project studies.

History

The concept of utilizing scientific techniques in locating clandestine graves originated in 1987 by a group of law enforcement investigators and scientists who were frustrated by conventional grave location methods such as large-scale ground searches and trial-and-error excavations employing heavy equipment (France, Griffin, & Swanburg et al., 1992; Haglund, Reichert, & Reay et al., 1990; Imaizumi, 1974). In 1986, law enforcement originated a search on a 2200-acre ranch located approximately 30 miles west of the Kansas border near Stratton, Colorado. According to information provided by an informant, up to a dozen bodies had been buried in an area of several square kilometers over the course of several years. A total of three bodies were unearthed and recovered through the use of backhoes, which unfortunately destroyed not only the crime scene but also much of the evidence. The remaining area was then arbitrarily trenched and plowed as investigators searched for further remains but turned up none. Due to the destructive and intrusive methods used in the search, further detection utilizing scientific methods proved ineffective. It was then and is still believed that additional bodies remain undiscovered on the property.

Because of the limitations found with traditional methods in the location and excavation of clandestine graves, the basis of the NecroSearch research began with Project PIG ("Pigs in Ground"). In 1988, a study of the relationships between buried pig carcasses and their surroundings was implemented utilizing various techniques from the scientific community and applying the results to actual cases of buried human remains. The multidisciplinary project involved law enforcement agencies, scientists, private businesses, and academicians (France, Griffin, & Swanburg et al., 1992). The information gained in this research had traditionally been obtained separately if at all. It should be noted that there is no singular technology that can determine if a body is buried beneath the surface; however, a compilation of all the techniques can identify a particular site or number of sites that are the most likely to be the location of a clandestine grave. In the same vein, compiling these techniques may also determine that there are no disturbances beneath the surface in a given area, saving time and unnecessary excavations (Hoving, 1986; Killam, 1989).

Key Point *38-1*

Success is not always measured in recovery of remains, but sometimes in knowing where not to dig.

Research Strategy

Pigs were originally used for burial at the research site, and they continue to be used for the following reasons. First, Colorado law does not allow human cadavers to be used for these types of studies. Second, pigs have a fat-to-muscle ratio similar to humans, and their skin is not heavily haired. The pigs used in this research were similar to humans in weight (70 kg/154 pounds), although some smaller pigs were included to simulate bodies of different ages or sizes. Third, pigs have been previously used in studies of patterns and rates of decay and scavenging because they have been considered to be similar to humans biochemically as well as physiologically.

The site of the original NecroSearch project was approximately 20 miles south of Denver, Colorado, on the Highlands Ranch Law Enforcement Training Facility property. The site was selected because it offered proximity to human and physical resources and yet had strict operating procedures and security barriers to control public access. Baseline data, including a series of black-and-white aerial photographs, geophysical measurements, and environmental observations of the site were carefully recorded before the burial of the first pig (Figs. 38-1 and 38-2). Aerial photography is the least destructive method, as it is virtually nonintrusive. It provides an excellent characterization of a particular site, including the access, culture, drainage, and topography. In addition, an extremely large area can be covered in a relatively short time. Preburial photographs may be available from a variety of sources including the US Geological Survey (USGS), county planning boards, utility companies, and railroads.

Best Practice *38-1*

Forensic death investigators should consider using dogs trained in finding pig remains when attempting to locate human remains because human remains are similar biochemically and physiologically to those of pigs.

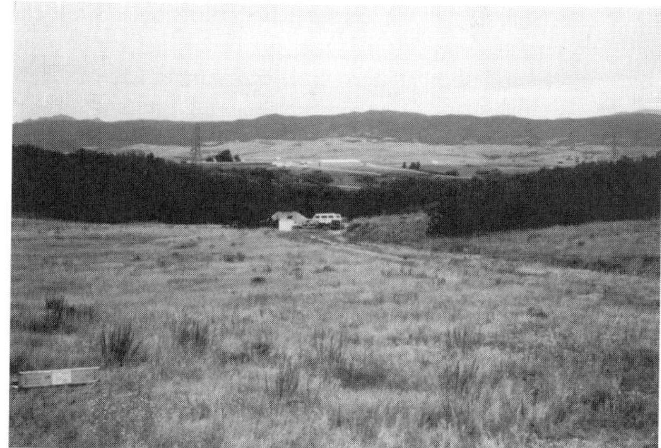

Fig. 38-1 View of the Project Pig site at Highlands Ranch Law Enforcement Training Facility located south of Denver, Colorado.

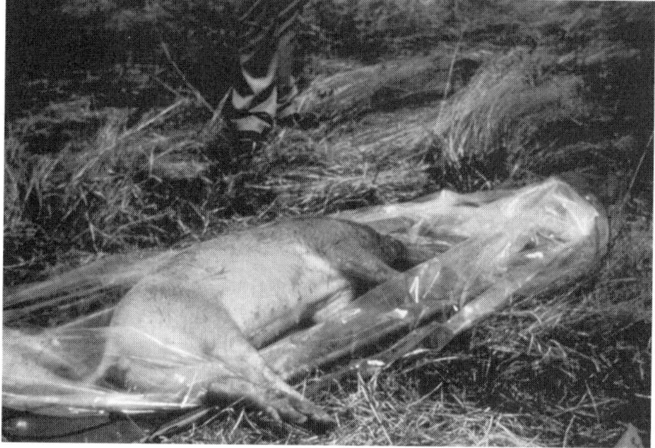

Fig. 38-2 A pig ready for burial at the research site.

Best Practice 38-2

Forensic death investigators should utilize aerial photographs to reveal the presence of clandestine graves because changes in vegetative growth patterns, anomalous soil marks, and other factors can be identified more readily from an aerial perspective.

Baseline Data

Near-field factors (i.e., interacting with the burial system) and *far-field* factors (i.e., uninfluenced by the burial system) were recorded before and after the burial of each pig carcass in order to appreciate physical site disturbances associated with the burial processes. Other research components included calibration pits (graves without an interred pig) and a control site (undisturbed at both the surface and the subsurface). The latter site is necessarily remote from where pigs have been interred. The *back dirt* (i.e., excess soil deposited near the perimeter of the grave or calibration pit) serves as a valuable marker of grave sites, useful even with aerial photography used to identify near-field characteristics. Vegetation growth patterns, soil markings associated with excavational boundaries, and snow settled in grave depressions were phenomena visible from the air (Fig. 38-3). Since an extended period must elapse before the grave site returns to its original state, pig burial sites continue to be monitored and photographed on a regular basis. Climatic conditions, seasonal changes, and freezing/thawing cycles affect soil properties and change the land's appearance when viewed from the air.

Best Practice 38-3

The best aerial photographs result from using a large film format to fully appreciate the details of vegetative or terrain changes.

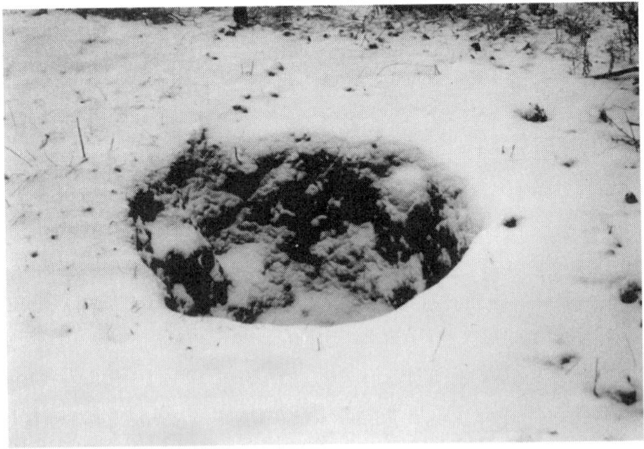

Fig. 38-3 Grave site after a fresh snowfall. Note the high visibility due to the contrast. Using aerial photography with the photographs taken in early morning or late afternoon also makes depressions and backfill more visible due to the shadows created.

Environmental Markers

Researchers prepared a list of all plants within the Law Enforcement Training Site including all plants growing on graves, calibration pits, and back dirt areas. When a grave has been created and a body buried, certain vegetation is destroyed and secondary successions are set into motion (Bass & Birkby, 1978). Five years after the pig burials, it was noted that undisturbed plots contained the greatest diversity in plant species, both weeds and wild flowers. After burials, the plots showed little species diversity. Although eventually other species invaded from the surrounding undisturbed areas, plots did not recover the plant mixture that they originally possessed. It should be noted, however, that even in graves that no longer contained pigs due to intentional disinterment or animal scavenging, revegetation characteristics were identical to those that still contained a pig. Warmth associated with a decaying pig in the ground and the presence of certain nutrients added to the soil did not seem to support or inhibit plant growth. It is evident from the NecroSearch findings that knowledge of native plants in an area can provide valuable clues to the site of a clandestine grave, particularly where the vegetation is largely otherwise undisturbed.

Burial of a corpse hinders the normal faunal succession of arthropods, many of which are useful as forensic indicators (Smith, 1983). Control sites with traps were created to study airborne and surface insects at 1, 2, 4, 7, 12, 25, and 30 days post–pig burial. There were no readily visible entomological indicators of the buried pigs, such as surface stains from saponification or liquefaction 30 days after the burial. The blowfly (*Calliphora vomitoria*) was noted in the Malaise trap within 24 hours of burial, and *Phormia regina* arrived 48 hours postburial. In two weeks, significant numbers of blowflies were trapped at the active graves compared to control sites. Pit traps did not capture any arthropods, typically considered to be forensic indicators (Payne, King, & Beinhart, 1968).

Evaluation Tools

Many methods, strategies, and resources are used to assist in detecting clandestine graves. They include photography; interpretation of the environment through geological, geophysical, botanical, and entomological sciences; and thermal imagery. Additional evaluation strategies include team augmentation using decomposition or scent-detecting dogs and the consultation of additional personnel, such as naturalists, archaeologists, and forensic physical anthropologists.

Geophysical

Three specific geophysical tools were selected for evaluation at the Project Pig site: magnetics (MAG), electromagnetics (EM), and ground penetrating radar (GPR). Of all of the methods applied at the Project Pig site, these have been the most useful (Davenport, Lindemann, & Griffin et al., 1998). Self-potential (SP) surveys have also been used at the NecroSearch site, but not as extensively as the other geophysical methods. These geophysical tools provide data about undisturbed areas, graves with buried pigs, and control pits. Their utility in finding clandestine graves has been confirmed, and after target areas have been designed, geophysical surveys can be efficiently run using portable equipment (Davenport, Lindemann, & Griffin et al., 1998). Portable computers in the field can be used to gather and store MAG and EM survey data for presentation as contour maps or individual profiles. Real-time GPR data are acquired in real-time formats and can be used immediately by field investigators. SP surveys seem to possess limited potential for finding clandestine graves due to the

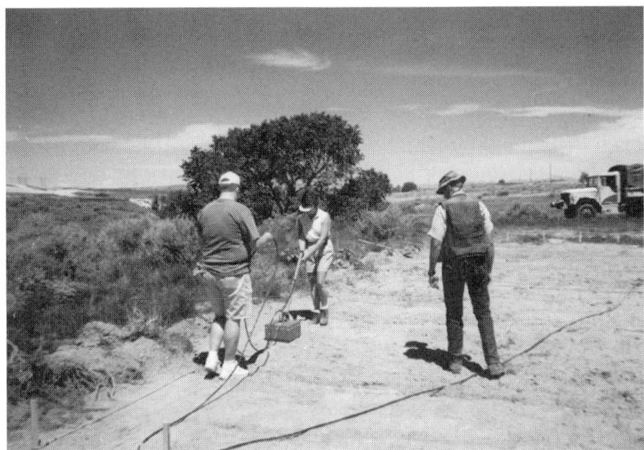

Fig. 38-4 Field study personnel on case site utilizing ground penetrating radar (GPR). (The box is the antenna of the GPR.)

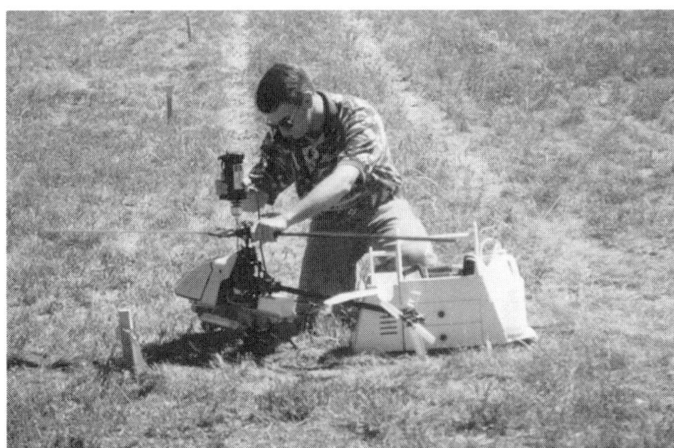

Fig. 38-5 Researcher preparing remote-controlled helicopter for flight. Attached underneath the helicopter is a 35-mm camera, also remote controlled.

fact that they are labor intensive and interpretation is ambiguous. EM surveys have proven to be more useful than MAG surveys, as the ground conductivity changes over graves as a result of the increased porosity of the backfill materials. EM surveys may be used to determine changes in ground conductivity and to detect ferrous and nonferrous metals in the soil. A GPR survey, however, seems to be the most useful method for finding and delineating grave sites because expert GPR technicians can readily identify soil changes and excavation patterns. Enhancements provided by color monitoring of the GPR systems allow investigators to easily identify changes in soil horizons over actual grave sites (Fig. 38-4) (Sheriff, 1983).

Best Practice *38-4*

Utility records for existing buried power lines, sewer lines, gas lines, and water lines should be obtained because these may produce artifacts and reduce the specificity of geophysical magnetic field readings.

Soil Gas

Soil gas surveys performed at the research site can be a useful technique for locating graves. However, this technique is labor intensive. Background levels of methane and other volatile compounds must be determined for the entire research site, and near-field readings must be taken directly over graves and calibration pits. Certain soil types and above-freezing temperatures provide the most favorable results when using gas surveys (Kelly, 1989).

Key Point *38-2*

Monitoring with MAG surveys after interment demonstrates that these surveys can be used at the site to detect areas of excavation, even when metallics are not present.

Thermal Imagery

Far-field thermal imagery of steady-state and dynamic scenes can be obtained by panning the camera across the terrain of the research site; aiming the camera toward and fixing it on each grave and calibration pit provides near-field information for researchers. Aerial photography combined with infrared photography (forward-looking infrared, or FLIR) has been successfully used in searches for buried bodies (Dickinson, 1977). A FLIR system offers high resolution but requires a helicopter or truck mount (Fig. 38-5). Experts believe that the use of infrared should not be limited to detecting heat-related changes associated with decomposition. It is also valuable for detecting compaction or density differences between the disturbed and undisturbed ground, and therefore it can be used to detect grave sites, even years after heat-generating decomposition has ceased (McLaughlin, 1974).

Scent-Detecting Dogs

The use of scent-detecting dogs or decomposition dogs, more commonly known as "cadaver dogs," is relatively nondestructive. Dogs can be effective over water as well as on land. NecroSearch uses bloodhounds because of their keen sense of smell. They are an excellent resource for locating bodies, whether above ground, buried, or even underwater. The dogs are tethered to a 15-foot lead, working over zigzag patterns downwind from a suspected area until the animal "alerts" to a scent. At this point, the dog is allowed to work its own search pattern to the source (Fig. 38-6). Note that the parameters for far-field and near-field investigations are essentially defined by the animal itself.

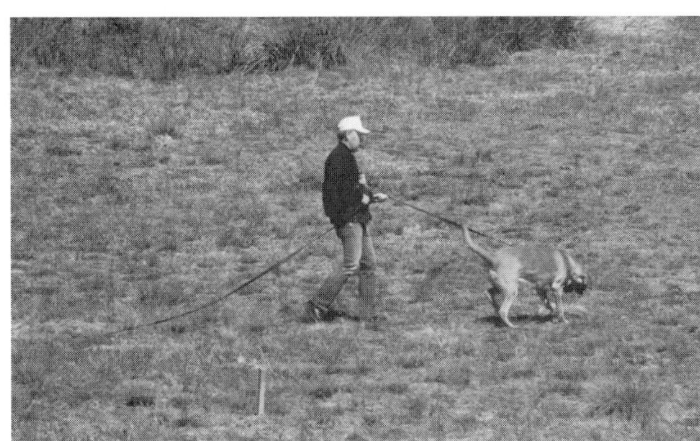

Fig. 38-6 Bloodhound on lead at research site.

The utility of scent-detecting or decomposition dogs is limited by high temperatures (temperatures above approximately 29° C, or 85° F) because of general animal discomfort; limitations are also imposed by extremely low temperatures, and in such conditions the dog must be within one meter to locate the source. When a pig is buried in snow or in the ground under snow with below-freezing temperatures, the dog may not locate the source at all (Tolhurst & Reed, 1984). The effects of temperature and wind on the dog's ability to locate the burial site have not been tested. Optimal conditions for the successful use of scent-detecting dogs include temperatures between approximately 4° and 16° C (40° to 60° F), 20% or higher humidity, moist or very moist ground, and a wind speed of at least 8 km (5 miles) per hour (Galloway, Birkby, & Jones et al., 1988). No upper limit for wind speeds has been established, although the scent cone becomes quite narrow and more difficult to detect with higher wind speeds. Meteorologists are helpful members of the team in determining optimum times for the dogs to be used.

Based on prior experience using scent-detecting dogs, researchers have found the trained animal will indicate the presence of decayed human scent when human blood, feces, urine, and other organic compounds are noted. Other materials that have been handled or worn by humans will also give rise to a false positive indication. Dog handlers involved in NecroSearch have reclassified their dogs as "decomposition dogs" rather than "cadaver dogs" because a positive reaction from the animal may not specifically indicate human remains. They also tend to "alert" on areas of a residual decomposing scent, even when the source had been moved. Double-blind tests have been recommended to determine conditions that will generate false results (Tolhurst & Reed, 1984).

Tests are being devised to determine the maximum time since death in which dogs can detect decomposition scents, since some decomposition dogs have indicated on archaeological remains that are 1400 years old (Hunter, 1994). Ordinarily, they have been recognized as successful in locating decomposed human tissue scents more than 170 years postburial (Hunter, 1994). As expected, the dogs are less likely to respond to pig burial sites where there has been a long interval since burial. However, in these latter situations, the dogs display atypical behavior and indicate on certain shrubs and trees, sometimes attempting to bite or chew this type of vegetation surrounding the grave site.

Animal Scavenger Effects

Naturalists helped NecroSearch personnel in understanding the habits of indigenous species and to track their behavior in relation to buried pigs. Patterns of bone modification related to scavenging were also studied (Haglund, Reay, & Swindler, 1989). There is considerable difficulty in defining standards for far-field and near-field investigation parameters related to scavenging since the terms are defined by the site of scavenged remains, scat, and other evidence of scavenging animals. At the Law Enforcement Training Facility, the animal population included coyotes, dogs, foxes, rabbits, deer, elk, skunks, raccoons, horses, cattle, porcupines, and rodents such as the wood rat and mouse. Searches within a 1-kilometer radius of the site were done, finding bones of deer, cattle, horses, canids, and rabbits. Fresh bone chips, teeth, and hair were also found, indicating scavenging. However, no large pig bones had been recovered within that search radius. The absence of large bones probably indicates that the pig remains were carried a greater distance than the approximately 0.2 kilometer maximum reported by Haglund et al. (1989). The ranges of coyotes vary considerably with differences in terrain and vegetation. Small VHF (very high frequency) transmitters designed for wildlife radio tracking have been attached to various parts of several new pig carcasses before burial to track the translocation of scavenged remains. Hawks, turkey vultures, and other birds of prey may be the first scavengers on the scene of shallow burials and are known to visit the remains at several intervals (Haglund, Reay, & Swindler et al., 1989). Field observations suggest that birds may remove the epidermis of the pigs in sheets, leaving straight surgical-like cut marks on the remaining tissue, which must be differentiated in forensic cases from tissue cut with other instrumentation.

Assets and Limitations of Detection Tools

When searching for clandestine graves, the team must consider many factors when choosing tools and other resources to aid in their work. The place, weather, and season are just a few of the factors that must be carefully considered. Methods used to detect clandestine graves include aerial photography, geology, botany, entomology, geophysics and magnetics, electromagnetics, ground penetrating radar, self-potential, soil gas, metal detection, thermal imagery, decomposition dogs, naturalists, archaeologists, and forensic physical anthropologists. The methods selected to aid in the search efforts maximize the team's efforts and minimize any impact on the environment.

Many methods are considered advantageous because they are nonintrusive; however, often these methods can also be limiting. For example, ground penetrating radar (Figs. 38-7 and 38-8) is nonintrusive, yet it is limited because the equipment is difficult to obtain. In the same way, a metal detector is relatively nondestructive and nonintrusive and can easily detect bullets, jewelry, and other metallic objects (Fig. 38-9). However, this method assumes there is metal on the body. Table 38-1 lists the advantages and disadvantages of principal searching methods.

Summary

Taphonomy, or the science of decomposition and dispersion of the body after death, is extremely important in the investigation of clandestine grave sites and other areas where the identity of the body, circumstances of death, and elapsed time since death are

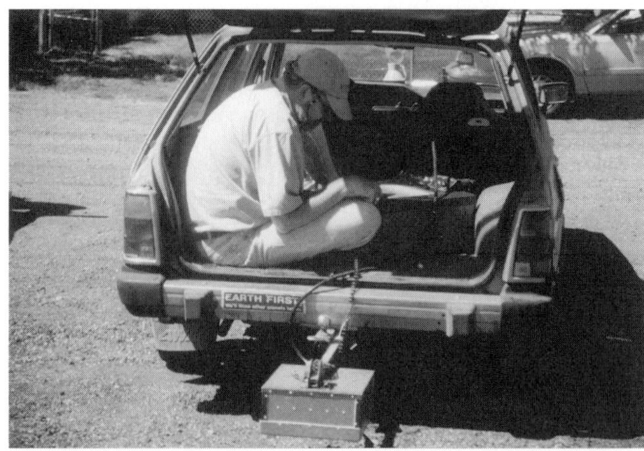

Fig. 38-7 Researcher logging data from ground-penetrating radar (GPR). Note the antenna attached to the bumper of the vehicle.

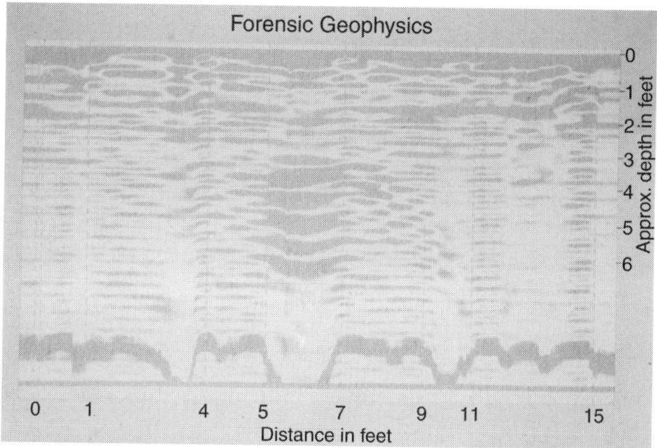

Fig. 38-8 Chart data from ground-penetrating radar (GPR).

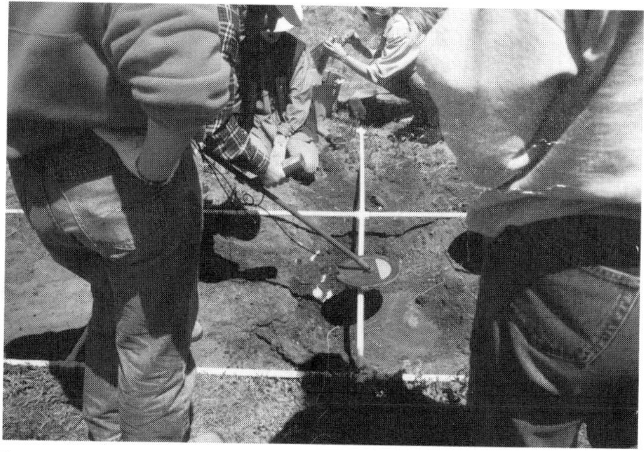

Fig. 38-9 A metal detector in excavation is useful for detection and recovery of metal objects such as bullets, belt buckles, or jewelry.

Table 38-1 Methods Used in the Detection of Clandestine Graves

METHOD	ADVANTAGE	DISADVANTAGE
Aerial photography	Least destructive Provides great overall characterization of a site; access, culture, drainage, topography	Best results with large film format (scale of readily available photography may be too small) May need to be performed at different times of growing season Natural (trees, etc.) and man-made (power lines, etc.) features may interfere with interpretations Requires trained personnel for interpretation May be moisture dependent
Geology	Relatively nondestructive Determination of site stratification through core samples "Real time" on site information about ground surface	Entire search area should be viewed
Botany	Relatively nondestructive Can be performed with photography and samples from area Can be performed years later	Similar succession patterns for any disturbance within ecosystem; not limited to burial
Entomology	Nondestructive Aids in narrowing site location Provides information about time since death	Requires limited area for searching Best for relatively fresh grave Different species for different geographical regions
Geophysics and magnetics	Relatively nondestructive Nonintrusive Equipment easily obtained Rapid coverage of large are Works over snow, fresh/salt water	Only for ferrous materials Target could be missed if search grid too large Data not in "real time"; values must be plotted and should be contoured Magnetic interferences (natural and man-made) confuse readings
Electromagnetics	Relatively nondestructive Nonintrusive Rapid coverage of large area Equipment relatively easily obtained For ferrous/nonferrous materials Records conductivity Works over/through snow	Subject to cultural (fences, etc) interferences Target could be missed if search grid is too large Difficult in rough terrain Data not in "real time"; values must be plotted and should be contoured
Ground penetrating radar	Relatively nondestructive Nonintrusive Fairly rapid coverage of large area "Real time" display Works over/through snow, fresh water	Equipment relatively difficult to obtain Most units require moderately smooth and level terrain
Self-potential	Relatively nondestructive "Real time" information	Intrusive No worthwhile information from our research
Soil gas	Relatively nondestructive "Real time" information	Intrusive Must be positioned relatively close to burial Site soil, ground moisture, climate, depth of probe critical Detection of decomposition product(s) time and temperature dependent

(Continued)

Table 38-1 Methods Used in the Detection of Clandestine Graves—Continued

METHOD	ADVANTAGE	DISADVANTAGE
Metal detector	Relatively nondestructive Nonintrusive Equipment easily obtained	Limited depth capability; detects only metal (ferrous/ nonferrous) objects; presumes metal objects on or with body Field application often improperly conducted
Thermal imagery	Nondestructive Can examine large area Handheld or attached to vehicle (land or aircraft) "Real time" data Videotaped for review	Requires little or no wind Requires special equipment and knowledgeable operators
Decomposition dogs	Relatively nondestructive Documented effectiveness even 170 years after burial Effective over water	Most effective when air/ground moist Dog may be trained for other uses and not properly trained for this type of work; handler may overstate qualifications
Naturalists	Excellent for information concerning scavenging cases and outdoor information	Ability to recognize animal scavenging may be altered by climatic conditions Tracking easiest in snow, med, soft sand, or dust
Archaeologists	Experienced in mapping, data collection, preservation of information from excavated materials, and is therefore extremely valuable for building court cases	Both destructive and intrusive Though data collection can be modified to meet most time demands, can be relatively slow
Forensic physical anthropologists (Figs. 38-10 through 38-13)	On-site interpretation of remains Locations of skeletal/body elements	Not all forensic physical anthropologists are trained in excavation techniques

From: Haglund, W. D., & Sorg, M. H. (1997). *Forensic taphonomy: the postmortem fate of human remains* (pp. 500-501). Boca Raton, FL: CRC Press.

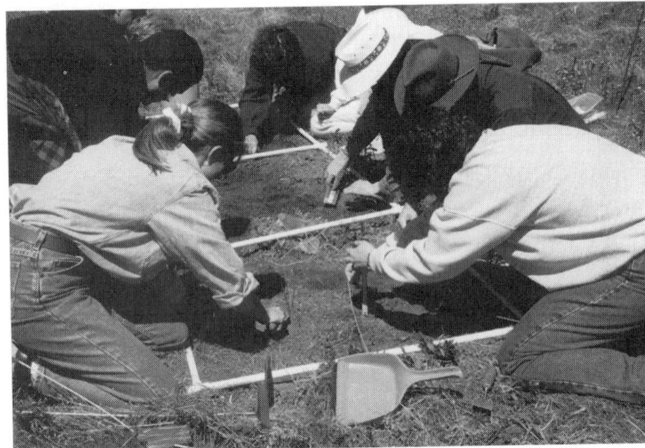

Fig. 38-10 NecroSearch students removing the top layer of soil in excavation. The grid is called the Rapid Archeological Grid System (RAGS), which permits precise measurements of where evidence is recovered.

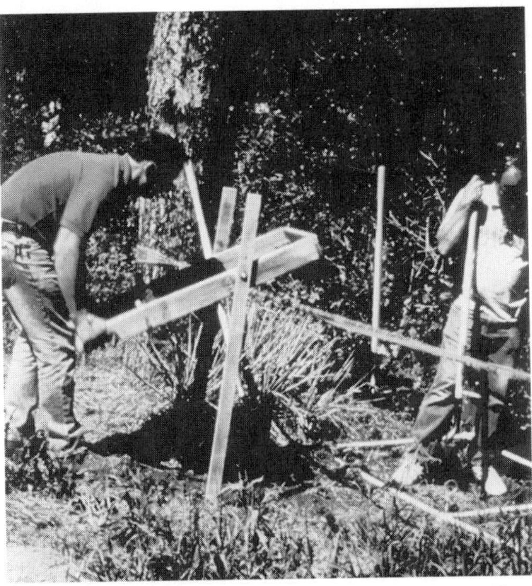

Fig. 38-11 Screening fill dirt from an excavation site allows recovery of evidential items that may have been missed during the excavation.

unknown. This relatively new subspecialty of forensic sciences and death investigation is dependent on an improved understanding of events that shape the fate of human remains in various locations and conditions. Unfortunately, research into this topic is influenced by the many factors that limit cadaver-related research. Fortunately, the ability to study certain elements using animal specimens has been facilitated by NecroSearch International. In addition to a research role, the organization has been beneficial in the investigation of more than 255 cases in 30 states and six countries. NecroSearch has grown from 15 members at its incorporation in 1992 to 35 members as of December 2004.

The membership has remained relatively low, as members are admitted by invitation only, and then only after a thorough background check and a presentation by the prospective member outlining additional skills that may be brought to the organization. It is not the number of persons in the organization but the quality of the individuals and their expertise that are paramount. Forensic nurses bring unique perspectives to the team by using knowledge from a professional acumen that includes medical, legal, and scientific education and training. Nurses have been invited to participate in NecroSearch endeavors, representing another opportunity for individuals interested in death investigation.

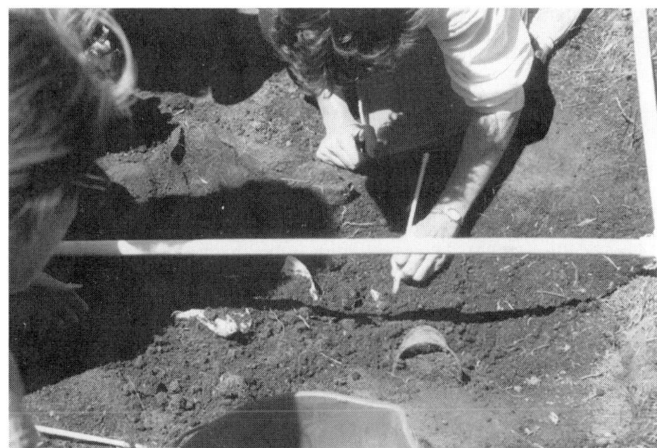

Fig. 38-12 This student is using a bamboo stick to carefully unearth evidence. Metal tools can cause damage to bones.

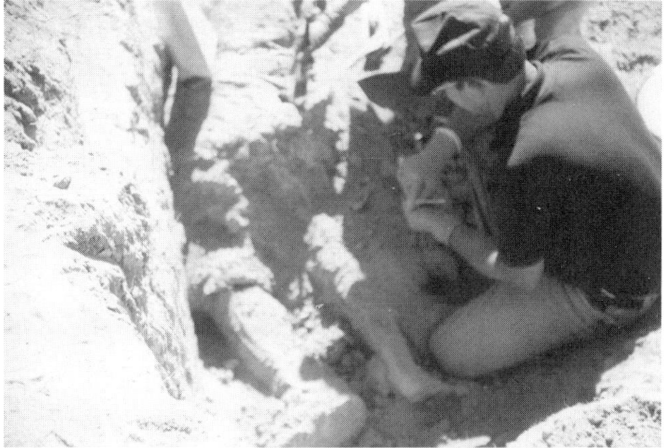

Fig. 38-13 A researcher sits in grave pit with remains that are being recovered.

Case Study 38-1 Missing Person–Homicide (Search)

Robert A. Madison was reported missing in mid-May 2000. He was last seen on the afternoon of April 24, 2000. The police department detectives conducted numerous interviews and located an individual who became an informant. According to the information gathered, the victim was shot near where the body was hidden and covered in the tumbleweeds for one to two days before the offenders arrived to move it. The informant assisted the suspect in loading the body in the bed of a pickup truck, transporting the body to a location on the west edge of the city limits, and dumping the body in a hole. They filled in the hole with the dirt that the suspect had previously removed with a backhoe, which was still at the scene. They dumped the body off the back of the truck where it "crumpled" at the bottom of the hole, then threw the white cotton blanket that had covered the body on top and filled in the hole with the dirt the subject had removed with the backhoe. The informant described the hole as being about 12 feet deep. He stated the hole was approximately two bucket widths at the bottom and flared out toward the top. He stated a mound of dirt was on his left and a tree was behind and off the side, which he was able to see in the lights of the backhoe.

The detectives took the informant to the described site on several occasions, and he picked an area that he thought was the location of the grave. Because a housing development had been started the previous year about the time of the burial and the area had seven new homes, the informant stated the area looked much different than when he had been there the previous year. The location he picked seemed about the right distance to the best of his recollection. Aerial photographs, taken prior to April 2000 and between May 2000 and the time the area had been leveled for development, were acquired. After review of the photographs, a mound or depression was visualized about 100 feet east of the trees, which correlated with the site described by the informant.

Two bloodhounds were brought to the chosen sight and gave a positive indication for decomposing human tissue. The areas indicated were marked and documented. This area was just north of the arroyo. The marked area was wet, and there had been no rain in the area for more than 48 hours. This was the only spot located that remained wet. According to the precipitation records, during the time period surrounding the burial the area received less than 0.5 inches of rain.

An employee with the construction company working in the area at the time of the burial stated that a backhoe matching the specifications had been moved and was tangled with barbed wire. The employee stated that he followed the tracks in the wet ground to an area where the backhoe had been used. Upon arrival at the site, investigators noted obvious evidence that the ground had been disturbed. There was a slight berm at the edges, and it was readily visible where old growth vegetation had ceased. Additional aerial photographs were reviewed and the newest photograph showed the possible primary burial site.

At this time this area, which was west of the area where the dogs indicated, was considered the primary location due to the additional information acquired. The area indicating a disturbance was outlined with pin flags. A botanical survey was the first priority before using other more invasive techniques. A survey was also taken of the secondary area. Ground penetrating radar (GPR) was used to search the outside of the disturbed area. The area was cleaned of vegetation and leveled approximately 2 meters past the edges of the disturbed area, to attempt to visualize the backfilled trench through color or texture changes in the soil. Next, the area was hand excavated in a series of shallow, narrow test trenches, which were shovel width and approximately 2 meters apart. Near the southern end of the marked area, a locality with less consolidated fill was discovered. However, the size or shape of the area could not be visualized. The GPR was utilized again within the marked area, but no anomalies were noted even after several passes. A cone penetrometer was used in an attempt to measure the approximate degree of compaction of the soil, and two separate areas of less compacted soil were found. This, coupled with shovel testing, led to probing using a surveyor's pin and actual excavation using a trowel. Through these methods, the north wall of the filled trench was located. Once the approximate limits of the grave trench were located, the trench was then excavated using shovels and trowels and passed through a quarter-inch mesh screen to allow recovery of any evidence missed in the excavation process.

Because of the available information indicating the victim was buried at a depth of 10 to 12 feet, limited personnel, and a vehicle observed circling the area that was thought to be associated with the suspect, it was decided that a backhoe would be used to dig approximately 5 to 6 feet into the trench before proceeding with hand excavation. The backhoe was used to excavate the material until a patch of dark color was observed in the trench. The backhoe was removed from the immediate site and hand excavation again resumed. The distal portion of the right humerus of a buried human body was located. The right ulna was located near the distal end of the humerus, but the right radius and hand could not be located. During the screening process, the left side of the mandible (with teeth intact) and several teeth were recovered. The left hand and arm were found to be intact and unharmed. Continued hand excavation revealed the remains were intact and were partially mummified, with the victim lying prone on a steeply sloping trench with the arms outstretched. The feet were lowest in the trench with the remains at approximately a 45-degree angle. The cranium was located in the spill dirt along with the right radius, right hand, and an earring. The remains were completely uncovered and the coroner's office was contacted to complete its investigation and to remove the remains. The area was screened for additional evidence, and a final mapping was completed. The site was then secured.

The victim had been missing for 14 months before his remains were located, and it took another 18 months for the perpetrator to be brought before a jury. That jury took only six hours to find him guilty, and he is currently serving 26 years in prison for murder in the second degree.

Case Study 38-2 Preserved Remains

A 35- to 45-year-old female's remains were sent to the National Museum of Health and Medicine in July 1992. The remains were found at a flea market entrance on August 20, 1989. The suspect was a man who was a rival in the flea market business. Following the suspect's death in 1990, friends and relatives provided information on the remains.

The body had supposedly been stored in a copper coffin in a funeral home for many years. After the sale of the funeral home, the body was placed on the rafters of what became a hardware outlet. A local historian remembered viewing the remains in 1939.

When the remains were examined, the ligaments, tendons, and muscle tissues were all preserved and evident in the legs, arms, and head. However, the tissue appearance differed from mummified remains. Internal organs had been injected with a red clay suspension in a paraffin base and a talc derivative comprised largely of carbonate. These hardened inside the organs and the organ tissues were dried and paperlike in texture. The appearance of the soft tissues and presence of organs represented an anatomical preparation similar to those done in the late 19th and early 20th centuries.

Modified from Sledxik, P. S., & Micozzi, M. S. (1997). Autopsied, embalmed, and preserved human remains: Distinguishing features in forensic & historic context. In W. D. Haglund and M. H. Sorg, *Forensic taphonomy: The postmortem fate of human remains*. Boca Raton, FL: CRC Press.

Resources

Organizations

NecroSearch International, Inc.

Box D, 9008 Highway 85, Littleton, CO 80125; Tel: 303-663-7205; www.necrosearch.org

Publications

Boyd, R. M. (1979). Buried body cases. *FBI Law Enforcement Bull, 48*(2), 1-7.

Haglund, W. D. (1991). *Applications of taphonomic models to forensic investigations.* PhD dissertation, University of Washington, Seattle. Ann Arbor, MI: University Microfilms.

Jackson, S. (2002). *No stone unturned: The true story of NecroSearch International.* New York: Kensington Books.

Mayo, K. (June 2004). Recovering human remains from clandestine graves, *Evidence Technology Magazine, 2*(3), 18-21; www.evidencemagazine.com.

Rodriguez, W. C., III, & Bass, W. M. (1985). Decomposition of buried bodies and methods that may aid in their location. *J Forensic Sci, 30,* 836-852.

Smith, K. G. (1972). *Insects and other arthropods of medical importance.* London: British Museum of Natural History.

References

Bass, W. M., & Birkby, W. H., (1978, July). Exhumation: The method could make the difference. *FBI Law Enforcement Bull,* 6-11.

Berryman, H. E., Bass, W. M., Symes, S. A., et al. (1997). Recognition of cemetery remains in the forensic setting. In W. D. Haglund & M. H. Sorg, *Forensic taphonomy: the postmortem fate of human remains* (Chapter 10). Boca Raton, FL: CRC Press.

Davenport, G. C., Griffin, T. J., Lindemann, J. W., et al. (1988, July). Geoscientists and law enforcement professionals work together in Colorado. *Geotimes,* 13-15.

Davenport, G. C., Lindemann, J. W., Griffin, T. J., et al. (1998). Geotechnical Application 3: Crime scene investigating techniques. *Geophysics: The Leading Edge of Exploration, 7*(8), 64-66.

Dickinson, D. J. (1977). The aerial use of an infrared camera in a police search for the body of a missing person in New Zealand. *J Forensic Sci Society, 16,* 205-211.

France, D. L., Griffin, T. J., Swanburg, J. G., et al. (1992). A multidisciplinary approach to the detection of clandestine graves. *J Forensic Sci, 37,* 1445-1458.

France, D. L., Griffin, T. J., Swanburg, J. G., et al. (1997). NecroSearch revisited: further multidisciplinary approaches to the detection of clandestine graves. In W. D. Haglund & M. H. Sorg, *Forensic taphonomy: the postmortem fate of human remains* (Chapter 32). Boca Raton, FL: CRC Press.

Galloway, A., Birkby, W. H., Jones, A. M., et al. (1988). Decay rates of human remains in an arid environment. *J Forensic Sci, 34,* 607-616.

Haglund, W. D., Reay, D. T., & Swindler, D. R. (1989). Canid scavenging/disarticulation sequence of human remains in the Pacific Northwest. *J Forensic Sci, 24,* 587-606.

Haglund, W. D. and Sorg, M. H. (1997). *Forensic taphonomy: the postmortem fate of human remains.* Boca Raton, FL: CRC Press.

Haglund, W. D., Reichert, D. G., & Reay, D. T. (1990). Recovery of decomposed and skeletal human remains in the Green River murder investigation: Implications for medical examiner/coroner and police. *Am J Forensic Med Pathol, 11*(1), 35-43.

Hoving, G. L. (1986, February). Buried body search technology. *Identification News,* 3, 15.

Hunter, J. R. (1994). Forensic archaeology in Britain. *Antiquity, 68,* 758-769.

Imaizumi, M. (1974, August). Locating buried bodies. *FBI Law Enforcement Bull,* 2-5.

James, S. H., Nordby, J. J., *Forensic science, an introduction to scientific and investigative techniques* (2nd ed.). Boca Raton, FL: CRC Press.

Kelly, D. P. (1989). *Postmortem gastrointestinal gas production in submerged Yucatan micro-pigs.* Unpublished MA thesis, Colorado State University.

Killam, E. W. (1989). *The detection of human remains.* Springfield, IL: Charles C. Thomas.

McLaughlin, J. E. (1974). *The detection of buried bodies.* Study of Andermac, 2626 Live Oak Highway, Yuba City, CA 95991.

Nawrocki, S. P. , Pless, J. E., Dawley, D. A., et al. (1997). Fluvial transport of human crania. In W. D. Haglund & M. H. Sorg, *Forensic taphonomy: the postmortem fate of human remains* (Chapter 34). Boca Raton, FL: CRC Press.

Payne, J. D., King, E.W., & Beinhart, G. (1968). Arthropod succession and decomposition of buried pigs. *Nature, 180,* 1181.

Schoenly, K., Griest, K., & Rhine, S. (1989). An experimental field protocol for investigating the postmortem interval using multidisciplinary indicators. *J Forensic Sci, 36,* 1385-1415.

Sheriff, R. E. (Ed.). (1983). *Encyclopedic dictionary of exploration geophysics* (2nd ed.). Tulsa, OK: Society of Exploration Geophysicists.

Smith, K. (1983). *A manual of forensic entomology.* Ithaca, NY: British Museum (Natural History) and Cornell University Press.

Spindler, K. (1994). *The man in the ice.* New York: Harmony Books.

Tolhurst, W., & Reed, L. (1984). *Manhunters? Hounds of the Big T.* Puyallup, WA: Hound Dog Press.

Chapter 39 Sudden Death during Acute Psychotic Episodes

Theresa G. Di Maio

Periodically, a forensic pathologist is presented with a case of sudden death during or immediately after a violent struggle where a complete autopsy fails to reveal either an anatomical cause of death or evidence of significant trauma. While most such cases are associated with the use of cocaine and methamphetamine, a number of cases involve individuals with endogenous mental disease not using the aforementioned drugs of abuse (Di Maio, 2001). Forensic nurse examiners who specialize in death investigation should be aware of acute psychotic episodes (APE) in cases of sudden death and consider these circumstances when gathering medical histories.

The concept of death due to "excited delirium" was introduced in 1849 by Dr. Luther Bell of the McLeon Asylum for the Insane in Somerville, Massachusetts (Bell, 1849). Bell thought that he was describing a new disease, a fatal form of delirium in the mentally ill. According to Bell, this unusual form of delirium presented with fever, a rapid pulse, and a lack of appetite and sleep. The patient was agitated and anxious, with increasing confusion that appeared suddenly. Any attempt to approach the patient resulted in a violent struggle regardless of the number who tried to restrain him or her. The physical and mental state of the patient continued to deteriorate over the course of weeks resulting in death. This entity became known as "Bell's mania." Today such deaths are described as those of "excited delirium" or "manic delirium" and limit deaths ascribed to it to those that occur minutes or hours after the condition becomes manifest (Di Maio, 2001).

The etiology of this condition and the mechanism causing death have been controversial. Bell attributed the deaths to a "malaise of the nervous system" (Bell, 1849). At the present time, such deaths almost always occur after restraint is either instituted or attempted, with the cause of death often attributed to the application of a "choke hold" or "positional asphyxia," even when there is neither testimonial nor physical evidence of these (O'Halloran & Lewman, 1993; Reay et al., 1992).

In deaths involving excited delirium in which the hogtie restraint has been used (a common method of restraint used by police in arresting violent individuals), it has been alleged that death was due to positional asphyxia (O'Halloran & Lewman, 1993; Reay et al., 1992). Research conducted by Chan and colleagues in 1997 essentially disproved "positional asphyxia" as the cause of deaths in such cases. Their research concluded that the "hogtie restraint" position does not cause hypoventilation or asphyxia in and of itself. This restraint position was not clinically significant in producing changes in respiratory or ventilatory functioning sufficient to be the sole causal factor in sudden death in normal cardiopulmonary functioning individuals.

Causal Factors

The usual presentation of an individual in "excited delirium" is one who is confused, irrational, delusional, and violent. It is the position of the author that sudden death from excited delirium is not a disease process, as first thought of by Bell, but rather a syndrome of common causal features cascading together and culminating in sudden cardiac death. Thus, this entity should more correctly be termed a sudden death due to "excited delirium syndrome." The common causal factors are as follows:

- The physiological manifestations of exhaustive physical exertion alone
- Exhaustive physical exertion in conjunction with preexisting disease
- Exhaustive physical exertion combined with medications

In fatal cases of excited delirium, death usually occurs immediately after the individual is restrained and struggling ceases. This post-struggle period corresponds to the time of "post exercise peril" defined by Dimsdale et al. (1984), a time where an individual is susceptible to developing a fatal cardiac arrhythmia. An understanding of the physiological changes that lead to "post exercise peril" is important in understanding excited delirium syndrome. These changes, resulting in cardiac dysfunction and arrest, are due to the physiological effects of the catecholamines, epinephrine, and norepinephrine, as well as potassium, on the heart.

Effects of Catecholamine on the Heart

Dimsdale et al. (1984) found that in the three minutes immediately following cessation of strenuous exercise, epinephrine, and norepinephrine continue to rise with norepinephrine at more than 10-fold baseline levels. Norepinephrine's action on the heart is stimulation of alpha-1 and beta-1 receptors (McCance, 1994). Stimulation of beta-1 receptors increases heart rate, contractility, and velocity of conduction. Alpha-1 receptors are found in the coronary arteries. Norepinephrine interacting with alpha-1 receptors causes vasoconstriction, thus decreasing the amount of oxygenated blood being supplied to the myocardium at a time when an increased amount is needed due to greater demand being put on the heart resulting from the stimulation of the beta-1 receptors.

Excessive levels of catecholamines, especially norepinephrine, can be cardiotoxic, resulting in catecholamine (norepinephrine) cardiomyopathy with impairment of myocardial contractility (Powers et al., 1994). Cardiac injury from excessive norepinephrine may be permanent. The lesions seen in catecholamine cardiomyopathy are myofibrillar degeneration, leukocyte infiltration, and focal necrosis. The pathogenesis of catecholamine-induced cardiomyopathy is disruption of myocardial calcium transport with resultant high levels of intracellular calcium. This results in a decreased rate of ventricular relaxation and an increased rate of diastolic tension, with resultant left ventricular dysfunction. Both diastolic and systolic functions are acutely impaired. Systolic function improves within 48 hours, while diastolic function remains depressed.

Effects of Potassium on the Heart

The effects of catecholamines and their role in sudden lethal cardiac arrhythmias were further expanded on by Young et al. (1992). They investigated not only the relationship between stress and catecholamine levels but potassium levels as well. Like Dimsdale et al. (1984), Young et al. (1992) found that the highest levels of plasma catecholamines occurred during the three minutes post--exercise. In addition, they found that during strenuous exercise, potassium increases dramatically. Post-exercise, while norepinephrine continues to rise, potassium levels fell at a maximum rate for one to two minutes to hypokalemic or near-hypokalemic levels.

Blood potassium concentrations have a very narrow range of safety. Fatal cardiac arrhythmias are associated with both hyperkalemia and hypokalemia. If sudden death occurs with increased levels of potassium, the question then arises as to why a fatal arrhythmia does not occur during the rising phase of potassium during exercise rather than post-exercise. Paterson et al. found that exercise-induced increases in circulating catecholamines have a cardioprotective effect to the rapidly rising potassium levels (Paterson et al., 1993). This cardioprotective effect is not known to occur for falling potassium levels.

Contributory Factors

Thus, changes in catecholamine and potassium levels, independent of each other, are potentially lethal. Post-struggle, however, the lethal potential of these changes converge, increasing the possibility of sudden cardiac death. The low incidence of cardiac death among the exercising population indicate that in most instances changes in catecholamine and potassium levels post-struggle, in and of themselves, rarely cause fatal cardiac arrhythmias. For death to occur in the post-exercise period, in most instances, there must be either underlying cardiac disease or the presence of medications or drugs that potentiate the action of the catecholamines to produce a cascade of biochemical actions that set a lethal course resulting in sudden cardiac death.

Case Studies

The following three cases present a range of factors that may contribute to the effects of elevated catecholamine levels and depressed potassium levels in causing death in the post-struggle period. These case studies represent a small portion of reported cases of sudden death in excited delirium syndrome.

Case Study 39-1 Sudden Death and Unsuspected Heart Disease

The deceased was a 45-year-old white male, manager of a company on the US-Mexico border, who for four to five days preceding his death had paranoid delusions and hallucinations. The day of his death, he ran hysterically towards the US Customs area on the border between Mexico and Texas. The agents attempted to calm him down. He became combative, was handcuffed, and was placed on the ground. He then developed seizures. On arrival of the emergency medical services (EMS) team, he had no vital signs. At autopsy, he was a slightly obese white male with minor contusions and abrasions of the body. The brain demonstrated a thin subdural film of blood over the right parietal and occipital lobes, no brain swelling, and some patchy subarachnoid hemorrhage. The brain was examined by a neuropathologist who concluded that the changes noted were either agonal or a postmortem artifact, of no significance and not contributory to the death. The rapidity of the death also negates attributing any significance to the findings in the head. The heart was slightly enlarged, weighting 430 g, with mild left ventricular hypertrophy and a single focus of 80% narrowing of the right coronary artery; 70% to 75% narrowing of a coronary artery is significant and can cause a fatal cardiac arrhythmia (Di Maio, 2001). Toxicology disclosed a low therapeutic level (0.06 mg/L) of amitriptyline.

It was felt that in this case a contributing factor to the death was the coronary artery disease.

Case Study 39-2 Sudden Death in an Apparently Healthy Teenager

The deceased was a 16-year-old black female with a history of recurrent depression. At the time of her death, she was a patient in a mental institution. She saw another patient being restrained and went to the patient's aid. She was described as extremely violent. The staff responded, placed her in a basket hold, and took her to the floor. She was given a 50-mg IM injection of thorazine. Approximately 10 minutes later, she stopped struggling. She was carried to her room. When checked on several minutes later, she was found unresponsive. At autopsy, there were no injuries. Her heart was slightly enlarged weighing 330 g (the mean heart weight in individuals 15 to 19 years old is 232 g with a standard deviation of 43 g). A complete toxicology screen was negative for any drugs or medications, including thorazine. A subsequent investigation revealed that her father had died of Wolfe-Parkinson-White syndrome at age 31.

In this case, the deceased had slight enlargement of the heart and a family history of a potentially fatal cardiac condition. In Wolfe-Parkinson-White syndrome, there are congenital conduction abnormalities of the heart that produce arrhythmias. Occasionally, the arrhythmias are fatal. This condition may have been present in the patient, as there is a hereditary tendency, and may have been a contributory factor in her death.

Case Study 39-3 Sudden Death of a Child on Prescribed Medication

The deceased was a 9-year-old white male with bipolar disease and attention deficit disorder who suddenly became violent while in a mental facility. He was brought to the floor and held there using a basket hold method of restraint for 20 minutes. He appeared to calm down and then was noted to be unresponsive. EMS was summoned and he was transported to a hospital. He survived approximately 21 hours in the hospital. At autopsy, there were minor abrasions and contusions. Toxicology on blood obtained at autopsy revealed blood levels of: 0.61 mg/L Venlafaxine and 0.20 mg/L amphetamine

Both of these drug levels are high therapeutic levels (Baselt, 2000). These drugs represent levels at the time of death—21 hours plus after arrest. The blood levels at the time of cardiac arrest would have been significantly higher. Venlafaxine, like cocaine, is a potent inhibitor of norepinephrine reuptake (*Physician's Desk Reference [PDR]*, 2004). Amphetamine causes release of norepinephrine from sympathetic fibers. Increased quantities of norepinephrine increase the heart rate, force of contraction, and conduction velocity while at the same time causing coronary artery constriction with resultant decreased perfusion of the myocardium (McCance & Huether, 1994). Thus, in this case, the elevated levels of the two medications present were felt to be cardiotoxic and contributory to the death.

We can conclude that changes in catecholamine and potassium levels post-struggle have the potential to cause sudden cardiac death, especially when there is underlying cardiac disease or the presence of medications or stimulant drugs. These factors clearly contribute to a series of biochemical actions that can result in death (Fig. 39-1).

Assessment and Prevention

Forensic nurse examiners can make a unique contribution to death prevention from excited delirium syndrome. Forensic nursing is not only involved in the medical-legal aspects of a death, but its impact is on families and the community as a whole. The forensic nurse examiners can educate healthcare providers and law enforcement officers (both of whom encounter this entity) about this syndrome so as to prevent such deaths.

Of critical importance in the prevention of death from excited delirium is the early identification of high-risk patients. As a tool for patient care, accurate nursing diagnoses have always been of fundamental importance. Assessment for prevention of sudden death due to excited delirium syndrome can now be another measure of patient care. Thus, a nursing diagnosis might be "potential for sudden death due to excited delirium syndrome, as evidenced by a history of endogenous mental disease with past violent behavior." Assessing characteristics for "high-risk patients" are as follows:

- A prior episode of excited delirium
- Violent and aggressive behavior
- Use of medication that increases the release or blocks reuptake of norepinephrine
- Cardiac disease
- Asthma or any pulmonary disease involving restriction of airway
- Epilepsy
- Use of stimulants such as cocaine and methamphetamine

Age is not an identifying factor, as these deaths can occur in the young as well as the old.

Early identification of behaviors predictive of violent activity requires immediate intervention measures to reduce escalating anger and aggression (Rawlins et al., 1993). Behavior characteristics for violence include the following:

- Verbal threats of violence
- Screaming, swearing, shouting at others
- Breaking or throwing objects
- Motor agitation, rigid/taut body expressions with poor concentration
- Projecting angry emotions onto another (e.g., blaming)
- Nonverbal behavior of rejecting others
- Pacing, restlessness, inability to sleep or eat, hyperactivity
- History of violent behavior with need for physical restraint
- Delusions and confusion of mental state
- Defiance
- Bullying others
- Using stimulants (e.g., cocaine, methamphetamine)
- Paranoid behavior with auditory hallucinations

Key Point *39-1*

The most critical time during excited delirium syndrome occurs when the staff engages in physically restraining the patient. It is the struggle between patient and staff that initiates catecholamine/potassium actions. Consequently, it is of extreme importance to prevent a struggle and the use of physical restraint.

When an individual's internal mechanisms for control are lost due to an acute psychotic episode, the person has lost his or her ability to perceive reality. These episodes are often extremely frightening to individuals having to care for such patients and require immediate attention to prevent violence to self or others.

Acute psychotic breaks can also occur from endogenous disease processes. MEND-A-MIND is a mnemonic for disorders that can cause an acute psychotic episode (Farrell et al., 1998):

- M–Metabolic disorder
- E–Electrical (convulsive) disorder
- N–Neoplastic disease
- DV–Degenerative (chronic) brain disease
- A–Arterial (cerebrovascular) disease
- M–Mechanical disease (actual physical structures of the brain)
- I–Infectious disease
- N–Nutritional disease
- D–Drug toxicity

Regardless of the cause of a psychotic break, prevention of violence and maintenance of the safety of the patient and staff are of direct importance.

The Use of Physical Restraint

The standard of care in behavioral emergencies is nonphysical and based on initial and ongoing assessment. These include knowledge of communicative techniques, verbal and nonverbal; the patient and families direct participation in care planning and the reduction of environmental stimulants that may trigger the escalation of violent behavior.

More restrictive measures (for example, physical restraint) should be used only in extreme behavioral emergencies. The use of

Best Practice *39-1*

Prevent a struggle during the use of physical restraint by reducing environmental stimulation that may trigger or escalate violent behavior.

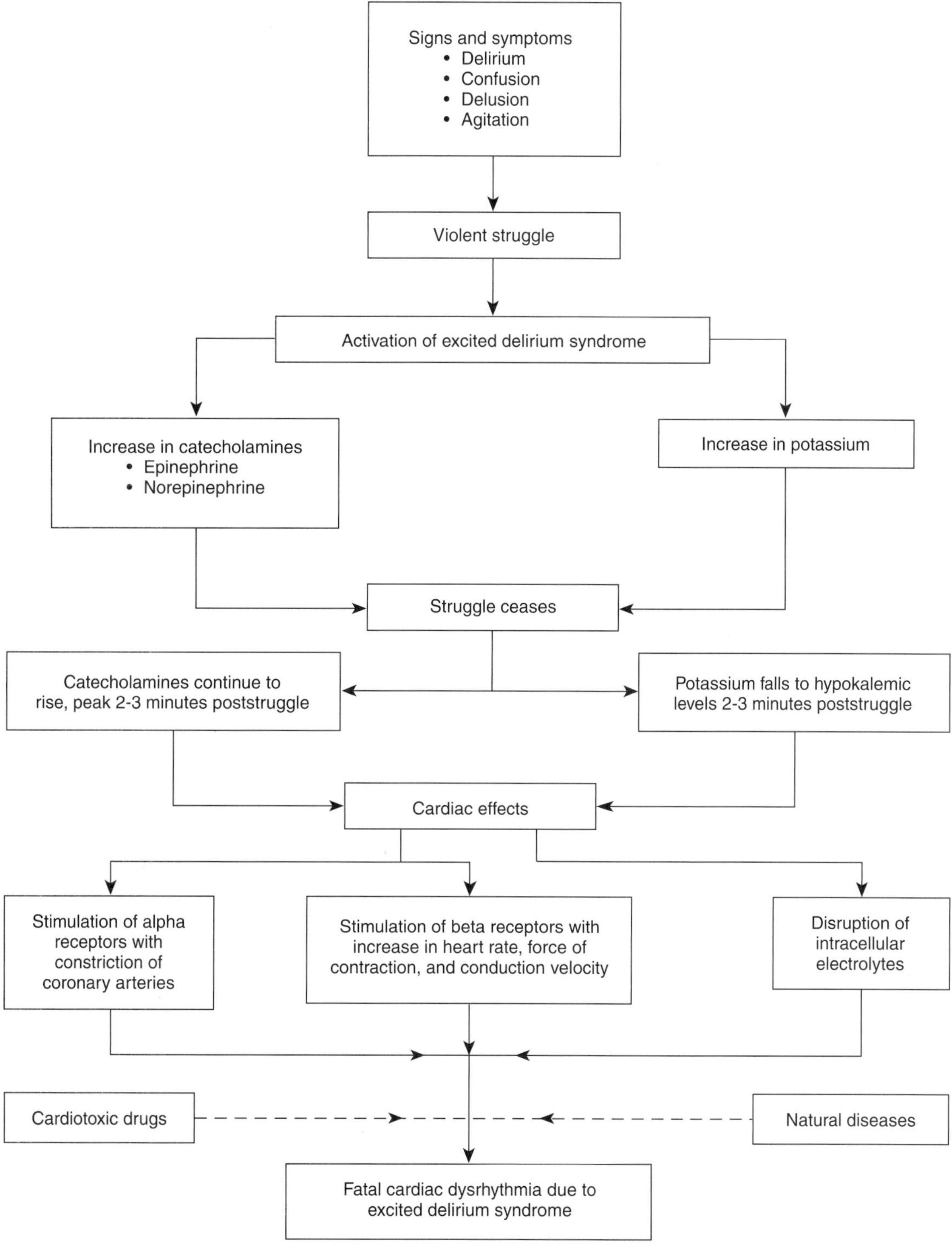

Fig. 39-1 Death during acute psychotic episodes.

physical restraint must be determined to outweigh the risk associated with it. Physical restraint should only be used when all other less restrictive measures have been used and failed to prevent the patient from harming self or others. The therapeutic benefit as well as the moral treatment of physically restraining patients has been debated frequently in the literature. While the elimination of physical restraint may not be possible in all situations, the least amount of time and points of restraint should be used to prevent the patient from harming self or others (American Psychiatric Nurses Association [APNA], 2000).

Management of Violence

Many theories have been written on the management of violence and aggression in mentally ill and violent patients. Planning to manage potentially violent situations before they occur should be the first component in providing care for the patient as well as staff. Identifying and avoiding "triggering" elements that may precipitate a violent behavior becomes crucial in care planning and risk management. A primary trigger in violent behavior can be provoking behaviors by staff and others in close proximity to the mentally ill patient. The mentally ill patient will often interpret behaviors of others as threatening and calling for legitimate retaliation (Whittington, 2000).

Best Practice 39-2

If the need for physical restraint becomes unavoidable, releasing the patient quickly and allowing the patient to pace or walk off anger will help prevent critical fluctuations of catecholamines and potassium levels during the post-struggle period.

Studies on treatment modules that may influence the success of reducing the need for restraint indicate that the training of staff in early assessment and intervention of alternative methods to defuse and deescalate aggression and violence can be successful in reducing the requirement for physical restraint (Mercer et al., 2000).

Summary

Sudden death due to excited delirium syndrome in individuals with acute psychotic episodes is not caused by positional asphyxia, choke holds, hogtie restraint, or physical restraint of patients in general. Death is due to a number of effects, cascading together, culminating in a lethal cardiac arrest. The clinical forensic nurse examiner who specializes in forensic mental health is in a key position to prevent death from this particular syndrome. Prevention involves knowledge of the mechanism of death for early initial identification of high-risk patients. Successful prevention requires alternative methods to reduce aggression and violence other than physical restraint. Mandatory teaching of these methods should be a standard of care for all individuals encountering aggressive and violent patients.

Resources

Books

Froede, R. (Ed.). (2003). *Handbook of forensic pathology* (2nd ed.). Northfield, IL: College of American Pathologists.

Organizations

National Association of Medical Examiners

1392 South Grand Boulevard, St. Louis, MO 63104; Tel: 314-577-8298; http://expertpages.com/org/name.htm

References

American Psychiatric Nurses Association (APNA). (2000). *Seclusion and restraints task force.* Position statement on the use of seclusion and restraint. Arlington, VA: Author.

Baselt, R. C. (2000). *Disposition of toxic drugs and chemicals in man* (5th ed.). Foster City, CA: Chemical Toxicology Institute.

Bell, L. V. (1849). On a form of disease resembling some advanced stages of mania and fever, but so contradistinguished from any ordinarily observed or described combination of symptoms, as to render it probably that it may be an overlooked and hitherto unrecorded malady. *Amer J Insanity, 6,* 97-127.

Chan, T. C., Vilke, G. N., Neuman, T., et al. (1997). Restraint position and positional asphyxia. *Ann Emerg Med, 30,* 578-586.

Di Maio, V. J., & Di Maio, D. J. (2001). *Forensic pathology* (2nd ed.). Boca Raton, FL: CRC Press.

Dimsdale, J. E., Hartley, G. T., Ruskin, J. N., et al. (1984). Post-exercise peril: Plasma catecholamines and exercise. *JAMA, 251,* 630-632.

Farrell, S. P., Harmon, R. B., & Hastings, S. (1998). Nursing management of acute psychotic episodes. *Nurs Clin North Am, 33,* 187-200.

McCance, K. L., & Huether, S. E. (1994). *Pathophysiology: The biologic basis for diseases in adults and children* (2nd ed.). St. Louis, MO: Mosby.

Mercer, D., Mason, T., McKeown, M., et al. (Eds.). (2000). *Forensic mental health care: A case study approach.* London: Churchill Livingstone.

O'Halloran, R.L. & Lewman, L.V. (1993). Restraint asphyxiation in excited delirium. *Am J Forensic Med Pathol, 14,* 289-295.

Paterson, D. J., Rogers, J., Powell, T., et al. (1993). Effects of catecholamines on the ventricular myocyte action potential in raised extracellular potassium. *Acta Physiol Scand, 148,* 177-186.

Physician's desk reference (PDR) (59th ed.). (2004). Montvale, NJ: Thomson Healthcare.

Powers, F. M., Pifarre, R., & Thomas, J. X. (1994). Ventricular dysfunction in norepinephrine-induced cardiomyopathy. *Circulatory Shock, 43,* 122-129.

Rawlins, R. P., Williams, S. R., & Beck, C. K. (Eds.). (1993). *Mental health-psychiatric nursing: A holistic life-cycle approach* (3rd ed.). St. Louis, MO: Mosby.

Reay, D. J., Fligner, C. L., Stilwell, A. D., et al. (1992). Positional asphyxia during law enforcement transport. *Am J Forensic Med Pathol, 13,* 90-97.

Whittington, R. (2000). Changing the environment in the management of aggression. In D. Mercer, T. Mason, M. McKeown, et al. (Eds.), *Forensic mental health care: A case study approach.* London: Churchill Livingstone.

Young, D. B., Srivastava, T. N., Fitzovich, D. E., et al. (1992). Potassium and catecholamine concentrations in the immediate post exercise period. *Am J Med Sci, 304,* 150-153.

Chapter 40 Mass Graves and Exhumation

Deborah Storlie

Mass casualty incidents can result from natural disasters or from human rights abuses. In either case, mass graves are often utilized to dispose of and hide remains. Forensic experts are often called on to exhume the bodies and to make positive identifications. In cases of human rights abuses, forensic experts are also requested to determine what happened, to help bring the perpetrators to justice, and to prevent similar events from occurring. Often these killings are deliberate, unlawful, and politically motivated. These deaths are considered homicides (Kirschner & Hannibal, 1994).

No legal definition of mass graves exists (Skinner, Alempijevic, & Djuric-Srejic, 2003). The United Nations has accepted the definition of *mass graves* as "locations where three or more victims of extra-judicial, summary or arbitrary executions were buried, not having died in combat or armed confrontations." The intent of conducting mass grave exhumations is to corroborate witness testimony, to recover evidence related to reported events of wrongful death, to document injuries, and to recover human remains.

Mass grave sites can support witness testimony and provide irrefutable evidence that crimes such as summary executions were committed. John Gerns, forensic expert of the United Nations' International Crime Tribunal for the former Yugoslavia (ICTY), stated, "Regardless of the reliability of the witness, testimonial evidence without corroborating physical evidence can be the most contentious and weak form of evidence in an investigation or during the subsequent trial" (United Nations: ICTY, no date).

Key Point *40-1*

"The main goals of postmortem examination are to determine the cause and manner of death and to collect and record data for identification of mortal remains" (Skinner, Alempijevic, & Djuric-Srejic, 2003).

Mass grave exhumations have been called "a milestone in the rendering of international justice" (United Nations: ICTY, no date). Prior to the 1980s, documentation of human rights abuses was almost entirely through witness and victim testimony. From 1984 to 1985, forensic scientists from the US, working under the auspices of the American Association for the Advancement of Science, exhumed skeletal remains for identification of disappeared persons in Argentina. "It became apparent that medical and forensic verification of torture and extra-judicial executions could provide irrefutable evidence that such activities had taken place" (United Nations: ICTY, no date). Such missions have been conducted in more than 30 countries including Bosnia-Herzegovina, Kosovo, El Salvador, and Guatemala, to name only a few.

Stages of Exhumation

Exhumation of mass graves is partitioned into four stages. Each calls on the skills of experts in a variety of fields including forensic anthropology, forensic pathology, and forensic botany. Forensic nurse examiners (FNE) offer knowledge and skills that complement or expand on those of other forensic professionals. Forensic nurses can be utilized in the field and can be a valuable asset throughout the entire exhumation process and post-exhumation analysis. Therefore, forensic nurses interested in this activity should present their skills and training to groups such as Physicians for Human Rights and make a place for themselves in the exhumation process.

The first stage is the identification and exhumation of a grave site utilizing forensic recovery methods. Following the careful, well-planned exhumation of the remains, the second stage, postmortem identification, is attempted using a variety of techniques. Autopsy and laboratory results, along with investigation reports, then allow for reconstruction of the crime scene and the criminal activities leading to death. This is the third stage. The ultimate goal, and final stage, is the identification and prosecution of the perpetrator(s). This chapter discusses the primary issues encountered at each stage, emphasizing the role of the FNE in contributing to the success of the mission.

No matter what the circumstances of exhumation, a chain of custody must be followed in order for recovered evidence to be admissible at trial. Dr. Clyde Snow, the world-renowned forensic anthropologist, emphasized the gravity of the forensic examiner role while exhuming a mass grave in Vukovar, Croatia: "It's not fun, you are the voice for the wronged. Lose one tooth or even a foot bone and you're an accomplice to the crime" (Stover, 1997).

The greatest injustice that can be done to the wrongfully executed and their family, second only to ignoring evidence, is the improper collection of evidence so as to make it inadmissible in court. Most mass graves exhumed by formal forensic teams are exhumed for forensic reasons relating to prosecution charges. Additionally, local governments may conduct exhumations for the primary purpose of identification of missing and disappeared persons. The physical exhumation usually takes about a month, depending on the number of bodies to be exhumed and extraneous circumstances. According to FBI special agent Tom O'Conner, who worked with teams in Kosovo to exhume mass graves, "on average a team of 8 or 9 investigators can exhume 5 or 6 bodies a day" (Lumpkin & Chang, 2002). The forensic and pathological examinations require considerably more time.

Key Point 40-2

The very existence of mass graves, alone, does not provide proof of criminality because many possible explanations may exist for their creation. Plagues, famine, and mass disaster in third world countries all produce dangerous health situations that demand rapid mass burial of victims to prevent further deaths from disease.

Stage 1: Exhumation Strategies and Forensic Recovery Methods

Primary Issues

Before beginning exhumation, preparatory work must be completed. This involves two stages: searching for the site and then preparing the site for exhumation. Searching for the site is often the first of many challenges. Investigation begins before exhumation is started through interviews with witnesses and a detailed survey of the area. The crime scene investigators incorporate witness statements, previous investigative and casualty data reports, alterations to the landscape, and evidence distribution to determine the area most likely to contain human remains (Hoshower, 1998). At times, the local government is asked to inform investigators of mass grave locations. Satellite photographs are also used to locate areas of disturbed earth and vegetation (Hoshower, 1998). Those trying to locate a mass burial site also rely on infrared film to detect heat emitted from a decomposing body as tissue begins to rot. The grave site should be identified and treated as a crime scene where homicides took place. This includes any location where physical or trace evidence may be found. Electronic mapping procedures precisely measure and map the entire grave area.

Key Point 40-3

The crime scene begins where the suspect(s) changed intent into action and continues through the escape route.

Upon recognition of a possible mass grave, aerial photographs should be taken of the area prior to disturbing the landscape (similar photographs should be taken at the completion of exhumation for comparison). Using a T-shaped steel rod and a probe to detect methane gas and measure temperature is useful when a possible grave site is discovered. The use of these techniques prevents unnecessary excavation at all suspected sites, which can be costly and time consuming (Boyd, 1979). Additionally, investigators must differentiate mass graves related to conflicts from those dating back to conflicts in the same territories during previous periods of violence (e.g., World War II). It is also important to distinguish between graves of combatants or civilians who were buried collectively for the purpose of sanitation or logistical reasons.

Best Practice 40-1

The forensic death investigator should arrange all logistical details before starting groundbreaking associated with exhumation.

A temporary autopsy site and forensic laboratory must be set up. Vehicles to transport the bodies and evidence should be arranged. Other details focus on funding and time constraints–funding is usually limited and deadlines are often very restrictive. Time constraints often create a challenge in utilizing proper scientific procedures, in recovering optimal data, and in closing the site in a timely manner. Time constraints include cultural pressures to rebury the bodies within a given period of time.

The grave site is now ready to prepare for exhumation. First, the scene must be secured from weather, wild animals, and people. The crime scene is most likely to be disturbed by suspects, witnesses, high-ranking officials, and investigators. The physical security of the exhumation team must also be considered at this time.

Key Point 40-4

Prevention of criminal activity and physical violence against the exhumation team are vital to deter any suspect groups from targeting members of the exhumation team and attempting to prevent or to influence the findings.

Complicating factors include heavily scavenged sites, unexploded ordnances, environmental and physical hazards, and time and budget constraints as well as demands made by foreign governments, cultural barriers, and a politically and emotionally charged atmosphere (Hoshower, 1998). "International incident scenes have often been subjected to concomitant cultural and natural transformations" (Webster, 1998).

Because each situation is unique, so must be the excavation strategies for each investigation. The situation includes physical, cultural, and resource limitations and is usually logistically complicated. Often, detecting and removing land mines are the first safety measures undertaken. Such mines are often buried with the bodies or on top of and around the site. De-mining and booby trap disposal is an activity that takes place throughout the exhumation process. During the reburial of victims from the Srebrinica massacre in the Bosnian War in August 1995, the Bosnian Serbs buried grenades and booby traps at multiple levels with the victims to deter exhumation efforts.

An excavation grid is placed around the area and excavation proceeds in gridded units (Fig. 40-1). On initiation of exhumation, investigators will begin documenting evidence and remains, noting the condition and relative position of each. Measuring distances to fixed objects that will remain long after the search ends is the best practice. Nearly all evidence is fragile and susceptible to contamination, breakage, or deterioration, so precautions should be taken to prevent such damage.

Best Practice 40-2

Never mark directly on the evidence; always mark on the container. Record specific information on each photographic exposure including date, time, and personnel involved.

After exhumation efforts have begun, collection, preservation, and analysis of evidence become the focus of the investigation. Soil is carefully removed in increments of whatever levels had

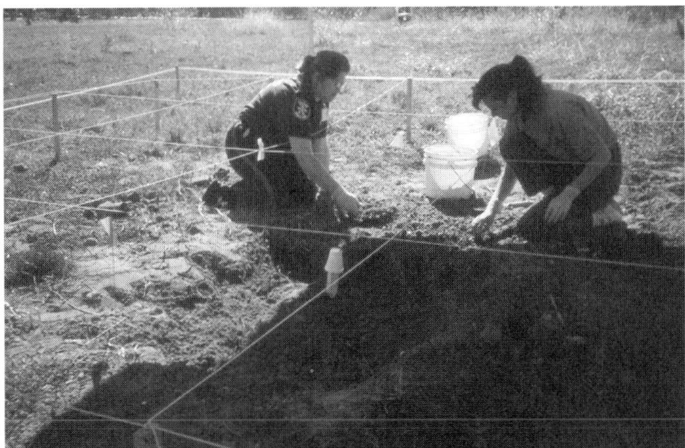

Fig. 40-1 A law enforcement officer and a forensic nurse collect evidence at a mass grave site.

been determined to allow the maintenance of three-dimensional control throughout the excavation. Three-dimensional control of artifact provenance is required to reconstruct the sequence of events (the focus of stage 3) in a mass grave with bodies superimposed over one another with shell casings and wadding scattered in, around, or between bodies (Hoshower, 1998). Throughout the investigation, several forensic experts from various disciplines are used. This group includes at least one forensic pathologist, archaeologist, anthropologist, odontologist, toxicologist, psychiatrist, entomologist, and botanist, along with the crime scene technician, detectives, and criminalistics laboratory personnel. At the grave site, forensic pathologists, forensic anthropologists, and forensic archaeologists are present along with workers. There may also be an investigating judge provided by the host government.

Physical evidence may be divided into three types: objects, body materials, and impressions. Objects include weapons, notes, letters, bullets, and cigarette/cigar butts. Body materials include blood, hair, tissue, urine, feces, and vomitus. Impressions can be in the form of fingerprints, tire tracks, footprints, bullet holes, and palm prints. Relevant evidence generally includes shell casings and bullets, and nonburied evidence (e.g., bullet hole patterns on nearby trees). It is important to remember that recovered items could bear latent fingerprints (Boyd, 1979). Plant and insect remains are also removed and studied to help identify the time of death more accurately.

The location and position of the bodies can be central to establishing how the victims were killed and their remains disposed of. The positions can also reveal whether victims were lined up and shot, and from what angle, and whether they were bulldozed into the site after being executed. "Spatial distribution of bones, teeth, and other items recovered in surface finds can help in determining the original location and position of the body" (Hoshower, 1998). An electronic locator, called a *surveying station*, has begun to be used to provide exact coordinates for recovered remains and evidence. If such technology is not available, a detailed diagram should be used. This diagram provides a record of the three-dimensional relationship between objects.

One of the golden rules of forensic investigations has been stated time and again in articles published on this subject: "Any item of evidence that has been moved, either accidentally or by mistake, must never be replaced for purposes of photographing" (Boyd, 1979). Items should be photographed with and without identifying numbers, a scale, and an arrow pointing to magnetic north (Boyd, 1979). All removed material should be sifted through two screens: the first with quarter-inch squares and the second with a standard window screen (Boyd, 1979). The condition of evidence depends on the presence of water and insects, as well as the pH of the soil. These factors can act to destroy or preserve evidence (Webster, 1998). Therefore, samples of the soil and water in the grave should be taken. This will allow forensic specialists to estimate the expected timing of degradation of evidence, including bodies, and therefore determine an approximate time of death.

Key Point *40-5*

When an item of evidence has been moved or altered, it is impossible to restore it to its original position or condition.

Role of the Forensic Nurse Examiner

Because forensic nurses are affiliated with multinational military units who are highly trained in de-mining pertinent areas, they bring this expertise, along with forensic skills, into human rights missions. For example, Captain Baldiv Adjula Singh is a forensic nurse examiner with the Singapore Armed Forces who is a specialist in removing land mines as well as other engineering skills. FNEs such as Singh would be an excellent addition to the human rights mission in the exhumation of human remains.

The proper collection and preservation of evidence from the crime scene, in this case the grave, serve several purposes. Primarily, the evidence is used to establish that a crime has been committed, that a certain person has committed a crime, and how the crime was committed. Most evidence collected in buried body cases is physical in nature, defined as any matter, material, or condition that may be used to determine the facts in a given situation. For each type of physical evidence, there is an appropriate collection technique that is to be followed by an appropriate preservation technique.

During this stage of investigation, the FNE can be of assistance in documenting location, condition, and removal of evidence. The forensic nurse may also be in charge of regulating the systematic numbering and tagging of remains and keeping the evidence and associated remains correlated. The FNE may also be a participant in the photographic documentation of the crime scene, both before and after the removal of objects. A chain of custody (evidence) form should be provided for each single piece of evidence and remains. The forensic nurse can take charge of this as part of the tagging system. A solid chain of evidence must be maintained to ensure the integrity of every specimen or piece of evidence seized. Failure to establish or maintain the chain of custody will prevent admissibility of the evidence in court.

During this stage, interviews may be conducted. Sexual assault investigation and examinations involving the documentation of evidence is one area of the FNE's expertise. Many victims, especially women, are more comfortable talking to other women about the crime, especially if rape is involved. This makes the FNE essential during the initial investigation of the crime when interviews are conducted.

Although several agencies and many people are involved, remember that everyone is working as a team and each participant is a vital link in the process. This is the first step in bringing closure and justice to survivors of the victims. It also allows the truth to be known.

FNEs have been trained in the exhumation of human remains at the Dade County Medical Examiner Metro Dade Police Department course in Miami, Florida. Other specialized courses in exhumation are available and are recommended for forensic nurses interested in working with human rights organizations. Greater numbers of nurses are becoming involved in forensic science and human rights organizations than ever before. This group of professionals represents a previously untapped resource to the forensic pathologist, anthropologist, and death investigative team. As the need for forensic services expands in the military forces, new roles and new responsibilities will be assigned to FNEs in death investigation, documentation of torture and abuse, and sexual assault of both living and deceased individuals. All forensic nurse death investigative (FNDI) personnel can be prepared with minimal training in minimal time due to their extensive background in death investigation and experience. This includes the postmortem examination of rape/homicide victims. The need for such personnel is at an all time high due to greater human rights investigations, the investigation of war crimes and crimes against humanity, and the number of prosecutions in the World Court, which require forensic specialists in these areas. The FNE is a well-recognized expert in many areas of consequence where healthcare, forensic science, and the law intersect.

Stage 2: Postmortem Identification of Remains

Primary Issues

Bodies and remains are transported to the lab where they are first radiographed before forensic autopsy. The goals of the autopsy are identification, documentation of injury, and determination of cause and manner of death. Primary identification is based on the estimated stature of the deceased, the gender, age, and whether the deceased was right- or left-hand dominant. These characteristics are based on forensic examination of bones. Bones can also indicate the cause of death. Entry and exit wounds or a pattern of bullet holes can show the manner of death and are often indicative of mass execution rather than death in combat. When there is commingling of skeletal remains, bones should be examined with shortwave ultraviolet light to segregate them (Kahana, 1999). After segregation, the bones should be arranged in anatomical order.

Buried body cases are complicated by mass numbers of bodies to compare with mass numbers of missing individuals. This makes a quick match nearly impossible. Personal effects are often recovered and can be returned to family members at the conclusion of the investigation. Clothing, dentures, and eyeglasses can aid identification if they have inscriptions or writing on them or if the eyeglass prescription is known for missing people. If complete decomposition has not occurred, tattoos or other skin markings are of considerable importance. Of course, fingerprints are useful, but only if fingerprints are available with which to compare them. In many countries where mass grave exhumation takes place, fingerprints are not often available.

No two sets of teeth are identical. Even if direct identification is not available, dentition can offer information on age, gender, racial affinity, and possibly socioeconomic status. "Dental identification is perhaps the primary method of identification in cases of mass disaster" (Weedn, 1998). "Positive dental identification can happen only when antemortem records are available for comparison" (Weedn, 1998). Along the same lines, medical records reveal a history of illness, injury, or surgical procedures. This can most easily aid in ruling out an identity or confirm whether a unique characteristic is noted.

Radiology is a common tool used to identify foreign matter in a body or the presence of illness. Sinus films provide good comparison tools, as they are highly variable between individual people. In cases of mass grave exhumation, anthropologic examination is one of the most powerful tools available to determine what happened, how it happened, and also to narrow the possible identities of the various remains. Analysis of hair for "characteristics such as color, length, and texture may be useful to exclude putative identifications and for investigation purposes" (Weedn, 1998). However, forensic anthropology alone "will not yield conclusive or positive, but presumptive, identification" (Weedn, 1998).

Given that the absence of dental and fingerprints records is common in these situations, DNA analytical methods are generally employed. Most tissue or fluid, including hair and bone, will permit DNA testing. Polymerase chain reaction (PCR)-based genetic testing allows testing on old, severely decomposed, and small samples. The advantages of DNA are that it is the same throughout the body (in all cells), throughout life, and it is unique in each person (with the exception of identical twins). Each cell contains the same DNA, which in humans contains 3 billion base pairs. Sets of thousands of base pairs code for one gene and generally each gene codes for a protein. Although proteins tend to be indistinguishable among most individuals, there are many regions on the DNA that do not code for proteins and vary considerably among people. These variations are exploited in the identification of individuals. All the genes in the body are passed on from the parents of the person. For this reason, if DNA from both the mother and the father can be collected and sequenced, then the identity of the individual can be confirmed or ruled out with a high degree of reliability. The type of DNA used for this process called *fingerprinting* is chromosomal DNA.

Another type of genetic testing is mitochondrial DNA (mtDNA) testing. There are thousands of copies of mitochondrial DNA for every copy of chromosomal DNA. Thus, when insufficient quantities of chromosomal DNA are available, an alternative exists. Mitochondrial DNA is more variable among individual people than chromosomal DNA. Additionally, because mitochondrial DNA is passed on only from the maternal contribution, an exact DNA sequence match can be found in a sibling, mother, aunt, or even distant maternal relatives.

Mitochondrial DNA is limited in its applications, however, because it cannot distinguish individuals from the same maternal line from each other, such as two siblings. Therefore, mtDNA should be used to confirm findings based on other clues such as height, gender, and medical history (Skolnick, 1993).

Teeth are optimal sources of DNA because the exterior surface of a tooth surrounds and protects soft pulp, which is composed of living cells. This DNA is therefore protected from the external environment and thus biological degradation (Weedn, 1998).

Evidence such as bullets, shell casings, and bullet fragments are also analyzed at the laboratory. These are compared with data on types of firearms and tool mark analysis of suspected weapons, specifically those well recognized as being associated with a specific group of military or paramilitary organizations suspected of committing the crime.

Role of the Forensic Nurse Examiner

The FNE may be called on to assist in the autopsy, especially in situations of mass body exhumation. Here the forensic nurse may need to rely on his or her forensic training and experience to identify trauma characteristics. For instance, the examining physician may request the forensic nurse to assist in distinguishing between blunt and sharp trauma or entrance and exit wounds from bullets. The forensic nurse may also be requested to make incisions or assist in specimen collection. The most common types of specimens to be collected in such situations are tissue and hair to be used for the purpose of assisting in identification of remains as well as identifying time of death and possibly means of death (if identifiable through toxicology). When investigating human-rights-abuse cases, the FNE can also be called on to interview living survivors. In this case, the nurse will employ interviewing, documenting, and examination techniques to collect evidence and witness testimony. Forensic pathologists, forensic anthropologists, and other forensic specialists, as well as laboratory technicians, do most of the work at this stage.

Forensic expertise helps families learn the fate of their loved ones (Kirschner & Hannibal, 1994). Emotional healing can finally be initiated for loved ones and family members at this time (Webster, 1998).

Stage 3: Reconstructing Crime Scene and Criminal Events Leading to Death

Primary Issues

A medicolegal autopsy will not only assist in identifying remains but also in determining the cause, manner, and mechanism of death. One of the challenges is often distinguishing between antemortem and postmortem injuries.

The cause of death is based on knowledge of the circumstances, history of the victim, and environmental factors. Circumstances are based on witness statements and physical evidence at the crime scene. If identification is made, the social and medical background of the victim is then considered. The investigation also includes an analysis of the environment where the body is found.

It must be determined whether the assault took place at the grave or if the bodies had been moved to the grave site after death occurred. This is generally easy to determine based on the presence of shell casings and the position of the bodies. If bodies are found wrapped around others, as though clinging to each other in their last moments or life, then they were probably killed at that site.

Forensic entomology aids in determination of manner of death, movement of a cadaver from one site to another, and the length of the postmortem interval. "The insects and other invertebrates colonizing corpses as decomposition progresses can provide valuable information concerning the time and manner of death" (Lord & Burger, 1983). Insects on, in, and below the corpse are collected. The insects should be kept in containers with the collection date and time, location of remains, area of body infested, and name of the collector on the container. Insects are helpful in determining time since death occurred, as well as the movement of bodies from other locations (Lord & Burger, 1983).

There are three stages of change after death: early, late, and tissue changes. Cessation of respiration, cessation of circulation, skin pallor, muscle relaxation, eye changes, and blood coagulation and fluidity characterize the early stage. The late changes after death are algor mortis, livor mortis, and rigor mortis. Algor mortis is the cooling of the body after death. Clothing, body size, and activity before death affect the rate of cooling. Livor mortis is a bluish-red discoloration of the dependent portions of the external surface of the body due to postmortem stasis of blood. (Norman, 1986). These spots are generally 4 to 5 mm or larger. Livor mortis indicates the position of the body soon after death. It can be used to indicate that the body was moved since initial burial. Rigor mortis is cadaveric stiffness. In the case of mass grave excavation, many postmortem markers have subsided as the death usually occurred months or years before.

Most important to such investigations are postmortem tissue changes. Decomposition occurs as the body degenerates as a result of natural cell enzymes and bacterial action. Insects soon migrate to the body and lead to skeletonization or removal of the soft tissue. Mummification is the drying of the body or its parts with leather-like changes, generally a finding that occurs in dry climates. *Adipocere* is the formation of a waxy substance due to hydrogenation of body fats. This occurs in moist environments. These stages of death are good indicators of the time of death, but time of death is always an estimate.

Plant life (i.e., flora) is examined by forensic botanists to indicate a range of time of burial and location change of bodies. Plants, seeds, or bark that grow in one area often do not grow in a neighboring area. Therefore, evidence of a plant foreign to an area of a grave indicates that it was brought there with the body from a different location (Lane, Anderson, & Barkley et al., 1990). This indicates that the body was moved from its original location.

Different types of cloth decompose at different rates. Clothes worn by a deceased person generally last two years or longer before total decomposition. Therefore, the level of decomposition of clothing can also be indicative of the length of time a body has been buried. The clothing can also be indicative of the social class and lifestyle of the victims (hospital workers versus farmers).

Role of the Forensic Nurse Examiner

The FNE has been an integral part of evidence collection and therefore has much to contribute to the reconstruction of criminal events. Forensic investigation into human-rights-related casualties serves as documentation to set the historical record straight. Therefore, it is important that all forensic experts be included in identifying the criminal events that led to the death casualties.

Stage 4: Identifying and Prosecuting the Criminal

Primary Issues

In cases of human rights abuses, the persons responsible for the abuses are generally known. Prosecutors require physical evidence in addition to eyewitness testimony to pursue justice. The numerous bodies exhumed and the manner of death determined for these people are used to construct the case against the suspected criminal(s). At the conclusion of the investigation, indictments for the arrest of suspected war criminals are issued. In Bosnia and Rwanda, the international community had to conduct extensive exhumation and crime scene investigations before issuing indictments for the arrest of war criminals.

Role of the Forensic Nurse Examiner

At this point, the FNE may become an expert witness and testify in grand jury or trial proceedings. The nurse may be called on to verify the chain of custody, initial collection, and location of evidence, and to describe exhumation methods used by the forensic team. The FNE can also be requested to give his or her expert opinion on trauma types, specimen collection procedures, and how the crime most likely occurred. This nurse may also be put on the stand to defend or explain his or her documentation during the investigation.

The primary purpose in the courtroom is to establish the corpus delecti, which is composed of three parts: identifying the deceased, determining that the death is not natural, and verifying that the death resulted from a criminal act and is thus not accidental or suicidal. Therefore, the FNE may participate in any or all of these efforts. It is hoped that such investigations will prevent such violations from occurring in the future by holding those responsible for the atrocities accountable for their actions.

Forensic missions to investigate deaths following human rights violations have traveled to Argentina, Bolivia, and many other countries (Kirschner & Hannibal, 1994). Legal obstacles often hamper these investigations. In addition, there is reluctance of eyewitnesses to testify because they fear reprisals. Sometimes the lives of investigators are subject to threats. The ultimate goal is to re-create as accurately as possible the circumstances of the crime committed, to identify and apprehend the perpetrator(s), and to guide the case successfully through the criminal justice system (Boyd, 1979).

Vukovar is a town on Croatia's eastern border. During the Balkan War of the 1990s, the Yugoslav National Army (Joint National Army [JNA]), composed primarily of Serbs, attacked Vukovar, a Croatian stronghold. That city quickly fell to the Serbs after an intense attack. The JNA soldiers took 200 patients and staff from the hospital and drove them to a farm complex called Ovcara. The JNA soldiers then brutalized these individuals by beating and mentally torturing them. At the time this grave was excavated, the Serbs held the territory. UN troops stood guard.

"The Ovcara grave had nothing to do with battlefield casualties" (Stover, 1997). Seventy-five spent cartridges of a caliber consistent with a standard JNA weapon were found mixed in with the bodies. Shortly after a forensic team visited the site for an initial analysis, the Serbs governing the area passed a resolution prohibiting work at the grave. This is an example of the tremendous influence local governments have on international exhumation efforts. There is potential for the FNE to have a vital and important role in the exhumation of mass graves. (See Fig. 40-2.)

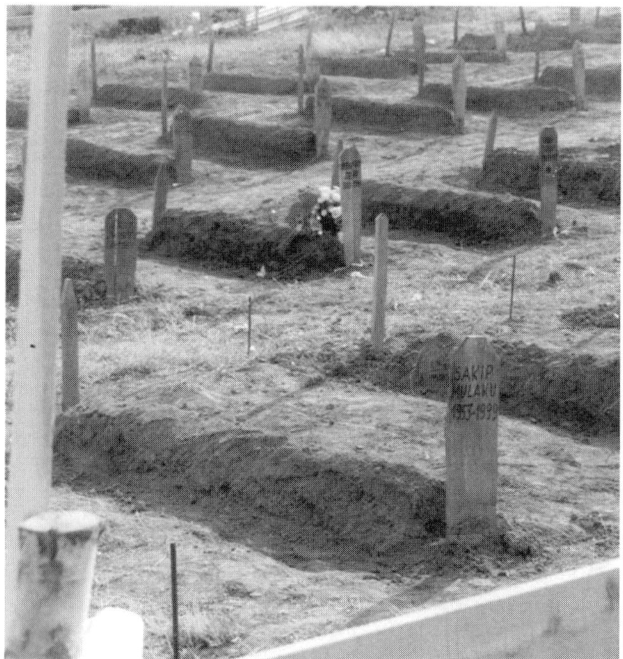

Fig. 40-2 Reinterred bodies recovered from a mass grave site in Kosovo.

Case Study 40-1 In Search of Clandestine Graves

During years of political strife and civil war in developing countries, mass executions are common where powerful groups attempt to persecute weaker, less organized groups or individuals of one country or a neighboring country. At the time of the "disappeared" in Argentina, men, both young and old, were taken from the streets never to be seen again. Thousands of these individuals simply disappeared. It is well known that the political powers use unnecessary and lethal force to reduce the number of potential soldiers who may one day fight for the opposing rebels. Those who had lost family members, friends, and loved ones sought help from the police, yet it is often the police who are used as an arm of the government to carry out mass murder as a means of instilling fear and threats among the population of minorities or noncombatants. The police did not assist in locating the "disappeared," nor did they assist in identifying any discovered human remains, which were brought out of shallow graves by the families.

The next cry for help went to the scientists at the universities in the departments of legal medicine. The scientists were afraid to get involved—knowing if they did, they would be next. However, a visitor to the university happened to be a forensic anthropologist from the US, Dr. Claude Snow. A mother of a young boy who had been missing was searching for help in identifying the remains of a small body suspected to be her son. Snow stated it was not his place to get involved in cases outside his country, but seeing the depth of grief in the mother, he agreed to identify this one case, which turned out to be her son. All the mothers and wives began to beg Snow to identify other remains, to relieve them of the ultimate question of life or death. He could not reject their pleas, but he needed help at a time when local forensic professionals feared for their lives. The students at the university volunteered to help and became forensic professionals under pressure. They were soon to identify hundreds of bodies buried in clandestine graves, 200 to 400 at a time. When Snow made his final visit, these impromptu forensic specialists had become the genuine specialists, unearthing remains alone and relying on the expertise they had learned. Ultimately, the numbers of bodies are documented for the prevention of such crimes against humanity, and identification of the remains helps to reduce human suffering among the survivors. Truth as the mantra of the forensic sciences has served both health and justice.

Summary

The exhumation process entails attention to detail, patience, cultural awareness, and an ability to extract the precise details of the criminal event. These are qualities innate in the forensic nurse through specialized education and training. This role is awaiting further development by forensic nursing pioneers and the exhumation teams who will benefit from inclusion of the FNE. The consequences of ignoring this area are not only a loss of scientific professional development but, more important, a loss to the greater cause of justice in the resolution of crimes against humanity.

Resources

Organizations

American Academy of Forensic Sciences (AAFS)

400 North 21st Street, Colorado Springs, CO 80904; Tel: 719-636-1100; www.aafs.org

Amnesty International, USA

5 Penn Plaza, 14th Floor, New York, NY 10001; Tel: 212-463-9193; www.amnesty.org

Armed Forces Institute of Pathology

6825 16th Street NW, Washington DC 20306-6000; Tel 800-577-3749; www.afip.org

NecroSearch International, Inc.

1713 Wilcox Court, Unit A, Fort Collins, CO 80524; 970-221-4044; www.necrosearch.org

Physicians for Human Rights

2 Arrow Street, Suite 301, Cambridge, MA 02138; Tel: 617-301-4200; www.phrusa.org

References

Boyd, R. M. (1979). Buried body cases. Published by the Federal Bureau of Investigation, U.S. Department of Justice, FBI Academy, Quantico, VA. Reprinted from the *FBI Law Enforcement Bulletin, 48*(2), 113-118.

Hoshower, L. M. (1998). Forensic archeology and the need for flexible excavation strategies: A case study. *J Forensic Sci, 43*(1), 53-56.

Kahana, T. (1999). Forensic radiology. *Br J Radiol, 72,* 129-133.

Kirschner, R. H., & Hannibal, K .E. (1994). The application of the forensic sciences to human rights investigations. *Med Law, 13,* 451-460.

Lane, M. S., Anderson, L. C., Barkley, T. M., et al. (1990). Forensic botany: Plants, perpetrators, pests, poisons, and pot. *BioScience, 40*(1), 34-39.

Lord, W. D., & Burger, J. F. (1983). Collection and preservation of forensically important entomological materials. *J Forensic Sci, 28*(4), 936-944.

Lumpkin, B., & Chang, A. (2002). *Old skills, new uses: Investigators in Mexico use techniques developed in Kosovo.* Retrieved from http://abcnews.go.com/sections/world/DailyNews/mexicojob991201.html.

Norman, W. C. (1986). *Death investigation bulletin: Glossary of terms and definitions commonly used in the investigation of death.* Quantico, VA: Behavioral Science Investigative Support Unit, FBI Academy.

Skinner, M., Alempijevic, D., & Djuric-Srejic, M. (2003). Guidelines for international forensic bio-archaeology monitors of mass grave exhumations. *Forensic Sci Int, 134,* 81-92.

Skolnick, A. A. (1993). Mitochondrial DNA studies help identify lost victims of human rights abuses. *Med News Perspect, 269*(15), 1911-1913.

Stover, E. (1997). The grave at Vukovar. *The Smithsonian, 27*(12) 7-25.

United Nations: International Criminal Tribunal for the Former Yugoslavia (ICTY). (no date). *Bulletin: Exhumations.* Retrieved from www.un.org/icty/BL/08art1e.htm.

Webster, A. D. (1998). Excavation of a Vietnam-era aircraft crash site: use of cross-cultural understanding and dual forensic recovery methods. *Forensic Sci, 43*(2), 277-283.

Weedn, V. 1998. (W). Postmortem identification of remains. *Clinics Lab Med, 18*(1), 115-137.

Unit Seven

Legal Standards and Practices

Chapter 41 Legal Issues for the Forensic Nurse

Susan Chasson

Every day new laws and new interpretations of existing laws are created. Forensic nurses must understand where to find the current sources of laws and how to apply those laws to their forensic practice. Because the law is constantly changing, a textbook should be used only as a reference source for legal information. When nurses require specific legal advice, they should consult with an attorney who is familiar with that area of the law. It is important to understand that the laws of each state may deal differently with the same issue or question. Federal laws may also be interpreted and applied differently in some states. This chapter will discuss state, federal, and international laws. The chapter will also examine the application of agency regulations and case law. Forensic nurses need to learn how the law affects decision making in forensic practice and how to protect the legal rights of the patients they serve.

Sources of Law

Forensic nursing practice is regulated and influenced by state and federal laws. Each level of government can create laws through the legislative process. Laws passed by state legislatures or the US Congress are called statutes. Most nurses are familiar with the process of legislative lawmaking, but they may be unaware of the process used by government agencies to create law. The purpose of legislation is to provide a framework for the government to create standards for regulating a subject. But many areas of government regulation require detailed descriptions of what and how a subject will be legally controlled.

Because elected officials often do not have the technical expertise to write regulations for a specific subject, they often delegate this task to governmental agencies. The process used by government agencies to make rules and regulations is called administrative rule making. In most states and within the federal government, administrative rule making follows strict guidelines. These guidelines are a way to protect the rights of citizens, because once these rules are made and approved, they become enforceable law. When an agency wants to create a new regulation it usually publishes a draft of the proposed rule. After the publication of a proposed rule the public is usually allowed to comment in writing. Sometimes the agency will open a public hearing to allow interested groups and individuals to make comments. Once the public has been given an opportunity to comment on the proposed rule, then a final rule is published and a date of enforcement is announced. This is a very simplified explanation of what at times can be a very complex process. If certain groups or individuals believe a rule or regulation is not properly promulgated, they may be able to challenge the agency in court to prevent enforcement of the rule.

Rules and regulations often govern details that may need to be modified or changed frequently. For example, the Nevada Nurse Practice Act gives the Nevada Board of Nursing the power to "adopt regulations establishing reasonable standards . . . of professional conduct for the practice of nursing" (Nev. Rev. Stat. § 632.120(1)(a)(2), 1985). Using this legislative mandate to regulate the professional conduct of nurses, the Nevada Board of Nursing can create regulations to control nursing practice as new areas of nursing practice develop. In 1996 the Nevada Board passed a regulation that determines how nurses will identify themselves to a client or patient when practicing telenursing (Nev. Admin. Code § 632.248, 1996). Because the Board has been granted the power to create rules, change can occur without involving the legislative process. This two-tiered approach to creating laws to regulate a practice or subject area allows the elected officials to create broad policies for regulating a field, while the details of the regulations are left to professionals with expertise in that subject area.

The federal government uses legislation and administrative rule making when there is a need for uniform application of standards across the nation. For example, Medicare is a national health insurance program for the elderly and disabled. The Social Security Act describes who qualifies for Medicare, but there are many pages of regulations that describe the details concerning what kind of care is covered and how healthcare providers must bill for their services. The law of the US is found in the US Code Annotated (U.S.C.A.), and federal regulations are recorded in the Code of Federal Regulations (C.F.R.).

In addition to laws created by legislators, and rules and regulations created by agencies, the state and federal courts can interpret existing law and create case law by making decisions in appellate cases. Both state and federal case law can have an impact on nursing practice. For example, in 1991 Richard Heinecke argued before the Utah Court of Appeals that having sexual relations with a patient was not unprofessional conduct and therefore was not a violation of the Utah Nurse Practice Act that should result in revocation of his license (*Heinecke v. Department of Commerce*, 1991). In this case the court interpreted the Utah Nurse Practice Act to prohibit sexual relations with a patient by looking at the clause that stated that a nurse can be charged with unprofessional conduct if he or she is ". . . guilty of immoral, unethical, or unprofessional conduct as it relates to the practice of nursing" (Utah Code Ann. § 58-31-14(1)(b), 1990). When a judge makes a decision in an appellate case, that decision becomes appellate case law. It is important to understand that case law may be used by attorneys to argue for a desired interpretation of the law in other legal cases.

For a judge to rule that a previous decision in a court case is the legal rule for another situation, the facts need to be similar. The Utah Board of Nursing did not want a different judge to decide that a different fact situation might allow a nurse to have sexual relations with a patient. As a result of this concern, in 1998 language was added to the Utah Nurse Practice Act to specify when sexual relations with a patient or former patient would be considered unprofessional conduct (Utah Code Ann. § 58-31b-502, 1998).

State laws are the source of regulation for most areas of health and safety for state residents. State laws that are important to forensic nursing practice include the practice acts for each healthcare profession, including both nurse and physician practice acts. A forensic nurse should also be familiar with state laws that regulate the licensing of healthcare facilities, laws that protect public health, and mandatory reporting laws for child or elder abuse.

Each state is also responsible for creating criminal codes. Criminal codes specify which acts are considered crimes and what the punishment will be if a person is convicted of a crime. Because a criminal conviction can result in the loss of liberty of an individual, these laws must be written in a manner that specifies what types of behavior are prohibited. Forensic nurses need to understand that criminal codes may define the same unlawful act differently in different states. Legal activity in one state may be illegal in another. For example, the age of consent for sexual intercourse varies from age 12 to age 18 in different states in the US (Sutherland, 2003). The federal government also creates criminal statutes. These laws deal with crimes that occur on federal property, or deal with criminal activity that crosses state borders. Federal criminal laws also deal with areas of the law that are enforced by federal agencies. For example, the US Security and Exchange Commission (SEC) regulates the trading of stocks and bonds. When a person illegally trades stocks or bonds, these criminal violations are prosecuted under federal law.

As standards for nursing become more global, there is also a need to understand the importance of international law. International law is created through treaties signed by two or more countries and through decisions made by international courts. The United Nations is the source of many international treaties that protect human rights and have potential application to nursing practice. The Universal Declaration of Human Rights (UDHR) is the document that provides the legal foundation for the protection of human rights throughout the world. On December 10, 1948, 48 of the 56 member nations of the United Nations General Assembly ratified this document that states in Article I, "All human beings are born free and equal in dignity and rights. They are endowed with reason and with conscience and should act towards one another in a spirit of brotherhood" (UDHR, 1948).

The Declaration goes on to state what rights are basic to both women and men, such as freedom to own property and the right to a standard of living that is adequate for health and well-being (UDHR, 1948). The Declaration also prohibits practices that deprive individuals of human rights, such as torture and slavery (UDHR, 1948). When looking at treaties as sources of international law, it is important to see if a nation that signs a treaty has created a reservation to a particular part of the document. A reservation allows a nation to opt out of any part of a treaty that it does not want to support or enforce. For example, the US has adopted the International Covenant on Civil and Political Rights but has reserved the right to not enforce Article 6, which prohibits the execution of persons who committed capital crimes prior to the age of 18 (International Covenant on Civil and Political Rights, 1966).

In recent years, there has been an increased use of international courts to investigate and prosecute war crimes and violations of human rights. Forensic nurses with training in death investigation and injury identification are in a unique position to provide assistance with these international proceedings (Weaver & Lynch, 1998).

Key Point *41-1*

The passage of new laws and the interpretations of existing laws are part of the constantly changing body of knowledge required in forensic practice. Creating a list of legal resources to update critical changes in regulations and case law interpretation is an important aspect of maintaining competence.

Two excellent sources of information are professional organizations and state bar associations. Professional organizations often publish newsletters and create online services informing members of the changes in the laws that apply to a specific area of practice.

The state bar associations are professional organizations for the attorneys of each state. The American Bar Association provides continuing education and updates about changes in state laws for attorneys. Information about continuing education offerings for attorneys is often accessible online and available to the public. When the forensic nurse needs to research a specific topic, most state government websites provide online access to state statutes and case law. Several Internet Web sites are dedicated to providing sources of legal information. Law libraries and their staffs can also offer valuable assistance in locating legal materials. Being able to locate statutes, regulations, and case law is a fundamental part of forensic nursing.

Forensic Nursing and the Nurse Practice Act

Nurses should begin practice with a thorough understanding of their state's nurse practice act. This state statute determines the scope of practice for nurses in each state. In many states forensic nursing is a relatively new area of practice. Nurses should examine their state's act to make sure that they can document that they are functioning within the scope of a registered nurse.

Best Practice *41-1*

Forensic nurses should possess a thorough understanding of their nurse practice acts to ensure that they are functioning within an acceptable scope and standard of practice for a registered professional nurse in the state.

The Alabama Nurse Practice Act states, "Additional acts requiring appropriate education and training designed to maintain access to a level of healthcare for the consumer may be performed under emergency or other conditions which are recognized by the nursing and medical professions as proper to be performed by a registered nurse" (Alabama Nurse Practice Act § 34-21-1(3)(a)). In Utah the practice of nursing includes "performing delegated procedures only within the education, knowledge, judgment and skill of the licensee" (Utah Code Ann. § 58-31b-102(12)(f)). These clauses allow for the expansion of nursing practice into new areas without redefining the role of nursing in the nurse practice act.

Nurses can request a ruling from their Board of Nursing to determine whether they are functioning within their scope of practice.

In Florida, sexual assault nurse examiners (SANEs) went before the Board of Nursing to discuss their forensic practice. The SANEs petitioned the Board to obtain a determination about whether performing evidence collection on adult and adolescent sexual battery patients was within a registered nurse's scope of practice. After examining national standards for the education and practice of SANEs, the Board voted to affirm that the role of the SANE was within the scope of practice of the registered nurse (Florida Board of Nursing Minutes, 2003).

Challenges to the expansion of nursing practice can come from nursing or other healthcare professions. In Missouri two nurses who worked for a family planning clinic were charged with the unauthorized practice of medicine (*Sermchief v. Gonzales*, 1983). In their jobs they performed pelvic examinations and provided contraception under standing protocols from the clinic's physicians. Many organizations and individuals felt these nurses were functioning beyond the scope of the Missouri Nurse Practice Act and the nurses were charged with the unlawful practice of medicine. The Supreme Court of Missouri examined the trend both nationally and within the state of Missouri to change nurse practice acts to allow for the expansion of responsibilities for professional nurses. The court determined that if the nurses had postgraduate training to perform family planning services and were using written standing orders and protocols, the nurses were well within the definition of professional nursing (*Sermchief v. Gonzales*, 1983).

Nurses who want to expand their scope of practice should maintain comprehensive records of education and training (*Hoffson v. Orentreich, M.D.*, 1989). They should also work closely with their professional organizations to create and follow standards of practice for their specialty area. In 1995 the American Nurses' Association recognized forensic nursing as a specialty and in collaboration with the International Association of Forensic Nurses published the *Scope and Standards of Forensic Nursing Practice* (McHugh & Leake, 1997). Collaborative relationships with other professionals in the field who value and support an expansion of nursing practice is another way to demonstrate the need for a change in nursing practice. Finally, nurses should collect data to quantify the increased access to care and the increased quality of care that results from the expansion of forensic nursing practice. Documenting the outcomes of forensic practice will help forensic nurses to continue to be pioneers in the field of providing care and improving the lives of victims of interpersonal violence.

Patient Confidentiality and the Forensic Nurse

The duty of confidentiality is a basic concept of ethical nursing practice. In the realm of forensic nursing, patient confidentially must be balanced with public and individual safety concerns. Both state and federal laws dictate how confidential patient information will be handled. Nurses who breach patient confidentiality can be sued for malpractice and lose their professional license. Under new federal privacy laws a nurse may face fines and possible prison sentences for breaching confidentiality. It is important for a nurse to know where to look for privacy information because different rules may apply in different states.

Each nurse should first look at the state's nurse practice act. Breach of confidentiality is usually considered unprofessional practice. State laws may create other privacy standards for patient information. State laws will also dictate specific circumstances when a nurse may be required to breach confidentiality.

The forensic nurse examiner will often be required to breach confidentiality as a result of mandatory reporting laws. In all 50 states there are mandatory reporting laws for both child and elder abuse. Under the elder abuse statutes of most states, the abuse of disabled adults is usually included. In addition to reporting elder and child abuse, 42 states require that healthcare providers report injuries that are the results of weapons, 23 states require the reporting of injuries that are the result of any crime, and seven states specifically require the reporting of injuries that are the result of domestic violence (Houry, Sachs, Feldhaus, et al., 2002).

The nurse should know who can make a report, what needs to be reported, and where reports should be made. By following the requirements of the mandatory reporting laws, the healthcare provider usually receives immunity from any liability that results from making a report. It is important to understand the extent of the immunity granted by law, because in each state that protection from liability may be interpreted differently. In California immunity is extended to both "required" and "authorized" reports of abuse (California Penal Code §§ 11172, 11172 (a)). Once a report is made, if a mandated reporter continues to provide information requested by an investigator of the abuse, those statements may also receive immunity (*Ferraro v. Chadwick, M.D.*, 1990). In Illinois an initial report made by a provider is protected by statutory immunity. If a provider gives negligent care after a report is made, then the provider may be held liable for malpractice (*Doe v. Winny*, 2002).

Failure to follow mandatory reporting laws is usually considered a misdemeanor criminal offense. Some states have refused to define failure to report as a cause of action for malpractice, and other states are allowing families or the legal representatives of patients to sue providers if an injury occurs after a provider should have reported suspected abuse (*First Commercial Trust v. Rank*, 1996). In Florida the courts do not allow victims of elder or child abuse to claim malpractice against a provider who fails to report suspected abuse (*Mora v. South Broward Hospital District*, 1998; *J.B. v. Department of Health and Rehab. Servs.*, 1991). However in Maryland the courts have taken the duty to report one step further, by stating compliance with a reporting statute does not necessarily preclude finding of negligence, if a reasonable person would take precautions beyond the statutorily required measure (*Bently v. Carroll, M.D.*, 1998).

In addition to laws that require the reporting of abuse or injuries, most states also have public health laws that require the reporting of communicable diseases such as tuberculosis or gonorrhea. The purpose of these laws is to provide public health officials with information about patients who could be spreading infectious diseases. When a patient with a communicable disease is identified, the public health worker contacts the patient. The public health worker then determines if there are other people at risk for infection who need to be notified, tested, or treated. It is important to remember that laws that require reporting of infectious diseases apply to all patients. For example, if the nurse is providing care to a sexual assault victim who is known to be HIV positive, a report needs to be made to the appropriate public health authorities. If possible, the suspect can then be contacted and notified of his exposure to an infectious disease.

In some states other diseases and health problems are reported in order to track and study other public health risks. Many states keep a record of patients with cancer in order to look for patterns that might indicate an environmental cause of the disease. In the state of Washington there is a mandatory reporting law for pesticide exposure (Washington Statutes 70.104.055). Nurses must be aware of the kinds of heathcare problems that are reportable in their community.

A nurse may also breach confidentiality when there is a direct threat to a specific person. On October 27, 1969, Prosenjit Poddar killed his former girlfriend. Two months earlier Mr. Poddar had informed his psychologist about his plans to kill Tatiana Tarasoff. The psychologist and his employers were sued by the parents of Ms. Tarasoff for failure to warn (*Tarasoff v. Regents of the University of California*, 1976). This case established a duty to breach confidentiality when a healthcare provider is made aware of a specific threat to a specific individual. Since the decision in Tarasoff (1976), many states have imposed a duty to warn either by statute or case law (Furrow, Greene, & Johnson et al., 2001). At this time only Virginia and Texas have upheld the duty of confidentiality when the life of another person is threatened (*Nasser v. Parker, M.D.*, 1995; *Thapar, M.D. v. Zezulka*, 1999).

Until recently privacy laws and regulations have been controlled by state statutes and state case law. In 1996 Congress passed the Health Insurance Portability and Accountability Act (HIPAA) (1996). Part of this law included a mandate from Congress to create privacy regulations for personal health information. As more individual health information is being placed into computers, there exists a real concern that private health information can be made readily accessible to the public. Incidents that reinforced this fear included the following: a Michigan-based health system accidentally posted the medical information of thousands of patients on the Internet, a truck in Connecticut dropped thousands of health insurance claims on the road on the way to the dump, and a patient in a Boston-area hospital discovered her medical record had been read by more than 200 of the hospital's employees (65 F.R. 82462, 82467). In an attempt to prevent future and more extensive disclosures of personal health information, on April 14, 2003, several hundred pages of new federal privacy regulations became effective (65 F.R. 82462). Under the new privacy regulation an unintentional disclosure can result in civil penalties of $100 per violation with a maximum fine of $25,000 in one calendar year. Intentional disclosure can result in fines of $50,000 to $100,000 and up to 10 years in prison.

It is important for the nurse to understand when HIPAA regulations apply to forensic practice. If a nurse is acting as a healthcare provider, then the rules and regulations of HIPAA apply. Under HIPAA three types of groups or individuals are classified as "covered entities." Covered entities include healthcare plans, healthcare clearinghouses and healthcare providers. Law enforcement officers are not considered to be covered entities under HIPAA (Podrid, 2003). Although HIPAA does impact how law enforcement can access healthcare information, police officers do not have to follow any of the HIPAA privacy regulations once they have obtained the personal health information of a patient.

If a forensic nurse is employed by a healthcare entity or provides healthcare as any part of the forensic role, then the privacy regulations apply to his or her forensic practice. Under HIPAA all patients are required to receive a written copy of their privacy rights. The patient is also entitled to a copy of all of his or her personal medical information, which may include the forensic record if it is created during the course of providing healthcare and includes personal health information. If a patient seeks care from a health provider, it is assumed under HIPAA that consent is given to the provider to share personal health information for the purpose of treatment, billing, and operating the business aspects of the provider's practice. This means that a forensic nurse may share a patient's confidential health information in order to consult with another healthcare professional about the treatment of the patient.

Best Practice *41-2*

The forensic nurse will release information to a non-healthcare provider only with the written authorization of the patient that specifically outlines the type of information to be released and to whom. The forensic nurse will keep a record of all disclosures.

If a forensic nurse needs to release personal health information to a non-healthcare provider, such as law enforcement or a prosecutor, the patient must first give written authorization. This authorization must give details about the type of information to be released and who will receive this information. The authorization should also include a disclaimer to the patient stating that once this information is released, it no longer carries any federal protection of privacy. The patient can revoke this authorization at any time, but the forensic nurse is not responsible for any release of information that occurs prior to the revocation. This revocation must be given in writing. The nurse is responsible for keeping a record of all disclosures so that a patient will know exactly who has received the personal health information. Forensic evidence that might be considered personal health information includes blood, urine, trace evidence swabs, photographs of injury, and any written records.

There are specific exceptions to HIPAA that deal with both victims and suspects of crime. HIPAA does not void any mandatory state reporting laws for the reporting of abuse, injuries, or communicable diseases (45 C.F.R. 164.512). Any state privacy laws that require stricter privacy standards than HIPAA override the federal regulations. Law enforcement may obtain personal health information from healthcare providers without the consent of the patient for the purpose of identifying and locating a suspect, fugitive, material witness, or missing person. Information that can be given to law enforcement includes name, address, social security number, date of birth, place of birth, type of injury, description of distinguishing physical characteristics, ABO blood type, Rh factor, and date and time of treatment (45 C.F.R. 164.512(f)(i)). Healthcare providers cannot release DNA, DNA analysis, dental records, or samples of body fluid or tissues without consent of the suspect or a court order (45 C.F.R. 164.512(f)(ii)).

Once a patient is deceased, his or her personal health information is still protected, except under the following circumstances. Covered entities may disclose information to coroners and medical examiners for the purpose of identifying a body or determining the cause of death (45 C.F.R. 164.512(g)(1)). State laws that require additional reporting when a death occurs are still enforceable under HIPAA. Forensic nurses can play an important role by understanding HIPAA and facilitating the release of information deemed permissible under the new privacy regulations.

Breach of confidentiality can be a complicated issue when working with adolescent patients. Forensic nurses need to be aware of any state or federal laws that entitle adolescents to confidential care. In many states adolescents may access confidential healthcare for reproductive health problems, drug and alcohol treatment, and mental healthcare. These laws vary from state to state and in some cases state laws determine which institutions can provide confidential care. For example, in Utah adolescents can receive confidential information about contraception unless they access healthcare at a state-funded facility (Utah Code Ann. § 76-7-322, 1988). In some states confidential reproductive healthcare can be received only at federally funded clinics.

Under HIPAA if a state law requires confidential care for an adolescent, then the adolescent must authorize any release of personal health information. In forensic practice an adolescent may be entitled to confidential care, but a nurse cannot guarantee that parents will not be made aware of what has happened to the child. Privacy laws prevent the nurse from contacting the parents without the child's consent. Yet, once information is released to law enforcement, under mandatory reporting laws, the police may contact parents.

In order to maintain confidentiality forensic nurses should create procedures that prevent unauthorized release of information. Patients should be asked how they want to be contacted by the nurse. Permission should be obtained to leave messages. Phone calls from an agency should not be identifiable by caller identification devices. Medical records should be kept in a secure area, and computerized information should be protected from unauthorized access.

Informed Consent

It is essential for a forensic nurse examiner to recognize the right of the patient to be given informed consent before providing care to a patient. The concept of informed consent is based on the right of the individual to make choices about what will happen to his or her body. This right of bodily self-determination was first acknowledged by Justice Benjamin Cardozo in 1914 when he stated, "Every human being of adult years and sound mind has a right to determine what shall be done with his own body" (*Schloendorff v. Society of N.Y. Hosp.*, 1914). For a patient to have control over what happens to his or her body, informed consent must be given before any treatment or procedure.

Key Point *41-2*

The forensic nurse must ensure that the patient has given informed consent prior to any evidentiary examination or related procedure. Informed consent comprises risks, benefits, alternatives to the recommended treatment, and consequences if the treatment or procedure is not performed.

Informed consent comprises four parts. First, the risks of the procedure or treatment must be explained. Second, the patient should be told about the benefits. Third, a patient should be informed of any alternatives to the recommended treatment. Finally, the patient needs to be told the consequences if the treatment or procedure is not performed.

Informed consent is an important part of any forensic examination and is particularly important when examining a victim of a crime. Most victims of crime perceive the crime as a loss of control and an invasion of their privacy. Informed consent allows the patient to regain control over the situation by explicitly permitting access to their body. Evidence collection usually consists of collecting specimens from different parts of the body. Although a patient may have given consent for the entire examination, the patient should be given an opportunity to consent during each new step of the examination.

If a victim of a crime is unconscious, collection of forensic evidence should be delayed until the patient can give consent. Forensic evidence can be collected if it is part of any required emergency care. For example, a women arrives with unexplained loss of consciousness to the emergency department. Under these circumstances it is routine part of the medical care to collect urine and blood for a toxicology screen. The primary purpose for collecting these specimens is to determine why the patient is unresponsive, but the specimens may be collected in a manner that preserves their value as evidence.

When deciding to collect evidence from an unconscious patient the forensic nurse should consider two things. First, will evidence be lost if the patient is allowed to regain consciousness prior to the evidence collection? Second, could the collection of evidence be considered an assault and battery by a patient who later becomes conscious and decides against having that evidence collected? If a nurse believes that critical evidence will be lost prior to a patient regaining consciousness, the prosecutor in charge of the case should be consulted. If the prosecutor wants the evidence collected, a court order can be obtained from a judge.

The care of children and adolescents creates unique concerns with informed consent. Before providing care to a child the informed consent of a parent or guardian is required. In cases of child abuse often the state will take temporary custody of the child and provide consent for the examination. In some states if abuse is suspected, a healthcare provider may be able to provide care without parental consent. Even if a child cannot give legal consent, the child's assent should be obtained before collecting forensic evidence.

Assent is the process of explaining a procedure to a child and requesting the child's cooperation. Even though a child is usually not capable of understanding the risks and benefits of a procedure, the child should be allowed to give permission, in order to obtain cooperation, before having a procedure performed. In forensic practice it is important to obtain the cooperation of the child. First, giving the child control will prevent further physical and psychological damage (Lynch & Faust, 1998). Second, a child who has been traumatized by a forensic examination may not be able to differentiate between the abuse and the medical examination when asked to testify at trial.

Adolescents may be allowed to give informed consent under several different types of circumstances. As mentioned earlier, in certain situations adolescents are entitled to confidential care. If an adolescent can receive confidential care, he or she can also consent to that care. In some states adolescents can be granted the rights of an adult, depending on their legal status. Some states consider minors to be emancipated and have the rights of adult if they are married or pregnant. Other states require a court order to establish that a child is emancipated (Office of Technology Assessment, 1991).

Nurses must also be aware that if an adolescent can consent to care, then he or she can also refuse care. Even when a child has a life-threatening illness or condition, some states recognize a mature minor exception. This exception allows a child to refuse lifesaving medical care if a court determines that the child is mature enough to understand the risks and benefits of refusing treatment. Nurses need to realize that they often hold the unique position of patient advocate. Informed consent should be an integral part of every forensic practice. Ultimately, the rights of patients need to be respected to enable them to make decisions about their healthcare.

When Should a Forensic Nurse Consult an Attorney?

The field of forensics requires the nurse to have a working knowledge of several areas of the law. Keeping informed of changes in state and federal laws and regulations is an essential part of forensic practice. Although the Internet provides an incredible ability for nurses to research legal issues online, the forensic nurse should know when it is important to seek the advice of an attorney.

Forensic nurses should be aware that there are several places to access legal advice. Nurses who work for the state or local government agencies can seek advice through city or county attorneys or their state attorney general's office. State and local governments usually employ both civil and criminal attorneys. Hospitals often have a risk manager or in-house counsel who can access or provide legal assistance for the nursing staff. The state Board of Nursing will usually be able to provide the forensic nurse with legal interpretations of the nurse practice act and other nursing regulations. The state bar association can make referrals to local attorneys, and sometimes state nurses' associations maintain a list of attorneys who are familiar with nursing issues and practice.

When a change in a law or regulation impacts forensic practice, a hospital or agency may need to change policies. An attorney who is familiar with that area of the law should review any changes in the policy and make sure they are appropriate and consistent with the new regulation. If a forensic nurse is dealing with a situation outside the standard procedures and protocols for collecting evidence, or is in conflict about evidence collection with a law enforcement agency, most jurisdictions have a prosecutor on call who can answer any questions or concerns. A nurse who is considering setting up a private practice should consider consulting a lawyer to review any contracts. Corporate lawyers can also provide consultation on tax issues and how to structure a business relationship.

Case Study 41-1 Patient Confidentiality

Karen Smith is a sexual assault nurse examiner (SANE). She has completed her second examination of the day and has gone into the examination bathroom to clean and restock. The toilet will not stop running, so she lifts the lid and in the back of the toilet is a plastic bag containing what appears to be a dried green leafy substance. Karen calls security to come and get the bag. Security notifies local law enforcement. The police determine that the bag contains marijuana and they want Karen to give them the names of all the patients who have received an examination during the last month. Karen is not sure what she needs to do to protect patient confidentiality. She contacts the hospital risk manager and the hospital's HIPAA privacy officer. The HIPAA privacy officer is the person designated by the hospital to train hospital employees about HIPAA and help the hospital enforce the federal privacy standards. After reviewing hospital policy and HIPAA regulations, Karen and the risk manager inform the police department that the patients' names cannot be released unless the patients agree to authorize the release of information or unless the police obtain a court order signed by the judge.

Summary

Forensic nursing is the intersection of nursing practice and the law. Nurses must maintain a working knowledge of the laws that apply to their specific area of practice. Updating this part of a practitioner's knowledge base should be a regular part of continuing education in order for the nurse to maintain competency in practice.

The forensic nurse should not hesitate to seek legal advice when a situation requires a comprehension or interpretation of the law that might best be provided by an attorney.

Resources

Organizations

American Association of Legal Nurse Consultants (AALNC)

401 North Michigan Avenue, Chicago, IL 60611; Tel: 877-402-2562; www.aalnc.org

A nonprofit organization dedicated to the professional enhancement of registered nurses practicing in a consulting capacity in the legal field.

American Bar Association

321 North Clark Street, Chicago, IL 60610; Tel: 312-988-5000; www.abanet.org

American Nurses Association (ANA)

8515 Georgia Avenue, Suite 400, Silver Spring, MD 20910; Tel: 800-274-4ANA; www.nursingworld.net

References

Alabama Nurse Practice Act § 34-21-1(3)a.

Bently v. Carroll, M.D., 734 A.2d 697 (Md. 1998).

Code of Federal Regulations. US Government Printing Office, Washington, DC.

California Penal Code §§ 11172,11172(a).

Doe v. Winny, 764 N.E.2d 143 (Ill. 2002).

Ferraro v. Chadwick, M.D., 221 Cal. App. 3d 86 (Cal. 1990).

First Commercial Trust v. Rank, 915 S.W.2d 262 (Ark. 1996).

Furrow, B. R, Greaney, T. L., Johnson, S. H., et al. (2001). *Health law cases and materials* (p. 336). St. Paul, MN: West Group.

Florida Board of Nursing. (Dec. 3-5, 2003). Minutes of meeting (p. 6).

Health Insurance Portability and Accountability Act of 1996. 42 U.S.C. §§ 201, et seq.

Heinecke v. Department of Commerce, 810 P.2d 459 (Utah 1991).

Hoffson v. Orentreich, M.D., 543 N.Y.S.2d 242 (N.Y. 1989).

Houry, D., Sachs, S. J., Feldhaus, K. M., et al. (2002). Violence-inflicted injuries: Reporting laws in fifty states. *Ann Emerg Med, 39*, 56-60.

International Covenant on Civil and Political Rights. (December 16, 1966). 999 U.N.T.S.171.

J.B. v. Department of Health and Rehab. Servs., 591 So.2d 317 (Fla. 1991).

Lynch, L., & Faust, J. (1998). Reduction of stress in children undergoing sexual abuse medical examination. *J Pediatr, 133*, 296-299

McHugh, J., & Leake, D. (Eds.). (1997). *Scope and standards of forensic nursing practice*. Washington, DC: American Nurses Publishing.

Mora v. South Broward Hospital District, 710 So.2d 633 (Fla. 1998).

Nasser v. Parker, M.D., 455 S.E.2d 502 (Va. 1995).

Nev. Admin. Code § 632.248 (1996).

Nev. Rev. Stat.§ 632.120(1)(a)(2) (1985).

Office of Technology Assessment. (1991). Washington, DC: US Congress

Podrid, A. (2003). HIPAA–Exceptions providing law enforcement officials and social service providers access to protected health information. *Am Prosecutors Res Inst Update, 15*, 4.

Schloendorff v. Society of N.Y. Hosp., 105 N.E. 93 (N.Y. 1914).
Sermchief v. Gonzales, 660 S.W.2d 683 (Mo. 1983).
Sutherland, K. (2003). From jailbird to jailbait: Age of consent laws and the construction of teenage sexualities. *William & Mary J Women Law, 9*, 313-339.
Tarasoff v. Regents of the University of California, 551 P.2d 334 (Cal. 1976).
Thapar, M.D. v. Zezulka, 994 S.W.2d 635 (Tex. 1999).
US Code Annotated. (2000). Washington, DC: US Government Printing Office.
Universal Declaration of Human Rights (UDHR). (Dec. 10, 1948). U.N.G.A. Res. 217 III.
Utah Code Ann. § 58-31-14(1)(b) (1990).
Utah Code Ann. § 58-31b-102(12)(f).
Utah Code Ann. § 58-31b-502 (1998).
Utah Code Ann. § 76-7-322 (1988).
Weaver, J. D. & Lynch, V. (1998). Forensic nursing: Unique contributions to international law. *J Nurs Law, 5*(4), 23-34.
Washington Statutes 70.104.055.
Washington Statutes 45 C.F.R. 164.512.
Washington Statutes 45 C.F.R. 164.512(f)(i).
Washington Statutes 45 C.F.R. 164.512(f)(ii).
Washington Statutes 45 C.F.R. 164.512(g)(1).
Washington Statutes 65 F.R. 82462, 82467.
Washington Statutes 65 F.R. 82462.

Chapter 42 Depositions and Courtroom Testimony

Belinda Manning Howell

One goal of the judicial system is to repair what has been damaged with an eye toward preventing further damage. In the criminal system, those found to be guilty of a crime are punished by a loss of liberty for a period of days to years. On the other hand, if found by a judge or jury to be liable, civil defendants are required to compensate the injured person, the plaintiff, by paying that person specific sums of money. Nurses may be involved in criminal actions by virtue of their contact with victims of crimes in a healthcare setting, or in civil actions through personal involvement with a patient who brings a lawsuit against another individual, usually without any allegation of a crime. In either situation, a nurse may be asked to tell the relevant facts to provide important pieces of the puzzle that must be reconstructed for a judge or jury. Typically, that fact finding will be done in a formal deposition of the nurse, often making a courtroom appearance at trial unnecessary.

Because forensic nurse examiners (FNEs) are very likely to be working in areas commonly associated with the litigation process, it is helpful for them to have a general understanding of the task of providing testimony, in deposition form or in the courtroom. FNEs may be involved with litigation because of knowledge of facts, either directly related to the event that led to the filing of the lawsuit, or concerning the damage resulting from the injury. Additionally, a forensic nurse may serve as an expert witness, either consulting or testifying. The consulting expert reviews documents and provides an opinion that is useful to the attorney in weighing the strengths and weaknesses of the claims; whereas the testifying witness provides written opinions followed by oral testimony in a formal deposition or on the witness stand, or both.

This chapter provides an overview of the roles of factual and expert witnesses, without an attempt to distinguish between relative federal laws and the various state laws.

Purpose of Depositions

In preparing to file a civil lawsuit, an attorney must consider the questions that ultimately will be posed to a jury relevant to the plaintiff's claims. Relevant factual information and the opinions of experts must be gathered. To accomplish that objective, the parties' attorneys will engage in the process of "pretrial discovery," a stage of the lawsuit that allows the story to unfold and gives the parties the tools to carve the most concise presentation of the facts and their relationship to applicable law.

Key Point *42-1*

The information obtained in a deposition constitutes evidence for attorneys who are either prosecuting or defending a client.

One critical step toward preparing an effective presentation of the events related to the plaintiff's claims in a civil matter is the taking of depositions. The purpose of a deposition is to elicit and preserve sworn testimony to rely on at all stages of the litigation (O'Keefe, 2001).

Best Practice *42-1*

A witness should seek legal counsel before complying with requests to furnish tangible items for use in an oral deposition.

A party's attorney can discover information pertinent to a legal claim or relative factual issue through this formal question-and-answer process, which, because the witness is under oath, is identical to the process of eliciting testimony in the courtroom. The opposing attorney will structure questions for the witness to determine their value to the case and to elicit the witness's position on key points. This pretrial deposition permits a preview of the witness's testimony and allows ample time for the opposition to engineer an effective rebuttal.

Key Point *42-2*

The testimony provided in an oral pretrial deposition and that given later in the courtroom must be highly consistent if the witness is to be perceived as highly credible.

To initiate the process, either party will serve a notice or *subpoena* to a witness to appear at a certain time and place to answer questions related to the issues of the case. The notice may include a list of documents or tangible items the witness is to bring, relevant to the subject matter of the action and within the witness's possession or control, such as records, anatomical models, instruments or equipment, books, or other materials that would amplify testimony. A witness should seek legal counsel before complying with such requests for documents or tangible items.

Oral Deposition

Various types of depositions exist, including written and electronic depositions; however, only standard oral depositions, the most common type, will be discussed here. An oral deposition consists of a series of questions posed by attorneys for the plaintiff and the defendant. Ordinarily, this type of deposition is accomplished in an attorney's office or conference space that will permit the formality and privacy required for the proceeding. In addition to the attorneys and the witness, a deposition officer, usually a court reporter, will attend to assure that every question, answer, objection, and statement made "on the record" is recorded verbatim.

The parties, spouses of parties, and employees of counsel may choose to attend the depositions, and with reasonable notice and by agreement, other individuals may be allowed to attend. If either party chooses to have a videographer present, a video recording is made, giving the attorneys the option of having the judge and jury see the witness during the trial, without the witness having to make another appearance. Videotaping will also be useful in the event of inconsistencies in testimony of parties to the suit or other witnesses who typically appear in person in the courtroom. The written record of testimony from a deposition may be read at trial instead of showing a video to the judge and jury, again saving a witness the inconvenience of making a second appearance.

Preparation

Generally, a witness will spend some time with one of the attorneys in the suit in order to be given an idea of the kind of questions to expect and an opportunity to ask questions about the process. Whether an attorney will meet with a witness prior to his or her deposition, and which attorney will meet with the witness, depend upon the role of the witness: if the witness is a party to the lawsuit, the attorney representing the party will prepare the witness; similarly, with expert witnesses, the party seeking that witness's services will spend time reviewing the expert's file and suggesting the kinds of questions the expert might expect to be asked. However, when a witness is an individual with knowledge of relevant facts, but not subject to the control of a party (for example, with an employer-employee relationship), either party's attorney may offer the witness an idea of what matters will be discussed at the deposition.

Witness Representation by Counsel

All deponents are free to bring an attorney to the deposition to represent them. Certainly if the witness is a party or is retained by a party, as in the case of an expert witness, the party's attorney, and the opposing party's attorney, will attend the deposition and represent their respective clients' interests. Fact witnesses may choose to bring their own counsel, depending upon the potential for a conflict of interest.

Professional Insurance Carrier Support

In the case of a nurse whose employer is a defendant, or potential defendant, the nurse should clarify with his or her professional liability insurance carrier that there is counsel available through the carrier; and if the carrier is the same as his or her employer's carrier, the nurse is well advised to request different counsel. This verification should take place well before any interviews or depositions, as sometimes the nurse's interests and the employer's interests do not coincide.

Although nurses encounter ongoing crises in their daily work, the stressors associated with legal proceedings are considerable. The experience is typically intimidating, and removes the nurse from a "zone of comfort." Although the ordeal is not unpleasant, it can be fatiguing because of its length and the intensity of the questioning process.

Length of Deposition

Rules vary by state and jurisdiction in regard to the length of the deposition. The attorneys should be able to give a witness a fair estimate of the time expected to obtain the deposition as well as an explanation of any rule limiting the time allowed for a deposition. A witness should receive a precise answer as to whether or not they may be required appear each day until the deposition is complete. The deposition officer, generally the court reporter, is the timekeeper.

Interrogatives

The attorney who initiated or "noticed" the deposition will most likely begin questioning the witness or *deponent*. At the completion of that direct examination, there may be further examination from attorneys representing other parties to the lawsuit. Cross-examination may or may not take place, but is generally reserved for the courtroom, if cross-examination is necessary at all.

Focus of Questioning

During depositions, the attorney may query the witness about anything as long as the question is reasonable and has been designed to lead to the disclosure of admissible evidence (Required Disclosures; Methods to Discover Additional Matter, 1998). The deponent should expect a series of questions about education, experience, credentials, and work experiences (O'Keefe, 2001). The majority of interrogatives, however, will be about the case or incident that is the subject of the lawsuit. A witness should expect both redundant and repetitive lines of questions that are extremely detailed. This is a tedious process, and the deponent must consciously guard against frustration that is often felt during this part of the deposition. Great care should be exercised by the witness to answer each question carefully and precisely without undue elaboration, which might reveal even the slightest of inconsistencies in the testimony. It is imperative for nurses to be prepared to answer precise questions about the state's nurse practice act, hospital policies, and procedures and nursing standards of practice that would impact the case (O'Keefe, 2002).

Composing Answers

In short, questions should always be answered truthfully. Answers should not be offered until, and unless, the question is understood in its entirety. Any hesitation due to possible misunderstanding should be addressed prior to a response. Once understood, a question should be answered clearly, but concisely. Avoid being forced into a "yes" or "no" answer when a qualified answer is required. A deponent has the right to explain or qualify an answer (Lanros & Barber, 1997). It is not wise to offer information not asked, as commonly done in conversations; the examiner should carry the responsibility of asking the questions. And it is very useful to remember that the truth includes "I don't know" and "I don't remember." A deponent should not feel pressured to come up with an answer or speculate on what would be most helpful to either party. Witnesses should remember that they have taken an oath to tell the complete truth, exactly as they would in a court of law. The deponent should guard against gamesmanship or attempts to outwit the questioning attorney. Not only are most trial lawyers very skilled at oral jousting, but it is the witness who will lose face and risk not being allowed to testify if inconsistencies or incompleteness are attempted. The best news is that there is no skill involved in truth telling.

Supporting Documentation

It is important to remember that typically each individual called to testify will be required by the court to produce any relevant

Best Practice 42-2

When making notes about unusual occurrences or sentinel events, the nurse should record only objective details, avoiding opinions and any reference to emotions surrounding the event.

documents or notes in the custody of the testifying individual. Emotional reactions and opinions should always be omitted if making personal notes following an incident. Merely recording facts that may be relative, such as the staff-to-patient ratio in the unit, the request by the laboratory technician to assist with lab work, the time of the admission, the charge nurses' duties other than patient care, and so on may be helpful to the nurse if litigation commences weeks, months, or even years later. There may be an earlier investigation by the hospital's counsel in anticipation of litigation by the family or by a peer review committee, and factual notes may be useful in preparation for those meetings. A witness may choose to bring *copies* of documents to the deposition; however, the originals must be available for inspection. The court reporter can make copies of documents for attachment to the deposition and return originals to the witness.

Objections to Questions

There is no judge in attendance at the deposition, so no one is authorized to rule on objections to questions. Generally, all questions asked must be answered if understood. In some instances, however, an attorney objecting to a question may be in a position to seek a ruling from the judge before allowing the witness to answer or to produce a particular document. It may be possible to get the judge's ruling immediately by telephone; but more often, the witness may be advised not to respond to that particular question and the deposition will continue until a hearing before the judge may be scheduled. It is safe to say that judges are not patient with attorneys or witnesses who attempt to restrict testimony, so most questions must be answered at the time of the deposition. Although opposing counsel has an interest in avoiding disclosure of information that is privileged, unless an objection can be made and is made, the question must be answered. Whether the testimony will be admissible at trial will be determined at a later date.

Completion of the deposition in the face of inappropriate questioning is not required. There may be a question asked that puts the witness at risk of self-incrimination or a question that appears to violate basic rights to privacy. In that event, a witness is wise to stop the questioning and request that the deposition be completed at a later date. Because the attorneys attending the deposition are representing their respective clients and not representing the witness, advice should be sought from an independent attorney before the scheduled date for completion of the deposition.

Best Practice 42-3

A deponent has the right the read and correct any errors in a deposition before presentation at trial. This right should not be waived (Aiken, 2004).

Postdeposition Procedures

After the examination process is complete, the deponent is usually given an opportunity to review the deposition in its written form, make minor corrections, and sign it. If answers are changed, such that the substance of an answer is revised, the witness will likely be recalled for a second deposition to address that issue. Witnesses who are nonparties, and not aligned with any party, whose depositions are not signed and returned will have effectively "waived" the signing; the deposition may still be used at trial, or it may be suppressed.

Testifying Expert

In any trial, the role of the judge is to rule on issues of law; in a "nonjury" trial, the judge will also serve as the trier of fact. However, when a case is tried to a jury, it is the jury's role to determine the facts. To assist the jury in understanding the evidence or in determining a vital fact issue, an individual with knowledge or experience who can assist the jury with fact finding is retained to be an "expert." An expert who is designated as one who will testify can count on being deposed in advance of trial. Questions will be focused on determining bias and weakening the expert's credibility. Attempts will be made to bolster the examining lawyer's own expert's opinions, for instance, by exposing flaws in the analysis utilized by the expert. The examining attorney must ascertain what the expert intends to say at trial and whether that testimony needs to be challenged for reliability in advance of allowing the fact finder(s) to hear the expert's testimony.

The expert is generally asked to review documents and, if named as a "testifying expert," to provide a written report describing opinions formed upon review of materials. That expert will be deposed so that the opposing party, or parties, may have an opportunity to ask questions about those opinions and the reliability of the bases for those opinions. The opposing party may assert that a particular expert should not be allowed to testify and may request that the court hold a hearing to review certain reliability criteria

The greatest disservice a nurse expert can provide to a party is to agree to consult or testify in a situation in which the nurse is not actually qualified or in a situation in which the nurse is professing to hold opinions or beliefs not actually held.

Jury Access to Oral Depositions

Specific question and *answer* segments of the deposition testimony may be presented at trial. Similarly, if a witness is called to testify live, the questions will be narrowed to present the evidence as briefly as possible. Much of the material that can be covered in a deposition may not be admissible in the courtroom for various reasons, including lack of relevance or a claim of privilege.

Case Study 42-1 Shift Change Confusion

It was a hectic but typical day in the medical intensive care unit at Metropolitan Hospital. Each nurse was assigned two patients, but Sara Ellis, the charge nurse, had to assume the additional responsibility for a newly admitted cardiac patient, Frank Benson, who was quite unstable when he arrived. There were two pages of orders to transcribe and a new IV line had to be started to accommodate the prescribed fluid and medications. Furthermore, the stat lab technician was overwhelmed and asked Sara to obtain the blood specimens that were needed. It was close to the end of the shift, and in addition to this work, Sara realized that she was way behind in her charting and certainly was not ready to give report to the oncoming shift. To make matters worse, there were several interruptions including phone calls from worried family members of the newly admitted patient and from nurses who were questioning the new shift schedule that had recently been posted. One nurse called in "ill" and indicated that she would not be on duty the following day. Just as Sara was racing among her three patients to manage all the "loose ends," she discovered that she had been carrying a syringe of medication with her that needed to be given "stat" (immediately). In fact, it should have been given upon the patient's arrival to the unit over an hour ago. She immediately stopped what she was doing, went to the patient's room, and emptied the syringe into the patient's IV line. Seconds later the patient experienced a cardiac arrest; a full code response was initiated, but all attempts at resuscitation failed. The incident was fully documented in the medical record and an incident report was written which outlined the sentinel event.

Several months later the five nurses who had been on duty during the shift were informed they needed to meet with the hospital attorney and would be expected to give a deposition.

Anticipation of Testimony

When an unusual occurrence or sentinel event occurs, nurses should immediately take steps to prepare for later legal proceedings that may follow. It is important to remember that typically each individual called to testify will be required by the court to produce any relevant documents or notes in the custody of the testifying individual. Emotional reactions and opinions should always be omitted if making personal notes following an incident. Merely recording facts that may be relative, such as the staff-to-patient ratio in the unit, the request by the lab technician to assist with lab work, the time of the admission, and the charge nurses' duties other than patient care may be helpful to the nurse if litigation commences weeks, months, or even years later. There may be an earlier investigation by the hospital's counsel in anticipation of litigation by the family or by a peer review committee, and factual notes may be useful in preparation for those meetings.

When nurses are involved in an unusual occurrence or sentinel event, it is imperative that they make prompt notification to their personal liability insurance carrier.

At this time, they will be advised about how to prepare for subsequent internal investigations or legal proceedings. For example, they will discuss with counsel whether or not to prepare written documentation and what should be precisely recorded for later reference. Nurses should communicate details of the event *only* to the attorney assigned by their insurance carrier and to the hospital's attorney. No discussion of the matter should take place with other individuals such as the patient's family, the other staff members, or any other attorney without consultation with the hospital attorney or the attorney assigned to the case by a personal insurance carrier.

All individuals who are involved in an unusual occurrence or sentinel event are potential fact witness (i.e., those with knowledge of relevant facts by virtue of having been present in the unit and seen or heard something related to the incident). There may be subsequent involvement of an expert witness, too, who possesses expertise in a specific area (e.g., relevant nursing standards of practice or hospital policies). These experts may be asked to testify by either the plaintiff's attorneys or the defendant's attorneys in order to shed light on issues unfamiliar to the lay person. There are a few occasions in which an individual may serve as both a fact witness and an expert witness in the same litigation.

It is common after unusual occurrences or sentinel events for the hospital's attorneys to meet with each staff person involved to ascertain who has relevant knowledge about the incident or the situation leading up to it. Each staff member will be asked to bring any notes made and retained. Additionally, each individual will be reminded not to discuss the facts, both for reasons of confidentiality and to avoid coloring the testimony of others. Fact witnesses often recall facts differently, but gathering and organizing the facts are the attorneys' responsibilities, not the witnesses'.

Witnesses in the Courtroom

It is common to feel uneasy in a courtroom, as there is a certain formality that must be followed. "All rise!" is heard as the judge enters or leaves the courtroom. The judge is always addressed as "Your Honor." Those wishing to speak may do so only with the court's permission when court is in session. The jury flows in and out as a group and only at the direction of the judge. Because the judge has complete control of the steady movement of the trial process, all participants in the courtroom are to give full attention to the judge and to assist in the orderly progression of the litigation.

Individuals, whether involved as a party or nonparty, need to observe and adhere to the "rules" of the courtroom regarding dress and demeanor. Most judges disallow beverages, food, newspapers, and chewing gum. Clothing should be conservative: dark suits for men; suits or long-sleeved dresses for women. Dresses that could be described as "revealing" should be avoided; judges have been known to halt a proceeding to ask an individual to leave the courtroom and return in clothing more suitable to the setting and the occasion.

The outside world is all but forgotten when court is in session as the trial proceeds with an eye toward completion and resolution. Attorneys, jurors, parties, and witnesses may be requested to remain in the courtroom into the evening to avoid disruption of testimony or arguments. The length of trial is typically estimated beforehand, but it is not unusual for unexpected circumstances to prevent adherence to predicted schedules. Although judges will attempt to accommodate any serious scheduling needs of jurors or witnesses, an individual called to testify as a fact or expert witness is well advised to consider the impact on all the participants in a trial before requesting any special considerations.

Summary

Providing testimony during trial, whether in an oral deposition or from the witness stand, is a valuable investment in the judicial system. The forensic nurse who is deposed should carefully prepare for the deposition by reviewing all pertinent documentation related to the case. The attorney representing the deponent should provide essential counsel regarding the expected line of questioning from the opposing attorney and offer advice on strategies appropriate to the deposition process.

During the deposition, the witness must carefully consider each question before answering it, seeking clarification when necessary. Many questions may be answered by "yes" or "no." The witness should not elaborate when responding to a query because such answers can provide valuable information to the opposition that otherwise might not have been elicited. If certain information or specifics are requested within a line of questioning, and the actual facts are vague or unknown to the deponent, speculation should be guarded against. Above all, a witness should always be truthful, despite the impact on the case.

Resources

Journals

Journal of Nursing Law
PESI HealthCare, L.L.C., 200 Spring Street, P.O. Box 1000, Eau Claire, WI 54702-1428; Tel: 800-843-7763;

References

Aiken, T. D. (2004). *Legal, ethical and political issues in nursing* (2nd ed.). Philadelphia: F. A. Davis.
Lanros, N. E., & Barber, J. M. (1997). Legal and forensic considerations. In *Emergency nursing* (4th ed., pp. 559-575). Stamford, CT: Appleton & Lange.
O'Keefe, M. E. (2001). *Nursing practice and the law: Avoiding malpractice and other legal risks.* Philadelphia: F. A. Davis.
Required disclosures; Methods to discover additional matter. (1998). Federal Rule of Civil Procedure 26(a), 30(b)(1).

Chapter 43 Testifying as a Forensic Nurse

Cari Caruso

Testifying in court can be a stressful experience. The anticipation of sitting before a judge and jury, being questioned by attorneys, can produce considerable anxiety, especially if it is a new experience. For a nurse who has never been in court, the local district attorney (DA) can usually arrange for the observation of a trial. Generally, this involves calling the DA's office and introducing oneself as a forensic nurse examiner, and explaining that it would be beneficial to see some court proceedings. The DA will usually be receptive to the request because if there is a chance that, in the future, the nurse may have a case that goes to trial, the DA would like to be assured that the nurse has some prior knowledge of how the court system works. Such an observation will also afford the nurse an opportunity to see the way the courtroom is set up, where witnesses will be seated, and where the jury, prosecutor, and the defense attorneys will be located. Forensic nurses should arrange to attend courtroom observations during a trial that has pertinent elements of their practice specialty. The day of the visit the DA will ask the judge for permission to admit an observer for the proceedings; typically, the judge will give approval if it can be ascertained that the observer has no connections with the case.

Normally, for a trial, an actual witness may not be allowed in the courtroom to hear anyone else's testimony (*Federal Rules of Evidence*, 2000). Witnesses should expect to be seated in the hallway or other adjacent area. Although pleasantries may be exchanged with others, it is inappropriate for a witness to speak to anyone about the case. There may be jurors, family members, or other witnesses in the area. It is a good idea for the nurse witness to bring a neutral kind of book or other activity to pass the time. The DA will attempt to schedule a witness as close as possible to the anticipated time that the nurse will go on the stand. However, it should always be expected that there may be waiting involved.

Witnesses who have had little experience with public speaking should keep in mind certain techniques that may help them to appear relaxed and comfortable while on the witness stand. It is recommended that a witness do a self-analysis of her or his own demeanor in order to pinpoint some basic areas for improvement. For example, if an individual has a tendency to fidget while sitting, conscious efforts to control this behavior may be employed. When a witness appears at ease, it is expected that this will have optimal impact with the jury. Soft, low voices may convey a lack of confidence and possibly detract from credibility. Additionally, it complicates proceedings if the court needs to request the witness to speak up or to repeat testimony. Practicing is an effective way to improve performance during testimony. For example, merely relating a story or event in front of friends or family members and requesting their critique may be a valuable tool. It may be helpful for a witness to ask someone to videotape such sessions in order to study the effectiveness of delivery, presence, and style. Was the event related accurately? Was the speech enunciated and distinct, or was there mumbling, stuttering, hesitation, or stumbling over certain words? Was the pace of speaking too slow or too fast? Was eye contact maintained with the audience? Were there meaningless phrases, such as "you know" or "and um"? Did the speaker maintain the audience's attention throughout the presentation? Some guidelines that may help convey a positive impression are outlined in Box 43-1.

Box 43-1 Guidelines for Effective Testimony

- Dress professionally. A professional appearance shows the jury that nurses take themselves and the proceedings seriously.
- Remember to breathe. When under stress, people tend to take shallow breaths. When getting tense, take a few deep breaths. Take normal breaths before speaking so that the voice will stay at a good level.
- Walk in to the courtroom with authority. Before arriving at the witness box, turn to the clerk, who will ask the witness to raise his or her right hand and recite, "Do you swear to tell the truth . . ." Say, "I do" in a clear and audible tone. Then sit in the witness box. It may be good to start by smiling and saying "Good morning" to the judge and jury.
- Sit up straight and look attentive. Don't fidget.
- Speak clearly and audibly.
- Make eye contact with those speaking, especially when replying to a question.
- Exude confidence.

Even though a witness may have limited experience in the forensic nursing field, he or she will typically have considerable experience as a nurse. These skills will serve the expert well during the testifying process, in which the major task is to educate the jury. Medical and nursing professionals employ their body of knowledge and clinical information to explain certain dynamics to a body of the public that must make sense of it in order to come to a reasonable conclusion. The lay public has little knowledge of medical terminology or physiology, so everything that is stated on the witness stand must be simplified and put into lay terms that can be readily understood. Nothing should be taken for granted in this arena. When most sexual assault nurses speak about the external genitalia they mean parts anterior to the hymen. However, the lay person may think that the reference is to the pubic area. The terms "external" and "internal" should be explained. Technical terms can be used if they have been thoroughly defined. Things that may seem second nature to a nurse may not have the same meaning to the jury, so it essential for the witness to assume the place of a teacher in order to ensure that there is an adequate understanding of the information that has been stated.

It may be strange, to a novice, that before the courtroom session begins, the prosecutor and defense attorney may be making plans for a golf game or amiably chatting about a recent sports event. They may not be rivals outside the court milieu; however, each has a job to do and they must maintain their professional facade during the proceedings.

Role of the Forensic Nurse Examiner

Forensic nurse examiners are called to testify because they have provided an important service that contributed to a particular body of evidence. Whether they function as a sexual assault nurse examiner (SANE), a death investigator, or any type of forensic nurse examiner, they have collected and evaluated information that furnishes data to a larger body of information. By the time of the trial, it is usually known whether or not the case is a viable one. The forensic nurse should have an opinion about whether findings during the forensic examination are consistent with injuries and the history given. However, it should be acknowledged that testimony of the SANE will not usually be the single hinge on which the verdict rests. It will be a supporting part, in a large body of evidence, but not necessarily the only consideration. The role of the forensic nurse examiner is to tell the unbiased truth. Without being present at the scene and not witnessing the event first hand, the intention of the nurse is to relay her or his findings of the examination in testimony. Although the forensic nurse does not want a guilty person to go free or a person who is not guilty to go to prison, a witness should avoid disparaging comments that condemn the defendant. It is inappropriate for the forensic nurse examiner to declare that a sexual assault occurred. The jury will be the force to evaluate the testimony and come to a verdict of guilty or not guilty. The forensic nurse should attempt to impress the court with professionalism, objectivity, and knowledgeable explanations of findings. Hopefully, the testimony will provide clear information to the jury in order for the jurors to reach a satisfactory decision.

Key Point *43-1*

The forensic nurse is a registered nurse who is an objective, nonbiased, skilled professional who has additional education and training in a forensic specialty.

A forensic nurse examiner may be called as a prosecution witness or a defense witness. However, most often, the nurse will appear as part of the prosecution's case. In essence, the forensic nurse examiner is testifying about the evidence that was collected and the truths that the findings reveal. The defense will often attempt to discredit the forensic nurse examiner and raise questions about the nurse's credentials, making it appear that the nurse is biased for the prosecution. However, this is the job of the opposing side and it should not be taken personally. Despite a sound education and outstanding credentials, the credibility of forensic nurses may be brought into question by the opposing attorney because the nurse's testimony will more than likely be damaging to the defense.

Key Point *43-2*

The forensic nurse examiner's objective is to relay the information about the evidentiary findings and to educate the court as to what those findings mean.

Curriculum Vitae

A curriculum vitae (CV) is an organized summary of employment and educational history. It functions like an extended résumé. It should include the nurse's legal name and contact information along with details regarding academic achievements, organizational affiliations, professional presentations, publications, and relevant work experiences.

There are many ways to design a CV, and some nurses choose to have a professional assist them in developing an exemplary record for use in the legal arena. It should be constructed to serve as a formal document that illustrates the education, training, and experience that contribute to the nurse's expertise.

Best Practice *43-1*

The forensic nurse should maintain an up-to-date curriculum vitae that outlines education, experience, and credentials including licensure and certification.

The forensic nurse examiner will be asked to furnish a CV to the prosecutor. It is imperative that it is current, including any classes, seminars, and conferences attended that may demonstrate expertise. It is beneficial to list the dates of individual meetings or conference sessions attended, including the names of the speakers. This will help in illustrating specific study topics along with venerable lecturers who taught them. Many nurses prepare both a comprehensive and an abbreviated format of their CV.

The nurse may want a thumbnail version for personal use to assist in organizing her or his thoughts prior to taking the stand and answering questions about qualifications. This shorter version would contain the elements from the full CV that are most important for the court to hear. It is advisable for the nurse to look over the brief form before going into the courtroom to ensure that all pertinent information can be relayed without hesitation. Although these suggestions may seem elementary, it is easy to overlook important elements of education and experience when sitting in the witness chair. Credentials should be listed first, followed by a work history, specialized training, other achievements, and publications. If there are numerous training sessions or conferences, the nurse may report, "I have attended all required annual training sessions at my employing institution and certain specific scientific assemblies for six consecutive years." Copies of the CV should be readily available upon request.

The CV will not be read in court, so what is said in the court regarding the nurse's qualifications may bear weight on whether the court will accept the nurse as an expert. The forensic nurse examiner should not allow her or his credentials to be stipulated. It is important for the jury to hear all the qualifications that the forensic nurse examiner possesses. Most likely, the prosecutor will have shared the CV with defense counsel to ensure the counsel's awareness of the individual's qualifications to be an expert. The CV may also be a tool to attempt to disqualify an expert when it is perceived that such a presence in the courtroom will be a powerful tool against the opposition.

Subpoena

When the forensic nurse receives a subpoena, certain details should be noted right away. Look at the date of the trial. In many jurisdictions, the subpoena comes shortly before the trial or preliminary hearing. The subpoena will usually list the name of the defendant and not the victim. If the work was primarily with the victim, the nurse may not know the name of the defendant. Look for the contact number of the witness coordinator's officer and make contact promptly. The nurse should state that she or he is the forensic nurse who conducted the evidentiary examination and has received a subpoena. The nurse will be asked to provide the case number, which may be found in a prominent site on the subpoena along with the name of the prosecuting attorney. The witness coordinator will confirm who the prosecutor will be and verify the identity of the victim. Ordinarily the coordinator will establish the nurse's availability for testifying within a certain time span and will ask whether the nurse will be on vacation or unavailable at certain times. At this time, the nurse should confirm the name and number of the prosecutor and make contact with the attorney as soon as the chart and other materials from the case have been located.

Generally, there are two boxes that can be checked that refer to the courtroom appearance: (1) be in court and (2) be on call. Once the witness coordinator has been contacted, the nurse should request to be placed "on call." If "be in court" has been checked, it is advised to contact the DA and be switched to "on call." This latter action will preclude being in court when the nurse is not needed and will avoid hours of waiting in the hall. The prosecutor will have a list of witnesses and will provide an estimated time for the nurse's appearance.

A subpoena may be issued for the preliminary hearing. Most of the time the forensic nurse will not be expected to appear at a preliminary hearing; however, there are exceptions. The preliminary hearing is a procedure to determine whether there was probable cause for the arrest of the suspect and if there is enough evidence for an indictment. There is no jury at this time. If an indictment is filed, then the matter goes to trial.

A pretrial conference may be held between the preliminary hearing and the trial. A subpoena may be received for that, too. A pretrial conference is used to review evidentiary issues prior to trial, but again, the forensic nurse may not be required to be present.

When a subpoena is received for the actual trial, the forensic nurse should contact the prosecutor and the witness coordinator, keeping in mind that trials may be continued and continued and continued. Maintain ongoing and consistent communication so there is no ambiguity about what is happening. It is possible that, somewhere along the line, the defendant will plead and there will be no trial at all. When such an outcome is ascertained, the information should be filed with nurse's other case records for subsequent reference.

Again, the on-call trial date status should be verified. The first day of the trial, listed on the subpoena, will not necessarily be for testimony but rather for jury selection. This may take a day or more, so the nurse's testimony will most likely not be on that day but a few to several days later. Once the jury has been selected the DA will have a better idea when the nurse will appear.

Best Practice *43-2*

Any potential expert should make sure that the DA and witness coordinator have all the pertinent contact information to facilitate communication regarding the date and time of appearance.

There is always a chance that the presence of the forensic nurse examiner may not be required. Photos and documentation will have been entered into evidence, and perhaps no further explanations or a court appearance will be necessary.

Potential witnesses should bring their subpoena to court on the prescribed day of appearance (it may even grant parking privileges in a restricted area). Even after the trial is over, the subpoena should be maintained. It is a useful document for recording the outcome of the case, including the details of sentencing. It should be filed with the chart.

Fact Witness versus Expert Witness

Different types of witnesses may testify in a trial. The two types that most often involve the nurse are "fact witness" and "expert witness." In either case, it is most important for the nurse to be nonbiased, objective, and scientific. The forensic nurse must be a witness, not an advocate. The role of a fact witness, as defined by *Webster's Revised Unabridged Dictionary* (1998), is, "To see or know by personal presence; to have direct cognizance of." These witnesses have firsthand knowledge of a particular event. That role may apply to nurses who are testifying regarding the observations and direct contact with the patient. A fact witness may testify to things that were heard, seen, touched, tasted, or smelled and may give an opinion related to those things perceived by his or her senses.

The expert witness, as defined by *Barron's Law Dictionary* (Giftis, 1996), is

> *a witness having special knowledge of the subject about which he is about to testify; that knowledge must generally be such as is not normally possessed by the average person. This expertise may derive from either study and education or from experience and observation. An expert witness must be qualified by the court to testify as such . . . but the court must be satisfied that the testimony presented is of a kind which in fact requires special knowledge, skill or experience.*

It is important to provide the court with a comprehensive, up-to-date curriculum vitae that will demonstrate accomplishments, experiences, skill, education, and training in a given subject area. The attorneys will question potential witnesses about qualifications, and the court will make a decision whether to accept that person as an expert witness.

Frye Rule

Forensic nurses should become familiar with the term "Kelly-Frye," also called the "Frye Rule," from *United States v. Frye* (1923). This case established, in the rules of evidence, that the results of scientific tests or procedures are admissible as evidence only when the tests or procedures have gained general acceptance in the particular field to which they belong. It clarified that an expert witness with knowledge, skill, experience, training, or education may offer an opinion in his or her area of expertise that is relevant to the case and will assist the court with its understanding of the matter at hand.

Daubert Test

Another important term is the "Daubert test." Under *Daubert* (*Daubert v. Merrell Dow Pharmaceuticals,* 1993) and *Kumho* (*Kumho Tire Company v. Patrick Carmichael,* 1999), "The opinion of the expert must be based on reliable methodology or analysis and not subjective belief or unsupported speculation. Reliability of expert testimony is as important as the relevance of the expert testimony." The *Daubert* decision caused much controversy because the scientific world had grown in leaps and bounds and some felt that the Frye rule was too weak, that because a proclaimed expert had made studies and observations and had come to a conclusion, even if it had gained acceptance in that field, if it was not supported by standardized scientific methodology and stringent controls, it could be challenged. All evidence can be challenged in court, but the *Daubert* decision made the criteria more rigorous. States have chosen to opt for either the Frye rule or Daubert test as their criteria, and other states have chosen methods of their own.

In 1993, the US Supreme Court replaced the Frye test with the Daubert test (*Daubert v. Merrell Dow Pharmaceuticals*). This decision was clarified by the Court in 1999 in *Kuhmo Tire Company, Ltd. v. Patrick Carmichael.* The Daubert test is now the standard for the admissibility of opinion testimony in federal courts. The criteria applied under *Daubert* and subsequent cases, as decided by lower federal courts, include the following:

> *The specific factors explicated by the Daubert Court are (1) whether the expert's technique or theory can be or has been tested–that is, whether the expert's theory can be challenged in some objective sense, or whether it is instead simply a subjective, conclusory approach that cannot reasonably be assessed for reliability; (2) whether the technique or theory has been subject to peer review and publication; (3) the known or potential rate of error of the technique or theory when applied; (4) the existence and maintenance of standards and controls; and (5) whether the technique or theory has been generally accepted in the scientific community.*

Still, the reliability of some issues thought to be valid under *Daubert* is wavering as a result of continuing controversies over techniques and new innovations in technology.

Hearsay Rule

Hearsay is a statement other than one made by the declarant while testifying at the trial or hearing, offered in evidence to prove the truth of the matter asserted (*Federal Rules of Evidence*, 2000). This means that the nurse may not testify to something that someone else told her or him. In other words, if the victim or suspect tells the nurse something during an interview or examination, it is considered hearsay.

There are many exceptions to the hearsay rule. For the most part, the exceptions are related to "trustworthiness" and "necessity." The Federal Rules of Evidence and the individual state evidence codes all have similar statutes, so it is advisable for the nurse to research the rules of hearsay exceptions for that state.

According to the California Evidence Code Section 1200:

> *1200. (a) "Hearsay evidence" is evidence of a statement that was made other than by a witness while testifying at the hearing and that is offered to prove the truth of the matter stated.*
>
> *(b) Except as provided by law, hearsay evidence is inadmissible.*
>
> *(c) This section shall be known and may be cited as the hearsay rule.*

Regardless, whether or not the rules of evidence, in a state, allow the nurse an exception to the hearsay rule, it is still up to the court and the judge to decide if those statements will be admissible.

Uniform Rules of Evidence Hearsay Exception, Rule 803(6)

Records in any form are admissible in evidence, if they are:

- Records of act or event
- Made at or near the time of the event
- By or from a person with knowledge
- Kept in the course of regularly conducted business activity

One exception is a deathbed confession. It is presumed that people don't lie when they are about to die. According to the California Evidence Code:

> *1243. Evidence of a statement made by a dying person respecting the cause and circumstances of his death is not made inadmissible by the hearsay rule if the statement was made upon his personal knowledge and under a sense of immediately impending death.*

Another exception refers to spontaneous utterances.

> *California Evidence Code:*
>
> *1240. Evidence of a statement is not made inadmissible by the hearsay rule if the statement:*
>
> *(a) Purports to narrate, describe, or explain an act, condition, or event perceived by the declarant; and*
>
> *(b) Was made spontaneously while the declarant was under the stress of excitement caused by such perception.*

Federal Rules of Evidence Rule 803, Section 4

Yet another exception refers to purposes of medical history:

> *(4) Statements for purposes of medical diagnosis or treatment. Statements made for purposes of medical diagnosis or treatment and describing medical history, or past or present symptoms, pain, or sensations, or the inception or general character of the cause or external source thereof insofar as reasonably pertinent to diagnosis or treatment.*

The following rule, in the California Evidence Code, states that it only applies to victims under the age of 12, describing any act or attempted act of abuse or neglect:

> *1226. Evidence of a statement by a minor child is not made inadmissible by the hearsay rule if offered against the plaintiff in an action brought under Section 376 of the Code of Civil Procedure for injury to such minor child.*
>
> *1228. Notwithstanding any other provision of law, for the purpose of establishing the elements of the crime in order to admit as evidence the confession of a person accused of violating Section 261, 264.1, 285, 286, 288, 288a, 289, or 647a of the Penal Code, a court, in its discretion, may determine that a statement of the complaining witness is not made inadmissible by the hearsay rule if it finds all of the following:*
>
> *(a) The statement was made by a minor child under the age of 12, and the contents of the statement were included in a written report of a law enforcement official or an employee of a county welfare department.*
>
> *(b) The statement describes the minor child as a victim of sexual abuse.*
>
> *(c) The statement was made prior to the defendant's confession.*
>
> *The court shall view with caution the testimony of a person recounting hearsay where there is evidence of personal bias or prejudice.*

(d) There are no circumstances, such as significant inconsistencies between the confession and the statement concerning material facts establishing any element of the crime or the identification of the defendant, that would render the statement unreliable.

(e) The minor child is found to be unavailable pursuant to paragraph (2) or (3) of subdivision (a) of Section 240 or refuses to testify.

(f) The confession was memorialized in a trustworthy fashion by a law enforcement official.

If the prosecution intends to offer a statement of the complaining witness pursuant to this section, the prosecution shall serve a written notice upon the defendant at least 10 days prior to the hearing or trial at which the prosecution intends to offer the statement.

If the statement is offered during trial, the court's determination shall be made out of the presence of the jury. If the statement is found to be admissible pursuant to this section, it shall be admitted out of the presence of the jury and solely for the purpose of determining the admissibility of the confession of the defendant.

1360. (a) In a criminal prosecution where the victim is a minor, a statement made by the victim when under the age of 12 describing any act of child abuse or neglect performed with or on the child by another, or describing any attempted act of child abuse or neglect with or on the child by another, is not made inadmissible by the hearsay rule if all of the following apply:

(1) The statement is not otherwise admissible by statute or court rule.

(2) The court finds, in a hearing conducted outside the presence of the jury, that the time, content, and circumstances of the statement provide sufficient indicia of reliability.

(3) The child either:

(A) Testifies at the proceedings.

(B) Is unavailable as a witness, in which case the statement may be admitted only if there is evidence of the child abuse or neglect that corroborates the statement made by the child.

(b) A statement may not be admitted under this section unless the proponent of the statement makes known to the adverse party the intention to offer the statement and the particulars of the statement sufficiently in advance of the proceedings in order to provide the adverse party with a fair opportunity to prepare to meet the statement.

(c) For purposes of this section, "child abuse" means an act proscribed by Section 273a, 273d, or 288.5 of the Penal Code, or any of the acts described in Section 11165.1 of the Penal Code, and "child neglect" means any of the acts described in Section 11165.2 of the Penal Code.

The hearsay rules may vary from state to state and even from trial to trial, so it will be the court's decision whether the nurse may quote a patient's statement during testimony. Many times a patient's statement may be on a form or document that has been entered into evidence. That may stand, or a part of the document could be construed as hearsay. For example, if a sexual assault nurse examiner has documented an injury, on a reporting form, which indicates a purple bruise to the left arm, this is permissible because the nurse examiner witnessed, first hand, the injury and its characteristics. If the nurse examiner states that the victim told her the injury was sustained by the suspect punching her, there may be an objection, citing hearsay. Even though the form may say, "Purple bruise to left arm where (s) punched her," the fact that the victim told the nurse how it happened may be considered hearsay. The jury will be able to examine documents so they will be able to see those entries during deliberation.

There is a familiar phrase that states: "You can't un-ring a bell." It refers to something said in court that may be stricken from the record, but the jurors have already heard it. It may be spoken unintentionally or intentionally. A question is asked and then answered. The opposition objects and the statement is stricken from the record and is to be disregarded by the jury. Then the questioning goes on. Let's use the preceding example: If the nurse is asked by the prosecutor what injury she observed on the left arm of the patient, suppose the nurse answers, "A purple bruise where the defendant punched her." The defense may then object and ask that the statement be stricken from the record, citing hearsay. If the objection is sustained, the court will ask the nurse to just answer the question as to what injury was observed. The question will be asked again, and the nurse's answer should be, "A purple bruise." The fact that the jury heard the nurse state that the patient said how the injury was sustained may not be easily forgotten by the jury. That is the bell that can't be un-rung. In this case, the nurse may not have known that such a statement would be stricken due to hearsay but in some cases litigators may use this as a tactic in their strategy. In other cases the nurse's statement would be appropriate, depending on what the court will accept in terms of hearsay.

Preparation for Trial

Preparation for trial should be done reasonably close to the actual time of trial. If preparation is done too early, it is possible that the nurse will have forgotten the details for which she/he has prepared and even may confuse one case for another.

The first thing would be to obtain the documentation that was prepared at the time of the nurse's encounter with the patient. Then, have any photographs duplicated that were taken, relating to the case. If the nurse has received a separate subpoena for records and photographs, these items should be prepared and delivered in response to the subpoena. These records may also be supplied to the DA in a manner that is customary in the local region. The forensic nurse may want to make some notes about the case but should remember that everything recorded, even brief notes, may be discoverable, meaning that it may be submitted as evidence to the court. That is not to say that notes should not be made; it means that if notes are made, the witness should be prepared to hand them over to the court. This implies that they should be written with the mindset that they are not for the writer's eyes only.

The forensic nurse should study all documentation thoroughly. It should be almost memorized. Although records may be accessed in courtrooms, it is preferred that the witness know all details prior to testifying. The focus should be on significant information, and the witness should be able to retrieve it promptly if a question about it arises during the testimony. Certain questions will surely be asked in nearly every case: when the examination was conducted, what evidence was collected, the demeanor of the patient, what injuries were observed, and so forth.

The nurse should not make notes on the actual documents to be submitted. For example, if an error is noted on the sexual assault documentation form, do not write "Uh-oh, problem" in the margin. In fact, no unofficial commentary should ever be written on a document. If the defense happens to ask to see a copy of the document or, even worse, a notation has been made on the document that will be duplicated for evidence, the nurse witness would have supplied great ammunition for the testimony to be attacked by the opposition. If an error has been made in documentation, the nurse should bring it to the DA's attention as soon as possible. Errors can be addressed in a manner that can avoid accusations that there are attempts being made to be deceptive, misleading, or untruthful. If it is explained to the DA that an injury was improperly labeled (right versus left arm, for example), the DA will have that information and will not be surprised if it comes up later. It may or may not be addressed in court, depending on how significant it is. The exchange could go like this:

Q: Ms. C., on diagram A you drew an injury to Ms. J.'s left arm; is this correct?

A: Yes.

Q: In your notes, you wrote, "Injury to right arm." Is this correct?

A: Yes.

Q: If you recall, Ms. C., was the injury to the right arm or to the left arm?

A: I do recall. The injury was to the left arm. Apparently, that was a clerical error.

Notes may contain certain pertinent bits of information that are located on several pages of an existing document. If the nurse places notes for these references on one page, it will prevent the need to rifle through many pages during testimony. Everything may be discoverable. It will not be possible to avoid having to refer to the original document at times. When witnesses must refer to written documents they should ask the court's permission. Before starting a search, just say, "Your Honor, may I refer to the document?"

Although the questions that a witness will be asked, by either the prosecutor or the defense, are difficult to predict, certain questions will be included among the interrogatives. Before the trial, it is helpful to prepare a series of questions for the DA to ask the forensic nurse. As knowledgeable as the DA may be about certain issues, the DA's field is not the nurse's field and the DA must be educated about what the forensic nurse does so that he or she will have a clearer picture of the witness's work as a forensic nurse. This information will help to educate the jury as well. Often, in court, a witness will wait for the DA to ask a pertinent question to facilitate expounding upon a point or providing support for a statement. The DA may have no idea to ask that particular question, so it may leave the witness feeling frustrated about not being able to bring out a very important issue regarding the case. As an expert in the field, the forensic nurse should assist the DA in making testimony demonstrable and illustrative.

It is very important to meet with the DA before the day in court. Because there is typically earlier communication after receiving a subpoena, nurse witnesses should ensure that it is made clear how important it will be to have an hour or so to meet before the court appearance. This is when the CV can be reviewed and the DA can be presented questions that the nurse has prepared for him or her to ask. Such a meeting is not a rehearsal for testimony. Counsel should not tell a witness what to say on the stand; however, there is always a strategy involved in a trial, and it is important to know what that strategy is. The DA will have a plan of action and will want to focus on certain characteristics of the case. If it is known where the DA is going with those characteristics, the parties will be able to communicate more effectively with one another. The nurse should ascertain the identity of any opposing expert and what that expert will be testifying about. It is also important to determine the strengths and weaknesses of the case, and what barriers, if any, might be present from the perspective of the prosecutor presenting the case.

A witness may, and should, speak to defense counsel, if asked. However, the DA should be informed about this action. When a witness avoids speaking with the defense, it appears that he or she is being uncooperative or hostile. Although as an expert the nurse is appearing as a neutral participant, testifying to the findings, the nurse should remain guarded about what kind of information that is disclosed to the defense because everything the nurse says could be used in court. Even though the conversation may seem informal, nothing is off the record. It would be improper to give strategic information to the defense that the prosecutor intends to use in trial to prove the case. Nevertheless, the truth is still the truth. Most often, the defense will request information regarding the meaning of medical terminology that was written on forms or questions about anatomy. Any given witness will not know everything about the case or what the devices are for either side, so staying conservative is a good approach. Rather, the witness should allow defense counsel to ask questions and not offer information that was not solicited.

The Court Appearance

After being sworn in, a witness will be asked to state and spell his or her name. The prosecutor will then begin the direct examination, followed by cross-examination by defense counsel.

"Direct examination" is the first direct questioning of a witness by the person who called the witness. "Cross-examination" is the questioning of a witness by someone other than the party who called the witness. "Redirect" is when the direct examiner asks questions after the cross-examination. "Re-cross–examination" is questioning after the redirect examination. This will continue, back and forth, until the questioning has been completed. At that time the nurse witness will be excused; however, there may be the potential for recall. This means that even though there are no more questions at the time, a witness may be asked to return at a later time for more questioning.

There will be questions about the nurse's credentials and qualifications as well as questions about the case, which are certain to be asked (Box 43-2).

There may be exhibits to describe. The prosecutor may have parts of a report, photographs, or diagrams enlarged and may request that the nurse describe certain details. There will be markers, pointers, and other tools to enhance the visual presentation. When a question is asked that refers to the diagram, the prosecutor will direct the nurse to the easel. At this point the witness should step down from the stand, go to the easel, and take a moment to look over the diagram. The nurse witness should always wait for a question to be asked and should not skip ahead and talk about things that are currently not being questioned.

The nurse should be aware of leading questions. "Leading questions" are those that suggest the answer sought by the questioner. They may be intended to elicit an answer that the nurse would not otherwise give or to guide the witness to a specific answer. The forensic nurse examiner must be very careful when interviewing patients, especially children, to not ask them leading questions; the nurse, as an expert witness, should be just as aware when leading questions are asked of the nurse. An example of a leading question would be, "Did he steal your $10,000 diamond ring?" A better question would be, "What items did the robber take from you?" or "What items did you find to be missing?" in the case of a burglary as opposed to a robbery.

Box 43-2 Qualifications as an Expert

The forensic nurse may be asked for the following information:

- Describe your current position and background as a nurse. How long have you been a registered nurse and in what areas have you practiced?
- How long have you been working as a forensic nurse? What education have you had to prepare for this specialty?
- What continuing education have you had in your specialty?
- What professional organizations do you belong to?
- Are you certified in your field?
- Have you published any material in your field?
- Please describe what you do as a forensic nurse.
- How does a forensic nurse conduct an examination (step by step)?
- The sexual assault nurse examiner (SANE) may be asked to describe the sexual assault response team (SART) and its members.
- How many cases have you done?
- What equipment is used, how does it work, and why is it used?
- How do you spell the name of the equipment and supplies that you use?
- Please describe other technical and procedural aspects of forensic work.
- Have you appeared as an expert witness in court before?
- Whether the nurse has ever been disqualified as an expert witness.
- The defense may ask, in cross-examination, whether the nurse always appears for the prosecution. If asked this question, you should remind the court that the nurse is appearing neither for the prosecution nor for the defense but as a witness for the truth and that the nurse may most often be called by the prosecution because of the nature of the work.
- If you have ever worked for defense counsel, as a consultant, let that be known in court. It will further your credibility as a nonbiased participant.

According to the California Rules of Evidence 767,

> *(a) Except under special circumstances where the interests of justice otherwise require:*
>
> *(1) A leading question may not be asked of a witness on direct or redirect examination.*
>
> *(2) A leading question may be asked of a witness on cross-examination or recross-examination.*
>
> *(b) The court may in the interests of justice permit a leading question to be asked of a child under 10 years of age in a case involving a prosecution under Section 273a, 273d, 288, or 288.5 of the Penal Code.*

Box 43-3 offers some important points that will maximize the impact of testimony and prevent mistakes from being made.

It may be wise to keep in mind that each attorney has an agenda. The nurse is a cog in the wheel of their plan. A witness should take care not to become too comfortable thinking that she/he will be protected from tough questioning or shielded from embarrassment and humiliation by the prosecutor. In fact, there may be times that a witness feels totally alienated and vulnerable. These bad experiences, as well as the good ones, are sources of important learning. Bad experiences may very well teach the witness more than the good ones ever will!

After the trial has concluded, a nurse witness should call the prosecutor and ask what the outcome was. The jury is often interviewed, after the trial is over, to see how conclusions were reached. It is important to ask what the strongest evidence appeared to be and what was the weakest. What helped the case the most, and what helped the least? Were there any shortcomings that failed to support the evidence? If the defendant was found guilty, ask what the most compelling evidence was for the jury. The sentencing will take place days or a few weeks after the conclusion of the trial, so if that has not taken place, the nurse should call and find out the results of the sentencing. If the defendant was found not guilty, what motivated the jury to acquit? What factors were lacking to convict?

Every time that a witness testifies, it is expected that there will be increased proficiency at anticipating the needs of the system. As comfort levels rise and stress levels fall, nurses may eventually look forward to court appearances. Good advice is to make every experience a learning experience and take nothing personally. Over time, the prosecutors will gain confidence in the adeptness of certain nurses and may even look to them for advice and guidance regarding other cases.

Consulting for the Defense

Forensic nurses may be asked, by a defense attorney, to consult on a case. Generally, this is most often done outside one's own immediate community. It may seem contrary to be working for "the other side," but as was discussed earlier, the nurse is testifying for the truth, and in the name of justice, the nurse can assist in the effort to get to that truth.

As a consultant, the nurse will be privy to certain aspects of the case that she/he normally would not be aware of while directly involved as a participant in the forensic examination. The nurse will be an outside surveyor and will have a unique overview of the event. The nurse will be supplied with materials such as police reports; victim statements, suspect statements, and witness statements; photographs of the scene, the victim, and the suspect; reports of analyzed evidence and medical reports; and possibly transcripts of the preliminary hearing. The task will be to evaluate the materials available and use experience and education to draw various conclusions regarding the findings. The nurse should stand back and try to look at the big picture. Conclusions may be based on the information that is available and information that is blatantly absent. There may be evidence that was collected but not analyzed and evidence that, perhaps, should have been but was not collected at all. Was the evidence collected and packaged correctly? Were the standards of forensic nursing practice followed? Were there any breaks in the chain of custody? Was there a chance of evidence contamination? Are the reports consistent with the statements? Are the statements consistent with previous statements? Are their any medical or psychological circumstances that may account for inconsistencies? Because the nurse is the expert in that particular field, the nurse should be aware of any procedural or technical breaches in the methods used.

The nurse will not be singling out any particular entity to criticize; the nurse examiner's work and the work of the police officers or detectives (unless it is obviously lacking) will be fitting together the pieces of a puzzle to see if the picture has continuity and cohesion. Any red flags that are spotted will come in to play when the findings are relayed to the attorney.

Make notes of impressions as the material is read. Keep in mind, as with any written material, that it may be discoverable. Attorneys make writings that are referred to as "work product." Work product refers to an attorney's notes, statements, theories,

Box 43-3 Case-Related Interrogatives

The forensic nurse may be asked the following questions:

- Do you recall the case on the date specified?
- Describe the demeanor of the subject.
- Describe the procedures that were conducted, how they were conducted, and who was present during those procedures.
- Describe specific aspects of evidence collection, such as how the evidence was packaged and preserved and what happened to the evidence after its collection.
- Were photographs taken? If so, describe their disposition.
- Describe the findings of your examination.
- What injuries were observed? What could have been the cause of said injuries? What was the age of the injuries?
- What are your opinions regarding the findings, and how did you come to have those opinions?
- Questions that further refine the possibilities: "Isn't it possible . . . ?" questions.

The following gives other pointers that may help the nurse:

- Pause before giving an answer to a question so that the attorney has a chance to object.
- Answer only the question that is asked.
- Do not answer until the question has been completely stated; do not interrupt to give an answer.
- If you don't understand a question, ask that it be restated.
- Be sure to answer the question asked.
- If you do not know an answer to a question, say that you don't know. Do not guess at answers.
- If there is silence after the answer is finished, do not fill the void with more talk or say, "That's it."
- If you don't remember something, do not guess. State that you don't recall.
- Keep the answers brief. Many questions cannot be answered by a simple "yes" or "no." If you must elaborate upon an answer, ask permission by saying, "Your honor, may I explain?"
- Beware of multifaceted or compound questions. For example, consider the question, "Did Ms. J. tell you that she was walking on Ninth Street at 12:00?" Perhaps Ms. J. told you that she was walking on Ninth Street, but it was at 9:00. The answer to that question cannot be "yes" because some of the information is incorrect. Ask the attorney to restate the question or answer the question with the statement, "Ms. J. told me that she was walking on Ninth Street at 9:00."
- Beware of rapid-fire questions, one right after another. Ask that the questions be asked one at a time.
- Avoid using medical terminology. Try to translate the medical words to simple terms that the jury can understand. Remember, the nurse witness is the jury's teacher.
- Do not show anger or frustration at the questions asked, no matter how elementary or how many times the same question is asked.
- Hypothetical questions may be asked. These questions are not based in the context of this particular case. They may take a variety of forms. They are often meant for the nurse witness to contradict herself. For example:
  "Is it possible that . . . ?"
  "Isn't it true . . .?"
  "In your opinion could . . . ?"
- Always answer truthfully, saying, "In this case . . . ," or follow the answer by saying, ". . . but in this case . . ." An attempt to answer may be struck down as unresponsive, but at least you tried to clarify. Perhaps the prosecutor will be aware that you had a point to make and address it on redirect.
- Never testify beyond your own scope of practice. If asked about a technique or process that is not within your field, even if you have some basic knowledge of it, do not attempt to answer. For example, if asked whether you collected samples for DNA analysis, answer that you did so, but if asked how the samples are analyzed, simply state that that is beyond your scope of practice and that you do not analyze the samples; they are sent to the crime lab. Let the person from the crime lab answer how the analysis is done.
- Be very cautious about bringing articles into court. You may be interested in citing a particular point from an article, but the defense could try to make you look foolish by exposing that you have not memorized every word of the article and may even ask you to discuss the authors in the bibliography. Rather, answers should be based on your experience and knowledge. If asked whether you are familiar with a study or an article, either you are or you aren't. Occasionally, you may be asked to take an article home, read it, and come back to give an opinion.
- If asked whether you are familiar with certain studies, answer; but studies have been done on certain subject matter that may be indicative of a particular region, population, or practice area, or they may be outdated and out of context.
- Never attempt do the jury's job. It is the jury's responsibility to pass judgment on the case. Although you may be asked, do not fall into the trap of stating whether someone is guilty or not guilty or something was consensual or nonconsensual. The nurse may state whether something is "consistent with" something or "not consistent with" something.
- The defense may take a "shot" by declaring that you are "only a nurse" or may say, "You are not a doctor, are you?" You should gracefully reply that you are a very good nurse.
- Be confident with things you know. Information doesn't always have to come from a book. Your experience as a nurse and a forensic examiner is valuable in and of itself.

tactics, and strategy that are anticipated to be used in trial. The attorney's work product is generally not discoverable. However, the nurse's work for the attorney may be discoverable. A consultant's confidential work product may become discoverable if the witness is designated to testify. Regardless of that, all writings should be formal with the idea that they may end up as evidence in court.

According to California Evidence Code Section 911-920 (1999):

915. (a) Subject to subdivision (b), the presiding officer may not require disclosure of information claimed to be privileged under this division or attorney work product under subdivision (c) of Section 2018 of the Code of Civil Procedure in order to rule on the claim of privilege; provided, however, that in any hearing conducted pursuant to subdivision (c) of Section 1524 of the Penal Code in which a claim of privilege is made and the court determines that there is no other feasible means to rule on the validity of the claim other than to require disclosure, the court shall proceed in accordance with subdivision (b).

(b) When a court is ruling on a claim of privilege under Article 9 (commencing with Section 1040) of Chapter 4 (official information and identity of informer) or under Section 1060 (trade secret) or under subdivision (b) of Section 2018 of the Code of Civil Procedure (attorney work product) and is unable to do so without requiring disclosure of the information claimed to be privileged, the court may require the person from whom disclosure is sought or the person authorized to claim the privilege, or both, to disclose the information

in chambers out of the presence and hearing of all persons except the person authorized to claim the privilege and any other persons as the person authorized to claim the privilege is willing to have present. If the judge determines that the information is privileged, neither the judge nor any other person may ever disclose, without the consent of a person authorized to permit disclosure, what was disclosed in the course of the proceedings in chambers.

The first contact with the attorney, after the nurse's review of the case, should not contain any written material. Instead, the nurse should relay opinions and comments verbally. If written material is required, it can be supplied later in a determined format. Most often questions will come up while reading the material. Prepare questions and discuss them with counsel. For example, a complainant has accused the defendant of sexually assaulting her, without a condom, and ejaculating in her vagina, yet the crime lab reports no semen or sperm was found during analysis. Although there may be several reasons that can account for this, one of them being that there was no sexual contact, consider asking counsel if he or she knows whether the client has had a vasectomy. This may be a point to consider for absence of sperm.

Create a timeline of the case to help map the events in order of their occurrence. The statements of witnesses and subjects will be in narrative form and can be compared while reading through each statement. Charting who was present and when can assist in reconstructing the scenario with better clarity and can also reveal inconsistencies.

The first step when consulting on a case is to negotiate the fee. If there are any other forensic nurses or legal nurse consultants in the area who have worked for defenders, the nurse may want to contact them to see what the going rate is for those types of services. Forensic nurses should not sell themselves short but also should not set too high a price. Set rates according to experience as a consultant in the forensic field. Fees don't have to be etched in stone. As a nurse progresses and grows as a consultant, she or he may want to adjust the rates on an annual basis. As a rule, one may want to set an initial fee for reviewing the documents and providing a verbal summary. Then an hourly fee may follow for any additional work. Some law firms will negotiate an offer for a fee with a limit of the number of hours. Because some of the work may take the nurse out of town, the nurse may also want to create a fee schedule that outlines a daily fee for travel plus expenses, accommodations, and miscellaneous charges. While traveling out of town, the nurse may have to pay for some reimbursable expenses up front, such as car rental. Keep meticulous records of meals, gas, and miscellaneous expenses so they can be itemized on the invoice sent to the client. Of course, keep records of time spent on work for that client.

After reviewing the case, the nurse may feel that she or he has nothing to add to enhance the defender's case; that is, the nurse's opinion of the material reviewed supports the prosecutor's case. That's perfectly fine. The nurse was hired to evaluate the case, not to invent something that may not exist to exonerate the defendant. Many times it is a required element that the defense counsel hire an expert to review the case. If everything seems to be consistent and nothing appears to be exculpatory, the nurse's work may be done. It is not the nurse's responsibility to manufacture loopholes to acquit the defendant. The truth is the truth. Send an invoice and offer services to them in the future.

The nurse is first hired as a consultant and expert witness to the defense counsel. Whether the nurse actually testifies as an expert witness will depend on many factors. For example, the nurse may be needed to oppose the prosecution's expert. That need may depend on what the opposing expert will be testifying to. If the opposing expert is going to testify that an injury can be sustained only in a certain manner and the nurse knows of other ways that the injury can occur, the nurse may be asked to take the stand to give that perspective.

As the consultant, the nurse may want to suggest other experts for the defense to secure for the trial. If the nurse has discovered, through review of the documents, that there are scientific evidence reports that may require explanation, the nurse may suggest that defense counsel find an analyst who is an expert in that field to explain the findings. The nurse may see that the DNA samples of the defendant did not match those found at the crime scene. The nurse can certainly see that from reading the reports, but the nurse, not being a criminologist, should not testify to those findings because the natural follow-up of questioning would be to explain how the criminologist came to that conclusion and how the testing was performed. It would not be appropriate for the nurse to offer testimony not in the nurse's area of expertise.

The job of a consultant is to give opinions, clarify the facts, and guide counsel toward a logical defense. The forensic nurse is in an excellent position for this task because his or her experience as a prosecution witness has exposed the nurse to the types of issues that will come into play.

Generally, the nurse will be doing most of the work long distance. Often the nurse will be in communication with the defender's assistants through paralegals or investigators. Once most of the information has been organized, the nurse may speak directly to counsel and relay the findings. The defender will let the nurse know if it will be required for the nurse to meet in person or appear as a witness in the trial.

The nurse should follow up, later, to learn the outcome of the trial and the verdict. The nurse should ask whether the jury was interviewed after the trial and how they perceived the case. If the client was found not guilty, the nurse will ask what the strongest issues were that brought them to that conclusion and gave them reasonable doubt. If the client was found guilty, ask what the specific weak spots were and what evidence was the strongest that precipitated their conviction.

If the client is found guilty, the sentencing will take place a few days to several weeks after the trial. The nurse should ask counsel to relay what sentence the client received.

Working for the defense will enhance the nurse's overall competency in being of service to the courts. It will increase her/his credibility as an objective, nonbiased witness, when called by the prosecution, and give the nurse a more balanced impression of the workings of the system.

Case Study 43-1 Sexual Assault of a Homeless Woman

In August 2000, a 37-year-old woman (W.M.) was brought in for a forensic sexual assault examination. She had a history of insulin-dependent diabetes, gallstones, and cesarean sections. She was gravida 5, para 5. At this time, W.M. was homeless and staying in a shelter. She was compliant with her insulin medication, alert, oriented, and cooperative. She was tearful at times while recollecting the events of the previous six days. A 41-year-old male, whom W.M. met at the homeless shelter, offered her a shower, food, cigarettes, and a place to sleep, if she wanted to go with him. After she arrived at his apartment, she took a shower and had some food. She slept there that night and when she thanked the male and told him it was time to leave, the male refused to let her go. He told her he would kill her, and he showed her a gun and threatened her with a knife. Over the next six days he held her hostage, hit her in the face (left cheek) with the handle of a knife, sexually assaulted and sodomized her multiple times, and threatened her with the gun and the knife. On the sixth day she told him that she badly needed her diabetes medicine and begged him to let her go to the clinic at the rescue mission. He went with her to the rescue mission to get her medication, but he threatened to kill her if she told anyone that he was keeping her against her will. At the rescue mission she told a security guard what was happening and the police were called.

The forensic evidentiary examination revealed evidence of a healing abrasion to the left cheek. There were no external vaginal injuries, but minor internal vaginal injuries (petechiae to the cervix) were found. There were anal injuries (abrasions and tears with positive toluidine blue dye uptake). Those finding were documented and photographed.

The case went to trial in January 2003. The forensic nurse examiner appeared by subpoena on the prosecution's witness list. After being qualified as an expert by the court, the nurse gave testimony regarding the case. The sexual assault nurse examiner described the injuries that the patient had sustained and testified that the absence of injury to the external vaginal area is not directly related to whether or not there was forced intercourse. She further stated that compliance does not necessarily imply consent in that the subject was threatened with harm if she did not cooperate. The subject was fearful that because the assailant had already hit her and caused her injury and pain, if she fought with him to resist the sexual assaults, he would hurt her more or even kill her. The nurse examiner stated that although the injuries appeared minor they could very well be consistent with the history given by the subject. When asked if the injuries could also be consistent with consensual sex, the nurse examiner stated that they could. The nurse was asked about the demeanor of the subject and the nurse replied that the subject was cooperative and anxious, verbalizing fear of retaliation from the male. The nurse examiner stated that the subject made good eye contact with the examiner and seemed sincere and relayed the history of the event in a concise, straightforward manner.

The defendant was found guilty and sentenced to several years in prison.

Ethics of Testifying and Malpractice Issues

The nurse's own personal and professional ethics should dictate the integrity and veracity in which one should approach testifying in court. The authenticity of everything from the validity of her or his credentials, experience, and knowledge to whether the testimony is completely truthful may come under scrutiny.

Expert witnesses were generally thought of as hard-working professionals who have taken time from their busy schedules to assist the court by shedding light on technical matters in which they have expertise. It is a well-known fact that some people have found that they can make a comfortable living by becoming professional witnesses. Physicians have left their practices behind to sell themselves exclusively as "hired guns." There shouldn't be anything wrong with that, except some unscrupulous characters have discarded their principles and will say anything, for a fee, to discredit the opposition's expert witness. This kind of behavior is tolerable unless there are issues of professional misconduct. If it is discovered that a person has lied about his credentials or strayed from acceptable parameters of treatment, there could be serious consequences. It could be professional malpractice. The nurse is accountable for the things she or he testifies to, and the facts that are presented are subject to peer review and standards of care in that profession. Medical malpractice is based on the fact that there are accepted methods of appropriate treatment.

One's professional organization would be the body to establish standards of practice and determine whether those standards have been violated. Each state has a Board of Registered Nursing that defines nursing practice in that state. Most nurses carry their own professional liability insurance. They know that they will be covered only if they abide by their scope and standards of practice. The International Association of Forensic Nurses (IAFN), with the support of the American Nurses' Association (ANA), has created and published the *Scope and Standards of Forensic Nursing Practice* (IAFN and ANA, 1997). The ANA *Standards of Clinical Nursing Practice* governs the fundamental practice of nursing. The IAFN *Scope and Standards* defines the role of the forensic nurse in this unique and independent specialty. It dictates the standards of care and the standards of professional performance. To deviate from these standards violates the trust and responsibility that is expected of all forensic nurses. Although forensic nursing is an ever-evolving specialty, which is constantly progressing with the advances of technology and innovations of science, the forensic nurse must demonstrate competency and exercise excellent judgment in her or his ability to deliver services that are based on the fundamental nursing process.

The expert witness was thought to have complete immunity from liability dating back to English common law. If witnesses could be held liable for their testimony, they would be less willing to testify. But, now, in some states, the expert witness may be held liable if he is negligent in forming his expert opinion, knowingly misleading the court or simply lying under oath. It was the advent of the "hired gun" witness that caused this to be true. Experts could get up on the stand and say anything without worrying about repercussions. Things have now changed and such witnesses may be held liable.

An expert witness can be held liable for testimony that deviates from the standard of care appropriate for their profession. The court often needs assistance with identifying inappropriate expert witnessing and it may depend on others in the same specialty to have it come to light. It is common for the prosecution and the defense to each have experts testify on the same subject. It may be up to one of those experts to report any improper testimony by the other to the professional organization to which he belongs.

A case in point is the ruling of the Seventh Circuit Court of Appeals, Chicago, Illinois, on June 2001, which allowed persons to be disciplined by their professional organizations when their testimony did not reflect the standards of those organizations. The case revolved around a 1995 malpractice suit against a neurosurgeon (Dr. D), a member of the American Association of Neurological Surgeons (AANS), who performed an anterior cervical fusion; the patient subsequently developed complications that led to the need for a tracheostomy. The neurosurgeon had performed more than

700 such operations, and this was his first adverse outcome. A second neurosurgeon (Dr. A), for opposing counsel, also belonging to the AANS, testified that the majority of neurosurgeons would agree that the only way such complications could arise would be if there was negligence and the doctor had been careless. Dr. A had performed approximately 25 to 30 of the same procedures in 30 years of practice. His testimony was based on two articles that he brought into court that outlined procedures for avoiding complications with the surgery. Neither article supported his testimony. Although rare (0.07%), this complication was a well-known risk of the surgery.

Dr. D reported Dr. A's testimony to the AANS and the AANS suspended Dr. A in 1997 for six months for irresponsible testimony, not conferring with other medical professionals in this matter, and having no basis for testifying as an expert. The AANS contended that the testimony in court did not reflect the view of the majority of neurosurgeons and violated provisions of the AANS's ethical code. It stated further that testimony that is one's personal opinion should be identified as personal opinion and not the consensus of the organization.

Dr. A attempted to sue AANS for lost profits as an expert witness, in 1998, stating that they were punishing him for testifying against another AANS member and that by suspending him they had caused his income to drop from $220,000 to $77,000. The ruling went against Dr. A owing to the fact that his membership in the prestigious organization was voluntary. He still had his regular practice, which afforded him adequate income, and his expert witness work was a side job. His testimony was ruled irresponsible and may have damaged the reputation of Dr. D.

Dr. A resigned from the AANS. He appealed his case, in 2001, but the judge dismissed it. The AANS was praised for upholding the standards of its organization and its peer review system. Because this was the first case of its kind, it set the precedent for this type of action. Now, most states acknowledge that absolute immunity cannot be granted to expert witnesses.

The issue of malpractice may confront the forensic nurse if the scope and standards of nursing practice and forensic nursing practice are not met. Additionally, if the standards of the professional organization are not met, the organization can take action if the organization's ethics were not upheld or if the behavior of the subject was not representative of the organization's integrity.

Summary

Always tell the truth. Forensic nurses represent not only themselves when testifying in court but also forensic nursing as a whole, along with their professional organizations. The nurse must abide by the standards set forth by his or her profession and the scientific standards that govern the practice. One can never go wrong if one approaches one's daily tasks by picturing oneself in the witness stand and being able to justify everything one does with pride. That means not cutting corners on even the most menial of undertakings. Do the best work possible . . . always. The nurse should develop organizational skills and routines so that when asked whether something was done, the nurse can confidently answer, "Yes, I always do that" or can state that something wasn't done because the occasion didn't warrant it. The idea of having to tell the court that something wasn't done because the nurse was in a rush to get to the next case or to a meeting can be devastating on the stand. Inconsistency is the spark that fans the flames to bring a case to court in the first place, so it would be unwise to furnish fuel for the fire.

Every time the forensic nurse goes to court her or his performance will improve. The nurse will be better at knowing what to expect and will be better at preparing for the trial. There are no shortcuts to excellence, but the path is exciting and rewarding. After all, this is what forensic nursing is about, by its very definition—connecting the nursing process to the law. Going to court is the ultimate responsibility, and the nurse may even learn to like it.

Resources

Web Sites

The American Association of Nurse Attorneys

www.taana.org

The American Society for Healthcare Risk Management:

www.hospitalconnect.com/DesktopServlet

Organizations

American Association of Legal Nurse Consultants

AALNC Headquarters, 401 North Michigan Avenue, Chicago, IL 60611; Tel 877-402-2562; www.aalnc.org

Nonprofit organization dedicated to the professional enhancement of registered nurses practicing in a consulting capacity in the legal field.

American Bar Association

321 North Clark Street, Chicago, IL 60610; Tel: 312-988-5000; www.abanet.org

American Nurses Association (ANA)

8515 Georgia Avenue, Suite 400, Silver Spring, MD 20910; Tel: 800-274-4ANA; www.nursingworld.com

References

Daubert v. Merrell Dow Pharmaceuticals, Inc. 509 U.S. 579 (1993).

Federal Rules of Evidence. (2000). Washington DC: US Department of Justice, US Government Printing Office.

Giftis, S. H. (1996). *Law dictionary* (Barron's Educational Series). New York: Barron's International Association of Forensic Nurses and American Nurses' Association. (1997). *Scope and standards of forensic nursing practice.* Washington, DC: American Nurses' Association.

Kumko Tire Company v. Patrick Carmichael, 526 U.S. 137, 1999.

State of California. (1999). California Evidence Code, Department of Justice, State of California.

United States v. Frye, 293 F. 1013 (1923).

Webster's revised unabridged dictionary. (1998). Plainfield, NJ: MICRA.

Chapter 44 Malpractice and Negligence

Alice Geissler-Murr and Mary Frances Moorhouse

Standards of Care

Nursing practice is based on the understanding and use of a body of knowledge, some of which is borrowed from other disciplines, some of which is unique to nursing. This body of knowledge is reflected in the various standards of care that have been adopted by professional organizations representing nurses (Aiken, 2004a).

The term *standard of care* is defined as "that degree of care, expertise, and judgment exercised by a reasonable and prudent nurse under the same or similar circumstances" (O'Keefe, 2001). The standard of care is established through use of the nursing process, as well as by facility policies, procedures, and protocols; by national accrediting agencies (e.g., Joint Commission on Accreditation of Healthcare Organizations [JCAHO]); and by national professional and clinical specialty organizations, (e.g., American Nurses Association [ANA], American Association of Critical-Care Nurses [AACN], Association of Operating Nurses [AORN]).

Standards of care are published in professional journals, nursing textbooks, and practice guidelines (e.g., care maps/clinical pathways, algorithms, protocols, technical bulletins). Standards may be implied in the advertising of any agency (e.g., "neonatologist on staff 24 hours a day" or "XYZ Hospital provides the best care in the Midwest") making a claim that can be held as a standard of care, particularly when a legal action is considered (Harvey, 2004).

In recent times, nursing practice and healthcare delivery have become highly technical, and nurses hold increasingly responsible positions. This expanding responsibility and independence is accompanied by a corresponding increase in accountability for the nursing treatment provided. The issue of accountability for nursing standards of care, particularly national standards of care, is becoming a factor in court rulings (O'Keefe, 2001).

Key Point 44-1

Forensic nurses must be familiar with several sources of standards that influence their professional practice, including those of professional organizations, state boards of nursing, and regulatory bodies.

Although all nurses at all practice levels are held to a standard of care, that standard of care varies somewhat according to geographical locale, practice setting (e.g., intensive care unit or medical floor), and type of practice (e.g., advance nurse practitioner versus staff nurse). Nurses and other healthcare providers must comply with established standards of care, which arise from the following:

- Regulations based on state and federal statutes. The clinician has an obligation to adhere to federal laws and her or his state's nurse practice act and scope of practice guidelines. State boards of nursing set the standards for entry into nursing practice, regulate licensure, enact regulations and standards, and adjudicate cases involving violations of professional standards or rules. Nurse practice acts contain general statements of appropriate professional nursing actions. They define nursing, set standards for the nursing profession, and give guidance regarding scope of practice issues. As such, the state nursing practice act is the single most important piece of legislation affecting nursing practice. The nurse must incorporate the nurse practice act with her/his educational background, previous work experience, institutional policies, and technological advancements. Violating any statute or regulation of the state automatically makes the nurse and her/his employing facility negligent.
- Professional practice guidelines. In the ANA *Code of Ethics* (2001), provisions are listed that state the ethical obligations and duties of nurses. The 11 elements describe the nurse's fundamental commitment and values, boundaries of duty and loyalty, aspects of duties related to advancing the profession, and collaborative efforts with other healthcare professions to shape policy and meet the health needs of society (O'Keefe, 2001; ANA, 2004). Nursing practice is also guided by protocols and practice guidelines written for specific practice areas (e.g., Barton-Schmitt protocols for pediatric telephone triage, or hospital accreditation standards) that are drafted in a general way so as to apply to nursing care in a variety of settings.
- Facility policies and procedures. Required by law and accrediting agencies, policies and procedures are used in court to establish standards of care. It is expected that the nurse's practice is consistent with these policies and procedures, and when a lawsuit has been brought, they are most likely the first documents examined when evaluating whether or not a standard of care was met. Failure to follow policy does not mean that the nurse is automatically negligent, but it can mean that it will be up to a jury to decide whether or not the nurse was negligent.

Nursing Malpractice and Negligence

The term *malpractice* is used to define professional negligence, and as such, it is a subset of negligence, although in general the terms are used interchangeably. Specifically, malpractice is negligence committed by a person in a professional capacity and differs from simple negligence in that it involves specialized skills and training not possessed by the average person.

Key Point 44-2

The most common legal charge brought against nurses is for an act of negligence that represents a deviation from a standard of care.

Although there are numerous legal claims that may be brought against a nurse, the most prevalent claim is negligence. Simply stated, nursing negligence is deviation from the standard of care. If the nurse acts in a way that a reasonably prudent nurse would not act, or fails to take action in a way that a reasonably prudent nurse would act, the nurse's actions (or omissions) are negligent (DeWitt, 2001).

The law touches on a wide range of possible nursing conduct that falls under the legal heading of negligence, including failing to render care that meets applicable standards and acting in a manner that is intentionally harmful to the patient (Janulis, 1997).

Expert witnesses are used by both prosecuting and defense attorneys to establish standards of care. The expert's role is to explain to the jury the standard of care based on her or his particular expertise. The question of who can testify to standards of care may depend on specific statutory or case law in any jurisdiction; but in general, a testifying expert must possess sufficient training, experience, and knowledge (as a result of practice or teaching in the clinical setting or specialty area where the incident occurred) as to satisfy the court that they are familiar with the accepted standard of care (Harvey, 2004). Although physicians have testified regarding nursing practice, it is being recognized that medicine and nursing have different philosophies and approaches, and physicians are not educated in nursing. Nurses should testify regarding nursing practice, and should not testify as a medical expert linking a breach of the nursing standard of care to medical complications suffered by the plaintiff (*Echard v. Barnes-Jewish Hosp.*, 2002). In the end, the jury will interpret the opinions of the expert witnesses and determine if negligence has occurred.

Whether the nurse's actions are intended to bring harm to the patient or not, the patient or representative can bring suit against the nurse for potential damages. Negligence per se is a situation in which no expert testimony is required to establish the applicable standard of care, and the defendant's conduct violates some law that is designed to protect the class of persons of which the plaintiff is a member. This could occur, for example, when a student nurse administers anesthesia, in violation of a state statute, and injures the patient (*Central Anesthesia Assoc., P.C. v. Worthy*, 1985).

Elements of Negligence

In order for a plaintiff to prevail in a suit against a nurse for negligence, the plaintiff must prove all four elements of the cause of action: duty, breach of duty, causation, and damages.

Duty

Duty is defined as acts or interactions required after the presumption of a relationship between the provider and a patient. Duty is established when the nurse (1) provides direct care to an individual, (2) observes an unattended person in need of care, or (3) observes/is aware of another provider performing care in a manner that may cause harm (O'Keefe, 2001; Brent, 1997).

Breach of duty

A breach of duty is defined as neglect or failure to fulfill, in an appropriate and proper manner, the duties of a job (O'Keefe, 2001). To determine whether or not a duty was violated, it is necessary to delineate the standard of care of a particular circumstance. It must be determined if the nurse (1) met the standard of care, (2) didn't do the right thing (misfeasance), (3) did nothing/did not act (nonfeasance), or (4) did the right thing in the wrong way (malfeasance) (Murr & Moorhouse, 2004).

Causation

The proximate cause (causation) is often the most difficult element to prove. The difficulty lies in the fact that the cause of an injury often cannot be easily identified. A nurse's negligence may be one of several possibilities. Foreseeability is a causation concept that can also apply, stating that the nurse has a responsibility to anticipate harm and eliminate risk. If *res ipsa loquitur* (the thing speaks for itself) applies to causation, four conditions have been met:

1. The act that caused the injury was exclusively in the nurse's control.
2. The injury would not have happened but for the nurse's negligence.
3. No negligence on the patient's part contributed to the injury.
4. Evidence of the truth as to what happened is unavailable (Brent, 1997; Morrison, 2000).

Damages

Damages are defined as monetary compensation that may be recovered in court if the plaintiff shows that the act or omission damaged or harmed him or her in some way. Actual or compensatory damages are losses sustained by the injured person and include relevant medical expenses, lost earnings, impairment of future earnings, and past and future pain and suffering. Punitive damages are designed to punish defendants. The character of negligence necessary to sustain an award of punitive damages must be of "a gross and flagrant character, evincing reckless disregard of human life, or of the safety of persons" (Brent, 1997). For example, a patient admitted to an extended care center for rehabilitation was left restrained in a bed or chair for extended periods of time until advanced pressure ulcers developed, ultimately leading to his death (Doherty, 1993).

Criminal versus Civil Law

Laws can be classified in a number of ways, based on whether they are substantive, procedural, civil, or criminal, and all types of law are intermingled in various ways and in different areas of litigation and practice. Civil law recognizes and enforces the rights of individuals and organizations. Criminal law defines crimes and punishment (Aiken, 2004b).

When it comes to guilt, the scales of justice are balanced in a civil trial, but weighted for the defendant in a criminal case. In a criminal case the defendant is presumed innocent until proved guilty. The winner in a civil trial need only move the scale a "feather's weight" (to 51%) to prevail, while in a criminal case guilt must be proved beyond a reasonable doubt (Murr & Moorhouse, 2004).

One of the two areas of civil law is tort law. A *tort* is a wrong that harms. The three types of torts include intentional torts, negligence (nonintentional torts), and strict liability. These wrongful acts, whether arising from intentional or negligent conduct, have as their common principle the idea that injuries are to be compensated. Differences between intentional and nonintentional torts can be characterized as differences in intent, injury, duty, and consent (Aiken, 2004b).

Although negligence can occur without harmful intent, an intentional tort is an action requiring a specific state of mind, usually an intention to do a wrongful act. In intentional tort actions, plaintiffs do not have to prove that any actual injury occurred, as the harm is in the invasion of a person's rights. Potential consequences of intentional torts include loss of reputation and esteem, exposure to criminal liability, loss of professional license, loss of insurance, and punitive damages (Standards of Care, 2004; Murr & Moorhouse, 2001; Springhouse, 2000).

Best Practice *44-1*

The forensic nurse must monitor direct nursing care measures to ensure that they do not constitute intentional torts, such as assault, battery, and false imprisonment.

Intentional Torts

These actions include acts that violate another person's rights or property. In the medical arena this includes assault, battery, and false imprisonment (O'Keefe, 2001; Harvey, 2004; Janulis, 1997; Morrison, 2000).

Assault

Assault is an act that is designed to make a person fearful or in apprehension of bodily harm. Assault does not require touching; it can be a threatening statement, such as, "If you don't stay in that chair, I am going to tie you down."

Battery

Battery is unlawful or offensive touching of another without consent. Examples of battery committed by a nurse are inserting an IV after the patient revokes permission, or inserting a feeding tube in a terminal patient who is refusing care.

False Imprisonment

False imprisonment is defined as unlawful, intentional, and unjustifiable detention of person against his/her will within fixed boundaries so that the person is conscious of or harmed by the confinement. An example of false imprisonment could be the use of direct physical or chemical restraints or detaining the person in a care setting against his or her will or desire for treatment.

Quasi-Intentional Torts

These actions include such elements as defamation, slander, invasion of privacy, and breach of confidentiality. The latter two have more implications in the healthcare environment of today (O'Keefe, 2001; Harvey; 2004; Janulis, 1997; Morrison, 2000).

- Invasion of privacy can occur in any medical setting where a patient's name or medical information are viewed by unauthorized individuals; these actions can involve public exposure of private facts, intrusion on the seclusion or private concerns of the person, or the patient's name or picture being used without express written consent.
- Breach of confidentiality is a legal and ethical concern for healthcare providers, especially in this day of electronic record keeping and transmission of medical information through various means, such as Email, the Internet, and facsimile (fax). For example, information can be left on a computer screen, faxes being sent to providers or payers can be viewed by many persons, and sensitive information can be unintentionally given to unauthorized individuals.

Liability Issues in Healthcare

Common sources of nursing liability include failure to notify the physician, making assumptions about following questionable orders, inadequate monitoring, failing to follow policies and procedures, medication errors, failure to safeguard against falls and other preventable injuries, using unsafe equipment or failing to use equipment correctly, and breach of confidentiality. Each will be discussed briefly here.

Failure to Notify the Physician

The nurse must communicate thorough, accurate, and timely information about the patient's condition to the physician and others as appropriate (e.g., other caregivers, family [if patient allows], and chain of command in nursing/facility staff). Some malpractice cases have hinged on whether the nurse was persistent enough in attempting to notify the physician or in convincing the physician of the seriousness of a patient's condition. Courts are likely to recognize that after-the-fact communication is "no communication" (Springhouse, 2000).

Making Assumptions and Following Orders

Assumptions cannot be defended in court, and neither can a nurse's assertion she/he was "just following orders." The standard of care requires that nurses question and clarify orders, especially when orders seem inappropriate, written orders are illegible, or the patient's life or safety is at stake. As a general rule, verbal and phone orders are acceptable only under acute or emergency circumstances when a doctor cannot promptly attend to the patient. Standing orders or protocols must be individualized and reviewed from time to time for accuracy and efficacy (Marden, 2000).

Inadequate Monitoring

Inadequate monitoring includes failure to adequately observe, especially when a patient's condition is undergoing change, if the patient possesses self-destructive tendencies, or if appropriate monitoring would have detected the complication or change in condition. As a nurse, one of the greatest responsibilities is to assess, monitor, and report to other healthcare providers, including notification of the physician (Springhouse, 2000). In *Harrington v. Rush Presbyterian, St Luke's Hospital*, a patient who was admitted for drug dependency began to suffer headaches and finally fainted. The nurses returned the patient to her bed. They did not contact a physician. Progress notes between 11:00 p.m. and 7:00 a.m. were not written. The patient died of drug toxicity. The verdict was $4 million awarded to the plaintiff's estate (*Medical Malpractice Verdicts*, 1989).

An additional concern in this area is failure to intervene when monitoring has revealed a problem with the patient. The nurse has an independent duty to act for the safety of the patient. Both failure to intervene and inappropriate interventions can result in liability.

Failure to Follow Policies and Procedures

Facility documents are used to guide nursing care and to orient and educate staff in the facility's expectations for employee conduct. Very often, not having a policy or not following an established policy can have legal consequences (Marden, 2000). In addition, being unaware of a policy is not deemed an excuse for failure to follow the standard.

Medication Errors

This problem encompasses the largest group of errors resulting in legal action. The major categories include the following:

- Not knowing or being unfamiliar with the drug that is ordered. Unless the order is questionable, the law expects the drug to be administered as ordered.
- Not administering what is ordered. Deviating from the "five rights" (right patient, right drug, right route, right dose, right time) is cause for nursing negligence.
- Not documenting what is administered. Poor record keeping is a common cause of duplicate and omitted medication doses.
- Awareness/documentation of allergies and at-risk populations (e.g., the very young, elderly, mentally ill, developmentally delayed, persons with limited or compromised communication). Ask and record client/caregiver response to allergies to drugs and document, using approved abbreviations (Springhouse, 2000).

Failure to Provide Safeguards

Lawsuits commonly arise from falls and from use of (or failure to properly use) restraints. The decision to use (or not to use) restraints must be made with caution and good judgment. Their intended purpose must be to protect either the patient or others who may be injured by the patient, including the staff caring for the patient. The ultimate determination of necessity is left with the physician, but often the moment-to-moment necessity is determined by the nurse. Safeguard the patient by careful, ongoing assessment of the condition necessitating the need for restraints and individual risks (e.g., circulation, skin condition) and by accurate documentation of safeguards used (e.g., side rails, adequate numbers of assistive personnel) (Marden, 2000).

Equipment Failures or User Errors

Equipment may be a central or peripheral issue in litigations. Malfunctioning devices as well as user errors must be considered in this category. For example, nurses may fail to set up or monitor equipment; they may also fail to note and correct a problem that causes harm to the patient (e.g., the patient could be burned from hot pack therapy, or may receive too much or too little fluid or medication through an IV pump).

Breach of Confidentiality

This area has recently become a popular ground for lawsuits because people are increasingly reluctant to reveal their health status and because of ease of access to medical data. Health information is typically considered confidential and privileged and cannot be disclosed without authorization or as otherwise provided by law (Marden, 2000). This is supported by the ANA *Code of Ethics* (2004) and by other documents, including the Health Insurance Portability and Accountability Act of 1996 (HIPAA Overview, 2004).

Reducing Risks of Malpractice

Perhaps the best defense against malpractice lies in the ethical practice of nursing. The profession founded on caring cannot afford to forget that patients are people. People generally don't sue people they like. So, treat patients better than they expect to be treated. Value them. Listen to their concerns. Bear in mind that attorneys report that people frequently complain to them that healthcare providers couldn't or wouldn't answer their questions.

Keep well informed. Continuing one's education, training, and certifications is key to keeping abreast of the knowledge and skills required to provide nursing care that falls well within standards of care. Although not all states require continuing education for relicensure, most nursing specialties have certification requirements to ensure that nurses are kept up to date on the latest healthcare information.

When it comes to patient care, recognize the importance of accurate clinical assessment data (and its absence). Identify actual and potential complications. Obtain additional data when not at ease about a patient's condition. Anticipate staffing needs and secure adequate resources to assure safe patient care, and document the patient's clinical status as well as provider actions and responses.

Value the nursing task of doing complete and accurate documentation in the patient's record. It has been said that "the best defense against lawsuits is a good documentation offense" (Wetter, 2004). Documentation forms the framework for all nursing activities, and documentation standards establish specific regulatory guidelines and policies (Aiken, 2004b). Nurses have been heard to say, "How could you possibly want to chart, let alone enjoy it, when it keeps you from giving direct patent care?" In reality, documenting *is* patient care (Springhouse, 2002). Certainly, the old saying, "if it's not documented, it was not done," has never been timelier as state and federal governments continue to enact legislation to protect healthcare consumers. Effective documentation is factual, accurate, complete, and timely (FACT). Failure to document or faulty or unfactual documentation is risky behavior that should be avoided (Aiken, 2004b).

In this day of nursing shortage and pressure associated with providing care for too many patients with too few resources, issues of quality are constantly arising. "It's not my job" reflects the view that raising issues of quality (e.g., inadequate staffing to do the job, operating obsolete or unsafe equipment) is simply too time-consuming and must be left to others with the energy and desire to pursue them. However, if the nurse fails to raise the issue with those who can effect change, and a patient sues for damages sustained as a result of the problem (e.g., inadequate staffing), the nurse as well as the facility could be found liable (DeWitt, 2001).

Another major issue relates to delegation of nursing tasks, and who is responsible for what. The nurse is directly responsible for her/his own actions, assignments, and supervision. The nurse has the right to rely upon other staff to competently carry out tasks within the scope of their employment. This is true for licensed and nonlicensed personnel. Each individual has certain responsibilities and will be held accountable for carrying out those responsibilities competently (Marden, 2000). There are, however, guidelines for what cannot be delegated by a nurse to an unlicensed person. These duties include assessments, formulating care plans, tasks to be done only by licensed individuals, patient teaching, and administration of medications (this last duty is not firmly decided yet and is being reviewed in a number of states as it relates to medication administration in certain care facilities) (Janulis, 1997).

It is vital for nurses to know their facility's job description for various categories of workers, as well as the state board's practice acts and limitations for licensed and unlicensed workers who might be under their supervision. All nurses should understand who can delegate and what tasks can be delegated and to whom and under what circumstances. All nurses should exercise their rights (e.g., right task, right person, right circumstances, right direction, right supervision) (Marden, 2000).

Common Malpractice Defenses

A specific time limit is allowed for bringing litigation. This is known as the statute of limitations. In many states the time period in which a malpractice suit can be filed has been set at two to three years. However, the statute of limitations may be extended if the individual does not know he/she was injured until after the statute has run, if fraud has been perpetrated, or if the individual was a minor (as defined by state law) at the time the injury occurred (Brent, 1997). For example, an individual injured at birth (a bad obstetrical outcome) may have until his/her eighteenth or twenty-first birthday to file suit.

Counterclaims can also be filed by a defendant nurse in some states. These counterclaims include (1) contributory negligence (by an injured plaintiff); (2) comparative negligence (when negligence is measured in a certain percentage against the defendant nurse and a certain percentage against the plaintiff); and (3) assumption of risk (e.g., patient signs himself out of the hospital against medical advice) (HIPAA Overview, 2004).

Best Practice *44-2*

Although employers may provide some insurance for nurses, forensic nurses should maintain their personal insurance coverage for professional liability.

Malpractice insurance is also considered a type of defense against malpractice, in that it can protect a nurse or employer by paying all or a portion of assessed damages when the court finds for the plaintiff. Although most facilities cover their nurses with malpractice insurance, there is a growing recognition of the importance of nurses carrying their own professional liability insurance. Reasons for this include (1) covering defense costs at the board of nursing hearings (not normally covered by the employer); (2) covering actions done as a volunteer (Good Samaritan actions); (3) being portable if a nurse has more than one job; and (4) allowing the nurse to obtain her or his own attorney, rather than depending on an attorney supplied by an employer and whose primary duty is to the employer, not the nurse in question (Marden, 2000).

Case Study 44-1 Complications and Negligence Involving an Intravenous Line

A patient came to the hospital with complaints of abdominal pain and was evaluated in the emergency department. The physician's orders included intravenous (IV) medications, for which a line needed to be inserted. The nurse assigned to the patient had difficulty finding veins in the woman's arms. He attempted to start a line in her hand, and was successful on the third attempt. For the remainder of the patient's treatment in the hospital, it was documented that the patient complained of discomfort at the IV site and tolerated it poorly. Although there was no indication that other symptoms of complication existed, there was also no indication that placement of another line was offered to, or refused by, the patient. Following her discharge, the patient filed a suit alleging negligence on the part of the nurse and the hospital. Specifically she claimed a poorly performed catheter insertion caused her to develop reflex sympathetic dystrophy (RSD) in her right hand. Severe burning pain, pathological changes in bone and skin, excessive sweating, tissue swelling, and extreme sensitivity to touch characterize this chronic condition.

Eventually when the case went to trial, after a review of the chart, and following expert testimony in the courtroom, no deficiencies in technique could be found in the placement of the catheter. By his employment record and training, the nurse was fully qualified to place IV lines as part of his scope of practice as a registered nurse. It was noted that the hospital's standards of care were breached as they allowed for a maximum of two attempts before calling for assistance. However, in further review, the "community" standard (which was the measure used in the case), allowed for four insertion attempts. By this standard of care the nurse was within reasonable limits by trying three times. Expert testimony addressed the issue of causation of the RSD. No direct causative links could be established between the starting of an IV and a diagnosis of RSD. In this case, summary judgment was entered for the hospital, finding that no negligence was evident. The client appealed and the appeals court affirmed the judgment of the lower court (*Coleman v. East Jefferson General Hosp.*, 747 S.2d 1044-LA [1999]).

Case Study 44-2 Use of Restraints

Following a head injury sustained in a motor vehicle accident, the patient was initially visibly confused, and for a long period of time, he was frequently agitated. During the course of his admission, an order for "soft" wrist restraints was obtained and implemented to protect the patient from injury related to his mental status changes. On the day of the incident, the nurse on duty had assessed the patient. In her professional opinion, based on her observation of the patient's mental and physical state and level of consciousness, restraints were not needed. Later in the shift the nurse was assisting the patient to get out of bed. In the course of this maneuver, the patient fell and claimed that an injury was sustained. A lawsuit was filed against the facility alleging negligence on the part of the nurse. The patient contended that the removal of the restraints breached the standard of care.

When the case was tried the plaintiff's arguments sought to convince the jury that poor judgment was exercised by the nurse, and that removal of the restraints and ambulation put him in harm's way. The nurse had assessed the patient to be calm. The purpose of the restraints was to prevent the patient from harming himself and not to "keep the patient from falling out of bed." This purpose was deemed to have been achieved. Thus, the removal of the restraints could not be deemed as negligent. There was no duty of care breached in allowing the calm patient to remain unrestrained. The court found there was not a causative relationship between removing the restraints and the patient's fall (*Gerard v. Sacred Heart Medical Center*, 937 P.2d 1104 [1997]).

Case Study 44-3 Catastrophic Cast

Nurses called the treating physician to report a patient's deteriorating condition involving that patient's upper extremity, which was in a cast. The physician initially did nothing about their concerns. The nurses failed to notify superiors or call the department chairperson. For three days the patient's temperature climbed. The patient's injured arm became swollen and black, and a foul-smelling drainage was seeping through the cast. The patient vomited his antibiotics. When action was finally taken, the damage was profound and the end result was amputation up to the shoulder.

As the judge stated to the jury, the nurses' failure to follow hospital policy (in failing to demand that the physician attend the patient given his deteriorating status and in failing to use chain of command to obtain assistance in getting attention from a physician) was the proximate cause of the patient's injury. This breach of the standard of care by the nurses points out what the various states' nurse practice acts have delineated: as a nurse, the nurse has a legal and ethical duty to use her or his own judgment when providing care (*Utter v. United Health Center*, 160 W. V. 703, 236 E.2d 213 [1977]).

Summary

The highly charged emotional and technical arenas in which forensic nurses practice compel them to be highly accountable for their activities. In fact, the definition of forensic nursing alone would imply that members of the discipline should have a high regard for the principles, standards, laws, and other regulatory guidance pertinent to the specialty. In addition to comprehension of the scope and standards of forensic nursing, it is imperative that practitioners be knowledgeable about their state's nurse practice act.

The immense responsibilities of independent forensic nursing demand a thorough understanding of nursing malpractice and negligence. In order for a plaintiff to prevail in a suit against a nurse for negligence, the plaintiff must prove all four elements of the cause of action: duty, breach of duty, causation, and damages.

Forensic nurses should have no ambivalence about what constitutes their roles and responsibilities to individuals and the community they serve. Exemplary documentation and supportive patient and family interactions are vital to a sound offense within the practice arena.

Resources

Organizations

American Association of Legal Nurse Consultants

AALNC Headquarters, 401 North Michigan Avenue, Chicago, IL 60611; Tel: 877-402-2562; www.aalnc.org

American Bar Association

321 North Clark Street, Chicago, IL 60610; Tel: 312-988-5000; www.abanet.org

American Nurses Association (ANA)

8515 Georgia Avenue, Suite 400, Silver Spring, MD 20910; Tel: 800-274-4ANA; www.nursingworld.org

References

Aiken, T. D. (2004a). Standards of care. In Aiken, T. D., Legal, ethical, and political issues in nursing (2nd ed.). Philadelphia: F. A. Davis.

Aiken, T. D. (2004b) Legal, ethical, and political issues in nursing (2nd ed.). Philadelphia: F. A. Davis.

American Nurses' Association. (2004). Code of ethics. Retrieved April 2004 from http://www.nursingworld.org/ethics/code/ethicscode150.htm.

Brent, N. J. (1997). Nurses and the law: A guide to principles and applications (pp. 41-46). Philadelphia: W. B. Saunders.

Central Anesthesia Assoc., PC, et al. v. Worthy, 333 S.E.2d 829 (1985), 254 (Ga.) 728.

DeWitt, A. L. (2001). The top 10 things you can do to get sued. Retrieved March 2004 from Advance for Nurses Web site: http://www.advancefornurses.com.

Doherty, 619 So.2d 367, Fla. 3d DCA (1993).

Echard v. Barnes-Jewish Hosp., S.W.3d(2002) (WL 1902103). August 20, 2002, Legal Eagle Eye Newsletter for the Nursing Profession, October 2002, p. 7.

Harvey, C. J. (2004). "Malpractice: What every nurse should know." Course for Nurses in Colorado Springs, CO. Outline published by HTA Consulting, Inc.

HIPAA Overview. Washington, DC: Department of Health. Retrieved April 2004 from http://dchealth.dc.gov/hipaa/hipaaoverview.shtm.

Janulis, D. (1997) Nursing law seminar. Houston: Southwest Seminars Association.

Marden, C. (2000). Nursing law update. Houston: Southwest Seminars Association.

Harrington v. Rush Presbyterian, St Luke's Hospital. In Medical malpractice verdicts. (1989). Vol. 5, No. 2, February 1989. Chicago: American Bar Association.

Morrison, C. A. (2000). Nursing malpractice, liability & your license. Altoona, WI: Medical Educational Services.

Murr, A. C., & Moorhouse, M. F. (May 24, 2001). Legal nurse consulting: You, too, can do it. Guest lecture, Forensic program. Colorado Springs: University of Colorado.

O'Keefe, M. E. (2001). Nursing practice and the law: Avoiding malpractice and other legal risks (p. 552). Philadelphia: F. A. Davis.

Springhouse. (2000). Nursing malpractice: Understanding the risks. Retrieved from SpringNet Web site (Springhouse Corp.): www.springnet.com/ce/nsoce2nso.htm.

Springhouse. (2002). Charting made incredibly easy (2nd ed., p. V.). Springhouse, PA: Springhouse Corp.

Wetter, D. (2004). The best defense is a good documentation offense. Online course. Washington, DC: Corexecel: Linking Learning to Performance.

Chapter 45 International Law

Jane E. Weaver

The Relevance of International Law to Forensic Nursing

Forensic practitioners are well aware of the partnership between law and forensic science that their profession entails. Usually, US forensic clinicians are enforcing municipal (local) ordinances or state laws. If a federal crime is being prosecuted, then federal statutes and the US Constitution are involved. In some countries, another origin of laws may be provincial or regional constitutions (e.g., European Union). It has also long been recognized that by harming a citizen of one nation, another state indirectly injures that citizen's nation. Thus, a nation state has an interest in protecting its citizens wherever in the world they may be, or wherever in the world a crime is committed against them. These latter two ideas extend certain legal rights and privileges, and the rule of national laws, beyond national boundaries. US jurisprudence, for instance, authorizes prosecution in the US for certain crimes committed abroad. US civil courts also allow causes of action to recover damages for wrongs alleged to have occurred abroad, often obtaining jurisdiction over non-US citizens and ordering them to pay monetary awards. Increasingly frequently, however, for both US and overseas forensic practitioners, an entirely separate body of international law may be involved.

Key Point *45-1*

International law involves agreements between two or more countries, formal bilateral or multilateral treaties, decisions of international courts, and universal norms as actually and consistently *practiced* from a sense of legal obligation by the majority of civilized nations (known as customary international law).

Although traditionally, international law encompassed relations between states, or treatment of groups vis-à-vis states, since the founding of the United Nations (UN), the individual has become a primary concern of international law. Indeed, the Preamble and Articles 55, 56, and 68 of the UN Charter indicate that the protection of human rights was to be one of the UN's highest priorities (Hannum & Fischer, 1993).

For example, a "domestic" legal case might involve a forensic nurse giving evidence in a hearing regarding the granting of asylum status by the US based on persecution by the applicant's home country under rules of the US Immigration and Naturalization Service. That same forensic nurse asked to testify before a regional international body human rights court, such as the European Court of Justice, or the Human Rights Committee of the UN, might be operating under international law originating outside the US (Buergenthal & Shelton, 1995).

Traditional Sources of International Law

International law emanates from a variety of sources. Two of the easiest to understand are laws or administrative regulations that originate in the international bodies of the Council of Europe and the European Union, because such entities parallel the legislative bodies found in most communities and treaties. A third source of international law, actually the oldest but perhaps the hardest to understand conceptually, is customary international law.

Treaties

Treaties are formal written agreements between two or more countries' governments intended to be legally binding by having the status of at least national law and national law enforcement behind them. Most international agreements and treaties into which the US entered before World War II are bilateral (between two countries) as compared to trilateral (among three countries) or multilateral. Bilateral agreements can be conceived of and entered into force within a week, whereas multilateral treaties can take decades of drafting, years of debate in the international organization(s) involved, and many more years to obtain enough countries' ratifications for them to finally enter into force. The Supremacy Clause of the US Constitution, Article VI, cl. 2, mandates that rights conferred by a treaty (ratified by the federal government) be honored by the individual states, and state courts are charged with remedying legal violations.

Even though a country has supported a particular treaty through the arduous ratification process, it does not mean it will then become a party to it. For instance, despite its often claimed leading role in advocating for human rights, by 1994 the US had become a party to only four major post-WWII human rights treaties (Box 45-1). Specifically, the US helped negotiate and draft the International Covenant on Economic, Social, and Cultural Right, which President Carter signed and sent to the Senate, but there it still remains pending (Article 12 recognizes the right of everyone to the enjoyment of the highest attainable standard of physical and mental health). The US was also instrumental in calling for the global improvement of the status of women and children worldwide which led to the Convention on the Elimination of All Forms of Discrimination against Women (CEDAW, or the women's convention of 1979), now ratified by at least 165 or more countries, as well as the Convention on the Rights of the Child (CRC, 1989), a multilateral treaty with which 193 countries, virtually every single recognized country in the world, have agreed to comply, save Somalia and the US.

CEDAW was signed by the US but never sent to the Senate until President Clinton sent it there when there was a Democratic majority. However, even with significant reservations, understandings, and interpretations designed to meet critics' objections added by the US State Department, the Senate failed to take a vote on CEDAW (Box 45-2). The children's convention (CRC) has yet to

Box 45-1 Key Conventions

The following list presents key conventions regarding human rights. The first date indicates the adoption, opening for signature of the treaty; the second date indicates the year the US ratified the treaty.

The Convention on the Prevention and Punishment of the Crime of Genocide (1945/1988)

The International Convention on the Elimination of All Forms of Discrimination (1965/1994)

The International Covenant on Civil and Political Rights (ICCPR, 1966/1992)

The International Convention against Torture and Other Cruel, Inhuman, and Degrading Treatment (CAT, 1984/1994)

In 1872, after five years of political lobbying and advocacy by Clara Barton, the US ratified one of the first multilateral treaties: the Geneva Convention. In 1949, the US ratified two additional Geneva Conventions, but it has not ratified further Geneva Conventions (circa 1967) that deal with situations such as the Vietnam War or treatment of refugees.

Box 45-2 Women's Convention: CEDAW

The UN's Convention on the Elimination of All Forms of Discrimination against Women (CEDAW) is a women's convention that reviews signatory countries' reports on activities to enforce the convention. Until 2000, CEDAW heard debate on an optional protocol to allow individual women's cases to be heard and penalties imposed similar to the enforcement schemes for other multilateral human rights instruments. In 1999, the UN adopted an optional protocol for CEDAW, which has since been ratified by a sufficient number of countries consenting to international jurisdiction to enter into force.

be sent to the Senate for ratification, ostensibly over parental rights issues. Because the US Senate has not given its advise and consent to either of these two treaties, the US has ratified neither.

A well-organized US National Committee for Ratification of CEDAW with representation from the American Nurses' and American Bar Associations would certainly welcome forensic practitioners' support (Box 45-3). Indeed, grassroots efforts to support the women's convention, without waiting for Congress to act, have resulted in many states and towns enacting legislation adopting the treaty within their own geographic jurisdictions. One problem with this approach is the US Department of State's opinion that CEDAW is not self-executing, usually limiting an individual's ability to enforce his or her rights under the treaty in US or other nations' courts.

A treaty that is self-executing takes effect immediately. If a treaty is not self-executing, each party intending to be legally bound must enact further domestic laws to see that the treaty is given full effect and enforced. An example of a self-executing international treaty would be the Geneva Convention of 1864. Thus, as soon as that treaty was ratified by the US (thanks to the efforts of Clara Barton), meaning that the US President had signed it and the US Senate had given its advise and consent, its terms became the equivalent of US federal law. On the other hand, the International Covenant on Civil and Political Rights (ICCPR, 1966), a multilateral treaty promulgated by the UN

Box 45-3 *Weaver v. Torres*

A refusal was experienced in *Weaver v. Torres* (No. WNN 00-1126 [Order of Dec. 27, 2000, D. Maryland]), a case against a state university administrator for violating a faculty member's freedom of expression. At that time, the court cited one federal appellate ruling and two federal district courts, in Georgia and Washington, as grounds not to allow an individual to sue under a treaty (i.e., international law). Since then, the Fifth, Sixth, Eighth, and Eleventh Circuits have followed suit, denying any obligation to enforce treaty provisions when the US executive branch asserts a treaty or provision is non-self-executing. Even when states admit violating a self-executing treaty, they often fail to provide a meaningful remedy. In *Faulde v. Johnson*, 81 F.3d 515, 520 (5th Cir. 1986), Texas courts refused to overturn a capital conviction/death sentence to remedy an admitted violation of an inmate's treaty rights.

General Assembly in the mid-1960s, is not considered by the US executive branch to be self-executing, and would require the US or individual states or municipalities to pass further laws internally before that treaty would be given full force and effect by US courts. When such further legislation has been enacted, US tribunals are more likely to grant individuals those treaty rights.

Because there are an increasing number of treaties governing almost every aspect of human behavior, from oceanic disposal of medical waste to creation of an international criminal court, the scope and origin of laws, rules, and regulations that forensic practitioners will practice under most likely will increasingly originate from international law. Although this may take more time in the US than elsewhere, the process has started. One example involves the definition of "refugee" in deportation proceedings. In the case of *INS v. Cardoza-Fonseca*, 450 U.S. 421, 441 (1987), the Supreme Court recognized that in writing legislation on refugees, Congress purposefully incorporated the definition of the UN Protocol on the status of refugees, which the US had ratified.

Another example involves foreigners arrested in US territory. Under Article 36(1)(b) of the self-executing Vienna Convention on Consular Relations, a foreign national is entitled to have his or her embassy informed and embassy staff allowed to visit them. However, until a federal statute and regulations implementing this treaty provision were enacted by Congress and relevant federal or state agencies, US courts hesitated to enforce this international right on behalf of individual arrestees, even though they clearly recognized the US had ratified and had become a party to this treaty. After numerous foreign nationals were sentenced to death or life imprisonment in US criminal proceedings, other countries complained to the International Court of Justice (a UN institution), which ruled against the US for not enforcing such treaty obligations and failing to give remedies to individuals whose rights under such treaties were violated. In the case of *Breard v. Pruett*, 134 F.3d 615, 622 (4th Cir. 1998), Fourth Circuit Judge Butzner wrote in support of US courts recognizing self-executing treaties as binding law under the Constitution and its Supremacy Clause. Yet, in numerous recent cases involving claims of violations of the International Covenant of Civil and Political Rights, which contains articles that the US Congress and State Department assert are non-self-executing, US courts have denied an obligation to enforce such rights (Box 45-3). Eventually, however, it seems US courts will increasingly decide issues of international law on their own merits (i.e., as enforceable without further parallel codification in domestic law), and US forensic practitioners will increasingly likely be involved in such international law cases.

International Law Originating in International Bodies

This source of international law includes both laws passed by regional governmental organizations such as the European Parliament or by international bodies such as the International Labor Organization (ILO, 1919). The ILO typifies many other specialty international bodies whose members have developed a considerable body of international law, as well as an effective global monitoring system (Mission of Inquiry, 1990). With some 200 international labor conventions now in operation, no doubt some of them govern working conditions, living standards, and equitable treatment for forensic practitioners.

Customary International Law

As certain truths, practices, or fundamental rules become recognized authority or generally and consistently practiced behavioral standards across a majority of territories or borders, they attain status as customary international law. Such laws are said to be "of custom" as opposed to being decreed or written by particular authorities. One example is the right of all nations' ships to sail the high seas, free from piracy. Although not initially written down as a legal decree, legal scholars have historically recognized this right as customary international law since at least the 1700s because the majority of civilized nations actually consistently practiced it and prosecuted pirates. Lip service to "universal" morality or norms is insufficient to attain status as customary international law; only actual consistent practice due to a sense of legal obligation, by the majority of civilized nations, meets the criteria. As the world becomes more interdependent, the body of customary international law must be expanded and clarified.

Key Point *45-2*

Customary international law refers to minimum standards as actually practiced from a *sense of legal obligation* governing relations between governments, between governments and certain citizens, and among human beings in general. In many societies, notions of universal justice or natural law support the concept of customary international law.

With increasing democratic national governance structures and more self-rule for groups of people, customary international law came to involve human rights. Often, there was debate as to whether some standards legal scholars were proclaiming as customary international law emanated too predominantly from Western cultural perspectives. Many arguments were made about cultural relativism and the possibility that the values of Western cultures and religions did not encompass the full range of human rights. Some of this debate has subsided since 1945 when the Universal Declaration of Human Rights (UDHR) was adopted by the UN General Assembly. A declaration is not intended to be legally binding and therefore is not the same as a treaty, but the UDHR is cited not only as evidence that nations representing numerous cultures, and all the major religions, recognize certain minimum standards or "inalienable" human rights, but also what those international standards are. Such universally recognized rights include certain rights to life and the humane treatment for prisoners. Having stood the test of 50 years' time within the 186 plus nation forum of the UN, the UDHR is usually now considered customary international law.

Since 1945, many detailed declarations, agreements, conventions, and numerous treaties to flesh out the human rights enumerated in the UDHR have been negotiated and come into force. This development is often referred to as the modern human rights movement (Stanley, 1997). One way devised to address philosophical, religious, and cultural differences, when it comes to codifying human rights into enforceable international law, is the reservations, declarations, and understandings mechanism. This allows nations becoming a party to a treaty to file certain legal interpretations, and reserve aspects of domestic law, even while ratifying a treaty. For instance, the Convention on the Elimination of All Forms of Discrimination Against Women has been ratified by over 165 countries. However, most of those signatory parties also filed reservations, some of which have been criticized as so extensive, and so incongruent, with the intent and spirit of the treaty as to effectively nullify the country's obligations to comply. The US often files an "understanding" that the US Constitution will prevail if there appears to be any conflict between it and the treaty. As nations file reservations to written international laws being created by multilateral entities like the UN, as international courts render decisions interpreting written treaties, and as sovereign nations comply with the findings and orders of international judicial forums by paying damages or changing certain behaviors, the body of customary international law is clarified and grows.

Global Opportunities for Forensic Nurses

Similarly, as professional associations adopt ethics codes and promulgate position statements (International Council of Nurses, 1995) that become recognized as the globally accepted standard within that profession, these documents become supporting evidence for customary international law. Kenneth Hoffman, Esq., is an authority on humanitarian law (the branch of international law governing armed conflict). Mr. Hoffman has stated that certain position statements accepted by the 120 national nurses association members currently making up the International Council of Nurses (ICN), and representing over 5 million of the world's professional nurses, are evidence that certain universal human rights exist, and because their recognition actually impacts professional nursing practice, such standards actually help clarify customary international law (Hoffman, 1997). So, even though international law may not be as easy to understand or interpret as local, domestic, or national law, this difficulty cannot be an excuse for forensic nurse practitioners to avoid becoming familiar with it.

Further, by working in concert with their colleagues across borders, forensic nurses are actually contributing to the formation and rule of international law. This results from helping investigate and prosecute violations of international law, by assisting in the enforcement of universal human rights laws, including those regarding prisoners, and by further delineating the ethical standards for clinical forensic practice and the role of forensic practitioners internationally (Box 45-4). One of the most important contributions of individual forensic nurses will be strengthening national capacities to collect morbidity and mortality data in UN priority areas such as violence against women and children (United Nations Non-Governmental Liaison Service, 1998a), human trafficking, and child prostitution and pornography (United Nations Non-Governmental Liaison Service, 1998b).

Box 45-4 Prisoner and Detainee Protection

The following sources give the international legal standards for prisoner and detainee treatment:

Standard Minimum Rules for the Treatment of Prisoners (Sales No. E 1956 IV. 4, annex I.A). United Nations. (1956). New York: United Nations Secretariat.

Principles of medical ethics relevant to the role of health personnel, particularly physicians, in the protection of prisoners and detainees against torture and other cruel, inhuman, or degrading treatment or punishment. Res 37/194. United Nations General Assembly. (1982, December 18). New York: Centre for Human Rights.

United Nations Convention against Torture and Other Cruel, Inhuman, or Degrading Treatment or Punishment, UN Document A/39/51. (1984). (Entered into force June 26, 1987.)

Most significantly, with the ratification by more than 80 countries of the July 17, 1998, treaty creating an International Criminal Court (ICC), demand for forensic clinicians in prosecuting international crimes should increase. The ICC treaty authorizes jurisdiction over genocide, crimes against humanity, and war crimes committed in both international or internal armed conflicts *if* national judicial systems are unwilling or unable to prosecute accused individuals (Winarick, 1998). ICC language defines many crimes against women and children, including rape, as a crime against humanity or war crime. Just as demand in most countries for domestic rape services is growing, with the global increase in internal armed conflict, the global demand for forensic nurses to treat rape victims from civil wars and refugee situations is expected to increase. If the US and Canadian experience with increased chances of successful domestic rape prosecution via forensic nursing (Weaver & Lynch, 1999; Esposito, 1998) is combined with a global reduction in impunity for war criminals, including rapists, due to the new ICC, it is hoped that forensic practitioners can deter potential perpetrators from committing such grave crimes.

Best Practice *45-1*

Forensic nurses should prepare a thorough study of the various regional and multilateral human rights international law instruments by searching the Internet, attending meetings on the topic, and reading legal cases mentioning them (again search the Internet for such cases) before contacting attorneys for potential roles as an expert witness in cases involving torture, rape, or human trafficking cases.

Forensic nurses should form professional contacts and network to advance forensic practice city by city, state by state, nation by nation, region by region. It is also advisable to apply for grants to conduct international forensic research and to publish the results, thus elevating the body of forensic knowledge. Grants may also be sought for introducing formal forensic nursing courses or continuing forensic education for nurses overseas. Finally, grant monies may be used to support the attendance of international law experts and ICC staff or judges to professional forensic nursing meetings.

Best Practice *45-2*

Forensic nurses should maintain contacts with international organizations and be prepared through education and training to assume roles in supporting human rights.

Forensic nurses should seek opportunities to volunteer to help international organizations and nongovernmental organizations (NGOs) add forensic services to their projects. Maintain contacts with leading UN, Interpol, and international human rights courts/tribunals' justices and policy makers to inform them about forensic issues relevant to their work; offer services to help them accomplish their stated aims. When seeing where a connection might have been made, but does not appear to have been, send a letter or Email, send some literature on the many forensic nursing roles, and keep the communications and networking going. Live the saying, "Success is the meeting of preparation and opportunity."

Case Study 45-1 ***Nwaokolo v. Immigration and Naturalization Service***

A Nigerian woman petitioned a court to stop her deportation on grounds that she and her four-year-old American citizen daughter would suffer irreparable injury if they were removed from the US and sent to Nigeria, and to insist that the Immigration and Naturalization judge reconsider evidence her daughter would be subjected to female genital mutilation (FGM) in Nigeria (*Nwaokolo v. Immigration and Naturalization Service*, No. 02-2964 [7th Cir. 2002]).

In the original deportation proceedings, the woman lost. In July 1999, she filed again, seeking protection under the Convention Against Torture and Other Cruel, Inhuman and Degrading Treatment or Punishment, as implemented through 8 C.F.R. Section 208.16(c).

This time she argued that both she and her 13-year-old daughter would face FGM. The Board of Immigration Appeals (Board) denied relief on grounds that she offered no evidence that she would be tortured upon return to Nigeria. The Board was silent about the 13-year-old American citizen daughter. In 2002, the woman filed again on grounds of changed circumstances, namely the birth of another daughter, now four, whom she claimed would also be tortured and subjected to FGM if the mother were forced to be returned to Nigeria. She cited new legal protections and remedies under the Convention Against Torture, and presented Department of State documents describing the serious physical and psychological injuries from FGM. Another State document confirmed that FGM remained "widely practiced" in 2000. The Board of Immigration Appeals issued another denial without addressing the risk to her four-year-old American daughter.

Upon appeal to federal court, the Seventh Circuit held that the Board abused its discretion in failing to consider the hardship to the US citizen children. The court took judicial notice of the official US government reports that 60% to 90% of the female population of Nigeria undergo FGM. The court also cited World Health Organization and United Nations documents concluding that FGM has serious effects on health including infection or hemorrhage, which can cause death, permanent disfigurement, and increased chance of death during childbirth. The court noted that previous

Board rulings recognized the prevalence and brutality of FGM in Nigeria and had allowed the threat of FGM as a basis for asylum (*In re Kasinger*, 21 I.N. Dec. 357, 361-62 (BIA, 1996).

Finally, the federal appeals court ruled that a stay of deportation would promote the US public's compelling interest in ensuring that US citizens are not forced into exile to be tortured. The court ordered the Board to give a full airing on its duty to consider notifying responsible state authorities of the departure of these minor American girls to Nigeria, a country where they would be in immediate danger of significant harm.

Testifying in International Forums

Be sure to know the legal framework of the forum and case (what is the governing law?), the exact nature of the proceeding (civil or criminal, fact finding or adjudicatory), and the standards for evidence (Pitts, 2001). Will they ask about training or experience, how evidence was collected, the science behind analysis of the evidence? Are scientific articles, documents regarding credentials, or equipment needed for court? What language will be used? How can the translator be trusted? Is it possible to import and export cameras, equipment, or graphic photographs into and out of another country without problems? What are the forum's rules on patient confidentiality? If allowed to accept compensation for work, how are work permits and taxes handled? Hopefully, if the suggestions in the preceding section were followed (i.e., heard speakers from international tribunals at professional meetings, and networked to establish and maintain contacts with staff or justices of such forums), one will be much better prepared to assist internationally. Once opportunities to practice internationally are found, be prepared and professional; know both ICN (ICN, 1995) and IAFN standards. After testifying, nurses should record and share their experiences with their colleagues and offer to serve as a mentor.

Summary

The role of the forensic nurse examiner domestically has been a success in strengthening the health of the individual crime victim, as well as the initially accused who benefit from better evidence. In addition, forensic nurse examiners within jails and prisons have contributed to improvements for the unjustly incarcerated and for actual perpetrators that forensic nurses seek to rehabilitate. Physicians and other providers, such as nurses, working for the US have been accused as well, though, of violating international law in regard to detainees of the "war on terror" (Singh, 2003). Eventually, better and more humane justice systems can lessen or prevent crime and thus improve the public health. Prevention of the most egregious human rights violations will allow for exponential increases of more constructively used human energy; thus, forensic practitioners have a major contribution to make by weaving the tapestry integrating domestic and international laws to produce a new global order of justice (Weaver & Lynch, 1999). Forensic nurses can help create a global future with less violence, less human suffering, and greater solidarity and achievement. In short, forensic nurses have a tremendous role to fulfill in the "big picture" concerning the health of the human family by contributing both healthcare and legal system expertise.

In his reflections on the Birmingham campaign, April 16, 1963, Dr. Martin Luther King stated, "The ultimate tragedy is not the brutality of the bad people but the silence of the good. Pessimism is a chronic disease. It destroys the red corpuscles of hope and slows down the powerful heartbeat of positive action."

Forensic nurses need to involve themselves with international issues, speak out, and use international law as a progressive tool for taking positive action to enhance global civil society.

Resources

Books

Bouchet-Saulnier, F. (2002). *The practical guide to humanitarian law.* New York: Rowman & Littlefield Publishers.

Gill, W. (2001). Global cooperation in international public health. In M. Merson, R. Black, & A. Mills (Eds.), *International public health: Diseases, programs, systems, and policies* (pp. 667-698). Sudbury, MA: Jones & Bartlett Publishers.

Kickbusch, I., & Buse, K. (2001). Global influences and global responses: International health at the turn of the twenty-first century. In M. Merson, R. Black & A. Mills (Eds.), *International public health: Diseases, programs, systems, and policies* (pp. 701-737). Sudbury, MA: Jones & Bartlett Publishers.

Merson, M., Black, R., & Mills, A. (Eds.) (2001). *International public health: Diseases, programs, systems, and policies.* Sudbury, MA: Jones & Bartlett Publishers.

Moir, L. (2001). *The law of internal armed conflict.* Cambridge, UK: Cambridge University Press.

Oulton, J. (2002). Nursing in the international community. In D. Mason, J. Leavitt, & M. Chaffee (Eds.), *Policy and politics in nursing and health care* (4th ed., pp. 711-722). Philadelphia: W. B. Saunders.

Weaver, J. (1998) Nursing, health, and healthcare in the international community. In D. Mason & J. Leavitt (Eds.), *Policy and politics for nurses* (3rd ed.). Philadelphia: W. B. Saunders.

Zwi, A. (2001). Complex humanitarian emergencies. In M. Merson, R. Black & A. Mills (Eds.), *International public health: Diseases, programs, systems, and policies* (pp. 439-513). Sudbury, MA: Jones & Bartlett Publishers.

References

Buergenthal, T., & Shelton, D. (Eds.) (1995). *Protecting human rights in the Americas: Cases and materials* (4th ed.). Arlington, VA: N. P. Engle.

Esposito, L. (1998, Sept. 21). SAFE RNs–Picking up the pieces after rape. *Nurs Spectrum, 8*, 19, 24.

Hannum, H., & Fischer, D. (Eds). (1993). *United States ratification of the international covenants on human rights* (p. 7). New York: Transnational Publishers.

Hoffman, K. (1997). International humanitarian law. In *Global migration.* Washington, DC: American Academy of Nursing.

International Council of Nurses (ICN). (1995). International Council of Nurses' Position Statements. Geneva: ICN.

Mission of Inquiry, American Association for the Advancement of Science. (1990). *Apartheid medicine: Health and human rights in South Africa: A report to the American Association for the Advancement of Science, American Psychiatric Association, American Public Health Association, Institute of Medicine of the National Academy of Sciences.* Washington, DC: American Association for the Advancement of Science.

Pitts, L. (2001, January). Beyond rhetoric: A civil rights approach to protecting children's due process rights. *Trial Briefs* (p. 3). North Carolina Trial Lawyers Association.

Singh, J. (2003). American physicians and dual loyalty obligations in the "war on terror." *BMC Medical Ethics, 4*, 4-12. Also retrieved from *http://www.biomedcentral.com/1472-6939/4/4.*

Stanley, R. (1997, October 23). Human rights in a new era. Muscatine, IA: The Stanley Foundation.

United Nations Non-Governmental Liaison Service. (1998a, April). 31st Session of the Commission on Population and Development. *NGLS Round-Up*, p. 1.

United Nations Non-Governmental Liaison Service. (1998b, April). 42nd Session of the Commission on the Status of Women. *NGLS Round-Up*, p. 2.

Weaver, J., & Lynch, V. (1999). Forensic nursing: A unique contribution to international law. *J Nurs Law, 5*(4), 23-34.

Winarick, S. (1998, August/September). Report from Rome: An international court is born. *U.N. Vision,* 7.

Chapter 46 Legal Nurse Consulting

Alice Geissler-Murr and Mary Frances Moorhouse

The title legal nurse consultant (LNC) has been recognized since the early 1980s. LNCs are registered nurses who use their clinical knowledge, expertise, and judgment in cases in which law and medicine overlap.

Legal nurse consulting is considered a subspecialty of forensic nursing and LNCs are the one group of forensic nurses whose expertise is used more often in civil, rather than criminal, cases (Wetther, 1993). In the course of their work, LNCs can be involved in a wide range of cases (Box 46-1), can perform many activities and functions (Box 46-2), and are bounded only by their creativity and risk-taking ability.

LNCs are not to be confused with nurse paralegals, who by virtue of formal legal training can perform the tasks of a legal assistant. The nurse paralegal does not provide testimony or function in the role of an expert witness. LNCs are retained for their expertise in a specific nursing field or specialty. They are paid for their expert nursing or medical knowledge and usually receive a higher rate of remuneration in the role of consultant.

LNCs cannot provide legal advice but they do work within a legal framework. For example, when dealing with a nursing malpractice case, LNCs provide opinions substantiated by data in the medical record, supported by reputable resources, and reflecting the four elements of negligence: duty, breach of duty, causation, and damages. Feutz-Hartner (1997) has defined these terms as follows: "*Duty* is a legal relationship between a nurse and a patient requiring the nurse to provide a certain standard of care to that patient." For example, a nurse establishes a duty to a patient or client, when an assignment to provide care is accepted or a telephone contact is made.

A *breach of duty* occurs when "the nurse's level of conduct falls below the standard of care required in that situation." For example, in a breach of duty, the nurse did not do the right thing (misfeasance), did nothing or did not act (nonfeasance), or did the right thing in the wrong way (malfeasance). Standards of care are the minimal requirements that define an acceptable level of care and are meant to protect and safeguard the public (Guido, 1988). In addressing nursing malpractice, the LNC relies on resources relative to the time frame of the incident, such as published professional standards of care, peer-reviewed journals, and textbooks in wide circulation as well as specific agency policies and procedures to support the opinion that a breach has occurred.

Causation implies that an adverse outcome is "a direct result of the nurse's negligence" or "it is more probable that the injury is attributable to the nurse's actions than to any other cause." For example, given action "a" (injecting 100 mg of morphine IV instead of the ordered 10 mg), effect "b" (respiratory arrest) could occur (foreseeability). Or the "loss of a chance" or "but for" rule may apply. Thus, "but for" the lack of timely assessments, the drop in the patient's blood pressure could have been recognized and possibly treated before the onset of shock. Causation is the most difficult element to prove (Morrison, 1999).

Damages "include physical, financial, and emotional injuries and may include both past losses and future losses." A breach of duty may cause an adverse outcome (nurse failed to apply the brakes on the wheelchair, resulting in the patient falling to the floor while

Box 46-1 Types of LNC Cases

- Nursing and medical malpractice
- Personal injury (e.g., motor vehicle crashes, falls)
- Worker's compensation/work-related injuries
- Product liability (drug and equipment)
- Environmental hazards/toxic exposure, drug or food tampering
- Probate, guardianship, child custody
- Healthcare/insurance fraud
- Americans with Disabilities Act (ADA)
- Federal civil rights
- Criminal law

Box 46-2 Services Provided by LNCs

- Interpret and screen cases for merit
- Review complaint and assist in determining strengths and weaknesses
- Summarize medical records, create timelines or chronologies
- Educate attorneys as to the medical facts and issues of a case
- Identify additional documents/data for document production requests
- Conduct literature searches and summarize findings
- Identify deviations from relevant standards of care or regulatory requirements
- Interview potential claimants or defendants; clarify information that is not evident in records
- Assist in preparing and responding to interrogatories
- Obtain and analyze medical, billing, employment, and other relevant records
- Assess damages/injuries and contributing factors
- Help develop evidence, coordinate use of demonstrative evidence
- Trace chain of custody of specimens/evidence
- Retain and consult with testifying experts
- Plan strategy with attorneys and experts
- Function as a liaison between parties (e.g., attorney, client, healthcare providers/experts)
- Assist in preparing for and attend depositions, trials, and mediation hearings
- Assist with preparing witnesses, developing questions for deposition or trial
- Assist with jury evaluation/selection
- Coordinate appointment, observe evaluation, and/or review reports of IMEs (Independent Medical Evaluations)
- Interpretation and modification of job descriptions and work environments for ADA (Americans with Disabilities Act)
- Prepare life care plans

Key Point 46-1

The American Association of Legal Nurse Consultants (AALNC) defines the LNC as "a licensed registered nurse who performs a critical analysis of healthcare facts and issues and their outcomes for the legal profession, healthcare professions, and others as appropriate. With a strong educational and experiential background, the legal nurse consultant is qualified to assess adherence to standards of healthcare practice as it applies to the nursing and healthcare professions."

transferring to the bed); however, if there is no injury to the patient or monetary loss, then no compensation is required. In lay language, "no harm, no foul."

Role of the Legal Nurse Consultant

LNCs are hired because of their expertise in nursing and medical issues. They come from a wide variety of clinical settings (e.g., medical-surgical, obstetrics, intensive care, emergency, long-term care, rehabilitation, psychiatry, or quality assurance). Their new practice arena is unlimited. For example, they can be private independent practitioners (working individually or in partnership), providing services to both plaintiff/prosecuting attorneys and defense attorneys in a wide variety of civil and criminal cases. They might work directly for a law firm or practice as in-house consultants for insurance companies who examine Medicare fraud, operate managed care companies, or provide professional malpractice coverage. LNCs can be found working in hospitals as risk managers. They may also function as expert witness or nontestifying experts doing behind-the scenes work. The LNCs' work is limited only by their creativity and marketing of their skills and services. For this reason the field continues to expand and LNCs are frequently identified as nurse entrepreneurs or individuals who create and maintain a successful business, making quality nursing care and services more available to the public (Brent, 1997).

Nurses bring many talents to the job at hand. Educated to provide services using the nursing process, LNCs are well grounded in assessment, diagnosis, planning, implementation, and evaluation. Because nurses are responsible for delivering, documenting, and analyzing a patient's healthcare and healthcare needs, it is easier to spot vital issues that could affect the outcome of a case, such as deviations from accepted standards of care, inadequate documentation, or alterations in the medical record. This interpretation of medical records and documents is an invaluable tool in participation in judicial process relating to medical and nursing malpractice.

It is important to note that despite an adverse outcome in a given case, there may not be evidence of negligence. In the screening of medical records, the LNC looks for errors of omission or commission, identifies discrepancies in timelines, or notes problems in the medical record, such as altered, incomplete, or missing records. Summarizing medical records, providing timelines or chronologies with involved-person charts, can identify and clarify legal issues or assist the attorney in comparing facts with allegations.

Key Point 46-2

The task for the LNC may be to identify primary medicolegal issues in order to determine the merit of a case, determine deviations and adherence to standards of care, or to educate attorney-clients of the relevance of the issues.

The LNC must be comfortable in and adept at medical literature searches in order to support or refute allegations and to educate attorneys, judges, or juries. This responsibility includes locating and interpreting relevant medical and nursing literature such as textbooks, articles, research studies, and relevant standards of care. This service is often enough to ascertain the merits of pursuing a case that may have some doubtful issues at the initial screening. Additionally, the LNC can aid in determining the validity of opposing theories or claims offered by experts with questionable qualifications, poorly conducted research, or anecdotal reports.

This step often leads to the identification of need for testimony from additional witnesses or experts who can support or refute certain issues. The LNC may provide expert witness testimony when qualified to do so, or may act strictly as a consultant, performing many behind the scene duties including locating, interviewing, and preparing expert witnesses for deposition and trial. It is vital that the testifying expert witness/LNC practice within the limitations of her or his own expertise and scope of practice in order to maintain credibility and avoid jeopardizing the outcome of the case.

Ethical Considerations

The focus for nursing has always been the patient and the patient's needs. In fact, nurses view themselves as advocates for their patients. However, for the LNC, the focus must be the intersection of medicine and the law. For example, in a nursing malpractice case the LNC must set aside concern for a patient who may have suffered an injury and incurred significant financial loss, focusing instead on the standard of care and whether the nurse in question met that standard. Therefore, LNCs do not speak for the patient but instead they speak for the nursing profession and educate others about the practice of nursing (Milazzo, 1993b).

Best Practice 46-1

The LNC focuses on the merits or facts of a case and works with both plaintiff and defense attorneys, rendering opinions that are free of compromising influences and loyalties.

In order to maintain credibility, the LNC must avoid conflicts of interest such as accepting a case for which she or he has confidential information about a party to the lawsuit (e.g., providing services for a plaintiff against a defendant the LNC consulted for during a previous case) (Milazzo, 1993a). Whatever the cause, if a conflict does exist, the LNC immediately informs the attorney without disclosing either the nature of the conflict or any confidential information.

Finally the LNC's practice is based on guidelines contained in the *Code of Ethics for Nurses with Interpretive Statements* (ANA, 2001) and the AALNC's *Code of Ethics and Conduct* (2002). These guidelines identify professional performance and behavior that help maintain the integrity and accountability of the LNC.

Educational Requirements

From the brief overview provided here, it becomes apparent that an inexperienced nurse cannot provide the services of an LNC. However, by background training and experience, a nurse can fit into the LNC category without a great deal of additional training. A nurse is already trained to be observant, objective, and detail oriented. The nurse knows how to explain disease processes, technical terminology, and complex medical procedures in terms that lay people can understand. The nurse can address issues related to healthcare based on first-hand experience.

Best Practice *46-2*

The LNC should seek education and training leading to certification to convey proficiency in a body of knowledge relating to medicolegal issues.

Knowledge and proficiency are job requirements. The nurse must be registered and licensed. Although not required, certification is desirable, as it is designed to show the LNCs proficiency and validation of a certain body of knowledge pertaining to medical-legal issues. The AALNC has identified legal nurse consulting as a specialty practice of nursing, and as such, their position is that "legal nurse consulting education should be developed and presented as specialty nursing curricula by nurse educators in partnership with legal educators."

Historically, the practice of legal nurse consulting was in place prior to any training, specialty organization, or certification programs. Nurses came to the specialty by being exposed to the legal field in some capacity, such as on-the-job training with attorneys or insurance companies, or by pursuing some avenue of nurse entrepreneurship. Although formal training was not required, many nurses sought the benefit of continuing their education and obtaining certification. Basic preparation for the job requires that the LNC be a registered (professional) nurse with an active license. Nursing education has traditionally (although not universally) been bachelor's degree or higher in the nursing field.

Over time, informal on-the job training, attendance at nursing-based legal seminars, and self-study courses have evolved into more formalized programs. Educational programs are currently provided in several settings such as universities, colleges, and for-profit and not-for profit organizations. Programs are being offered by schools of nursing, continuing education companies, and paralegal programs. Information regarding training programs is widely available in journals and online.

Credentialing and Certification

Certification may be offered at the completion of some educational programs and is issued upon successfully passing a certification examination. At this point in time, it should be noted that several certifications are offered and that certification granted by one body may not be recognized by another. A certified legal nurse consultant may use the "C" (to designate certification), which can appear before or after the LNC, depending on the certifying agency. In 1997, the AALNC established the American Legal Nurse Consultant Certification Board to administer the Legal Nurse Consultant Certified program, which is accredited by the American Board of Nursing Specialties. Their certification is signified by the letters LNCC. Another nationally recognized training and certification program (and the oldest formal training program in the US) is offered by the Medical-Legal Consulting Institute, a founding company in the National Alliance of Certified Legal Nurse Consultants. The letters CLNC signify their certification. Certification programs are of varying lengths and may be attended in person, or by means of home study packages, often including audio or video instructions. Ongoing education and experience in the field of nurse consulting is required to extend certification periods. Information may be obtained about any or all programs at online Web sites, as well as in many professional journals. Fees for training and certification vary widely.

Case Study 46-1 Arthritis and a New Career

J.D. was a 54-year-old nurse who had worked over three decades in emergency departments and critical care units. She developed severe, degenerating arthritis that made it impossible to work as a staff nurse or manager in the clinical area. However, she wanted to continue to work. She desired both the professional challenge and the social stimulation inherent in the workplace and began to search for pathways to a second career. On a nursing Web site she discovered information about "legal nurse consulting" and noted that one of the criteria was a solid base in clinical nursing practice. She enrolled in an online course and attended several seminars to prepare herself for certification as a legal nurse consultant. Fortunately, during this time she was able to attain a position in a local law firm reviewing and analyzing medical records associated with medical malpractice cases. Her outstanding work resulted in several referrals to other law firms and soon she was as busy as she had been working full time at the hospital. J.D. had found a perfect new career that utilized her extensive nursing experiences and permitted her to work at her own pace, usually without even leaving her home. She joined the American Association of Legal Nurse Consultants and became actively involved with its educational and professional development programs and volunteered to teach the medical-legal aspects of nursing documentation to nursing students and staff nurses within the community.

Summary

Legal nurse consulting is included in the realm of forensic nursing and as such offers opportunities and challenges with unlimited potential for professional growth. LNCs function in a variety of roles, perform a wide range of activities, and have many employment options that are limited only by the individual's nursing expertise, imagination, and business skills. Furthermore, ever-changing healthcare issues and advancing technology help ensure the continued need for competent LNCs.

Resources

Web Sites

American Association of Legal Nurse Consultants

www.aalnc.org

The American Association of Nurse Attorneys

www.taana.org

American Society for Healthcare Risk Management

www.ashrm.org

Institute for Legal Nurse Consulting (Vickie Milazzo Institute)

www.legalnurse.com

References

AANA. (2003). A comprehensive guide to legal consulting: The nurse expert. Conference papers of the American Association of Nurse Attorneys. Ellicott City, MD: Author.

American Association of Legal Nurse Consultants (AALCN). (1995). *Standards of legal nurse consulting practice and professional performance.* Glenview, IL: Author.

American Association of Legal Nurse Consultants (AALCN). (2002). AALCN position statement of education and certification in legal nurse consulting. Retrieved from: www.aalnc.org/scope/scope-3.cfm.

American Nurses Association (ANA). (2001). *Code of ethics for nurses with interpretive statements.* Silver Springs, MD: Author

Brent, N. J. (1997). *Nurses and the law: A guide to principles and applications.* Philadelphia: W. B. Saunders.

Feutz-Hartner, S. A. (1997). *Nursing and the law* (6th ed.). Eau Claire, WI: Professional Education Systems.

Guido, G. W. (1988). *Legal issues in nursing: A source book for practice.* Norwalk, CT: Appleton & Lange.

Milazzo, V. L. (1993a). Conflicts of interest. *National Medical-Legal J, 4*(4), 5.

Milazzo, V. L. (1993b). Who does the legal nurse consultant speak for? *National Medical-Legal J, 4*(4), 2.

Morrison, C. A. (1999). Legal aspects of forensic nursing. *On the Edge, 5*(1), 5.

Wetther, K. L. (1993). Forensic responsibilities of the legal nurse consultant. *J Psychosoc Nurs, 31*(11), 21.

Unit Eight

Opportunities and Challenges in Forensic Nursing

Chapter 47 Suicide Risk Assessment

Karolina E. Krysinska and Paul T. Clements

Assessment of suicide risk continues to provide challenges for forensic nurses. There is a high probability in a variety of clinical settings that forensic nurse examiners (FNEs) will encounter a patient who may be at risk for suicide. In such circumstances, the knowledge concerning risk factors for suicidal behavior, basic tools, and methods for suicide risk assessment, as well as the role of clinical judgment, can be of great help and importance.

Key Point 47-1

Beware of a seeming "flight into health" by victimized and traumatized patients. This apparent elevation of mood and affect is often not actually the result of an alleviation of the related intrapsychic or psychosocial stressors. Rather, it is potentially the acceptance that an overarching "solution" (i.e., a determination to commit suicide to end the problems) has been attained. Such a decision to commit suicide can actually bring significant relief to patients, as there is now a measurable end point to their distress and suffering.

Assessment of suicide risk includes identification of individuals with a potential for suicide and the assessment of an individual's intent. This implies that although it may be possible to make a clinical judgment concerning the *probability* of suicidal behavior in a given individual, it precludes the accurate *prediction* of suicide attempts or completed suicide. Although this seems to be a subtle distinction, it highlights that based on current knowledge it is practically impossible to determine whether a patient will engage in suicidal behavior; it is only possible to judge the relative probability. Maris (1992) wrote, "Of course, suicidal hindsight is 20/20. But before the fact of suicide, everything is usually not so obvious. . . . One may cynically conclude that only suicide predicts suicide" (p. 3).

Suicide risk assessment can be analyzed on two levels: individual and social. Although this chapter only reviews the individual level, it should be remembered that the assessment of suicide risk in the level of the general population and specific groups (e.g., occupational, economic, ethnic) is of great importance for setting mental healthcare goals related to suicide prevention, organization of mental health systems, and healthcare budgets.

Typically, assessment of suicide risk is a first step toward prevention, intervention, and therapy for at-risk individuals. A systematic and thorough suicide risk assessment is crucial in making proper decisions concerning the type of intervention necessary in a given case: whether the patient should be referred to intensive outpatient or community-based care, whether the patient should be voluntarily or involuntarily hospitalized and treated in a psychiatric inpatient setting, whether pharmacotherapy is indicated, or whether suicide watches or a no-suicide contract should be applied.

Assessment of suicide risk may be necessary in various settings and situations (Jacobs, Brewer, & Klein-Benheim, 1999; Maris, 1992). It may be conducted within the context of forensic or other outpatient assessment and intervention (e.g., when any suicidal ideation or behavior is noticed or whenever suicidality becomes an issue for the patient), and in the psychiatric inpatient setting (e.g., during the initial psychiatric assessment during admission and again predischarge, or before initiating or altering patient psychopharmacologic regimes). The assessment of the risk for repetition of suicidal behavior by patients with previous suicide attempts who are treated in general hospitals is a basic component of postvention with this significantly vulnerable population. It is also an important tool in suicide prevention in schools and workplace settings, where counselors, teachers, peers, and other gatekeepers are trained to identify and refer at-risk individuals to mental health professionals (Clements, DeRanieri, & Fay-Hillier et al., 2003). Forensic nurses are also uniquely positioned to assess and identify at-risk patients.

As previously mentioned, suicide assessment is not an easy task or an accurate science. The inherent difficulty is related to numerous factors. Most significantly, suicidal behaviors are rare events. According to the American Association of Suicidology (AAS) (American Association of Suicidology, 2004a), since the mid-1980s the overall completed suicide rates in the US have been relatively stable, and as recently as 2001, the national suicide rate was 10.8 per 100,000. Although there are no official statistics on attempted (nonfatal) suicide, it is estimated that there are approximately 8 to 20 attempts for each completed suicidal death. Although, from clinical and ethical perspectives, it is impossible to minimize the impact and consequences of suicidal behaviors on individual and societal levels, from the statistical perspective, completed suicides continue to represent a rare event, occurring at a rate of 1 (completed suicide) to 20 (attempted suicide) cases for every 10,000 people in the general population in the US.

According to the results of a study by Pokorny (1983), suicide risk assessment scales typically produce such large numbers of false positives (cases in which suicide was predicted but did not happen) that they cannot be distinguished from true positives (suicide correctly predicted). In the study, 4800 psychiatric patients who were monitored over a five-year period reported a significantly small number (n = 67) who died by suicide. Using the best available predictive tests, the study correctly identified 35 of 63 individuals who completed suicide (true positives) and 3435 as not being at risk of suicide (true negatives). However, of note, 1206 individuals were incorrectly identified as being at risk of suicide (false positives), and 28 patients who committed suicide were judged as being at low risk (false negatives). These results led to the conclusion that the assessment of long-term suicide risk is practically impossible, particularly because current tests or scales do not have the expected sensitivity (proportion of correctly identified positive cases) and specificity (proportion of correctly identified negative cases).

Another difficulty in suicide risk assessment stems from the basic question: What type of suicidal behaviors are being predicted and prevented–specifically, completed suicides or attempted suicides? Although the distinction between these two types is often blurred, they represent two distinct categories of direct self-destructive behaviors and subsequently require different types of assessment and intervention within different clinical settings (O'Carroll, Berman, & Maris et al., 1996).

Short-term and long-term suicide risk factors are often not identical. For example, in a study conducted by Stelmachers and Sherman (1992), it was noted that clinicians considered different sets of variables while making a judgment on short- versus long-term suicide risk. It was also discovered that there was a low consensus among clinicians concerning the estimation of suicide potential (as well as recommended crisis management and clinical interventions). This was particularly evident in cases of long-term and low to moderate short-term suicide risk. This led the authors to conclude that "there is higher consistency in judgments about cases that are more emergent, critical, or extreme" (p. 263). In addition, the changeability of protective and risk factors, as well as the unpredictability of changes in an individual's life situation, may make the long-term suicide risk assessment practically impossible and lead to many false positives and negatives (Pokorny, 1983).

Ultimately, the assessment of suicide risk must be based on a thoughtful consideration of the unique and dynamic constellation and interaction of protective risk factors observed in a specific case. It is never enough to mechanically use standardized suicide screening checklists and other tools that have been created on the basis of general knowledge surrounding the characteristics of high-risk groups. The suicide risk assessment procedure should be based on clinical judgment, supported by data obtained from prediction scales, medical files, clinical history, and a thorough interview with the individual who is considered to be at risk, as well as collateral contacts such as relatives and significant others.

Best Practice *47-1*

The assessment of suicide risk must be based on a thoughtful consideration of the unique and dynamic constellation and interaction of protective and risk factors observed in a *specific case*. It is never enough for the forensic nurse to mechanically use standardized suicide screening checklists and other tools that have been created on the basis of general knowledge surrounding the characteristics of high-risk groups..

Risk Factors for Suicidal Behavior

Suicide is a complex, multidimensional phenomenon that has been associated with many correlates, antecedents, and risk factors. Although there are still some controversies among researchers and clinicians regarding predictors of suicidal behaviors, there are some risk factors that almost everyone agrees are present in most suicides (AAS, 2004b; Jacobs, Brewer, & Klein-Benheim, 1999; Maris, 1992). These are discussed next and represent risk factors identified in the populations typically seen in various mental health practice settings.

Demographic Characteristics

Demographic factors (e.g., sex, age, marital status, race, geographic location) provide a general indication of those groups in the general population that are at the highest risk of suicidal behaviors (AAS, 2004a, 2004c; Garrison, 1992). It has been identified that demographic profiles of suicide attempters and completers are different.

In the US, males *complete suicide* at a rate four times that of females (in 2001: accordingly, 17.6/100,000 and 4.1/100,000). Suicide rates are the highest among the elderly (age 65 and older), the divorced, the separated, and the widowed. In regard to race and ethnicity, whites die by suicide twice as often as nonwhites, and Native Americans have the highest overall suicide rate, although there are differences between tribal groups. Blacks and Hispanics exhibit low risk of suicide; however, the suicide rate is increasing faster among African-American youth than among Caucasians. White men over the age of 85 are at the greatest risk of all demographic groups. In 1999, the completed suicide rate in this population was 59.6 per 100,000, which is almost six times the overall national suicide rate in the US. Geographically, suicide rates are the highest in the Mountain states (in 2001: 16.2/100,000).

Nonfatal suicidal behaviors are more frequent among the young and among females, who make three to four times as many attempts as males. African-American females are more likely to attempt suicide, but males in this ethnic group are more likely to die by suicide. Although the elderly make suicidal attempts less frequently than individuals in other age groups, their attempts are more lethal. For example, in this group, the ratio of attempted to completed suicide is 4:1, while for all ages combined the ratio is 20:1.

Although demographic factors reflect high-risk groups in the general population, there is little reliability in the predictive probability that a particular person will engage in suicidal behavior. Therefore, the consideration of other types of information is necessary to improve the sensitivity and specificity of suicide risk assessment.

Mental Disorders

Psychological autopsy studies (i.e., a postmortem examination of decedent presuicide risk factors, behaviors, and method of death) indicate that more than 90% of persons completing suicide have one or more mental disorders. These results are supported by data obtained using other methods of research (i.e., prospective follow-up studies and retrospective reviews of medical records). Suicide and nonfatal suicidal behaviors occur more frequently than expected among individuals with the diagnosis of mental disorder, and when coexisting disorders are identified, the risk is even greater (Jacobs, Brewer, & Klein-Benheim, 1999; Tanney, 1992).

Harris and Barraclough (1997) conducted a meta-analysis of 249 reports (published between 1966 and 1993) and found that 36 of 44 diagnoses (according to the *DSM-III-R* or ICD systems) had significantly raised standardized mortality ratios for suicide. These data led them to the conclusion that "if these results can be generalized, then virtually all mental disorders have an increased risk of suicide excepting mental retardation and possibly dementia, and agoraphobia" (p. 222). Although persons with practically any mental disorder engage in suicidal behaviors more often than individuals in the general population, the completed suicide risk is the highest among individuals diagnosed with affective disorders (major depression, bipolar disorder) and schizophrenia. The risk for nonfatal suicidal behaviors is significantly increased in case of depressive neuroses (dysthymic disorders) and personality disorders (especially Axis II diagnoses of borderline, antisocial, and narcissistic personality disorders). Many researchers and clinicians point out that *comorbidity* of mental disorders (e.g., panic disorder and affective disorder, schizophrenia and comorbid depressive disorder/substance abuse, co-occurrence of personality disorders and depression/schizophrenia) makes the risk of suicide even greater. The suicide risk factors in affective disorders and schizophrenia are discussed next.

Lifetime risk of suicide in *affective disorders* is 15%, and patients with these diagnoses constitute 50% to 70% of suicides. Among factors associated with an increased suicide risk in patients with the diagnosis of *major depressive disorder* are the severity of depression (the more severe clinical depression, the more acute suicide risk), increasing agitation and worsening melancholic symptoms, early course of illness before diagnosis and treatment, the recovery period and the period following hospitalization, as well as the co-occurrence of other psychiatric and substance abuse disorder.

Long-term suicide risk factors connected with the diagnosis of depressive disorders are high hopelessness, suicidal ideation, and previous suicide attempts. There is no consensus among researchers concerning increased suicide risk in delusional versus nondelusional depression (Jacobs, Brewer, & Klein-Benheim, 1999).

Significant risk factors for suicide in the *manic-depressive illness* include the increased severity of symptoms, family history of suicide, and history of patient's previous suicide attempt. The suicide risk is raised early in the course of the illness, in mixed states (the combination of morbid depressive thoughts with high energy and agitation), in the depressive phase, the recovery period, and following hospitalization (Jamison, 1999).

Individuals with the diagnosis of *schizophrenia* account to 10% to 15% of completed suicides, and the lifetime suicide risk in this population is 10%. The risk of suicide is greater in case of comorbidity (e.g., depressive disorder or substance abuse) and in paranoid schizophrenia with numerous positive symptoms, while it is lower in patients with negative (deficit) subtypes of the illness. The majority of researchers point out the fact that suicide in patients with the diagnosis of schizophrenia is most often related to the painful awareness of the deterioration of their abilities, and the discrepancy between the future envisioned in the past before the onset of the illness and the likely degree of chronic and incurable disability in the future (especially in young males with good intellectual functioning and good premorbid school or work progress). Additionally, the suicide risk is heightened during early stages of the illness, in periods of clinical improvement after relapse and during periods of hopelessness and depressed mood (Jacobs, Brewer, & Klein-Benheim, 1999).

The causal relationship between the diagnosis of a mental illness and suicidal behaviors is not clear. Tanney (1992) suggested several mechanisms, ranging from direct causes or consequences (e.g., command hallucinations and depressive delusions) and indirect complications (e.g., iatrogenic toxicity of medication, and hopelessness of chronic disorder) to additive and releasing effects (e.g., alcohol abuse in depression leading to psychological disinhibition) and common etiology (e.g., isolation or loneliness may lead both to suicide and depression).

Substance Abuse

Numerous studies have found a strong relationship between suicidal behavior and substance abuse (Jacobs, Brewer, & Klein-Benheim, 1999; Lester, 1992). There is consistent evidence of elevated suicide rate among alcoholics. Of note, approximately 18% of alcoholics commit suicide, and 21% of all suicides involve patients diagnosed with a substance abuse disorder involving alcohol. The evidence for the association between alcohol abuse and nonfatal suicidal behavior is less consistent, although some studies have found a high incidence of suicide attempts (up to 24%) in alcoholics (Lester, 1992).

Several factors have been linked to suicide in alcohol abusers. The prominent risk factors are comorbid depression, communication of suicidal intent, continued drinking (suicide in alcoholics usually is related to late stages of the addiction), serious medical illness, unemployment, living alone, and poor social support, as well as a recent loss of an important interpersonal relationship.

The pathways between suicidal behavior and alcohol abuse are numerous and variegated. For example, substance abuse can be considered a "chronic suicide," and abused substances can be used as means of suicide (e.g., cocaine and heroine overdoses, a lethal concoction of alcohol and medications). Addictions and abuse often disrupt individuals' interpersonal networks and their professional performance, which may cause isolation and social decline. Alcohol and drugs may lower restraints against suicide, impair judgment, and increase impulsivity and risk taking, as well as increase an individual's self-depreciation and depression. Some people planning suicide use alcohol and other drugs to achieve such mental state to "get the courage to die." There is also a possibility that substance abuse and suicide stem from the same predisposing factors (e.g., personality disorder, mood dysregulation) and chronic alcohol abuse may directly change the brain neurochemistry through its impact on the serotonergic system. Paradoxically, in the early stages of abuse, when alcohol and other drugs are used as self-medication, they may lower the suicide risk in depression or replace direct suicidal behavior.

Much more research has been done on alcoholics than on drug abusers; however, the available data point out that individuals addicted to drugs have higher incidence of suicide, nonfatal suicidal attempts, and suicidal ideation than individuals in the general population. An increased suicide rate was found in narcotic and opioid addicts; for example, results of studies showed that up to 7% of cocaine abusers and 11% of methaqualone users died of suicide, and more drug abuse was noted in a sample of military trainees who attempted suicide than in the control group (Lester, 1992).

Physical Illness

Medical disorders are associated with suicide in various ways (Harris & Barraclough, 1994; Kelly, Mufson, & Rogers, 1999). For example, some medical disorders may be caused by self-injury or substance abuse stemming from preexisting mental disorders, and a medical disorder and treatment (e.g., medication) may affect brain functioning, leading to personality disorders and mood disturbances. Additionally, disfigurement or disability caused by medical illness may result in mood dysregulation, and stigmatized diagnoses may contribute to social isolation and withdrawal of diseased individuals.

Numerous medical diagnoses have been related to increased suicide risk. For example, Harris and Barraclough (1994) noted that suicide risk increases with the following diagnoses (note that the number in parentheses means increased suicide risk in patients with the given diagnosis over the general population risk): HIV/AIDS (6.6), Huntington disease (2.9), malignant neoplasms (all sites, 1.8; head and neck, 11.4), multiple sclerosis (2.4), peptic ulcer (2.1), renal disease (hemodialysis, 14.5; transplantation, 3.8), spinal cord injuries (3.8), and systemic lupus erythematosus (4.3).

Suicide risk is increased in epilepsy (fivefold) and in chronic pain syndrome and traumatic brain injury, which are associated with depression and suicidal ideation (Kelly, Mufson, & Rogers, 1999).

Suicidal Ideation

Suicidal thoughts range from harmless, transient fantasies that may help one to cope with life problems–as exemplified by Nietzsche's famous words: "The thought of suicide is a great consolation; by means of it one gets successfully through many a bad night" (Nietzsche & Zimmern, 1989)–to recurrent suicidal ideation and concrete plans of self-destruction (Kerkhof & Arensman, 2001; van Heeringen, 2001).

Adolescent population surveys show that considering suicide as an alternative problem solution is a rather normal and prevalent way of coping in this age group, and a study by Meehan et al. (1992) reported that 54% of college students have thought about suicide, including 26% of subjects who thought about it in the previous 12 months. Although still common, adult subjects report less suicidal ideation. Epidemiological studies have shown that the 1-year prevalence for suicidal thoughts ranges between 2.3% and 5.6%, and the lifetime prevalence is 13% to 15% (Kerkhof & Arensman, 2001).

Although suicidal ideation in the general population may be a quite frequent phenomenon, it should be remembered that suicidal ideation may evolve into a suicide plan, leading to self-destructive behavior that may result in death. A general population study by Kessler, Borges, & Walters (1999) showed that the transition from ideation to plan occurred in 34% of individuals who thought about suicide, and further transitioned into an attempt in 72% (specifically, 26% of subjects proceeded from ideation to an impulsive attempt).

Therefore, an essential part of any suicide assessment procedure should be asking the interviewed individual about her or his suicidal ideation and plans. One of the most serious warning signs of high suicide risk, which calls for an immediate intervention, is a well thought-out and detailed suicide plan (including a place, time, and method), which is to be carried out in circumstances excluding the possibility of discovery and intervention by others. Any activities that show that an individual is preparing for death (e.g., writing a suicide note, making a will, giving away possessions) are other warning signs of suicide (Jacobs, Brewer, & Klein-Benheim, 1999).

Of course, a lack of a detailed suicide plan or denial of any suicidal ideation by a patient does not mean that there is no risk of suicide; in such cases other means of assessment of suicide risk are recommended (e.g., the clinical judgment, risk assessment scales, and checklists).

Previous Suicidal Behavior

Maris (1992) has stated that "any individual with a history of one or more prior nonfatal suicide attempts is at much greater risk for suicide than most of those who have never made a suicide attempt" (p. 11). Results of his psychological autopsy study showed that 30% to 40% of suicide completers had made at least one prior nonfatal suicide attempt, and about 15% of suicide attempters eventually died by suicide.

Several factors associated with risk of suicide after attempted suicide have been identified. These include older age (only females), male gender, unemployment or retirement, marital status (widowed, divorced, or separated), living alone, poor physical health, psychiatric disorder (especially depression, alcoholism, schizophrenia, and sociopathic personality disorder), high suicidal intent in current episode, violent method in current attempt, leaving a suicide note, and previous attempt(s) (Hawton, 2000).

A history of a suicide attempt is also correlated with the risk of repetition of nonfatal suicidal behavior. A classification of suicide attempters based on the history of repetition of their behavior has been proposed by Kreitman and Casey (1988): "first evers," "minor repeaters" (lifetime history of two to four attempts), and "major/grand repeaters" (five attempts and more). A study conducted in Great Britain indicated that 48% of males with a history of nonfatal suicidal behaviors were first evers, 36% minor, and 16% grand attempters (for women, accordingly, 53%, 35%, and 12%). Factors that are associated with risk of repetition of attempted suicide have additionally been identified. These include a previous attempt, previous psychiatric treatment, personality disorder, substance abuse, unemployment, lower social class, criminal record, history of violence, age 25 to 54 years, and marital status (single, divorced, or separated) (Hawton, 2000).

Marzuk and colleagues (1997) have described a category of an "aborted suicide attempt" in which an individual has intent to kill himself or herself, changes his or her mind before making the attempt, and there is no physical injury. Their study on the prevalence of suicidal behavior among psychiatric inpatients showed that 46% of subjects made a suicide attempt, and 29% had a history of at least one aborted suicide attempt (which, in the case of almost one third of the patients, would be of high lethality, i.e., gunshot, jumping from heights). The authors concluded:

> *The finding that many individuals who made aborted attempts have also made actual suicide attempts suggest that aborted attempts lie closer to the actual attempts than ideation does on the spectrum of suicidal behaviors. . . . Some aborted suicides might have occurred before actual attempts and, in effect, served as a rehearsal. . . . Given the high lethality of some of these aborted attempts, it is possible that aborted attempts are predictive of actual completed suicide. (p. 495)*

Although Marzuk and colleagues admitted that the relationship between aborted attempts, actual attempts, and suicidal ideation is not clear, they suggested that suicide risk assessment should include inquiries about aborted attempts and reasons for abandoning the suicidal behavior.

Although the acts of self-mutilation (defined by the lack of conscious suicidal intent) are usually distinguished from suicidal behaviors, they should also be considered as suicide risk factors. Research shows that more than 50% of self-mutilators attempt suicide by a drug overdose, usually as a result of demoralization related to their inability to control self-mutilating behaviors (Favazza & Simeon, 1995).

Access to Lethal Means

Although practically all methods used by individuals engaging in suicidal behaviors may lead to death or serious injuries, the statistical lethality of different means ranges from high to low risk of death (McIntosh, 1992). The likelihood of death is the highest in case of gunshot, carbon monoxide, hanging, drowning, suffocation by plastic bag, physical impact (jumping from heights, in front of a train, etc.), fire, poison, drugs, gas, and self-cutting. At least two factors contribute to the probability of death when using a particular method: the amount of time between the initiation of the suicidal act and death (e.g., drugs and poisons allow for the possibility of changing one's mind and seeking help, and detection and intervention by others) and availability and effectiveness of medical intervention related to the method.

The choice of means of suicide depends on several factors: availability of the method and familiarity with it, suicidal intent and motivation of the individual (although there is no direct relationship between the medical lethality of the method and the desire to die, it is mediated by the attempter's knowledge of the lethality of the method), and the cultural/ethnic factors (e.g., the gender socialization, social acceptability of suicide, the symbolic meanings of particular methods, and sites of suicide).

A specific suicide plan including an available and highly lethal means of suicide is a major risk factor of suicidal behavior and calls for a prompt and decisive intervention. Reducing access to means of suicide (e.g., legislations limiting access to firearms, careful dispensing of over-the-counter and prescription medications, detoxification or reduced toxicity of domestic gas and car exhaust, reduced access to high buildings, bridges, and legendary "suicide sites") has been proven to reduce the incidence of suicide on both individual and population levels. It has to be kept in mind that many suicidal behaviors are impulsive and involve ambivalent attitudes toward life and death; in such cases, limited access to highly lethal methods increases the probability of survival and the effectiveness of medical intervention.

Family History of Psychiatric Illness and Suicidal Behavior

Roy (1992) observed that "suicide, like so much else in psychiatry, tends to run in families" (p. 578). Since the mid-1980s, results of numerous studies have led to the conclusion that there may be familiar or genetic determinants of suicidal behavior. Different lines of evidence point out to this possibility (Roy, 1992). For example, clinical and follow-up studies (including Amish studies) show that individuals with a diagnosis of a mental illness (mostly affective disorders, especially depression) and a history of (fatal or nonfatal) suicidal behavior and affective disorder among the first- and second-degree relatives have increased risk of engaging in suicidal behavior themselves. These data are supported by results of twin studies showing the statistically significant higher incidence of suicide and psychiatric disorder in monozygotic pairs than among dizygotic twins.

Several explanations concerning the familial vulnerability to suicide have been offered. Genetic factors related to suicide may mostly represent a genetic predisposition to psychiatric problems associated with suicide. These include affective disorders, schizophrenia, and alcoholism, as well as the inability to control impulsivity. Besides, the mechanism of social modeling may play an important role: the family member(s) who die by suicide may serve as role model(s), pointing to suicide as the best "solution" to life problems (Krysinska, 2003).

Biological Factors in Suicide

Biochemical studies of individuals with a diagnosis of depression, schizophrenia, and personality disorders show that a reduced metabolism of serotonin (5-TH; 5-hydroxytryptanine) and a lower concentration of its main metabolite, 5-hydroxyindoleacetic acid (5-HIAA), in the cerebrospinal fluid (CSF) are linked with disturbances in regulation of anxiety and inward- and outward-directed aggression (van Praag, 2001). Suicide attempters with a low CSF 5-HIAA level show an increased risk of repeated suicidal behaviors. On the basis of these results, van Praag concluded:

> *The association between 5-XT disturbances and states of increased aggression, suicidality and anxiety is not surprising if one takes into account, first, that in humans these affective states are highly correlated across diagnoses, and second, that both in animals and humans serotonergic circuits play an important role in the regulation of both anxiety and depression. (pp. 59-60)*

Economic Factors

Although suicidal behaviors are present in all occupational groups and social classes, epidemiological data show that certain economic factors are correlated with high suicide risk (Stack, 2000). Poverty increases the risk of suicide through its association with financial stress, unemployment, fear of job loss, family instability, and mental problems (e.g., alcoholism, depression, crime victimization). Sociological studies have consistently found a negative correlation between socioeconomic status and suicide rates (for example, in 1985 the US suicide rate for laborers was eight times higher than the overall national rate; Stack, 2000), although there are some high-status occupations with increased suicide risk (e.g., dentists, physicians, veterinarians) stemming from high job stress and easy access to lethal medication and other means of self-destruction. Another factor connected with the increased suicide risk among the disadvantaged economic groups is the relative deprivation related to the income gap between the rich and the poor, making the latter more frustrated and suicide prone.

Unemployment has often been mentioned as a major suicide risk factor, especially among men. Although the nature of the relationship between those two phenomena has not been fully explained, many correlational or causal pathways have been described. These explore how unemployment may heighten the suicide risk directly through eroding an individual's income, economic welfare, and self-esteem, or it may affect dependent family members by lowering their financial capabilities. Psychologically disturbed persons may be at risk of both losing their jobs (and not being able to find another one) and being suicidal. High unemployment rates in the general population may lead to one's fear of losing his or her job and may be related to smaller wages and underemployment.

Stress and Coping Potential

Many studies have shown that individuals who attempt or commit suicide experience more stressors and negative life events than individuals in the general population. For example, in the study by Paykel, Prusoff, & Myers (1975), subjects who attempted suicide reported four times as many life events (especially negative and uncontrollable stressors) as subjects from the general population and 1.5 as many as depressed patients, with a peak in a month prior to the suicide attempt. Among the life stressors most often found in life histories of suicidal individuals are family and relationship problems, mental and physical health problems, bereavement, unemployment, imprisonment, loss of status, abuse, and trauma (Yufit & Bongar, 1992). According to Maris (1992):

> *Most stress is chronic and accumulates slowly. There can be a few intense, acute, "triggering" events preceding a suicide, but without a history of stress most of us can tolerate time-limited, single, dramatic episodes of stress without resorting to suicide. Triggering events are usually not substantially different from the chronic stressors in one's life. (p. 15)*

Other studies concentrate on the relationship between life events and an individual's coping potential, following the premise that "although recent (as well as long-standing) life stresses can be important catalytic events in an individual's subsequent suicide, these stressful events must be contextualized within the larger picture of the individual's personality structure and life-long characterological ability to cope with (or to be vulnerable to) stress, failure, and loss" (Yufit & Bongar, 1992, p. 557). The coping potential is usually understood as ego strengths, self-trust, problem-solving skills, sense of mastery and control, and the capacity to adjust to life changes.

An essential part of suicide risk assessment should be collecting information about the individual's past responses to stress, particularly to losses, because, as Shneidman (1996) described, the common pattern in suicide is consistency of lifelong styles:

> *We must look to previous episodes of disturbance, dark times in that life, to access the individual's capacity to endure psychological pain. We need to see whether or not there is a penchant for constriction and dichotomous thinking, a tendency to throw in the towel, for earlier paradigms of escape and egression. . . . The repetition of tendency to capitulate, to flee, to blot it out, to escape is perhaps the most telling single clue to an ultimate suicide. (pp. 135-136)*

Social Isolation

Isolation and the lack of social support has been related to many aspects of psychopathology, including ineffective coping with stress and life crises (Bonner, 1992). Individuals at high risk of suicide are often described as isolated and alienated from their families and communities, and bereft of social support and resources related to it (i.e., the emotional and instrumental help). Loneliness may lead to depression and emotional distress, as well as exacerbate the effects of negative stressors, as social support is often described as a buffer against life adversities. Besides, isolated and lonely individuals are at higher risk of death when they engage in suicidal behaviors, as the chances of lifesaving intervention by others are severely reduced or nonexistent.

Hopelessness and Other Cognitive Factors

Research by Beck and his colleagues (1985, 1990) proves that hopelessness (a state of negative expectancies concerning oneself and one's future life) is a better predictor of suicidal ideation and behavior than depression. This notion has been strongly supported by prospective studies of psychiatric inpatients and outpatients, in which individuals' self-reports, as well as clinicians' ratings of hopelessness, were used. According to Beck's cognitive theory of depressive schemata, in some individuals the level of hopelessness escalates during the depressive episode, later subsides with the course of the illness, and is indicative of the level of hopelessness during subsequent episodes. However, there is another group of individuals in whom high hopelessness seems to be a trait characteristic (e.g., individuals with personality and alcohol abuse problems) and who may be chronically prone to suicidal ideation and behavior.

Other cognitive risk factors of suicide are dysfunctional assumptions (lack of reason for life, depressiogenic attitudes, and irrational beliefs), problem-solving deficits, perfectionism, and cognitive rigidity (dichotomous "all-or-nothing" thinking) (Ellis, 1998).

Other Risk Factors

The suicide risk factors described earlier in this chapter are correlates of suicidal behaviors that are widely described in the literature and agreed on. However, other factors have been examined in the contemporary literature that may increase suicide risk in vulnerable individuals. These have not been considered to be common predictors of suicide, although there is mounting evidence to the contrary. These include a history of trauma (and a diagnosis of post-traumatic stress disorder [PTSD]) and homosexuality.

History of Childhood Trauma

Numerous studies have demonstrated that there is a relationship between an individual's history of childhood physical or sexual abuse and psychopathology (e.g., depression, substance abuse, dissociation, eating disorders, personality disorders), as well as direct and indirect self-destructiveness (Chu, 1999). For example, a study by Read and colleagues (2001) showed that the outpatients who reported at least one form of child abuse (sexual or physical) were more likely to have attempted suicide than subjects who have experienced one form of abuse or none. Besides, current suicide risk of subjects was better predicted by past child sexual abuse than by a present diagnosis of depression. The authors concluded that "the taking of abuse histories should be a routine part of assessment process so as to ensure accurate formulation and appropriate treatment planning" and added "knowledge of abuse history of adult patients will enhance the accuracy of suicide assessment" (pp. 370-371).

PTSD

Of note, an experience of adult trauma and the diagnosis of PTSD may be related to elevated suicide risk. For example, in a group of women with a history of sexual trauma (rape), almost 20% of subjects attempted suicide, and among Vietnam combat veterans, 19% reported a suicide attempt, while 15% of subjects were chronically thinking about suicide (Herman, 1992). Chu (1999) pointed out that suicide risk among traumatized persons may be increased as a result of trauma-related comorbidity (e.g., depressive disorders, substance abuse, anxiety, eating disorders), which should be addressed in treatment before actively working on trauma issues.

Sexual Orientation

Research on psychological and social functioning relating to *sexual orientation* shows that although completed suicide rates do not appear to be increased among homosexual men and women, there is a greater lifetime prevalence of nonfatal suicidal behavior in these populations (especially in gay men) when compared to heterosexuals (Catalan, 2000). Research in this field is scarce due to methodological (e.g., small samples, self-identification of sexual orientation) and cultural (e.g., published reports are limited to developed countries with liberal attitudes toward sexuality) limitations. The discussion on the relationship between homosexuality and suicidality is further complicated by association with HIV infection, which is a known suicide risk factor.

Interactions among the Risk Factors

The predictors of increased suicide risk listed and discussed here typically do not occur in mutual exclusivity. Suicide is often a result of a constant dynamic interaction and comorbidity of risk factors encompassing the entire life span of an individual ("a suicidal career"). The complexity and multidimensionality of suicide has been a serious challenge to all researchers and clinicians working in the mental health profession.

Best Practice 47-2

A forensic nurse facing the challenging task of the assessment of suicide risk has to find guidelines that will help her or him to conduct this procedure in a systematic and consistent manner, which will reduce the likelihood of missing important risk factors.

Protective Factors Lowering the Risk of Suicide

The assessment of an individual's suicide risk requires a careful consideration of both risk and protective factors. The following variables have been associated with reduced risk of suicide (Maris, Berman, & Maltsberger, 1992; Sanchez, 2001):

- Family and nonfamily social support
- Significant relationships (including marriage)
- Children under the age of 18 living at home
- Physical health
- Hopefulness, problem-solving and coping skills, cognitive flexibility
- Plans for the future
- Constructive use of leisure time
- Treatment and medication
- The propensity to seek treatment and maintain it when needed
- Religiosity, culture, and ethnicity
- Employment

Suicide Risk Assessment Tools

A clinician estimating patient level of suicide risk may use several tools. These may include both general personality tests and specific suicide risk assessment scales. However, usually these are not free from methodological flaws and never should be considered the only sources of information for the clinician, as no suicide prediction tool offers a level of accuracy that would encourage decision making on the basis of its score alone.

Direct Assessment of Suicidal Ideation, Intent, and Behavior

Numerous standardized psychological test instruments, suicide risk scales, and other estimators have been designed to assist a clinician in the difficult task of suicide risk assessment (Bongar, 1991; Rothberg & Geer-Williams, 1992).

Suicide Potential Scales

Several scales have been constructed to identify an individual's suicide potential (the likelihood that the individual will engage in suicidal behavior):

- *Los Angeles Suicide Prevention Center Scale* (by Beck, Brown, & Berchick et al., 1985): 65 items in 10 categories focusing on demographic and clinical characteristics of a patient; this scale, along with *Suicide Potential Scale* and the long and short forms of *Suicidal Death Prediction Scale* are popular tools used by crisis intervention centers and hot lines
- *Clinical Instrument to Estimate Suicide Risk* (by Motto, Heilbron, & Juster, 1985): a 15-item checklist of clinical and demographic variables
- *Suicide Screening Checklist* (by Yufit & Bongar, 1992): a 60-item inventory of clinical and social variables
- *Index of Potential Suicide* (by Zung, 1974): a self-report 69-item scale including clinical and social-demographic variables
- *Suicide Risk Measure* (by Plutchik, Van Praag, & Conte et al., 1989): a self-report, 14-item scale
- *Depression Inventory* (by Beck, Ward, & Mendelson et al., 1961): a widely used and accepted 21-item inventory to measure the severity of depression in adults and adolescents
- *Hopelessness Scale* (by Beck, Weissman, & Lester et al., 1974): self-report, 20-item scale, measuring the severity of the individual's negative attitudes about the future; a score of 9-plus is predictive of high short- and long-term suicide risk
- *SAD PERSONS* (by Patterson, Dohn, & Bird et al., 1983): a 10-item scale of demographic suicide risk factors: sex, age, depression, previous attempts, ethanol abuse, rational thinking loss, social supports lacking, organized plan, no spouse, sickness
- *Reasons for Living Inventory* (by Linehan, Goldstein, & Nielson et al., 1983): a 48-item self-report inventory, measuring protective factors

Suicide Risk Assessment in Adolescents

Some scales are designed specifically for suicide risk assessment in adolescents. They include the following:

- *Hilson Adolescent Profile* (by Inwald, Brobst, & Morrissey, 1987): 310 items
- *Suicidal Ideation Questionnaire* (by Reynolds, 1991): 15, 25, or 30 items
- *Suicide Probability Scale* (by Cull & Gill, 1982): a 36-item self-report measure that can be used both with adults and adolescents

Suicide Ideation Scale

The following scale can be used to measure the current levels of suicidal ideation and intent:

- *Scale for Suicidal Ideation* (by Beck, Kovacs, & Weisman, 1979): 19 items measuring the intensity, duration, and specificity of a patient's wish to commit suicide; a score of 10-plus is indicative of high short-term suicide risk

Scales for Those Who Have Attempted Suicide

A number of scales have been designed to identify individuals who attempted suicide and are at risk of completed suicide or repetition of suicidal attempt:

- *Scale for Assessing Suicide Risk* (by Tuckman & Youngman, 1968): 14-item checklist of demographic variables, used to identify suicide attempters at risk of committing suicide
- *Neuropsychiatric Hospital Suicide Prediction Schedule* (by Farberow & McKinnon, 1974): 11 items useful to identify individuals who attempted suicide and are at high risk of subsequent suicide
- *Instrument for the Evaluation of Suicide Potential* (by Cohen, Motto, & Seiden, 1966): 14 items, used to predict subsequent suicides among hospitalized attempters
- *Short Risk Scale* (by Pallis & Sainsbury, 1976): 6 items discriminating individuals at high risk of future suicide from individuals at high risk of future suicide attempts

Scales to Evaluate Degree of Lethality of Suicide Attempt

Four scales can be used to evaluate the degree of lethality of the suicidal attempt:

- *Risk-Rescue Scale* (by Weisman & Worden, 1972): 10 items: 5 risk and 5 rescue factors
- *Lethality of Suicide Attempt Rating Scale* (by Smith, Conroy, & Ehler, 1984): an 11-point scale
- *Suicide Intent Scale* (by Beck, Kovacs, Weisman, 1979): 20 items
- *Intent Scale* (by Pierce, 1977): 12 items, combined self-report, situational and medical data

A clinician willing to use these suicide risk assessment tools should remember that they are not free from methodological flaws and further research in this field is required. Bongar (1991) and Rothberg and Geer-Williams (1992) pointed out that in some scales there is a serious lack of detailed psychometric descriptions (no available data on their reliability, validity, specificity, and sensitivity) and their utility is not clearly defined; for example, it is not clear whether the tool can be used in any clinical context or only in a particular environment (e.g., suicide risk assessment in an emergency room versus inpatient treatment planning), if they should be used to assess acute or chronic risk, whether they are easy to use, and what amount of information can be gained from them. The considerable variation of risk estimates obtained using different tools leads to questions relating to the confidence that can be placed in their results.

Risk factors listed in the tools are rarely weighted (the noteworthy exceptions are the Los Angeles Suicide Prevention Center Scale, the Clinical Instrument to Estimate Suicide Risk, and the Suicide Screening Checklist), usually do not permit interactions between risk correlates, and exclude subtle factors that may play a decisive role in the individual case (Stelmachers & Sherman, 1992).

Key Point *47-2*

Victimization from interpersonal violence or other crime may potentially result in or increase suicidal ideation. Victimized patients should be assessed regarding their perception of the perpetrator and the related violent events. Any patient who expresses self-blame or guilt regarding his or her victimization must be assessed for self-safety and suicidal ideation, and appropriate intervention or referral should be initiated as indicated.

Case Study 47-1 Sexual Assault Victim and Suicidal Thoughts

As Betsy arrived to work the day shift at the sexual assault response clinic, she was stunned to hear that one of her patients from the previous day, "Suzy," had committed suicide by polypharmacy overdose. Betsy had been the sexual assault nurse examiner who had completed the forensic examination of Suzy after the police brought her in. Suzy, a 22-year-old student at the local college, had reported that her "date" had raped her at a frat party a few hours earlier. Suzy had consented to the forensic examination and had been quiet but cooperative throughout the evidence-collection procedure: behaviors that were not unusual within the circumstances.

It had been a long week with many complicated patients to manage. Betsy had been getting ready to leave the clinic just as Suzy arrived with the police. Betsy remembers that Suzy seemed exhausted as well, and that her answers to the examination questions were minimal and at times yielded nothing more that monosyllabic responses. Looking back, Betsy recalls that near the end of the examination, Suzy commented, "I had a friend who was date raped a few years ago. She has never been the same. I don't know how she does it. . . . I don't think I could do it." At the time, Betsy did not think much of the comment, as Suzy was minimally responsive to the medicolegal inquiries throughout the examination; Betsy remembers thinking that the comment was likely an early attempt by Suzy to "normalize" the current situation by describing a similar situation experienced by one of her peers. However, such a comment, within the context of otherwise minimal communication, warranted additional inquiry and exploration by the forensic nurse as it was more likely indicative of risk for self-harm.

Suicide Risk Assessment Guidelines

A clinician facing the challenging task of the assessment of suicide risk has to find guidelines that will help him or her to conduct this procedure in a systematic and consistent manner, which will reduce the likelihood of missing important risk factors. In the professional literature, many (overlapping) models of suicide risk factors have been proposed. In this chapter, three of them will be described: the seven-step decision model proposed by Fremouw and colleagues (1990), the suicide assessment protocol guidelines developed by Jacobs and colleagues (1999), and the risk factor model for suicide assessment and intervention by Sanchez (2001). It has to be kept in mind that the guidelines presented here have a heuristic value only, and even a strict adherence to them does not guarantee accurate estimation of suicide potential of an individual.

The Seven-Step Decision Model

This decision model provides guidance for clinicians utilizing the following seven steps (Fremouw, de Perczel, & Ellis, 1990):

1. *Collection of demographic information*: Identification of demographic factors associated with high suicide risk (e.g., male sex; age 65-plus; divorced, separated, or widowed marital status).
2. *Examination of clinical and historical indicators*: Questions about general historical-situational factors, clinical indicators and warning signs of suicide risk (i.e., having a specific plan), and psychological indicators (e.g., recent loss, hopelessness, substance abuse, change in clinical features).
3. *Initial screening for risk*: On the basis of the first two steps, a decision should be made if the suicide risk is elevated and further assessment is recommended. If there is no risk, the clinician should proceed in the routine fashion; in case of identification of risk factors, he or she should process to the next step (direct assessment of risk).
4. *Direct assessment of risk*: Through clinical interview (including questions about reasons for patient's suicidality) and (if suicide risk is unknown, mild, or moderate) the patient's self-report using the standardized assessment instruments (e.g., Beck Hopelessness Scale, Reasons for Living Inventory).
5. *Determination of the level of risk and the implementation of a response*: If direct assessment of risk leads to the conclusion

that the risk is none to low or mild, the clinician should continue monitoring the patient; if the risk is moderate or high, the imminence of suicide risk should be assessed.
6. *Determination of the imminence of risk*: Includes questions about a specific suicide plan and availability of lethal methods; in case of imminent danger, the decision should be made whether intensified outpatient treatment will be appropriate or the option of voluntary/involuntary hospitalization should be considered.
7. *Implementation of treatment strategies*: On the basis of determination of risk, the outpatient treatment should be continued or contact with the hospitalized patient should be maintained and followed up. Besides, the clinician is advised to notify supervisors, document the actions taken, and indicate the rationale for his or her decisions.

Suicide Assessment Protocol Guidelines

According to this model, the following steps should be considered when assessing the patient's suicidality (Jacobs, Brewer, & Klein-Benheim, 1999):

1. *Identification or detection of predisposing factors*: Diagnosing the Axis I disorders (affective illness, schizophrenia, alcohol and drug abuse) and evaluating the category and course of disorder, its clinical features, and diagnostic comorbidity
2. *Elucidation of potentiating factors*: Gathering information about the patient's social and family environment, his or her biological vulnerability, personality disorders (especially borderline, narcissistic, and antisocial personality disorders) and traits, physical illness, life stress or crisis, and availability of lethal means
3. *A specific suicide inquiry*: Determining the level of the patient's suicidal ideation and intent and the history of suicidal behavior and current suicide plans
4. *Determination of the level of intervention*: Estimating acuteness versus chronicity of the patient's suicidality; evaluating his or her competence, impulsivity, and acting-out potential; assessing the therapeutic alliance; and planning the nature and frequency of reassessment
5. *Documenting the suicide risk assessment*

Risk Factor Model for Suicide Assessment and Intervention

Sanchez (2001) designed a detailed method for collecting important data from various sources. The order of inquiries depends on the specific case and available time:

1. Review record(s).
2. Conduct clinical observations.
3. Conduct clinical interview.
4. Conduct mental state evaluation.
5. Diagnose all mental disorders.
6. Assess suicidal ideation.
7. Assess suicide-homicide risk.
8. Examine prior self-injurious and suicidal behavior.
9. Request prior treatment records and collateral information.
10. Conduct psychological testing and administer rating scales.
11. Incorporate the data to develop a risk profile: identify acute and chronic suicide risk factors and temporary and permanent protective factors.

The Empirical Approach and the Clinical Approach

There are two approaches to the assessment of suicide risk: empirical and clinical (Motto, 1992). The former, which was presented earlier in this chapter, is based on the premise that an inquiry about a number of items derived from the results of epidemiological studies of individuals who committed/attempted suicide will help to identify the suicide potential of the assessed individual. The clinical approach "in pure form is a time-honored interview method that elicits detailed information about a person's life experience, character structure, and adaptive needs; when effectively carried out, it enables the examiner to recognize the circumstances under which a suicidal act is likely to occur in a given individual" (Motto, 1992, p. 626). Both have certain advantages and disadvantages. For example, the former is quicker and requires less training and experience, although it is inflexible, mechanical, and static. The latter is individualized and specific, but it is relatively time consuming and calls for an experienced and well-trained professional, as well as an undisturbed environment.

Motto (1992) pointed out that the clinical approach enables the clinician to take into consideration the protective factors and the individual's strengths, which may be overlooked while using the standardized assessment tools. It concentrates on the unique characteristics of the patient's life circumstances and personality, which sometimes may lead to paradoxical conclusions–for example alcohol abuse (statistically one of the major suicide risk factors) in the case of a particular individual may be a protective factor enabling him or her to cope with psychological pain and providing an escape from unbearable life circumstances. Besides, it is a valuable source of information derived from the nonverbal messages given by the patient: the tone of voice, demeanor, and subtleties of manner and speech.

Although some clinicians are highly skeptical about the usefulness of the empirical approach, the optimal and thorough assessment of suicide risk should encompass both categories. The proportion of clinical versus empirical methods used in a particular case should depend on the specific circumstances of the suicide risk assessment procedure: the amount of time available, the type of clinical setting, the patient's condition and his or her willingness to cooperate with the clinician, and the clinician's experience, training, and style.

In some cases, the clinician's judgment based on the empirical approach may contradict his or her intuitive sense–for example, when there is a discrepancy between the intuitive assessment and a score on a risk scale or the content of the patient's responses. In such circumstances Motto (1992) advised the mental health professionals to review the situation again, but "if this does not reconcile the difference, the subjective judgment deserves precedence" (p. 628). Other suicidologists (e.g., Maris, Berman, & Maltsberger, 1992) do not agree with Motto and give a warning that "there are also bad clinicians with poor insight and inferior training. Thus, clinical judgment is not always the answer to our suicide prediction problems" (p. 652).

Critical Points in Suicide Risk Assessment

According to Motto (1999), there are several critical points in assessment and management of suicidal individuals that are potential sources of difficulties and mistakes made by clinicians.

Eight of them pertain to the subject of this chapter and are listed here:

1. No one is invulnerable to suicide.
2. The absence of a diagnosable psychiatric disorder, especially depression, does not imply the little or no risk of suicide.
3. Every person is unique, therefore the applicability of epidemiologically based risk factor scales is limited.
4. The use of alcohol and other drugs can be a short-term suicide preventive factor; therefore, discontinued use should be closely monitored, and the individual's support systems at such times should be strengthened.
5. Remission of a psychotic disorder (especially schizophrenia) may paradoxically increase the suicide risk, as it is the time when an individual may realize the catastrophic consequences of the illness and the relative futility of treatment, as well as be lured to discontinue taking the antipsychotic medication, which will lead to another episode of the illness.
6. Sometimes suicidal behaviors stem from chronic stress and emotional exhaustion; in such cases the identification of the triggering event ("the last straw") is practically impossible and the assessment of suicide risk is more difficult than usually.
7. Personality structure and personality disorders that temper the significance of traditional risk factors (e.g., impulsivity, need for a feeling of control) are major considerations in suicide risk assessment.
8. Protection against legal liability requires documentation of recognition, assessment, and management of suicide risk, which should follow the standards of ordinary and reasonable care to the patient.

Summary

Assessment of suicide risk continues to provide challenges for forensic nurse examiners. There is a high probability in a variety of clinical settings that forensic nurses will encounter a patient who may be at risk for suicide. In such circumstances, the knowledge concerning risk factors for suicidal behavior, basic tools, and methods for suicide risk assessment, as well as the role of clinical judgment, can be of great help and importance.

Assessment of suicide risk includes identification of individuals with a potential for suicide and the assessment of an individual's intent. This implies that although it may be possible to make a clinical judgment concerning the *probability* of suicidal behavior in a given individual, it precludes the accurate *prediction* of suicide attempts or completed suicide. Although this seems to be a subtle distinction, it highlights that based on current knowledge it is practically impossible to determine whether a patient will engage in suicidal behavior; it is only possible to judge the relative probability.

Resources

Organizations

American Association of Suicidology

5221 Wisconsin Avenue NW, Washington, DC 20015; Tel: 202-237-2280; www.suicidology.org

The National Suicide Prevention Lifeline

800-273-TALK(8255)

Provides access to trained telephone counselors, 24 hours a day, seven days a week.

American Foundation for Suicide Prevention

International Headquarters, 120 Wall Street, 22nd Floor, New York, NY 10005; Tel: 888-333-AFSP(2377), 212-363-3500; www.afsp.org

National Institute of Mental Health (NIMH)

Office of Communications, 6001 Executive Boulevard, Room 8184, MSC 9663, Bethesda, MD 20892-9663; Tel: 301-443-4513, 866-615-6464 (toll-free); www.nimh.nih.gov

References

American Association of Suicidology [AAS]. (2004a, May 25). Some facts about suicide in the U.S.A. Retrieved from www.suicidology.org/associations/1045/files.

American Association of Suicidology [AAS]. (2004b, May 25). Understanding and helping the suicidal person. Retrieved from www.suicidology.org/associations/1045/files.

American Association of Suicidology [AAS]. (2004c, May 25). U.S.A. suicide: 2001 official final data. Retrieved from www.suicidology.org/associations/1045/files/2001datapg.pdf.

Beck, A. T., Brown, G., Berchick, R. J., et al. (1990). Relationship between hopelessness and eventual suicide: A replication with psychiatric inpatients. *Am J Psychiatry, 147*(2), 190-195.

Beck, A. T., Kovacs, M., & Weisman, A. (1979). Assessment of suicidal intention: The scale for suicidal ideation. *J Consult Clin Psychol, 47,* 343-352.

Beck, A. T., Steer, R. A., Kovacs, M., et al. (1985). Hopelessness and eventual suicide: A 10-year prospective study of patients hospitalized with suicidal ideation. *Am J Psychiatry, 142,* 5, 559-563.

Beck, A. T., Ward, C. H., Mendelson, M., et al. (1961). An inventory for measuring depression. *Arch Gen Psychiatry, 4,* 561-571.

Beck, A. T., Weissman, A., Lester D., et al. (1974). The measurement of pessimism. The hopelessness scale. *J Consult Clin Psych, 41,* 861-865

Bongar, B. (1991). The suicidal patient. *Clinical and legal standards of care.* Washington, DC: American Psychiatric Association.

Bonner, R. L. (1992). Isolation, seclusion, and psychosocial vulnerability as risk factors for suicide behind bars. In R. W. Maris, A. L. Berman, J. T. Maltsberger, et al. (Eds.), *Assessment and prediction of suicide* (pp. 398-419). New York: Guilford Press.

Catalan, J. (2000). Sexuality, reproductive cycle and suicidal behaviour. In K. Hawton & K. van Heeringen (Eds.). *The international handbook of suicide and attempted suicide* (pp. 293-307). Chichester: Wiley & Sons.

Chu, J. A. (1999). Trauma and suicide. In D. G. Jacobs (Ed.), *The Harvard Medical School guide to suicide assessment and intervention* (pp. 332-354). San Francisco: Jossey-Bass.

Clements, P. T., DeRanieri, J. T., Fay-Hillier, T., et al. (2003). The benefits of community meetings for the corporate setting after the suicide of a co-worker. *J Psychosoc Nurs Ment Health Serv, 41*(4), 44-49.

Cohen, E., Motto, J. A., & Seiden, R. H. (1966). An instrument for evaluating suicide potential. *Am J Psychiatry, 122*(8), 886-891.

Cull, J. G., & Gill, W. S. (1982). *Suicide Probability Scale.* Los Angeles: Western Psychological Services.

Ellis, T. E. (1998). Rethinking suicide: Toward a cognitive-behavior therapy for the suicidal patient. *Behav Therapist, 21,* 196-201.

Farberow, N. L., & McKinnon, D. (1974). A suicide prediction schedule for neuropsychiatric patients. *J Psychiatr Ment Health Nurs, 6*(1), 9-14.

Favazza, A. R., & Simeon, D. (1995). Self-mutilation. In E. Hollander, D. J. Stein (Eds.), *Impulsivity and aggression* (pp. 185-200). Chichester: Wiley & Sons.

Fremouw, W. J., de Perczel, M., & Ellis, T. E. (1990). *Suicide risk: Assessment and response guidelines.* New York: Pergamon Press.

Garrison, C. Z. (1992). Demographic predictors of suicide. In R. W. Maris, A. L. Berman, J. T. Maltsberger, et al. (Eds.), *Assessment and prediction of suicide* (pp. 484-498). New York: Guilford Press.

Harris, E. C., & Barraclough, B. M. (1994). Suicide as an outcome for medical disorders. *Medicine, 73*(6), 281-296.

Harris, E. C., & Barraclough, B. M. (1997). Suicide as an outcome for mental disorders. *Br J Psychiatry, 170,* 205-228.

Hawton, K. (2000). General hospital management of suicide attempters. In K. Hawton, & K. van Heeringen (Eds.), *The international handbook of suicide and attempted suicide* (pp. 519-537). Chichester: Wiley & Sons.

Herman, J. L. (1992). *Trauma and recovery.* New York: Basic Books.

Inwald, R., Brobst, K., & Morrissey, R. (1987). *Hilson Adolescent Profile.* St. Mary's University of Minnesota: Hilson Research.

Jacobs, D. G., Brewer, M., & Klein-Benheim, M. (1999). Suicide assessment: An overview and recommended protocol. In D. G. Jacobs (Ed.), *The Harvard Medical School guide to suicide assessment and intervention* (pp. 3-39). San Francisco: Jossey-Bass.

Jamison, K. R. (1999). Suicide and manic-depressive illness: An overview and personal account. In D. G. Jacobs (Ed.), *The Harvard Medical School guide to suicide assessment and intervention* (pp. 251-269). San Francisco: Jossey-Bass.

Kelly, M. J., Mufson, M. J., & Rogers, M. P. (1999). Medical settings and suicide. In D. G. Jacobs (Ed.), *The Harvard Medical School guide to suicide assessment and intervention* (pp. 491-519). San Francisco: Jossey-Bass.

Kerkhof, J. F., & Arensman, E. (2001). Pathways to suicide: The epidemiology of the suicidal process. In K. van Heeringen (Ed.), *Understanding suicidal behavior: The suicidal process approach to research, treatment and prevention* (pp. 15-39). Chichester: John Wiley & Sons.

Kessler, R. C., Borges, G., & Walters, E. E. (1999). Prevalence of risk factors for lifetime suicide attempts in the National Comorbidity Survey. *Arch Gen Psychiatry, 56,* 617-626.

Kreitman, N., & Casey, P. (1988). Repetition of parasuicide: An epidemiological and clinical study. *Br J Psychiatry, 153,* 792-800.

Krysinska, K. (2003). Loss by suicide: A risk factor for suicide. *J Psychosoc Nurs Ment Health Serv, 41*(7), 34-41.

Lester, D. (1992). Alcoholism and drug abuse. In R. W. Maris, A. L. Berman, J. T. Maltsberger, et al. (Eds.), *Assessment and prediction of suicide* (pp. 321-336). New York: Guilford Press.

Linehan, M. M., Goldstein, J. L., Nielson, S. L., et al. (1983). Reasons for staying alive when you are thinking of killing yourself: The reasons for living inventory. *J Consul Clin Psychol 51,* 276-278.

Maris, R. W. (1992). Overview of the study of suicide assessment and prediction. In R. W. Maris, A. L. Berman, J. T. Maltsberger, et al. (Eds.), *Assessment and prediction of suicide* (pp. 3-22). New York: Guilford Press.

Maris, R. W., Berman, A. L., & Maltsberger, J. T. (1992). Summary and conclusions: What have we learned about suicide assessment and prediction? In R. W. Maris, A. L. Berman, J. T. Maltsberger, et al. (Eds.), *Assessment and prediction of suicide* (pp. 640-672). New York: Guilford Press.

Marzuk, P. M., Tardiff, K., Leon, A. C., et al. (1997). The prevalence of aborted suicide attempts among psychiatric inpatients. *Acta Psychiatrica Scandinavica, 96,* 492-496.

McIntosh, J. L. (1992). Methods of suicide. In R. W. Maris, A. L. Berman, J. T. Maltsberger, et al. (Eds.), *Assessment and prediction of suicide* (pp. 381-397). New York: Guilford Press.

Meehan, P. J., Lamb, J. A., Saltzman, L. E., et al. (1992). Attempted suicide among young adults: Progress toward a meaningful estimate of prevalence. *Am J Psychiatry, 149*(1), 41-44.

Motto, J. A. (1992). An integrated approach to estimating suicide risk. In R. W. Maris, L. Berman, J. T. Maltsberger, et al. (Eds.), *Assessment and prediction of suicide* (pp. 625-639). New York: Guilford Press.

Motto, J. A. (1999). Critical point in the assessment and management of suicide risk. In D. G. Jacobs (Ed.), *The Harvard Medical School guide to suicide assessment and intervention* (pp. 224-238). San Francisco: Jossey-Bass.

Motto, J. A., Heilbron, D. C., & Juster, R. P. (1985). Development of a clinical instrument to estimate suicide risk. *Am J Psych, 142*(6), 680-686.

Nietzsche, F. M., & Zimmern, H. (Translator). (1989). Beyond good and evil (Great Books in Philosophy). Amherst, NY: Prometheus Books.

O'Carroll, P. W., Berman, A. L., Maris, R. W., et al. (1996). Beyond the Tower of Babel: A nomenclature for suicidology. *Suicide Life Threat Behav, 26,* 237-252.

Pallis, D. J., & Sainsbury, P. (1976). The value of assessing intent in attempted suicide. *Psychol Med, 6,* 487-492.

Patterson, W. M., Dohn, H. H., Bird, J., et al. (1983). Evaluation of suicidal patients: The Sad Persons Scale. *Psychosomatics, 24,* 343-349.

Paykel, E. S., Prusoff, B. A., & Myers, J. K. (1975). Suicide attempts and recent life events. *Arch Gen Psychiatry, 32,* 327-333.

Pierce, D. W. (1977). Pierce Suicide Attempt Scale. *Br J Psychiatry, 130,* 377-385.

Plutchik, R., Van Praag, H. M., Conte, H. R. et al. (1989). Correlates of suicide and violence risk: The suicide risk measure. *Compr Psychiatry, 30*(4), 296-302.

Pokorny, A. D. (1983). Prediction of suicide in psychiatric patients: Report of a prospective study. *Arch Gen Psychiatry, 40,* 249-257.

Read, J., Agar, K., Barker-Collo, S., et al.(2001). Assessing suicidality in adults: Integrating childhood trauma as a major risk factor. *Prof Psychol Res Pr, 32*(4), 367-372.

Reynolds, W. M. (1991). *Adult Suicidal Ideation Questionnaire.* Odessa, FL: Psychological Resources.

Rothberg, J. M., & Geer-Williams, C. (1992). A comparison and review of suicide prediction scales. In R. W. Maris, A. L. Berman, J. T. Maltsberger, et al. (Eds.), *Assessment and prediction of suicide* (pp. 202-217). New York: Guilford Press.

Roy, A. (1992). Genetics, biology, and suicide in the family. In R. W. Maris, A. L. Berman, J. T. Maltsberger, et al. (Eds.), *Assessment and prediction of suicide* (pp. 574-588). New York: Guilford Press.

Sanchez, H. G. (2001). Risk factor model for suicide assessment and intervention. *Prof Psychol Res Pr, 32*(4), 351-358.

Shneidman, E. S. (1996). *The suicidal mind.* New York: Oxford University Press.

Smith, K., Conroy, M., & Ehler, P. (1984). Lethality of suicide attempt rating scale. *Suicide Life Threat Behav, 14,* 215-242.

Stack, S. (2000). Suicide: A 15-year review of the sociological literature part I: Cultural and economic factors. *Suicide Life Threat Behav, 30*(2), 145-162.

Stelmachers, Z. T., & Sherman, R. E. (1992). The case vignette method of suicide assessment. In R. W. Maris, A. L. Berman, J. T. Maltsberger, et al. (Eds.), *Assessment and prediction of suicide* (pp. 255-274). New York: Guilford Press.

Tanney, B. L. (1992). Mental disorders, psychiatric patients, and suicide. In R. W. Maris, A. L. Berman, J. T. Maltsberger, et al. (Eds.), *Assessment and prediction of suicide* (pp. 277-320). New York: Guilford Press.

Tuckman, J., & Youngman, W. A. (1968). Scale for assessing suicide risk of attempted suicide. *J Clin Psychol, 24,*17-19.

van Heeringen, K. (2001). The suicidal process and related concepts. In K. van Heeringen (Ed.), *Understanding suicidal behavior: The suicidal process approach to research, treatment and prevention* (pp. 3-14). Chichester: John Willey & Sons.

van Praag, H. M. (2001). About the biological interface between psychotraumatic experiences and affective dysregulation. In K. van Heeringen (Ed.), *Understanding suicidal behavior. The suicidal process approach to research, treatment and prevention* (pp. 54-75). Chichester: John Willey & Sons.

Weisman, A. D., & Worden, W. (1972). Risk rescue rating in suicide assessment. *Arch Gen Psychiatry, 26,* 553-560.

Yufit, R. I., & Bongar, B. (1992). Suicide, stress, and coping with life cycle events. In R. W. Maris, A. L. Berman, J. T. Maltsberger, et al. (Eds.), *Assessment and prediction of suicide* (pp. 553-573). New York: Guilford Press.

Zung, W. W. (1974). Index of Potential Suicide (IPS): A rating scale for suicide prevention. In A. T. Beck, H. L. Resnick, & D. J. Lettieri, (Eds.), *The prediction of suicide* (chap. 12, pp. 206-221). Bowie, MD: Charles Press.

Chapter 48 Motor Vehicle Collision Reconstruction

Kristine M. Karcher

Motor vehicle collisions are considered a medicolegal event. The accurate investigation and reconstruction of motor vehicle collisions is important in determining the cause and events involved in a crash and provide valuable information and statistics that are used in producing safety changes, such as vehicle and roadway engineering, as well as information that may be useful in criminal or civil prosecution. The annual production of vehicles continually integrates new features to improve the safety of occupants based on the information obtained. Roadway engineers will improve dangerous sections of highway based on the frequency and cause of crashes at a certain location. The importance of a thorough investigation and collision reconstruction cannot be overestimated. The forensic nurse examiner (FNE) can contribute significantly in the investigation through knowledge of injuries and injury causation, and the understanding of the biomechanics of impact.

Laws of Motion

It is important to have an understanding or the basic physics that govern the behavior of all moving objects, including vehicles. Newton's first law of motion states that if in rest, one tends to remain in rest, while if in motion, one tends to remain in motion, unless one is acted upon by an unbalanced external force. This describes inertia. If a vehicle suddenly stops, the inertia of the occupants' bodies tends to resist the stopping, and the occupants tend to slide forward against the seat belts. Newton's second law of motion states that the acceleration of any body is directly proportional to the force acting on the body, while it is inversely proportional to the mass or weight of the body. If an occupant in a vehicle is traveling 50 mph, his or her body within the vehicle will be traveling at the same rate of speed. Newton's third law of motion states that for every force exerted on a body by another body, there is an equal but opposite force reacting on the first body by the second. Another way to say this is for every action, there is an equal but opposite reaction. In the field of motor vehicle collision investigation, acting and reacting forces are found when a vehicle skids to a stop.

The Biomechanics of Impact

The science that helps investigators to understand the mechanism of injury and the tolerance of the human body is known as the *biomechanics of impact* and links medicine with science. In vehicle crashes, the injuries generated are related to both the speed of the vehicle and how suddenly it stops. This sudden change in velocity is known as delta V, and it measures the severity of the crash or impact. This change in velocity may occur to the occupant's entire body or effect specific blows to certain areas and is dependent on the varying deceleration that occurs to anatomical structures, such as the head (for example, impacting the windshield), chest (impacting the steering wheel), or lower extremities (striking the dashboard) within the vehicle. The human response to these various forces and the change in vehicle velocity contribute to the science of biomechanics (Association for the Advancement of Automotive Medicine [AAAM], 1992).

Key Point 48-1

A collision involves a series of three impacts:(1) when the vehicle impacts something that changes or stops its speed; (2) when the occupant is thrust toward the direction of the impact, striking the interior of the vehicle; and (3) when the occupant's various internal organs collide within the body's bony structures (Besant-Matthews, 1998).

The human body, observing the laws of motion, continues to move forward at the same rate of speed that the vehicle was traveling. The shorter the time and distance to stop, the greater the force required in bringing motion to a halt. The opposite is true when the time and distance to stop deceleration are delayed; the force is reduced. Consequently, the more rapidly a person decelerates, the greater the likelihood that bodily injury will occur. (Besant-Matthews, 1998). The slower the deceleration, sometimes by just a few feet or a fraction of a second, improves occupant outcome enormously.

Automotive Engineering Improvements

Automotive engineering improvements include seat belts, air bags, auto safety glass, and changes in dashboards.

Seat Belts

The development and implementation of seat belt use has proven the most effective device in the prevention of serious injuries and fatalities. Seat belts were designed to provide a longer ride down (deceleration) within the vehicle, allowing riders to avoid impact with the interior of the car. The longer the ride down, the less chance of injury. This is accomplished by actual stretching of the seat belt, as much as 6% to 14%, to allow the occupant to decelerate slower and ride down the collision (Besant-Matthews, 1998) (Fig. 48-1). The seat belt should be examined during the vehicle inspection for evidence of stretch. Seat belts also prevent ejection from the vehicle, holding the occupants in their seats, and distributing the force more evenly over the body surfaces (Besant-Matthews, 1998).

The forces in a serious crash are such that parts of the human body are still going to contact the steering wheel, dashboard, or windshield. The average forward motion in an abrupt collision at

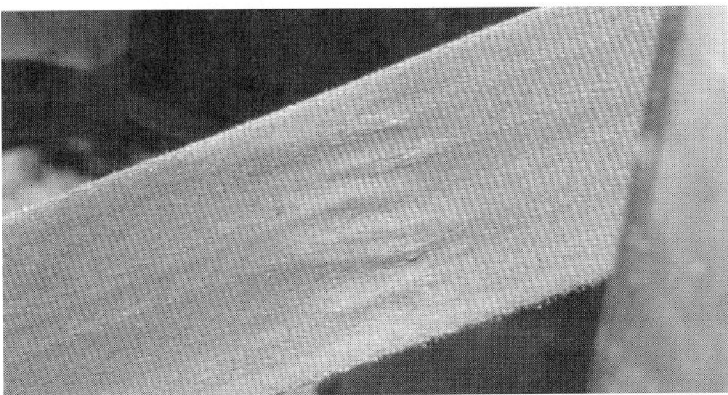

Fig. 48-1 Characteristic appearance of "stretched" seat belt.

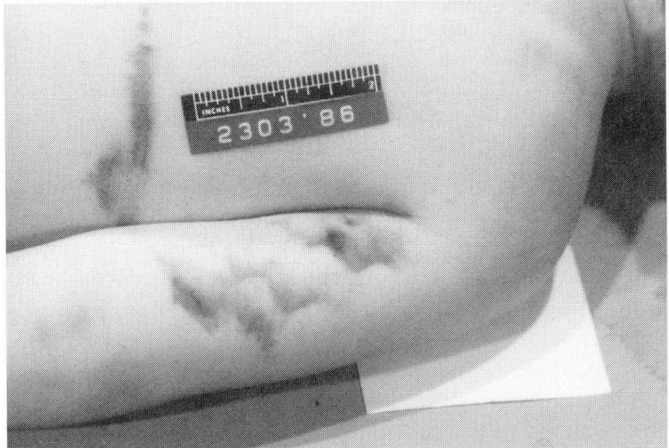

Fig. 48-2 Contusions and abrasions from shoulder harness and lapbelt restraints.

34.2 mph can result in forward movement of the head 22 inches, forward movement of the chest $15^3/_4$ inches, and forward movement of the pelvis $14^1/_2$ inches (Besant-Matthews, 1998). This forward motion is due to seat belt stretch, seat belt slack, improper use of the seat belt (i.e., wearing it too loose or in the wrong position) (Besant-Matthews, 1998), and momentary flexing of vehicle parts. The ride down of properly worn seat belts has reduced death and injury by 45% (AAAM, 1992).

Injuries associated with seat belt use range from superficial abrasions in minor collisions to major internal injuries in high-impact collisions. Lap belts may cause lacerations or injury to the liver, spleen, omentum, and mesentery, whereas shoulder belts are often the cause of injuries such as fractures to the spine, clavicle, sternum, and rib cage (Fig. 48-2).

Air Bags

To improve and supplement seat belts, air bags were developed. Not only do they protect the chest from the steering wheel and column, they provide gradual deceleration of the head and neck, preventing the whiplash motion of frontal impact (Fig. 48-3). The use of air bags has significantly decreased injuries to the neck, face, and head that only a few years ago were commonly seen when drivers impacted steering wheels. As with seat belts, air bags also have associated injuries (see Chapter 15).

Commonly made of a nylon-type material, air bags are kept folded in a container until sensors detect a frontal collision of sufficient force, causing them to deploy. Air bags deploy at speeds up to 150 to 200 mph in 24 to 45 milliseconds. Bursting through the flaps that cover them, air bags deploy with enough force to dislocate, fracture, and even amputate thumbs (Spitz, 1993). They are capable of causing an array of injuries including fractures to the forearms, abrasions and contusions to the face, corneal abrasions, and head injuries (Spitz, 1993). As with seat belts, air bags need to be examined and collected for potential evidence, such as saliva or blood. With the increased use of side air bags, related injuries will be observed including rib fractures and related contusions and abrasions. In spite of related injuries, air bags and seat belts have played a major role in decreasing the fatalities associated with motor vehicle collisions.

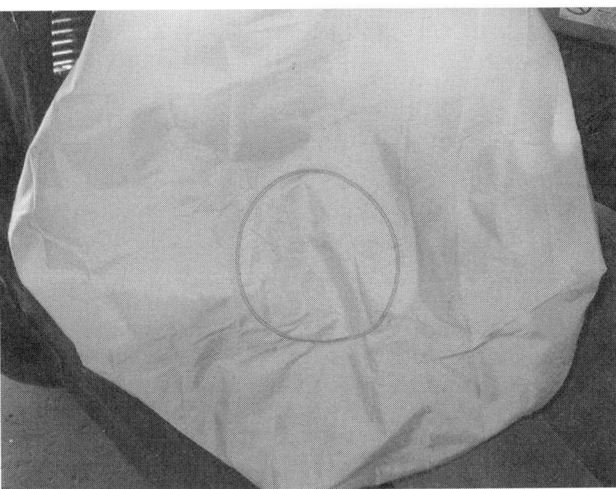

Fig. 48-3 Automotive air bag.

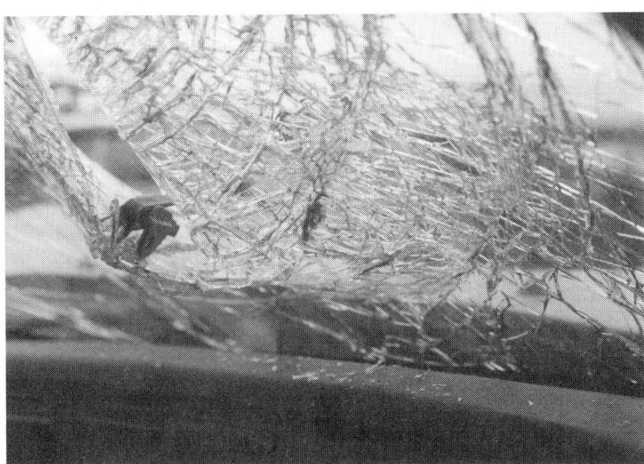

Fig. 48-4 Safety windshield glass is fractured and stretched from force of impact, but it retains its integrity due to a shatter-proof design.

Auto Safety Glass

Another safety improvement to vehicles was to the material content of windshields. They are made of two layers of glass, separated by a thicker interlayer of polyvinyl butyral. This allows the windshield to absorb more energy and freely bulge (as much as 5 inches) before the plastic interlayer tears (Fig. 48-4). In a high-speed collision, the body is thrust forward, and the head arches forward and downward,

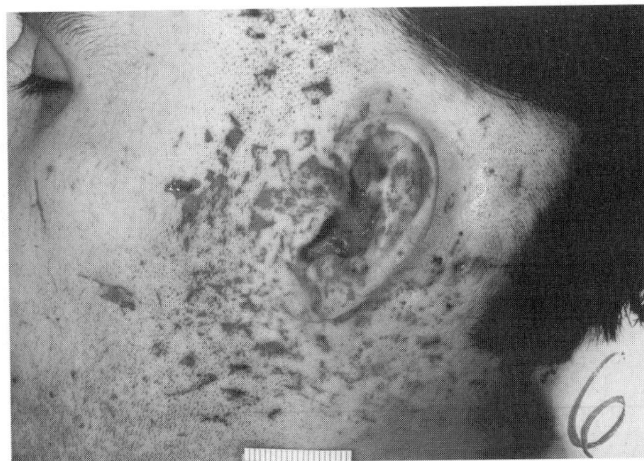

Fig. 48-5 Dicing injury to side of face due to impact with side-window glass.

making contact with the windshield and often resulting in large, deep cuts. These cuts may be horizontal, diagonal, or parallel to the face, scalp, and neck, due to head bobbing after impact. In less severe impacts, the incisions to the face will be more superficial. These injuries can be seen on the nose and forehead and are caused as the head slides down the sharp edges of broken glass (Spitz, 1993).

Side windows differ in construction and are not laminated as windshields are. Injuries associated with impact to the side windows are very identifiable. When side glass is broken, it disintegrates into numerous quarter-inch cubes with sharp edges. These produce right-angled superficial cuts to the skin and are referred to as dicing injuries (Spitz, 1993) (Fig. 48-5). Dicing injuries are easily recognized and can usually be located on the side of the face, scalp, shoulder, or arm nearest to the involved side window. The presence of dicing injuries can assist investigators in determining where an occupant was seated in the vehicle at the time of impact. In the clinical setting (hospital, emergency deptartment), pieces of glass that remain embedded in the wound would be secured as evidence.

Best Practice *48-1*

The forensic nurse should carefully document and preserve evidence associated with dicing injuries because it will be valuable in determining the location of the individual in the vehicle at the time of impact.

Dashboards

Change of dashboard contour is another safety feature development that is worth discussion. Dashboards have the capability of changing form up to 3 inches, contributing to a slower deceleration. The knees commonly contact the dashboard in frontal, head-on collisions. The severity of injuries to the knees depends on the amount of contact that occurs with the dash and may range from a bruise or minor abrasion to a large laceration or dislocation/fractures. It is important to examine both knees for even subtle injury. The steering wheel column has undergone safety features as well and is constructed to collapse when impacted by an occupant, allowing for a slower ride down.

Probably the most overlooked pieces of evidence on the body at a collision scene are patterned injuries. These usually arise from contact with something within the vehicle, such as a knob or handle, and may be subtle or very impressive. As with other injuries, they may be helpful in determining the position of the occupant, as well as the direction of impact.

Collisions

Types of collisions to consider include frontal, side angled, motorcycle, and automobile versus pedestrian crashes.

Frontal

Frontal collisions account for 50% of all motor vehicle crashes. The force to a unrestrained occupant in a frontal crash of a vehicle traveling 30 mph and impacting a rigid object resulting in a 2-foot intrusion to the bumper is equivalent to falling from a third-story window onto concrete. This intrusion to the front of the vehicle occurs in 90 to 100 milliseconds or one-tenth the time it takes to blink (AAAM, 1992). Vehicles do not have structures that crush uniformly. Front structures, such as the bumper or grill, are much less rigid and do not actually slow a vehicle as much as contact with more rigid structures such as the vehicle frame, engine, or suspension. As previously mentioned, an unrestrained front seat occupant of a vehicle traveling 30 mph would strike the dashboard, steering wheel, or windshield with different parts of the body. The injuries would then relate to the structures within the front of the vehicle that were impacted and the amount of localized deceleration of each. For instance, was the occupant's head experiencing a slower ride down due to windshield bulge, or were chest injuries lessened because the steering wheel column collapsed?

Side or Angled

Side or angled collisions account for approximately 20% of motor vehicle crashes. The occupant moves toward the point of impact and often makes contact with the windows, A-pillars (roof supporters between the windshield and front door), or roof. Even in 90-degree side impacts, lap belts will restrain the occupant. The rotation of vehicles after impact will often complicate the injuries observed to the occupant. Common injuries that result from lateral or side impacts include rib fractures, lung contusions, hemothorax, pericardial damage, and aortic rupture or tears. If the vehicle rolls over and makes no contact with a solid object, the injuries observed may be minor, but if the vehicle strikes a solid object, the injuries will be more severe (Fig. 48-6). Ejection of occupants through the door or windows of a vehicle is not uncommon in rollovers.

Key Point *48-2*

Ejected occupants often have severe neck, head, or brain injury. Research has shown that most injuries to occupants are sustained *prior* to being ejected.

Motorcycle

Motorcycle collisions account for about 8% of motor vehicle crashes, and the rider is 10% to 25% more likely to be killed or injured based on a comparison of miles traveled. The injuries sustained by their riders are usually more extensive because they

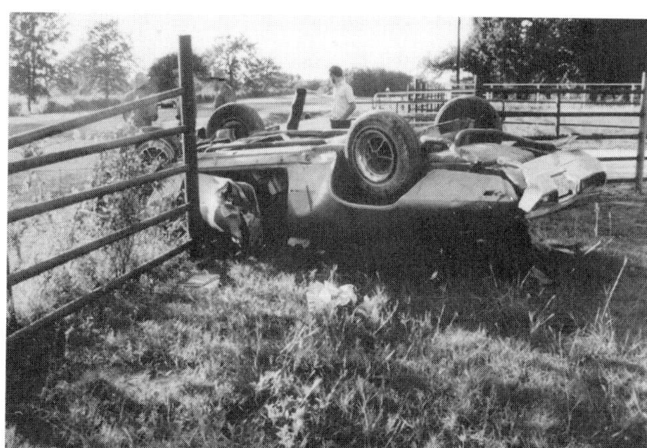

Figure 48-6 Injuries of occupants will be compounded by impact with fence and rollover forces.

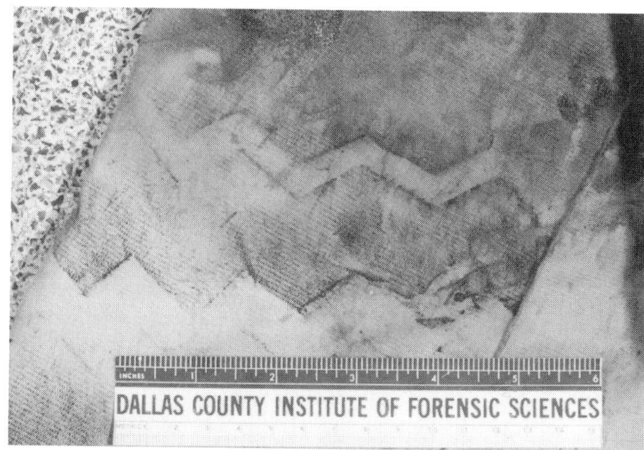

Fig. 48-7 Tire tread marks on clothing.

basically ride unprotected. Helmets offer limited protection, with head injuries still remaining the cause of 75% of motorcycle deaths. Leather outerwear provides protection of the body surface, but it offers no reduction in the injuries to the skeletal or internal organs.

Common injuries observed with frontal impact when bikes collide with a stationary object result in injuries to the head, chest, pelvis, and lower extremities. As the motorcycle impacts, the rider slides forward onto the gas tank and the pelvis lifts, thrusting the chest and head forward, usually striking the object. In addition, the internal organs are subject to injury from the violent turning of the handlebars. Patterned injuries may occur from the chain, muffler, or bike parts if the bike falls on the rider.

Other recreational vehicles, such as ATVs, snowmobiles, and jet skis, produce injuries similar to those seen with motorcycles, but potential environmental complications need to be considered. As with any motor vehicle collision, it is important to examine the scene, vehicles, and any equipment that might have been used or worn. The helmet is especially useful in determining the exact location and direction of impact.

It is important to be aware that if the rider has consumed alcohol, his or her ability to maintain balance is considerably impaired. Serious accidents can occur with lower blood alcohol levels than are seen with motor vehicle drivers.

Auto versus Pedestrian

Pedestrians account for 16% of road deaths, which usually occur in urban areas at speeds less then 22 mph. An adult is impacted at knee level and may sustain fractures or ligament and joint injury; these are commonly referred to as bumper injuries and increase with severity as the vehicle speed/impact increase. Bumper injury is located at the level of the most protuberant section of the bumper, and the pattern of the bumper may be evident on the pedestrian (patterned injury). If the vehicle was braking, the bumper will be at a lower level when it contacts the pedestrian. On impact, the pedestrian is rotated onto the hood of the vehicle, frequently fracturing the femur. As the pedestrian continues onto the hood of the vehicle, his or her body is accelerated to the speed of the vehicle and will be thrown onto the roadway where rolling and sliding injuries will be sustained. At this point, the pedestrian may actually be run over by the vehicle. Injuries to pedestrians struck by vehicles have tremendous potential, often extensive, and may include fractures to the skull, spine, pelvis, ribs, or extremities, as well as multiple contusions, abrasions, and lacerations.

The higher bumper, such as a truck impacting an adult pedestrian, usually results in the pedestrian being thrown directly down on to the roadway. The pedestrian may be carried on the front of the vehicle and dropped to the ground due to inertia as the vehicle slows down; it is not unusual for the pedestrian to be run over by the vehicle if the brakes are not applied. A child struck by a car is comparable to an adult being struck by the height of a bumper on a truck. However, as one might imagine, injuries are most often to the head and pelvis.

Bumper injuries provide valuable information about the position and movement of the pedestrian at the time of impact. Questions regarding standing, walking, running, or being struck from behind must be in the foreground of the investigator's thoughts. Comparison measurements must be made between the height of the bumper injury and the height of the bumper of the vehicle in determining whether the driver was braking. Tire tread marks may be evident on the clothing or skin, and glass or paint transfer should not be overlooked (Fig. 48-7).

Reconstructing Motor Vehicle Collisions

The reconstruction of a motor vehicle collision determines how the crash occurred and is based on evidence gathered at the scene. The absence of a thorough investigation will limit *and* compromise the outcome of the reconstruction. The evidence collected combined with the thoroughness of the investigation is critical to a reconstruction.

Scene and Vehicle

The scene of the collision will provide additional roadway evidence that will be measured and examined by the reconstructionist and includes skid marks, yaw tire marks (markings from a sliding vehicle), gouges, or scrapes in the pavement, the final positions of the vehicles, and debris from the vehicles themselves. The area of the initial impact will be determined (Fig. 48-8).

Damage to the vehicles is examined for the amount and direction of intrusion or crumple, and secondary impact. This will occur when several vehicles are involved or if the vehicle impacted a roadway object, such as a road sign, before or after the initial impact of the collision. The amount of intrusion is measured and will assist in

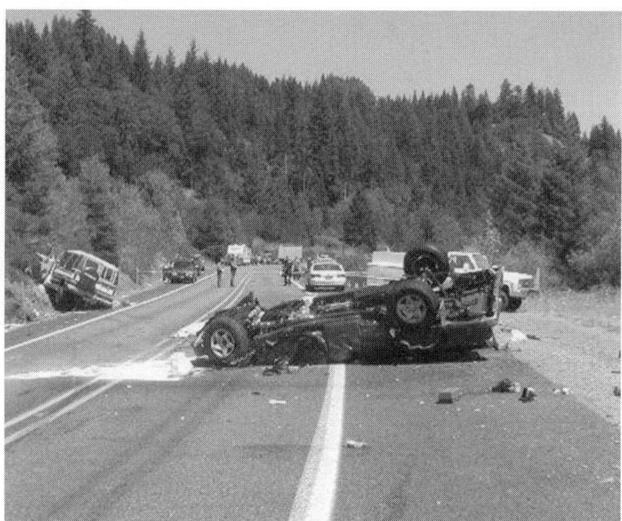

Fig. 48-8 Scene of highway accident where reconstructionist work begins to decipher the biomechanics of the collision.

determining the rate of vehicle speed at the point of impact. Vehicles crush differently–for example, newer vehicles with safety features such as crumple zones are designed to slow deceleration. Engineers have designed the engines of vehicles to collapse down and back during a collision, which will increase the amount of visible distortion to the front of the vehicle. The damage may appear severe when in actuality it was responding the way it was designed to, by providing a slower deceleration to the occupants. The amount of tire tread, tire pressure, brakes, steering, and the overall mechanical wellness of the vehicle should be assessed. If there is a question whether vehicle lights were in use at the time of impact or if a vehicle was braking, light filaments will be examined. If the lights were in use, the filaments would be hot on impact causing them to stretch. If the lights were off, the filaments would be cool on impact and break easily. Obstructions that would have interfered with the driver's view, such as weather or a dirty windshield, must be considered in the investigation by the reconstructionist when determining additional details of the collision.

Witness Accounts

Information should be obtained surrounding the drivers of the vehicles including witness statements regarding the collision and observations of the vehicles prior to the collision. Were they observed driving erratically or otherwise unsafe? Investigators will seek information about the driver's driving experience, where and when the driver started his or her travels, where the driver was traveling to, whether he or she stopped to eat, whether the driver was fatigued, under stress, emotionally upset, preoccupied (using a cell phone), or under the influence of alcohol or drugs (illegal or prescription). The FNE can assist in collecting blood or urine from the driver, following the guidelines of the state or hospital. Every attempt should be made to gather as much information as possible.

Vehicle Interior Details

The interior of the vehicles will be examined for evidence, such as seat belt use and air bag deployment. Seat belts will be examined for stretch, as well as transfer from the clothing of the occupants. If the air bag deployed, DNA evidence should be available from saliva or blood. The brake pedal is examined for the possible imprint of the driver's shoe, and the entire interior, especially the interior windshield, dashboard, A-pillars, roof and steering wheel, will all be carefully checked for blood, tissue, and hair transfer. Any evidence found within the interior of the vehicle will be collected, preserved, and placed into evidence.

Role of the Forensic Nurse Examiner

The forensic nurse examiner is a member of the investigative team and works closely with the multidisciplinary members. At the scene of a motor vehicle collision, the FNE should make contact with the reconstructionist to receive as much detail surrounding the dynamics of the crash as possible, learning where and how the occupants rode down the collision. The direction of impact is information that will assist the FNE in assessing and predicting occupant injuries. The FNE will take several photographs, including the overall scene from a distance first, and then continue to take pictures while walking toward the collision. This should be done from both directions. Photos of each vehicle should be taken individually, including photos from the middle, all four sides, and the license plates of the vehicles involved. Pictures should include roadway evidence, debris, and numerous photos of the intrusion and damage to the vehicles.

Injury Assessment and Documentation

With the information that has been obtained from the scene, the FNE can better assess injuries of all the vehicle occupants. By knowing the direction of impact, the FNE should first assess for injuries that would be expected. For example, if the vehicle sustained frontal impact, associated injuries might include lap and shoulder restraints, air bag deployments, knees contacting the dashboard, or windshield and dicing injuries. The shoulders of the occupants should be examined carefully. Contusions or abrasions from the shoulder restraint may be subtle and difficult to visualize, but there is usually at least a small area of erythema over the anterior shoulder or clavicle. Assess for patterned injuries (Fig. 48-9).

Carefully document every visual injury observed, either with photography or completion of a traumagram. Also, examine the shoes of the known drivers for possible imprints of the vehicle pedals on the soles, as well as the clothes worn by the occupants when the collision occurred. These should be described and documented, and in some cases they may need to be seized as evidence.

Any glass or other foreign bodies found on victims' clothing or bodies–for example, in hair or wounds–should be documented and seized. All evidence that is seized must be maintained with a chain of custody.

Best Practice *48-2*

The forensic nurse should elicit as much information as possible about the mechanics of the crash, including the use of passive restraints and air bag deployment to assist health team members in predicting resultant injuries.

Vehicle Inspections

With the injuries of all known occupants, it will be most beneficial to then perform vehicle inspections. This will be the most important assessment to determine the biomechanics of impact.

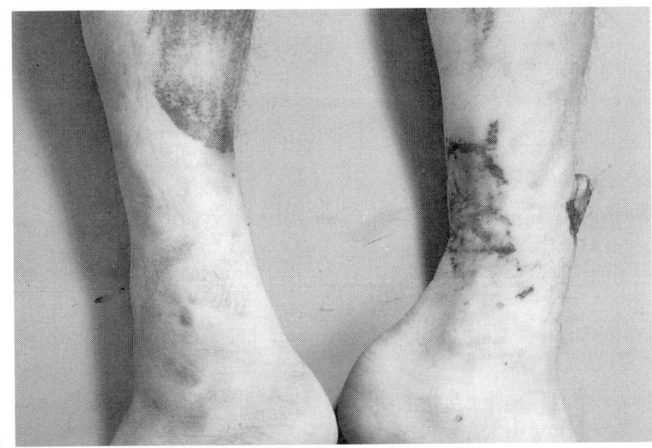

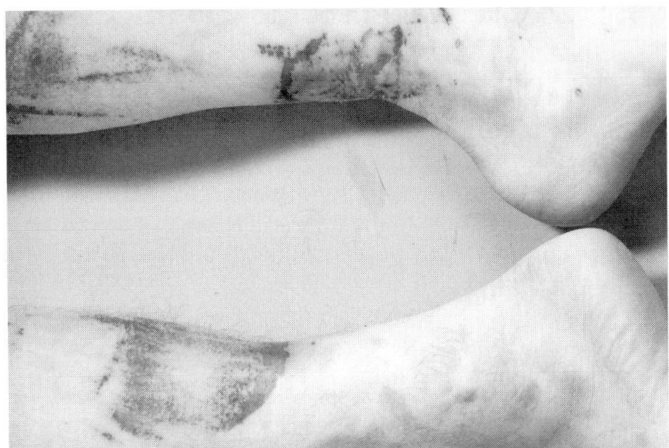

Fig. 48-9 Occupant injuries of lower extremities from impact with car's interior. When viewing the injuries from two planes (*A* and *B*), the reconstructionist can appreciate the biomechanics of the accident.

This is when all injuries are known and the interior of the vehicle can be examined to identify the direction of forces and structures that caused each specific injury. It is the role of the FNE to understand and describe the mechanism of all injuries that were sustained. The interior of the vehicle should also be examined for evidence, such as clothes, hair, blood, or tissue transfer. The location of such evidence will be made much easier due to the knowledge of injuries sustained and the expected location based on that knowledge. For example, if the driver has a large facial laceration located on the left side of his or her forehead, examine and expect to find evidence of impact on the steering wheel, door, or A-pillar.

The results of the information, evidence, and findings of the FNE's investigation must then be written in report form. The report will include all times, dates, locations, names of the individuals contacted, a list of the evidence seized, including photographs or traumagrams, and, most important, a narrative of the FNE's entire investigation. The report will include the findings, the biomechanics of impact. It should describe the mechanism for every injury to every occupant, as well as identify each occupant's seating position. It should be complete and thorough. A copy of this report will go to the investigative officer, and in cases that are to be prosecuted, a copy will go to the district attorney.

Summary

The FNE provides an ideal addition to the multidisciplinary investigation of motor vehicle collisions. It is critical for the FNE to conduct a thorough investigation that includes documentation, photos of injuries, injury causation, and securing relevant evidence that will assist the reconstructionist in determining the cause of the motor vehicle collision. The reconstructionist brings a knowledge that enhances the science of biomechanics of impact and can act as a liaison that bridges law enforcement, district attorneys, and the medical profession.

Case Study 48-1 Intoxicated Pedestrian and Hit-and-Run

S. D. was intoxicated and had left a nearby party stating he was going to walk home. Several passing motorists witnessed him walking/marching along the shoulder of the highway. Sometime after midnight he was struck by a southbound vehicle, which did not stop. At approximately 0300 hours, an anonymous caller reported a male body lying off the shoulder of the road. The body was found a short time later by a county deputy. The weather was cold, in the low 30s, and there was a torrential downpour of rain mixed with snow. Visibility was very poor.

The busy, paved, two-lane highway ran north/south. The body was located approximately 10 feet from the fog line off the west shoulder of the highway. The victim was in mud and tall grass at the edge of a thick brushy bog. The victim's left shoe was lying near the fog line, approximately 30 yards south of the body. His lower left leg had been amputated and was lying another 10 yards from the shoe off the shoulder of the road. Evidence collected at the scene included three pieces of red plastic from a vehicle air dam, a square corner from the headlight, and pieces of side window glass. The pieces of plastic and the piece of headlight were taken to a local automotive shop, and they determined that the suspect vehicle was a late 1980s or early 1990s red Chevrolet.

Further examination of the body at the morgue a short time later revealed additional information. There were deep linear, avulsion-type injuries to the left side of the face and left temple. Several pieces of glass, which appeared to be from a vehicle side window, were removed from these wounds. Windshield glass was removed from the front of the victim's shirt. A very large 10-cm flap-type laceration was located over the right occipital scalp, exposing the skull. Over the dorsal left shoulder was a reddened abrasion with numerous linear scrapes leading from the larger abrasion. The left posterior shoulder had a large 8-cm, reddened abrasion with a linear reddened contusion that extended from the posterior shoulder to the waist. The left shoulder was unstable, and several fractures were palpated, including the left humerus. There was a large, deep laceration to the right groin at the base of the penis. This was approximately 12 cm by 2 cm. No stretch marks to the skin were noted. The left lower leg had been amputated above the ankle, with approximately 8 inches of bone and muscle tissue pulled out from the upper lower leg. The left tibia and fibula had numerous fractures. The posterior left leg had horizontal linear reddened contusions of different widths. The first contusion, midcalf, was noted at 15 inches from the foot, a wide contusion at 20 inches above the foot, and a linear contusion at 27 inches. There was a reddened contusion over the front left knee. The right leg was without visible injury. No other injury or trauma was noted to the body. The blood alcohol level was 0.26%.

Based on the location of the abrasions to the victim's left leg and additional evidence found on the body and at the scene, it was determined that the victim was walking with his back to the vehicle and was struck in the back of the left leg. His weight was on his left foot, which resulted in the amputation of the lower leg. This was also evidenced by the lack of injury to his right leg, in addition to the deep laceration to the right groin resulting from the right leg being thrown out from the body when he was impacted. After impact he was thrown up and onto the hood of the vehicle where his left shoulder struck the A-pillar and broke the windshield, continuing onto the roof of the vehicle where his head struck the passenger door window.

The media were contacted and requested the public's assistance in locating the suspect's vehicle, a late 1980s or early 1990s red Chevrolet, with passenger side damage to the front bumper, hood, windshield, and door window. Approximately one week later a citizen reported the location of the suspect's vehicle. The vehicle was identified as a 1987 Chevrolet Cavalier with damage to the passenger side front bumper, air dam, hood, A-pillar, windshield, and passenger door window. In addition, blood, tissue, and clothing were collected from the vehicle, which was identified as belonging to the victim.

Resources

Books

Anderson, W. (1998) *Forensic sciences in clinical medicine. A case study approach.* New York: Lippincott-Raven.

Daily, J. (1988) *Fundamentals of traffic accident reconstruction.* Jacksonville: Institute of Police Technology and Management, University of North Florida.

Rivers, R. (1997) *Technical traffic accident investigators' handbook* (2nd ed.). Springfield, IL: Charles C Thomas.

Organizations

National Highway Traffic Safety Administration

400 Seventh Street, NW, Washington, DC 20590; Tel: 202-366-0123, 888-327-4236; www.nhtsa.dot.gov

National Institute for Occupation Safety and Health (NIOSH)

Centers for Disease Control and Prevention, 1600 Clifton Road, Atlanta, GA 30333; Tel: 404-639-3311; www.cdc.gov/niosh

"NIOSH Alert: Preventing Worker Injuries and Deaths from Traffic-Related Motor Vehicle Crashes," DHHS (NIOSH) Publication No. 98-142, available from NIOSH; Tel: 800-35-NIOSH (800-356-4674).

References

Association for the Advancement of Automotive Medicine. (1992). *Traffic injury: The medicine-engineering link.* Video.

Besant-Matthews, P. (1998). *Injury and death investigation* (pp. 1-48). Colorado Springs, CO: Beth-El College of Nursing.

Spitz, W. (1993). *Medicolegal investigation of death: Guidelines for the application of pathology to crime investigation* (3rd ed., pp. 528-584). Springfield, IL: Charles C Thomas.

Chapter 49 Psychiatric Forensic Nursing

Judith W. Coram

The names of small towns float together in a haze of stunned confusion amid the fading sound of sirens: Moses Lake, Washington; Paducah, Kentucky; Jonesboro, Arkansas; Columbine, Colorado.

President Clinton attempted to frame the string of killings in schools by referring to the events as "symptoms of our changing culture." The apparent increase in violence among youth is alarming. The US attorney general's office reports that in the 1996-1997 school year, six thousand kids were expelled for taking a gun to school. The National Institute of Justice reports that most robbery victims are boys age 12 to 14 and that youth constitute 25% of murder victims and half of serious crime victims. Juvenile arrests for major violent crimes rose 150% between 1983 and 1992. The murder rate in this age group increased 165%.

Along with schoolyard shootings, there are other events in American society that were unheard of in the 1960s: satanic graffiti is scrawled across a storefront, churches are burned to the ground, a woman is killed by her stalker, a family-planning clinic is bombed, a neo-Nazi compound readies for a public parade, a newborn is left in a dumpster by its teenage parent, a young gay man is severely beaten, a gang shooting leaves a 12-year-old dead.

Has violence increased, or has media coverage made people more aware? Is it the type of violence that appalls us, frightens us, or repulses us? Does the violence, or the not understanding of why, abhor us? Is culture changing in the values of the masses to one of violence? Is it a younger generation, those known as Generation X or the Echo Boomers, who seemingly have no social values? To what is this increase in violence attributed?

The National Institute of Justice reports that a quarter of the general population believes drugs are the cause of crime. Another 22% blame the collapse of the American family. Eleven percent believes the cause can be found in economic reasons (loss of jobs, lack of work). Declining moral values, as portrayed by television, movies, and rap music, are also blamed. Over 6% believe that flaws in the US criminal justice system or lax law enforcement contribute to criminal behavior. Access to weapons is a factor. Approximately 70% of murders are committed with firearms, whereas the use of knives accounts for only 7%.

Why is there interpersonal violence in society? Some believe that violence is a male prerogative. History has illustrated man's inclination toward clan struggles and war over territory. Man has been celebrated for his stamina and strength in the folklore of all cultures. Although it is argued against, Western society condones aggression in men, as evidenced by the use of violence in entertainment. However, the reaction is still revulsion to violent behavior by women.

Some believe men are socialized to violence. This is promoted by encouraging roughhousing in young boys and holding up to them heroes and role models that are physical. Despite advances, there is still a message that men need to reduce or eliminate their emotional responses. If men cannot deal with frustration through hurt and sadness, then only anger is left. Violence results as a consequence of restricting emotions.

Some attribute changing cultural standards to the promulgation of violence. Americans applaud competitiveness. Entertainment confuses sexuality with violence in video games and movies. Some look to a biological need to express strength or stamina and the fact that society has changed dramatically in its technological revolution. Heavy physical work for men has been replaced with mental fatigue and no outlet for the physical need for exertion.

Social scientists are struggling to make sense of the increase in crime and violence. Many theoretical explanations have been proffered. Box 49-1 describes the seven major schools of thought as contained in Ohlin and Farrington (1991).

Box 49-1 Seven Major Schools of Thought

1. **Individual Development Theory** predicts that conduct disorders and early delinquency lead to crime. Temperamental and developmental deficiencies are predictors of a career in crime and are disproportionately common among adolescents who continue criminal activity into adulthood.
2. **Social Control Theory** predicts that when the social constraints on antisocial behavior are weakened or absent, delinquent crime emerges. Socially acceptable behavior is more likely if the individual maintains an attachment to others, shares their values, and shares involvement in law-abiding activities.
3. **Social Learning Theory** predicts that those who persist in criminal activity continue to increase the frequency, duration, and intensity of contact with other offenders, whereas those who desist from crime decrease contact with offenders and increase contact with nonoffenders. Individuals learn how to break the law in the same way they learn other types of behavior; therefore, criminal behavior is learned. This learning is communicated in intimate groups of family and peers. The learning includes motives, attitudes, and rationalization, as well as technique.
4. **Social Disorganization Theory** predicts that crime results when community life becomes disorganized, when high mobility and a heterogeneous population cause a breakdown in conforming controls over criminal conduct. Community consensus on norms, values, and beliefs cannot develop. Residents encounter cultural conflict, loss of control, and an increase in organized illegal activities.
5. **Network Theory** predicts that when network ties are weak, social sanctions against crime will work. People become offenders by being recruited into networks and socialized to crime.
6. **Rational Choice Theory** predicts that individuals choose crime when the benefits outweigh the costs of disobeying the law. Crime will decrease when opportunities are limited, benefits reduced, and costs are increased. Criminal behavior is more than a response to social pressures or upbringing. It is also a choice.
7. **Deterrence Theory** predicts that when punishment is swift and certain, incidence of crime is reduced. A study indicated that 30% of Americans believed that crime could be reduced by emphasizing punishment, and 71% supported greater use of the death penalty.

Data from Ohlin, M. & Farrington, D. (1991). *Human development and criminal behavior: New ways of advancing knowledge*. New York: Springer-Verlag.

Theories of determinism are also used to explain responses given by a perpetrator who blames his own attitude and behavior on things he thinks he cannot control. He ascribes his behavior to one of three sources of determinism: genetics ("It's my grandparents' fault"), psychological upbringing ("It's my parents' fault"), or environment and surroundings ("It's my spouse's fault," "It's my boss's fault," or "It's my culture's fault").

The forensic examiner will factor these influences in, and take them into consideration, but realize they are not fully responsible. The accused still made a choice at the particular moment of the crime. The difference is an explanation of motive based on *influenced by* rather than *determined by*.

All these theories have merit in given situations. Their tenets help comprehension, in a broad sense, of human beings' criminal nature and wend to violence. However, they do little to explain why a specific criminal act occurred at a specific time and place.

Psychiatric forensic nursing is psychosocial in two ways: (1) the interaction with individuals, groups, and the community and (2) the understanding of social and cultural factors influencing a perpetrator's motivation and behavior just prior to and during a criminal act. Of these theories, psychiatric forensic nursing holds most to rational choice theory.

Key Point *49-1*

Psychiatric forensic nursing holds to free will, an individual's ability and right to make a decision, even if it is a poor one.

The Role of Dignity and Personal Values

People tend to make the best decision they are capable of making at a given time. There is always an explanation for behavior. It just may not be readily evident. It is not necessary to see a perpetrator as completely rational in the sense that he is making the best or most efficient choice. Perpetrators can show limited rationality in a given circumstance by drawing on their own value systems (the way they see it). It has been said, "All behavior is meaningful." One's behavior illustrates personal expression of one's values.

Key Point *49-2*

The forensic psychiatric nurse believes that all individuals possess the capability of committing a criminal act, given the right circumstances.

The patients of the forensic nurse specialist demonstrate criminal patterns and lifestyles that must be examined in their own light. Mechanic and colleagues (2003) believe that individuals are viewed as dynamic beings functioning and interacting at multiple system levels, developmental stages, and interrelationship patterns, and manifesting adaptive and maladaptive responses. They must be considered in the context of their family, environment, and lifestyle. Physical and emotional health practices, attitudes, and individual responses to illnesses are understood and acted on by interrelating the influence of all these various psychosocial, cultural, spiritual, and physiologic dimensions. Z. G. Standing Bear believes forensic nursing brings together the necessarily neutral and detached arena of law enforcement with the empathetic, involved, and accepting dimensions of psychosocial nursing (Lynch, 1997).

Best Practice *49-1*

The forensic nurse must be disciplined to examine a person's motivation for a particular act in an objective, nonjudgmental fashion and be capable of personally communicating with the patient to gain the patient's perspective, which is essential for understanding *the patient's* actions through *the patient's* value system.

Implications for the Forensic Nurse

The nature of psychiatric nursing is defined by society and by nurses. Peplau (1987) called for an expansion of psychiatric nursing skills. The authority of nursing knowledge comes not from its source but from its application to phenomena that society decides is within the purview of nursing.

Defining Psychiatric Forensic Nursing

Psychiatric nursing continues to be an area of changing patient profiles. Nurses working in this area have expanded their knowledge to meet the changing needs of the individuals, groups, or communities they serve. Psychiatric nursing has increasingly been involved with patients whose chronic illnesses and behavior occasionally involve them in the legal system. Jails and prisons have long used registered nurses with physical assessment skills to treat minor illness and injury (American Nurses Association [ANA], 1985). Since the 1980s, changing social problems have demanded that these nurses incorporate more teaching about substance abuse, AIDS prevention, and wellness into their care.

Increased substance abuse, gang involvement, easy access to weapons, and diverse social pressures have resulted in an explosion in the crime rate, with a growing number of people requiring assessment and evaluation after their arrest. Most of these people have had no previous contact with the mental health system (Bencer, 1989).

Psychiatric forensic nursing shares many of the same medicolegal aspects of physiologic forensic nursing. The essential difference is the nature of their patients.

The number of practicing physiologic forensic nurses has grown substantially since 1992. The focus of their work is to apply forensic aspects of healthcare in the scientific investigation and treatment of trauma and/or medicolegal issues (Lynch, 1997). Physiologic forensic nurses work as coroners, death investigators, sexual assault nurse examiners, child abuse specialists, elder abuse specialists, battered woman specialists, or legal nurse consultants. Their patients are the alleged victims, either living or dead.

Key Point *49-3*

Psychiatric forensic nursing is the psychiatric nursing assessment, evaluation, and treatment of individuals pending a criminal hearing or trial. The defendant is the client, and the client's thinking and behavior prior to, and during, the commission of the crime are the primary focus of the nurse-client relationship (Coram, 1993b).

Prior to 1993, there was no literature defining the characteristics of psychiatric nurses who also overlap into forensic areas. Nor could one find written work describing the expanded role of a clinical nurse specialist (CNS) who chooses to practice in an area that contains elements of physiologic nursing, psychiatric nursing, correctional nursing, law enforcement, and the criminal justice system.

In 1993, a study was undertaken as part of a master's thesis to collect data on the number of registered nurses providing psychiatric forensic nursing services in the US (Coram, 1993b). The study was important because there had been no previously published work identifying either the number of psychiatric forensic nurses in the US or what forensic role functions were being performed.

Survey forms were sent to registered nurses working in all facilities listed in the *Directory of Programs and Facilities for Mentally Disordered Offenders* as published by the National Institute of Mental Health (1992). Survey forms were returned from 45 states. The response rate was 45%. The data suggested that master's-prepared nurses are more likely to perform forensic functions involving assessment, consultation, or courtroom testimony. This reinforced the position that forensic nurses view their intersections of practice outside their own discipline.

The study brought to light the confusion between the terms *forensic* and *correctional*. Many nurses claimed identification as a forensic nurse because of the location of their work or the legal status of their patient, rather than the role functions performed. For example, nurses may perform only psychiatric or correctional nursing functions and call themselves forensic nurses because their patients are incarcerated. This was illustrated by a study in Canada (Niskala, 1986), which focused on the competencies and skills of registered nurses working in correctional healthcare. Although the title suggested the nurses were "working in forensic areas," none of the actual duties involved were forensic role functions.

Role Functions

Forensic nursing is not determined by the location or the patient, but by the nurse-patient relationship and the role functions performed. Role functions are the nursing acts, behaviors, and skills performed by the role occupant, which are related to categories of practice. Role functions only partially identify practice. Defining the role of a forensic nurse means incorporating role behaviors with values and attitudes. Boxes 49-2 and 49-3 list role functions within the separate subspecialty areas of physiologic and psychiatric forensic nursing.

Box 49-2 Role Functions within Physiologic Forensic Nursing

- Forensic photography
- Bite mark identification
- Identification of sharp or blunt trauma
- Assessment of sexual assault trauma
- Identification of patterned injury
- Establishing chain of custody
- Evidence identification, collection, documentation, and preservation
- Assessment of pattern of injury in abuse
- Provision of fact witness testimony

Data from Lynch, V. (1997). *Handbook of clinical forensic nursing: A new perspective in trauma.* Colorado Springs, CO: Beth-El College of Nursing.

Box 49-3 Role Functions within Psychiatric Forensic Nursing

- Legal sanity evaluation
- Competency evaluation
- Assessment of capacity to formulate intent
- Assessment of violence potential
- Prediction of dangerousness
- Parole/probation considerations
- Assessment of racial/cultural factors in crime
- Consultation on countermeasures to violence
- Assistance in jury selection
- Investigation of criminal history
- Assessment of personality disorders
- Sexual predator screening
- Courtroom consultation to attorneys
- Provision of competency therapy
- Provision of formal written reports to court
- Provision of expert witness testimony

Expanding the Scope of Psychiatric Nursing Practice

A theoretical foundation for psychiatric forensic nursing comes from King's theory for the patient-nurse relationship. She holds that the patient is a personal system within an environment, coexisting with other personal systems. The nurse and the patient perceive one another and the situation, act and react, interact and transact. King defined nursing as a process of human interactions between nurse and patients, who communicate to set goals, explore means for achieving the goals, and then agree on the means to be used. King speaks of nursing as a discipline and an applied science, with emphasis on the derivation of nursing knowledge from other disciplines.

Systems theory from the behavioral sciences led to the development of her dynamic interacting systems (King, 1971). She identified three distinct levels of operation in this system: (1) individuals, (2) groups, and (3) society. The patient-nurse interactions in psychiatric forensic nursing affect each level. For example, the psychiatric forensic nurse evaluates a felony defendant prior to a competency hearing (individual level). The expert witness testimony is given during the trial (group level). The opinion rendered on dangerousness subsequently affects the patient's sentence (society level).

Expanded roles in nursing are defined by their practice. The *Social Policy Statement* of the American Nurses Association (ANA) describes scope of practice as multidimensional and characterized by four major elements: a core of professional practice common to all members of a discipline, "dimensions" or characteristics of practice, intra- and inter-professional intersections, and practice boundaries (ANA, 1980). Intersections are practice areas that interface or overlap with the professional domain of practitioners in other clinical specialty areas. A discipline's boundaries mark the outer edge of practice for which it is responsible (ANA, 1980). This demarcation is flexible and expands in response to changing societal needs (Mechanic, Weaver, & Resnick, 2003).

Forensic nursing intersections are within other disciplines, rather than other specialty areas of nursing. The psychiatric forensic nurse's scope of practice is greatly affected by the practice setting, which can vary among a crime scene, a courtroom, a forensic hospital, or a correctional facility. The dimensions of practice in psychiatric forensic nursing are affected by the nature of the patient and the patient's current involvement with the criminal justice system. The core of practice is psychiatric nursing, but the relationship between patient and nurse is affected to a greater degree by the alternative social context of the situation precipitating their interaction.

Differentiating Correctional Nurses and Psychiatric Forensic Nurses

There is a commonality between physiologic forensic nurses and psychiatric forensic nurses in that the nurse-patient relationship is predicated on the possibility that a crime has been committed. The role functions performed contribute data toward answering the question of whether or not a crime has been committed. There is an investigative quality to the nursing assessment that does not exist in other areas of practice. Elsewhere, the RN may be expected to describe and report findings, but not to interpret them. For example, a school nurse may observe and document the design of marks upon a child's back, but the forensic child abuse specialist would take the data further and make an assessment of patterned injury that includes speculation about the type of weapon used in the suspected battering. Where a pediatric nurse treats the immediate injury, the forensic nurse sees the possibility that a crime has been committed and collects evidence that may help to determine facts of the case. Similarly, whereas the pediatric nurse without forensic training takes a history of repeated apneic spells, the forensic nurse specialist may look further for suspected Munchausen's syndrome by proxy.

Evidence collection is central to the role of all forensic nurses. One way evidence collection is performed within psychiatric forensic nursing is in the finding of intent or diminished capacity in the perpetrator's thinking at the time of the crime. This aids in determining the degree of crime and may later impact the perpetrator's sentencing. Psychiatric forensic nurses who work as competency therapists demonstrate evidence collection in another manner. They spend many hours with a defendant, and much of the dialogue related to the case is documented carefully.

Although both correctional nurses and psychiatric forensic nurses interact with the perpetrator, the nature of their relationship, and the timing, differentiate their roles. Correctional nurses care for the patient's *present* medical or mental health needs. Correctional nurses care for inmates without knowing the nature of their crimes. This is a philosophy of treatment based on the premise that such blinders promote more objective care. Correctional nurses do not play a role in determining future dangerousness of the patient. For the most part, correctional nurses care for the inmate after the charge has been adjudicated.

Role functions within correctional nursing include (1) determining need for restraint, (2) conducting a body cavity search, (3) assessing risk for custodial suicide, (4) collecting evidence with a sexual assault kit, among others.

A Model for the Nurse-Patient Relationship

A model has been developed to illustrate the differences among correctional nursing, physiologic forensic nursing, and psychiatric forensic nursing, all of which overlap in the criminal justice system (Fig. 49-1).

There is a timeline that begins when an interaction between the victim and perpetrator violates a law or may be criminal in nature. The physiologic forensic nurse interacts with the victim, and the nature of their relationship is based on the possibility that the interaction between victim and perpetrator was a criminal one. For this same alleged action, the future patient of the psychiatric

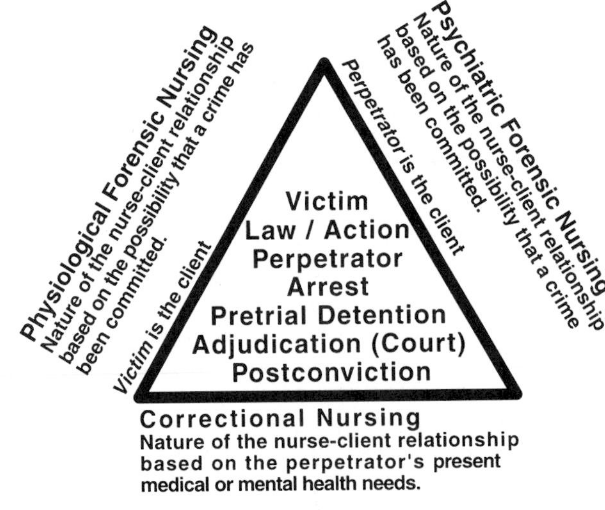

Fig. 49-1 Model for nurse-patient relationship.

forensic nurse is arrested. That person is detained in a correctional facility or on a forensic unit in a mental hospital. Eventually there is a hearing or trial, and the person is adjudicated. If convicted, the period in incarceration continues (most likely at a different facility than where pretrial detention took place).

Both the physiologic forensic nurses who work with victims and the psychiatric forensic nurse working with the perpetrator time their nurse-patient relationship before adjudication. Correctional nurses may care for the perpetrator both before and after the trial, but the nature of their relationship differs from that of the psychiatric forensic nurses who provided part of the investigatory information prior to trial. The correctional nurse deals with the perpetrator's day-to-day medical or mental health needs.

Correctional nursing is defined by the nature of the patient, an inmate. Nurses who work on long-term psychiatric units housing patients who have been acquitted by reason of insanity also define their role by the nature of the inmate. They are more accurately described as correctional mental health nurses. It is misleading for a nurse to self-identify as forensic merely because she or he works in a building with that label. Predominantly, correctional nurses do not perform forensic role behaviors. An exception would be the prison nurse who conducts a rape exam or collects a sample for DNA testing.

Roles within Psychiatric Forensic Nursing

Successful role development must include clearly defined purposes, goals (Barrett, 1971), and role responsibilities; mutual agreement of role expectations; and self-confidence of clinical knowledge and ability (Ball, 1990).

Clinical Nurse Specialist

The role functions of a clinical nurse specialist have been categorized in a variety of ways: clinician, educator, researcher, consultant, executive, change agent, role model, implementer, advocate, manager, and mentor. Hirst and Metcalf (1986) pointed out that it takes considerable time to integrate every role function into one's repertoire.

Table 49-1 Evaluation Issues

CLINICAL ISSUE	MENTAL HEALTHCARE PROVIDER	FORENSIC EXAMINER
Person is the patient/client of:	The practitioner	The attorney
Nature of the privilege	Therapist-patient	Attorney-client or attorney-work product
Cognitive set of evaluator	Supportive, accepting, empathetic	Neutral, objective, detached
Area of expertise	Therapeutic techniques	Psychologal evaluation standards
Standards	Diagnostic criteria/treatment	Legal criteria for adjudication
Structure of the evaluation	By patient, less structured	By evaluator, more structured
Evaluation completeness	Based on information from patient	Checked for accuracy of sources
Nature of the process	Rarely adversarial	Frequently adversarial
Advocacy of evaluator	For the patient	For issues or results of evaluation
Outcome of evaluation	To benefit the patient	To aid the legal process

The psychiatric forensic nurse must be highly skilled in interpersonal relations and in developing and maintaining channels of communication. Developing collegial relationships with other disciplines is central to the role because of its intersections of practice with those areas that overlap with the professional domain of other disciplines.

Roles performed within psychiatric forensic nursing include forensic examiner, competency therapist, consultant to law enforcement or the criminal justice system, etc.

Forensic Nurse Examiner

The role of the forensic examiner is to conduct an evaluation, answer specific medicolegal questions as directed by the court, and render an expert opinion. There are marked differences between the purpose, techniques, and goals of psychiatric interviews performed by mental health treatment counselors and forensic examiners. Table 49-1 highlights these differences.

The cognitive set of the forensic examiner differs from that of mental health personnel. Whereas treatment staff members strive to be supportive, accepting, and empathetic, the forensic examiner strives to remain neutral, objective, and detached. A treatment intake interview is usually patient structured (nonconfronting or probing), mostly based on information from the patient, and for the purpose of treatment. The purpose of the forensic evaluation is legal adjudication. The forensic examiner controls the interview, which is frequently adversarial, and does more checking of the accuracy of information given by the patient. Mental health personnel advocate for the patient, whereas the forensic examiner advocates for the issues or the results of the evaluation.

A thorough and complete forensic evaluation must include a face-to-face interview, review of contents of the police reports, and a thorough social/psychiatric history. The ethical forensic examiner will decline a request for an examination or expert opinion when denied access to any of the three.

The formation of an expert opinion is based on the following steps:

1. The forensic examiner will collect pertinent clinical data, including observed behaviors of the patient, forensic evidence in the police reports, lab reports, psychological testing results, and a thorough social/psychiatric history.
2. The examiner will process all the information based on her or his education and training, experience, and scientific/clinical knowledge and expertise.
3. The examiner will skillfully interview the patient, noting all related clinical findings, including symptoms of mental disorder, behavior, past diagnoses, personality traits, emotions, cognitive abilities, and the psychodynamics of interpersonal relationships.
4. A mental state reconstruction will be based on both behavior exhibited and affect expressed. An evaluation of behavior will include evidence at the scene, witness statements of observed symptoms, retrospective self-report of symptoms, and disclosed motivation. An assessment of the patient's affect will be based on the patient's cognitive processing and reasoning ability, presence of drugs or medical conditions, the social/interpersonal context of the crime, and any causation explanations offered by the patient.
5. The forensic examiner will apply legal standards to all the assessment data. The jurisdiction's statutes and definitions of mental state/sanity/competency will be compared to applicable case law and published expert legal interpretation (in law reviews, articles, books).

Traditionally, the role of forensic examiner has been only within the scope of practice of the psychiatrist or psychologist. The prerequisite to the expanded role of a forensic examiner by a forensic nurse specialist is educational preparation and experience. Nurses cannot practice in this expanded role if they hold narrow conceptualizations of the issues confronting patients or if they perceive motivation primarily within a cause-and-effect framework. Clinical role development requires not only skill in data gathering from a multisystem perspective, but also critical thinking skills in interpreting and using information for problem solving (Murphy, 1986). Membership or certification in such organizations as the American Academy of Forensic Sciences or the American College of Forensic Examiners substantiates credibility in the role. The forensic nurse specialist is encouraged to seek board certification in areas previously represented only by psychiatrists or psychologists.

It is paramount that the forensic examiner verbalizes an exceptional understanding of major mental illness and personality disorders. The forensic examiner must keep abreast of theories being developed on social deviancy and interpersonal violence and must keep current on societal trends (for example, changes in drug use, growth of gang activity, participation in cults), both nationally and in the nurse's own jurisdiction.

A successful forensic examiner is able to separate personal opinion from professional opinion. Personal opinion is based on one's background, upbringing, education, and values. Professional opinion is based on scientific principle, advanced education in a specific field of endeavor, and the unbiased standards set by research in that area.

Best Practice 49-2

Forensic nurse examiners must be able to isolate their personal value systems in dealing with cases of criminal violence, sexual deviancy, ethnic norms, or cultural behaviors.

Legal Insanity

Legal sanity differs from clinical sanity. Legal sanity is defined as the person's ability to know right from wrong with reference to the act charged, the capacity to know the nature and quality of the act charged, and the capacity to form the intent to commit the crime. Legal sanity is determined for the specific time of the act, which may range from the split second the accused trains a weapon and fires or over a long weekend, during which several criminal acts are committed. Clinical sanity is the presence of a major mental disorder currently and at the time of the crime.

In most states, a major mental disorder is a prerequisite for a finding of legal insanity. State insanity laws may have wording variations, but they will cite the *presence of mental disorder or defect.* The term *mental disorder* usually refers to major mental illness, whereas *mental defect* usually refers to developmental disability or some physiologic condition affecting cognition (e.g., head injury, meningitis, brain tumor, dementia).

The general public frequently misconstrues insanity hearings as manipulation by the defense, a current political ploy, or an aberration of the criminal justice system. Although history has shown that a sudden change in legislation frequently follows a widely publicized violent event, the foundation for such hearings was laid long ago. For example, Aristotle's writing stated that one is morally responsible if, with knowledge of the circumstances and in the absence of external compulsion, he deliberately chooses to commit a specific act. Ancient Roman law did not hold a child or insane person accountable if they committed homicide, based on a premise that one is excused by the innocence of his intentions and by the act of misfortune. Seventh-century Mohammedan law was probably the first to formally recognize criminal responsibility. It specified that unintentional murder committed by "a child or lunatic" was to be "repaid by compensation, not punishment."

In 1732, a paranoid and disturbed man named Ned Arnold believed that Lord Onslow had entered his body. He was charged with attempted homicide after shooting and wounding him. Judge Tracy charged the jury with what has become known as the Wild Beast Test. This means that a person must be completely deprived of understanding and memory so as not to know what he or she is doing—"no more than an infant, a brute, or a wild beast." The jury rejected Arnold's insanity defense after listening to lay witnesses testify that, despite his mental illness, he took care of himself and got along fairly well.

There was no expert witness testimony in the Arnold trial. The first time a psychiatrist testified was in 1760. At that time, psychiatrists were called to court only for the purpose of educating the court or jury about insanity.

The best known insanity case is that of Daniel M'Naghten, a Scottish carpenter who believed he was being harassed by Catholic priests and Jesuits. He told his family that spies for the Tories were following him night and day, laughing at him. He was evicted from his boarding house due to his loud moaning, yelling, and walking about naked at night. In 1843 he stalked Prime Minister Sir Robert Peel and eventually shot Peel's secretary. The victim's wounds were treated with leeches "to let out the bad blood." This caused further blood loss, and the man died. M'Naghten was charged with murder.

Nine psychiatrists testified at M'Naghten's trial—three for the defense, three for the prosecution, and three who listened to the evidence and watched the defendant in the courtroom. All nine agreed that he suffered from "Monomania" (probably called paranoid schizophrenia today). All nine agreed he was not legally sane according to the legal tests at that time. The jury huddled for two minutes, not even leaving the room. They found him to be legally insane.

The public was outraged, believing his confinement at Bethlehem Hospital too lenient. A task force in the House of Lords reviewed the case and came up with a new legal standard. So the M'Naghten rule was not applied in this famous case but was a result of its conclusion. Daniel M'Naghten was later transferred to the Broadmoor Criminal Lunatic Asylum. He died at the age of 49 and was buried in an unmarked grave on hospital grounds.

Prior to 1843, the legal standard was "irresistible impulse." It dealt with *volition*—the capacity to will or not will to do an act. M'Naghten deals with *knowledge*: (1) knowing the nature and quality of the act and (2) knowing the wrongfulness of the act. Today approximately half the states use M'Naghten as the legal standard, and half use irresistible impulse in some form or another.

When the issue of legal sanity is raised in a high-profile case, the public reacts with outrage. It is a popular myth that the plea is overused. A study by Sales and Hafemeister in 1984 indicated that less than 10% of all criminal cases raise the issue of insanity. Another study (Cirincione, Steadman, & McGreevy, 1995) found that the rates for insanity pleas and successful acquittals varied widely by state.

The burden of proving legal insanity is on the defense. Proof of criminal action must be determined "beyond a reasonable doubt" (that is to say, it is about 90% likely that the defendant committed the act). Need for civil commitment is based on "clear and convincing" evidence (somewhere between 51% and 90%, maybe 70% to 80%). Legal insanity is determined by "a preponderance of the evidence" (the least, at 51%). The court does not restrict the reasons an insanity plea is entered. Examples of issues commonly raised are discussed in the following sections.

Psychosis or Chronic Mental Illness. Perhaps the defendant has a history of psychiatric hospitalizations, with a previous or current diagnosis of any major mental disorder. The defendant may be claiming command auditory hallucinations at the time of the alleged act, or perhaps witness statements include evidence of delusional thinking at the crime scene.

People with mental illness are quite capable of goal-oriented, reality-based decision making. The presence of a mental disorder does not automatically indicate the person was also legally insane. Case Study 49-1 illustrates the difference.

Case Study 49-1 Paranoid Joe and Delusional Behavior

Joe was first diagnosed with paranoid schizophrenia 20 years ago. He had been hospitalized 12 times. After discharge, he remained compliant with case management and prescribed medication for several months; however, he subsequently discontinued treatment and his mental state deteriorated. Part of his delusional system was the belief that orbiting satellites were sending him coded information from the CIA. He said the rays occasionally zapped him in the jaw, causing pain.

Joe discovered that lining the ceiling and walls of his trailer with aluminum foil prevented the rays from getting to him indoors. He spent his entire Social Security check for foil. Three days later, leaks in the foil led to continued electric shocks to his jaw. In his rage against the pain and harassment, Joe destroyed the inside of the trailer. His landlord became involved when others complained of the noise of breaking glass, yelling, and pounding. The landlord was unhappy with the damage. The police were called, and Joe was arrested for malicious mischief.

Six months later, after release from the state hospital, Joe was again living in the same trailer park. He became upset when his Social Security check did not arrive. He had not been attending the mental health center and did not want to contact his case manager for assistance. The nearest Social Security office was 70 miles away. Because he had no funds, he could not buy a bus ticket to get there. Despite the probability that he would be zapped repeatedly by the rays en route to the city, Joe took the landlord's car. He knew stealing a car was wrong, but he believed the urgency of his business justified his actions.

In both cases, Joe was acutely ill, paranoid, and experiencing somatic delusions. In the first scenario, his delusional beliefs directly influenced his criminal behavior. In the second, although he was again psychotic, Joe was legally sane for the act of stealing his landlord's car. His motivation was reality based. He needed transportation to the Social Security office and made a decision to risk arrest.

Developmental Disability. There are many reasons a person may be labeled as disabled. A disabled person may display cognitive difficulties only in a particular area. Many disabled people live independently. It is important to examine the defendant in terms of his or her mental age and level of functioning, rather than just simply an IQ number.

Sexual Deviancy. Either in a case involving criminal sexuality or when the defendant is revealed as practicing paraphilic tendencies, the forensic examiner may be required to explain to a jury that such behaviors do not presume the defendant to have a mental disorder. Because the general public does not consider some sexual practices normal, the jury may assume the defendant is mentally ill.

Post-Traumatic Stress Disorder. Post-traumatic stress disorder is described in the *Diagnostic and Statistical Manual of Mental Disorders* with such symptoms as hypervigilance, flashbacks, nightmares, anger, exaggerated startle response–all of which may be indicators of psychological distress at the time of the crime.

Medical Issues. Examples of physiologic problems that may prompt a request for a forensic evaluation include temporal lobe epilepsy, cerebral vascular accident (stroke), diabetic instability, a history of head injury, brain tumors, sleep anoxia, or other sleep disorders.

Malingering. A marked indicator for a diagnosis of malingering is that the person is facing a forensic evaluation. Aside from attempting to portray psychosis or mental retardation, creative malingerers invent self-described disorders such as Barnyard Animal Disease (only speaks with moos, quacks, oinks, and braying), Alternate Dimension Traveler (can snap one's fingers and go into a space-time continuum), victim of Alien Abduction, or My Evil Twin.

Munchausen's Syndrome by Proxy. Patients demonstrating factitious disorder are less likely to be seen on a forensic unit, unless arrested for fraudulent procurement of services. Their goal is to be the patient, rather than achieve other external incentives. But when the self-induced symptoms are produced in another, under one's care, and the other is seriously injured or dies, the defendant may rely on a defense of factitious disorder by proxy.

Medications. Many prescribed medications can alter cognition. Examples of presentations in court include "Prozac made me do the crime," "Steroids made me do the crime," and "Halcion made me do the crime." These defense strategies tend to be trendy. What's next? "Viagra made me do the crime"?

Personality Traits. It is a misnomer that all criminals are sociopathic. Only half the inmate population could be diagnosed as having an antisocial personality disorder, whereas about 15% of the general public would qualify. There are too many reasons why people commit crimes. As a defense, any personality disorder could be proffered (see Case Study 49-2).

Case Study 49-2 Obsessive-Compulsive Behavior and Violence

The inmate claimed to have obsessive-compulsive personality disorder. He stated he liked his cell orderly, with his shoes lined up at the door. "The guard was messing with me. He moved my books and shoes around. I had to hit him."

Erotomania. Stalking crimes have increased. Motivation behind such crimes can vary from the delusional thinking in schizophrenia to the narcissistic injury in the personality-disordered patient. Another possibility, though less common, is a delusional disorder, in which the theme is the unrequited love of someone who may not even be aware of the perpetrator's existence.

Cultural Issues. America is a land of immigrants and their descendants. Becoming a more mobile society since the 1960s has meant the loss of ethnic neighborhoods, where new immigrants could adjust slowly. Since the 1990s, immigrants have been thrown into an ethnically mixed society with abruptly different values and social behaviors. They may have difficulty assimilating. A defendant may attempt to present the clash and confusion of his or her value system against accepted American conduct as a basis for a criminal defense. Some examples are (1) an immigrant from an eastern European communist country believes he is being watched by the government and his cultural paranoia results in the stabbing of his sponsor; (2) an Arabic national misinterprets an American female's behavior and eye contact and stalks her, believing she has betrothed herself to him; or (3) a man whose homeland averred that a man's wife and children are his property is displeased by his teenage daughter's modern American ways and feels justified in ending her life.

Culture can mean a frame of reference for a value system, rather than ethnic background. For example, there are codes of behavior within gang structure that include respect, honor, belonging, and acceptable or unacceptable behavior. Groups of individuals come together under the banner of religious freedom while using illegal drugs (e.g., the Church of the Peyote) or forming a "church" that supports sex with children.

Other Issues. Depression is another commonly raised issue relative to legal insanity. Questions to consider include was the crime motivated by suicidal thought? Or was it motivated by a desire for "suicide by police"? (See Case Study 49-3.) Other issues include drug- or alcohol-induced blackout, amnesia, or dissociative states, including a claim of multiple personality disorder. (See Case Study 49-4.)

Case Study 49-3 Failed Marriage and Suicidal Ideation

The defendant explained, "My life was over when my wife left me. She flaunted the new boyfriend in public. The humiliation and shame was too much for me. I wanted to punish her for her sinful ways. I wanted her to find my body, so she could know how much I suffered for her. I wanted to die in that house where we had so many happy years together. I planned to shoot myself. At some point I called 911 and told them what I was going to do. They sent the cops over. Her new boyfriend is a cop. I figured it would be final irony to have one of them shoot me, so I started firing at the car when they drove up."

Case Study 49-4 Drug Abuse and Rape

The defendant explained that although he had used a variety of street drugs over the past 20 years, he had not abused Merazine before last summer. On the date of the alleged act, he drank approximately six beers and took 30 Merazine tablets. He claimed to have no memory for the events leading to his arrest. His girlfriend reported they went to bed around 10 p.m. At 2 a.m., the defendant got out of bed, dressed, and went out the front door. He returned two hours later. He is accused of entering the mobile home across the street, taking the six-year-old from her bed, carrying her outside, and raping her in the field next door.

Diminished Capacity

Diminished capacity is an element of the insanity law that refers to the defendant's capacity to form the intent to commit a specific act. There are four levels of intent (purposely, knowingly, recklessly, or negligently), and a court may order an evaluation specific to one level, depending on the crime charged. The criteria for a finding of diminished capacity are based on a legal standard in each state. In Washington *(Edmon v. Washington)* the cause of the inability to form intent must be a mental disorder, not amounting to insanity, and not emotions like jealousy, fear, anger, or hatred. The mental disorder must be causally connected to a lack of specific intent, not just reduced perception, awareness, understanding, or overreaction. A "crime of passion" would not qualify. For example, it is not uncommon for people with drug or alcohol intoxication to initiate a defense of diminished capacity, especially if a blackout occurred. The defendant will exclaim, "How can you hold me responsible for doing something I can't remember doing?" However, having a blackout only means one cannot remember, not that one was unable to make decisions at the time. It is true that judgment is impaired and sensibilities are deadened while intoxicated; however, altering one's own cognition voluntarily should not excuse criminal behavior. Many states have case law stipulating that voluntary consumption or intoxication precludes the defense (for example, *State v. Wicks,* 1983). On the other hand, if a person is drugged involuntarily and then, while under the influence, commits a criminal act, the behavior may be excused. Potentially eligible diminished capacity defenses are illustrated in Case Studies 49-5, 49-6, and 49-7.

Case Study 49-5 Bipolar Mischief

The defendant had an undiagnosed bipolar disorder. She visited her family physician, complaining of difficulty sleeping. He interpreted her complaints as worry from marital problems and prescribed an antidepressant medication. Her hypomanic behavior escalated. On a follow-up visit, the doctor increased the dosage. She went into a manic state and decided to redecorate the downtown businesses. After painting brick walls pink and removing several windows, she was arrested for malicious mischief.

Case Study 49-6 Depression and Shoplifting

The defendant was referred to an HMO for depression. He was prescribed an antidepressant. Because he did not feel better soon, he saw a different doctor, who prescribed another medication. The defendant did not tell the physician he was already taking a medication that was contraindicated. Three days later, he became confused and disoriented. He wandered aimlessly in a strange neighborhood, eventually walking into a small grocery store. He picked up some items at the front counter and ambled out, seemingly oblivious to the clerk's calls to stop. Police followed a trail of dropped items to find him sleeping under a tree.

Case Study 49-7 Alcohol and Drugs Don't Mix

The defendant attended a fraternity party, planning on a few beers before going home. While there, someone slipped LSD into his drink. The defendant had never used LSD and would not choose to use it. While under the influence, he became aggressive and delirious. He damaged property and furniture in the building and was later charged with assault and destruction of property. A blood test in the ER following arrest confirmed a high level of the drug in his system.

Competent to Proceed

Another issue to be answered is whether or not the person is competent to proceed. The question of competency to stand trial is considered the most important mental health inquiry pursued within the criminal law system (Stone, 1978). An estimated 25,000 defendants are evaluated annually in the US (Winick, 1995). Criminal insanity is a test of culpability. Competence to stand trial is an issue of "try-ability."

As far back as the eighteenth century, courts were concerned about a person being able to make a well-informed plea and establishing a defense. In the *Frith* case of 1790, the court stated, "No man shall be called upon to make his defense at a time when his mind is in that situation as not to appear capable of so doing, for however guilty he may be, the inquiry into his guilt must be postponed to that season when by collecting together his intellects, and having them entire, he shall be able so to model his defense as to ward off the punishment of the law."

At the turn of the nineteenth century, the circuit court judge hearing a famous case involving an assault on Andrew Jackson remarked that if a mad man is placed on trial, the judge may use discretion, discharging the jury, and sending him to jail to be tried after the recovery of his understanding.

In 1899, the Sixth Circuit court held that "It is not due process of law to subject an insane person to trial upon an indictment involving liberty of life" *(Youtsey v. US,* 1899).

By the turn of the twentieth century, a test for competency was developing. The ruling in *US v. Chisholm* (1901) alluded to the cognitive powers and communication capabilities of the defendant. Sixty years later, such capacity and skills were specifically stated in a Supreme Court ruling *(Dusky v. US,* 1960). American law elevated the competency rule into a constitutional principle *(Drope v. Missouri)* in 1975.

Whereas legal sanity issues are framed at the time of the alleged act, competency is in the future: "Will the defendant be competent on the day of the hearing/trial?" *Competent to proceed* is defined as having the capacity to assist one's attorney and to understand the proceedings. The legal standard in most jurisdictions for competence to stand trial is *Dusky v. US.* This case brought forth the question, "Does the defendant have sufficient present ability to consult with his lawyer with a reasonable degree of rational understanding and whether he has a rational and factual understanding of the nature of the proceedings against him?"

Mental retardation does not in itself result in incompetency to stand trial. Developmental disabilities occur in many varied forms and may impact the capacity of the accused to comprehend the proceedings. A disabled person may experience short attention spans, poor memory, difficulty following direction, poor reading and comprehension, and other problems. Reasoning may be deficient or illogical. One does not need to be literate to be deemed competent.

"The presence of a mental illness does not mean that an accused is not mentally competent to stand trial" *(Feguer v. US,* 1962). It is the degree to which the symptoms affect the abilities and skills needed to be competent. The presence of delusions may or may not have an impact (Goldstein & Burd, 1990).

Because it is a determination of mental state in the future, a defendant's competency must be determined anew each time the defendant goes to court. A prior finding of incompetency, even when due to developmental disability, does not preclude a subsequent finding of competency in a later, unrelated case *(State v. Minnix,* 1991). Box 49-4 lists some typical questions a defense attorney might be asked.

The national standard for competence is the McGarry checklist. The 13 criteria are intended to cover all possible grounds for a finding of incompetency. The court may weigh each item differently, or selectively weigh items differently for individual defendants. A serious mental disability arising out of psychosis or mental retardation, even at the moderate level, does not rule out competency. A disability is relevant to the determination of competency only if it results in malfunctioning in one or more of the specific items of the checklist (Brooks, 1974). Box 49-5 lists and explains the 13 criteria.

Box 49-4 Determining Client Competence

In determining whether a client is competent to proceed, one should ask the following questions:

Can the defendant consult with someone rationally?

Does the defendant have a factual and rational understanding of the proceedings?

Does the defendant understand the defense to be used?

Does the defendant understand the plea options?

Will the defendant be able to help pick a jury?

Will the defendant be able to follow the evidence presented?

Will the defendant be able to advise counsel during adverse evidence?

Can the defendant help locate witnesses?

Does the defendant understand he or she may testify? If the defendant agrees to testify, could he or she do so relevantly?

Occasionally the court will request an evaluation on a specific competency issue, such as "competent to act as one's own attorney." To waive the right to representation requires a higher level of competence than that required to stand trial (*State v. Hahn,* 1985). Other specific evaluations include "competent to give the confession," "competent to be sentenced," or "competent to receive the death penalty."

A number of structured interview/assessment tools address competence. These include the Competency Screening Test developed by McGarry and his colleagues (Laboratory of Community Psychiatry, 1973; Lipsitt, Lelos, & McGarry, 1971), the Competency Assessment Interview (ref), the Competency to Stand Trial Assessment Instrument (Laboratory of Community Psychiatry, 1973), the Interdisciplinary Fitness Interview (Golding, Roesch, & Schreiber, 1984) and the Georgia Court Competency Test (Wildman, Batchelor, & Thompson et al., 1980). Further studies have indicated that there is no correlation between diagnosis of psychosis and performance on these tests. The tests can be used as an adjutant in determination, but they should not be used as the sole qualifier.

Competency Therapist

A conviction of an incompetent defendant is considered a violation of the Fourteenth Amendment–the right to due process. When a defendant is determined to be incompetent, the court can order the defendant to "a suitable facility," usually a secure location, for "treatment to regain competency." Another specialized role performed by the psychiatric forensic nurse is to work as the competency therapist with such patients.

In most locations across the country, treatment to regain competency is limited to the prescribing of psychotropic medications. Such an approach equates psychosis with incompetence and presumes that stabilization returns the defendant to competence. However, many of the 13 items listed in Box 49-5 are not directly related to mental illness.

The author has developed a bio-psycho-social treatment program that has been lauded by hospital accrediting agencies for its comprehensive treatment of such individuals. Within this program is a series of 24 classes in three phases that address the 13 items on the McGarry checklist. In the first phase, the patient may present with active symptoms of psychosis. In the second phase, the patient may still be delusional, but his or her contact with

Box 49-5 McGarry Checklist

1. Appraisal of available legal defenses:
   Is the defendant aware of the possible legal defenses? Are they consistent with the defendant's particular circumstances? Ask, "How can you explain your way out of these charges?" "What should your lawyer do to defend you?"
2. Unmanageable behavior:
   Will the defendant's verbal or physical behavior disrupt the courtroom? If the defendant is disruptive or inappropriate, it must be due to a substantial degree of mental disorder.
3. Quality of relating to an attorney:
   Does the defendant have the ability to trust and communicate relevantly? Ask, "Do you have confidence in your lawyer?" "Do you think your lawyer is doing a good job for you?" "Do you agree with the way your lawyer is handling your case?"
4. Planning of legal strategy including guilty pleas to lesser charges where pertinent:
   Can the defendant understand, participate, and cooperate with counsel in planning strategy? Issues may include plea bargaining, change of venue, consideration of an insanity defense, or decision to testify. Cooperation can be passive, but does the defendant accept the attorney's strategy, or does the defendant give irrational instructions to his or her attorney or insist on defending himself or herself on the basis of an irrational theory?
5. Appraisal of the role of the principals involved in the courtroom:
   The defendant should be able to describe the courtroom process as adversarial. The defendant should be able to identify the prosecutor and prosecution witnesses as being against him or her, his or her attorney as being for the defense, the judge as neutral, and should know that the judge or jury determines the verdict.
6. Understanding of the court procedure:
   Does the defendant understand the basic sequence of events in a trial? Ask what is a cross-examination? Must a person testify? If one decides to testify, what happens after the lawyer finishes asking questions?
7. Appreciation of the charges:
   Does the defendant have a concrete understanding of the charge against him? And the seriousness of the charge?
8. Appreciation of the range and nature of possible penalties:
   Does the defendant have a simple, concrete understanding of the conditions and restrictions that could be imposed?
9. Appraisal of likely outcome:
   How realistically does the defendant perceive the likely outcome of the case? Does the defendant irrationally perceive that there is little to no peril against him or her when the case is strong? Does the defendant accept the jurisdiction of the court? Ask, "What do you think your chances are of being found not guilty?" "Does the court have authority over you?" "How strong a case does the prosecution have against you?"
10. Capacity to disclose to attorney available pertinent facts surrounding the offense, including the defendant's movement, timing, mental state, and actions at the time of the offense:
    Can the defendant give a consistent, rational, relevant account of fact, including motivation? Take into consideration honesty, memory, and intelligence, as well as a possible disparity between what the defendant is willing to share.
11. Capacity to realistically challenge the prosecution's witnesses:
    Can the defendant recognize distortions in the prosecution testimony? Can he or she be attentive? Does the defendant have memory problems that would interfere in his or her ability to follow the courtroom drama? Does the defendant have the initiative to notify his or her attorney if he or she disagrees with the accuracy of testimony?
12. Capacity to testify relevantly:
    Does the defendant have the ability to testify coherently and relevantly? What are the defendant's verbal communication skills?
13. Self-defeating versus self-serving motivation:
    Is the defendant motivated to adequately protect himself or herself? Is he or she pathologically seeking punishment? Is the defendant deliberately failing to avail himself or herself of appropriate legal protection? Are active self-destructive behaviors present?

Data from Brooks, A. (1974). *Law, psychiatry, and the mental health system* (pp. 351-361). Boston: Little, Brown.

Table 49-2 Three Phases

	PHASE I	PHASE II	PHASE III
Patient presents as	Having active symptoms. May be psychotic, confused, disoriented, uncooperative, and refusing medications or treatment.	May be psychotic, but is cooperative. Delusional but oriented. Argumentative, but willing to participate.	Stable. Has achieved maximum potential. Awaiting court hearing.
Focus of treatment	Reality orientation. Trust issues. Stabilization. Accepting treatment.	Interpersonal skills. Ability to work with attorney. Behavior in court.	Symptom management. Recognition of mental illness. Preparing for discharge.
Competency issues	Name of legal charge. Nature of the charge. Attorney name. Oriented × 3. Roles of the principals in the courtroom. Understanding of court order and purpose of hospitalization.	Plea choices. Consequences. Plea bargains. Ability to testify relevantly. Behavior in the courtroom.	Higher level competency issues: that is, diminished capacity, competent to be sentenced or give confession, or act as own attorney.
Competency therapy modalities	Video consent. 1:1 rather than group. Fitness game. Worksheets. Timelines.	Supplemental rights. Role play. Worksheets. Puzzles. Board games. Mock courtroom.	Review police reports. Review patient video. Worksheets. Mock courtroom.

reality and socialization skills have improved. The patient is able and willing to attend groups or classes, although the content of his discussion may not always be relevant. The third phase is one of reintegration. The patient has achieved his maximum potential emotionally, cognitively, and in competence. Table 49-2 summarizes the three phases.

In Phase I, the therapist focuses on concrete information and a rudimentary understanding that the patient is now involved in the criminal justice system. Classes center on the defendant's ability to understand some basic information: that he or she has been arrested and on what charge, the jeopardy for the charge, the name of his or her attorney, and the roles of the courtroom participants. Because patients in this phase may be acutely psychotic, it is sometimes necessary to meet briefly (5 to 10 minutes) with individuals, instead of attempting the 30-to-40-minute group. The content of these meetings is repetitive because retention of the information may be poor. As an example, objectives for a Phase I class on arrest, booking, incarceration, and trial may include the following:

- Patient will demonstrate an ability to place events in proper sequence on a timeline.
- Patient will be able to identify where he or she is now on the timeline.
- Patient will be able to complete a more detailed timeline without assistance.

The patient will advance to Phase II when he or she has mastered the concepts in Phase I and is able to participate in group discussion (usually two weeks). It is not necessary that the patient be free of delusional thinking. In Phase II, the patient is given a prepared packet of information and is expected to attend classes, complete worksheets, and participate in group activities (games, role-play, mock courtroom activities). The patient's written work, as well as the therapist's documentation of the patient's participation, becomes part of the evidence of competence when the patient returns to court. Boxes 49-6 and 49-7 are a sample class outline and a worksheet for Phase II.

Patients move to Phase III when they have mastered the concepts on Phase II. In Phase III, personal issues are discussed privately with the therapist (i.e., reviewing contents of the police reports). The patient continues group classes and activities. Together they review a videotaped interview recorded when the patient was in Phase I and use it as a learning tool during medication teaching.

Throughout the course, it is important for therapists to emphasize to patients that the therapist is not an attorney and is not giving legal advice. Information given to the patient, such as "You are entitled to use an insanity plea, but you have other options. That is a choice you will make with your attorney," is based on case law (in this case, *State v. Jones*).

At the end of the court-ordered hospitalization, a formal letter to court will offer an expert opinion on competency. The therapist may be called to testify as to the basis for the opinion. The therapist's opinion gives the court information on which to base its finding. Not all states require a specific court hearing and testimony before finding the defendant competent. The court may make its finding on competency based on the written report. Both defense and prosecution attorneys in the expert's jurisdiction will know the reliability of the expert's report, based on previous patients, and may be willing to defer to its conclusions. Therefore, the reputation of the therapist/expert and the descriptive writing of the letter become emphasized. For rural areas, this may also be important because it will decrease the number of court appearances required by the expert.

Consultant to Prosecution or Defense

The psychiatric forensic nurse may be asked by prosecution attorneys to assist in preparing for trial by providing education: "How can the psychologists' report of testing be more easily explained to a jury?" "Do you have suggestions on questions I should ask

Box 49-6 Phase II Class Evidence Worksheet

RELATED COMPETENCY ITEMS

- Understanding of arrest process
- Understanding of legal process/evidence
- Capacity to disclose to lawyer
- Appraisal of available legal defenses

OBJECTIVES

1. Client will verbalize understanding that evidence is used to convict.
2. Client will attempt to recall receiving his or her rights at arrest.
3. Client will discuss the various kinds of evidence that are presented in a criminal trial:
    - Weapon
    - Eye-witness account
    - Videotape
    - Fingerprints
    - Footprints
    - Tire prints
    - Voice recording
    - Clothing
    - Confession
    - Police reports
    - Urinalysis
    - Location
    - Ballistics report
    - Handwriting
    - Photographs
    - Property damage
    - Physical injury
    - Medical reports
    - Blood type
    - DNA
    - Tools
    - Serial numbers
    - Breathalyzer
    - Other

CONTENT/ CONCEPTS

- Evidence
- Confession
- Statement
- Miranda rights
- Probable cause

LEARNING ACTIVITY

- Worksheet Q (see Box 49-7)

Box 49-7 Evidence Worksheet

WORKSHEET Q

Pretest:____ Posttest:____ Other ____

Patient's Name:____________________ Date: ________

The following situations led to an arrest. What items might be presented as evidence at the trial?

1. A stereo is stolen from a house:________________
2. A man is beaten up behind a bar: ________________
3. A threatening message is left on an answering machine: ________________
4. A garage is set on fire:________________
5. A bank is held up: ________________
6. A woman is sexually assaulted in a park: ________________
7. A drive-by shooting leaves holes in a front door: ________________
8. A plastic baggie full of white powder is found in a pocket: ________________
9. Headlights and the rear window are shattered: ________________
10. The car runs into a telephone pole: ________________

the defense psychiatrist?" "What information is needed to counter the psychiatrist's testimony?" The psychiatric forensic nurse may be used as a resource for education and information about mental illness and may be asked to testify on her or his opinion regarding the dangerousness of the patient in the community.

Defense counsel may also consult with the psychiatric forensic nurse: "How can I teach the jury about the defendant's mental illness?" The psychiatric forensic nurse may be used as a resource for information about mental health treatment options, medications, and community resources and may be asked to testify on the defendant's amenability to treatment.

Either side may request the forensic psychiatric forensic nurse to attend the hearing as a courtroom observer who listens to other witness testimony and makes observations about the defendant's behavior or testimony for the purpose of guiding further cross-examination.

Consultant to Law Enforcement

Since the 1980s, there has been an increase in interagency cooperation between law enforcement and community mental health agencies. The functions of mental health personnel in those situations are deescalation, civil detention, and referral of the patient to a hospital or into agency care. The mental health worker summons advocates for the patient, and the patient's well-being becomes consultant's focus. This is a needed and appropriate interagency cooperation for the mentally ill or suicidal patient.

The new area of practice for psychiatric forensic nurses is the expansion of their expertise into the realm of the behavioral sciences and to act as a consultant to law enforcement (Coram, 1993a). This is a forensic role function that differs in skill and philosophy from the role of mental health personnel who may be present at the same scene.

In the late 1970s, the Federal Bureau of Investigation (FBI) began expanding hostage negotiation team structure by recommending the use of consultants regarding the mental status of the perpetrator and appropriate negotiation strategies (Fuselier, 1981). In the next decade, police agencies began to develop specialized teams and use consultants (Fuselier, 1988). In most agencies, the consultant is a police psychologist.

As a consultant to law enforcement, psychiatric forensic nurses use many of the same skills and techniques they use as forensic examiners. In this role, the nurse is not an advocate of the patient (perpetrator), but of the process.

The consultant is called on-scene with negotiators and tactical teams. The duties typically include the following:

- Consultation regarding specific negotiation techniques
- Assessment of the perpetrator
- Interview of others for background information
- Interview of released hostages
- Liaison with mental health agencies/caregivers involved with the perpetrator
- Incident counseling for police and victims after the incident
- Participation in post-incident critique (Fuselier, 1988)

It may be difficult for some law enforcement agencies to accept someone outside the department. "I needed to know if she was pro-cop. I mean, can I trust her? Is she going to put me in a position where I might get killed?" It is necessary for the consultant to have an understanding of police culture, from the language to the devotion to duty. Acceptance into this role may be tested; but once given, it is long honored.

The consultant has no supervisory power or authority and must be willing to accept the idea that after hours of negotiation it may become necessary to attempt to capture or even kill the hostage taker. The line officers, tactical team, and command post need to believe that the consultant accepts that possibility and would be willing to assist.

To be contributive as consultants, psychiatric forensic nurses should have characteristics similar to those of successful negotiators (Fuselier, 1981). They must be able to think clearly under stress, possess emotional maturity, and to maintain a clear head when those around them are anxious, frightened, or confused. They must be able to accept abuse, ridicule, and insults without responding emotionally and should have the ability to use logical arguments and communicate with people from all socioeconomic classes. Psychiatric forensic nurses should have common sense and be "street wise." They should be able to cope with uncertainty (time, location, weather, outcome) and be willing to accept responsibility with no authority. They should express a total commitment to the negotiation process, but understand clearly their potential role in any plan to assault in a rescue. It is essential that the consultants receive the same negotiator training as the officers.

Information from the FBI Academy indicates that more than half of all hostage incidents involve people classified as mentally disturbed. This includes people with a thought disorder, mood disorder, or personality disorder. Although it is essential that the consultant have knowledge about psychiatric illness, a forensic background is more congruent to the goals of negotiation than is a profession in mental health. Most mental health professionals have a lack of experience dealing with armed individuals making threats, and they are reluctant to play a role in manipulating the perpetrator into a position that would facilitate an attack by the SWAT team.

A study by Butler, Leitenberg, and Fuselier (1993) found that police agencies that use a consultant in hostage incidents reported significantly more negotiated surrenders, significantly fewer incidents ending with tactical team assault, and fewer incidents in which the perpetrator killed or seriously injured a hostage.

Criminal Profiling

For centuries there have been attempts to describe physical or psychological attributes that indicate criminal types. The actual origins of criminal profiling are obscure (Pinizzotto, 1984). In 1971 the FBI first used the psychological profile when it assisted local law enforcement in solving a murder case. The formal process has been renamed as criminal investigation analysis, but the more common term continues to be used, perhaps because it is reinforced by the media and in entertainment. Unlike its portrayal on television, psychological profiling is only one investigative tool among many. It is not magic or ESP. It is not a substitute for a thorough and well-planned investigation. The purpose of profiling is to provide law enforcement investigators with information that will help eliminate suspects or narrow leads.

The method of developing a profile is similar to the nursing process. The profiler will collect all the data, attempt to reconstruct the situation, formulate hypotheses, develop a profile, test it, and check the results. The first step consists of an examination of the crime scene (including photos of body positioning), review of autopsy results or medical records (including toxicology and wound description), and study of the victimology apparent.

In the second step, the profiler will generally be looking at three points in time: preoffense behavior, during the offense, and post-offense behavior. The hypothesis is formed when the psychopathological elements are identified. This is the point at which the profiler's knowledge becomes useful. Whereas a background in behavioral science is fundamental, other specialized education is not as important as having investigative experience. Profilers come from a variety of backgrounds: law enforcement, psychology, psychiatry, criminal justice, sociology, and nursing. A profiler with common sense, "street sense," and intuition is more valuable. Intuition cannot be learned, but it is enhanced by experience.

In testing the hypothesis, the skilled profiler will isolate his or her own emotions and attempt to reconstruct the crime using the criminal's reasoning process. Attempts to analyze the situation based on one's own values or logic will result in a misinterpretation of the behavior. Skilled profilers are patient and reserve conclusions while examining the data. When frustrated or puzzled, skilled profilers keep in mind that there is an explanation for the behavior–it may just not be apparent yet.

Profilers can be used in ways other than investigation. Law enforcement may ask profilers for suggestions regarding how to interview and interrogate suspects. Profilers may be called on to assist prosecutors by suggesting techniques in cross-examining defendants.

Consultant to the Community

Psychiatric forensic nurses have entrepreneurial opportunities similar to those available to forensic mental health nurses. Examples are providing education/training to correctional staff and responding to requests by private businesses for assessment of potential for workplace violence. Ball (1990) identified the principle of market segmentation, which is simply to identify and define the target group that requires CNS services and then develop services to meet the demands of the customer. This marketing strategy claims service promotion is essential to role success.

Forensic nurses who strive to expand the influence of their pioneering roles participate in public forums that address violence as a healthcare issue. Psychiatric forensic nurses can become catalysts and attempt to effect social change by participating on local or statewide task forces examining needed changes or amendments in the law. They are activists when petitioning the legislature for new law. Examples of practice in this area include interagency work on a diversion program for mentally ill misdemeanants, drafting legislation affecting legal sanity commitment, or proposing law to allow prosecution of psychiatric inpatients for serious assault on staff.

Key Court Testimony Considerations

All forensic nurses are in positions that may require court appearance as a fact witness. The psychiatric forensic nurse, however, is in the unique position of being called to court as an expert witness.

Role of the Expert Witness

A fact witness testifies to direct observations made. She or he does not offer expert opinions or draw conclusions from the reports of others. An expert witness has facts directly related to some body of knowledge that is beyond the scope of the layperson. An expert witness may offer opinion. Nurses, by their license and responsibilities, have been called to court as fact witnesses for decades. It is an expansion of the RN scope of practice to be considered as an expert in a court of law alongside surgeons, clinical psychologists, psychiatrists, and others.

Once on the stand, the psychiatric forensic nurse undergoes a three-step process to be deemed an expert. The attorney asks questions regarding training, experience, and specialized knowledge. The witness answers the questions, and the judge concludes acceptance as an expert. It is helpful to take a copy of one's current curriculum vitae to court and to offer it to the attorney prior to the hearing as an aid in chronological questioning. The psychiatric forensic nurse who has testified repeatedly in her or his jurisdiction may find that steps 1 and 2 are waived. When the attorney calls the forensic nurse to the stand, the judge may reply, for example, "Yes, Ms. Smith is well-known to this court. I will stipulate to her acceptance as an expert witness."

To establish credibility as an expert and to have one's opinion assigned equal weight in court opposite a psychiatrist, the forensic nurse specialist must have expertise, trustworthiness, and presentational style. Expertise is established by one's credentials, including academic background, professional training, experience, and professional association. Rule 702 of the Federal Rules of Evidence states, "If scientific, technical, or other specialized knowledge will assist the trier of fact to understand the evidence or to determine a fact in issue, a witness qualified as an expert by knowledge, skill, experience, training, or education, may testify thereto in the form of an opinion or otherwise."

Trustworthiness, as perceived by the judge or jury, is the degree of honesty in one's demeanor and opinion. Research (Birnbaum & Stegner, 1979) demonstrates that testimony from an unbiased source will be given more weight than biased sources with the same perceived expertise. The jury perceives the witness as trustworthy if he or she remains calm, unruffled, and cooperative.

Presentational style includes dress, demeanor, and the ability to communicate to a jury. Although the two responsibilities of the expert witness are to be authoritative in the area of specialization and to be of value to the judge or jury, it is imperative that the forensic examiner be an effective communicator (Bank & Poythress, 1982). One can have the foremost authority, but without the ability to communicate in a concise and convincing fashion, the value of the testimony will be severely limited.

Skill is necessary in the verbal communication of testimony, as well as the written report completed and submitted prior to the hearing or trial. The ability to explain one's legal opinion succinctly, and with justification, is of more value than a lengthy, verbose document filled with terminology of the profession. The written report should be self-sufficient. If other documents were used to reach the opinion, they should be briefly summarized within the report.

The courtroom is theater. It has been said that 80% of jurors make up their minds during the opening statements. Possibly more than anywhere else, the power of a positive first impression is played out in a courtroom. An effective expert witness understands the impact of dress and demeanor on the psyche of a jury and has prepared in this way also. The forensic nurse specialist will wear clothing that projects the same expert power as others being called to testify. Briefly, guidelines for dress are a conservative suit (gray or dark blue), with understated jewelry, hair, and makeup. Cell phones, umbrellas, lab coats and stethoscopes, fur coats, or sunglasses are absolutely not carried to the witness stand. Those who are new to expert witness testimony will be well advised to follow the simple rules described in Box 49-8.

Ethical Standards

Forensic nursing is predicated on the search for truth. Forensic nurses are not tools of the prosecution. It is important for the pioneers within psychiatric forensic nursing to hold firmly to professional ethics. Those that provide expert witness services should

Box 49-8 Rules for Expert Witnesses

1. When approached by an attorney, the fees and terms (if any) should be clearly established. Discuss the case in enough detail to unveil any possible conflict of interest. If there is any, acknowledge it now.
2. Remember to educate the court or jury. The expert is not there to convict or defend or to justify the defendant's actions. State what is known to be fact, and only offer opinion when asked. The jury will decide if it wants to accept or reject the opinion.
3. Have a current and accurate curriculum vitae, and be able to elaborate on it if asked. Never inflate your professional background.
4. Be prepared. Reread the case the night before. Know the report. Be able to explain how the opinion was formed. Meet with the attorney prior to the hearing.
5. Don't develop a "star witness" fantasy. Don't get carried away on the stand. Never give an opinion about things in which you are not trained. Never give an opinion you cannot support. Know when to state, "That is outside my scope of practice."
6. Tell the truth, always. Remember it is permissible to say you have not formed an opinion. Likewise, it is all right to say you were wrong or that you don't know.
7. Watch out for absolutes. Watch for traps during cross-examination; for example, statistics related to dangerousness (Standing Bear, 1999).
8. Speak in simple terms. Define technical words, and make them easy to understand. Stay away from jargon and "psychobabble". When the attorney requests a "yes or no" response, the expert may ask the judge if she can qualify her answer. It is permissible to refer to written records to refresh your memory.
9. During testimony, try to state your opinion three times in three different ways.
10. Appear genuine and sincere. Be yourself. Do not try to copy someone else's style. Appear dignified and confident, yet humble.
11. Listen to the questions and think before answering. Structure the thought. Avoid appearing defensive. The expert may ask the judge if he or she has a concern about how to answer the question posed. The expert may ask the judge if the material requested is privileged. The expert can refuse to answer a question not understood or can ask the attorney to clarify the question.
12. Look at the jury members. Don't talk down to them. Smile, if appropriate. Watch humor. If you stumble, shrug it off (for instance, spilling your water glass). A jury will appreciate the expert showing he or she is human.
13. Do not offer information. There may be a valid reason why a certain question was not asked. For example, the answer may violate a prior court order limiting testimony and the volunteered response may result in a mistrial.
14. Pay attention to your vocal patterns, body language, and mannerisms. Avoid appearing defensive. Handle your emotions. Don't lose patience or your temper. If interrupted, continue to speak through the interruption or protest, calmly. You have a right to complete your answer.
15. When finished testifying, leave the courtroom. Staying to listen suggests one might be personally involved, rather than emotionally removed, from the proceedings.
16. After the trial, meet with the attorney to debrief. Ask what you did well. Bring up questions that were not asked that should have been to get the most out of your testimony. Reflect on the experience. Use this as education in your professional growth. For example, learn about note-taking practices, interviewing style, or something that will make you a better witness next time.

never be viewed as "hired guns"–those that proffer testimony at a purchase price. Forensic nurses take pride in the integrity of their opinions. Psychiatric forensic nurses will not allow themselves to be swept up by the human need to be identified with their opinions. They will never sacrifice truth for the sake of persuasion ("We won!" or "We got him!").

Best Practice *49-3*

Forensic nurses will tenaciously guard their professional ethics and the integrity of their opinions, never sacrificing truth for the sake of persuasion.

Personal Safety

Due to the nature of the nurse-patient relationship in psychiatric forensic nursing, the interaction is usually involuntary on the part of the patient. The patient is not seeking the services of the nurse and is not necessarily going to cooperate with any proceedings by actively participating. Although it is true that everyone is capable of committing a crime given the right circumstances, and that not all criminals are bad people, some are.

In working with violent perpetrators, predators, and those who are mean just for the sake of continuing a lifetime of being threatening, intimidating, harassing, overbearing, or profane, it will be a natural occurrence to feel afraid–for oneself, one's family, one's property. All may be threatened. Acknowledge the feeling when it happens and be willing to talk about it. It is worrisome when individuals are not afraid, since being scared is self-protective.

The Department of Corrections provides the Victim-Witness Notification Program. It notifies participants when a violent, sex or serious drug offender moves through the system. The forensic nurse specialist becomes eligible after being identified as a witness for the prosecution if the offender was found guilty. The FNE is notified when these offenders are approved for furlough from a prison or work-release facility, approved for parole, complete their sentences, transfer from prison to work release or community supervision, escape from custody, or are recaptured.

Summary

Holt (1984) proposed that every clinical nurse specialist articulate a conceptual framework for nursing practice in her or his own specialty to organize key concepts used in that practice and to provide for a conscious framework for decision making. Professional development should be planned at all levels of nursing. Each registered nurse must structure and implement an individualized professional plan to reach his or her highest career potential. "If each CNS fulfills this role within her own particular specialty, the authority and power of that expertise will echo across the nation, the quality of healthcare will change . . . and the CNS will achieve her mission of excellence in the quality of nursing care for all patients" (Holt, 1984, p. 448).

McGivern (1986) claimed that the expanded role is as much a way of thinking as it is a set of functions. To push the limits of one's scope of practice requires personal gumption and a commitment to the future of the profession. Nursing places high value on its traditions. Challenge to those who push the boundaries will come as much from within the profession as from the outside.

Ball (1990) pointed out that facilitation of the CNS role to its highest potential will include role acceptance by nursing, medicine, and other professionals. Successful introduction of the role of the psychiatric forensic nurse specialist will set a precedent for other nurse specialists who will follow. Anyone who meets the challenge of developing a new CNS role must have justifiable confidence in one's own knowledge and ability and in one's self as an individual. One needs to have strong convictions about the value of the CNS role in which one is functioning and an appreciation of the far-reaching effects it can have on the professional practice of nursing (Barrett, 1971).

Nursing is a career still predominantly held by females. Psychiatric forensic nursing overlaps into areas that are not only new for nursing, but also for women. Traits necessary to succeed in this area are aggression, autonomy, and assertiveness. These are less tolerated in women (Ednie, 1996). Ednie wrote, "Women in forensic psychiatry must confront obstacles imposed by predominantly male systems and patients, and learn to cope with dangerous situations and hostile environments" (p. 43). The challenges are being identified as professional, finding mentors, breaking into the "good old boy network," not being viewed as having the same amount of "expert power" as men, working in a predominantly male atmosphere, communicating in an effective manner, and the issue of danger and the threat of violence.

So why do it? Personal happiness and career satisfaction come when there is congruence between one's personality, life's mission, and work role. Psychiatric forensic nursing appeals to a particular type of nurse, whether male or female. These nurses thrive on the opportunities to work in a stimulating intellectual environment; they seek opportunity to apply clinical skills to complex legal problems. For those who seek entrepreneurial openings, there is a chance for independent practice. For the nurse who strives to make a difference, this subspecialty holds the opportunity to affect individuals, groups, and the community and to be a force for change in the response to violence as a healthcare issue.

Resources

Organizations

American Academy of Forensic Sciences

410 North 21st Street, Colorado Springs, CO 80904; Tel: 719-636-1100; www.aafs.org

American Board of Forensic Nursing and American College of Forensic Examiners

ACFE Institute of Forensic Science, 2750 East Sunshine, Springfield, MO 65804; Tel: 417-881-3818, 800-423-9737 (toll-free); www.acfei.com

American Psychiatric Nurses Association

1555 Wilson Blvd, Suite 602, Arlington, VA 22209; Tel: 703-243-2443; www.apna.org

International Association of Forensic Nurses

East Holly Avenue, Box 56, Pittman, NJ 08071-0056; www.forensicnurse.org

References

American Nurses Association (ANA). (1980). *Nursing: Social Policy Statement (Publication No. NP-68A).* Kansas City, MO: Author

American Nurses Association (ANA). (1985). *Standards of nursing practice in correctional facilities.* Kansas City, MO: Author.

Ball, G. (1990). Perspectives on developing, marketing, and implementing a new clinical specialist position. *Clin Nurse Spec, 4*(1), 33-36.

Bank, S., & Poythress, N. (1982). Persuasion and ethics in expert testimony. *Kentucky Defense Counsel Newsletter, 2*(2), 2-6.

Barrett, J. (1971). Administrative factors in development of new practice roles. *J Nurs Adm,3,* 25-29.

Bencer, B. (1989). Caring for clients with legal charges on a voluntary psychiatric unit. *J Psychosoc Nurs, 27*(3), 16-20.

Birnbaum, M. H., & Stegner, S. E. (1979). Source credibility in social judgment: Bias, expertise, and the judge's point of view. *J Pers Soc Psychol, 37,* 48-74.

Brooks, A. (1974). *Law, psychiatry, and the mental health system* (pp. 351-361). Boston: Little, Brown.

Butler, W., Leitenberg, H., & Fuselier, G. (1993). The use of mental health professional consultants to police hostage negotiation teams. *Behav Sci Law, 11,* 213-221.

Cirincione, C., Steadman, H., & McGreevy, M. (1995). Rates of insanity acquittals and the factors associated with successful insanity pleas. *Bull Am Acad Psychiatry Law, 23*(3), 399-408.

Coram, J. (1993a). Forensic nurse specialists: Working with perpetrators and hostage negotiation teams. *J Psychosoc Nurs, 31*(11).

Coram, J. (1993b). *Role development within a new sub-specialty: Forensic nursing.* Master's thesis. Spokane, WA: Washington State University.

Drope v. Missouri, 420 US 162 (1975).

Dusky v. US, 362 US 402 (1960).

Ednie, K. (1996, Spring). Challenges for women in forensic psychiatry. *New Dir Ment Health Serv, 69,* 43-48.

Feguer v. US, 302 F 2 d 214 (CA8), cert. denied, 371 US 872. (1962).

Frith, 22 Howell St. Tr. 307, 311 (1970).

Fuselier, G. (1981, June/July). A practical overview of hostage negotiations. *FBI Law Enforcement Bull,* 1-11.

Fuselier, G. (1988). Hostage negotiation consultant: Emerging role for the clinical psychologist. *Prof Psychol Res Pr, 19,* 175-179.

Golding, G., Roesch, R., & Schreiber, J. (1984). Assessment and conceptualization of competency to stand trial. *Law Hum Behav, 8*(14), 321-334.

Goldstein, A., & Burd, M. (1990). Role of delusions in trial competency evaluations: Case law and implications for forensic practice. *Forensic Rep, 3,* 361-386.

Hirst, S. P., & Metcalf, B. J. (1986). Learning needs of caregivers. *J Gerontol Nurs, 12,* 24-28.

Holt, F. M., (1984). A theoretical model for clinical specialist practice. *Nurs Heath Care, 5*(8), pp. 445-449.

King, I. (1971). *Toward a theory for nursing.* New York: John Wiley & Sons.

Laboratory of Community Psychiatry, Harvard University. (1973). *Competency to stand trial and mental illness.* DHEW Pub. No. (HSM) 73-9105. Rockville, MD: National Institute of Mental Health, Center for Studies of Crime and Delinquency.

Lipsett, P., Lelos, D., & McGarry, A. (1971). Competency for trial: A screening instrument. *Am J Psychiatry, 128,* 105-109.

Lynch, V. (1997). *Handbook of clinical forensic nursing: A new perspective in trauma.* Colorado Springs, CO: Beth El College of Nursing.

McGivern, D. (1986). The Evolution of Primary Care Nursing. In. M. Mezney & D. McGiven (Eds.), *Nurses, nurse practitioners: The evolution of primary care* (pp. 3-14). Boston: Little, Brown.

Mechanic, M. B., Weaver, T. L., & Resnick, P. A. (2003). Intimate partner stalking behavior: Exploration of patterns and correlates in a sample of acutely battered women. *Violence Vict, 15*(1) 55-71.

Murphy, K. (1986). Primary care in an undergraduate curriculum. In M. D. Mezey & D. O. McGivern (Eds.), *Nurses, nurse practitioners: The evolution of primary care* (pp. 78-85). Glenview, IL: Scott, Foreman, and Co.

National Institute of Mental Heath. (1992). Directory of Programs and Facilities for Mentally Disorders Offenders. Dept. of Health and Human Services, Washington, DC.

Niskala, H. (1986) Competencies and skills required by nurses working in forensic areas. *West J Nurs Res*, *8*(4), 400-413.

Ohlin, M., & Farrington, D. (1991). *Human Development and Criminal Behavior: New Ways of Advancing Knowledge.* New York: Springer-Verlag.

Peplau, H. (1987, January). Tomorrow's world. *Nursing Times*, 29-32.

Pinizzotto, A. (1984). Forensic psychology: Criminal personality profiling. *J Police Sci Adm, 12*(1), 32-40.

State v. Hahn. (1985).

State v. Jones, 99 Wn.2d 735, 664 P.2d 1216. (1983).

State v. Minnix, 63 Wn. App 494. (1991).

State v. Wicks, 98 Wn.2d 620, 657 P.2d 781. (1983).

Stone, A. (1978). Psychiatry and the law. In A. Nichols (Ed.), *The Harvard guide to modern psychiatry.* Cambridge, MA: Harvard University Press.

US v. Chisholm, 149 f. 284, 5th Cir Ct. (1901).

Wildman, R., Batchelor, E., Thompson, L., et al. (1980). *The Georgia competency test: An attempt to develop a rapid quantitative measure for fitness to stand trial.* Unpublished manuscript, Forensic Services Division, Central State Hospital, Milledgeville, GA.

Winick, B. (1995).The side effects of incompetency labeling and the implications for mental health law. *Psychol Public Policy Law, 1*, 6-42.

Youtsey v. US. (1899).

Chapter 50 Forensic Mental Health Nursing and Critical Incident Stress Management

Judith W. Coram

Psychiatric forensic nurses assess perpetrators on issues of mental status, competency, legal sanity, and dangerousness (see Chapter 49). The term *psychiatric* denotes examination, diagnosis, discernment, and discovery, whereas the term *mental health* denotes care, restoration to optimal functioning, and psychological treatment for mentally ill people, as well as for the mentally well during a crisis (for example, grief counseling). Psychiatric forensic nursing differs from forensic mental health nursing, then, in the type of patient and the goals of the nurse-patient interaction.

Physiologic forensic nursing addresses the victims of trauma and violence, providing medicolegal exams, trauma care, and documentation of injury. Examples of roles within physiologic forensic nursing are the sexual assault nurse examiner, death investigator, nurse coroner, child abuse specialist, elder abuse specialist, battered woman specialist, and legal nurse consultant.

Forensic mental health nurses also provide care to victims of violence. They may specialize in disaster counseling or workplace violence, assist in preparing child witnesses for court, or provide psychological counseling for male and female victims experiencing rape trauma syndrome.

All subspecialties within forensic nursing are psychosocial. Although it focuses predominantly on direct care to victims, forensic nursing understands that the impact of crime is frequently much broader than the personal interaction between victim and perpetrator. There is often a wider circle of victims. The psychological aftermath of crime affects family, witnesses, emergency responders, trauma teams, and may continue to violate others months later within the criminal justice system.

Historical Perspective

Procedures for crisis intervention have evolved from the work of such people as Erich Lindemann (1944), who conducted studies on grieving in the aftermath of a major conflagration at a nightclub. Kardiner and Spiegel (1947) devised three basic principles in crisis work: (1) immediacy of interventions, (2) proximity to the occurrence of the event, and (3) the expectancy that the victim will return to adequate functioning. There are many models of crisis intervention in general agreement about the principles: (1) to alleviate the acute distress of victims, (2) to restore independent functioning, and (3) to prevent or mitigate the aftermath of psychological trauma and post-traumatic stress disorder (PTSD) (Everly & Mitchell, 1999).

The concept of critical incident stress was identified by Jeffrey Mitchell, a former fireman in New Jersey. He identified a psychological response in other emergency responders who witnessed horrifying situations during traumatic accidents or disasters. He noted that paramedics, firemen, or police officers left to deal with the psychological aftermath of trauma were developing symptoms of PTSD (nightmares, anxiety, concentration problems, and increased drug and alcohol use, among others). Only 4% to 10% of those who experience a critical incident develop PTSD, but studies indicate that more than 86% of emergency personnel do experience some kind of reaction (Mitchell, 1986b). He discovered it was not uncommon for those affected by a distressing event to have health and marital problems, increased substance use, and a higher rate of leaving their job. Returning to graduate school, Mitchell wrote about the concept of critical incident stress (CIS) among emergency workers. He began teaching response units across the country to address the symptoms in order to avoid burnout and to keep their responders functioning at optimal levels.

The Stress Response

Stress is the nonspecific, physiologic or psychological, response of the body to any prolonged demand made upon it. It is nonspecific because individuals react differently to the same stressor. A stressor is any event that is perceived by the body as being harmful or a threat. Over time, if the stress continues, it becomes a strain to cope day to day.

There are four basic types of stress that differ in their precipitation and duration; however, our bodies do not differentiate between these types of stress. With an acute stress response, physical, emotional, or cognitive symptoms can occur at the scene of the event or within 24 hours of the event. A delayed stress response is present when the symptoms occur 48 hours to several months later. In extreme cases, it may occur up to one to two years later. Accumulative stress is a mixture of all of life's stresses lumped together. This would include a person's childhood experience, his or her present home life, and the routine day-to-day stress of living. Post-traumatic stress disorder is a clinical diagnostic category that starts from the same cause as acute stress, but it has a pathological end state.

Post-Traumatic Stress Disorder

The *Diagnostic and Statistical Manual of Mental Disorders (DSM-IV)* defines post-traumatic stress disorder (PTSD) as the "development of characteristic symptoms following a psychologically distressing event that is outside the range of usual human experience. The event is usually experienced with intense fear, terror, and helplessness. The characteristic symptoms involve re-experiencing the dramatic event, avoidance of stimuli associated with the event or numbing of general responsiveness, and increased arousal." (American Psychiatric Association, 1994, p. 427) Commonly disclosed traumatic events include "a serious threat of harm to one's close friends, or seeing another person who has recently been, or is being, seriously injured or killed as a result of an accident or physical violence."

Critical Incident Stress

Critical incident stress is also precipitated by a specific event and may cause symptoms that last two to six weeks. The person may have a tremendous fear of repetition of the event and experience physical, cognitive, or emotional reactions.

Implications for the Forensic Nurse

While this chapter will focus on critical incident stress management applications by the forensic mental health nurse, it should be recognized that forensic nurses working in all subspecialty areas may be exposed to situations that could cause psychological trauma. This section provides examples of such potential situations.

Failed Resuscitation Efforts

Emergency response personnel, critical care staff, and other medical professionals measure their worth on an ability to control the outcome during the precarious balance between life and death. Each life, each incident, requires a 100% success. Less is failure. It is a professional and personal expectation to win every time. When these efforts do not result in meeting this high standard, staff members have difficulty accepting their sense of powerlessness. (See Case Study 50-1.)

Case Study 50-1 Failed Resuscitation Efforts

A child took a shotgun and stuck it under his chin, blowing his face off, but the shot did not kill him instantly. The EMTs got a line started and kept his airway open, but he eventually died at the hospital. Some people thought that might be best, given what he had to look forward to.

It wasn't the dying that got the nurses. It was the fact that while they were working on the patient, he was still conscious. He could hear and follow their directions. He held the monitor on his chest when he was asked to.

The best part about this debriefing was having a big picture of the kid in the room. The team just needed to see a face. So many people are already gone by the time the nurses get to them. This kid was *alive!*

Traumatic Death of a Patient

Nurses are trained to accept physiological death under certain circumstances. Death, under expected circumstances, is usually not a critical incident for medical personnel. However, when factors are present that make the death unexpected or unusual, the fact of death becomes heightened and difficult to accept.

The Unexpected Death of a Child

The human instinct to protect the young and vulnerable often seems more acute among those who choose to serve their communities. Police, firemen, paramedics, and medical personnel have an innate desire to shield and care for children. A child's accidental death is nearly always a critical incident for the emergency responders and medical personnel who work on the child. CIS symptoms are frequently exacerbated by these events (Knazik, Gausche-Hill, & Dietrich et al., 2003). (See Case Study 50-2.)

Case Study 50-2 Family Mass Murder and the Death of Children

Bart and Nancy were EMTs that volunteered on their rural county's ambulance squad. Married 10 years, they had recently been told they were unable to bear children of their own. This week they had spent many hours discussing adoption.

The call came in to 911 after 2 a.m.: a distressed elderly father concerned that his 40-year-old son may have tried to commit suicide. The name and address were familiar to Bart and Nancy. Living in a small town means knowing when neighbors are having trouble. They had heard Mark had become despondent over his wife's recent request for a divorce. Increased alcohol use was precipitating heated arguments between them over custody of their two preschool children.

Bart and Nancy arrived in the ambulance only moments after the sheriff's deputy pulled into the gravel driveway. They later reported that they would never forget that scene. Mark's wife was dead in her bed with a single gunshot to her head. It looked like her husband was sleeping peacefully next to her until they turned his head to find half his brain inside the pillow.

Mary kept saying to Bart, "Where are the kids?" She was worried that they heard the noise and hoped they were spending the night elsewhere. She didn't want to think of them being without a mom and dad at such a young age

Then they saw the little sleeping bags on the living room floor. Both kids had been shot and killed while they slept, their little angel faces still cuddled inside the bag.

Patient Suicide

The taking of one's own life is taboo in many cultures and religions. American society has seen a marked increase in suicide since the 1980s, as high as quadruple among adolescents. Healthcare workers who strive to find cure or care options have difficulty accepting a patient's evident refusal to continue care. The response to such surrender is more pronounced when the suicide is dramatic, unusual, or traumatic. (See Case Study 50-3.)

Bartels (1987) reported that suicides on inpatient units occurred 5 to 30 times more frequently than among the general population,

Case Study 50-3 Patient Suicide

A forensic patient was missing at the 10 p.m. head count. Attendant staff checked all doors again. Every exit was secure, and rooms that should have been locked were locked. Staff members were systematically checking inside those locked rooms when they found the missing patient in a full tub of water with his head inside a plastic bag.

The nurse couldn't get that image out of her mind, "his eyes staring at me through the bag, like he was saying, 'It's your fault I wasn't found soon enough.'"

although half occurred while the patient was on pass or after elopement. However, Smith & Munich (1992) reported that there has been an increase in the rate of suicides occurring on inpatient units. Because a staff person interprets the meaning of the death based on her or his own values, there will be differing levels and displays of grief shown by the staff members that shared the incident (Joyce & Wallbridge, 2003). Without an opportunity to come together and discuss those feelings, the staff response to the suicide can split the interdisciplinary team. (See Case Study 50-4.)

Case Study 50-4 Child Suicide

The teenager couldn't face his father's anger and disappointment. When Brian's teacher told him he was cut from the team, Brian went home and shot himself in his father's bedroom.

The nurse was just a friend of the family, but when she found out what had happened, she knew she had to be part of the debriefing.

Because the event occurred in such a little town, word of the accident spread quickly. The nurse thought to herself that she didn't want the parents to go home from the hospital after losing their son and have to face that mess. She took it upon herself to go back to the house alone. She wiped blood off the walls and cleaned up the bedroom. She kept talking about picking up all the "brain bits," little pieces of Brian's brain tissue, off the wall, the carpet, everywhere.

While staff attempt to deal with their own emotions following a patient suicide, they also need to continue providing care to other patients on the unit. Occasionally, hearing of a suicide exacerbates self-destructive behavior. Decisions need to be made about how much information to give patients, possible visitor restrictions, and the need for increased staff on the ward. Having a policy on such events in advance assists staff when decision making is difficult and provides for continuity between events. It also helps ensure that the responsibility for post-suicide interventions does not fall entirely on the nursing staff. Box 50-1 outlines a suggested policy for guidelines following inpatient suicide.

Box 50-1 Hospital Policy and Procedure Manual

Guidelines for Assistance Following Completed or Life-Threatening Suicide Attempts

PURPOSE

An inpatient population is at greater risk for suicide than the general population. The suicide of another patient exerts a powerful influence on suicidal or depressed patients. Patients with prior history of attempts are most at risk. Following a completed suicide or life-threatening suicide attempt or after an unusual or unexpected death, direct care staff need to be alert to signs and circumstances that might indicate increased risk for suicide in other patients on their ward. Steps will be taken to deal with the highly charged feelings of both staff and patients. Staff (those with patients and those without) will attend the meetings described as follows. This will assist in the resolution of the crisis.

PROCEDURE

1. The hospital will follow its patient death policy.
2. The hospital will contact the critical incident stress management team, if the event was a critical incident for staff, within 24 to 72 hours after the incident.
3. The treatment team will review the privileges and level of observation of all patients, with the patients' knowledge and participation. Off-ward privileges may be temporarily suspended. Privileges will be reviewed again in three to five days.
4. The clinical director will ensure that the following events occur:
   - An informational, interdisciplinary staff meeting to inform the team of the circumstances of the suicide, for the purpose of minimizing confusion and rumors.
   - A patient-staff meeting to give patients information about the death. As many staff members as possible should attend so that they can observe the reactions of patients, especially those considered to be at risk. Staff should indicate they are available to meet with patients who have questions or would like to talk.
   - A memorial service, arranged by the hospital chaplain and to be held in the hospital. Patients and staff will be encouraged to attend. Memorial services help bring closure and facilitate mourning.
   - A formal review of the incident.
   - A psychological autopsy.

Suicide of a Colleague

Mental health personnel and other healthcare providers, although capable of giving others permission to grieve or be angry at a colleague's suicide, frequently are harder on themselves, perpetuating the fallacy that mental health professionals do not have psychological problems and do not require assistance from others. "We believe we are different because we are educated to be caregivers," noted Mericle (1993, p. 11). A study by Thompson and Brooks (1990) indicated that the issue of "stigma" is an unspoken understanding that mental health professionals are not supposed to have problems. This can be a major factor in a colleague's decision to not seek help for suicidality.

Handling Bodies after Violent Death

Ursano and McCarroll (1990) reported that the profound sensory stimulation associated with the corpses, the shock of unexpected events associated with death, identification or emotional involvement with the dead, and the handling of children's bodies were significant stressors. McCarroll et al. (1993) studied the stressors and coping strategies at three different periods: before, during, and after exposure to bodies. In the period *before exposure*, the stressor was anticipation of one's reaction and the lack of information on the nature of the tasks to be performed, even for experienced workers.

For the period *during exposure*, it was the sensory stimuli associated with the dead. These include the sight of grotesque, burned, or mutilated bodies and the sounds that occur during autopsy, such as heads hitting tables and saws cutting bone. In addition, there are the smells of decomposing flesh and burned bodies and the tactile stimuli experienced as bodies are handled throughout the process. (McCarroll, Ursano, & Wright et al., 1993). The process of emotional involvement with the dead seems to occur naturally.

Even a nonhuman body can produce discomfort. When a worker found a dead dog in the luggage compartment of a commuter plane crash, he said that he couldn't handle it and that he was distressed because he feared ridicule from others. (McCarroll, Ursano, & Wright et al., 1993).

The handling of personal effects can lead to identification with the deceased. During the Vietnam War, handling personal effects of the dead was more stressful for soldiers than was working in the mortuary (McCarroll, Ursano, & Wright et al., 1993).

For *after exposure*, many of the personnel expressed the need for a debriefing or some kind of transitional event back to the real world. Stressors in this phase included strong personal reactions, problematic responses from spouses, and increased alcohol use (Peterson, Nicolas, & McGraw et al., 2002).

Severe Injury to Staff from Patient Assault

Although many staff have wanted to prosecute the patient following assault, the reason to do so did not include self-blame, belief that their anger was inappropriate, or fear there would be no conviction (Morrison, 1987/1988). Staff-victims of patient assault may find themselves being held at fault. Administration may tell staff-victims to perform better, thus denying the frequency of assault or that an assault problem even exists (Lanza, 1992). Administration may attribute the assault to some staff characteristic; however, Lanza (1988) showed there were no significant differences in assaulted staff and nonassaulted staff based on experience, position, race, sex, amount of time spent with the patient, or amount of limit setting. The study did show that women are held accountable more often than men, however. In less severe situations, nurses often shoulder the blame, as do those who have minor injuries (Lanza, 1992).

According to Janoff-Bulman (1989), most people base their worldviews on three basic assumptions: the world is benevolent; the world is meaningful; and they are invulnerable as long as they are cautious and honorable. To preserve these assumptions after an incident, coworkers blame the victims and the victims blame themselves (Dawson, Johnston, & Kehiayan et al., 1988). The symptoms of PTSD following an assault can be exacerbated by the administration's reactions and the staff's own counter-transference issues. (See Case Study 50-5.)

Case Study 50-5 Patient Assaults

A helicopter medic crew sped away to pick up an inmate who was being held in an out-of-state jail. The crew was aware of the added security measures despite the report that the inmate had cardiac problems. Once inside the chopper, handcuffed and strapped to the board, the inmate appeared to be resting comfortably. The crew expected a routine flight back to the medical center. An hour later, a frantic call came through to staff waiting in the ED. Somehow the inmate had loosened the restraints and attempted to take control of the chopper. A struggle was occurring, then the radio became silent. A wave of grief and shock rippled through the medical center as word came that the chopper had inverted and plummeted. There were no survivors. The CISM team convened at the medical center and divided into paired teams to conduct defusings in all departments.

Staff Taken Hostage

Forensic nurses and correctional nurses who choose to work with inmate populations are aware that there are risk factors inherent in their work due to the nature of their patients. Hostage takers are repeat offenders. The forensic patient is frequently being confined involuntarily. This is a population that has demonstrated poor decision-making skills and is likely to use desperate measures in an attempt to procure immediate gratification. (See Case Study 50-6.)

Case Study 50-6 Staff Taken Hostage

The four-person night staff on the forensic unit became victims when two patient-inmates used curtain cords to tie up the male staff. A "shiv" (a homemade knife made by melting a razor blade into a toothbrush) was held to a nurse's throat so that the inmates could bargain for the supervisor's security key to escape from the locked unit. The nurse was held at knifepoint and her life was threatened as the inmate used her as a shield as they escaped down the stairwell, out the building, and off the hospital grounds.

Although both inmates were later apprehended, prosecuted, and convicted, the incident had not ended. Reliving that trauma caused one attendant to display cardiac symptoms. One nurse left her job, abandoning more than 20 years' worth of accrued retirement. Another sold her house and moved, fearful the perpetrator would return.

Theoretical Foundation

An event may not be a critical incident for all involved. Critical incident stress is impact specific. If the personal impact is not there, then the incident is probably not a critical incident for that individual. The entire group may not require a formal debriefing.

Key Point *50-1*

A critical incident is any situation faced by normal, healthy people that causes them to experience strong emotional reactions and potentially interferes with their ability to function at the scene or later.

Death of victims of violent crime is not uncommon in emergency departments or intensive care units. It is not just the death of the patient that causes critical incident stress symptoms. It is intrinsic that there be a momentary thought, a flash, if only for a second, through the person's mind that the person or one next to him or her could die. This may not be a conscious thought. All that is required is one tiny connection. (See Case Study 50-7.)

Case Study 50-7 Mass Murderer and Spree Killer

In late December 1987, a 47-year-old man murdered 14 members of his family in his rural home outside Dover, Arkansas, and buried most of the bodies in shallow graves on his property. A few days later, his actions not yet discovered, he appeared in the nearby town of Russellville and went on a shooting spree that lasted 35 minutes. He methodically visited four local businesses and shot individuals against whom he held a grudge, as well as others who happened to be in his way. Before surrendering to authorities, he killed two people and injured four more. A study by North et al. (1989) reported the psychopathology in eyewitnesses of the shootings evidenced by high rates (80%) of PTSD symptoms.

Mitchell gave the theoretical explanation for why CIS occurs. When a situation happens that is too intense to be emotionally resolved promptly, an individual will suppress or store away part of that experience, in order to continue to function effectively in the present crisis. Common signs and symptoms of a stress reaction in a traumatized person are summarized in Boxes 50-2, 50-3, 50-4, and 50-5.

How each person deals with stress symptoms is based on early learning and one's individual coping style. Which symptoms are experienced, and how they are expressed, will be different for everyone.

Box 50-2 Physical Symptoms of Critical Incident Stress

Chest pain	Hyperventilation
Chills	Muscle aches
Diaphoresis	Nausea
Diarrhea	Sleep disturbances
Dizziness	Tachycardia
Dyspepsia	Thirst
Fatigue	Tremors
Feeling uncoordinated	Vision disturbances
Headaches	Vomiting
Hypertension	Weakness

Box 50-3 Cognitive Symptoms of Critical Incident Stress

Slowed thinking	Distressing dreams
Difficulty making decisions	Poor attention span
Confusion	Difficulty naming objects
Disorientation	Flashbacks/nightmares
Difficulty in problem solving	Hypervigilance
Memory problems	Change in awareness
Difficulty calculating	Poor abstract thinking
Poor concentration	

Box 50-4 Emotional Symptoms of Critical Incident Stress

Agitation	Guilt
Anger	Irritability
Anxiety	Limiting contact with others
Apprehension	Panic
Depression	Sadness
Fear	Shock
Feeling abandoned	Startled
Feeling isolated	Suspiciousness
Feeling lost	Uncertainty
Feeling numb	Wanting to hide
Feeling overwhelmed	Worry about others
Grief	

Box 50-5 Behavioral Signs of Critical Incident Stress

Blames others easily	Emotional outbursts
Change in appetite	Erratic movements
Change in level of activity	Increased drug or alcohol use
Change in sexual functioning	Pacing
Change in speech patterns	Restlessness
Change in usual communication	Withdrawal
Easily startled	

Formal Critical Incident Stress Debriefing

A critical incident stress debriefing (CISD) is a structured group process that uses a psychological and educational format with the aim of reducing the impact of the incident. It is not a critique of any procedures used or of the individuals involved. Predominantly, it is a cognitive process that focuses on wellness and puts the blame on the event, not the personnel involved (Mitchell, 1986a). CISD helps to accelerate normal recovery of people experiencing strong reactions to the event.

The Role of a Critical Incident Stress Management Team

Most debriefings will be conducted by a two-person critical incident stress management (CISM) team–a peer chosen to coincide with the profession of the group (firemen, law enforcement, critical care nurse, etc.) and a mental health person specifically trained in PTSD or CIS and skilled at group dynamics. The mental health person is designated as the leader of the debriefing.

Best Practice *50-1*

The CISD leader will use active listening skills and demonstrate concern and caring for each person's experience by eliciting involvement of all group members.

The leader should strive to create an atmosphere of acceptance and understanding by using active listening. The leader will be cognizant of voice tone and body language as she or he tries to validate participants' feelings. She or he will attempt to elicit openness in the group by including everyone and by conveying concern and caring for each person's experience. When technical language is used, the peer co-leader can translate terminology so the leader can paraphrase each participant's reactions.

The leader must be viewed as being honest, genuine, and open to disclosure. The leader's feelings and words must be congruent. Sarcasm must be avoided. Humor may be selectively appropriate. It will be extremely important for the leader to avoid expressing approval or disapproval for any actions taken at the scene. The leader should avoid appearing to be judgmental either way by using such phrases as "You did a good job" or "I agree—you screwed up." It would be more supportive and nonjudgmental to say, "Sometimes we're not sure of the choices we make."

Mental health personnel new to CISM will become aware of a desire to make the participants feel less bad. There is an urge to fix the problem for them. The leader needs to learn that the actual healing is internal and that it takes time. Instead of attempting to take away participants' sorrow and guilt, she or he will encourage participants to acknowledge the emotion that is present and accept it.

Best Practice 50-2

The CISD leader will avoid self-disclosure, center on the event that precipitated the debriefing, and avoid reference to other critical incidents or debriefings.

The level of emotionality during the debriefing is tightly controlled by the group leader, who will call upon certain aspects of Glasser's reality therapy and Gestalt therapy during the process. The type of approach used will depend on the types of people involved. Most emergency response personnel respond to a very direct approach that allows them as much control as possible. Use of overly emotionally laden words is not effective, but a very cognitive approach will be (Jones, 1988). If, for example, the participants are a group of psychiatric staff dealing with the aftermath of a patient suicide, the process may be more impassioned, as these people are accustomed to emotional interactions. At this time the group process may take on a more Gestalt approach as the leader requests participants to relive their memories of the event. (See Case Study 50-8.)

Case Study 50-8 CISM Teams and the Mental Health Nurse

A mentally disturbed adult male threatened to kill his elderly mother, his brother, and himself. He started the family home on fire and then lay on his bed with a loaded rifle. When the police and fire crews arrived, the house was nearly engulfed in flames. A rainstorm assisted fire crews, but the man prevented the rescue of his family members by shooting at officers from the upstairs windows. An officer was hit and lay in the yard calling for help. Across the street, children in a daycare watched the flames and felt the heat of the fire. They heard the shots and watched the confusion and noise of the sirens, smoke, and fire trucks.

It is customary for the police chaplain to go door to door after such an event to check on the well-being of those in the neighborhood and thank them for their cooperation. The woman running the daycare expressed concern over some of the comments and behaviors exhibited by the children since the fire. The chaplain contacted the CISM team to request a specialty debriefing for the children.

The mental health nurse met with the eight children, ages three to seven. They drew pictures of the house fire, rain, fire trucks, and police and talked about their memories of that day. In age-appropriate conversation, they discussed what was "scary" about the fire and about the dreams and fears they have had since. The nurse left a written note for parents, letting them know about her contact with the children and offering to speak with them individually if they had any concerns.

The Purpose of Critical Incident Stress Debriefing

Humans have the need to believe that life is not random and that they have control. The more "normal" one is, the more one believes she or he is in control. Most feel they are 70% in control, while depressed people think they are only 20% in control. After a psychological trauma, victims continue to feel vulnerable and at risk. They blame others, themselves, and outside sources in order to get back that sense of control. One purpose of a debriefing is to recognize the feelings of vulnerability and longing for control. By resolving that internal conflict, the symptoms of PTSD are less likely to increase. Choosing healthier coping strategies for the short term is a way of regaining a sense of control.

Another purpose of the debriefing is to let those people experiencing very strong reactions hear that their responses are normal. Participants will express versions of the *fallacy of uniqueness* and the *fallacy of abnormality*. The fallacy of uniqueness is expressed in such comments as "I am the only one having trouble" or "I am the only one that was upset." The fallacy of abnormality is heard in "I am having symptoms that are crazy" or "I am more whacked out than anyone else. There must be something wrong with me." By teaching about the range of CIS symptoms, the leader can reduce or eliminate participants' belief in the fallacies and prevent an increase in symptoms. She or he will also be able to assess those who may require further mental health intervention and refer them accordingly.

A debriefing also provides a move back toward group cohesiveness. An event that caused participants to question their skills and abilities, equipment or procedures, or purpose for being can strike hard at the bonds that tie the team together. Intershift blaming can shatter a team's unity. By keeping the blame on the event, not the individuals, the leader can be effective in decreasing a major cause of long-term burnout–distrust of one's peers.

A formal debriefing allows the participants to relive the event, first cognitively and then emotionally. Ideally the formal debriefing is held 24 to 72 hours after the incident. Attempting to hold a debriefing too early does not allow the participants to reflect on or process any of their feelings. They may still be in shock.

The co-leaders will avoid being used as a tool of administration. A CISD should not be used as a disciplinary tool. For example, to be effective, the debriefing process must be voluntary. Co-leaders should be cautious if the request for debriefing indicated that participants' attendance was mandatory. A CISM team should transcend all jurisdictional, labor-management, or disciplinary issues.

The Seven Phases of a Critical Incident Stress Debriefing

Once the meeting time and place is set, CISM team debriefers should meet one hour beforehand. This allows time to meet people informally, arrange seating and get the coffee going, and make sure the paging system is off for that room. Debriefers should remember they have been invited and should not take over the location.

A minimum of two CISM members will lead the debriefing: a peer and the mental health professional. There is less credibility if only the mental health professional responds. Mitchell maintains that the most important ingredient to a CISD is the presence of the trained peer.

The peer is there to add credibility and to role model. He or she may be able to comment on the reality of feeling abandoned by administration or experiencing lifestyle changes. The peer co-leader should be honest and genuine ("I'm here to help if I can"). He or she should try to connect emotionally with the participants. The co-leader can help to identify the situation by using the jargon and terminology of the group. Trust will increase if the debriefers speak the same language. During the reentry phase, the peer co-leader will make positive comments about participants or their department. It may be the peer co-leader who is assigned to check back with administration ("Is there anything else we can do?").

The Introductory Phase

Because trust of outsiders is difficult for some groups, it is important that the mental health leader establishes credibility. She or he will give a brief introduction of the co-leaders, without using ranks or titles and explain that they are there as volunteers. The leader will express appreciation at being invited. She will give an explanation of the purpose for the debriefing (For example, "because you want to speed up the healing process" or "We will do teaching regarding stress reactions"). The leader will explain these are the kinds of events that can be a precursor to PTSD. At this point, the mental health leader introduces the co-leader, who establishes himself or herself as a peer person.

The co-leader explains the ground rules and stresses confidentiality. The following is an example of ground rules given during this phase:

- No breaks, if possible. "We ask that nobody leaves the room. A debriefing usually takes two to three hours; some are shorter, some longer. If you do have to leave the room, one of us will go after you to check and see if everything is okay."
- "Is there anybody here who was not involved in the scene? If so, what is your interest?" The debriefing cannot be performed if it is not limited to people who were directly involved. "Any media here?" Media personnel are absolutely restricted due to confidentiality requirements. Occasionally administrative or supervisory personnel attend out of a sense of responsibility. They need to be pulled aside and told that the debriefing will not be as effective if they are present.
- "There is no rank in this room."
- "You do not have to talk. We do ask that everyone listens. We will ask everyone the facts. Just being here is showing support for others."
- "This is not a critique. If you know certain facts that you are afraid may jeopardize your job, keep them to yourself. That information may not be pertinent to what we are trying to accomplish."
- "Speak only for yourself. Don't talk for someone else or relay information for others."
- Stress confidentiality. Emphasize there can be no note taking or recording.
- Acknowledge the record keeping of the team. "We do make a record of the number present and where we met, but there are no names or quotes in the information."
- Ask, "Are there any questions? If not, then we will go into the fact phase."

The Fact Phase

The leader initiates the conversation by asking the participants to re-create their involvement at the scene. This can be done in a structured pattern, such as going around the circle, or chronologically by those who arrived at the scene first. The process should start with the dispatchers, if any were involved. The leader elicits contributions from the participants with such comments as: "I was not there. Tell me in as much detail as you can what you saw, heard, felt, or smelled. Where were you when you heard the alarm? How did you respond (on foot or by car)? What did you see when you first arrived?"

If the group is large, the debriefing can be streamlined by each participant telling his or her sequence of events just getting to the scene, and then starting again with who was first at the scene to describe what happened there. The leader attempts to get a clear picture of what happened through the eyes of the participants.

While it is not mandatory that every participant talk, the leader can attempt to involve those who are quiet by asking them questions. "I'm still unsure. When did you get there?"

After the last person has described his or her involvement, the leader will give a brief summary of the event. "It sounds like everyone got a call from dispatch and was on-scene in 10 to 15 minutes. Two of you handled the victims in the blue car, while the other crew worked on the kids that were thrown out of the other vehicle. Everything went well until you were aware that a third car was involved."

The Thought Phase

The leader will initiate this phase with, "Tell me at what point in time you realized this event was different" and then will ask each participant to respond. Emergency responders and critical care nurses have referred to this as the "lightbulb" moment.

The Reaction Phase

The leader will ask, "If you could erase one part of this event, which would it be? What was the worst moment for you? What went on with you at that time?" Each participant will be asked to respond. This is the moment at which the event became a critical incident for each participant. The skilled leader will extract fine details of this moment and attempt to get the participant to identify for himself or herself the personalization of the moment and the flash of thought connected to the participant's mortality.

The Symptom Phase

The debriefers will have brought with them copies of three handouts:

1. A list of symptoms of critical incident stress
2. A list of coping strategies for stress management
3. A list of suggestions for family and friends

The symptom list is distributed first. The leader explains that symptoms of critical incident stress can be cognitive, physical, or emotional and denotes that these symptoms can cause behavioral changes that may have been noticed by family or coworkers. There are three sets of symptoms to identify: those at the scene, those occurring in the next few hours or the next day, and those appearing later. It is not necessary to go around the circle. The leader will ask participants to reflect on their own experience. "Would anyone like to share any symptoms they have experienced since the event?" The debriefers will allow time for silence as people reflect.

Responses may include such comments as "I've lost my appetite and I'm having trouble sleeping." "I get nightmares. I keep seeing the same scene over and over." "My wife says I'm drinking more." "I can't concentrate at work. I just stare at the wall."

Occasionally the group may be resistant to acknowledging any problems. The leader will not confront or probe. There may be

Box 50-6 Coping Strategies for the Suicidal Patient

- Get more rest.
- Eat a well-balanced diet. Eat regular meals. Avoid drug and alcohol use.
- Contact friends. Have someone stay with you for a while.
- Reestablish a normal schedule as soon as possible and try to maintain it.
- Try to keep a reasonable level of activity. Exercise is helpful.
- Spend time with people you care about. Express your feelings.
- Reoccurring thoughts, dreams, or flashbacks are normal. Don't try to fight them. They will decrease with time.
- If symptoms are severe or last longer than six weeks, speak with a counselor or physician.

Box 50-7 Coping Strategies for Family and Friends

- Listen carefully. Don't say, "It could have been worse." Say, "I want to understand."
- Spend time with the traumatized person. Give private time when requested.
- Offer assistance. Help with everyday tasks.
- Give reassurance. Tell the person you are sorry the event occurred.
- Don't take the person's anger or other feelings personally.

trust issues among the participants of which the debriefers are not aware. If the group is quiet, it can be turned into an educational format. The leader will allow for quiet time. After a period of time, the leader will ask if anyone wants to add any thoughts or reflections. After ensuring that all have been included, the group can move to the next phase.

The Teaching Phase

The debriefers will distribute copies of the remaining two handouts. Examples of guidelines for coping with stress or assisting another who is coping are listed in Boxes 50-6 and 50-7. Information given in this phase is significant for healing after psychological trauma. After validating the examples of symptoms that had been offered, the leader will nullify the fallacy of abnormality by repeating that the responses heard in the group were normal. Experiencing abnormal reactions to abnormal events is normal. The leader will negate the fallacy of uniqueness by emphasizing that stress responses occur in almost everyone who is exposed to a critical incident. The leader will reassure the participants that although the symptoms may be extreme, they are time limited. The leader will make statements such as "Continue to expect these things to happen to you over the next few days. If we had a magic wand that could take away your pain, we would use it. But the truth is, it just takes time, usually two to four weeks. We can tell you that because you participated in this debriefing, you will have substantially shortened the amount of time you will need."

The Reentry Phase

At this point, the leader will begin to close the debriefing by saying, "A terrible thing has happened. Your lives will be different now." There should be a chance for participants to ask further questions. If there are none, the leader will ask the group (no matter how awkward) if anything positive can come from this. "What about this event was a strong point? Is there something we learned, something we will be better for?" Often the responses will be something like an agreement on doing something for family survivors of the victim, changing a protocol, getting new equipment, or making a personal connection with a neighboring EMT group. The focus in this phase can be on learning: "I realize now the first call needs to be to the shift supervisor." "I found out my crew will work to the end to save a child." It is important for healing to find something positive, no matter how small or under what horrendous circumstances. This rekindles a sense of hope and allows participants to think in terms of the future, rather than continue to dwell on the past.

It is not unusual for a group to slip back to a previous phase, especially if much grief has been expressed (more likely when debriefing the death of a child or peer). The leader does not announce that the group is going back. She or he will continue to emphasize normalcy and group cohesiveness. There may be laughter as the group begins to normalize. Participants may express caring and concern for each other. After a while, the conversation will ebb to a close. At this point, the leader will make a brief summary of what has been said and end positively. It is important that the debriefers thank the group for allowing them to be there. "We appreciate being invited."

A formal CISD is not a disciplinary tool. The process will lose all effectiveness if attendance is mandatory or the process is used to point out the foibles of one person. It is not a critique of either the procedures or people involved. The content of the discussion is not discussed later with administration. Participants are told the debriefing is not psychotherapy. People experiencing severe reactions can be referred to outside resources for ongoing intervention.

Critical Incident Stress Management

Critical incident stress management is the all-inclusive list of services offered by certified teams. People interested in volunteering can call the local fire dispatch office for the location of the nearest team.

There are now more than 300 organized teams nationwide structured to include the roles of coordinator, clinical director, mental health team members, peer support personnel, communications, and selection committee. Prospective members attend a 16-hour course and are expected to have annual continuing training. National certification is available. One such organization is the American Critical Incident Stress Foundation, Inc.

The International Critical Incident Stress Foundation, Inc., has a coordination center with a 24-hour hotline. Request for services can come from anywhere in the US and the closest team will be notified. The center also provides coordination between teams in the event of a large-scale disaster.

Critical incident stress management is the umbrella term for the range of services offered by organized teams. These services include the following:

1. On-scene support.
2. Defusing (mini-debriefing using same seven steps): Defusings are performed immediately after the incident, ideally within one to four hours, but at least by the end of the shift. If a defusing cannot be done in this time frame, a recommendation for a formal debriefing is made. The key is immediate intervention. The purpose of this brief (15 to

30 minutes) meeting is to allow initial ventilation of feelings, to establish if a formal debriefing is needed, to offer support or information, and to stabilize personnel who need to remain on duty.

A trained peer support person (PSP) who was not directly involved in the incident can perform a defusing. The PSP should be aware of his limitations and should call for support from a mental health team member if the situation warrants.

The format for a defusing is similar to that of the formal debriefing. There will be a brief introduction. The leader will then ask the group to tell her or him what happened and will ask, "What was the worst part?" After allowing for initial ventilation of feelings and validating the feelings, the leader will move on to educate and give information on signs and symptoms of stress. It is not appropriate to probe or dwell. It is too early after the incident for any confrontation. The leader will keep the session informal, but to the point. The staff will not be allowed to lapse into a critique. The closing will include an announcement of the date, time, and location of the (voluntary) formal debriefing.

3. Large-scale demobilization (multiple casualties or natural disasters).
4. Formal debriefing: The American Critical Incident Stress Foundation (ACISF) reports that 95% of all debriefings involve one or two victims and 95% involve children. Rural teams are busier than urban teams, because rural teams know 60% of the victims. Once personalized, the event is more likely to be a critical incident.
5. Follow-up services: This is generally performed several months to a year after the incident. If the event was personal in some way, the actual anniversary may be very important to the participants and a good time for the team coordinator to call. The main purpose is to touch base and identify any unresolved issues. It is an opportunity to assess for delayed stress responses. This can be done with a phone call to the person originally requesting the formal debriefing, or with a recall of all participants or only a portion of that group.
6. Individual consults: This is a debriefing with one or two people. If more than three are being addressed, it should be considered a formal debriefing. This is appropriately used for supervisors, administrative staff, or safety officers who may have been present at the incident but should not be included in the formal debriefing.
7. Specialty debriefing: Occasionally, requests come from groups in the community, usually through emergency responders. Each team decides if and how to handle such requests. If the group includes children, it is important to have mental health professionals who specialize in the care of children lead that debriefing.

Jeffrey Mitchell has advised hospitals not to form their own team for the following reasons:

- The debriefing must be done by personnel outside the chain of command. Supervisory staff cannot perform an effective debriefing.
- Debriefings need to be confidential. This may be difficult to maintain within a department. Unit staff members know each other too well. It is impossible to debrief friends.
- Too often there is confusion regarding the difference between a critique and a debriefing. The organization's safety officer wants to be part of the CISM team or attends debriefings because he or she was on-scene.

Box 50-8 Use of CISD Team

Utilization of the Critical Incident Stress Management Team at __________ Hospital

POLICY

It is the policy of __________ Hospital to provide CISD services to its employees. Contact with the team and request for debriefing may be made by any employee.

SCOPE

CISD services are available to staff in all departments and on all shifts.

CISD services are to be provided only by people specifically trained in CISD.

In the event of a large-scale incident or disaster, the hospital team will contact the regional team for assistance.

PROCEDURE

1. Current team membership and home phone numbers are available at the switchboard.
2. Contact the team at work or home to notify them that an incident has occurred and to determine if CISD services are appropriate.
3. The CISD team will contact the appropriate supervisor to arrange time and place for a debriefing. A formal debriefing is most effective if held within 24 to 72 hours of the incident.
4. The supervisor will be asked not to participate with the individual or group unless directly involved in the incident. The supervisor may be debriefed separately.
5. Team members are exempt from obligatory reporting of disclosed information while performing CISD activities, which are outside of regularly assigned duties.
6. Department heads may arrange for staff to participate on their day off by paying them for that time.
7. An annual summary of team contacts and the number of debriefings will be submitted to the CEO. The report will not contain any names, identifying information, or disclosures.

Members agree to provide a CISD on the shift of the staff involved within 24 to 72 hours.

The __________ Hospital team will be available to all departments and shifts.

The __________ Hospital CISM team will maintain strict confidentiality regarding debriefings held, including topics discussed and personnel involved. Any breach in confidentiality will result in immediate removal from the team.

Team members are exempt from obligatory reporting of disclosed information heard during performance of CISM duties (which are outside of regularly assigned duties).

Hospital teams can be formed, and be effective, under strict guidelines. Box 50-8 highlights policies adhered to by the first state mental hospital to adopt such a service for their employees.

All agencies that may have situations involving unexpected death or trauma should have a plan in place. Dr. Robyn Robinson in Australia did a study on the perceived effect of CISD on emergency department (ED) personnel (Robinson, 2000). Three quarters of those involved in the CISD found it "helpful to extremely helpful"; another 25% reported, "It wasn't needed by me, but it was all right for others." Not a single one reported harmful effects and there was a marked reduction of stress symptoms within 24 hours following the debriefing, as compared to others involved in the same event who did not have the debriefing.

Applications within Forensic Mental Health Nursing

The theoretical framework of CISD lends itself to other specialized events. The same seven-stage process can be used in one-to-one counseling situations or other group situations. This section provides specific examples of the application of the seven-stage process.

Child Witnesses of Violence and Domestic Abuse

It has been estimated that 3.3 million children in the US each year see or hear at least one incident of physical conflict between their parents (Carlson, 1984). There is mounting evidence that exposure to this type of family violence has a negative psychological effect on children (e.g., Fantuzzo & Lindquist, 1988; Jaffe, Wolfe, & Wilson, 1990; McDonald & Jouriles, 1991). Early exposure to such events does more than model poor conflict resolution strategies (intergenerational transmission of marital violence); it appears to traumatize children in a way that is similar to other forms of childhood abuse (Henning, Leitenberg, & Coffey et al., 1996). The trauma for a child witness is likely to be greatest when the child was within the danger zone emotionally or physically.

Ornitz and Pynoos (1989) conducted a study of the changes in startle response in children who had been under fire during a sniper attack at their school playground that resulted in many injuries and two fatalities. The results suggested that the traumatic experience had induced a possible long-lasting brain stem dysfunction and vulnerability to future stress.

Juries after Murder Trial

Feldmann and Bell (1991) described a debriefing session for jurors after the murder trial of a man whose truck had collided with a school bus, killing 27 people. The graphic evidence of the accident, the high levels of emotion of the survivors and the victims' relatives, and the intense community and national attention to the trial placed the jurors under considerable stress. Their stress became evident when frequent recesses in the trial were required because the jurors appeared visibly shaken and emotionally distraught.

The judge requested the debriefing, which was held immediately after the sentencing. Although none of the jurors had been directly involved in the accident, their reactions were as intense as that of rescue workers and law enforcement officers.

Forensic mental health nurses have the entrepreneurial opportunity to contract with court systems for the purpose of providing a needed service. The legal system in the US expects honorable and competent service from empanelled jury members. When the trial is long, the crime violent, and the evidence presented especially chilling or graphic, the effect on the jurors can be profound and long lasting. It is not enough to thank them for their time. They deserve the opportunity to ventilate their experiences in a controlled environment, among those who can understand empathetically what they have just been immersed in and with someone who is specially trained.

Prison Staff Following an Inmate Execution

Corrections staff interact daily with the same inmates for many consecutive years. Policies that prohibit correction staff from knowing the inmate's background, criminal history, or the details of the evidence behind the current conviction contribute to the development of counter-transference and ease inhibition from forming caring relationships. Staff may have personal opinions regarding capital punishment that cannot interfere with their duties, one of which may be the officially sanctioned taking of an inmate's life.

Vasquez (1993) outlined a pretrauma prevention program tied to critical incident stress debriefings held after the execution of Robert Alton Harris, California's first execution in more than 25 years. Training was held for all correctional staff who interact with death row inmates, chaplains, medical staff involved in the execution's aftermath, and the victim's relatives who were scheduled to witness the execution.

Other correctional situations potentially leading to critical incident stress include being held hostage, exposure to a riotous situation, and use of lethal force on an inmate (Fix, 2001).

It would not be appropriate for correctional nurses working at the prison conducting the execution to conduct debriefings. However, networking between facilities would provide for a roster of CISD-trained correctional nurses to act as the peer support person in the debriefing at a different facility.

Hostage Negotiators

It is clear that law enforcement officers are exposed to psychological and traumatic events, generally outside the range of usual human experience as described in the definition of PTSD proposed by Martin and colleagues. Recurrent and intrusive recollections of the event are among the most frequently reported symptoms (Martin, McKean, & Veltkamp, 1986). The least frequently reported symptom is "avoidance of activities that arouse recollection of the event." Officers are not always given the opportunity to avoid similar situations. While law enforcement agencies do have protocols for officer-involved shootings that include counseling, the officers are sometimes hesitant to avail themselves of the service, especially if the same psychologist also provides administration of the fitness for duty evaluation.

Some regional CISM teams have developed relationships with local law enforcement and are invited to conduct a CISD for incidents other than shootings. Trust is often hard won with line officers. The team must not breach confidentiality. It is paramount that a trained officer (who can be from another jurisdiction) be present as the peer support person for credibility.

An area of expertise newly developed within forensic nursing is that of consultant to law enforcement on hostage negotiation teams. A role function of the consultant is to provide debriefing to officers after prolonged negotiation or following an incident that resulted in serious harm or death to hostages or officers. When a negotiation team is called to the scene of a barricaded subject, similar stress responses can occur if the incident results in suicide. (See Case Study 50-9.)

Case Study 50-9 Hostage Negotiators

A patrol officer responded to a routine call of a suspicious car in the parking lot of a motel. When he ran the plate, he was startled to hear the car was stolen and most likely being driven by a fugitive wanted in connection with a kidnapping and three murders in Texas. The officer called for backup. Suddenly the blast of an automatic weapon slammed into the seat beside him. The fugitive yelled for the officer to "Leave, or the boy will die!" The SWAT team and hostage negotiators were summoned while the fugitive was held at bay.

Law enforcement discovered the man had killed his estranged wife and mother-in-law and kidnapped their young son. He had driven out of state and ditched his car. The 72-year-old owner of the car he was now in was presumed dead.

By comparison, this incident was short—only three hours of negotiating—but most of it over a bullhorn. The fugitive refused to use a radio or phone. He refused to give up the boy and continued to threaten his life. Desperation turned to resolve.

Suddenly a shot rang out. The negotiation team waited while SWAT crept up to the car, where they discovered the man had killed himself. The toddler had his father's blood on his face and shirt. The negotiator lifted him out of the car and carried him safely away, covering him from the press.

It took a couple of hours to locate grandparents in Texas. CPS was called to care for the child until the family could fly up to retrieve him. The team's consultant, a psychiatric forensic nurse, held the toddler, rocking him gently until he fell asleep in her arms. What a rough few days. The child was filthy, cold, and hungry. How much of this would he remember?

One team member thought this was probably the most difficult incident the team had ever worked, yet it was the shortest. They knew at the outset that this could end badly. The man was desperate, and he knew that they knew about the three murders.

The focus was on keeping the child alive. This was rough on the primary negotiator. When he heard the gun go off in the car, he thought the boy was dead.

The most important thing done that day was insisting that CPS not take the toddler until the negotiators could hold him again—to have those last minutes of providing shelter, being the one who kept him safe. Doing this also helped the officer overcome the emotional trauma he felt the moment he thought the boy had been killed.

Workplace Violence

Along with making workplace assessment and recommendations regarding safety procedures and policies, the forensic mental health nurse working as consultant to businesses and corporations concerned about employee safety can impact the acceptance of debriefings following a critical incident by citing the cost-effectiveness of employee well-being and retention (Antai-Otong, 2001). A study of ED staff in Canada underscored the need for hospital administrators to be aware of the extent of PTSD symptoms in their employees, as 20% of those involved in the incident considered changing jobs as a result of their trauma (Laposa, Alden, & Fullerton, 2003).

Key Court Testimony Considerations

Forensic mental health nurses cannot be seen as interfering with witness testimony. It is unlikely, however, that a debriefer would be called to testify, because repeating statements heard during a debriefing would be considered hearsay and as such would not be admissible as evidence. Not keeping notes or recordings of debriefings is conveniently protective then for the debriefer. It would also be a safeguard to develop a very short retention period for what was discussed.

Key Point *50-2*

The nurse who reported details from a debriefing would be violating confidentiality. Trust is sacrosanct in CISM, or the value of the program is lost.

As to conducting a critical incident debriefing with victims or witnesses of violence, it may be appropriate to delay the debriefing until after their testimony is given so that memories are not altered. Although CISDs are ideally conducted 24 to 72 hours after the incident, Mitchell states that the process still has therapeutic application up to three months after the incident.

In the case of child witnesses, Loftus and Davies (1984) suggested that children's greater difficulty in retrieving information from long-term memory makes them more prone to rely on new information to fill in blanks. Dale and associates (1978) found that asking leading questions increased the likelihood that subjects would incorporate new information into answers given two weeks later.

From a prosecution standpoint, it may be desirable that a witness appear as traumatized as possible. In some cases, witness testimony can be preserved on videotape, allowing time for intervention.

Mental health personnel have become increasingly aware that a child victim may be victimized a second time by being subjected to the court proceedings (Benedek & Schetky, 1986). Some children freeze and are unable to remember the event, some children cry, others are visibly shaken. Under the stress of cross-examination, children may recant previous testimony. Confronting the defendant and talking about the horror of victimization may be similar to reliving the crime.

Forensic mental health nurses may become part of a multidisciplinary team consisting of a prosecutor, police, and social services personnel in the investigation and prosecution of cases involving child witnesses or victims. Such teams would have specialized training, education, and experience. Using the team would ensure the child deals with people he is familiar with throughout the traumatic courtroom experience.

A role for the forensic mental health nurse, who has had specialized training with child victims of sexual assault, would include assisting the child through the prosecution of the case and dealing with the traumatic aftermath. The nurse professional would prepare the child for testimony and the abuse of cross-examination, educate and support the child's family through the symptomatology the child may demonstrate during a lengthy trial, and assist counsel in formulating questions understandable to the child.

Summary

Addressing violence as a healthcare issue means not only bandaging wounds and x-raying broken bones of the victim in the nurse's care, but also identifying the unseen victims. Forensic nursing is psychosocial. It understands that victimization extends past the patient in front of you to the family, emergency responders, witnesses, and others within the criminal justice system.

While psychiatric forensic nursing seeks an explanation for the criminal act, forensic mental health nursing seeks to prevent further trauma by identifying potential victims. One application is critical incident stress management. Forensic mental health nursing can utilize the concepts in CISM to restore optimal functioning to victims of violence and the greater circle of victims—the emergency responders, juries, and witnesses who have also been victimized.

Forensic nursing is inherently a difficult emotional role, due to the types of patients and scenarios faced. Those who choose the profession need to learn how to cope with the stress of the specialized role so they can continue to be present and effective for their patients. Forensic nurses can benefit as recipients of the therapeutic and educational applications of critical incident stress management.

Resources

Organizations

American Academy of Forensic Sciences

410 North 21st Street, Colorado Springs, CO 80904; Tel: 719-636-1100; www.aafs.org

American Board of Forensic Nursing and American College of Forensic Examiners

ACFE Institute of Forensic Science, 2750 East Sunshine, Springfield, MO 65804; Tel: 417-881-3818, 800-423-9737; www.acfei.com

International Critical Incident Stress Foundation

3290 Pine Orchard Lane, Suite 106, Ellicott City, MD 21042; Tel: 410-750-9600; www.icisf.org
(Formerly called the American Critical Incident Stress Foundation)

American Psychiatric Nurses Association

1555 Wilson Blvd, Suite 602, Arlington, VA 22209; Tel: 703-243-2443; www.apna.org

International Association of Forensic Nurses

East Holly Avenue, Box 56, Pittman, NJ 08071-0056; www.forensicnurse.org

References

American Psychiatric Association. (1994). *Diagnostic and statistical manual of mental disorders* (4th ed.). Washington, DC: American Psychiatric Association.

Antai-Otong, D. (2001). Critical incident stress debriefing: A health promotion model for workplace violence. *Perspect Psychiatr Care, 37*(4), 125-134.

Bartels, S. (1987). The aftermath of suicide on the psychiatric inpatient unit. *Gen Hosp Psychiatry, 9*(3), 189-197.

Benedek, E., & Schetky, D. (1986). The child as witness. *Hosp Community Psychiatry, 37*(12), 1225-1229.

Carlson, B. E. (1984). Children's observations of interpersonal violence. In A. R. Roberts (Ed.), *Battered women and their families* (pp. 147-167). New York: Springer.

Dale, P., Loftus, E., & Rathburn, L. (1978). The influence of the form of the question on the eyewitness testimony of preschool children. *J Psycholinguist Res, 7,* 269-277.

Dawson, J., Johnston, M., Kehiayan, N., et al. (1988). Response to patient assault: A peer support program for nurses. *J Psychosoc Nurs Ment Health Serv, 26*(2), 8-15.

Everly, G., & Mitchell, J. (1999). Critical incident stress debriefing: A meta analysis. *Int J Emerg Ment Health, 1*(3): 169-174.

Fantuzzo, J., & Lindquist, C. (1988). Violence in the home: The effects of observing conjugal violence on children. *J Fam Violence, 4,* 77-90.

Feldmann, T., & Bell, R. (1991). Crisis debriefing of a jury after a murder trial. *Hosp Community Psychiatry, 42*(1), 79-81.

Fix, C. (2001) Critical incident stress management program: Responding to the needs of correctional staff in Pennsylvania. *Corrections Today, 63*(6), 94-97.

Henning, K., Leitenberg, H., Coffey, P., et al. (1996). Long-term psychological and social impact of witnessing physical conflict between parents. *J Interpers Violence, 11*(1), 35-50.

Jaffe, P., Wolfe, D., & Wilson, S. (1990). *Children of battered women.* Newbury Park, CA: Sage.

Janoff-Bulman, R. (1989). Assumptive worlds and the stress of traumatic events: Application of the schema construct. *Soc Cogn, 17,* 113-136.

Jones, C. (1988). Fatal feelings. *Police, 2,* 26-49.

Joyce, B., & Wallbridge, H. (2003) Effects of suicidal behavior on a psychiatric unit nursing team. *J Psychosoc Nurs Ment Health Serv, 41*(3), 14-23.

Kardiner, A., & Spiegel, H. (1947). War, stress, and neurotic illness. New York: Hoeber.

Knazik, S., Gausche-Hill, M., Dietrich A., et al. (2003). The death of a child in the emergency department. *Ann Emerg Med, 42*(4), 519-529.

Lanza, M. (1988). Factors relevant to patient assault. *Issues Ment Health Nurs,* 9, 239-257.

Lanza, M. (1992). Nurses as patient assault victims: An update, synthesis, and recommendations. *Arch Psychiatr Nurs, 6,* 163-171.

Laposa, J. M., Alden, L. E., & Fullerton, L. M. (2003). Work stress and post-traumatic stress disorder. In ED nurses/personnel. *J Emerg Nurs, 29*(1), 23-28.

Lindemann, E (1944) Symptomology and management of acute grief. *Am J Psychiatry, 101,* 141-148.

Loftus, E., & Davies, G. (1984). Distortions of memory in children. *J Soc Issues, 40,* 50-52.

Martin, C., McKean, H., & Veltkamp, L. (1986). Post-traumatic stress disorder in police and working with victims: A pilot study. *J Police Sci Adm, 14*(2), 98-101.

McCarroll, J., Ursano, R., Wright, K., et al. (1993). Handling bodies after violent death: Strategies for coping. *Am J Orthopsychiatry, 63*(2), 209-214.

McDonald, R., & Jouriles, E. (1991). Marital aggression and child behavior problems: Research findings, mechanisms, and intervention strategies. *Behav Therapist,, 14* 189-191.

Mericle, B. (1993). When a colleague commits suicide. *J Psychosoc Nurs, 31*(9), 11-13.

Mitchell, J. (1986a). Living dangerously. *Firehouse* 8, 50-52.

Mitchell, J. (1986b). Teaming up against critical incident stress. *Chief Fire Executive, Vol 1:*24, pp 36-84.

Morrison, E. (1987/1988). The assaulted nurse: Strategies for healing. *Perspect Psychiatr Care, 3,* 120-126.

North, C., Smith, E., McCool, R., & Shea, J. (1989). Short-term psychopathology in eyewitnesses to mass murder. *Hosp Community Psychiatry, 40*(12), 1293-1295.

Ornitz, E., & Pynoos, R. (1989). Startle modulation in children with posttraumatic stress disorder. *Am J Psychiatry, 146*(7), 866-870.

Peterson, A., Nicolas, M., McGraw, K., et al. (2002). Psychological intervention with mortuary workers after the September 11 attack: The Dover Behavioral Health Consultant Model. *Mil Med, 167* (9 supp), 83-86.

Robinson, R. (2000). Debriefing with emergency services: Critical incident stress management. In Raphael, B. and Wilson, J. *Psychological debriefing: Theory, practice and evidence.* (pp. 91-107.) Cambridge: Cambridge University Press.

Smith, T., & Munich, R. (1992). Suicide, violence, and elopement: Prediction, understanding, and management. In A. Tasman & M. Riba (Eds.), *American Psychiatric Press review of psychiatry: Vol 11.* (pp. 239-252). Washington, DC: American Psychiatric Press.

Thompson, J., & Brooks, S. (1990). When a colleague commits suicide: How the staff reacts. *J Psychosoc Nurs, 28*(10), 6-11.

Ursana, R., & McCarroll, J. (1990). The nature of a traumatic stressor: Handling dead bodies. *J Nerv Ment Dis, 178,* 396-398.

Vasquez, D. (1993, July). Helping prison staff handle the stress of an execution. *Corrections Today,* 70-72.

Chapter 51 Caring for Offenders: Correctional Nursing

Pamela J. Dole

Correctional care nursing integrates the principles of nursing, forensic, psychiatric, primary care, and public health knowledge during the care of prisoners and parolees. Violence is increasingly visible within the US and around the world. The booming incarceration rate in the US leads the industrialized nations, is fourth in the world, is a very political and controversial topic, and is tied to complex social problems. Offenders are in need of nurses with medicolegal knowledge as well as compassion and caring, irrespective of whether we support the current social milieu regarding offenders.

Correctional nursing in this chapter refers to the job of nurses who work "behind bars" or with detained individuals. These settings may include penitentiaries, prisons, jails, detention centers, holding cells, work camps, work release programs, court programs, drug rehabilitation centers, or forensic psychiatric institutions. Individuals accused of breaking laws are confined with sanctions specific to this custody and will influence the practice of nursing. All rights are lost during confinement, and privileges must be earned. It is challenging for nurses to maintain caring and human rights under the sanctions of custody. Thus, the phrase "custody and caring" has been coined to depict this contradiction of terms (Peternelj-Taylor & Johnson, 1998).

Professional debate exists as to whether correctional care nursing and forensic nursing can be viewed in the same vein (Maeve & Vaughn, 2001). If one considers forensic nursing as being limited to the collection of medicolegal evidence, then the answer is no. However, if forensic nursing is considered within the broader context where law and medicine (nursing) intersect, then it is within this purview. Offenders have been convicted of a crime (law) and receive healthcare (medicine). Forensics provides for legal arguments that can be used to advocate for the health and well-being of offenders. Forensic nurses also comprehend the importance of detailed, unbiased documentation that protects both the institution and the offender. Correctional nursing will be viewed within the broader context of forensic nursing and as practicing within all of these institutions, both correctional and forensic psychiatry.

In 1998, America incarcerated a million nonviolent prisoners (Irwin, 2000). This hallmark represented a threefold increase in prison and jail populations over two decades, a direct response to escalating stringent sentencing laws culminating in 1994. These laws provide for mandatory sentencing for first-time offenses. Approximately 75% of the prison populations are not violent offenders. The Rockefeller laws or the "Two Strikes" 1994 law applies to individuals who commit violent crimes a second time who are then required to serve a life sentence. Only 25% to 33% of prisoners have committed violent crimes, such as murder, rape, kidnapping, armed robbery, aggravated child molestation, aggravated sodomy, and aggravated sexual battery.

Healthcare becomes a by-product of institutional responsibilities to incarcerated individuals, as it must protect prisoners from harm. Penal and psychiatric institutions for the offender and criminally insane respectively are potentials for major public health problems because large aggregates of people are living together in small, confined, and overcrowded quarters. Approximately 95% of inmates will be released back into the community carrying whatever they came to prison with or acquired within prison (*Washington Times*, 2002). Minimum standards of healthcare for prisoners lack consensus among the laws governing human rights and correctional facilities, as well as among professional organizations. The issue of public health risks to incarcerated individuals and lack of consensus regarding the institutional responsibility for healthcare has a long history that has reached a pinnacle.

Key Point 51-1

The primary objective of a correctional institution or psychiatric correctional facility is to provide safety to the public by incarcerating those individuals who have committed crimes against society. The institution is responsible for its own needs and safety, as well as the safety and the needs of the prisoners and patients.

Forensic nursing has much to offer correctional facilities, which this chapter addresses in detail. In summary, forensic nurses can do the following:

- Consult and advocate on human rights issues
- Perform medicolegal examinations (not where employed)
- Teach and perform detailed, unbiased documentation
- Provide nursing care that is free of bias and judgment
- Advocate for healthcare and healthcare education
- Inspire self-care for offenders
- Assist nursing and other professionals in creating protocols with the highest ethical standards
- Assist in providing an impartial and secure environment for offenders and staff
- Develop and implement initiatives that decrease the roots of violence

Nurses, as well as other healthcare providers, are often confronted with situations that raise ethical and professional dilemmas while caring for offenders. Additionally, the issue of power and the questionable ability to consent while incarcerated demand strong moral and ethical convictions by all correctional care nurses and healthcare providers caring for offenders or the criminally insane. Advocacy, prisoner rights, health education, standards of care, and caring are often defined very differently "behind bars." Forensic nurses should utilize guidelines for care developed by professional organizations. These guidelines come include the following:

- ANA's Scope and Standards of Nursing Practice in Correctional Facilities (1985, updated 1995)

- American Nurses Association and International Association of Forensic Nurses (ANA, 1997), Scope and Standards of Forensic Nurse Practice
- United Nations (UN, 1982), Principles of Medical Ethics and Standard Minimum Rules for the Treatment of Prisoners
- International Council of Nurses (ICN, 1989), The Nurse's Role in Safeguarding Human Rights, Nurses and Torture, and The Nurse's Role in the Care of Detainees and Prisoners
- American Correctional Health Services Association (ACHSA), Code of Ethics (1999)

Integral to correctional healthcare are many disciplines and agencies. These include nurses and other medical personnel; psychiatrists; pharmacists; social workers; nutritionists; correctional officers; parole officers; Department of Corrections (DOC) administrators; local, state, and federal officials; managed care agencies; and peer educators. Nursing is an integral component of prison life, as nurses constitute 19% of overall correctional staff. The official federal government agency is the National Institute of Law Enforcement and Criminal Justice, currently referred to as the National Institute of Justice (NIJ).

Correctional care nursing is an exciting opportunity to practice community health nursing, primary care, psychiatric nursing, and forensic nursing, to name a few specialty areas. The majority of prisoners have a history of poverty, substance abuse, and mental illness with episodic healthcare. Many offenders are illiterate or poor readers and often have learning disabilities. Incarceration may represent the first time an offender receives comprehensive healthcare, continuity of care, and has the opportunity to develop a relationship with the nurses and primary healthcare providers (Flanigan, 1999). Correctional facilities offer excellent opportunities for nurses to practice all their skills including the therapeutic use of the self (Miller, 1999). Correctional care nursing provides an excellent opportunity for nurses to apply the art and science of nursing and the principles of public health and forensics while providing caring, health education, health promotion, injury prevention, and community health initiatives.

The relationship between incarceration and violence is also dependent on the social and political milieu. The current climate is punitive or vindictive. It is a major public health concern and will challenge every correctional care nurse. Violence has direct and indirect costs on the healthcare system and the victims affected by it. To improve health outcomes, *Healthy People 2010* (US Department of Health & Human Services, 2000) lists the reduction of violence as imperative to reduce morbidity and mortality-related injuries. Correctional care nurses will be challenged to create and initiate models that heal the mind, body, and spirit of traumatized survivors of violence.

Societal Factors Contributing to High Incarceration Rates

Most incarcerated individuals are disproportionately affected by acts of violence and are overwhelmingly from poor communities. Although many factors contribute to violence, being poor places an individual at high risk for being affected by violence and its sequel. Offenders are often members of vulnerable populations and lack access to healthcare, placing a heavy burden on correctional institutions when individuals are incarcerated.

The World Health Organization (WHO) defined violence in (2002) as the following:

> *Violence is the intentional use of physical force or power, threatened or actual, against oneself, another person, or a group or community, that results in or has a high likelihood of resulting in injury, death, psychological harm, maldevelopment, or deprivation.*

WHO further categorizes violence into three types, which is also used by the Centers for Disease Control (CDC). They are self-inflicted violence (suicide, mutilation), interpersonal violence, and organized violence (generally organized around political, social, or economic agendas, such as with war, gangs, or mobs).

Better crime prevention is generally related to the "War on Drugs," which was stepped up in 1994 to deflect soaring crime rates that in fact had not dropped in the preceding years. Several studies have demonstrated that increasing imprisonment does not reduce crime (Irwin & Austin, 1987, 2000). Crime rates during the past three decades have remained relatively constant.

The 1997 annual household telephone survey conducted by the Department of Justice (DOJ) reported the following about victims:

- There were more victims with an income greater than $7,500 than with an income greater than $75,000.
- Only 37% of crimes were reported, and even fewer rapes and sexual assaults were reported.
- Victims reported 80% of automobile accidents secondary to insurance requirements.
- Half the crimes were perpetrated by known assailants, and in sexual assaults the majority of assailants were known.
- More than half the victims were between 12 to 24 years old.
- A greater number of victims were male (46% versus 33%).
- Blacks were most vulnerable (49%) compared to Hispanics (43%) and whites (38%).
- Crime was higher in urban areas.
- Crimes against the elderly are increasing.

If the statistics are carefully examined, it becomes clear that the majority of crimes occur in poor communities, disproportionately among blacks and young people. This profile has remained fairly constant according to the CDC (1997). Researchers and professionals experience the effects and affects of crime, poverty, and racial discrimination daily. Their experience is that things are getting worse. There are fewer initiatives to remedy or even to stabilize poor communities. The money is being spent on warehousing the poor behind bars rather than improving services that benefit the neighborhoods. Unfortunately, incarceration has the rippling effect of further deteriorating individuals, families, and communities who have the fewest resources.

Children arrested for a violent crime revealed a significant history of abuse. (National Center on Child Abuse and Neglect, 1996). There are many public health concerns that the money would be better spent rehabilitating individuals and communities rather than incarcerating low-level crime offenders who are not rehabilitated by being incarcerated. Rehabilitation would also include universal healthcare. Change can only occur when justice is a key principle in public health and economic inequality is viewed as injustice (Drevdahl, Kneipp, & Canales et al., 2001).

Many researchers agree that vulnerable aggregates experience increased exposure to risk factors and that this greater and prolonged exposure directly impacts the higher levels of morbidity and mortality (CDC, 1997; Magura, Kang, & Shapiro et al., 1993; Wallace, Fullilove, & Flisher, 1996). Morbidity and mortality are further compounded by limited resources such as income, jobs, education, and housing; aggregates with decreased social connectedness or integration that are heightened with stigmatized discrimination and decreased social status and power; and populations with decreased environmental resources such as healthcare and quality care (Flaskerud & Winslow, 1998). Women and children are especially vulnerable and will be discussed later in this chapter.

Cohen and colleagues (2000) reported an example of compounded environmental and social influences on morbidity and mortality, which was the high correlation between neighborhood disorder and high-risk sexual behavior (which was measured by increased gonorrhea rates). This study was based on several other prevailing theories that the environment (broken windows, litter, and graffiti) contributes as much to violence as poverty by sending a message to the community that no one cares. Ellickson and McGuigan (2000) found that adolescents in middle school who had few bonds, poor grades, and deviant behavior were the same teens who later committed acts of aggression and violence in high school. These teens displayed additional risk behaviors represented by cigarette and marijuana use.

Health outcomes must be expanded to encompass the environment and social needs of the individual and their aggregates. Researchers at Columbia University stated that risk-taking behavior is reflective of an interwoven social network in low socioeconomic communities and that community initiatives must be comprehensive:

> *We suggest that violent acts in particular may emerge as key behavioral symbols for "sending a message" in socially disorganized communities, implying that school-based or other individual-oriented harm reduction strategies for violence prevention, in the absence of a comprehensive, multifactorial reform program, cannot significantly reverse the effects of continuing economic and social constraints or of public policies of planned shrinkage and benign neglect, factors primarily responsible for the disorganization of urban minority communities with the United States. (Wallace, Fullilove, & Flisher, 1996, p. 533)*

Initiatives must be holistic and include all needs related to disorganized and disenfranchised communities. In addition to access to quality healthcare, initiatives must include employment (with income that will provide power, housing, and educational opportunities) as well as violence prevention initiatives at all levels that include decreasing racism, gender bias, cultural indifference, and lack of respect.

Researchers of disorganized communities, many social and religious leaders, as well as ghetto survivors support public health initiatives within communities and not "behind bars." Recommendations by these groups are for alternatives to incarceration for first time nonviolent crime offenders, especially women with children. Their philosophy is that warehousing the poor without rehabilitation only further disorganizes the communities and families they have come from. There are individuals who do commit horrific crimes and need to be separated from society. Several decades ago the majority of prisoners fell into these categories. Distinction must be made between the violent offender and the nonviolent offenders. Drug law reforms are emerging in the form of legislative laws supported by voters in various states. Twenty-five states enacted new mandatory minimun sentencing laws in 2003 as a response to pressure from social justice groups (Drug Policy Alliance, 2003). While the Rockefeller Drug Laws have not been repealed, Michigan, Washington, Kansas, Texas, and New York have significantly reduced the harshness of these laws. State prisons in California, Texas, Kansas, and Indiana have instituted drug treatment in place of prison for nonviolent offenses related to substance abuse, and governors of other states are considering plans for similar programs (VonZielbauer, 2003b). Federal penitentiaries have not instituted such programs, and, in fact, former Attorney General John Ashcroft gave federal prosecutors orders to reduce plea bargaining and tighten prosecution for serious crimes. The forensic nurse should apply critical thinking when a simple solution or theory is offered for this immensely complex public health concern.

Who Is Incarcerated?

The faces behind bars have always been disproportionately from minority, poor, vulnerable, and disenfranchised populations. Minority groups within the prison population have risen significantly over the past decade. Of black (non-Hispanic) males age 25 to 29, 13.1% were in prison or jail. In the same age group, only 4.1% of Hispanic males and 1.7% of white males were jailed. Male inmates make up 88.6% of local jail populations (Beck & Karlberg, 2001).

Female prisoners have doubled since 1990 and now account for 6.7% of jailed prisoners (Beck & Harrison, 2001; Beck & Karlberg, 2001). Among incarcerated females in 2000, black (non-Hispanic) women were three times more likely than Hispanic females and six times more likely than white women to be in jails or prisons. For black women, the highest rate of incarceration was among those 30 to 34 years old.

The highest number of arrests in the US (21.9%) occurred in the 15- to 19-year-old age group (Department Justice–FBI, 1999). The 20 to 39 age group followed in the most numbers of arrests with rates decreasing with age (Department Justice–FBI, 1999).

More minority youth were also incarcerated in the late 1990s and early twenty-first century. The majority of juvenile offenders were male (86.5%) and black (40%) (Office of Juvenile Justice and Delinquency Prevention [OJJDP], 1999). The balance for racial/cultural breakdown of youth offenders includes 37.5% white, 18.5% Hispanic, 1.5% American Indians, 1.8% Asian Americans, and 0.3% Pacific Islanders (OJJDP, 1999). Private facilities (nongovernmental organizations) provided 27.8% of the assigned beds, as compared to 5.6% for adult incarcerations (Beck & Harrison, 2001; OJJDP, 1999). Serious personal or property offenses constituted 42.4% of crimes. This breaks down into 25% aggravated assault, a kidnapping, or a robbery; 20% serious property offenses including arson, auto theft, and burglary; and 2% were charged or adjudicated for homicide or murder (OJJDP, 1999). Another 6.5% of status offenses included running away, underage drinking, truancy, curfew violations, and other offenses that would not be classified as offenses for adults (OJJDP, 1999).

Federal prisoners sentenced for violent crimes declined from 17% to 11% (Beck & Harrison, 2001). Robberies, however, had increased 81% with a 21% decrease in other offenses such as assault and sex offenses. (Beck & Harrison, 2001). In the federal penitentiaries, 92.5% of offenders are male. Within penitentiaries, men who committed violent crimes constitute 60% of the population, and 58.4% are incarcerated for drug offenses. Women have similar drug offense crimes rates in federal prison; however, only 25% to 33% are violent offenders. By the end of 2000, all state and federal prisons were operating above capacity, 15% and 31%, respectively (Beck & Harrison, 2001).

Rockefeller drug laws have contributed to the 6% annual increase in state and federal prisons (Beck & Harrison, 2001). Jail populations have grown at a slightly faster rate. In 1999, 61% of federal prisoners had drug-related offenses (Beck & Harrison, 2001); 71% of prisoners were tested for drugs in 1998, and only 25% of prisons were testing prisoners in 2000. Fifty-one percent of prisoners were using alcohol or drugs when they committed their offense, and 57% were using drugs in the month before their offense; 83% of prisoners reported past substance abuse. Only 25% of offenders in federal prison and 33% of offenders in state prison had participated in substance abuse programs since admission (Mumola, 1999). For offenders who had used substance during the month prior to committing the offense, only one in seven had received treatment. Another 33% had enrolled in other drug abuse programs such as Alcoholics Anonymous (AA) or peer education programs.

Since the late 1990s and early twenty-first century, offenders have reported increased use of alcohol while committing offenses. These rates have increased from 10% to 20%. State and federal prisons had treated 14% of these offenders. A third of these offenders had enrolled in other alcohol programs such as AA or peer education programs (Mumola, 1999). Arrests for drinking while intoxicated (DWI) decreased 18%, whereas applicants for drivers licenses increased 15% (Mumola, 1999).

Lack of social and environmental attainments combined with physical impairments and poor access to care contribute to increased risks for incarceration (Flaskerud & Winslow, 1998). Approximately 10.7% of offenders have learning disabilities, two fifths of inner city youth read at a fifth grade level or less, and most offenders have not completed high school (Persersilia, 2000). Another 4% to 10% of offenders are mentally challenged. Seventh graders who got into trouble in school were significantly more violent five years later (Ellickson & McGuigan, 2000). Predictors of adolescent violence included poor grades, poor self-esteem, rebelliousness, early tobacco and marijuana abuse, moving frequently and not being bonded to the school, and attending schools that were located in poor socioeconomic communities (Ellickson & McGuigan, 2000). Approximately 10% of the jail populations are supervised in alternative programs (Beck & Karlberg, 2001). Many activist groups believe that treating substance abuse and alcoholism would be a better alternative for nonviolent offenders.

Historically, sheriffs and correctional officers have underrepresented minority populations. This has been problematic for other departments who care for offenders, including departments of nursing and medicine. Since the late 1990s and early twenty-first century, employment of sheriffs' and correctional officers has risen, as has the representation of racial and ethnic minorities within correctional departments. In sheriffs' departments, 19% of full time officers were minorities compared to 13.4% in 1987 (Bureau of Justice Statistics [BJS], 2000). Increasing minority representation at all levels of employment may have the benefit of decreasing racial disparities and tensions behind bars.

History of Prison Care

Prisons and jails have historically gone between the philosophies of punishment and rehabilitation. During the earlier periods of punitive philosophies, poor diets, hygiene, sanitation, and healthcare placed prisoners at risk for plagues, tuberculosis, typhus, sexually transmitted infections (STIs), gangrene, and scurvy. Prison reform has impacted the living conditions and healthcare of prisoners.

Following numerous typhus outbreaks in 1775, prisons began delousing prisoners upon arrival to prison and began issuing clean clothing. Prisoners started receiving examinations by a physician, and moral and medical crusades urged improved diets.

In the 1800s, Louis René Villerme of France was the first to do epidemiological studies in institutions (King, 1998). Reform issues began to include rehabilitation of prisoners and with it came education, exercise, reduced crowding, increased lighting and ventilation, green vegetables, work, and fair treatment of inmates. Making these reforms was thought to improve the mental outlook of prisoners and contribute to their rehabilitation.

It was also Villerme and others who began to question the role of the physician in correctional care. Should physicians be independent of the institution or employees of the institution? As independent practitioners, they would be unbiased; however, the prisoners would not have the continuity and physical presence of a doctor within the institution. If employees of the institution, who would they report to and what would they be responsible for? These questions persist.

Physicians during this time period began seeing prisoners with more regularity. This effort included reexamining inmates prior to release, a practice that has continued, although it has become more of a medicolegal issue taken to protect the institution from lawsuits from the prisoner.

The Walnut Street Jail was the first detention center in the US, opening in 1776 in Philadelphia (May, 2000). The Quaker belief in redemption through penitence was a revolutionary departure from European institutions and embraced the new "nationalistic" philosophy of the founders of the US government. Unfortunately, reading the Bible in isolation did little to rehabilitate prisoners who were not ready to be saved.

By the 1800s, redemption would again be replaced by a philosophy of punishment. Inmate labor became a popular method to redeem inmates. In 1851, a Texas prison constructed a cotton mill within the prison walls and offenders were used as laborers. Chain gangs in the Texan and southern prisons resembled slavery as 75% of the inmates were black and the guards were primarily white (Edgardo, 1995). Imbalance of ethnic diversity among prison staff continues to plague the penal system. In the later part of the 1800s, prisoners were employed to build railroads, public utilities, iron mines, and foundries.

Today incarceration is viewed as punitive with little rehabilitation offered. Even if the social milieu were more favorable, it is doubtful that many rehabilitation efforts will be realized due to the incredible prison growth occurring since the mid-1990s. Most penal facilities find it challenging enough to keep up with standard healthcare. Prisoners have few rights, no privacy, and sometimes endure maltreatment. They have limited exercise and only basic hygiene.

In 1929, the US published two reports that would not be acted upon for nearly five decades. The first was a report of the National Society on Penal Information, which gave rise to correctional care as it is known today. President Herbert Hoover appointed the National Commission on Law Observance and Enforcement (also known as the Wickersham Commission), which published 14 reports endorsing parole, probation, and incarceration treatment to be individualized for prisoners. The Wickersham Commission reports were the first national and comprehensive survey of the American criminal justice system. These two sources of reports laid the foundation for significant future correctional care reform.

In 1975, the National Institute of Law Enforcement and Criminal Justice published another report. *The Prescriptive Package–Health Care in Correctional Institutions,* authored by Edward Brecher and Richard Della Penna, was a historic landmark with several original foundations laid for correctional healthcare as it is practiced today. The authors called for social and medical reform in what they viewed as "the typical chaos of healthcare delivery in most prisons and jails at that time" (King, 1998, p. 8). The *Prescriptive Package,* as it came to be known, provided guidance on organizing medical services within prisons and jails. It endorsed the following topics:

- Utilization of outside healthcare agencies to provide medical care to inmates as an effort to increase the variety of services needed, decrease the isolation of medical personnel within correctional care, and make prison care affordable.
- Community liaisons and collaboration in all aspects of healthcare.
- Locked secure units in community hospitals.
- Designing a system of care that offered consistently good healthcare was the antidote for the numerous class-action suits plaguing prison administration, which the authors noted as being a highly effective method in this instance for change.
- Utilization of physician assistants to decrease staffing problems.
- Improved medical record systems.
- In the areas of quality of care and issues of recidivism among healthcare workers, the community ties were again addressed (increase compensation and support staff; increase ties to professional organizations, continuing education, academic faculty appointments, and relationships with schools of medicine and nursing) (Brecher & Della Penna, 1975).

In retrospect, the *Prescriptive Package* has significantly influenced healthcare reform since the 1970s. The end result has been improved and more humane care for prisoners with increases in contractual medical arrangements. While a for-profit agency and some private managed care agencies specializing in correctional healthcare have been under attack for their profit margin, they have provided increased autonomy to healthcare providers within correctional healthcare that is viewed as an advantage for prisoners. The 1975 *Prescriptive Package* has been criticized for its lack of rehabilitative and mental health issues that were found in the earlier 1929 reports.

Correctional healthcare continues to improve. The relationship between healthcare providers and respective correctional institutions is often poorly defined. The federal courts have articulated some questions. Correctional institutions and professional organizations continue to improve and standardize care. Prisoners lose their rights for public healthcare through Medicaid and Medicare. The custody and healthcare of offenders is the financial responsibility of local communities and state and federal budgets. The doubling and tripling of offenders nationally since the mid-1980s, with increasing numbers of HIV-infected prisoners, has heightened the financial, healthcare, and public health concerns once again. The "one strike and you're out" law is responsible for the current rise in correctional populations, and of those incarcerated as a result of this law, the numbers are disproportionately higher among blacks and Hispanics, especially women. Increased numbers of HIV-infected prisoners have added costly healthcare visits and medications. At no other point is the health education of prisoners and correctional staff, including guards, so necessary to reduce mortality, morbidity, and escalating financial costs.

The current attitude toward prisoners and their advocates is less than positive and is reflected in the Violent Crime Control and Law Enforcement Act of 1994 (refined from the 1987). In 1987, the US responded to the frustration of citizens and law enforcement by enacting stiffer prison sentences as part of the questionable "War on Drugs." These laws are commonly referred to as the War on Drugs laws, the Rockefeller laws, or the 1994 Crime Bill. Under the state and federal drug laws, crack possession carries a mandatory prison sentence for a first-time offense. This law was strengthened with the 1994 federal crime bill after financial incentives were added to state budgets when certain offenders served 85% of their sentence. Unfortunately, this law has barely affected high-level drug dealers.

The 1994 Crime Bill law also added Title 42, US Code, Section 14141, which empowers the Department of Justice (DOJ) to enforce the constitutional rights of incarcerated individuals through civil suit. Built on the 1980 Civil Rights of Institutionalized Persons Act (CRIPA), it enabled the US government to investigate and bring legal action against state institutions when there is a question of civil rights (constitutional) violations. CRIPA will be important when prisoner abuse and medical issues are examined.

The 1994 Crime Bill was weakened two years later when Congress passed the 1996 Prison Litigation Reform Act (PLRA) as part of the Balanced Budget Down Payment Act II of 1996. This law significantly decreases the ability to intervene in class-action suits pertaining to medical and prison conditions (including abuse) by the federal courts, nongovernmental organizations, or individuals. This law provides some check and balance for prisoners requiring correctional institutions to be responsible for the quality of healthcare and healthcare providers.

The Violence against Women Act passed by Congress in 1994 was a long-waited bill to increase prosecutions of perpetrators, to provide organizations with startup and educational money, to reduce some of the humiliation and embarrassment for women by shielding their past during courtroom proceedings, and to prompt research (Crowell & Burgess, 1996). This act has slightly increased the number of people (primarily men) serving longer sentences for domestic violence, stalking, and sexual assault.

Prison Life and Organization

Most correctional facilities are organized utilizing a military or police force model. The warden or superintendent is the highest position, followed by captains, lieutenants, sergeants, and correctional/custody officers. Until recently these have been male-dominated organizations.

Employment reflected gender-based dualism, and men were employed as correctional officers for both men and women. Integration of women into the workforce was afforded under the 1972 amendments to Title VII of the Civil Rights Act of 1964. However, not until *Dothard v. Rawlinson* in 1977 did integration of women into the workforce of correctional institutions actually occur. The amendment carried height and weight restrictions, and women correctional officers were restricted to female prisons and were not allowed to have contact with offenders. In 1979, *Gunther v. Iowa State Men's Reformatory* ruled that women could not be excluded from training and contact with offenders. It also marked the beginning of the divide regarding privacy rights accorded to male and female offenders.

Fourth Amendment rights for reasonable privacy were upheld only if they did not jeopardize the security of the institution.

Reasonable cell searches were clarified in 1979 by *Bell v. Wolfish* and 1981 by *Hudson v. Palmer*. *Turner v. Safely* clarified reasonable body cavity searches in 1987.

The viewing of naked female bodies by male correctional officers was perceived as a violation of elemental self-respect and personal dignity. Female prisoners have a right to privacy in their housing units, in showers, and during other periods of surveillance. *York v. Story* in 1968 and *Forts v. Ward*, restricting male correctional officers from areas where women undress, upheld these conditions.

Even the handling and viewing of the clothed female body during cross-gender searches or patdowns came under question. In 1991, with *Ellison v. Brady* and in 1992 *Jordan v. Gardner*, courts upheld the right of female prisoners for same-gender searches, thus protecting women from inappropriate touching by male corrections officers.

Maintaining Human Rights during Incarceration

Forensic nurses in the area of correctional care are not well organized in a collective manner through professional institutions. Therefore a unified voice in the areas of healthcare, ethics, and advocacy for human rights is often lacking. The nursing profession lacks or has limited position statements in many areas related to caring for detained individuals. The majority of the available position statements have been listed throughout this chapter.

Human rights issues have become an even greater concern for nurses and healthcare professionals employed by correctional facilities. Understanding these rights requires some familiarity with the Constitution and its interpretation, knowledge that forensic nurses should possess on a limited basis. The Office of the Attorney General on both state and federal levels can guide questions about interpretation. Prisoners are afforded human rights even when their freedom has been taken away. In fact, healthcare is the *right* of an incarcerated person, whereas members of the general population, including the underinsured, have no entitlements to healthcare.

Issues Related to Incarcerating Prisoners

In 1966, the American Correctional Association (ACA) developed guidelines for the minimum conditions of confinement. These conditions included minimum access to outdoor exercise, adequate clothing, and minimum square footage of space per prisoner. Acceptable levels of violence were also defined. *Jeldness v. Pearce* (1994) provided the equal protection theory. Programs and services available to male prisoners such as education must also be available to female prisoners.

The Fourth Amendment of the US Constitution provides protection against sexual abuse while incarcerated. It states, "The right of the people to be secure in their persons . . . against unreasonable searches and seizures, shall not be violated." This raises issues with respect to body searches and bodily privacy while showering and toileting. Whereas sexual misconduct between prisoner and prison guards is expressly prohibited within the federal system, states are not bound to this law. Many states have enacted laws that prohibit sexual abuse and misconduct during incarceration; however, 23 states still have no such laws (Human Rights Watch, 1996).

Human rights for detained people are also guided by global history. In 1998, the United Nations (UN) celebrated the 50th anniversary of the adoption of the Universal Declaration of Human Rights. It was the belief that the adoption of this proclamation by all UN member countries (including the US) would preserve and define human rights and freedoms. The action followed the post–World War II Nuremberg Nazi war crime trials, which had produced the Nuremberg Code stating that "the voluntary consent of human subjects is absolutely essential" for medical research. Other international standards are guided by the International Covenant on Civil and Political Rights (ICCPR); the Convention against Torture and Other Cruel, Inhumane or Degrading Treatment or Punishment (Convention against Torture, or CAT); the Convention on the Elimination of All Forms of Discrimination against Women (CEDAW); and the International Convention on the Elimination of All Forms of Racial Discrimination (CERD). All of these standards seek respectful, reasonable, and compassionate interactions between facilities that detain individuals and the incarcerated individual. Women and ethnic minorities generally carry a disproportionate burden of abuse and incarceration (see the sections on substance abuse and violence), further complicated by the fact that the US has ratified and abides by ICCPR, CERD, and CAT but has failed to ratify CEDAW, which might assist in decreasing crimes against women especially while incarcerated. Many of these rights were challenged in the post-9/11 detainment of 5000 foreigners (Eviatar, 2003).

Many of the aforementioned international standards have their foundations in the First United Nations Congress on the Prevention of Crime and the Treatment of Offenders adopted in 1955 and updated in 1977. This document outlines the standards for minimum rules for the treatment of prisoners (United Nations, 1982). It includes guidelines on accommodation, personal hygiene, clothing and bedding, food, exercise and sport, medical services, discipline and punishment, instruments of restraint, handling complaints of prisoners, contact with the outside world, books, religion, retention of prisoners' property, notification of death, illness and transfers to families, removal of prisoners, behavior of institutional personnel, inspection of the prison, separation of prisoners by offenses, privileges, work, education and recreation, social relations and aftercare, treatment of insane and mentally abnormal prisoners, treatment of prisoners under arrest or awaiting trial, treatment of civil prisoners, and treatment of people arrested or detained without charge. The fundamental thread throughout this document is humanity and dignity for all prisoners or detainees regardless of race, religion, color, creed, gender, or economics.

During this same period, federal courts were hearing *Ruiz et al. v. Estelle*. In 1980, the courts found that widespread "pernicious conditions" were serious enough to be unconstitutional. The major issues that came out of this ruling included deficient healthcare, sanitation, access to courts, employee brutality, vague and unconstitutional disciplinary procedures, overcrowding, other general conditions of confinement, and correctional guards who may "build tenders."

In 1978, Human Rights Watch began to monitor human right abuses internationally, especially in three categories: arms transfers, children's rights, and women's rights (www.hrw.org). Other nongovernmental organizations such as Amnesty International have similar goals. Box 51-1 highlights organizations that monitor human rights internationally and nationally as well as humanitarian and social justice organizations.

Human rights within correctional institutions have come to the forefront as jail and prison overcrowding has reached its highest point to date. In March 1999, Amnesty International released its report "Not Part of My Sentence" as part of its human rights violations campaign on the custody of female offenders. Numerous examples of misuse of power, humiliation, sexual

Box 51-1 Professional Organizations Contributing to Correctional Healthcare Standards

American Correctional Health Care Services Association (ACHSA)—established as a result of the *Prescriptive Package*, position statement available
American Medical Association: Standards for Health Services in Prisons
American Nurses Association (ANA)—position statement
American Public Health Association's (APHA), Jail and Prison Health Council, position statement available
Association of Nurses in AIDS Care (ANAC)
National Commission on Correctional Health Care (NCCHC)
Society of Correctional Physicians (SCP)
World Health Organization (WHO)

Box 51-2 Human Rights, Humanitarian, and Social Justice Organizations

ORGANIZATIONS THAT MONITOR HUMAN RIGHTS INTERNATIONALLY AND NATIONALLY

Amnesty USA and International—Rights for All Campaign
Human Rights Watch—Women's Rights Project
United Nations

HUMANITARIAN AND SOCIAL JUSTICE ORGANIZATIONS

Critical Resistance Organizing Committee
Justice Policy Institute
Justice Works (interfaith efforts by community churches, citizens, ex-offenders, and attorneys on a local and national basis)
National Prison Project—American Civil Liberties Union

assault, and inappropriate conduct of male guards with female prisoner during patdowns and body searches were reported. The findings were so appalling that ABCs *Nightline* featured a six-part series titled "Crime & Punishment: Women in Prison," which aired beginning October 29, 1999 (Koppel, 1999). CNN also featured correctional care stories in February 2000. Twenty-seven percent of incarcerated women and 20% of incarcerated men reported sexual abuse (*Washington Times*, 2002). The Prison Rape Reduction Act was introduced to the US Senate and House with the goal of establishing a national commission to set standards that would reduce and eliminate prison rape (*Washington Times*, 2002).

Nurses can advocate for offenders when they suspect improprieties. However, they must be careful not to be labeled a "snitch" by offenders or a troublemaker by prison or jail authorities. Nurses must also understand that advocacy and empowerment are not highly valued behind bars and must be offered with care to provide for the safety of the entire facility. Institutions fear that prisoners will become agitated and create safety issues such as riots or other behavior problems.

Issues Related to the Healthcare of Prisoners

The Eighth Amendment of the Constitution provides the right of prisoners to a safe and humane environment. The *Spicer v. Williams* Supreme Court case (191 N.C. 487) in 1926 stated that the public must care for prisoners who, because they are deprived of their liberties, cannot care for themselves. This ruling fell short of recognizing the prisoners' constitutional rights under the Eighth Amendment. Many correctional healthcare practices originated from the 1975 *Prescriptive Package* that incorporated Eighth Amendment considerations. The 1976 US Supreme Court *Estelle* decision further clarified that correctional facilities could not deliberately show indifference to serious medical needs, upholding the Eighth and Fourteenth amendments of the US Constitution (*Estelle v. Gamble*, 429 US 97, 1976; McNally, 1998). This decision initiates rights of prisoners to healthcare and begins to set minimum standards of healthcare for prisoners. In 1975 and 1976, community standards for healthcare were applied within the correctional institutions. In 1983 (*Revere v. Massachusetts Gen. Hospital*, 463 US 239, 244), pretrial detainees under the Fourteenth Amendment were also provided legal rights to healthcare. More and more lawsuits, legal decisions, and professional organizations are applying community standards to correctional healthcare. In lawsuits, prisoners must prove that correctional facilities purposefully intended to provide inadequate treatment (*Wilson v. Seiter*, 111 S. Ct. 2321, 1991). A 1994 ruling (*Farmer v. Brennan*, 511 US 825) stated that prison officials must ensure that prisoners receive "adequate" food, clothing, shelter, and medical care but that "deliberate indifference" requires a culpable state of mind.

The consequence of these decisions, however, is disproportionate to the rights of those in the general public, to whom the government is not required to pay for healthcare. Correctional facilities were not prepared for escalating populations that are sicker than in the past and aging prisoners who develop chronic illnesses sooner than those their age in the general population. HIV issues are costly and complex, and when the disease is managed with appropriate antiretroviral therapy (ART), costs of medications are less than the costs of opportunistic diseases and their sequelae (Bozzette, McCaffrey, & Leibowitz, et al., 2001; DeGroot, 2000). Costs for healthcare within correctional facilities have skyrocketed. These costs are the subject of many debates.

Box 51-2 highlights examples of professional organizations that contribute to correctional healthcare standards.

Ethical Issues

The forensic nurse can be beneficial within correctional facilities by assisting nurses and staff in developing guidelines and protocols regarding ethical issues. The principle of justice is the area where issues of ethics and human rights intersect. Forensic nurses must deliver care that is distributed fairly and equitably. It should be free of discrimination with rules enforced equally, be free of exploitation, and be free of derogatory statements about others. Nursing care should be consistent among all prisoners; social action should increase the availability and access to care for all prisoners and protect human rights through education allowing for informed choices (ANA, Ethics and Human Rights Position Statement, 1991; International Council of Nurses, 1998). Many nurses and healthcare providers choose to not know the particulars of an individual offender's conviction in an effort to remain unbiased. This is easier to accomplish for healthcare providers who are subcontracted by the correctional institution for specific work.

The correctional care nurse must define the relationship with offenders with respect to advocacy, confidentiality, care and special needs of disabled inmates, codes of ethics as they relate to informed consent, the right to refuse care, the right to die, participation in executions, the use of pharmaceuticals to restrain prisoners, and hunger strikes that may be dictated by the employment arrangement. If a healthcare professional is an employee of the institution, then often nonmedical professionals such as the warden significantly affect medical ethics. Nurses and other healthcare professionals must often rely on the judgments of correctional officers (COs), who have no medical knowledge yet are with offenders most of the time, to suggest that a prisoner attend sick call when there is a medical problem. Nursing must be proactive and should not expect COs to assess prisoners or disburse medications.

Correctional care nurses often get caught between the needs of the institution and ethics with respect to safety and security, including body cavity searches, patdowns, collecting forensic evidence, use of restraints and force, writing up offenders, and segregation. Most professional organizations prohibit healthcare professionals from participating in *executions*, which presents a catch-22. Who will ensure compassion and appropriate doses of medications, and who will certify the death? Presently, 38 states have death penalties, including the US government and the military, and more than 400 deaths by execution have occurred since the late 1970s. Fifteen of those states have women on death row, and four women have been executed since the death penalty was reinstated in 1976. Present DNA technology is becoming more available to inmates, especially those on death row, which will help to decrease wrongful executions (Clines, 2000). Nurses can advocate for the use of DNA to reduce prosecution's errors. Both the International Council of Nurses and the American Nurses Association have position statements that state that participating in the taking of a life is a breach in the ethical code of nursing (American Correctional Health Services Association, 1999; American Nurses Association, 1994; International Council of Nurses, 1998).

Best Practice *51-1*

The forensic nurse should ensure that medicolegal examinations of prisoners are done in accordance to strict protocols to avoid breaching Fourth Amendment rights.

The skills and knowledge of forensic sciences can assist in the proper collection of forensic evidence. When body searches are required, the forensic nurse can be instrumental in developing relationships with consultant forensic nurses who can be called to do such examinations, thereby maintaining the relationship with offenders and their facility nurses. Forensic nurses must insist that during patdowns and body cavity searches women offenders are examined by women professionals to avoid breaching Fourth Amendment rights. Developing protocols that utilize an independent forensic nurse for medicolegal examinations would provide one solution to this conflict.

In 1997, the National Commission on Correctional Health Care (NCCHC) clarified the issue of nurses and healthcare providers collecting medicolegal evidence. It called for written policy and procedures for the collection of medicolegal evidence and prohibited facility-employed healthcare providers from doing the collection (NCCHC, 1997). This policy provides benefits to both the nurses and the offenders. Impartial medicolegal evidence collection can benefit offenders who are wrongly accused or who are trying to document an assault that occurred while being incarcerated. The caring and trusted relationship between nurses and offenders can be preserved.

Debate regarding clinical research/trials in correctional institutions goes in and out of favor. During the 1960s and 1970s, prisoners tested over 90% of FDA drugs, which brought significant financial rewards to the prison (DeGroot, Bick, & Thomas, et al., 2001). Coercion of prisoners to participate in research studies and several deaths prompted the development of the Belmont Report (National Commission for the Protection of Human Subjects, 1978). This was followed by the code of federal regulations in correctional care that stipulates that only the following types of research can be conducted (HHS Regulations 45 CFR 46, 45 CFR 46.306, 45 CFR 46.306):

1. Low-risk studies of "the possible causes, effects, and processes of incarceration, and of criminal behavior"
2. Low-risk studies of "prisoners as institutional structures" or of "prisoners as incarcerated persons"
3. Research on conditions particularly affecting prisoners as a class (e.g., vaccine trials and other research on hepatitis, which is much more prevalent in prisons than elsewhere)
4. Research that demonstrates "the intent and reasonable probability of improving the health or well-being of the subject" (Department of Health and Human Services, 1978)

Access to clinical trials for HIV drugs has raised the issues of inmate rights to standard healthcare afforded under the Eighth and Fourteenth US amendments. With the increase in the number of HIV-infected individuals behind bars, shouldn't inmates be able to access HIV medications available to HIV-infected individuals in the community? This is especially critical for offenders who are resistant to many of the HIV medications. Clinical trials and research in correctional institutions were banned because of coercion and the inability of inmates to freely consent. Some prisons have begun to allow HIV clinical trials back into their systems in order to provide medications that are available in the community.

Privacy

For safety reasons, privacy in correctional facilities does not exist. Hiring more female correctional officers would reduce the humility and embarrassment associated with daily dressing and showering, menstrual care, and during required isolation. Prior to 1975, few female COs were employed in prison facilities. It is the belief of many human rights groups that increasing the number of female COs would decrease violations of the Fourth and Eighth Amendments.

Confidentiality

Confidentiality is another difficult issue, as privacy virtually does not exist within a prison or jail. However, nurses are responsible for being careful as to where and when they speak about confidential issues. For example, specialists often provide HIV care in a specialty clinic, and everyone knows who attends the clinic; however, the nurse cannot reveal in front of other offenders the fact that an offender attends an HIV specialty clinic. This issue of confidentiality is further strengthened by the Health Insurance Portability and Accountability Act of 1996 (HIPAA) regulations.

Informed Consent

Prisoners are unable to give informed consent because they lack true freedom of choice. This raises many ethical considerations related to sexual activity, participation in research protocols, and healthcare. It is generally accepted that the inmates most at risk for coercion are those with the fewest resources both economically and socially. This is especially true for women who often participate in sexual activity or other activities to buy favors or status. Forensic nurses can establish proactive support groups that empower these women and decrease the risk of damage to their self-esteem.

Advocacy

Advocacy for offenders is often a delicate matter behind bars. If the forensic nurse is an employee or consultant to the correctional facility, safety of all prisoners must be the first concern. Empowering prisoners is sometimes viewed by administration as a threat to security. Assisting prisoners to heal their emotional wounds requires empowerment during the process. This process must be well thought out and planned so as not to encourage aggression or create agitation. "You are a guest in the warden/supervisors house" is a phrase that reminds all employees, visitors, and offenders who enter a facility who has the last word. Communication with all levels of staff is important to the success of implemented programs. Human rights violations are serious and need solutions that provide for the safety and compassion of all concerned.

Scope of Practice

Since the 1970s, prison reform has improved standards of community life and healthcare within correctional facilities. NCCHC is now the national accrediting agency. Standards of care are beginning to emerge after the court ruling mandating that community standards are met behind bars (NCCHC, 2003). The prison environment is a minisociety complete with healthcare; however, it is not a free society. It is important to set boundaries for the safety of all. Failure to do so can jeopardize lives and human rights.

Key Point *51-2*

Professional conduct with appropriate behavior and the ability to set boundaries are essential when working with forensic and incarcerated individuals.

Professional dress codes and interpersonal relationships must be respectful and therapeutic. Mental illness and disease often present as antisocial, manipulative, aggressive, impulsive, or angry behavior requiring nurses to exercise restraint and caution. Destructive manipulation is oriented for the sole purpose of the individual with no regard for the feelings of others, and others are often treated as dehumanized objects. Correctional nurses must be careful not to be manipulated into providing personal information, granting favors for specific offenders, or participating in sexual or erotic interpersonal relationships (Love, 2001).

Individuals who find themselves in hostage situations often exhibit the Stockholm syndrome as a survival mechanism. This bizarre syndrome, characterized by emotional bonding between captors and captives, was first documented in 1973. Hostages fearing for their lives who perceive some act of kindness from their captor, defend the captor and refuse to prosecute after the situation is resolved. Conditions that must be met for the Stockholm syndrome to occur include the following (Trigiani, 1999):

1. A perceived threat to survival with the belief that the captor will act on it
2. Within the context of terror, a perceived act of kindness from the captor
3. Isolation that restricts the hostage's perceptions to that of the captor
4. Perceived inability to escape

The hostage-captor bond phenomenon exist in other scenarios as well. Other victims of this phenomenon include concentration camp prisoners, prisoners of war, cult members, pimp-procured prostitutes, incest victims, physically or emotionally abused children, battered women, and victims of hijackings. This codependency is manipulated for the captor's advantage. The captives deny the stress, terror, and anger related to the incident. Often, self-destructive behavior follows. For women, recovery from the Stockholm syndrome includes developing strong friendships and political alliances with feminist women (Trigiani, 1999). Given the high level of lifetime victimization, including sexual and emotional abuse, experienced by individuals behind bars, offenders are at high risk for manipulation and may already suffer from the Stockholm syndrome. Correctional nurses must be aware of these phenomena in the event they also find themselves in hostage situations.

Nurses account for 19% of all correctional staff and have the same types of professional responsibilities within correctional facilities with the added concern of safety. Learning to be caring while being cautious is often a challenge. All equipment, supplies, and pharmaceuticals must be locked. Used needles, instruments, gloves, and other materials can be used as contraband and must be accounted for. There are no newspapers, magazines, and other such material to read on breaks. There are no beepers or cell phones. Health education material must be evaluated for appropriateness before it can be dispensed.

Nursing personnel must develop working relationships with correctional officers who have their own issues and responsibilities for the safety of the institution. It is imperative to understand and work within their policies and procedures regarding security. Lockdowns, counts, passes, etc., often interfere with the flow of nursing care. However, these impositions are necessary to protect the integrity of the institution.

Healthcare professionals approve many privileges for prisoners. These include work restrictions, shoe passes, slow eating passes, air conditioning, lower bunk status, special diets, sunglasses, special soaps, blankets, and special clothing. Offenders often try to manipulate this perceived power.

Some facilities have complete medical accommodations including hospitals, radiology departments, and laboratories, and some facilities provide essential surgery. Other facilities will have a physician several hours per day and a small infirmary. Work release programs may offer no healthcare, expecting prisoners to seek care in the community. In most facilities, sick call requests are answered within 24 hours.

Correctional care nurses suffer from isolation on several levels. Prisons are often located in geographically undesirable places outside of mainstream society. This often precludes nurses from attending local professional meetings or from pursuing continuing education. Presently this problem has been remedied by telemedicine conferences, Internet conferences, or public health initiatives designed to bridge this gap by affiliating with colleges and universities. There is stigma associated with being employed by a correctional facility, decreasing available applicants. Failure to meet competitive salaries has also decreased the diversity and availability of the working pool.

Applying the art and science of nursing itself can be utilized to develop areas of offender advocacy that benefit everyone.

Correctional care facilities can be a nurse's paradise if the individual enjoys health education. Many offenders have never had an opportunity to develop a relationship with any healthcare provider. Basic anatomy and physiology, self-care strategies, anger management, parenting, pharmacology, health promotion, and health prevention are all potential teaching opportunities behind bars. Health education in these areas empowers offenders and improves health outcomes that are beneficial to the offender and the institution. Educating offenders about the medication system and sick call procedures is also valuable. Many institutions require prisoners to notify the medication nurse when they are low on medications and need refills (for "on person" medications). Refills often take a week, as they go to an outside vender. Creating charts and calling offenders to sick call at times when medications should be running low would provide an opportunity for health education, evaluation of adherence, and mutual participation in creating a plan of care. Teaching offenders to follow self-care practices, to appropriately utilize healthcare, and to journal concerns (including symptoms) benefits both offenders and correctional healthcare providers.

Stress and anxiety increases for most offenders during incarceration. Any method to decrease stress would contribute to the overall well-being of the offender. Some facilities offer poetry or writing programs, meditation, music, and art therapy as means to manage stress. Stress reduction methods learned and practiced during incarceration will also benefit offenders when they are released back into the community.

Overall education for correctional officers on issues of universal precautions, reporting changes in the conditions of offenders, not withholding medications or sick calls as punishment, and general health education is also beneficial to the prisoners and the institution. This education is particularly necessary for informing all of those within the correctional facility about the transmission of communicable disease including hepatitis, tuberculosis, and HIV. Basic anatomy and physiology as well as women's health including reproductive issues, vaginal and sexual health, and mental health issues including depression and suicide are useful topics. Dispelling myths and providing accurate information is beneficial for everyone.

Nurses have an opportunity to apply *Healthy People 2010* behind bars. In addition to topics already mentioned, programs in the following areas are needed and would benefit offenders:

- Violence prevention
- Anger management
- Parenting skills
- Coping strategies
- Skills building and social support enhancement
- Injury prevention
- Smoking prevention
- Substance abuse rehabilitation
- STI harm reduction
- Increased literacy and assistance in obtaining a general equivalency diploma (GED)
- Increased social skills
- Job training

Nurses can play a key role by assessing offenders for functional (low) illiteracy and learning disabilities, which are pervasive among incarcerated populations. Failure to adequately screen and identify illiteracy results in offenders not understanding prison protocols, medical regimens, informed consent, and ultimately the inability to perform self-care practices (American Medical Association [AMA], 1999; Perdue, Degazon, & Lunney, 1999). Low literacy can also result when English is not an offender's first language (Collins, Gulette, & Schnept, 2005). Many offenders with low literacy have learned to compensate and hide it very well (Doak, Doak, & Root, 1996; Schultz, 2002). Nurses must be alert to offenders who only use visual cues and demonstrate difficulty adhering to medical regimens.

Illiterate youth and adults are also at risk for future incarceration if they are not identified early. Sixty-five percent of offenders in state prisons have not completed high school (Health Resources and Services Administration, 2000). Incarcerated people must be supported in the hope that they are worthwhile and can accomplish their goals. Providing the desire to overcome illiteracy combined with a program to do so requires educators who are gentle, have a positive outlook, are forgiving of offenders' shortcomings and their own, and interact with unconditional caring (Carrera, 1996). Until incarcerated individuals are helped to attain skills to overcome low literacy (and other deficits), they will remain at risk for recidivism and marginalization as they generally lack employable skills or a high school diploma. Box 51-3 highlights additional references that address issues related to literacy and learning disabilities.

Box 51-3 Resources Related to Literacy and Learning Disabilities

Hayes M. Social skills: The bottom line for adult LD success; www.ldonline.org/ld_indepth/social_skills/social-1.html

"Improving Patient Education for Poor Readers"; http//nsweb.nursingspectrum.com/ce/ce195.htm

Literacy behind Prison Walls. (1994). National Center for Education Statistics.

Literacy Volunteers of America, www.literacyvolunteers.org

Parker, R. M., Baker, D. W., Williams, M. V., et al. (1995). The test of functional health literacy in adults: A new instrument for measuring patients' literacy skills. *J General Internal Med, 10,* 537-541.

Schultz, M. (2002). Low literacy skills needn't hinder care. *Regist Nurse, 65*(4), 45-48.

Nurses in Cascade County, Montana, created the first correctional healthcare services, which opened in January 1998 and is run by the Montana State University–Bozeman College of Nursing at Great Falls. Nurse practitioners (NP) on the faculty provide 95% of the healthcare to offenders, thereby reducing transportation and overall costs to Cascade County (Boswell, 2000). In addition to the two nurse practitioners, there are three full-time nurses, an administrative assistant, a medical records assistant, and nursing students. The nurses contract physician services. Early reports from jail administrators, offenders, and nurses have been positive. The program received awards from the National Organization of Nurse Practitioner Faculty (NONPF). Some examples of other non-nursing creative programs to empower and heal offenders are displayed in Box 51-4.

Nurses can create healing environments within the chaos of prison life. Nursing leader Martha Rogers supported holistic nursing practice where individuals work, play, and live. Campbell (1992) stated that nursing education in the area of interpersonal violence would be more beneficial if it were rooted in "ways of knowing" rather than pathology and taught "advocacy, mutuality, critique, and transformation" as tools of empowerment for both practitioners and patients. Both of these nursing leaders recognize

Box 51-4 Non-Nursing Creative Programs to Empower and Heal Offenders

- *Cell Block Art* (Princeton Publishers, 2001) by Joyce is a collection of work done by offenders. This art therapy program is designed to empower the human spirit through art, thus providing the mind with the freedom to escape the pain.
- Girl Scouts behind Bars serves to bring mothers and daughters together to develop service, values, and healing.
- *Jesus Hopped the 'A' Train*, written by Stephen Adly Giurgis as part of the Hospital Audiences, Inc. (HAI), Violence Prevention Program, is a play about two inmates, religious cults, and life in prison. Shown to offenders at Ryker's Island, the play provided dialogue between actors, correctional officers, and offenders. The play moved to a London theater after receiving "Fringe" Edinburgh Festival awards.
- Training Seeing Eye Dog Program in New York State. Offenders earn the right to evolve responsibility and improve self-esteem.
- The Wild Animal Rescue Project at the Maryville Prison in Ohio affords women inmates the opportunity to develop self-worth by caring for injured animals until the animals can be released back into nature.

the power of nursing to affect their environment and patients. It is important to not revictimize offenders by being critical and judgmental. Compassion, caring, and programs that empower and educate are needed behind bars.

Health Problems of Inmates

General Health Status of Inmates

Escalated morbidity and mortality rates are secondary to earlier lives in poverty and poor access to healthcare prior to incarceration (Hammett, Harmon, & Rhodes, 2002; McLaughlin & Stokes, 2002). Minority groups, especially African Americans, are overrepresented within the prison systems and generally enter the prison system in the poorest of health secondary to disparity in healthcare while in the community (Davis, Liu, & Gibbons, 2003; Nelson, 2002). Twenty percent of offenders report health concerns other than injuries at the time of admission. Approximately 5% to 7% of offenders have more than one medical impairment or mental condition. Another 26% to 28% of offenders in state and federal prisons report injuries secondary to accidents or fights while incarcerated (Maruschak & Beck, 2001). Injuries increase with time served and double after 72 months of incarceration. The likelihood that inmates will require surgery also increases with length of time incarcerated from 2.5% of offenders confined less than 6 months to 21% of offenders confined 120 months or greater.

Table 51-1 highlights common medical problems of state and federal inmates. It should be noted that some physical and mental impairments are three times higher in prison than in the general populations. These include learning and speech impairments and mental impairments. Box 51-5 highlights types and number of deaths in state prisons.

Healthcare Costs for Inmates

Offenders lose federal and state-funded medical care benefits such as Medicaid and Medicare. Healthcare for offenders is therefore passed on to taxpayers through DOC budgets. Costs for healthcare are often escalated if medical charts are not electronic. This occurs during transfers to hospital locked wards for care or more often when offenders are transferred to other correctional facilities. Transfers to other correctional facilities occur frequently for a variety of security and medical reasons. For security reasons, transports generally occur in the middle of the night and are on a need-to-know basis, generally leaving medical personnel out of the loop. This is problematic for offenders who may wait days or weeks for medical records to follow without needed medications. Approximately 18 to 20 state and federal institutions have electronic medical records that can easily follow offenders, thereby reducing the chance for missed medications, repeated procedures, or the need for additional laboratory tests and healthcare provider

Table 51-1 Medical Problems

CONDITION	STATE	FEDERAL
Learning (including dyslexia and attention deficit disorder)	9.9%	5.1%
Speech (including lisp/stutter)	3.7	2.2
Hearing	5.7	5.6
Vision	8.3	7.6
Mental impairment	10.0	4.8
Physical impairment	11.9	11.1
Mental illness	16%	7%
Significant psychiatric problems	12.5%	Combined
Colds/flu/virus	19.0	21.9
Medical conditions	21.4	21.7
HIV infection	7.5% Northeast (especially New York and Florida), 1.1% Midwest, 0.8% West	5%

Data from Maruschak, L. M., & Beck, A. J. (2001). *Medical problems of inmates,* 1997. US Department of Justice, Bureau of Justice Statistics, January, NCJ 181644. www.ojp.usdoj.gov/bjs; Health Resources and Services Administration (HRSA). (2000). *Incarcerated people and HIV/AIDS.* US Department of Health and Human Services, Washington, DC, August/September. www.hrsa.gov/hab; Hammett, T. M., Harmon, P., & Maruschak, L. M. (1997). *1996-1997 Update: HIV/AIDS, STDs, and TB in Correctional Facilities.* Washington, DC: US Department of Justice, NCJ 176344, July; Ditton, P. M. (1999, July). Mental health and treatment of inmates and probationers, Bureau of Justice Statistics Special Report, NCJ US Department of Justice, 1-12.

Box 51-5 Types and Number of Deaths in State Prisons

Total = 3095
Natural (not HIV/AIDS) = 55%
AIDS = 29% (slightly ↓ over the past several years secondary to HAART, except in women)
Suicide = 5%
Accident = 1.3%
Execution = 1.3%
By another person = 1.95%
Other/unspecified = 5.19%

Data from Bureau of Justice Statistics (BJS); National Prisoner Statistics, 1996; and CDC. (1999). Decrease in AIDS-Related Mortality in a State Correctional System. New York, 1995-1998. *MMWR,* 47(51), 1115-1117.

Table 51-2 Approximate Incarceration Costs per Offender Each Year*

TYPE OF OFFENDER	YEARLY COST
Average offender	$38,500
Geriatric offenders	$69,000
HIV-infected offenders	$80,000–$106,600

*Costs vary from location to location.
Data from Health Resources and Services Administration (HRSA). (2000). *Incarcerated people and HIV/AIDS.* US Department of Health and Human Services, Washington, DC; August/September. www.hrsa.gov/hab; and Pelosi, A. (1997, May 5). Age of innocence: A glut of geriatric jailbirds. *The New Republic, 216,* 15-18.

visits. Table 51-2 highlights approximate incarceration costs per offender each year.

With healthcare costs soaring and as many as 90% of offenders abusing tobacco, applying *Healthy People 2010* can reduce morbidity and mortality behind bars. Smoking cessation programs can benefit correctional institutions by reducing healthcare expenditures related to smoking. Fraser Regional Maximum-Security Prison in British Columbia was the first of six correctional institutions in Canada to require a smoke-free environment (*Edmonton Sun,* 2000). Legal battles between offender rights and employees being exposed to secondhand smoke ensued. It is reasonable to expect smoking regulations to increase in prison systems.

Healthcare costs, as previously mentioned, come out of public health budgets that are designated for the department of corrections on local, state, and federal levels. Private healthcare companies specializing in correctional healthcare often participate in healthcare delivery to prisoners at various levels. This may involve providing physicians, nurse practitioners, or physician assistants to provide most of the healthcare within a facility, or it may be limited to specific specialties such as gynecology or infectious disease/HIV care. Perhaps several facilities share a pharmacist or contract those duties out to a private agency. Some hospitals contract to provide HIV care to correctional institutions in the area.

The advantage of private agencies is that highly specialized areas like HIV care is furnished by healthcare providers with that expertise. The down side is that offenders may not see the same person from visit to visit, further contributing to fragmented care and preventing offenders from developing lasting or trusting relationships. For the institution, the use of private agencies reduces transfers to outside medical facilities, a costly and potentially unsafe venture. Correctional care nurses can benefit by being intellectually stimulated by outside healthcare providers. Offenders often prefer or take joy in the fact that their "doc" is from the "outside." It is unclear if this method of healthcare delivery is cost-effective.

Telemedicine has increased utilization behind bars. Prisoners can sit and speak with an outside specialist in the presence of a correctional physician or nurse practitioner who has already performed an examination. This method of healthcare delivery is especially suited for specialty areas such as dermatology, urology, otolaryngology, orthopedics, general surgery, and the treatment of infectious diseases. It also is very helpful in states with rural correctional facilities. Initiated in the late 1990s, telemedicine has become a viable system in many states including Texas, Florida, California, Iowa, and New York, to name a few. Telemedicine decreases the need to transport a prisoner outside of the facility, which decreases cost and increases security/safety. Eliminating the need to transport a prisoner in shackles and chains reduces the humiliation many offenders experienced during clinic appointments.

Geriatric Offenders

It is estimated that by 2010, one third of the incarcerated population will be over the age of 51, representing a significant increase over the decades since the 1970s (Drummond, 1999; Neeley, Addison, & Moreland-Craig, 1997). One state reported that among offenders over the age of 60, two thirds were incarcerated between 1996 and 2001 for violent or sexual offenses. These offenders did not grow old behind bars from youthful offenses but rather had committed crimes as elders.

The primary problems with aging offenders include elder abuse and reduced housing safety, increased chronic illness and health needs, increased costs to the department of corrections (DOC), and end-of-life issues. Offenders over age 45 reported having medical problems other than common colds or injuries since admission. In federal penitentiaries, rates for older offenders were approximately 48%, and in state prisons approximately 40% of those incarcerated entered prison with medical problems (Maruschak & Beck, 2001). This is two times higher than for younger offenders.

Seventy-five percent of elder offenders (50 years old or older) have chronic illness suffering from hypertension (40%), myocardial infarctions (19%), emphysema (18%), and gross physical functional impairment (42%) including missing teeth (Colsher, Wallace, & Loeffelholz et al., 1992). They suffer from hearing and visual impairments that decrease their quality of life and place them at higher risk for elder abuse from other offenders. They require skilled nursing care, physical therapy, special diets, and increased pharmacy needs. Some will require surgery including cardiovascular interventions.

The needs of aging offenders are more complex within correctional institutions. Accessibility and safety issues are often difficult to accommodate. Doors in prisons may not be the required three feet wide to accommodate wheelchair access; doors may be very heavy, sometimes more than five pounds; and there may be insufficient space for ramps or handrails (Carroll, 2001). Frail elders may not be able to defend themselves and are therefore vulnerable to physical abuse and may lose commodities including food.

Many offenders will face dying behind bars without the support of family and friends. End-of-life issues must be met with compassion and caring, qualities not always fostered behind bars for fear of institutional security. Whether or not to release older offenders with life-threatening illnesses continues to be debated. Several states have dealt with this dilemma by developing special needs facilities for those offenders that would never qualify for release such as first- and second-degree murderers. In some states, offenders over age 50 who have served at least the average time for their crime and are terminally ill may be released under various programs to halfway houses or other post-release housing arrangements. Project for Older Prisoners (POPS) has been one such program releasing half of those who qualify to relatives and other to church-run low-cost apartments (Himelstein, 1993). The National Institute of Justice provides program guidelines for release of offenders with chronic diseases. Canadian correctional programs parallel guidelines used in the US for release of older offenders. Risk of recidivism does decrease with age, an argument often used to encourage compassionate release programs.

Correctional institutions will then have to decide what the policy is for those not eligible for release. Is it plausible to adapt a hospice program behind bars? Many correctional nurses and administrators have negative attitudes toward offenders, and this is exhibited by professional inattention that must first be addressed (Cohn, 1999). The National Prison Hospice Association provides guidance for implementing such programs without sacrificing the safety of the institution. Utilizing other offenders as hospice volunteers can be done with discretion, careful planning, and good organization with a multidisciplinary team of physicians, nurses, social workers, chaplains, correctional officers, and offenders (Rold, 2002). Coordinators generally choose from offenders in good standing with no infractions in the past six months. They attend educational sessions and ongoing meetings.

Offenders often have mixed feelings about utilizing hospice programs. Many individuals are in denial about their illness, whereas others fear being vulnerable and exploited if they are in a hospice program. Some offenders refuse palliative care including pain medication for fear of being out of control and therefore vulnerable to other inmates. Offenders who utilize the hospice program have the opportunity to experience community, compassion, and dignity behind bars (Beck, 1999; Mahon, 1999).

Communicable Diseases

Offenders have all the same medical concerns as the general population. At the time of incarceration, they often have undiagnosed or poorly managed chronic diseases, sexually transmitted infections (STIs) including human immunodeficiency disease (HIV), pregnancy, and mental illness secondary to the social conditions previously mentioned. As offenders age, increased rates of cancer and chronic disease require increased medical services and nursing care.

After the issue of safety, public health issues pose the most significant problem to correctional facilities. Confined space with overcrowding, poor ventilation, and increased community rates of tuberculosis (TB) and HIV have set the stage for several outbreaks of tuberculosis (TB) that peaked in 1991 (New York), again in 2000 (South Carolina) (Maddow, Vernon, & Pozsik, 2001); and again in 2004 (Florida) (Ashkin, Malecki, & Thomas, 2005). TB remains the single most communicable disease behind bars and occurs five times more frequently than in the general population (Hammett, Harmon, & Maruschak, 1997; Maddow, Vernon & Pozsik, 2001). The initial outbreak prompted mandatory TB testing in 73% of all correctional facilities with slightly higher rates of mandatory testing in state prisons and lower rates of required testing in jails. TB prevalence is 7% to 10% of correctional facilities with the highest rate seen in local jails where offenders often enter the correctional system. Correctional facilities account for one third of all cases of TB in the US (Nicodemus & Paris, 2001). Multidrug-resistant TB (mTB) is especially problematic behind bars where higher rates of HIV exist as well. The nurse can play an important role by developing proactive screening programs and policies that increase awareness of all communicable disease.

Other communicable diseases are also higher among offenders. Concern about confidentiality, combined with fear and denial, often affect whether an offender seeks care. Substance abusers often report not seeking care prior to incarceration and are at the highest risk for STIs. Rates of communicable diseases are difficult to estimate without routine testing policies.

Hepatitis was found in 155,000 offenders (Bureau of Justice Statistics, 2000). Compared to the general population, hepatitis B (HBV)/hepatitis C (HCV) is the second communicable disease that disproportionately affects incarcerated individuals at higher rates. Vaccinating offenders who do not test positive would reduce healthcare costs in the long run. Treatment for hepatitis C may not be readily available behind bars and remains controversial. Cost of treatment may still outweigh the limited outcomes from treatment. In an effort to reduce viral hepatitis, the National Commission on Correctional Health Care (NCCHC) has produced a CD titled "The ABC Hepatitis Education" as a resource for both inmates and prison staff (888-4-HEP-CDC).

An estimated 558,000 offenders had syphilis in 1999 (Bureau of Justice Statistics, 2000). Alabama experienced an outbreak of syphilis in three male prisons during 1999. New York City reported a 25% syphilis rate among incarcerated women (Nicodemus & Paris, 2001). This is alarming given the decreasing syphilis rates in the general population. Outbreaks of syphilis in prisons have been linked to mixing of offenders with unscreened jail prisoners, transfer of infected offenders to other prisons, and multiple concurrent sexual partners (Wolfe, Xu, & Patel et al., 2001).

Chlamydia rates among offenders are approximately 13%, and gonorrhea rates are 9%; 1% have both diseases (Bureau of Justice Statistics, 2000; Centers for Disease Control, 1999). Not unsurprisingly, chlamydia rates were higher among juveniles with females having a 22.2% rate of infection and males having an 8.7% rate in several Texas juvenile detention centers.

Incarcerated individuals also acquire sexually transmitted infections (STIs) while behind bars. Sexual relations are prohibited in correctional facilities, considered a felony in many states and federal prisons, and therefore not widely discussed. Rape and HIV in prison are reported to be eight to ten times that of the general population (*Washington Times*, 2002). Harm reduction strategies such as distributing bleach kits, condoms, sterile needles, and methadone can reduce transmission of STIs (Gaiter, Jurgens, & Mayer et al., 2000). Condoms are considered contraband, and bleach is not available to clean syringes. In addition to sexual acquisition of communicable diseases, shared needles for tattooing, body piercing, and injecting drugs also contribute to the spread of disease. Only seven correctional facilities distribute condoms: New York City jail, Los Angeles County jail, Philadelphia jail, San Francisco jail, Washington jail, Vermont prison, and Mississippi prison (Nerenberg, 2002; Sallot, 2002). In some of these facilities, the offender must self-proclaim to be homosexual to receive condoms. This does not help men who have sex with men (MSM) who do not identify as gay. This has raised civil liberties questions.

Condoms have been widely available in correctional institutions outside the US. As of 1997, 81% of European prison systems distributed condoms (Nerenberg, 2002). For the past decade, Canadians have provided condoms to incarcerated individuals. Ralf Jürgens, who represents the Canadian HIV/AIDS Legal Network, stated that researchers had found that 82% of correctional facilities had not found problems related to safety or security since the distribution of condoms (Nerenberg, 2002). The 18% reporting problems stated that their concerns were related not to safety or security but to using too many. The experience of other industrialized nations poses questions as to why US policies have not been updated.

HIV-Infected Offenders

The World Health Organization (WHO) reported that the US was one of four industrialized nations lacking a national policy regarding correctional care for the HIV-infected inmate (Harding &

Schaller, 1992). The rate of HIV within prison is seven times higher than that found in the general population. HIV, substance abuse, and mental illness are the leading medical conditions within prison.

HIV rates differ geographically and between genders behind bars (see Table 51-1). In Northeast areas, 30% to 40% of incarcerated women are HIV infected–nearly double that of men in the same area. The majority of women learn their HIV status while incarcerated or during pregnancy.

Often, incarcerated individuals have not had continuous healthcare when they enter prison, so viral loads (HIV-1 RNA) are frequently high and these individuals are generally sicker. Offenders not on highly active antiretroviral therapy (HAART) with elevated viral loads are more susceptible to opportunistic infections (OI), including tuberculosis, and experience reduced treatment outcomes with a higher risk for end-of-life complications. Offenders with high viral loads are potentially more contagious and pose a safety threat to others during sex, needle exchange, or altercations (including biting). HIV-infected offenders present a multitude of challenges for prison administrators ranging from housing, medical care delivery, administration of medications (including special dietary requirements), and increased economic burdens in an already constricted financial picture.

Maintaining confidentiality behind bars is complicated by several issues. Offenders often fill roles where they either hear or handle information related to healthcare. Word of mouth behind bars is a highly efficient means of transmitting information among prisoners. This often places offenders at risk for not disclosing a health concern, as they fear stigmatization and subsequent abuse. Fear of stigmatization may include choosing not to be tested for HIV. HIV-infected offenders who enter prison knowing their status may choose to defer treatment so as not to be identified. Many prisons contract out for specialty care such as infectious disease and HIV care. Care may occur in special clinics inside or outside the prison. Attending these special clinics also labels the prisoner. Choosing to "take care of yourself" in prison is not always a simple choice.

As in the general population, offenders seek to interact with professionals who can provide competent, trusting, and respectful services (Abercrombie, 2001; Altice, 1998; Flanigan, 1999; Parker & Paine, 1999; Stone, 1999). Confidentiality is a component of this therapeutic relationship as well. Healthcare provider relationships, as previously mentioned, are somewhat dictated by the administration and safety boundaries that cannot be broken. There is an overriding distrustful paranoia in prison that is increased by a number of factors, such as the power structures, mental illness and substance abuse issues, the history of prisons, the history of medical research inside prison (including the Tuskegee experiments in Georgia), disenfranchised communities of origin, and the discrepancies ethnically with respect to who is incarcerated and who has the power. Healthcare professionals have a responsibility to provide information for informed consent and to reduce refusal for treatment. These issues have medicolegal repercussions.

Many prisons do not have mandatory testing or optimal voluntary testing, so the HIV rates reflected are low. Only 16 states in the US have mandatory HIV testing at admission. Developing nations in particular often omit testing unless requested by offenders. If the HIV status of an offender is unknown, healthcare costs are reduced.

HIV testing is an important component to diagnosis and treatment. Providing voluntary testing that has the support and confidence of the inmates is imperative to a good program. Sufficient education and counseling is required to prevent increased anxiety and possible suicide, increase hope, replace myths with facts, and establish a plan of action that adequately addresses treatment options. The issue of partner notification must be explored as well. It is important to understand before the results are back whether inmates fear retribution from partners or family members or have economic concerns that make dealing with this issue sensitive. Women are at increased risk for abandonment upon returning to the community, and they risk domestic violence when partners have been notified of their HIV status (Rothenberg & Paskey, 1995). Incarcerated women may also fear for their children if those children remain in the care of violent partners. Most public health departments have anonymous mechanisms for notifying individuals of risk from exposures to STIs, including HIV, without linking the exposure to a specific person.

Disclosing HIV results is an opportunity for education. The inmate needs to hear about the hope surrounding HIV and that it is not a death sentence but considered a chronic disease. Discussing the natural disease of HIV can dispel myths and provide exploration with the prisoners to assess readiness to commit to the rigorous medication regime. It is important not to start individuals on medications until they have had time to internalize the information and make a reasonable decision. Stopping and starting HIV medication is a worse scenario than waiting to start medication, as it can contribute to ART resistance. The correctional care nurse is invaluable in this role, which can be expanded to include HIV peer educators.

The majority of prisons are in a difficult position with respect to drugs and sex, neither of which is supposed to occur. Yet it is widely known that both sex and substance abuse occur behind bars. Unfortunately this dualistic problem is a major health concern. If sex is prohibited, then possessing condoms or using oral contraceptives is prohibited, which is the policy of most prisons. That policy is under review because of the rising number of HIV cases in prison. Clean needles and bleach policies for injection drug use (IDU) lag even further behind and reflect not only the positions of prison officials but the philosophical debate in the US regarding needle exchange policies (Burris, Lurie, & Abrahamson et al., 2000). Conservative estimates are that approximately 3.2% of offenders are becoming HIV infected from sex and IDU during incarceration (Human Resources and Services Administration, 2000; Taylor, Goldberg, & Emslie et al., 1995). One ex-prisoner in New York City said that he and 50 other known prisoners who were part of an inmate "drug-shooting" circle and shared one needle had become infected while incarcerated in a state prison. The correctional care nurse can routinely teach about modes of HIV transmission, universal precautions, safer sex, and how to clean a needle properly. Post-exposure protocols (PEP) should be in place for altercations between individuals and needle sticks that pose the threat of HIV infection.

Increasingly, the treatment of HIV infection has become more complex. It is the belief of many professional organizations that HIV care should be left to those healthcare providers who specialize in treating HIV-infected individuals (DeGroot, Hammett, & Scheib, 1996). This has been a challenge for prisons, with safety the primary concern. Many larger state institutions utilize telemedicine to bring state-of-the-art-treatment to inmates infected with HIV.

In other states such as Alabama, Mississippi, Georgia, and South Carolina, HIV populations are housed in one facility, creating a much-debated human rights issue. Offenders complain that they are being stigmatized; prison officials state this is the only way they can provide quality of healthcare in a cost-effective man-

Box 51-6 Key Cases Related to HIV/AIDS in Correctional Facilities

1997–*Nolley v. Johnson* (US Dist. LEXIS 17651. S.D.N.Y.) ruled that the prison did not show "deliberate indifference" when an inmate was off HIV medication for a week during transport between facilities. This was of concern to healthcare providers because of the high resistance patterns that occur when there is not a 95% adherence rate (missing one dose a week).

1999–*Perkins v. Kansas Dept. of Corrections* (165 F.3d 803) upheld correctional facilities' decision to treat HIV with two (no protease inhibitor) rather than three antiretroviral medications even though three medication regimens had been the community standard of care for several years. The ruling stated that the offender had received care and there was no "deliberate indifference."

2000–*Sullivan v. County of Pierce* (US App. LEXIS 8251) upheld the complaint of "deliberate indifference" when the offender's protease inhibitor was withheld because the prison did not stock it. The court felt that this was far from the medical norm.

2000–*Leon v. Johnson* (96 F. Supp. 2d 244. WDNY) upheld that the prison did not show "deliberate indifference" when a Spanish-speaking-only offender missed picking up medications because directions were written in English even though his condition worsened.

2000–*Edwards v. Alabama Dept. of Corrections* (81 F. Supp. 2d 1242) upheld that the prison was not liable for damages resulting from delivering HIV medication three to four days late, basing its decision on the fact that Alabama was poor and care did not differ from that in the community.

ner and keep non-HIV-infected prisons safe from HIV transmission. It should be noted that aggregate HIV housing was shown to contribute to TB outbreaks (Nicodemus & Paris, 2001). Prison policy to segregate HIV-infected inmates from the rest of the prison population was upheld by the US Supreme Court, on January 18, 1990, when the court stated that the policy did not violate the Rehabilitation Act of 1973. The ruling further denounced that this policy discriminated against offenders testing positive for HIV. Prisoners who were assigned to segregated prison housing for HIV-infected offenders are then identified by association.

Specific laws related to HIV/AIDS have evolved since the 1990s. Circuit courts applying Eighth Amendment rights to HIV have been divided in their rulings, leaving HIV management to healthcare providers in the various correctional facilities (Sylla & Thomas, 2000). Most ruling to "deliberate indifference" has failed to set HIV standards of care to which offenders are entitled. Box 51-6 highlights key cases related to HIV/AIDS in correctional facilities.

The second most problematic area in the treatment of HIV-infected offenders is medications. HIV is a complex disease with a high resistance. Drug resistance can occur in a number of ways and combinations. The first combination of medications used to treat newly diagnosed HIV cases is the most important step. If not carefully chosen, a number of treatment options are lost when resistance to them develops. Triple combination ART is the recommended therapy for HIV, and other therapies such as monotherapy are considered substandard and may contribute to drug resistance. Resistance can develop via sexual intercourse where the resistance of one person is transferred to the other person via body fluids. Missing doses or not taking medications properly also increases the likelihood that resistance to medications will develop. This is the single most perplexing problem for those who care for HIV-infected people. Inmates and staff need education on resistance, preferably before they begin therapy. Medication adherence is further complicated in prisons by the food/no food restrictions that many of the HIV medications carry. Some prisons find allocating extra foods necessary for medications or disease states difficult to accommodate.

Medication resistance with HIV is further complicated while a person is incarcerated. There are a multitude of situations that may leave the offender without medications for days and weeks at a time. Diminishing missed HIV medication doses is the primary goal of healthcare providers and an area where correctional nurses can take a leading role. Educating prison administration and correctional officers regarding the importance of this policy is imperative in the fight against HIV. Correctional officers often possess the least amount of knowledge regarding HIV disease and express the most negative attitudes about HIV-infected people (Kantor, 1998; Soubik & Frank, 1999).

The areas that remain problematic are transferring offenders for healthcare appointments, paroling and releasing inmates from prison, refilling medications in a timely manner, lockdowns and searches, and safety transfers to other facilities that occur in the middle of the night with no notice to healthcare professionals and without medications. Unfortunately, upon arrival at the second institution a transferred inmate has no medications and must wait to see a physician. Upon seeing the healthcare provider, the offender must often wait from one to two weeks to receive the medications as most facilities contract out to management and pharmaceutical companies.

On a day-to-day basis, adherence to medications and withholding medications as a form of punishment are ongoing challenges, and community health nurses can best address these issues through education at a variety of levels. Whether to allow prisoners to hold medications "on person" or to require directly observed therapy (DOT) is often determined by prison policy, and both options have their strengths and weaknesses (Babudieri, Aceti, & D'Offizi et al., 2000; Lucas, Flexner, & Moore, 2002). Triple combination therapy and the advent of protease inhibitors has significantly reduced AIDS-related mortalities in prisons (Wright & Smith, 1999). A study in Florida compared DOT with on-person therapy with respect to viral suppression. The findings revealed that 85% of the DOT and only 50% of the matched self-administered group had a viral suppression (plasma HIV RNA) of less than 50 copies/mL at week 48 (Fischl, Rodriguez, & Sceppella et al., 2000). This study may greatly affect the decisions of correctional facilities regarding medication administration and the reintroduction of clinical trials behind bars. The primary objection by offenders regarding DOT is that it labels them as HIV-infected because no other chronic disease has the number and frequency of doses that HIV carries. With newer improvements to decrease the number and frequency of doses, HIV medications may begin to resemble medication patterns similar to those of other diseases.

Adherence to medications is generally related to a number of factors including knowledge of the medications and HIV together with a good rapport with healthcare providers. Because adherence is vital to decrease resistance to HIV medications, it is important that institutions examine treatment outcomes. Research has shown that adherence and acceptance of medications depend on three factors: trust in the medication, trust in the healthcare system, and good interpersonal relationships with providers and peers (Abercrombie, 2001; Altice & Buitrago, 1998; Holzemer, Corless,

& Nokes et al., 1999; Mostashari, Riley, & Selwyn et al. 1998; Roberts, 2002). Additional barriers in medication administration behind bars include frequency of dosing, being asymptomatic, stigmatization, correctional issues related to safety and administration, and fear of side effects. A study reported that institutions find accommodating HIV medication regimes difficult; nurses are often not knowledgeable about all the food-related timing issues required and the drug-to-drug interactions; and observation about the overall needs of the facility and staff must be examined when trying to increase adherence (Finlay & Jones, 2000; Frank, 1999; Miller & Rundio, 1999). A suggested tool to improve medication ordering, administration, and delivery is to do periodic, retrospective chart reviews (Ungvaraski & Rottner, 1997). Nurses can collectively develop a process for addressing these issues that will in the long run help offenders to be more successful in the medication regime. For recommendations regarding treatment options, a number of publications are available including two that are specific to correctional care and HIV.

Nurses can foster a caring attitude within the prison system. This can be a motivating factor in prisoners choosing to be tested for HIV, receiving adequate healthcare, being receptive to learning about HIV and their medications, adhering to HIV medications, and decreasing stereotypes and myths about HIV. An onsite weekly or daily HIV nurse practitioner can contribute to continuity of care, education, and adherence of complex HIV medications (Miller & Rundio, 1999). Educating correctional officers, prison administrators, and other offenders about HIV is the first step in empowering inmates to take care of themselves as well as decreasing tension by debunking myths. As noted earlier, several studies report correctional officers as possessing the most negative attitudes toward HIV-infected inmates, as well as being the least informed about HIV transmission and prevention (Allard, April, & Martin, 1992).

Educational opportunities within prison are limitless. One study showed education was the single most important element for improving the quality of life for HIV offenders (Hammet, Harmon, & Maruschak, 1999). Prisons and jails have significantly increased HIV rates. However, only 10% of state/federal prison systems and 5% of jail systems have comprehensive programs. A comprehensive program includes the following elements:

- Orientation
- Peer education
- Community-based prevention and education
- Individual prevention and education, on request
- Written and audiovisual materials
- Prevention and education in prerelease, day reporting, and pretrial populations
- Gender-specific programs at facilities housing women
- Expansion of HIV curriculums to cover other communicable diseases
- Programs and materials in Spanish and English (Hammett, Harmon, & Maruschak., 1999, p. 27)

In order of the most prevalent, the following methods have been utilized to promote education in prisons and jails: pre-/post-test counseling, written material, inviting lecturers to do educational programs, use of audio-visual materials, peer-led education, and health fairs. A comparison of the 1994 to 1997 National Institute of Justice/Centers for Disease Control surveys shows that educational programs about HIV have increased from half the federal and state prisons surveyed in 1994 to 61% in 1997 (CDC, 1996; Hammett, Harmon, & Maruschak, 1999). In the 1997 survey, jails reported that approximately 66% had educational programs. It should be pointed out that having an educational program does not mean that offenders attend or utilize the program.

Women in Prison

The number of women behind bars has increased 23 times since the 1980s. Minority women have been hardest hit with a 132% increase (eight times) among blacks, whereas the number of Hispanic women inmates has increased four times, and the number of Caucasian women inmates has increased 109% (Human Rights Watch, 1996). Offenses by females include violent crimes (25% to 33%), and drug-related offenses such as loitering, possession, and burglary accounted for 40% to 70% of the crimes. The majority of drug-related offenders were using drugs within the 30 days prior to incarceration, and less than 10% will receive drug treatment while incarcerated.

Gender Differences in Corrections

The natural question would be why is the population of women in prison growing in such large numbers? Women in general have the least amount of power, which is often represented by economic power or gender inequality. Most single parents, generally women, live in poverty. Economic power buys better legal advice, which translates into reduced sentences for crimes. Women for the most part lack high-level knowledge about their crimes. Lack of knowledge results in little information to trade for reduced sentences. Women of color often lack respect among their peers and society in general, so they may be viewed as castaways or incidentals. Women may lack political power in general and are often underrepresented by their elected officials. This lack of power means more severe sentences than their male counterparts.

This lack of power extends to the correctional facilities. Studies have indicated that one of the most stressful problems for women related to incarceration is their lack of power with prison guards, the majority of whom are men. Studies have shown that anxiety and depression escalate during incarceration by this lack of power combined with fear of retribution, including sexual assault.

Sexual assaults and harassment were found in 50 states in America, reported Congresswoman Eleanor Norton (Geraldo Rivera special, *Women in Prison: Nowhere to Hide,* September 10, 1999). The code among prisoners is to keep their mouths shut and submit to sexual assault or shakedowns. Shakedowns or patdowns are often viewed as authority to "feel up" prisoners. Sexual assault is often termed "consensual sex with intimidation" or viewed as "trading favors." Offenders may be "traded" to other prisoners or to correctional staff for sex (Human Rights Watch, 1996). The power imbalance while incarcerated makes consent between prisoner and guards impossible, and it is also illegal in federal prisons. There are prisoners, especially women, who lack family and social support and find themselves in a position of swapping favors as their only means for attaining money. Here again is the imbalance of power from an economic and psychological perspective. Offenders who have access to money can negotiate more favorable conditions for themselves while incarcerated. Prison staff and guards retaliate by placing feces in the offenders' food, urinating on the person, forced hanging, and refusing medical care. Offenders in isolation or "segs" are often more vulnerable to sexual misconduct. A federal judge found the progressive, prolonged, and prurient observation in dressing areas is considered sexual misconduct.

Most women enter prison with a long history of victimization resulting in anxiety, depression, and post-traumatic stress disorder

(PTSD). One study reported that in the year prior to incarceration, women experienced 10 stressful life events, and 90% of women suffered from severe anxiety and depression (Keaveny & Zausznieski, 1999). Researchers have estimated that 75% of incarcerated women have a history of childhood or adult sexual abuse (Browne, Miller, & Maguin, 1999; Haney & Kristiansen, 1998; Harris, Sharps, & Allen et al., 2003; Human Resources and Service Administration, 2000; Maeve, 1999). The majority of women (90%) have come from homes where there was violence in the form of hitting, striking, and slapping (Bond & Semaan, 1996; Browne, Miller, & Maguin 1999; Fogel, 1993). Forty-four percent of women behind bars were beaten by one or both parents (Bond & Semaan, 1996). Many women have seen violence in their environment on a daily basis, which contributes significantly to PTSD (Wallace, Fullilove, & Flisher, 1996). Although men in the impoverished areas also experience daily violence, their rates of PTSD are not as high. Researchers postulate that it is the long history of victimization, secondary to power inequities, that occurs in conjunction with physical and sexual abuse that contributes to the higher rates of PTSD in incarcerated women. Another compounding factor to the increased rates of PTSD is the fact that approximately 50% of prisoners have some form of mental illness and that the combined effect of mental illness with PTSD contributes to the criminal behavior leading to the incarceration of women (Jordan, Schlenger, & Fairbank et al., 1996).

PTSD and the related anxiety and depression also contribute to the inability of female offenders to cope, both prior to incarceration and during incarceration (Kupers, 1999). A high correlation exists between alcohol and substance abuse following sexual abuse, either as a child or as an adult (Blume, 1998). While not all women who are victims of sexual abuse rely on substances to numb their feelings, it is more prevalent among women who have fewer family and social resources. Additionally, women who have been beaten about the head during interpersonal violence may suffer from post-concussion syndrome (PCS) placing them at risk for poor decisions and inability to multitask, thereby placing them at risk for further abuse (Fullilove, Fullilove, & Smith et al., 1993). Leenerts (1999, 2003) reported that the experience of abuse significantly decreased the offenders self-care practices. The constellation of PTSD, substance abuse, and possible post-concussion syndrome places women at risk for overall poor decisions and at risk for behavior that contributes to their arrest.

Physical and sexual abuse are problematic within prisons and are further complicated by the poor state of mental health described earlier. Female inmates often develop PTSD. Women with PTSD are unable to return and reintegrate into their communities and as mothers. They become paralyzed by their state of mental distress.

Correctional nurses can assist prisoners and facilities in developing confidential anonymous reporting systems for offenders to disclose sexual misconduct and sexual assaults. Georgia and California have either confidential anonymous hot lines or reporting boxes. Georgia prison reform now requires that 85% of guards in female prisons are women and forbids male correctional officers to do pat-downs, strip searches, or frisks. Nurses must be able to identify symptoms of anxiety, depression, and PTSD in prisoners and provide intervention strategies.

Women enter prison in overall poor health, both physically and psychologically. Up to 21% of women in prison are HIV infected, and those who are not infected are at significant risk for acquiring HIV (DeGroot, 2000). Those women who are HIV infected were less likely than men to have accessed healthcare with any regularity and entered prison with more advanced stages of HIV disease than men. HIV is highest among black women who were less likely to have accessed healthcare (Lynch & Pugh, 2000). Nearly half of the incarcerated women were sexually active with a drug-injecting partner. Few practiced any form of safe sex. The combined effects of substance abuse, mental illness including PTSD, few socioeconomic resources, and increased risk-taking behavior place women at a very high risk for acquiring HIV (DeGroot, Hammett, & Scheib, 1996; El-Bassel, Ivanoff, & Schilling et al., 1995; Wyatt, Myers, & Williams et al., 2002). Many studies have shown a high correlation between domestic violence/childhood sexual abuse and the risk of acquiring HIV (Dilorio, Hartwell, & Hansen et al., 2002; Flitcraft, 1995; Fogel & Belyea, 2001; Hartwell et al., 2002; Magura, Kang, & Shapiro et al., 1993; Manfrin-Ledet & Porche, 2003; Mullings, Marquart, & Brewer, 2000; Schwab-Stone, Chen, & Greenberger et al., 1999; Stevens, Zierler, & Dean et al., 1995b).

Prison therefore presents a unique opportunity for HIV prevention. Subgroups of detainees greatest at risk for acquiring HIV include injecting drug users, people whose arrests were associated with drug charges (either misdemeanors or felonies), people who had several prior arrests for less serious charges especially related to drug charges, and people with severe mental illness (McClelland, Teplin, & Abram, et al., 2002). Providing substance abuse rehabilitation is an important aspect of HIV prevention. Teaching condom use is not especially helpful in this population due to fears of retribution from their partners (Bond & Semaan, 1996; Manfrin-Ledet & Porche, 2003). Female condom education, however, has proved to be more accepted by some women (VanDevanter, 2002; Witte, Wada, & El-Bassel et al., 2000). Teaching empowerment skills may contribute to reducing risk-taking behavior. Many women released from prison felt this type of risk reduction was not met while they were incarcerated (Fickenscher, Lapidus, Silk-Walker, et al., 2001; Young, 2000).

Reproductive and Sexual Health Issues

Many women currently in prison are incarcerated for the first time. Eighty-five percent are mothers, and three quarters of their children are under the age of 18. It should be noted, however, that only one third of these children were living with them at the time of the arrest. Many children had been removed from the home for substance abuse related problems previously. Some children live with relatives, whereas others are in foster care or have been adopted. Other incarcerated women leave children behind and are concerned about their safety and who is taking care of them. Family members or the father (who may have been abusive) often watch these children. Mothers who don't keep in touch with their children often lose them to adoption. It is therefore important for incarcerated mothers to write regularly to children. Nurses can assist offenders in this process.

Women generally suffer from *empty nest syndrome*. Many women have already lost their children because of substance abuse issues that have forced placement of their children in foster care or because of a lack of continued contact with children in foster care. A number of HIV-infected inmates may have lost children who were also infected. Children visit their mothers less frequently than fathers who are incarcerated, with only 50% of women ever seeing their children (Maeve, 1999). Prisons are often geographically a distance from families, and the families may be unable to travel due to economic constraints. Many women spend the long hours being locked up thinking about their children and longing for improved scenarios. Many women are guilty and ashamed that they were not better mothers. Many women are angry at the bureaucratic system for the mess they are in. As most women are in their reproductive years when incarcerated, many think about starting new families upon release.

The correctional care nurse can do much in this area. Many women do not understand basic anatomy and physiology and would benefit from education in this area as well as being taught basic fertility awareness and being provided with contraception information. Parenting classes are very important. Women would benefit from support groups that allow them to express their feelings regarding their children and offering some healing to this deep wound. It is not until women can heal from these emotions, including the guilt and shame, that they can begin to set healthy plans for their release. Offering suggestions as to how to begin to heal the pain of their loss and supporting them as they reach out to children they have harmed are necessary steps that will help to prevent these women from repeating old patterns.

Few prison systems have provisions for children to accompany their mothers while incarcerated; those that do have long waiting lists. Fragmenting families has become a social and economical issue as more women are being incarcerated for nonviolent crimes. Most pastoral groups are calling for alternatives to incarceration that promote family unity rather than further destroying already fragile family units. They argue that these alternatives are cheaper than the current system. Some states have also begun to introduce special programs, such as Girl Scout programs at prison to promote interaction among mothers and daughters. Such programs typically transport the children to prison and conduct structured family programs.

Approximately 6% to 10% of women entering prison are pregnant. Some women may not have known that they were pregnant and may choose a pro-choice option if they can afford it. Some correctional facilities may not offer therapeutic abortions. Other women choose to continue their pregnancies, with approximately 1300 live births per year (Richardson, 1998). This is often a more difficult choice for prisons that find it problematic to provide additional nutritional food. Transporting shackled offenders to and from prenatal appointments and for delivery of the baby has been the source of much criticism nationally. Stories of women delivering while shackled to the bed have raised numerous issues ranging from human rights to medical complications (Siegal, 1998). The end result for the offender has been generally little time with her newborn infant, who will typically be shuttled off to foster care.

New York State's Bedford Hills is one of a few model programs offering comprehensive services to offenders and allowing mothers to keep their babies following delivery. Federal prisons have the Mothers and Infants Together (MINT) program for women who qualify. These offenders are placed in halfway houses three months prior to delivery and for two months after delivery.

These programs offer an opportunity for mother-child bonding. Parenting classes offer an opportunity for offenders to build relationships with each other. Nursing staff reports that women with PTSD often have difficulty bonding with their infants. Being touched and touching are often associated with abuse, and women with PTSD have fears related to physical touch and intimacy. Women often avoid breast-feeding, rocking, or cuddling their babies. The correctional nurse who is aware of these possibilities could utilize prenatal visits to explore these concerns and issues with mothers and provide educational and emotional support. Appropriate psychiatric counseling would be beneficial in altering old patterns of childcare that have their roots in past traumatic events and violence.

It is also important to remember that pregnancy may not have occurred within the framework of a loving relationship. One lesbian woman said that her only heterosexual coitus occurred as the result of being raped. At the same time she became pregnant for the first time, she also became HIV-positive and was exposed to human papillomavirus (HPV) and Neisseria gonorrhea, which resulted in pelvic inflammatory disease (PID) and continual abdominal discomfort. Eventually she also developed cervical disease from the HPV, which could progress to cervical cancer. In addition to the medical complications of this assault, she suffered emotionally with PTSD, issues related to her body image, and sexual orientation identity issues related to being a lesbian and being pregnant. Her mother agreed to care for her child until the woman was emotionally able to bond with the child. Portions of this scenario were common to many incarcerated women.

Many people might ask, what benefit is having family-oriented programs in prison if women are not bonding with their children? Case Study 51-1 demonstrates the importance and raises the issue of whose standards are being used to measure program success. This example stresses the amount of education and support women often require when they are arrested for a drug-related charge. Studies have shown that women lacking social support and who come from families where physical and emotional abuse were present are more likely to then abuse their own children (Hall, Sachs, & Rayens, 1998). Bedford Hills and the MINT programs provide an opportunity to break the cycles of violence by providing education and counseling to mothers and babies. Without this intervention, the women would be at risk for continuing in the same lifestyle.

Case Study 51-1 Breaking the Cycle

An inmate and mother of two delivered her third baby at Bedford Hills in New York. Both of her other children were in foster care and slated for adoption. The inmate had a long history of substance abuse and stated that this was the first delivery she had experienced while not high on crack cocaine. She appreciated the opportunity to turn her life around and begin a new life with supervision. Upon release she was in a halfway house with her newborn where emotional support and parenting skills were provided. She eventually went back to using drugs but stated that she was able to place the baby in responsible hands before doing so. She would have just abandoned the baby in the past. She was also able to get back on track within a few weeks rather than being incarcerated again.

Women with a history of sexual abuse and who experience PTSD find childbirth and gynecologic exams, including colposcopy, extremely difficult. These medical exams trigger memories of sexual abuse and cause these women to dissociate from the examination. Dissociation may become out-of-control behavior and extreme anxiety. It is important to screen for sexual abuse histories so care can be taken to guide women through the process. This may be the first time that someone has made the association with them–between exams, anxiety, and sexual abuse–and the new awareness often generates many tears. Many women will not disclose sexual abuse the first time they are asked but will wait until they feel there is respect and trust between themselves and the healthcare provider. Admission gynecological screening for concealed contraband or weapons may revictimize women with a history of sexual abuse.

An inmate experiencing difficulty with a gynecological exam could receive a digital exam only, which would satisfy prison staff that nothing is concealed within the vagina. At this point, the gynecological examination could be broken into smaller steps to allow the inmate to begin dealing with her anxiety surrounding the vulnerability of this process. This gentle stepped process of providing gynecological care to traumatized inmates is described elsewhere (Dole, 1996, 1999). A stepped process is especially helpful with women who have HIV and HPV diseases that require colposcopy and gynecological examinations every six months. Approximately half the women offenders who have HIV also have cervical disease, which is a rate approximately double that of women not incarcerated (DeGroot, 2000; Dole, 1999). Non-HIV-infected offenders have much lower rates of HPV infection; however, the rates are still considerably higher for this population compared to nonincarcerated women.

Taking the additional time with inmates who experience difficulty with gynecological examinations is imperative if healing the painful wounds of sexual abuse is to occur. Prison affords healthcare providers this opportunity as many inmates are incarcerated for several years. Not taking the time to assist inmates with this concern further victimizes and traumatizes these women. The correctional nurse can do much in this area to identify women who may suffer from PTSD and alert healthcare providers of the problem. Whenever possible, sensitive female providers should exam offenders with PTSD who are anxious about gynecological exams. As many as 50% to 75% of female offenders may suffer from PTSD. Support groups and education would benefit this population. Offenders suffering from PTSD may repeatedly seek excuses or refuse to have a gynecological exam. Another tip to PTSD is chronic abdominal pain or dysmenorrhea without apparent pathology (Golding, Wilsnack, & Learman, 1998; Keamy, 1998). Lifestyle and high-risk behavior prior to incarceration place women at higher risk for STIs including cervical disease, making pap smears an essential component of incarcerated women's healthcare.

Nurses working in corrections also have the unique opportunity to effect change through education and policies related to female products carried in the commissary. Many women douche regularly, feeling that this is required for cleanliness. Data suggest that douching can actually facilitate pelvic inflammatory disease (PID) by pushing bacteria further up the reproductive track, and douching may facilitate the acquisition of STIs including HIV (Koblin, Mayer, & Mwatha et al., 2002; Vermund, Sarr, & Murphy et al., 2001; Visser, Moorman, & Irwin et al., 1995). Offenders require information about the relationship between various vaginal secretions and the menstrual cycle. Education about vaginal cleanliness and debunking the douching myth would reduce gynecological complications and benefit offenders by saving money for the institutions while empowering the inmates with knowledge.

Education is also beneficial with respect to sexual health. Many women prisoners have traded sex for money or drugs and possess little knowledge about sexuality or their bodies. Feminine hygiene products (including douches), deodorant sanitary napkins and tampons, perfumed powders, and the relationship between these products and contact dermatitis and ovarian cancer risks needs to be taught (Cook, Kamb, & Weiss, 1997). This topic also provides the healthcare provider with an excellent opportunity to discuss human sexuality issues, the menstrual cycle, reproduction, and the human sexual response cycle. This discussion often leads to disclosures of dyspareunia and lack of sexual fulfillment. Decreased sexual functioning is sometimes associated with PTSD, providing nurses with an opportunity to further explore these concerns. Male offenders would also benefit from similar discussions, which would offer healthcare providers the opportunity to substitute myths with facts. Knowledge is power and the foundation for change.

For HIV-positive inmates who are considering pregnancy, nurses may also discuss how these women can protect their babies from HIV and neural tube deficiencies (folate acid education). Education can alleviate fears and dispel myths that many women hold regarding use of zidovudine (AZT), the CDC-recommended medication to reduce horizontal transmission (Vittiello & Smeltzer, 1999). Education about not breast-feeding with HIV infection is also helpful. These discussions of pregnancy and infant care may also present the opportunity for nurses to discuss smoking cessation prior to pregnancy and the impact of smoke on the mother's health and the health of her baby. Men should also understand this relationship and how secondhand smoke increases a child's risk for asthma.

Women also need assistance in redefining their sexuality, as the majority have been sexually abused and have used their bodies to acquire money or drugs. For many of these women, love often equaled sex, whereas intimacy and empowered relationships were unknown. While incarcerated, 80% of women will participate in sexual relationships with other women, including half the women who self-identified as heterosexual (Maeve, 1999). Women seek relationships that provide love, caring, and support.

Best Practice *51-2*

Nurses can assist in redefining concepts of sexuality by being nonjudgmental about this behavior and using relationships to explore definitions of loving relationships.

Mental Illness

Poor mental health is a significant contribution to incarceration rates. Mental illness, including serious psychiatric conditions, substance abuse, physical and sexual abuse, and poor coping skills, contributes to high-risk behavior and poor decisions making. Offenders with mental illness were more likely to be incarcerated for a violent crime, were more likely to have used alcohol or drugs during the offense, and were twice as likely to have been homeless prior to arrest (Ditton, 1999). Low literacy, poor social skills, and being mentally challenged also contribute to poor mental health and increased risk for incarceration. Mental illness also contributes to higher rates of recidivism and longer sentences. Approximately 60% of offenders with mental illness receive psychiatric services while incarcerated. One study found the majority of the mentally ill were in local jails (Cox, Banks, & Stone, 2000).

It should be noted that psychopathy or antisocial behavior is the extreme end of the serious mental disease continuum. Offenders have lifelong patterns of exploitive behavior, including manipulation (see "Scope of Practice"). Psychopathic offenders are devoid of anxiety or depression, which differentiates them from people suffering from other mental illnesses. As many as 50% of sexual offenders (especially rapists) may be psychopaths as measured by the Hare Psychopathy Checklist, Revised (Hare, 1998; Hare, Cox, & Hart, 1994). Interventions are rarely successful with individuals who lack a conscience and are unable to be compassionate.

It is clear from the literature that there is a strong link between the cycles of violence, poverty (poor access to care), and mental illness, although there is no consensus on the interrelationship. Seventy-eight percent of female offenders and 30% of male offenders have experienced physical and sexual abuse (Health Resources and Services Administration, 2000). Physical and sexual abuse is often given as the reason youths have run away, placing them in unsafe places and often leading to incarceration. Correlations have shown increased alcohol and substance abuse among individuals who are abused, especially among women (Singer, Bussey, & Song, et al., 1995). As previously addressed, higher rates of depression are related to PTSD and its related sequel of sexual abuse. Is it possible that the victims of crime have now become the incarcerated?

Over half of the individuals incarcerated stated that they had used illegal drugs in the month prior to being arrested. However, the majority of offenders had used illegal drugs at some time in their past: 73% of federal offenders, 83% of state offenders, and 66% of people in jail (CDC, 2001b). Substance abuse places individuals at increased risk for incarceration. Substance abuse also places individuals at increased risk for health-related problems, such as HIV (especially for IDUs), hepatitis, STIs, acquired brain injury, renal impairment, cardiovascular complications, poor nutrition, and poor self-care.

The CAGE diagnostic instrument is an easy screening tool for alcoholism based on the answers to four questions.

Cut down on drinking (Have you ever felt you should cut down on your drinking?)
Annoyed by criticism about drinking habits
Guilty feelings about drinking
Eye opener drink needed in the morning

Based on CAGE screening, one third of the mentally ill also have a history of alcohol dependence. Untreated alcoholism contributes to incarceration despite the fact that 22% of mentally ill offenders and 11% of other offenders had been in a detoxification unit at some time prior to arrest. Most offenders admit to negative consequences of drinking prior to arrests such as lost jobs and scrapes with law enforcement. Alcoholics Anonymous (AA) is available in most correctional facilities offering a peer program for recovery. AA has been the most successful program overall for individuals who are no longer in denial about their alcoholism. Society has failed to develop adequate strategies for reducing denial. Many offenders often admit years later that incarceration forced them to deal with their substance abuse denial, allowing for successful rehabilitation.

Treatment for substance abuse (including alcoholism) behind bars is available. In addition to AA, Narcotics Anonymous (NA) provides self-help and recovery for substance abusers. Additional interventions available to offenders include the following (CDC, 2001a):

- Detoxification when needed upon admission
- Education and counseling
- Therapeutic communities (TC) (long-term, highly structured residential treatment programs have been shown to reduce recidivism)
- Methadone maintenance offered in some correctional facilities
- Diversion programs (including drug courts): Sentences are reduced if the individual successfully completes treatment
- Intermediate sanctions: Short incarceration with mandated substance abuse program
- Coerced abstinence: Mandatory frequent drug testing during probation

Despite available treatment for substance abuse, it is clear that more offenders need treatment. Many community advocates, such as Justice Works (an interfaith organization) support increasing community programs and decreasing incarceration for substance abuse in nonviolent offenses. Some of the innovative programs that are beginning to address this problem include the following (CDC, 2001a):

- California's Proposition 36: Requires substance abuse treatment, not jail, for drug possession or use
- The National Compendium of Local and State Interventions for Substance-Abusing Persons Involved with the Justice System: A federal collaborative program that will provide online information for the most promising public health and criminal justice programs
- The Residential Substance Abuse Treatment for State Prisoners Formula Grant Program (RSAT): Funding from Department of Justice (DOJ) for correctional residential facilities operated by state and local
- Breaking the Cycle: Demonstration project from DOJ for early identification and evaluation of offenders for substance abuse; provides early individualized treatment with intensive supervision, and strong judicial oversight may reduce crime
- Treatment Accountability for Safer Communities (TASC): A program that integrates the criminal justice and substance abuse treatment programs to increase effective criminal processing, correctional supervision, and aftercare

Healthcare professionals also have a significant role to play in community efforts to screen and identify alcoholism and substance abuse, and to refer individuals for treatment. This is difficult to accomplish with inadequate mental health insurance and detoxification programs. Untreated mental illness or continuing treatment for those who are diagnosed is also problematic. Community and family support are vital. It is essential for healthcare professionals to screen and identify substance abuse, including alcoholism. Ongoing missed opportunities contribute to the larger problem of untreated mental illness and increasing incarceration rates (Lovell & Jemelka, 1998). One study showed a high association with marijuana use prior to incarceration (Braithwaite, 2004). Substance abuse is often viewed as a psychosocial problem and therefore omitted as a priority during healthcare appointments.

Ninety percent of offenders with schizophrenia, bipolar disorder, and antisocial personality disorder were also found to have addictive disorders, often in the form of alcohol or substance abuse. In one study 2% to 4.3% of offenders were found to have bipolar disorder, and another 2.3% to 3.9% of offenders have schizophrenia (Greifinger, 1999).

Inmates displaying psychotic, suicidal, or violent behavior are housed in forensic psychiatric units (Moran & Mason, 1996). Nurses must be astute to crisis intervention, good history, and assessment skills while developing therapeutic relationships. Offenders must be closely supervised for self-mutilation, suicidal attempts, anger outbursts, and swallowing contraband including sharps. Providing patient-centered care to these prisoners while maintaining a secure environment can be a challenge. Nurses have an opportunity to offer individual counseling, leading therapeutic groups that include assistance with anger management, and teaching coping and problem-solving strategies (Melia, Moran, &

Mason, 1996; Perez & Batong, 2003). Nurses can model and foster self-esteem, hope, and positive outlets.

It is important to distinguish between depression (previously discussed) and neurocognitive disorders that are particularly prevalent in patients with AIDS, as well as those who have Parkinson's disease and Huntington disease. Distinguishing between subcortical signs (HIV) and cortical signs (depression) will aid in the differential diagnosis. Screening tools that test subcortical signs include the Johns Hopkins HIV Dementia Scale or the Center for Epidemiologic Studies-Depression Test (CES-D) for patients who display symptoms such as being irritable, forgetful, disorganized, apathetic and slow, and distractible (Herfkens, 2001).

Bridge Programs with the Community

The role of the correctional nurse is vital in this area of correctional care. Few model programs at this time utilize nurses in their discharge or release plans. Yet recidivism is highest in the first 24 hours and first days upon release. Many release plans lack proper coordination to ensure success. The primary resources needed are housing, a job, and continuity in medical care (CDC, 2001a). One example is the Doe Fund in New York City's Harlem, which provides released prisoners with shelter and a job while building self-sufficiency (Richardson, 2003; VonZielbauer, 2003a). Providing these necessities actually decreases public costs by decreasing substance abuse and poor access to healthcare. The benefit of comprehensive prerelease programs is that they decrease recidivism by half (Flanigan, Kim, & Zierler et al., 1996; Freudenberg, Willets, & Greene, et al., 1998). Recidivism rates vary but are approximately 35%.

Four types of prevention programs have been shown to be effective in reducing transmission, morbidity, and mortality related to HIV. They include peer education, discharge planning, transitional case management, and technical assistance outreach models (AIDSAction, 2001). These models can also be applied to other medical problems. HIV education and prevention is important as approximately 25% of all HIV cases pass through jails and prisons at some time (Spaulding, Stephensen, & Macalino et al., 2002). HIV prevention in prison should include mandatory HIV testing (including oral tests), continuity of care for HIV-infected inmates, and access by community-based groups to provide AIDS-based education and prevention programs (Braithwaite & Arriola, 2003). Programs that have received grants to implement such programs are being evaluated by the Corrections Demonstration Project of the Centers for Disease Control and Prevention (Arriola, Kennedy, & Coltharp et al., 2002; Bauserman, Ward, & Eldred et al., 2001).

Few correctional facilities utilize peer education programs (7% prisons, 3% jails, and 3% penitentiaries) to provide information to offenders and to develop skills that can be applied on the outside (Hammett et al., 1999). The Bedford Hills ACE (AIDS Counseling and Education) program is probably one of the original models to be implemented nationally on a limited basis (Dubik-Unruh, 1999; Members of the ACE Program at Bedford Hills Correctional Facility, 1998). New York has expanded the program to the other state prisons under the name PACE (Prisoners AIDS Counseling and Education). The curriculum tenets outlined by ACE (1998) include the following as well as the suggested comprehensive components outlined previously:

- Harm reduction through intention to engage in safer behavior
- The examination of life situations that create stressors, gender-based imbalance, or aggression
- The concept of taking care of oneself first
- Groups of at least three sessions
- Advisory boards to include inmate planning
- HIV knowledge
- HIV prevention
  - Female and male condom utilization (O'Leary, Jemmott, & Goodhart et al., 1996)
  - Issues of love and cultural consideration
  - Issues of abuse and condom utilization (Amaro & Hardy-Fanta, 1995)
- HIV transmission
  - Relationship to viral load (Lurie, Miller, & Hecht et al., 1998)
  - Sexual
  - IDU
  - Perinatal and breast milk
  - Occupational and incarceration altercations
- Confounding belief systems
- African American concerns
  - Tuskeegee backlash
  - HIV origination in chimpanzees of west central Africa
- Duesberg theory: HIV-is-not-the-cause-of-AIDS theory

HIV peer education programs may increase voluntary testing for HIV and adherence to HIV medications (Fink, Walker, & Dole et al., 2001). Most offenders preferred peer-led groups to groups led by professionals (Grinstead et al., 1997, 1999).

Release programs utilize a systematic approach to release and network with community organizations and halfway houses to maximize a successful transition back into the community. The two oldest programs are found in Rhode Island (Project Bridge) and New York (ETHICS, founded 1967) (Flanigan, Kim, & Zierler et al., 1997). These programs as well as nine others were funded by Ryan White CARE Act federal funds (Health Resources and Services Administration, 2000). Connecticut has also added a program. The program objectives are to provide continuing comprehensive care to HIV-infected inmates upon release. In New York these programs network with others designed for released prisoners including the Fortune Society and ETHICS (Empowerment through HIV Information). Both New York programs are run and operated by ex-offenders. Common to these programs are substance abuse treatment, mental healthcare, and comprehensive medical care including HIV care, social support with constructive ties to the community, job readiness training, and court advocacy. Several comprehensive residential programs are being evaluated for recidivism and successful reentry back into the community. Study findings from Healthlink, a research demonstration grant at Hunter College that networks with Fortune Society and other community programs, support this type of comprehensive residential model.

Building community partnerships by developing a personal link with healthcare providers is imperative for the success of any program (Rich, Holmes, Salas et al., 2001). Healthcare providers who will come into the prisons and assist prisons with first appointments help to promote ideal situations. Most offenders have difficulty maneuvering the healthcare system, and this allows offenders to make contact with their providers prior to release (Mitty, Holmes, & Spaulding et al., 1998). It is helpful to schedule a drop-in policy for offenders initially and to schedule an appointment for the second week post-release. This time can be utilized to familiarize offenders with the clinic, and it gives them a sense that their transition is being carefully managed by a staff that cares

Box 51-7 Additional Resources on HIV in Correctional Facilities

PUBLICATIONS

Albany Medical College HIV educational series for corrections in Spanish and English; includes special tapes on women's issues; 518-262-6864, santosm@mail.amc.edu

Cell Wars by Bristol-Meyers Squibb is distributed free; in comic book format appropriate for low literacy; basic HIV information

Get Tested (video geared toward correctional populations—Glaxco Welcome)

Infectious Diseases in Corrections Report, formerly *Hepp* (HIV Education Prison Project), distributed by Brown University AIDS Program for Corrections and HIV Health Care Providers; www.idcronline.org

HIV Inside, distributed free for healthcare providers

HIV Invading T-cell Model—Merck

HIV Medication Guide—Glaxco Welcome of Canada (can be downloaded from www.jag.on.ca)

My Gramma Has HIV—Agouron

WEB SITES

amfAR Global Link: HIV information source
www.amfar.org/td

Association of Nurses in AIDS Care (ANAC)
www.anacnet.org

HIV InSite: information on HIV/AIDS treatment, prevention, and policy
http://hivinsite.ucsf.edu

Kaisernetwork.org: Daily HIV/AIDS report
www.report.kff.org/aidshiv

Medscape: HIV
www.hiv.medscape.com

about them and their successful transition. Providing a business card and encouraging offenders to call for help with any problem increases their confidence and provides them with a safety net as well as social and medical support. Offenders are anxious upon release, because they must now deal with many life stressors concurrently. Having a safe place to drop in to may often mean the difference between success and reincarceration. Box 51-7 provides additional resources for information on HIV in correctional facilities.

Summary

Caring for offenders involves many important forensic issues. Among the roles and responsibilities of correctional nurses are advocacy and protection of the offender's human rights. Unbiased documentation is vital for both the facility and its incarcerated population. The healthcare of prisoners is a critical element that requires an understanding of major public heath problems and their management within a confined population. The correctional nurse must possess knowledge, skills, and attitudes consistent with advocacy, health education, and prisoner rights as outlined in key documents of federal and state agencies as well as professional nursing organizations.

Resources

Books

Scope and standards of nursing practice in correctional facilities. (1995). Waldorf, MD: American Nurses Publishing.

Organizations

The Academy of Correctional Health Professionals (ACHP)

PO Box 11117, Chicago, IL 60611; Tel: 877-549-ACHP (2247); www.correctionalhealth.org

American Correctional Association

4380 Forbes Boulevard., Lanham, MD 20706-4322; Tel: 800-ACA-JOIN (800-222-5646), 301-918-1800; www.aca.org

American Correctional Health Services Association

250 Gatsby Place, Alpharetta, GA 30022-6161; Tel: 877-918-1842; www.achsa.com

Correctional News Online

1241 Andersen Drive, Suite N, San Rafael, CA 94901; Tel: 415-460-6185; www.correctionalnews.com

The Corrections Connection Network

159 Burgin Parkway, Quincy, MA 02169; Tel: 617-471-4445; www.corrections.com

Criminal Justice Institute, Inc. (CJI)

213 Court Street, Suite 606, Middletown, CT 06457; Tel: 860-704-6400; www.cji-inc.com

National Commission on Correctional Health

1145 West Diversey Parkway, Chicago, IL 60614; Tel: 773-880-1460; www.ncchc.org

References

Abercrombie, P. D. (2001). Improving adherence to abnormal pap smear follow-up. *JOGN Nurs, 30*(1), 80-88.

AIDSAction. (2001). *What works in HIV prevention for incarcerated populations.* Retrieved from www.aidsaction.org. Washington, DC: Author.

AIDS Counseling and Education Program (ACE). (1998). *Breaking the walls of silence: AIDS and women in a New York state maximum security prison.* New York: Overlook Press.

Allard, F., April, N., & Martin, G. (1992). Knowledge and attitudes of correctional staff towards HIV and HBV-infections. In *Program and Abstracts of the VIII International Conference on AIDS.* Amsterdam. Abstract PUD 3003.

Altice, F. L. (1998). Overview of HIV care. In M. Puisis, *Clinical practice in correctional medicine* (pp. 141-163). St. Louis: Mosby.

Altice, F. L., & Buitrago, M. I. (1998). Adherence to antiretroviral therapy in correctional settings. *J Correctional Health Care, 5,* 179-200.

Amaro, H., & Hardy-Fanta, C. (1995). Gender relations in addiction & recovery. *J Psychoactive Drugs, 27*(4), 325-337.

American Correctional Health Services Association's (ACHSA) ACHSA Code of Ethics. (1999).

American Medical Association (AMA). (1999). Health literacy, report of the Council on Scientific Affairs. *JAMA, 281,* 552-557.

American Nurses Association (ANA) and the International Association of Forensic Nurses (IAFN). (1997). *Scope and standards of forensic nursing practice.* Waldorf: American Nurses Publishing.

ANA. (1991). Ethics and Human Rights Position Statement.

ANA. (1994). ANA's Nurses' Participation in Capital Punishment.

Arriola, K. R. J., Kennedy, S. S., Coltharp, J.C., et al. (2002). *Development and implementation of the cross-site evaluation of the CDC/HRSA Corrections Demonstration Project.* AIDS Education & Prevention, 14(suppl A), 107-118.

Ashkin, D., Malecki, J., & Thomas, D. (2005). TB outbreaks among staff in correctional facilities, Florida, 2001-2004: lessons re-learned. *Infectious Diseases in Corrections Report, 8*(2), 1-7.

Babudieri, S., Aceti, A., D'Offizi, G. P., et al. (2000). Directly observed therapy to treat HIV infection in prisoners. *JAMA, 284*(2), 179-180.

Bauserman, R. L., Ward, M. A., Eldred, L., et al. (2001). Increasing voluntary HIV testing by offering oral tests in incarcerated populations. *Am J Public Health, 91*(8), 1226-1229.

Beck, J. A. (1999). Compassionate release from New York state prisons: Why are so few getting out? *J Law, Med Ethics, 27*(3), 216-233.

Beck, A. J., & Harrison, P. M. (2001, August). *Prisoners in 2000.* Washington, DC: US Department of Justice, Bureau of Justice Statistics.

Beck, A. J., & Karlberg, J. C. (2001, March). *Prison and jail inmates at midyear 2000.* Washington, DC: US Department of Justice, Bureau of Justice Statistics.

Blume, S. B. (1998). Addictive disorders in women. In R. J. Frances & S. I. Miller (Eds.), *Clinical textbook of addictive disorders* (2nd ed., pp. 413- 429). New York: Guilford.

Bond, L., & Semaan, S. (1996). At risk for HIV infection: Incarcerated women in a county jail in Philadelphia. *Women Health, 24*(4), 27-45.

Boswell, E. (2000). Nurses in jail keep inmates in prison. *Montana State University Communications Services.* Retrieved on June 26 from www.montana.edu/wwwpb/univ/jailone.

Bozzette, S. A., Joyce, G., McCaffrey, D. F., et al. (2001). Expenditures for the care of HIV-infected patients in the era of highly active antiretroviral therapy. *N Engl J Med, 344*(11), 817-823.

Braithwaite, R. L., & Arriola, K. R. J. (2003). Male prisoners and HIV prevention: A call for action ignored. *Am J Public Health, 93*(5), 759-763.

Braithwaite, R., Stephens, T., Conerly, R. C., et al. (2004). The relationship among marijuana use, prior incarceration, and inmates' self-reported HIV/AIDS risk behaviors. *Addictive Behaviors, 29*(5), 995-999.

Brecher, E. M. & Della Penna, R. D. (1975). *Health care in correctional institutions.* Washington, DC: National Institute of Law Enforcement and Criminal Justice, US Department of Justice.

Browne, A., Miller, B., & Maguin, E. (1999). Prevalence and severity of lifetime physical and sexual victimization among incarcerated women. *Int J Law Psychiatry, 22(2-3)*, 301-322.

Bureau of Justice Statistics (BJS). (1998). Sheriffs' departments, 1997. Washington, DC: US Department of Justice.

Bureau of Justice Statistics (BJS). (2000). *HIV in Prisons and Jails, 1999.* Washington, DC: US Department of Justice.

Buris, S., Lurie, P., Abrahamson, J. D., et al. (2000). Physician prescribing of sterile injection equipment to prevent HIV infection: Time for action. *Ann Intern Med, 133*(3), 218-226.

Campbell, J. (1992). Violence demands nursing solutions. *Am Nurse, 24*(4), 4.

Carrera, M. A. (1996). *Lessons for lifeguards: Working with teens when the topic is hope.* New York: Donkey Press.

Carroll, L. A. (2001). *Geriatrics in the prison system.* York College of Pennsylvania. Retrieved from www.ycp.edu/besc/Journal2001/Article_1.htm.

Centers for Disease Control (CDC). (1996). HIV/AIDS education and prevention programs for adults in prisons and jails and juveniles in confinement facilities. *MMWR, 45*(13), 268-227.

Centers for Disease Control. (1997). Mortality patterns-preliminary data US, 1996. *MMWR, 46*(40), 941-944.

Centers for Disease Control. (1999). High prevalence of Chlamydial and gonococcal infection in women entering jails and juvenile detention centers–Chicago, Birmingham, and San Francisco, 1998. *MMWR, 48*(36), 793-796.

Centers for Disease Control. (2001a). *Helping inmates return to the community.* Washington, DC: Author. Retrieved from www.cdc.gov/idu/facts/cj-transition.

Centers for Disease Control. (2001b, August). *Substance abuse treatment fo[r] drug users in the criminal justice system.* Atlanta, GA: Divisions of HIV/AIDS Prevention.

Clines, F. X. (2000, December 19). Access by inmates to tests for DNA gains ground. *New York Times,* A22.

Cohen, M., Deamant, C., Barkan, S., et al. (2000). Domestic violence and childhood sexual abuse in HIV-infected women and women at risk for HIV. *Am J Public Health, 90*(4), 560-565.

Cohn, F. (1999). The ethics of end-of-life care for prison inmates. *J Law Med Ethics, 27*(3), 252-259.

Collins, A. S., Gulette, D., & Schnept, M. (2005). Break through language barriers. *Advance Practice Nurses,* 30, 19-20.

Colsher, L. P., Wallace, B. R., Loeffelholz, L.P., et al. (1992). Health status of older male prisoners: A comprehensive survey. *Am J Public Health, 82,* 881-895.

Cook, L. S., Kamb, M. L., & Weiss, N. S. (1997). Perineal powder exposure and the risk of ovarian cancer. *Am J Epidemiol, 145*(5), 459-465.

Cox, J. F., Banks, S., & Stone, J. L. (2000). Counting the mentally ill in jails and prisons. *Psychiatr Serv, 51*(4), 533.

Crowell, N. A., & Burgess, A. W. (Eds.). (1996). *Understanding violence against women.* Washington, DC: National Academy Press.

Davis, S. K., Liu, Y., & Gibbons, G. H. (2003). Disparities in trends of hospitalization for potentially preventable chronic conditions amo[ng] African Americans during 1990s: Implications and benchmarks. *Am J Public Health, 93*(3), 447-455.

DeGroot, A. S. (2000). HIV infection among incarcerated women: Epidemic behind bars. *AIDS Reader, 10*(5), 287-295.

DeGroot, A. S., Bick, J., Thomas, D., et al. (2001). HIV clinical trials i[n] correctional settings: Right or retrogression. *AIDS Reader, 11*(1), 34

DeGroot, A. S., Hammett, T. S., & Scheib, R.G. (1996). Barriers to ca[re] of HIV-infected inmates: A public health concern. *AIDS Reader, 6* 78-87.

Department of Health & Human Services. (1978). *Code of federal regulations.* Title 45, part 46. Washington, DC: Author.

Department of Justice (1997). *Criminal victimization.* Washington DC Author

Department of Justice–FBI. (1999). *Crime in the United States.* Washington, DC: Author.

Dilorio, C., Hartwell, T., Hansen, N., et al. (2002). Childhood sexua[l] abuse and risk behaviors among men at high risk for HIV infecti[on] *Am J Public Health, 92*(2), 214-219.

Ditton, P. M. (1999, July). Mental health and treatment of inmates a[nd] probationers, Bureau of Justice Statistics Special Report, *NCJ* US Department of Justice, 1-12.

Doak, C. C., Doak, L. G., & Root, J. H. (1996). *Teaching patients with literacy skills* (2nd ed.). Philadelphia: J.B. Lippincott.

Dole, P. J. (1996). Centering: Reducing rape trauma syndrome anxie[ty] during a gynecologic examination. *J Psychosoc Nurs, 34*(10), 32-37.

Dole, P. J. (1999). Examining sexually traumatized incarcerated wom[en] *HEPPNews, 2*(6), 3.

Drevdahl, D., Kneipp, S. M., Canales, M. K. et al. (2001). Reinvesti[ng in] social justice: A capital idea for public health nursing? *Adv Nurs* 24(2), 19-31

Drummond, T. (1999). Cellblock seniors: they have grown old and fr[ail] in prison: Must they still be locked up? *Time,* 153, 60.

Dubik-Unruh, S. (1999). Peer education programs in corrections: Curriculum, implementation, and nursing interventions. *J Am Nur[ses] AIDS Care, 10*(6), 53-62.

Edmonton Sun. (2000). Edmonton, Alberta, Canada, March 2, p. 3.

Edgardo, R. (1995). The failure of reform. In N. Morris & D. Rothman (Eds.), *The Oxford history of prison.* New York: Oxford University Pres[s]

El-Bassel, N., Ivanoff, A., Schilling, R. F., et al. (1995). Preventing HIV/AIDS in drug-abusing incarcerated women through skills building and social support enhancement: Preliminary outcomes. *So Work Res, 19*(3), 129-192.

Ellickson, P. L. & McGuigan, K. A. (2000). Early predictors of adolescent violence. *Am J Public Health, 90*(4), 566-572.

Eviatar, D. (2003, October 4). Foreigners' rights in the post 9/11 era: A matter of justice. *New York Times,* Arts & Ideas, B7, B9.

Families against Mandatory Minimums (FAMM). (2003, October). Positive Trends in State-Level Sentencing and Correcions Policy. www.smartoncrime.org

Fickenscher, A., Lapidus, J., Silk-Walker, P., et al. (2001). Women behind bars: Health needs of inmamtes in a county jail. *Public Health Rep, 116,* 191-196.

Fink, M. J., Walker, S., Dole, P., et al. (2001, November). Educational videotapes for incarcerated women: Using focus groups to learn and teach. Paper presented at the 25th National Conference Correctional Health Care, and the Academy of Correctional Health Care Professionals, Albuquerque, New Mexico.

Finlay, I. G., & Jones, N. K. (2000). Unresolved grief in young offenders in prison. *Br J Gen Pract, 50*(456), 569-570.

Fischl, M., Rodriguez, A., Sceppella, E., et al. (2000). Impact of directly observed therapy on outcomes in HIV clinical trials. *Programs and Abstracts of the Seventh Conference on Retroviruses and Opportunistic Infections,* (abstract 7).

Flanigan, T. P. (1999). HIV behind bars: *The challenge of providing comprehensive care.* Women and HIV Conference, Los Angeles, CA. October 12.

Flanigan, T. P., Kim, J. Y., Zierler, S., et al. (1996). A prison release program for HIV positive women: Linking them to health services and community follow-up. *Am J Public Health, 86*(6), 886-887.

Flanigan, T. P., Kim, J. Y., Zierler, S., et al. (1997). A prison release program for HIV-positive women: Linking them to health services and community follow-up. *J Correctional Care, 4,* 1-9.

Flaskerud, J. H., & Winslow, B. J. (1998). Conceptualizing vulnerable populations health-related research. *Nurs Res, 4*(2), 69-78.

Flitcraft, A. (1995). From public health to personal health: Violence against women across the lifespan. *Ann Intern Med, 123,* 800-801.

Fogel, C. I. (1993). Hard time: The stressful nature of incarceration for women. *Issues Ment Health Nurs, 14,* 367-377.

Fogel, C. I., & Belyea, M. (2001). Psychological risk factors in pregnant inmates. *Am J Matern Child Nurs, 26*(1), 10-16.

Fortinash, K. M. & Holoday-Worret, P. A. (1996). Psychiatric mental health nursing. St. Louis, MO: Mosby–Year Book.

Frank, L. (1999). Prisons and public health: Emerging issues in HIV treatment adherence. *J Assoc Nurses AIDS Care, 10*(6), 25-31.

Freudenberg, N., Wilets, I., Greene, M. B., et al. (1998). Linking women in jail to community services: Factors associated with rearrest and retention of drug-using women following release from jail. *J Am Med Womens Assoc, 53*(2), 89-93.

Fullilove, M. T, Fullilove, R. E., Smith, M., et al. (1993). Violence, trauma, and post-traumatic stress disorder among women drug users. *J Trauma Stress, 6*(4), 533-543.

Gaiter, J., Jurgens, R., Mayer, K., et al. (2000). Harm reduction inside and out: Controlling HIV in and out of correctional institutions. *AIDS Reader, 10*(1), 45-52.

Golding, J. M., Wilsnack, S. C., & Learman, L. A. (1998). Prevalence of sexual assault history among women with common gynecologic symptoms. *Am J Obstet Gynecol, 179*(4), 1013-1019.

Greifinger, R. (1999). An interview. *HEPPNews, 2*(12), 4.

Grinstead, O., Faigeles, B., & Zack, B. (1997). The effectiveness of peer HIV education for male inmates entering state prison. *J Health Educ, 28,* s31-s37.

Grinstead, O. A., Zack, B., & Faigles, B. (1999). Collaborative research to prevent HIV among male prison inmates and their female partrners. *Health Educ Behav, 26*(2), 225-238.

Hall, L. A., Sachs, B., & Rayens, M. K. (1998). Mothers' potential for child abuse: Roles of childhood abuse and social resources. *Nurs Res, 47*(2), 87-95.

Hammett, T. M., Harmon, P., & Maruschak, L. M. (1999). 1996-1997 update: HIV/AIDS, STDs, and TB in correctional facilities. Washington, DC: US Department of Justice, NCJ 176344, July.

Hammett, T. M., Harmon, P., & Rhodes, W. (2002). The burden of infectious disease among inmates of and release from US correctional facilities, 1997. *Am J. Public Health, 92*(11), 1789-1794.

Haney, J., & Kristiansen, C. (1998). An analysis of the impact of prison on women survivors of childhood sexual abuse. In J. Harden & M. Hill (Eds.), *Breaking the rules: Women in prison and feminist therapy.* New York: Harrington Park Press.

Harding, T. W., & Schaller, G. (1992). *HIV/AIDS and prisons: Updating and policy review.* A survey in 31 countries. Geneva: University Institute of Legal Medicine for the WHO Global Programme on AIDS.

Hare, R. (1998). Psychopaths and their nature: Implications for the mental health and criminal justice systems. In Millon, T., Simonsen, E., Birket-Smith, M. and Davis, R. D. (eds.) *Psychopathy: Antisocial, Criminal and Violent Behavior.* New York: The Guilford Press.

Hare, R. D., Cox, D. N., & Hart, S. D. (1994). *Manuel for the psychopathy check-list: Screening version.* Toronto, Ontario: Multi Health Systems.

Harris, R. M., Sharps, P. W., Allen, K., et al. (2003). The interrelationship between violence, HIV/AIDS, and drug use in incarcerated women. *J Am Nurses AIDS Care, 14*(1), 27-31.

Hartwell, T., Hansen, N., & NIMH Multisite HIV Prevention Trial Group. (2002). Childhood sexual abuse and risk factors among men at high risk for HIV infection. *Am J Public Health, 92*(2), 214-219.

Health and Human Services Regulations. (1978). Sections 45 CFR 46.305 and 45 CFR 46.306. Additional DHHS Protections Pertaining to Biomedical and Behavioral Research Involving Prisoners as Subjects. National Institutes of Health, Office for Protection from Research Risks, Part 46. Protection of Human Subjects, Washington, DC.

Health Resources and Services Administration (HRSA). (2000, August/September). Incarcerated people and HIV/AIDS. Washington, DC: US Department of Health and Human Services. Retrieved from www.hrsa.gov/hab.

Herfkens, K. M. (2001). Depression, neurocognitive disorders and HIV in prisons. *HEPPNews, 4*(1), 1-9. Retrieved from www.hivcorrections.org.

Himelstein, L. (1993, August 16). The case for not letting 'em rot: Freeing old cons may make sense. *Business Week,* 89.

Holzemer, W. L., Corless, I. B., Nokes, K. M., et al. (1999). Predictors of self-reported adherence in persons living with HIV disease. *AIDS Patient Care and STDs, 13,* 185-197.

Human Rights Watch Women's Rights Project. (1996). *All too familiar: Sexual abuse of women in U.S. state prisons.* New York: Human Rights Watch. Retrieved from www.hrw.org.

International Council of Nurses (ICN). (1989). Death Penalty and Participation by Nurses in Executions. Geneva, Switzerland: Author.

Irwin, J. (2000). America's one million nonviolent prisoners. Justice Policy Institute, 2/26. Retrieved from www.cjcj.org/jti/one million.

Jeldness v. Pearce. (1994). 30F. 3d 1220 (9th circ).

Jordan, K., Schlenger, W. E., Fairbank, J. A., et al. (1996). Prevalence of psychiatric disorders among incarcerated women. *Arch Gen Psychiatry, 53,* 513- 519

Joyce, B. (2001). *Cell block art.* Princeton, NJ: Princeton Publishers. Aired on AMC, We Entertainment, Cool Women, November 4.

Kantor, E. (1998, May). AIDS and HIV Infections in Prisoners, *The AIDS Knowledge Base,* HIV InSite. Retrieved from www.hivinsite.ucsf.edu.

Keamy, L. (1998). Women's health care in the incarcerated setting. In M. Puisis, *Clinical practice in correctional medicine* (pp. 188-205). St. Louis, MO: Mosby.

Keaveny, M. E., & Zauszniewski, J. A. (1999). Life events and psychological well-being in women sentenced to prison. *Issues Ment Health Nurs, 20,* 73-89.

King, L. N. (1998). Doctors, patients, and history of correctional medicine. In M. Puisis, *Clinical practice in correctional medicine* (pp. 3-11). St. Louis, MO: Mosby.

Koblin, B. A., Mayer, K., Mwatha, A., et al. (2002). Douching practices among women at high risk of HIV infection in the US: Implications for microbicide testing and use. *Sex Transm Dis, 29*(7), 406-412.

Koppel, T. (1999). Crime & punishment: Women in prison (six-part series). *Nightline ABC,* October 29. ABCNewsstore.com or 1-800-CALL-ABC for transcripts.

Kupers, T. A. (1999). *Prison madness: The mental health crisis behind bars and what we must do about it.* San Francisco: Jossey-Bass.

Leenerts, M. H. (1999). The disconnected self: consequences of abuse in a cohort of low-income white women living with HIV/AIDS. *Health Care Women Int, 20,* 381-400.

Leenerts, M. H. (2003). From neglect to care: A theory to guide HIV-positive incarcerated women in self-care. *J Assoc Nurses AIDS Care 14,* 25-38.

Love, C. C. (2001). Staff-patient erotic boundary violations. *On the Edge, 7*(4), 4-8.

Lovell, D., & Jemilka, R. (1998). Coping with mental illness in prisons. *Fam Community Health, 21*(3), 51-66.

Lucas, G. M.; Flexner, C. W.; Moore, R. D. (2002). Directly administered antiretroviral therapy in the treatment of HIV infection: Benefit or burden? *AIDS Patient Care and STDs, 16*(11), 527-535.

Lurie, P., Miller, S., Hecht, F., et al. (1998). Post-exposure prophylaxis after non-occupational HIV exposure: Clinical, ethical, and policy considerations. *JAMA, 280*(20), 1769-1773.

Lynch, M., & Pugh, K. (2000, January). Uneven ground: HIV in women of color. *Adv Nurse Pract,* 45-50.

Maddow, R., Vernon, A., & Pozsik, J. (2001). TB and the HIV-positive prisoner. *HEPP News.* Retrieved on March 2001 from www.hivcorrections.org.

Maeve, M. K. (1999). The social construction of love and sexuality in a women's prison. *Adv Nurs Sci, 21*(3), 46-65.

Maeve, M. K., & Vaughn, M. S. (2001). Nursing with prisoners: the practice of caring, forensic nursing or penal harm nursing. *Adv Nurs Sci, 24*(2), 47-64.

Magura, S., Kang, S. Y., Shapiro, J., et al. (1993). HIV risk among women injecting drug users who are in jail. *Addiction, 88,* 1351-1360.

Mahon, N. B. (1999). Death and dying behind bars–cross-cutting themes and policy imperatives. *J Law Med Ethics, 27*(3), 213-215.

Manfrin-Ledet, L., & Porche, D. J. (2003). The state of science: Violence and HIV infection in women. *J Am Nurses AIDS Care, 14*(6), 56-68.

Maruschak, L. M., & Beck, A. J. (2001). *Medical problems of inmates, 1997.* Washington, DC: US Department of Justice, Bureau of Justice Statistics. January, NCJ 181644. Retrieved from www.ojp.usdoj.gov/bjs.

May, J. P. (2000). *Building violence.* Thousand Oaks, CA: Sage.

McClelland, G. M., Teplin, L. A., Abram, K. M., et al. (2002). HIV and AIDS risk behaviors among female jail detainees: Implications for public health policy. *Am J Public Health, 92*(5), 818-825.

McLaughlin, D. K., & Stokes C. S. (2002). Income inequality and mortality in US counties: Does minority racial concentration matter? *Am J of Public Health, 92*(1), 99-104.

McNally, P. (1998). Offenders who have a learning disability. *Br J Nurs, 5*(13), 805-809.

Melia, P., Moran, T., & Mason, T. (1996). Triumvirate nursing for personality disordered patients: Crossing the boundaries safely. *J Psychiatr Ment Health Nurs, 6,* 15-20.

Members of the ACE Program at Bedford Hills Correctional Facility. (1998). *Breaking the walls of silence.* New York: Overlook Press.

Miller, S. K. (1999, November). New directions for nurse practitioners: Correctional health care. *Patient Care Nurse Pract,* 53.

Miller, S. K., & Rundio, A. (1999). Identifying barriers to the administration of HIV medications to county correctional facility inmates. *Clin Excell Nurse Pract, 3*(5), 286-290.

Mitty, J. A., Holmes, L., Spaulding, A., et al. (1998). Transitioning HIV-infected women after release from incarceration: Two models for bridging the gaps. *J Correctional Health Care, 5*(2), 239-251.

Moran, T. & Mason, T. (1996). Revisiting the nursing management of the psychopath. *J Psychiatr Ment Health Nurs, 3,* 189-194.

Mostashari, F., Riley, E., Selwyn, P. A., et al. (1998). Acceptance and adherence with antiretroviral therapy among HIV-infected women in a correctional facility. *J Acquir Immune Defic Syndr Human Retrovirol, 18*(4), 341-348.

Mullings, J. L., Marquart, J. W., & Brewer, V. E. (2000). Assessing the relationship between child sexual abuse and marginal living conditions on HIV/AIDS-related risk behavior among women prisoners. *Child Abuse Negl, 24*(5), 677-688.

Mumola, C. J. (1999, January). *Substance abuse and treatment, state and federal prisoners, 1997.* Washington, DC: US Department of Justice.

Naegle, M. A., Richardson, H., & Morton, K. (2004). Rehab instead of prison. *Am J Nurs, 104*(6), 58-61.

National Center on Child Abuse and Neglect. (1996). *Third national incidence study of child abuse and neglect.* Washington, DC: US Government Printing Office.

National Commission for the Protection of Human Subjects. (1978). *The Belmont report: Ethical principles and guidelines for the protection of human subjects of research.* Washington, DC: Author.

National Commission on Correctional Health Care (NCCHC). (1997). *Standards for health services in prison.* Chicago: Author.

National Commission on Correctional Health Care (NCCHC). (2003). *Standards for health services in prison.* Chicago: Author.

Neeley, L. C., Addison, L., & Moreland-Craig, D. (1997). Addressing the needs of elderly offenders. *Corrections Today, 59,* 120-124.

Nelson A. (2002). Unequal treatment: confronting racial and ethnic disparities in health care. *J Natl Med Assoc, 94*(8), 666-668.

Nerenberg, R. (2002). Condoms in correctional settings. *HEPPNews, 5*(1).

Nicodemus, M., & Paris, J. (2001). Bridging the communicable disease gap: Identifying, treating and counseling high-risk inmates. *HEPPNews. 4*(8 & 9). Retrieved from www.hivcorrections.org.

Office of Juvenile Justice and Delinquency Prevention (OJJDP). (1999). *Fact Sheet #96.* Washington, DC: National Institute of Justice.

O'Leary, A., Jemmott, L. S., Goodhart, F., et al. (1996). Effects of an institutional AIDS prevention intervention: Moderation by gender. *AIDS Educ Prev, 8*(6), 516-528.

Parker, F. R., & Paine, C. J. (1999). Informed consent and the refusal of medical treatment in the correctional setting. *J Law Med Ethics, 27*(3), 240-251.

Perdue, B. J., Degazon, C., & Lunney, M. (1999). Diagnoses and interventions with low literacy. *Nurs Diagn, 10*(1), 36-39.

Perez, J. C., & Batong, J. (2003, September 1). Patients and prisoners. *Advance for Nurses, 3*(19), 14.

Persersilia, J. (2000, November). When prisoners return to the community: Political, economic, and social consequences. *Sentencing & Corrections: Issues for the 21st Century.* Washington, DC: USDOJ, National Institute of Justice.

Peternelj-Taylor, C. A., & Johnson, R. (1998). *Custody & caring: A challenge for nursing.* (Video documentary). University of Saskatoon, Saskatchewan.

Rich, J. D., Holmes, L., Salas, C., et al. (2001). Successful linkage of medical care and community services for HIV-positive offenders being released from prison. *J Urban Health, 78*(2), 279-289.

Richardson, L. (2003, June 4). A blue jumpsuit and a path to self-sufficiency. *New York Times,* Section B, p. 2.

Richardson, S. Z. (1998). Preferred care of the pregnant inmate. In M. Puisis, *Clinical practice in correctional medicine* (pp.181-187). St. Louis, MO: Mosby.

Rivera, G. (1999). *Women in prison: Nowhere to hide.* NBC. Aired on September 10.

Roberts, K. J. (2002). Physician-patient relationships, patient satisfaction, and antiretroviral medication adherence among HIV-infected adults attending a public health clinic. *AIDS Patient Care & STDs, 16*(1),43-50.

Rothenberg, K. H., & Paskey, S. J. (1995). The risk of domestic violence and women with HIV infection: implications for partner notification, public policy, and the law. *Am J Public Health, 85*(11), 1569-1575.

Rold, W. (2002). End of life care. *CorrectCare, 16*(3), 1-21.

Sallot, J. (2002). You can have the right to remain safe: Las Correct HELP goes behind bars to save lives. *Posit Living, 11*(1), 24-28.

Schultz, M. (2002). Low literacy skills needn't hinder care. *Regist Nurse 65*(4), 45-48.

Schwab-Stone, M., Chen, C., Greenberger, E., et al. (1999). No safe haven II: The effects of violence on urban youth. *J Am Acad Child Psychology, 38*(4), 359-367.

Scope and Standards of Nursing Practice in Correctional Facilities (1995). Waldorf, MD: American Nurses Publishing.

Siegal, N. (1998, September/October). Women in prison. *MS,* 64-73.

Singer, M. I., Bussey, J., Song, L. Y., & et al. (1995). The psychological issues of women serving time in jail. *Soc Work, 40*(1), 103-113.

Soubik, L., & Frank, L. (1999). Peer education program educates inmates. *Corrections,* 8.

Spaulding, A., Stephensen, B., Macalino, G., et al. (2002). Human immunodeficiency virus in correctional facilities: A review. *Clin Infect Dis, 35,* 305-312.

Stevens, J., Zierler, S., Dean, D., et al. (1995b). Prevalence of prior sexual abuse and HIV risk-taking behaviors in incarcerated women in Massachusetts. *J Correctional Health Care, 2*(2), 137-149.

Stone, V. (1999). Considerations for special populations with HIV infection. *HIV Physicians Strategic Treatment Initiative–Medscape,* December, program 5. Retrieved from www//:hiv.medscape.com.

Sylla, M., & Thomas, D. (2000, November). The rules: Law and AIDS in corrections. *HEPPNews,* 1-2.

Taylor, A., Goldberg, D., Emslie, J., et al. (1995). Outbreak of HIV infection in a Scottish prison. *Br J Med, 310,* 289-292.

Trigian, K. (1999). Societal Stockholm syndrome. *Women's Web Ring.* Retrieved from http://web2.iadfw/ktrig246/out_of_cave/sss,

Ungvarski, P. J., & Rottner, J. E. (1997). Errors in prescribing HIV-1 protease inhibitors. *J Assoc Nurses AIDS Care, 8*(4), 55-61.

United Nations (UN). (1982). *Principles of medical ethics and standard minimum rules of the treatment of prisoners.* Washington, DC: United Nations General Assembly.

US Department of Health and Human Services. (2000). *Healthy people 2010*–2 volumes (November 2000). Washington, DC: Authors. Retrieved from www.health.gov/healthpeople.

VanDevanter, N., Gonzales, V., Mertel, C., et al. (2002). Effect of an STD/HIV behavioral intervention on women's use of the female condom. *Am J Public Health, 92*(1), 109-115.

Vermund, S. H., Sarr, M., Murphy, D. A., et al. (2001). Douching practices among HIV infected and uninfected adolescents in the United States. *J Adoles Health, 29*(3S), 8-86.

Visser, E., Moorman, A. C., Irwin, K., et al. (1995, January 14). The influence of douching on the severity and microbiology of acute pelvic inflammatory disease. *Women's Health Weekly,* 13-17.

Vitiello, M. A., & Smeltzer, S. C. (1999). HIV, pregnancy, and zidovudine: What women know? *J Assoc Nurses AIDS Care, 10*(4), 41-47.

VonZielbauer P. (2003a, September 20). City creates post-jail plan for inmates. *New York Times,* Metro section, B1-2.

VonZielbauer, P. (2003b, September 28). Rethinking the key thrown away. *New York Times,* Metro section, 41-42.

Wallace, R., Fullilove, M. T., & Flisher, A. J. (1996). AIDS, violence and behavioral coding: Information theory, risk behavior and dynamic process on core-group sociogeographic networks. *Soc Sci Med, 43*(3), 339-352.

Washington Times. (2002, July 26). Prison rapes spreading deadly diseases. *Washington Times.* Available online CDC News Updates, HIV/AIDS Sexually Transmitted Diseases, and Tuberculosis Prevention News Update.

Witte, S., Wada, T., El-Bassel, N., et al. (2000). Predictors of female condom use among women exchanging street sex in New York City. *Sex Transm Dis, 27*(2), 93-100.

Wolfe, M. I., Xu, F., Patel, P., et al. (2001). An outbreak of syphilis in Alabama prisons: correctional health policy and communicable disease control. *Am J Public Health, 91*(8), 1220-1225.

Wright, L. N., & Smith, P. F. (1999). Decrease in AIDS mortality in a state correction system: New York State 1995-1998. *MMWR,* 47(51-2), 1115-1117.

Wyatt, G. E., Myers, H. F., Williams, J. K., et al. (2002). Does a history of trauma contribute to HIV risk for women of color? Implications for prevention and policy. *Am J Public Health, 92(4),* 660-665.

Young, D. S. (2000). Women's perceptions of health care in prison. *Health Care Women International, 21*(3), 219-234.

Chapter 52 Forensic Nursing in the Hospital Setting

Mary K. Sullivan

One forensic nursing subspecialty that is underrepresented and not yet formally recognized within the general hospital setting is clinical forensic nursing. This role requires nurses with a broad range of forensic knowledge and skills that may be applied to any patient care area within a healthcare facility. The clinical forensic nurse serves as a role model in clinical situations by increasing staff awareness of the potential for forensic implications in everyday patient care as well as working hand in hand with those charged with investigating patient complaints, suspicious patient events, unexpected death, questionable trends, and emergency/traumatic patient admissions. In addition to fulfilling another critical link between the clinical arena and the judicial system, the clinical forensic nurse is in a position to provide vital protection to victims of foul play when they are at their most vulnerable. "The importance of evidence recognition, collection, and accurate documentation is a means to an end for giving patients who are victims of violence, true holistic care, all of which are components of forensic nursing" (McCracken, 1999, p. 213).

Clinical Forensic Nursing Roles

The clinical forensic nurse is an essential part of any hospital team and has responsibilities that include monitoring and studying adverse events through a root cause analysis process. Adverse patient events range from accidents and therapeutic errors to the willing abuse and neglect of patients. Adverse events may cause serious harm to patients or personnel, but the vast majority are not criminal in nature. Regardless, the precise identification, collection, and management of facts, data, and medical evidence are critical, criminal or not. It is the duty of every healthcare provider to ensure a high level of quality patient care and accurate delivery of such services. This means all healthcare providers must have some level of awareness of what constitutes medicolegal significance. In addition, patients deserve a safe environment in which to receive healthcare, and healthcare providers deserve a safe place to practice.

Another important responsibility occurs in the clinical arena. Forensic issues range from trauma and wound pattern evaluation to proper evidence collection and management and even the evaluation of the level of care provided and the timeliness of treatment (Anderson, 1998). The role of the clinical forensic nurse is critical in each area of patient care delivery in that the nurse is most often the first to see the patient, whether in triage, as first responder in a code arrest, before the patient sees the primary care provider in clinic, or before the elderly patient is formally admitted into the nursing home care units that some healthcare facilities are still fortunate to offer. The nurse is also the one most likely to observe interactions and nonverbal communication between the patient and significant other or parent/guardian.

Recognition of both overt and subclinical abuse and neglect, as well as situations where artificial means are used to create illnesses (i.e., Munchausen's syndrome by proxy), is often obscured by the mindset of the healthcare provider, who is focused on "natural" illnesses (Anderson, 1998). The astute forensic nurse practicing in a clinical setting is able to maintain a professional balance between the nursing assessment of "natural" illness and the willingness to consider all possibilities, no matter how distasteful. Consideration of all angles and maintaining a heightened awareness does not mean the clinical forensic nurse focuses only on the next investigation, but instead the nurse provides a more thorough assessment of any given patient situation.

Best Practice 52-1

The clinical forensic nurse must perform an objective investigation of all unexpected deaths or untoward patient events, ensuring a balance of considerations of "natural" phenomena while maintaining an open mind about the possibilities of malfeasance.

Suspiciousness Factor

Winfrey and Smith (1999) said it best when describing "the suspiciousness factor" of a forensic nurse. "When an individual nurse masters forensic content and incorporates it into clinical practice, forensic science can also serve as a framework for honing intuition by increasing the 'suspiciousness factor' " (Winfrey & Smith, 1999, p. 3). No individual enters a medical facility diagnosed as either a victim or offender. It is the legal system that, after due process, affixes these labels. The nurse must at times help make that identification in order to activate the justice system. In some cases, it is only a hunch that compels the nurse to act. This hunch or intuition is the suspiciousness factor within the experienced clinician (Winfrey & Smith, 1999). The importance of the rapidity of nursing response inherent in intuition cannot be overlooked or dismissed, especially as it pertains to potential forensic cases. This intuition results in definitive action and timely nursing intervention (Brenner, Tanner, & Chesla, 1992).

Winfrey and Smith (1999) acknowledged that critics of this theory question the legitimacy of intuition in the doctrine of nursing. Easton and Wilcockson (1996) concluded that intuition involves the use of a sound, rational, relevant knowledge base in situations that, through experience, are so familiar that the person has learned how to recognize and act on appropriate patterns. Further, Paul and Heaslip (1995) stated that the thinking nursing practitioner has learned the art of "critically noticing" and is on the alert for unusual circumstances or deviations form the norm.

For example, over time and with experience nurses develop the ability to detect the most subtle signs and symptoms that a patient is not doing well. This includes patients who are not able to verbalize in a normal manner, (e.g., patients who are comatose, anesthetized or heavily sedated, mechanically ventilated, or in a psychotic state). It is the experienced clinician who detects the subtle changes that indicate serious problems or herald deterioration. Usually, the sooner these changes are noticed, the better the chances that medical staff may respond with timely and appropriate treatment. Sometimes a nurse will state, "I had a gut feeling something was wrong, but I just couldn't pinpoint it." This "gut feeling"or suspiciousness often leads to lifesaving interventions as a result of critical thinking. The associated decision-making processes that are honed through repeated experiences emerge when situations call for prompt and decisive actions. Combining this clinical savvy with a firm knowledge base in forensic science further enhances the nurse's acumen and effectiveness in the hospital setting.

Cognition and Intuition

Forensic science adds to the cognitive base from which the nurse draws for intuitive action. If suspiciousness is understood as part of intuition, the resulting actions and interventions are immediate and tailored to the unique features of the clinical situation. The forensically trained nurse is unique in that this nurse has a realistic set of responses that assumes the justice system is an established part of the multidisciplinary response to patient needs as reflected in the care in which evidence is collected and how documentation accurately reflects the situation (Winfrey & Smith, 1999).

Forensic Nursing and Patient Care

As this specialty continues to evolve within hospital and clinical settings, the impact of clinical forensic nursing practice is being felt in many of the patient care areas to which nurses are routinely assigned. These nurses put on their "forensic caps" and apply this expertise to a practice that might have become routine or second nature. They now see routine patient care assessment and healthcare delivery in a whole new way. A nurse does not have to leave the bedside, the outpatient clinic, the nursery, or nursing home care unit to be a legitimate forensic nurse. Although specific titles and position descriptions have not been established, several roles appear to be emerging that constitute specific forensic nursing responsibilities. Some of these roles overlap.

Forensic Nursing Specialties

In the traditional practice of nursing, some nurses emphasize specialties and focused interests of practice, whereas some nurses prefer to be generalists, gaining expertise in variety of settings. In the specialty of forensic nursing, the same dynamics are observed. Many nurses are trained and certified as sexual assault nurse examiners (SANEs) and their forensic nursing practice focuses on adult or pediatric sexual assault. The sexual assault nurse examiner is trained to recognize and collect physical evidence from both living and deceased victims and to elicit sensitive information from distraught individuals. The procedures require nurses not only to do a thorough head-to-toe physical assessment but to identify, document, collect, and preserve evidence, maintaining a flawless chain of custody. Sexual assault nurses frequently assume this role in addition to their regular duties in other clinical settings such as the emergency department, maternal and child health services, or an outpatient clinic.

There are also nurses who are employed as death investigators working with law enforcement and the medical examiner. Many of these individuals also maintain employment in a more traditional nursing role during other hours. The medicolegal death investigator (which is not a nurse-only position) is trained to recognize what constitutes a crime scene as well as operate within the boundaries of such a scene with a multidisciplinary forensic team. Duties and responsibilities include collecting, preserving, and documenting all types of evidence, including physical and biological evidence (see Chapter 34).

There are as many combinations of how nurses fulfill their traditional and forensic nursing practices as there are individual nurses. The clinical forensic nurse (CFN) who chooses to practice exclusively in the patient care setting brings together a combination of expertise that includes traditional nursing knowledge as well as skill sets that borrow from the SANE, death investigator, and legal nurse consultant. Skill sets include specific techniques for evidence collection and safeguarding as well as an understanding of the essential steps for maintenance of the chain of custody. There are also documentation requirements that include fundamentals of forensic photography. Forensic personnel must also be facile in the use of medical records and other source documents and may need to interpret their relevance to nonmedical personnel involved in the investigation.

The nursing profession has many levels of expertise, licensing, and certification designations, as well as myriad specialty areas of practice, permitting many options for the nurse. Likewise, within the clinical forensic nursing field there are variations in education, training, credentialing, and experience that determine potential areas of practice. It appears that four distinct roles are evolving: the clinical forensic nurse provider, the clinical forensic nurse examiner, the clinical forensic nurse specialist, and the clinical forensic nurse investigator.

Clinical Forensic Nurse Provider

The clinical forensic nurse provider works on a regular basis in a caregiver role. Additionally, however, this nurse has obtained education and training in the forensic science disciplines and applies this expertise in patient care scenarios. Forensic science principles and the art of "critically noticing" is applied to every patient encountered, whether it be in the emergency department, operating room, outpatient clinic, or an inpatient unit such as geriatric care, psychiatric, critical care, pediatric or obstetrics and gynecology. At this point it is very important to note that simply providing patient care and having the ability to recognize a potential forensic implication does not make one a clinical forensic nurse. The CFN not only recognizes what constitutes a medicolegal case, but knows what chain of events need to be set in motion and is able to do so. The CFN keeps current on rules and regulations for reporting, evidence collection techniques, and legal requirements of the justice system.

The clinical forensic nurse provider is essentially an experienced clinician in any patient care area who has continued the education process with forensic training opportunities such as medicolegal investigation, sexual assault examination training, legal nurse consulting courses, or formal graduate or undergraduate university programs. This nurse is "forensically influenced" in all patient assessments and documentation of findings and is up to date on the latest information and procedural techniques in a particular nursing area. This nurse is self-directed and self-motivated, staying informed on how forensic science can be applied in the clinical arena while continuing to refine suspiciousness and intuition. While the "forensic antennae" are up, this nurse serves as an ideal role model for other staff in detecting inconsistencies and identifying what is potential forensic evidence in day-to-day patient care activities. This nurse provides accurate and concise documentation while maintaining objectivity and avoiding the temptation to infer associations or draw conclusions about causes and effects. The clinical forensic nurse provider must be proactive in recognizing the forensic implications of any patient case where there are potential liability-related injuries. These include the victim as well as the victimizer (McCracken, 1999). The clinical forensic nurse provider must also be prepared to function as a fact witness through oral depositions or testimony in a courtroom.

Collateral Duties

Ideally, collateral duties of the forensic nurse provider would include providing assistance to the quality management department by monitoring all resuscitations or code events and assessing the events surrounding them, as well as critically assessing all patient deaths that occur in the hospital, *in real time*.

Code Events

The clinical forensic nurse provider would respond to all codes called whether the patient survives or not. This nurse does not participate in providing treatment during the code, but instead monitors events and accounts for all treatments provided. The nurse ensures that ECG strips are preserved along with the sequential records of medications, airway management, and other interventions such as defibrillation. In addition, all circumstances that immediately preceded the code are documented, including the names of family and staff members present before and during the code. A standard set of laboratory specimens are typically collected, especially if the patient does not survive the resuscitation attempt. This information is archived and if a suspicious trend is later identified, more complete information is available for root cause analysis or other investigation processes.

Other examples of code responses might include bomb threats, fire alarms, infant abduction, environmental security breaches, or hostage scenarios. The forensic nurse might assume certain duties in both responses and investigations in such incidents.

Clinical Deaths

Another responsibility would involve responding to every patient death, whether it is expected or not. When using the term *expected,* it is important to clarify that while a patient may be slowly succumbing to terminal illness, the exact moment of death cannot be predicted. At times, caregivers or family members may choose to hasten death as a way to end suffering, perhaps by administering a medication to depress respirations enough to cause death. This is an example of what a clinical forensic nurse may evaluate when looking at circumstances of any given death.

Ideally, upon each death, a standard set of laboratory work is collected and circumstances surrounding the patient's demise are documented. The laboratory specimens that would yield the most helpful information are blood gases, complete blood counts with differential, pertinent drug levels (these may vary from patient to patient), and EEG/ECG, as well as whatever would be appropriate for the circumstance (e.g., amniotic fluid, vitreous, gastric contents, hair or nail clippings). Notations are made of the last physician order changes, medication and treatments received in last 24 hours, any visitors, and other pertinent data. All information, including the laboratory results, is archived and reviewed. If a suspicious trend is later identified, more complete information is available for root-cause analysis or investigation. (Personal communication, Brian Donnelly, PhD, Federal Bureau of Investigation, 2001).

This idea is not really new, but rather a different take on an activity that clinical pathologists routinely utilize–that is, utilizing data relating to a specific illness or disease process, gathered through anatomic and clinical laboratory evaluation in the postmortem setting, to be able to better assess the course and outcome of patients with similar pathology in the clinical setting (Anderson, 1998). The clinical forensic nurse, in collaboration with the quality management (QM) staff, may utilize specific data not only to conduct a more thorough root-cause analysis should there be a complaint or concern about the care provided, but also to enhance future patient care delivery and process improvement systems for patients with the same illness or disease process.

Best Practice *52-2*

The clinical nurse should immediately secure the scene, collect baseline laboratory specimens, and preserve other clinical data when a sudden, unexpected death occurs.

If the death is suspicious or completely unexpected, the clinical forensic nurse provider may opt to "freeze" the scene until further consultation with the supervisor or law enforcement. Fortunately, these events happen rarely, but it is important to have someone who realizes what may be vital evidence and to assign that person to maintain the integrity of this potential crime scene. An example of a suspicious circumstance that should capture the attention of a clinical forensic nurse is illustrated in the case of nurse Kristen Gilbert, Northampton VA Medical Center. When Gilbert reported for evening shift duty on February 2, 1996, in the intensive care unit (ICU), there was only one patient. Gilbert would be the only nurse on duty in ICU during that shift. The patient was a 41-year-old male with multiple sclerosis who had been a patient for five days. His health status had remained unchanged that afternoon and death was not imminent. After her 6:00 p.m. dinner break, Gilbert asked her supervisor if she could leave early if her patient died. The supervisor said yes. At 7:10 p.m., the patient experienced ventricular fibrillation and expired. Gilbert transported his body to the morgue and reported off-duty by 9:00 p.m., in time to keep her social plans, as she later testified (Farragher, 2001). Had a clinical forensic nurse been available to evaluate the general circumstances of this patient's death, the red flags of this case would have been brought to the attention of the hospital management much sooner (Sackman, 2001).

Further, had a clinical forensic nurse been in a collaborative role with the QM staff, perhaps the suspicious pattern of Gilbert being on duty for half the total number of patient deaths occurring on her ward over seven years would have indeed come to the attention of administration much sooner than it did. This type of thought process, one that at least considers the suspicious or unthinkable, is routine with a clinical forensic nurse. A statistical study used by the prosecution said that the odds that Gilbert attended so many deaths simply by chance was 1 in 100 million (Farragher, 2001). Gilbert was ultimately found guilty of four counts of first-degree murder and three counts of attempted murder.

There are several contributing causes to this type of caregiver malfeasance. The reality is that most medical facilities across the country are in a crisis mode when it comes to who provides hands-on patient care and how well it is accomplished. In hospitals across the US, units are filled to capacity and those patients are sicker. A high patient census with equally high acuity levels combined with fewer licensed registered nurses (RNs) to share the workload makes for a dangerous situation. Rarely do RNs have time to help each other because of their own workloads and supervisor positions have been cut back in efforts to downsize. Additionally, some new applicants are not always completely honest with background histories, and screening efforts do not always catch the discrepancies. Further, there is an overall failure to discipline or terminate marginal employees, and because of short staffing it is often felt that a "warm body" is better than nobody showing up for work. These all contribute to setting the stage for those who may have something other than the best intentions of patients in mind. History has certainly shown that individuals such as former nurse Gilbert and many other former licensed healthcare professionals who have been successfully prosecuted for criminal acts against patients have taken advantage of these dynamics. These are additional reasons to increase the number of healthcare providers who are indoctrinated in forensic science in hospitals and clinics.

Key Point *52-1*

The change of shift, with its confusion and ambiguities in roles and responsibilities, is a "window of opportunity" for visitors and hospital personnel to engage in malfeasance.

Shift Change Vulnerabilities

Another situation where the clinical forensic nurse provider's antenna is invaluable is at change of shift. Barber (2001) believes that the time frame between the change of shifts offers the ideal "window of opportunity" for the individual who has designs for performing malicious or illegal acts. Such acts may include tampering with infusions or life support equipment or pilfering narcotics or other medications not routinely accounted for. This remains true for any specialty area in any healthcare facility. There are several dynamics of both the behavior of the healthcare providers and the overall workplace setting that should raise red flags among managers and investigators alike.

For example, staff members who are getting off duty, especially after a busy shift, may disengage from responsibilities too early, leaving loose ends and incomplete reports. Documentation and oral reports often take precedence over hands-on care activities, increasing the risks for omissions or duplications of tasks, medication administration, or specifically timed one-to-one checks on patients in leather restraints or seclusion. There is often a tendency to assume that "it will be done" by the next staff or "it has been done" by the previous staff. The oncoming staff will often have the need to "get organized" (e.g., make a fresh pot of coffee) before beginning their shift and will only engage in work duties after the preceding shift has departed. Social interactions may take precedence over professional communications when shift workers merge. Patients as well as visitors are often aware of the confusion and chaos that may occur at change of shift, and some may take advantage of these opportunities to engage in behavior not conducive to the health and welfare of other patients on the unit. Those caregivers who have ideas other than providing healthcare on their minds will also realize that the change of shift provides an optimum time for inappropriate, illegal, or otherwise dangerous behavior (Barber, 2001). The clinical forensic nurse provider may encourage and reinforce the heightened awareness of all staff at these particular times.

Essential Forensic Competencies

There are basic competencies that all clinical forensic nurses should be able to demonstrate in the hospital setting. These include the basic tasks necessary to ensure that evidence and trace evidence are properly collected, preserved, and documented. Nurses already utilize the principles of clean versus sterile in the operating room or in the administration of patient treatments of various types. Nurses already know why it is important to clean an exam table after seeing a patient in a clinic, why instruments are wiped down or sterilized, why needles are never reused, and why numerous other tasks are completed in the course of patient care–the reason is to prevent contamination. Many tasks a nurse performs and takes for granted as part of delivering good patient care form much of the basis for good medical evidence collection and preservation. Specific forensic techniques can be added to this nursing skill set. These forensic techniques may be learned in SANE training courses, through medicolegal practicums with the medical examiner/coroner, or by attending courses designated for a specific skill. Box 52-1 contains a list of basic knowledge and skills that should be included in any competency checklist for the clinical forensic nurse provider practicing in a patient care area.

Clinical Forensic Nurse Examiner

This role often overlaps with the *provider* role. The forensic nurse examiner is the nurse who is credentialed as a sexual assault nurse examiner or a medicolegal death investigator and may perform these functions as a second job. These credentials are separate from the patient care function and other nursing board certifications. However, the nurse who is able to apply the knowledge, skills, and abilities of either of these second functions to the patient care arena is a very special resource indeed. Keep in mind that the forensic nurse *provider* is one who is *actually providing* the patient care and is constantly assessing for potential forensic implications in any given case, initiating the appropriate chain of events as necessary. Part of this necessary chain of events may include collecting and preserving medical evidence. The forensic nurse provider, if trained appropriately, may now wear the nurse examiner hat. Ideally, however, and depending on the circumstances, the forensic nurse *examiner* is not involved in providing patient care, unless perhaps it is in the emergency department and evidence is being collected during the course of providing treatment (removing a bullet; photographing a stab wound and then removing the clothing without cutting through the hole made by the wounding instrument).

The forensic nurse examiner (FNE) is called onto the scene and focuses completely on identifying, collecting, preserving, and documenting the evidence. This is a completely unbiased approach–whereas in the traditional nursing role, the caregiver is often viewed as the patient advocate. This approach would apply especially in an unexpected patient death or serious adverse patient events. It would not be appropriate for the same nurse involved in the care of the patient who expires unexpectedly to be evaluating the circumstances. Another example of when it would be appropriate for

Box 52-1 Basic Competencies: Knowledge and Skills

KNOWLEDGE

The nurse possesses the following points of knowledge:

- Understands chain-of-custody procedures and related issues
- Understands federal guidelines and jurisdictional issues
- Recognizes what constitutes potential medical evidence in one's own area of expertise
- Knows the reporting and referral regulations in one's own jurisdiction (i.e., vulnerable adults, children, neglect of elderly, domestic violence)
- Understands the forensic implications of tissue and organ donation
- Knows legal requirements and procedures for obtaining consent for an autopsy, including religious beliefs that may conflict with legal issues
- Understands which deaths require notification of the medical examiner or coroner and knows the related procedures for initiating the process
- Knows procedures for making referrals to appropriate hospital and community services

SKILLS

The nurse can properly demonstrate the following forensic techniques:

- Obtaining both a wet and dry swab
- Air-drying wet, damp, or bloody material/clothing
- Scraping dried blood and packaging for preservation
- Assisting patient to remove clothing without losing trace evidence
- Bagging and storing forensic evidence in recommended types of containers
- Photographing evidence using the three basic shots, employing a grayscale or similar reference tool
- Obtaining forensic specimens of blood, urine, sputum, or stool
- "Freezing a scene" in a patient care unit or clinical area
- Documenting evidence with medical record entries
- Preparing a body for the medical examiner/coroner postmortem without compromising evidence
- Interviewing and eliciting sensitive information from a distraught/impaired individual
- Restraining a patient within hospital guidelines for behavioral or custodial purposes
- Preserving products of conception (stillbirths, abortions, placental fragments), especially under suspicious circumstances
- Exercising precautions for individuals in custodial restraint
- Securing the environment in threatening or hostage-taking scenarios

staff to call in a forensic nurse examiner would be in the operating room. Consider an unconscious trauma patient being prepared for lifesaving surgery and as the nurse inserts the catheter, it is observed that the patient may have been sexually assaulted. Then nurses involved with the preparation of this patient have enough insight to recognize that an evidentiary examination is needed and that it should be conducted by someone who can focus on that examination without distraction of other patient care requirements. Forensic nurse examiners are trained to conduct evidentiary examinations of victims of violence in and out of the hospital setting and are knowledgeable about preservation techniques when it comes to physical, medical, or trace evidence. These nurses have expertise in a specialty area such as sexual assault or death investigation and responding to crime scenes. These nurses can be qualified as fact or expert witnesses in a court of law.

Clinical Forensic Nurse Specialist

These nurses function as nurse scientists, researchers, teachers, and consultants and can be qualified as expert witnesses in a court of law. Within the hospital or clinical setting, the forensic nurse specialist has a broad range of nursing knowledge and can analyze patient care events in a variety of specialty areas. The forensic nurse specialist is adept in performing forensic medical record reviews and is the appropriate liaison to hospital risk management and legal personnel. The forensic nurse specialist is an ideal adjunct to quality management with regard to analyzing trends and performing root cause analyses to adverse patient and sentinel events.

When analyzing an incident, it is important to determine the time of the occurrence. An unusually high number of incidents occur in and around the change of shifts (Barber, 2001).

A clinical forensic nurse specialist assisting the QM staff or other authorities in an investigation may reconstruct the event within the context of the hospital's schedule of activities. Tools that assist in pinpointing personnel presence and timelines of activities include the following: medical and pharmacy records, equipment sign-out sheets, housekeeping log, Email files and computerized medical record entries, records of charges billed to patients, monitoring records from bedside recording devices, and the supervisor's report. Others include the personnel schedule or time clock records and telephone paging logs (Barber, 2001).

Key Point *52-2*

The clinical forensic nurse investigator and the hospital's quality management team share roles and responsibilities in performing root cause analyses that result in care delivery improvements.

Clinical Forensic Nurse Investigator

These nurses evaluate, review, or otherwise investigate patient care programs, patient care delivery systems, and patient complaints. This role, even though listed as a different position title, is well established in some federal healthcare systems. In some instances, this nurse will work as a member of a multidisciplinary team consisting of administrative, law enforcement, or legal personnel to provide essential subject matter expertise in cases involving suspicious, unexpected patient death, or other sentinel events that have occurred in a healthcare facility.

The term *evidence* describes data presented to a court or jury to prove or disprove a claim. Evidence is any item or information that may be submitted and accepted by a competent tribunal for the purpose of determining the truth of any matter it is investigating (Federal Bureau of Investigation, 1993). Evidence may be informational or physical.

Although the QM staff of any medical facility may not play the same role as a court of law or jury, they do share at least one responsibility. QM staff must review a set of data or collection of facts and decide on a course of action based on these particular facts. This course of action usually involves a change in processes that should result in improved patient care delivery. It may also entail recommendations to monitor staff competency or to notify appropriate authorities when a suspicious trend of events is identified. Whatever the plan, decisions and recommendations must be based on facts, data, and good evidence.

However, the problem is that attempts to collect the necessary facts and evidence are often made by those without the appropriate training to do so, or the critical information reaches the QM staff long after the event has occurred. Opportunities to capture specific details about the scene and circumstances as well as the immediate recall of those involved no longer exist (i.e., the trail is cold). Further, in these litigious times healthcare providers in all specialties are usually hesitant to admit to or discuss any activities observed that could be viewed as an error.

So how appropriate is the plan of action if the collection of facts on which the decision was made is not accurate or complete? Dr. George Wesley of the Veterans' Affairs Office of Inspector General has pointed out the link between clinical quality management activities and forensic medicine/nursing. In a review conducted by the Office of Healthcare Inspections of more than 1000 cases over 11 years, forensic issues emerged prominently (Christ, Wesley, & Schweitzer, 2000). These forensic issues fall into several major categories including patient abuse/neglect, assault, suicide, homicide, medication or delivery system tampering, improper medication administration/error, and medical equipment or device tampering (Wesley, 2001).

Recognizing the link between forensic nursing and QM may greatly facilitate patient safety activities. The clinical forensic nurse is the crucial link between effective QM activities and the increased recognition of potential forensic cases by healthcare providers. Improved awareness will lead to increased sensitivity to the importance of preserving potential medical evidence for both QM and jurisprudential purposes (Christ, Wesley, & Schweitzer, 2000). Any of the specific roles of the clinical forensic nurse previously described contributes to more effective QM review and investigation efforts by assuring that real-time information/data/evidence is identified, collected, and preserved. This process should result in quicker identification of problem areas via a more thorough root cause analysis.

Case Study 52-1 Accidental Death or Change of Shift Disaster?

A 32-year-old man with recurrent kidney stones arrived in the emergency department (ED) at 10:30 p.m. The problem was diagnosed and medication ordered at 11:15 p.m.; orders were written for admission to the medical-surgical floor. Morphine bolus was given but *not* documented. The patient was rebolused on the floor and placed on a patient-controlled analgesia (PCA) pump. There was superficial monitoring throughout night. The patient was found lifeless when the day shift arrived.

When reviewing the medical record after the patient's death, the CFN noted that timelines pointed to poor communication at the change of shift, both written and oral. The ED nurse gave the analgesic medications but failed to chart that they was administered, resulting in duplication of the order on the medical-surgical floor. The case illustrated that change-of-shift times are vulnerable periods for omissions or duplication of care components if communication is not flawless. During forensic investigations, the CFN should carefully analyze events occurring immediately before or after personnel changes since this is a likely time for misadventures.

Case Study 52-2 Improper Restraint Application or Homicide?

An 82-year-old woman was an inpatient at a nursing home care facility. She was doing well until the nurse making rounds found the patient to be unresponsive in bed. Evidentiary findings included areas of contusions and petechiae, but the mechanism of injury was not immediately determined. The presence of injuries on the patient did not correspond with the medical history given by staff. Subsequent testimony revealed the patient was initially found suspended by her neck by the "Posey" vest she was in and the vest had not been fitted/secured properly on the patient. It appears the original scene was altered so that the nurse making rounds would find the patient placed in bed. Many factors may be responsible for altering a scene, including an attempt to cover up negligence on the part of the provider (Anderson, 1998).

Issues in Role Implementation

One barrier to be recognized within the hospital structure is that of possible turf issues with nurse colleagues in the quality management (QM) or risk management (RM) departments. The clinical forensic nurse role is complementary to the roles of staff in QM and RM. The clinical forensic nurse provider has an opportunity to participate in frontline patient care on a frequent if not daily basis and is not as focused in the same way in overall patient care improvement processes as is the QM nurse. But understanding the QM process, the clinical forensic nurse recognizes potential landmines in real time as well as identifying suspicious trends that beg for action.

Another possible barrier–and this will vary widely–is that of the law enforcement attitudes toward the role of the clinical forensic nurse in an investigation process. Standing Bear (1995) described very well the concept of community policing and the fact that police officers cannot do it alone. He further explained the reciprocal exchange of information between community members and the officers assigned to protect that community.

The role of the clinical forensic nurse is that reciprocal arm of the community that happens to be located within the hospital walls. It has been established that police officers or criminal investigators are not trained to navigate through a complicated medical or surgical area, nor do they comprehend the medical/nursing jargon commonly used within medical facilities. It is rare that the officer or investigator can speak "the language." The practice of clinical forensic nursing, with its broad focus on healthcare expertise, the ability to apply forensic science to the hospital setting, and knowledge of justice system requirements, is the critical link behind the white curtain. Nurses, whether they have a forensic background or not, are key players with immediate access to the principals of events that occur in hospitals. Nurses know other key players, the environment, the language, and modus operandi of many daily scenarios that occur within any given hospital and are most likely to recognize irregularities in any routine pattern of activity. A nurse that is able to utilize forensic nursing thought processes and the previously described suspiciousness factor and apply these to everyday patient care activities and hospital routines will have the edge in spotting even the most subtle inconsistencies. This shared insight into a world that is foreign for most police officers has gradually won the respect and cooperation of law enforcement throughout the US in all forensic nursing subspecialties.

It is also possible that in some instances the administration of any given healthcare facility would prefer to keep some forensic cases or specific aspects of these cases under wraps and delay reporting to the appropriate authorities, preferring to handle problems quietly and discreetly. It is during these circumstances that the clinical forensic nurse must know what regulatory guidance applies with regard to reporting. The forensic nurse must be unbiased, consistent, and objective in taking actions in order to ensure the integrity of the forensic case.

JCAHO Regulatory Guidance

The Joint Commission on Accreditation of Healthcare Organizations (JCAHO) has laid the groundwork for the roles of forensic nurse providers and examiners within hospitals in its published scoring guidelines for patient care assessment. Additionally, the Joint Commission includes the review of organizations' activities in response to sentinel events in its accreditation process that opens the door for an important role to include the clinical forensic nurse specialist or investigator.

The first standard to be addressed is PC.3.10, which states that victims of sexual molestation, domestic abuse, elder neglect or abuse, and child neglect or abuse are identified using criteria developed or adopted by the hospital (Joint Commission on Accreditation of Healthcare Organizations, 2004). The paragraph on the intent of this standard acknowledges that victims of abuse or neglect arrive at hospitals in many ways and are often not obvious to the casual observer. It is the responsibility, therefore, of each hospital to have objective criteria for identifying and assessing these patients throughout each department, and all providers are to be trained in the use of these criteria. When the assessment has been made, the provider makes the appropriate decision regarding treatment or referral. The criteria focus on observable evidence and not on allegation alone. These include physical assault, rape or other sexual molestation, domestic abuse, and abuse or neglect of elders or children.

With the influence of forensic science on nursing assessments made by the clinical forensic nurse provider, it is more likely that a patient who is a victim of domestic abuse or neglect will be discovered. With this discovery, the appropriate assessments, documentation, and referrals will be made in a timely manner. If the assessment uncovers an injury or an admission of physical or sexual abuse in which an evidentiary examination is appropriate and accurate photography is required (i.e., a bite mark on the breast or genital area), this nurse is ideal for identifying and setting into motion the events that will establish the appropriate treatment and referrals for this patient and, if necessary, activate the justice system.

Patients who are thought to be possible victims of abuse or neglect have special needs relative to the assessment process. Hospitals must conduct assessment within the context of legal requirements to preserve evidentiary materials and support future legal actions. Further, the hospital policy must define these activities and specifiy who is responsible for carrying them out (JCAHO, 2004).

The clinical forensic nurse examiner is the ideal person to collect and preserve all evidentiary material in these clinical situations. This nurse is particularly knowledgeable about the safeguarding of evidence and chain-of-custody requirements that are paramount in all cases that involve legal action. Further, this nurse should be involved in writing all policies and procedures that define these activities within the hospital setting.

JCAHO defines a sentinel event as an unexpected occurrence involving death or serious physical or psychological injury, or the risk thereof. Serious injury specifically includes loss of limb or function. Such events are called *sentinel* because they signal the need for immediate investigation and response (JCAHO, 2004).

Each hospital is to establish mechanisms to identify, report, analyze, and prevent these events and is expected to identify and respond appropriately to all sentinel events. Response includes conducting a timely, thorough, and credible root cause analysis; implementing improvements to reduce risks; and monitoring the effectiveness of those improvements (JCAHO, 2004). Utilizing the expertise of a clinical forensic nurse will assist hospitals with fulfilling these standards.

Assid and Barber (1999) provided a complete checklist as to what any medical facility needs to do to ensure compliance with JCAHO standards. See Box 52-2.

Legal Implications of Clinical Forensic Nursing

The clinical forensic nurse is on the cutting edge of new ways to improve patient care delivery as well as strengthen quality assurance

Box 52-2 JCAHO Forensic Nursing Checklist

- Screening tools are available for personnel in clinics; the emergency department; or inpatient, geriatric, or critical care units to identify patients who have been abused or neglected.
- All personnel are trained in the use of specified criteria for detecting abuse or neglect using objective assessments, not allegations alone, to identify cases for further management by appropriate authorities.
- Orientation and annual training programs include information and procedures useful in detecting forensic cases and referring them to appropriate individuals or services for treatment, required interventions, and follow-up.
- Personnel are skilled in the appropriate techniques required for identification, collection, preservation, and safeguarding of evidentiary items outlined in the facility's policy and procedure manual.
- Patient standards of care include the recognition of forensic patients.
- Policy and procedures outline management of sudden, unexpected deaths; sexual assault; and human abuse and neglect.
- Personnel training folders incorporate required training and skills validation associated with the management of human abuse and neglect.
- The facility has a clear plan for managing victims of sexual assault of all ages and both genders.
- The facility has a dedicated space for examining forensic patients, which is equipped with locked units for storage of forensic evidence.
- Forensic reference resources are available to providers who may need guidance in identifying signs and symptoms of human abuse and neglect.
- The communication and reporting system within the facility is designed to maintain a high degree of patient privacy and discretion when forensic cases are being managed (short chain of reporting, dedicated phone lines, locked files, record security, release of information, etc.).
- Mechanisms are in place to accomplish various types of photodocumentation and to manage these photos with high level of security and flawless chain of custody.

and risk management efforts in any hospital or clinical setting. But as new ground is broken, there are serious questions that must be answered before this specialty can comfortably move ahead in establishing itself within healthcare. Answers to these questions will vary somewhat in the many jurisdictions across the US or in the type of healthcare system in which the issue occurs (public versus private), but there needs to be a standardized way of handling suspicious patient events while examining what precedence has already been set and under what circumstances.

Fortunately, the vast majority of adverse patient events are not criminal in nature or intent, but whether it is due to an increased vigilance or the improved ability of forensic investigators to identify these, there seems to be a rise in the number of healthcare providers who are charged or convicted of serial murder. In addition, more patients are victims of some type of violence or criminal activity that requires forensic diligence on the part of the healthcare provider. Given the increasing numbers of opportunities for the healthcare provider to participate in the justice system (whether the provider wants to or not), clinical forensic nurses will find themselves in the middle of patient care events that will benchmark the practice of all licensed providers in the years to come.

Some issues to carefully consider involve the CFN who suspects something suspicious or inconsistent in the course of a normally routine course of therapy. Perhaps the nurse suspects that a patient is slowly being poisoned but does not know whom the perpetrator is. When reported to a physician, these suspicions are disregarded as "impossible." What is the legal position of the nurse who, thoroughly convinced that someone is poisoning the patient, collects lab specimens without a physician's order? What if the patient gives consent for the specimens to be drawn, but has not been informed about the reason they are being obtained? Would law enforcement directives take precedent over the physician's directives if the nurse gathered enough documentation to warrant their involvement? How much information should be documented in the medical record? At what point should hospital administration, risk management, hospital security, and the hospital's attorney be notified?

Case Study 52-3 Suspiciousness Factor in the OR

A young woman was found in a roadside ditch after a passing motorist notified police. She had multiple injuries and was unconscious. There was evidence of multiple ant bites and severe "road rash." Due to unstable vital signs and apparent abdominal and chest injuries, she was taken from the ED directly to the OR for surgical exploration and intervention. While prepping the woman for surgery, the nurse who was about to insert a Foley catheter noticed extensive perineal injuries (bleeding, bruising, tears, etc.). The staff suspected she had been sexually assaulted and then thrown out of a car. Now realizing the body was actually a crime scene, a forensic nurse examiner was called to collect vital evidence before it was contaminated by surgical procedures. The woman survived this experience and testified that she had been gang-raped and then thrown from a moving vehicle being left for dead. The physical evidence corroborated the history given. Thanks to the wherewithal of the nurse in the OR who recognized the potential forensic implications of this case and the subsequent physical evidence collected, the perpetrators were eventually identified and successfully prosecuted.

Case Study 52-4 Stroke on the Medical Unit

A 70-year-old male was admitted to a medical ward and continued to be in a near vegetative state as a result of a stroke. Several years prior to this, he had signed a living will in which he expressed his wishes that in the event of a catastrophic medical condition, he should not be kept alive by artificial means. He requested comfort measures only.

The patient's wife, who was approximately 20 years younger, had never agreed with this request and continued to argue with hospital officials that her husband needed to be kept alive by any available means and that the living will should not apply. The wife contacted the media to complain about the situation, and stories began appearing in the local newspaper. The stories defended her position, and she appeared as a heroine for trying to keep her husband alive.

One day the wife visited her husband, who was in a private room. The nurse had just hung the feeding bag prior to the wife's arrival. When the wife left a short time later, the nurse returned to the patient's room to check on the feeding bag and noticed both the bag and tubing had changed from the clear coloring to a yellowish tint. The nurse did make note of it in the patient's record but discarded the bag and tubing. There was no noticeable change in the patient's condition.

Two days later the same scenario occurred, but this time the bag and tubing were saved. The patient continued unchanged.

Data from Sackman, B. (2003). Personal communication, October.

Position Descriptions

As the different roles and responsibilities of the clinical forensic nurse continue to evolve in the many specialties of patient care, it is unrealistic to expect that one generic position description in any given medical facility will be adequate. However, there are several recommended requirements that should be included on every position description for a forensic nurse who wishes to practice in a hospital or clinical setting (Box 52-3).

Educational Requirements

With regard to educational preparation, it depends on the role the nurse plays in the medical facility. The expert clinician with many years of nursing experience and a high level of interest in the medicolegal aspects of nursing but without a formal degree should not be disregarded. The nurse who is willing to maintain a heightened awareness of what may constitute a potential forensic case is invaluable, degree or not. This includes the forensic nurse examiner with demonstrated expertise in forensic evidence identification, collection, preservation, and documentation. However, as roles and responsibilities of a clinical forensic nurse increase with more complex cases encountered more frequently, it is highly desirable for a nurse to have the advanced formal education of a master's of science in nursing, as well as a clinical specialization in forensic nursing along with that expertise in a given clinical area.

Organizational Relationships

These relationships will vary from the private medical center to public/government healthcare facilities. Most clinical forensic nursing positions will interface with quality assurance and risk

Box 52-3 Position Description

- Is a registered nurse (RN) with an unrestricted, unencumbered license
- Has a minimum of three to five years of clinical experience, noting that experience does not necessarily equal expertise (Easton & Wilcockson, 1996).
- Demonstrates strong assessment, documentation, and communication skills
- Exhibits impeccable integrity and uses good judgment and discretion when communicating sensitive patient information
- Displays a high level of interest in the medicolegal aspects of nursing
- Is thoroughly familiar with all regulatory guidance regarding management of forensic cases within the medical environment of a private, state, or federal facility
- Maintains current knowledge of case law, legal evidence collection procedures, and investigative responsibilities of medicine and law enforcement
- Maintains currency in the science of forensics and the emerging trends in clinical practice that affect the medicolegal management of victims and perpetrators of violence
- Maintains current knowledge of forensic nursing through literature, continuing education courses, workshop attendance, formal university education, and the use of sound benchmark practices

management staff, but these nurses should never report to these departments. In fact, when wearing the "forensic hat" within a medical facility, the clinical forensic nurse should ultimately report to a top administrator or director, given the fact that sensitive information may need to be relayed and the shorter chain of command is always preferred. Until the role of the clinical forensic nurse is firmly established in medical facilities, it is imperative that nurse managers and supervisors be educated and kept informed of why the job of a forensic nurse varies from that of the nonforensic nurse provider. Turf issues and management problems may be avoided with the sharing of information and continuing education.

Domain of Practice

Most nurses have been trained both formally and informally to believe that the practice of *traditional* nursing is providing the absolute best care possible for one's patient. As all nurses know, this often involves much more than just providing treatments, bedside care, and medication. Being a patient advocate involves interacting with a multidisciplinary team of healthcare providers and ancillary services as well as family members. The patient is counting on the nurse to be biased for his or her needs.

The International Association of Forensic Nurses proudly displays in its logo "Beyond Tradition." This may be interpreted to mean that a nurse who puts on the forensic hat is no longer a patient advocate in the traditional sense, but is an advocate for the kind of care that promotes the best possible outcome for the patient, including protecting the patient's legal rights. This nurse is an advocate for truth and justice, even if it means a patient is identified as a serious offender who is entitled to quality healthcare delivery or psychiatric evaluation, even if it means exposing a colleague whose practice puts people's lives in danger, even if it means someone in a managerial position has been abusing his or her authority in some way. This nurse has no bias toward any one element of a patient's case and will protect the rights of all patients no matter whom the patient is, as well as uphold the law no matter what the politics of the institution are. Therefore, it is important for the nurse who is willing to pursue clinical forensic nursing beyond a provider or examiner role to have a clearly identified chain of command involving as few people as possible.

Functional Relationships

These include relationships with law enforcement agencies, the medical examiner's office, organ donor/transplant coordinators, the district attorney's office, and community social services. For federal and military institutions, relationships include but are not exclusive to the Federal Bureau of Investigation, the US Attorney's Office, the Office of Inspector General, Regional Counsel, and the Office of Special Investigations.

Specific Responsibilities

These responsibilities should be tailored to the primary role/function of the clinical forensic nurse. For example, a clinical forensic nurse provider's position description should take into account that the primary assignment is patient care delivery. The collateral duties should not be so overwhelming as to prevent the nurse from fulfilling patient care responsibilities. It is not unreasonable to expect that the forensic nurse provider be able to assist QM with monitoring all patient deaths and codes as described previously, especially if more than one forensic nurse provider is on staff. This may also involve occasional meetings or consultations with QM staff; however, it should not be the forensic nurse provider's responsibility to interpret data or trends on a frequent basis. And, of course, it is the responsibility of the clinical forensic nurse provider to "freeze" a scene and notify appropriate people if a suspicious circumstance occurs that warrants this type of action. The idea of being paged or called when a patient dies or when there is a code taking place is similar to the duty of the IV nurse who will leave the unit to assist with IV insertion elsewhere in the facility or the duty of the code team member who is paged for a code and returns to duty afterward. It is also unreasonable to expect this nurse to be on call for every sexual assault examination or to assist in critical stress debriefing processes of other professionals.

Other roles and responsibilities will become common for all clinical forensic nurses, and some will be appropriate for only specific specialties (Boxes 52-4 and 52-5).

Summary

The clinical forensic nurse is an essential part of the continuous efforts to improve healthcare delivery. The CFN role is crucial in all dimensions of patient care including the frontline, hands-on care of all patient groups in all specialty areas as well as after the fact, when the quality of care is evaluated or investigated. In addition, the CFN is in an ideal position to ensure that the rights of victims of foul play are protected within the domain of the hospital or clinical setting.

As the specialty continues to evolve, roles and responsibilities are becoming more defined and essential competencies more clearly identified. However, several important questions must be confronted before the CFN can be comfortably established within the healthcare arena, and many of the answers will depend on the jurisdiction in which the CFN wishes to practice. There must be a standardized way of handling suspicious patient events and managing medical evidence. The pioneers of this specialty

Box 52-4 Roles and Responsibilities

- Provides direct services to individual patients and family
- Provides consultation services to the nursing and medical/surgical departments as well as to law enforcement agencies and legal departments
- Serves as a preceptor for students and staff members seeking additional knowledge or skills related to the medicolegal management of patients
- Applies knowledge and skills of biomedical/medicolegal investigation in the immediate interventions and follow-up care of victims of violence (e.g., nonfatal assault, accidents, self-inflicted wounds, poisoning, suspicious/adverse in-house patient events)
- Establishes mechanisms for providing forensic education and training within the medical facility as outlined by JCAHO regulatory guidelines
- Ensures that forensic nursing assessment and referral services, mandated by JCAHO guidance, are offered within the medical facility
- Participates in the review, revision, or updating of medical center policies and procedures that include medicolegal content.
- Creates and directs the implementation of a forensic care plan in response to episodic crisis situations (e.g., internal disasters, bioterrorism, sudden or violent death)
- Participates in patient care multidisciplinary team meetings relating to human abuse or maltreatment issues as the forensics-oriented representative for this team
- Initiates/participates in research related to clinical forensic science
- Collaborates with quality assurance personnel in collecting information and identifying questionable/suspicious trends within the medical center
- Monitors/evaluates clinical, forensic activities as an integral part of the medical facility's risk management program
- Performs periodic audits of medical records from all departments to ensure that potential forensic cases have been identified and managed in compliance with regulations and JCAHO guidelines
- Provides information and guidance for medical personnel relating to organ donation/procurement
- Reports, as appropriate, medicolegal cases to law enforcement, the medical examiner's office, or other identified agencies
- Supports, assists, or serves as a liaison for the local (or onsite) sexual assault nurse examiner team leader
- Provides sexual assault examination as an expert practitioner for male and female, child or adult victims
- Educates personnel in techniques of critical incident stress debriefing

will most likely find themselves in the center of patient care events, which will benchmark future nursing practice.

Resources

Publications

Journal of Clinical Forensic Medicine
Official Journal of the Association of Police Surgeons, Journal Subscription Department, Harcourt Publishers Ltd., Foots Cray High Street, Sidcup, Kent DA14 5HP, UK

Journal of Forensic Sciences
Official Journal of the American Academy of Forensic Sciences, Michael A. Peat, PhD, Editor, 7151 West 135th Street, PMB 410, Overland Park, KS 66223

Box 52-5 Examples for Clinical Applications

DELIVERY ROOM OR NURSERY

- Infant is born addicted to dangerous drugs or with fetal alcohol syndrome
- Infant is delivered prematurely as a result of trauma incurred in a motor vehicle accident or act of domestic violence
- There are many new infants in the nursery and the hospital/clinic is short on staffing, creating the optimum conditions for infant abduction
- Infants are misidentified and associated with the wrong mother, or identifications are intentionally altered to effect a "baby swap"

THERAPEUTIC MISADVENTURES (IATROGENIC ISSUES)

- Bedside procedures performed on wrong patient
- Medication errors resulting from any cause
- Failure of critical equipment, such as infusion pump, ventilator, or oxygen supply
- Wrong patient receives diagnostic test such as x-ray or CT scan

ALLEGED SEXUAL ASSAULT

- Nursing home care unit patient
- Any private/single patient room
- Psychiatric unit assaults (psychotic female on a primarily male unit)
- Late weekend ER admit—date rape/substance abuse involved

TRAUMA WITH THIRD-PARTY PAYOR

- Multiple vehicle traffic accident with trauma to victims and involving several insurance policies

UNEXPECTED DEATHS

- Assisted suicides
- Homicides
- Psychopathic caregiver
- Real accident due to medication error
- Negligence on long-term care unit

OPERATING ROOM

- Wrong-site surgeries
- Failures of critical equipment and main power
- Loss of dissected body organ or part

MEDICAL RECORD TAMPERING

- Patient continues to complain of pain despite increased medications charted
- ECG strips are removed from monitor or chart
- Alteration/removal of death certificates
- Removal of pages in paper chart/delayed entries
- Misappropriation of computer records (certain sections deleted; data of another patient entered)
- Destruction of automatic documentation—destruction of memory chips

DRUG TAMPERING

- Drug diversion for staff's own use
- Increase in medications to hasten death
- A hazardous substance is mixed with an intended medication (IV or PO) and given

NONACCIDENTAL INJURIES TO PATIENTS OR CAREGIVERS

- Poison (injectables, inhaled substances, food, drink, etc.)

- Posey vest not applied properly resulting in asphyxiation
- Patient improperly restrained during behavioral emergency
- Negative or positive airflow is improperly secured in isolation area or operating room, respectively
- Needle sticks (nonaccidental)
- Instruments or sponges left inside surgical patient post-wound-closure
- Cancer medication diverted from IV drug solution supply
- Elderly, confused patient wanders off unit and is "lost" within hospital

SCREENING FOR HUMAN ABUSE, NEGLECT, AND VIOLENCE

- Primary care: Routine visits when the nurse sees the patient before the physician
- Emergency department: Child presents with suspected nonaccidental injuries
- Nursing home admission: Upon intake—assessment reveals gross neglect, bruises

CAREGIVER-ASSOCIATED DEATHS (MUNCHAUSEN BY PROXY)

- Death in the operating room or procedure room
- Restraint or accidental death (psychiatric unit/nursing home)
- Leather restraints improperly applied—suicidal patient is able to asphyxiate himself or herself

OTHER SCENARIOS

- Computer fraud
- An individual is court-ordered to receive a 30-day psychiatric evaluation in a locked facility; a staff member may see the vulnerability of this patient and attempt to gain something from this situation by threatening to enter notes in the medical record about this patient that would not lead to a fair or just outcome.
- Investigation of employee-related extortion (e.g., workers' compensation fraud)
- Foodborne illness outbreaks (food poisoning)

On the Edge (official newsletter of the IAFN)
East Holly Avenue, Box 56, Pittman, NJ 08071-0056; www.forensicnurse.org

Organizations

American Academy of Forensic Sciences

410 North 21st Street, Colorado Springs, CO 80904; Tel: 719-636-1100; www.aafs.org

American College of Forensic Examiners International

2750 East Sunshine, Springfield, MO 65804; Tel: 800-423-9737, 417-881-3818; www.acfei.com

International Association of Forensic Nurses

East Holly Avenue, Box 56 Pittman, NJ 08071-0056; www.forensicnurse.org

References

Anderson, W. R. (1998). *In forensic science in clinical medicine: A case study approach.* Medicolegal implications in clinical patient evaluation and treatment (pp. 223-234). Philadelphia: Lippincott-Raven Publishers.

Assid, P., & Barber, J. D. (1999, August). 10th Medical Group, US Air Force Academy Hospital Checklist.

Barber, J. D. (2001). *Cause of death: Change of shift.* Paper presented at Forensic Nursing Clinical Update 2001, August 27-28: Death Investigation, Adverse Patient Events, and Evidence Collection in the Hospital Setting, Phoenix, AZ.

Brenner, .P, Tanner, C., & Chesla, C. (1992). From beginner to expert: Gaining a differentiated clinical world in critical care nursing. *Adv Nurs Sci, 14*(3): 13-28.

Christ, P., Wesley, G., & Schweitzer, A. (2000). *Quality assurance program oversight on a large scale often reveals forensic issues.* Poster session presented at the 107th Annual Meeting of the American Military Surgeons of the US, November 6-8, Las Vegas, NV.

Donnelly, B. (2001). Federal Bureau of Investigation. Personal communication, February 13, 2001.

Easen, P., & Wilcockson, J. (1996). Intuition and rational decision making in professional thinking: A false dichotomy? *J Adv Nurs, 24,* 4, 667-673.

Farragher, T. (2001). Death on ward C: She liked to play the star. *Boston Globe.* Retrieved from www.boston.com/globe/metro/packages/nurse/part2.htm.

Federal Bureau of Investigation (FBI). (1993). *Crime in the United States, 1992.* Washington, DC: US Department of Justice.

Joint Commission on Accreditation of Healthcare Organizations (JCAHO). (2004). Joint Commission 2004 Hospital Accreditation Standards. Oakbrook Terrace, IL: Author.

McCracken, L. M. (1999). Living forensics: A natural evolution in emergency care. *Accid Emerg Nurs, 7,* 211-216.

Paul, R. W., & Heaslip, P. (1995). Critical thinking and intuitive nursing practice. *J Adv Nurs, 22,* 1, 44-47.

Sackman, B. (2001). *Profile of a VA serial killer: Red flags for health care inspectors.* Paper presented at Forensic Nursing Clinical Update 2001: Death Investigation, Adverse Patient Events, and Evidence Collection in the Hospital Setting, Phoenix, AZ.

Standing Bear, Z. G. (1995). Forensic nursing and death investigation: Will the vision be co-opted? *J Psychosoc Nurs, 33,* 9, 59-64.

Wesley, G. (2001). *Forensic aspects of medical quality assurance: Is "forensic quality assurance" a new medical discipline?* Unpublished manuscript. Washington, DC: Office of Healthcare Inspections.

Winfrey, M. E., & Smith, A. R. (1999). The suspiciousness factor: Critical care nursing and forensics. *Crit Care Nurs Q, 22,* 1, 1-7.

Chapter 53 Evidence Collection in the Emergency Department

Deborah R. Fulton and Pamela Assid

The emergency department (ED) is typically the point of entry into a medicolegal environment for both victims and perpetrators of violent crime and other accidental injuries having related forensic issues. According to the Bureau of Justice, in 1994, US hospital ED personnel treated 1.4 million people for injuries from confirmed or suspected interpersonal violence (CDC, 1996). Approximately 92% of these individuals were released after initial treatment in the ED, making it virtually impossible to have subsequent opportunities to capture forensic evidence.

Key Point 53-1

During the course of ED evaluation and treatment, evidence can be overlooked, lost, or destroyed unless members of the healthcare team, especially nurses, are aware of what constitutes evidence and are facile in the procedures and techniques to capture and preserve it.

It is essential that all ED nurses have the basic skills to gather evidence effectively, and it is preferable to have a forensic nurse examiner available for the collection of evidence whenever possible. Emergency departments must establish guidelines for consistent documentation and preservation of forensic evidence. This chapter will outline the types of forensic cases typically encountered in the emergency department, along with guidelines for documentation and proper collection of evidence. There are, of course, many variables in protocol, depending on the jurisdiction. When questions arise regarding the laws or practices within a particular area, the FNE should review the applicable statutes for the subject matter and be informed about the local laws regarding search and seizure. Legal problems regarding evidence collection and preservation can usually be avoided if the nurse is following established hospital policies and procedures that have been based on the recommendations or counsel of the local crime laboratory, medical examiner, or coroner. Without such attention to details, important evidentiary items or findings may not withstand the scrutiny of the courts for admissibility in criminal or civil proceedings. The information in this chapter is not intended to meet specific requirements of various jurisdictions or to override existing hospital policy. Instead, it provides fundamental guidance consistent with recommended standards of forensic sciences.

Identification of Forensic Cases

Forensic cases include those that potentially involve criminal or civil liability. Box 53-1 lists the categories of forensic cases that may present in the ED. It is not all-inclusive, but serves as a guideline to identify commonly encountered forensic cases.

Box 53-1 Forensic Cases in the Emergency Department

- Domestic violence, abuse, or neglect (child, spouse, partner, elder abuse)
- Trauma (nonaccidental or suspicious, and accidental injuries with third-party payer implications)
- Vehicular and automobile versus pedestrian accidents
- Substance abuse
- Attempted suicide or homicide
- Occupational injuries
- Environmental hazard incidents (fire, smoke inhalation, toxic chemical exposures, etc.)
- Victims of terrorism or violent crime
- Illegal abortion practices
- Supervised care injuries
- Public health hazards
- Involvement of firearms or other weapons
- Prominent individuals or celebrities
- Unidentified individuals
- Damaged or improperly used equipment
- Poisoning, illegal drugs, or overdose
- Anyone in police custody for any reason
- Sudden, unexpected, or suspicious deaths
- Sexual assault and abuse

In 2000, more than 40 million injury-related visits to the emergency department were reported in the US (CDC, 2002). The most common causes of these injuries included traffic accidents, falls, and violence. Furthermore, it is estimated that up to 25% of ED visits involved alcohol or drug abuse (CDC, 2002). What does this mean to a forensic nurse examiner? Simply, there is an abundance of evidence that needs to be collected to ensure that objective information is available to those who make critical decisions.

Responsibilities in Evidence Collection

When the victim of violent crime or liability-related injuries is treated by ambulance or emergency department personnel, valuable forensic evidence is often lost because personnel are not aware of its presence or potential value. The problem of gathering evidence in the clinical setting is not restricted to the failure to recognize or collect forensic evidence; often there is a failure to properly preserve fragile or perishable evidence. The accurate documentation of medicolegal evidence is essential as well. Literature suggests the causes of this deficiency are due, in part, to poor communication between medical and law enforcement personnel and a lack of forensic education among medical personnel (Lynch, 2001). One approach might be to designate a hospital property custodian to retain evidentiary items for collection by medical examiner's investigators or law enforcement officers. Clinical forensic nurses, whose education prepares them for gathering facts and preserving evidence that would help reconstruct the circumstances of death or injury, could ideally fill this vital role.

Basic evidence is used to establish the facts of a crime: (1) that a crime has been committed; (2) that a certain person has committed a crime; and (3) the modus operandi (how a crime was committed).

Types of Evidence

Black's Law Dictionary identifies several types of evidence. Examples include admissible, circumstantial, documentary, and real evidence. For the purposes of this section, the discussion will be limited to physical evidence.

Physical evidence can be defined as any matter, material, or condition, large or small, solid, liquid, or gas, which may be used to determine facts in a given situation. Therefore, items such as clothing, hair, nails, bullets, contusions, lacerations, and other wounds are classified as physical evidence. What is critical in medicolegal cases is to ensure that any and all evidence is appropriately managed using precise forensic procedures.

Physical evidence is the concern of the criminalist, who will identify and analyze the materials submitted to the crime laboratory. For the evidence to be used, it is imperative that it has been properly collected and preserved. It is hoped that the evidence will link a victim to a suspect, link a suspect to a crime scene, identify an assailant, establish an element of a crime, or corroborate or disprove an alibi.

Emergency personnel need to understand the legal procedures required in handling physical evidence, the types of physical evidence, and the value of that evidence. They must also know proper methods for collecting, documenting, and preserving forensic evidence. Education should include the identification of specific wounds and how their interpretation may provide critical information regarding the type of weapon and circumstances surrounding the injury. In the absence of a specially educated forensic physician or nurse clinician, potential liability exists. Search and seizure become complex. It is recommended that healthcare professionals seek legal counsel or information about forensic procedures when questions arise concerning the legality of evidence recovery. Once medical personnel are taught the value of physical evidence and the proper procedures for handling it, they generally support police requests for assistance and do not inadvertently hinder progress of the investigation.

Most trauma EDs have some type of cooperative program established with the local police when evidence collection is required. However, many rural or smaller EDs do not handle evidence collection often and therefore may not be aware of the specifics regarding collection and documentation. Forensic nurse examiners can assist patients and other ED personnel through sharing their education and training and assisting in the development of policies, procedures, and protocols for other facilities. It is recommended that the FNE work in conjunction with the local crime lab and district attorney's office to ensure strict compliance to guidelines within the jurisdiction. Other recommendations are outlined in Box 53-2.

When to Collect Evidence

Accidents that involve trauma are potential forensic cases until intent has been confirmed or ruled out. It is not always possible to predict if an accident will have medicolegal implications. Yet, almost all accidents result in some type of litigation, whether civil or criminal. All non-vehicular trauma should be considered abuse until proven otherwise. Equal consideration must be afforded trauma cases to rule out or confirm abuse. The term *accident* must be used with great caution in nursing documentation. For example, if a patient offers information to the triage or other emergency nurse that suggests a condition or injury is the result of an accidental event, the statement should be placed in quotation marks. The term *accident* implies a nonintential injury, which cannot be proven without an investigation. The terms *intentional* or *nonintentional* injury refer to a conclusion, which must be drawn after the investigation of circumstances and evidence are recovered. (Lynch, 2001).

A medicolegal case is defined as a treatment situation with legal implications (Middleman, Goldberg, & Waksman, 1983). When a patient dies in the emergency department or is "dead on arrival," personnel should refrain from following customary procedures often employed in hospital deaths. The body should not be washed; tubes, drains, and appliances should be left in place; and all personal clothing and other items should be carefully packaged and retained with the body, not returned to the family or significant others. These typical procedures are not suitable for medicolegal cases, and often it is impossible to initially determine if a case has medicolegal implications, even when the death appears to be "natural" or easily explained.

Box 53-2 Forensic Nurse Responsibilities in the Emergency Department

- Investigate what resources are available for victims of violent crimes. Some communities might have domestic violence programs or safe houses. If discharging a victim of violent crime from the ED, make sure she/he has someplace safe to go where the attacker cannot find him/her.
- Create an evidence collection educational program for the ED staff. Also consider annual refresher training, especially if these are skills the staff is not likely to use often.
- Be sure to advocate for the patient. A forensic nurse must be objective and sometimes will care for victims and perpetrators. Don't let personal judgments cloud professional actions.

Clothing

If the individual is able to undress, place a sheet on the floor, then place clean white paper on the sheet. Have the patient disrobe while standing on the paper. The paper will catch trace evidence that may fall from the clothing. Trace evidence consists of very small particles such as hair and fibers. For obvious reasons and because of universal precautions followed by all healthcare facilities, the person collecting evidence must wear gloves. Fold the paper inward and secure. Place this in a small paper bag or envelope, and then seal the envelope with evidence tape and a patient label. Initial, including date and time, both the evidence tape and the patient label. Do not use gummed envelopes because they may contaminate the evidence. When sealing the packaging, do not use staples. They present the potential for injury to the person opening the evidence package. Complete and attach a chain of custody form. In the area on the chain of custody for a description of package contents, write "clothing paper." Lock the envelope in a secured area that has controlled access. If the patient arrives by ambulance, preserve the gurney cover in a similar manner.

After the patient is undressed, place each item of dry clothing in a separate paper or cardboard container. Always use paper to prevent breakdown of the integrity of biological evidence such as blood, semen, or saliva that may be present on clothing. Biological evidence is subject to decay and mildew because of its inherent moisture content. Seal, label, and secure the package as previously described. In the area marked "contents" or "description" describe the article, including defects such as tears, gunshot residue, burns, and stains.

Place wet or damp clothing in a paper container and label appropriately. Stand this container inside a waterproof, nonpermeable receptacle. If placing in a plastic bag, do not seal the bag. Whenever biological evidence is placed in a nonpermeable container, bear in mind that there is a limited length of time before the evidence begins to degrade. Contact the appropriate law enforcement personnel to collect the evidence as soon as possible. Indicate the exact time that the evidence was collected on the chain of custody form. As with dry evidence, secure the evidence in an area with controlled access.

If the patient is unconscious or severely ill or injured and cannot assist in removing clothing, the FNE must remove clothing from the patient, maintain as much garment integrity as possible. Ensure packaging of all garment pieces. Do not shake the clothing. When cutting garments off a patient, do not cut through defects in the clothing such as bullet holes, tears, or stab entry areas. Package and label as appropriate any linen that has come in direct content with the patient (e.g., top and bottom sheets, EMS gurney covers, pillowcases). Process all items as previously described. The greatest universal error made by ED staff during treatment of a trauma case is throwing clothing on the floor in the trauma room. This egregious error results in the cross contamination of critical evidence as it comes in contact with debris such as hair, fibers, dust, drops of solutions, soil, and other contaminants, as well as blood and bodily fluids, commonly present during emergency trauma treatment. Consider what may be tracked into the hospital and into the trauma unit on the soles of the paramedics directly from the crime scene. Is the evidence adhering to the clothing from the victim, the perpetrator, from the first responders or the doctors and nurses within the trauma environs?

It is not uncommon to hear the response from emergency personnel that "we are trying to save a life; we don't have time to provide a clean field for clothing or other evidence. That is not our job." Clearly, forensic evidence should never take priority over lifesaving interventions under any circumstances. However, this is the role of the forensic nurse examiner, who is not part of the trauma team but responds to the emergency to serve as the evidence custodian, that extra pair of hands historically absent in times such as these. One may attempt to justify the absence of an FNE on the hospital staff as impossible (due to cost) based on a specific job description for forensic services alone. When hospital administration is faced with the liability issues afforded the patient whose evidence has been lost or destroyed by the hospital employees it may be worth far more than the funds necessary to recover, preserve and secure forensic evidence. One example is the major lawsuit filed against a New York hospital for the failure to protect the patient's legal, civil, and human rights through the proper collection of evidence related to sexual violence. The loss of evidence in a criminal case precludes the state, not only from successful prosecution of the perpetrator, but also diminishing the possibility of filing a civil case.

However, from the justice perspective, not taking the opportunity to prevent further crimes committed by the suspected offender is an injustice to us all. The following are simple steps to ensure proper handling of clothing during a trauma case:

- Place a clean white sheet on the floor, empty gurney, mayo stand, or cabinet top.
- Place the clothing on the sheet rather than the floor, out of the way of human traffic.
- After the crisis, place each garment in individual paper bags following recommended labeling.
- Fold and place the sheet in a separate paper bag and send to the crime lab along with the clothing and other evidence. If stains are present, put clean paper over the stains before folding to avoid cross contamination. If stains are wet, notify the police of the damp clothing so they will transfer it to the crime laboratory for urgent air-drying.

Although any staff member may certainly be able to perform such duty, one must also accept the responsibility of custody and security of evidence until the time it is handed over to the proper legal agency and be prepared to testify in court as necessary. The role of the FNE provides the ideal clinician to assume these responsibilities and to reduce the risk of liability to the institution as well as to ensure the victim and the community have not been denied social justice from the healthcare perspective.

Good quality photographs should be made that adequately depict the location of the injury. Photographs should be made with and without a scale (ABFO #2 gray scale is preferred). The scale used should be rigid and not obscure the wounds. A coin may be placed near the wound to establish a reference perspective if no scale is available. Always retain the coin or scale with other evidence. Whenever possible photographs should be made prior to suturing or other procedures in the area of injury. Infrared and/or ultraviolet photography may be used to elicit bruises or bite marks at a later date as the patient's condition warrants.

If prehospital personnel have taken on-scene photos or have drawn laboratory samples in the field for ED use, these items along with clothing or other personnel should be transferred with a formal chain of custody documentation (see Chapter 32).

Best Practice *53-1*

The forensic nurse should not dispose of *any items* collected from the patient or return any personal items to the family during the course of ED care and treatment because such items may have evidentiary value.

Do not dispose of *any items* collected from the patient. Do not return any personal items to the family. Personal items belonging to the victim may have evidentiary value. Family can obtain personal items from the appropriate law enforcement agency at a later time. If the patient expires in the ED, the family can obtain collected items from the medical examiner's office when they have been properly documented, examined, and released.

Missiles and Other Debris

This type of debris refers specifically to items removed from the victim during the course of treatment. Some examples are bullets, glass, bags of unknown substances, pills, and weapons. Items that are imbedded in the victim (e.g., bullets) or entangled in the clothing or hair (e.g., glass) should be removed with rubber-tipped forceps to maintain the integrity of the item by preventing potential damage, alteration, or destruction of the item.

Place small items in clear, rigid plastic containers (urine specimen containers or sputum cups may be used). Before placement of the item in the container, punch a few small holes in the lid to allow the item to "breathe" and place gauze or cotton batting loosely in the container. This prevents the degradation of residual biological evidence that may be on the item. After the item has been placed in the container, cover it loosely with cotton batting or other soft material. Seal the container with evidence tape. Label the container with a patient label. Initial the seal and the label. Place the container in a paper bag. Seal the bag with evidence tape and a patient label. Initial both seals. Attach and fill out the chain of custody form. In the area marked "contents" or "description," describe the packaged item. It is also essential to indicate where the item was retrieved from. Secure the item appropriately in accordance with evidentiary safeguarding procedures.

Place large items such as knife blades and firearms in an appropriate-sized cardboard box. Handle these items with *extreme* caution. Pad the item with cotton batting or similar material. Seal the box as previously indicated and attach a chain of custody form.

Body Fluids

When collecting blood, the earliest drawn specimens are of the greatest evidentiary value. Collect one red top (without preservative), one purple top, and one gray top Vacutainer as soon as possible. When preparing the skin for venipuncture, do not use alcohol. Cleanse the site with povidone-iodine followed by saline. After collection of the blood, put it in appropriate tube(s), place evidence tape across the top of the tube(s). Place a patient label on the tube(s) and initial each one. Wrap tube(s) in protective material and place them in an appropriate package. Seal package with evidence tape and a patient label. Initial both seals. Attach and fill in a chain of custody form. In the area marked "contents" or "description," write "blood" and the time of collection. Many healthcare facilities have premade packages for the purpose of collecting evidentiary blood alcohol levels. It is suggested that the nurse review the statutes pertaining to evidentiary blood alcohol testing for the jurisdiction in which the nurse practices.

All other body fluids, such as gastric contents, chest tube drainage, peritoneal tap fluid, urine, may also be collected. Place fluids in clean plastic containers, such as empty saline bottles. Seal the neck of the bottle with a waterproof sealing tape, such as Parafilm. Place evidence tape across the top of the bottle so that it extends beyond the waterproof seal. Place a patient label on the specimen. Initial the evidence tape and label. Place the specimen in a paper bag. Seal the bag with evidence tape and a patient label. Initial the tape and the label. Attach and complete a chain of custody form. In the area marked "contents" or "description," state the type of fluid, and other pertinent factors (e.g., gastric contents + 1500 mL NaCl 0.9% used for instillation).

Photographic Documentation

When photographing patients, the FNE is required to get informed consent. Make sure that the patient understands the purpose of the photographs. Although 35-mm cameras provide superior pictures, many EDs and law enforcement agencies use the Polaroid Spectra camera. This camera is user-friendly, and therefore, every nurse in the ED will be able to use it when necessary. Further, it eliminates the chain of custody problem that may arise with developing 35-mm film. The FNE can also be sure that the photographs are usable because they are immediately viewable. Photographs for documentation purposes in the ED are usually limited to domestic violence cases, child abuse, and sexual assault. However, current policies indicate that photo documentation of any injury is the best method of memorializing the wound for liability, medical malpractice, worker's compensation, or any case that may go to court. This includes most accidental injuries.

Do not write directly on the photographs. Place a patient label on the photograph. Indicate time and date on the label prior to placing it on the photograph. The photographer must initial the label. Document the number of photographs taken on the patient record. In cases of domestic violence, do not give copies of the pictures to the patient. If the batterer finds them, the victim will be in more trouble for going to the hospital and revealing the abuse. If photographs are taken in the ED, they do not leave the department with the police. The pictures become part of the medical record and are the property of the hospital. If law enforcement officials need photographs for an investigation, they must come with their own film and cameras unless otherwise designated by hospital policy and a predetermined agreement between the forensic nursing services unit and the police.

Other Documentation

Meticulous documentation is vital not only in patient assessment data but also in providing medicolegal protection for the patient's legal, civil, and human rights. Proper documentation can also keep FNEs out of court or provide strong support if they are required to testify. The widespread lack of knowledge about and noncompliance with medicolegal protocol supports the need for greater awareness and forensic education for ED staff and first responders involving reportable cases.

Physical Findings

All physical findings should be documented precisely, using correct terminology. These notations should include the exact location, size, and characteristics of injuries. Both narrative notes and body diagrams should be used (see Appendix C). ED personnel should refrain from making forensic interpretations of wounds, such as "entrance wound, anterior chest." Instead use objective terminology of injuries, such as, "3-cm circular wound with abraded edges at fifth intercostal space, midclavicular line."

All procedures, even minor ones, should be documented. If the patient expires in the ED, make a list of all treatment-related skin defects or alterations. Use a skin-marking pen to annotate these. Cover each wound with a dry dressing and label as a treatment site. The medical examiner will need this information to make an accurate determination as to cause of death. Include names of visitors (if any) and any law enforcement officials and their badge numbers. Document the demeanor and appearance of involved parties as objectively as possible. Do not paraphrase statements. Directly quote the statements as much as is possible. Do not document things such as "alleged" or "smells of alcohol." Nurses do not "allege" someone has chest pain! The smell of alcohol is highly subjective. Document statements made by the patient and describe all behaviors in objective terms.

Verbalizations

Statements of the victim and other involved parties as well as nursing observations become part of the medical record. Meticulous and accurate documentation will make the record a valuable piece of evidence. It is critical that documentation is accurate and objective. The possibility always exists in medicolegal cases that the FNE might have to go to court to defend his or her documentation. It is essential that the FNE not only defend but also accurately depict events that might have transpired months or years prior to the time they are presented in court.

Security of Patients in the Emergency Department

Victims of serious crime should be kept in a private room with access limited to an identified few. Anyone visiting such a patient must check in with the nurse assigned to that patient or a law enforcement officer, and the visitation will be noted on the chart. Many hospital EDs now have "airport-like" screening procedures of both patients and visitors in the ED to assure a safe environment.

The Body as Evidence

When sending a body to the medical examiner's office, the body itself becomes evidence. Maintain chain of custody as with any other piece of evidence.

Do not cut any lines or remove any tubes prior to releasing the body. If there is any indication that gunshot residues may soil the hands, or, following an altercation, if there might be hair or fragments of skin beneath the fingernails, then each hand should be enclosed in a small paper bag. Place the hands of the decedent in the paper bags and secure at the wrist with tape. This is especially important in cases that involve firearms or sexual assault. Send all collected specimens, clothing, and linen with the body. Do not return any personal belongings to the family. The office of the medical examiner will determine what to release to the family. If the patient has died of a violent crime or under suspicious circumstances, the body should not be viewed without attendance of emergency department personnel to ensure that there is no opportunity to alter potential evidentiary sources.

Best Practice *53-2*

Nurses in the ED should use extreme caution when working with patients in police custody and should not permit the offender to distract or manipulate them during the course of assessment or treatment.

Patients in Police Custody

Forensic nurse examiners should possess considerable knowledge about the policies and procedures relevant to patients in police custody. Although caring for the challenging patient becomes routine in some EDs, the nurse should avoid becoming comfortable with the situation. These patients always pose a certain hazard in the ED. Remember that individuals in custody have an intense desire to regain their freedom, which often involves manipulation of a well-meaning healthcare worker. FNEs should not expect custodial officers to "step out" during procedures or to release the prisoner for trips to the bathroom. They should never be left unattended despite their seemingly benign behavior.

They may become agitated, volatile, and physically aggressive with little provocation and without warning. Recently apprehended offenders in custody may be undergoing detoxification from drugs or alcohol, or may be in the midst of a psychotic behavior pattern with delusions, hallucinations, and extreme paranoia. Bearing these factors in mind, the ED nurse should always assume that prisoners can be "violent at a moment's notice" and therefore should be approached with this factor in mind.

Assessment of patients in custody is frequently complicated by their reluctance to be forthright and direct when answering healthcare questions in the presence of a police officer. The FNE should also recall that offenders might have underlying health, alcohol-related, and drug-related issues that are unknown to the police. It may be extremely difficult to "rule out" certain medical conditions in the presence of the secondary issue of custody and the manipulative behavior that is often displayed by these individuals. It is well known among correctional personnel that offenders feign illness and injury in order to go to the hospital, where they believe that they can "make a break" during the process of triage, medical observation, or diagnostic procedures. Additional complications such as excited delirium may be present and even life-threatening for the patient.

Restraints

Restraints will be employed for the overwhelming number of patients in police custody. When patients arrive with restraints in place, the ED physician should be promptly notified in order to accomplish a prompt screening history and physical examination and to determine the type of restraining procedures or confinement that is required for safety in the ED. Jail patients may have leather restraints and locked ankle cuffs upon arrival, and such restraint placements should be confirmed and authorized by the physician in writing to establish periodic nurse monitoring associated with restraint safety. Additional chemical restraints may be ordered if indicated. Offenders should not be restrained in a prone position with wrists and ankles tied together behind the back, (i.e., "hog-tied" or "hobbled") because this position can lead to positional asphyxia (McCarron & Challoner, 1999). Should any marks or injuries be observed related to the restraints (handcuffs, ligatures), the marks should be photodocumented and reported. The stun belt (remote electronically activated control technology, or REACT) has been used since 1993 in some settings to control jail and prison inmates. The belt is worn by the prisoner and controlled as far away as 300 ft by an officer who can activate the belt by pressing a button, resulting in a 50,000-volt low-current shock lasting about 8 seconds. The REACT produces pain and incapacitation, sometimes including involuntary urination and defecation. Amnesty International and other organizations have objected to the utilization of such a device because it is considered a weapon of terror (McCarron & Challoner, 1999). The FNE should avoid modifying any restraints without direct consultation and support from an attending police officer.

Medical devices, plastics, sharps, compressed gases, cords, and instruments should not be left within reach of prisoners. There is ample evidence of an offender's ability to use such items to fabricate weapons or to otherwise gain some control over others (Mallon & Perez, 1999).

ED personnel who are not vigilant in the presence of prisoners or other individuals in custody can easily become involved in a hostage-taking scenario, endangering themselves, the police officer, and others in the department. Be firm, direct, vigilant, and focused at all times. Appearing indifferent, tolerant, tired, or distracted permits the offender to entertain the possibility that one could be taken easily as a hostage. The nurse should maintain a businesslike attitude at all times, avoiding socialization with either the officer or the offender. Behavior should be deliberate and purposeful to ensure that the officer is not distracted and that the offender is not incited to react or respond.

Care should be planned to ensure that prisoners and their custodians receive high-priority management. All required assessments and interventions should be expedited and accomplished without delay to minimize the time that the offender is in the ED environment. The FNE is trained to maintain a high index of suspicion and to be alert to possible circumstances that could result in hostage taking. This training is invaluable in the ED where a clear and rapid response within the first five to ten minutes of a threatening situation or assault can reduce harm to the staff or patient and increase the chances of survival.

Key Point 53-2

The ED nurse should not reveal to the offender the date, time, or place of any follow-up care. This information could be used to take advantage of a low-security site for escape attempts or other counterproductive moves against law enforcement.

Body Searches

Emergency personnel may be requested to participate in body cavity searches for contraband. These searches must be court-ordered or done with the written consent of the offender. Exceptions may be made for contraband that might be immediately life-threatening to a patient (Mallon & Perez, 1999). Cavity searches must be fully documented with the signatures of two physicians and accomplished in the presence of a witness of the same gender as the patient. Recovered items or contraband must be accounted for, using the ordinary chain of custody procedure. Depending on the law in individual state statutes, the FNE must either turn contraband over to the police or have the destruction of the materials witnessed according to hospital policy. This is important information that may protect the patient's constitutional rights or protect the FNE from being sued by the patient for giving away his or her personal property. A hospital forensic protocol should address this situation according to the legal statutes that will indicate when to act and when not to act. This forensic protocol should also include rules of evidence applicable to the specific state regarding search and seizure in the ED.

Blood Alcohol and Drug Testing

Emergency nurses may become involved in obtaining blood for alcohol levels, or blood or urine samples to detect the presence and levels of other substances, usually illegal drugs. In most jurisdictions there is a specific procedure that must be followed (Box 53-3).

Blood alcohol is a complicated subject with an important medicolegal significance, frequently resulting in confusion and misconception. Alcohol is a small molecule; 25% is absorbed directly into the bloodstream on ingestion, with the balance being absorbed through the small intestine. Alcohol is widely distributed, following water, and appears anywhere in the body where there is water. Alcohol can be measured after ingestion in organs, muscles, brain, blood, urine, saliva, and perspiration; once absorbed into the bloodstream, 5% is eliminated through saliva, urine, and sweat, with the other 95% being eliminated by means of oxidation in the liver. Blood alcohol is a "picture" of the extent to which the body's capacity to metabolize and get rid of alcohol has been exceeded. A single drink (1 oz) is absorbed in about 20 minutes and the drug remains in the body normally for approximately 1 hour, oxidizing at the rate of 15 mg/100 ml per hour.

One ounce of 80-proof whiskey will register a blood alcohol level of 20 mg/100 ml, proportionately, depending to a greater or lesser extent upon body weight. A 70-kg man (154 lb), given 1 oz of 80-proof whiskey, will show a blood alcohol level equivalent to 0.02% or 20 mg/100 mL. In the same man, a 12-oz can of beer will show a blood alcohol level of 25 mg/100 mL, and the rate of oxidation (or disappearance from the blood) will be about 15 mg/100 mL per hour, as with the 80-proof whiskey (Besant-Matthews, 2004).

Consider the following rule of thumb:

20 to 50 mg/100 mL (0.02 to 0.05%), within legal limits
50 to 80 mg/100 mL (0.05 to 0.08%), nearing legal limit
450 to 500 mg/100 mL (0.45 to 0.50%), toxic and lethal!
(Besant-Matthews, 2004)

In recent years the trend has been to establish lower legal limits for blood alcohol levels. A level of 80 mg/100 mL (0.08%) has been adopted by England and Canada, and at this time Germany and Scandinavian countries observe a legal limit of 50 mg/100 mL (0.05%) (Besant-Matthews, 2004). Most states currently recognize the legal limit at around 100 mg/100 mL (0.1%), but there is a trend to reduce this to a range of 50-80 mg/100 mL in many states. If there has been a negligent homicide involving a motor vehicle accident, an alcohol blood level must be obtained to submit essential proof to a jury. Therefore, it is necessary to get a blood alcohol sampling if at all possible; otherwise, there may not be any enforcement action available.

Effects of Alcohol

The effects of alcohol are irregular and progressive, descending depression of the central nervous system. Low doses decrease attentiveness to the task at hand (an example is careless driving after two or three drinks), although chronic alcoholics currently drinking may tolerate higher blood levels before they begin deteriorating.

The first things affected are the higher centers of the brain, the most skilled task abilities, and the most recently learned tasks. As the blood alcohol level climbs higher, more of the brain's functions become depressed, and the effects become obvious. Alcohol does tend to be a self-limiting overdose with coma or sickness limiting further intake, and for this reason fatality from alcohol alone is rare.

Most states now have an implied-consent law, whereby, as a condition of accepting a driver's license, the applicant agrees to give a sample of blood or breath if an officer of the law has reasonable grounds to suspect the person has been drinking and driving. The driver has the option either to submit a sample or to accept a six-month suspension of the driver's license if cooperation is refused.

Box 53-3 Blood Alcohol Specimens for Legal Purposes

- A written request from law enforcement must be submitted to the ED. For the evidence to be admissible, a qualified laboratory duly authorized by the state jurisdiction must do the blood alcohol determination.
- The blood test must be related to a lawful arrest with probable cause that a crime was committed while the offender was under the influence of alcohol or while intoxicated.
- ED personnel should provide necessary medical care and treatment without consideration of the forensic laboratory specimen that has been or will be ordered.
- Usual laboratory collection procedures are followed. Alcohol is typically not used to cleanse the skin, however. Povidone-iodine or other agents are preferred. The nurse who obtains the sample should document on the label that alcohol was not used to clean the skin. *Note:* Offenders who are on anticoagulant therapy or who are hemophiliacs are typically exempt from an ordered phlebotomy.
- Hospital policy should clearly articulate the procedure for obtaining blood alcohol samplings and the conditions of consent. The consent of the patient is necessary, and it should be *informed consent.*
- Blood should be drawn in the police officer's presence so that he or she can so testify, eliminating the need for other witnesses to appear and testify.
- Blood drawn must be given to the officer requesting it, who then takes it to an authorized laboratory, preserving the chain of evidence.
- A notation of blood drawn, by whom, and the time must be documented in the ED record of the patient, and the blood so labeled before it is sealed with tape, cross-initialed, and given to the officer.
- If a blood alcohol determination is needed for medical purposes, separate samples must be drawn.
- The skin preparation for drawing a blood alcohol sample should be done with aqueous benzalkonium (aqueous Zephiran) rather than alcohol.
- Draw 10 mL, and label with the name, date, time drawn, and initial. If it is a case of negligent homicide, draw two samples, one hour apart, to demonstrate the curve as firm legal evidence. Either the blood alcohol level will have peaked and started down, or it will be higher, indicating that the subject took more alcohol immediately prior to the incident. It is estimated that the blood level will fall 15 to 20 mg/100 mL per hour, so if, for instance, a blood alcohol is drawn four hours after an arrest and tests at 0.18% (180 mg/100 mL), it can be assumed that the subject's blood level at the time of arrest was 0.26%, or 260 mg/100 mL (Lanros & Barber, 1997).

Guidelines for Obtaining Evidentiary Blood Alcohol Specimens

Interpretation of the statutes relating to obtaining blood alcohol levels for evidentiary purposes varies from state to state, but Box 53-3 offers some basic guidelines that can well apply anywhere.

Mandatory Reporting Laws

The forensic nurse should be aware of the mandatory reporting laws for forensic patients: Emergency Medical Treatment and Active Labor Act (EMTALA) or the Consolidated Omnibus Budget Reconciliation Act (COBRA), coroner's cases, infectious diseases, adverse drug reactions, sexual assault, child and elder abuse, domestic violence, workplace violence, and impaired physicians or nurses (Mallon & Kassinove, 1999). In some states or jurisdictions, additional reportable cases may exist. It is essential that specific provisions of these laws are immediately available for staff reference if reportable cases are encountered. There are in some areas additional reportable events such as seat belt violations, medical device failures, foodborne illness, and acute lapses in consciousness. The failure to report is usually the result of lack of knowledge that a report is required, or personnel making the assumption that someone else will take the responsibility to initiate the report. Neither of these reasons for nonreporting reduces the responsibility of any staff member to make reports or negates

Case Study 53-1 Nonaccidental Trauma: Abuse

A 38-year-old female comes into the ED stating that her ribs hurt. The triage nurse suspects that something more is going on with the patient.

When asked how her ribs got hurt, the patient avoids eye contact and mumbles something about falling into a counter. The nurse asks if someone hit her (research has shown that victims of domestic violence are more likely to answer affirmatively to direct questioning versus having them tell the story without prompting). She looks at the nurse, and as tears fill her eyes, she says yes.

The nurse writes down what she says in quotation marks. Her spouse (who is 8 inches taller and 100 lb heavier) had "grabbed her upper arms and threw her into a kitchen counter." The nurse explains to the physician what has occurred and lets him read her notes to alleviate the need for the patient to tell her story again.

The physical examination reveals huge purpling contusions on her upper arms that appear consistent with large hands grabbing her. On the left biceps, a hematoma and significant swelling are already forming under the contusion. On the anterior side of her right chest wall, below her breast at approximately the sixth through eighth intercostal spaces, there is a large linear contusion with some abrasions around the edges. These marks are consistent with hitting a solid object such as a counter. Using a body diagram, the nurse documents these findings. The nurse discusses photographing her injuries and contacting law enforcement. The patient consents to photography and, although reluctant, consents to report the incident to the police.

The nurse takes a full-body photograph, which includes her face, and then photographs the specific injuries. Two sets of pictures are taken—one for the patient's ED record and one for the police. The pictures are properly labeled in accordance with the facility policy. One set is given to the law enforcement officer upon her arrival to the ED.

Eventually, it is determined that the spouse will be arrested because the patient agreed to press charges.

Before the patient leaves the ER to stay with a friend, the nurse provides her with both written and oral information about community support programs for victims of domestic violence.

legal actions for failing to report. Mandatory reporting laws must be understood and respected by forensic nurses in the ED. When there are doubts about reporting any event or condition, consult hospital administration or its legal team for guidance.

Summary

The recovery of evidence, in concept, is little different from maintaining aseptic technique. The goal is to prevent contamination. Evidence collection in the ED by skilled forensic nurse examiners fills a void from the time of injury or death until the time of trial.

As trends in social violence change, so must nursing knowledge change in order to recognize the most recent forms of criminal acts, weapons and designer drugs that produce the patients we seek to serve. It is essential that healthcare professionals work with law enforcement in an effort to decrease and prevent violence. This is not a shift in duties. Mutual cooperation between law enforcement and healthcare professionals will better serve communities, making them as safer placer for everyone.

Resources

Publications

American College of Emergency Physicians. (1997). Mandatory reporting of domestic violence to law enforcement and criminal justice agencies. *Ann Emerg Med, 30*(4), 561

Bureau of Justice Statistics. (2002). *National crime victimization survey.* Washington DC: US Department of Justice.

Joint Commission on Accreditation of Healthcare Organizations (JCAHO). (2004). *Comprehensive accreditation manual for hospitals.* Oakbrook Terrace, IL: Author.

References

Besant-Matthews, P. (Sept. 30, 2004). Autos and Alcohol. Unpublished papers, Dallas, TX.

Black's Law Dictionary. (6th Edition). St. Paul, MN: West's Publishing.

Centers for Disease Control (CDC). (May 17, 1996). *Hospital ambulatory medical care survey: 1994 emergency department summary advance data* (p. 275). Atlanta: CDC.

Centers for Disease Control (CDC). (2002). *Special report: Violence-related injuries treated in hospital emergency departments, Atlanta, GA.* Atlanta: CDC.

Easter, C., & Muro, G. (1995). An ED forensic kit. *J Emerg Nurs, 21*(5), 440-444.

Lanros, N., & Barber, J. (1997). *Emergency nursing* (4th ed.). Stamford, CT: Appleton & Lange.

Lynch, V. (2001). *Forensic nursing: A new perspective in trauma and the medicolegal investigation of death* (5th ed.). Divide, CO: Bearhawk Consulting Group.

Mallon, W. K., & Kassinove, A. (1999). Mandatory reporting laws and the emergency department. *Top Emerg Med, 21*(3), 63-72.

Mallon, W. K., & Perez, J. F. (1999). Weapons fabrication from medical supplies. *Top Emerg Med, 21*(3), 55-62.

McCarron, M. M., & Challoner, K. R. (1999). Emergency department treatment of patients in custody. *Top Emerg Med, 21*(3), 39-48.

Chapter 54 Occupational Health and Safety Issues

Janet Barber Duval

Forensic nurse examiners work in many environments that can pose occupational health and safety hazards. As forensic evidence is identified, documented, collected, and preserved, there are imminent dangers of injury and contact with infectious or toxic agents, from either living or deceased individuals. Open wounds, undiagnosed disease conditions, decomposing tissue, blood, stool, semen, wound drainage, and poisonous substances are a few examples of occupational hazards in the everyday workplace of the forensic nurse. Sexual assault nurse examiners, death investigators, clinical forensic specialists, and correctional nurses each have their own risk factors for injury and contacts with infectious or toxic agents. Without adequate personal barrier protection, harmful exposures can occur by inhalation or by making direct contact with harmful substances when handling body fluid and tissues. This chapter highlights infection control principles and practices that are vital to all environments where nurses encounter living and deceased individuals. Nurses and those who choose forensic nursing or other aspects of the forensic health sciences as a career path are often "breaking new ground." They may be viewed by some as risk-takers or mavericks, operating "outside the box." Henderson offers an indirect warning to "risk-taking" groups to be especially vigilant (Henderson, 2001). Staff members who perceive themselves at risk (for occupational injuries) are likely to be more compliant in observing standard precautions. Forensic nurse examiners need to well versed in infection control practices and occupational health issues and should appreciate that they are indeed quite vulnerable to several life-threatening conditions that can be contracted easily in one shortcut or one careless practice. Prevention is a more advanced science in infection control than either treatment or cure (Henderson, 2001). Primary prevention is the mainstay of safe, injury-free practice in forensic nursing science. Routine PPD (purified protein derivative) antigen skin tests for tuberculosis and current status for hepatitis B and tetanus immunization should be assured.

Well-educated forensic nurses appreciate the implications of Locard's principle, that is, whenever two surfaces come into contact with one another, there is an exchange of material. If one takes time to consider the parallel with the transfer of microorganisms or toxins from one surface to another, there should be little need to elaborate on the use of barrier protection in the clinical or other work environment. However, forensic nurse examiners are often so intently focused on the needs of the client or victim that they fail to appreciate the looming perils that surround them as they examine bodies, collect specimens, and work with scientific equipment. As a common starting point, the next section considers the forensic examination rooms in hospital settings serving both the living and the deceased and identifies several ways that occupational health and safety risks can be minimized.

Forensic Work Environments

In order to establish this ideal environment, some specific guidelines should be followed in the design and equipment of the examination room.

Key Point 54-1

The forensic examination room should be considered "ultra clean." That term implies that every potential foreign material that could result in contaminated evidence or infectious risks to personnel is either contained or eliminated.

Dedicated Space

The forensic nurse often is required to share space with other clinical functions in an emergency department or outpatient area. Obviously, when other nonforensic patients share the space with those requiring evidentiary examinations, there is a risk of "foreign" biological materials that could potentially confuse findings in specimens. Hair, clothes fibers, body fluids on surfaces of an examination table that has been inadequately cleaned are potential culprits. It is imperative to have a dedicated space.

Minimal Equipment and Supplies

Because of the need to have materials at hand quickly, many nurses become "hoarders" and tend to want to have a "year's supply" of everything in the cabinets or drawers within the examination room. However, having only the supplies required for the examination at hand will ensure that cross-contamination episodes are unlikely. In-room supplies ideally should be limited to those needed for a single examination. A few back-up supplies, of course, may be prudent, but be advised that clean and sterile items must be separated and reside within closed drawers and cabinets. Avoid placing any medical supplies in the drawers on the examination table itself. Frequently identify the need for additional supplies or special equipment during the examination and ensure that they are individually packaged. As in all clinical settings, inventory control procedures should include monthly checks on expiration dates on medical and laboratory supplies.

Equipment Barriers

Flexible or movable light sources, cameras, and the colposcope should be sheathed in plastic at the point of contact for adjustments. All protective barriers or covers must be discarded after each examination. Ideally, blood pressure cuffs, linens, and patient gowns should be individually wrapped and disposable. Avoid having the patient retrieve a gown from a stack of linens, as this could result in cross-contamination.

Cabinets and Drawers

All cabinets should have doors and locks (as appropriate) to protect supplies and equipment used in the forensic evidentiary examination. Table and counter surfaces should be smooth, nonporous, and free of nonvital equipment and supplies to ensure a thorough cleaning after each examination. Toxic laboratory supplies, cleaning agents, and all aerosols should be stored in locked cabinets. Ensure that no items from a previous examination or patient remain in the room after the examination is completed. This cleaning includes the emptying of all trash containers and linen receptacles.

Air Management

Avoid drafts and direct air currents in and around the zone where forensic examinations are occurring. High-efficiency particulate air (HEPA) filtration units may be used to remove allergens and particulates from the room air. In autopsy suites or laboratories, hoods are suggested for the removal of foul odors and noxious fumes. If a patient has a known or suspected contagious illness or toxic exposure that might be spread via air currents, negative airflow should be assured.

Hand-Washing Sinks

There should be a hand-washing sink in the room, preferably one that has wrist, knee, or foot controls. Antimicrobial soap should be supplied at this sink. An automated sink, with an electronic sensor, is an option in some facilities and ensures a true hands-free operation. Due to the high potential of biological contamination during evidentiary examinations, alcohol-based hand-washing agents should not be used as a substitute for a "soap and water" scrub. Alcohol-based products are ineffective in the presence of organic materials. Alcohol also degrades DNA and therefore is not recommended for any forensic examination in which biological evidence is to be collected (Bjerke, 2004). A liquid soap dispenser and paper towel holder should be installed at the sink to minimize risks of water splash contamination (Larson, 1995).

Gloves

Individually wrapped, powder-free gloves should be used for evidentiary examination. Do not use boxes of gloves, which invite cross-contamination when retrieving or replacing gloves. The few gloves used for forensic examinations should not pose a budgetary strain on the facility, and the costs are well-justified in principle and practice (see later discussion on latex allergies).

Communication Systems

Each forensic examination room should be equipped with routine and emergency communication equipment. A panic button or other emergency call system is highly desirable. If a computer is used for data entry or recovery, or for the printing of postdischarge instructions, the forensic nurse must ensure that all transmissions are "secure" to ensure patient privacy. Keyboard "skins" may be used to minimize contamination and cross-contamination that may be associated with keyboard use. Forms and other required stationery for documentation should not be stored in the examination room because they can be easily contaminated by the examiner.

Wall and Floor Coverings

Carpeting, upholstered furniture, and draperies are not recommended for the forensic examination setting, even in the interview or visitor areas. Such items may be easily soiled and may convey obvious opportunities for cross-contamination. Achieving a comfortable environment does not require carpeting and upholstering. Such effects may be achieved by sound, lighting, and other décor, such as artificial plants. Avoid aquariums, fountains, or live plants that carry inherent risks in the clinical arena.

Sharps and Biological Waste Containers

All rooms must be equipped with a sharps container and a receptacle for biological waste. Each hospital's infection control program will specify the requirements for these items. Liquid waste should not be discarded in the sink that is used for personnel hand washing. Soiled speculums and other instruments should not be deposited, even temporarily, in the sink after use. They should be placed in dedicated waste containers and removed from the room during postprocedure cleanup. Red bag and routine trash receptacles should be available and used in accordance with standard procedures of the facility.

Disinfection and Cleaning

All surfaces on the examining table must be thoroughly cleaned after each examination with an approved hospital-grade disinfectant agent. Aerosol disinfectants may be used only after organic materials (blood, body fluids, excreta) are completely removed from surfaces. They should be applied only to the clean surface and permitted to air-dry before another patient occupies the room. Disposable exam-table paper and sheets do not circumvent the requirement for cleaning and disinfecting!

Best Practice *54-1*

It is imperative that the room is carefully cleaned *after each patient use* to ensure that biological and trace evidence do not remain and create the potential for compromising subsequent forensic examinations. Hair, fiber, and biological materials may be easily missed if the cleaning routine is not thoroughly accomplished.

Waste receptacles and linen hampers should be emptied after each examination, primarily to prevent cross-contamination of potential forensic evidence. Occasionally, although certainly not planned, important evidentiary items may have been accidentally discarded and must be retrieved from waste receptacles. Again, like other disposables, trash cans and linen bags are relatively inexpensive compared to a compromised forensic examination.

Cameras, colposcopes, flexible light sources, and other equipment should have been protected with disposable coverings, to be removed after each examination. If such coverings were not used, or if some parts of the equipment were touched with a gloved hand, the contacted surfaces must be cleaned or disinfected according to the facility's infection control policies and procedures.

Floors should be damp-mopped and sinks cleaned after each examination. Disposable mop pads are easy to use and facilitate cleanup.

Personal Attire and Hygiene

The forensic nurse examiner should wear a clean laboratory coat or disposable gown for each examination to prevent cross-contamination from previous patients. Long hair should be restrained with a clip, barrette, or disposable head covering (bonnet). Nails should be short to prevent puncturing the gloves. Acrylic wraps, nail polish, and artificial nails are not appropriate in the forensic examination environment because they invite infectious risks to the nurse. Jewelry, other than a smooth band ring, should not be worn because it is likely to create tiny defects in the gloves that obliterate their protective value as a barrier. They also are ideal repositories for soap residue and other soil that could harbor microorganisms. Because rings with stones are likely to damage gloves and are not adequately and regularly cleaned, they should not be worn during forensic procedures.

The forensic nurse examiner should don protective barriers for procedures that may result in splash contamination. Obtaining samples of fluids from body cavities using a bulb syringe or other aspirating device can result in such splashes. Protective eye shields and masks are appropriate attire in such instances.

Hand Washing and Use of Gloves

Every healthcare worker is well educated about the value of hand washing, and yet compliance with hand-washing standards is less than 70% (O'Boyle, Henley, & Larson, 2001).

Key Point *54-2*

> Hand hygiene should occur when hands are visibly soiled, before and after patient contact, after contact with body secretions or excretions or inanimate objects likely to be contaminated, before donning gloves, and after removing gloves.

The appropriate technique is simple: Use an approved agent on the surfaces of the hands and rub vigorously for 10 to 15 seconds. Soap and water should be used when there is potential for organic soiling from blood, body fluids, tissue, or other similar agents incurred with direct patient contact. Glove use does not substitute for hand washing! Microscopic holes in gloves may permit penetration of certain materials. Although frequent hand washing may be irritating and tends to dry the skin, petroleum-based lotions should not be used in conjunction with some gloves because they tend to break down the glove's base materials, releasing organic compounds into the wearer's skin. This phenomenon has been linked to latex allergies. Oil-based lotions also tend to weaken latex and should not be used in conjunction with gloving. Remember, hand washing must always be done before donning gloves and again, right after removal. If required to use powdered gloves, residual powder should be removed to decrease the potential for powder contamination of wounds, cuts, or body cavities. Gloves must be changed after touching any contaminated site if they come in contact with acids, alkalies, solvents, oils, disinfectants, or sterilants. When gloves are in prolonged contact with body fat, they must be changed frequently to prevent swelling (ballooning) of the glove fingertips. During lengthy procedures, the forensic nurse should change gloves often because they become fatigued. When removing gloves, never put them on a clean surface; place them at once into a waste receptacle.

Gloves should be stored in a cool, dry place with frequent rotation of stock. They should never be placed near fans, air-conditioning units, or electric motors. Keep glove supplies away from direct sun or fluorescent lights and x-ay equipment, all of which can contribute to glove deterioration. Use glove liners or wire-mesh gloves for high-risk situations (autopsies, crime scene searches, etc.).

Powdered latex gloves are not appropriate to use in the forensic examination setting. The powder not only can serve as a medium for microbial growth, it can transmit latex allergens within the environment, potentiating the risk of latex allergies. Latex-free gloves should be readily available for all nurses and other forensic personnel who require them.

Cover Coats or Gown

Laboratory coats or cover gowns must be worn over clothing when performing forensic activities. Such garments protect personal clothing and provide a barrier to blood and body fluids. Remember, the point of interface between the gloves and gown is the weakest point in the chain of protection. Gowns should be promptly changed when contaminated with body fluids. When the gown is removed, it must be promptly discarded. It is never appropriate to use a cover gown or laboratory coat for more than one patient examination due to the potential for cross-contamination of evidence as well as microorganisms. When using clinical head cover devices, it is inappropriate to wear these outside the forensic examination rooms to other locations within the facility.

Masks, eye coverings, and face shields should be worn for any procedure that has an inherent risk of splash contamination. They should be one-time use items for forensic examinations to guard against potential for cross-contamination.

Smoking, Eating, and Drinking

Smoking, food, and beverages are inappropriate in the forensic examination room at any time. Hand-to-mouth contact is ill-advised in the clinical environment, and residues from food and drink could support the growth of microorganisms and encourage environmental pests.

Occupational Health Hazards in Forensic Nursing

The subjects of forensic investigations represent almost all the health-related occupational risk factors. They may bring in and on their bodies blood-borne illnesses, infectious diseases, toxins, antibiotic-resistant organisms, and infestations of scabies and lice. The forensic examiner must be able to appreciate that all patients should be treated as "infectious" and as a "biohazard." Standard precautions must be employed at all times during contact with the subject and the materials or equipment that contacts the patient, including linens. Donning of protective barriers is not an optional practice.

Blood-Borne Pathogens

The opportunity to contact blood-borne pathogens is very high in forensic nursing encounters. Considering the types of clients, the settings for practice, and the presence of unknown factors in subject's history, such as chronic illness, intravenous drug use, and other high-risk behaviors, every patient must be managed with attention to all precautions designed to protect against occupational illnesses and injuries.

The infection control practitioner in the institution or affiliates should be consulted if there are questions or issues that the forensic nurse does not fully understand. Occupational health and safety standards should be readily available for review and study. Risks are higher than average for forensic settings because they often operate in quasi-healthcare settings, outside the protective realm of the typical healthcare regulatory guidance and supervision of infection control professionals. Forensic personnel should consult their medical directors or an infection control practitioner regarding immunization requirements for the forensic work environment.

Hepatitis

There are several hepatotropic viruses, but only five are currently of high importance. Heptatis types A and E are contacted by stool and saliva. B, C, and D hepatitis forms are essentially blood-borne.

Hepatitis A is primarily found in saliva and feces but can be transmitted by blood at a certain point within the incubation cycle. There are suitable vaccines for exposed healthcare workers.

Hepatitis B is blood-borne. Healthcare workers are considered at high risk for this type and typically receive protection via vaccine.

Hepatitis C is also referred to as non-A, non-B hepatitis. It, too, is blood-borne and is more prevalent among certain patients. For example, individuals who have been tattooed, are intravenous drug abusers, have had body piercings, or are on hemodialysis are likely victims. There is confirmation that the virus can be spread through eye splash accidents and direct contact with organs or tissues. This type of the virus is difficult to diagnose and treat and is considered cytotoxic. The body mounts an immunological response against virally infected hepatocytes (i.e., circulating immune complexes produce activation of the complement cascade; the host's own cyctotoxic T-cells and natural killer cells also attack the infected liver). The resulting damage includes necrosis, scarring, obstruction of bile ducts, and cholestasis. Currently the screening for hepatitis C is imprecise and there is no prophylactic vaccine. Standard precautions are vital because there is no definitive therapy (Barber, 1996).

Hepatitis D coexists with hepatitis B and is blood-borne. The risk factors and transmission modes are similar to those of B and C types.

Hepatitis E is non-A, non-B enteric hepatitis and commonly associated with poor sanitation. It is rarely found in the US, but can be found among travelers returning from endemic areas including Asia, Africa, and the Middle East, as well as Central and South America. There is no vaccine currently available for this type.

Human Immunodeficiency Virus (HIV)

Blood and body fluid precautions normally protect against the threat of HIV. However, recent findings suggest that *Pneumocystis carinii* behaves like a fungus and may exist in certain environmental reservoirs. This particular virus replicates both sexually and asexually, and in today's culture in the US, approximately 78% of the population have been exposed to it by age 10. In high-risk patient groups, airborne spread has been demonstrated (i.e., smokers, transplant and oncology patients). It is commonly associated with tuberculosis, aspergillosis, and hepatitis B, C, and D.

Antibiotic-Resistant Organisms

Forensic nurses, especially those dealing with individuals with long-term hospitalizations and illnesses, should be aware of the risks posed by antibiotic-resistant organisms. Four organisms are of major importance.

Methicillin-resistant Staphylococcus aureus (MRSA) has several reservoirs. It can be found in the vagina, especially during menstruation, and in the nose, on skin, in wounds, and throughout the respiratory tree. Pulmonary secretions, suction catheters and canisters, and ventilators are common places that the organism is found. Although these patients are not typically isolated in the clinical setting, barrier precautions and careful hand washing are required to prevent the spread.

Vancomycin-resistant Enterococcus (VRE) is prevalent in the bowel, and once the patient is infected, colonization of the organism is indefinite, despite antibiotic therapy. VRE may be found in the drainage of colostomies, vaginal secretions, wounds, urine, and stool. Common environmental items such as equipment, chart backs, electronic thermometers, and point-of-care testing instruments (e.g., glucometers) have been implicated in the spread of the organism. Death investigators and clinical forensic personnel should appreciate that the best protection against the spread of the organism is the judicious use of standard precautions and careful disinfection of environmental surfaces.

Multiple drug-resistant tuberculosis is most prevalent among institutionalized or incarcerated persons. Alcoholics, IV drug abusers, residents of nursing homes, the homeless, and persons living in shelters are likely reservoirs. The organism is fueled by poor compliance with antituberculosis agents. Correctional nurses, forensic psychiatric nurses, and death investigators, particularly, should use masks when dealing with the living individual or the respiratory tissues or secretions of the recently deceased.

Clostridium difficile is an organism that resides in the bowel, usually after antibiotic therapy. It can be easily transferred on the hands of personnel and via environmental reservoirs. Telephones, rectal thermometers, bathrooms, blood pressure cuffs, privacy curtains, and chart backs are common sites where the organism is found.

VRSA (vancomycin-resistant *Staphylococcus aureus*) and VISA (vancomycin-intermediate-resistant *Staphylococcus aureus*) cases have also been confirmed in the US within the past few years. However, they should pose little or no threat to the forensic examiner who is essentially healthy and observes standard precautions.

Latex Allergies

Although latex gloves have been most effective in preventing transmission of many infectious diseases among healthcare workers, they pose an allergic risk to some workers. Skin rashes, hives, flushing, itching, and irritations of the eyes, nose, and sinuses are among common complaints of sensitive personnel. More serious reactions include asthmatic crises and, rarely, anaphylaxis. Although many hospitals and other clinical facilities have become "latex-free" in terms of gloves and other routine supplies, latex continues to be a threat to forensic nursing personnel from unsuspected sources.

Latex allergies stem from the allergy-causing proteins found in the rubber tree's (*Hevea brasiliensis*) milky fluid that is used in the production of latex. In the hospital environment there may be many products that contain latex other than gloves. Blood pressure cuffs, stethoscopes, oral and nasal airways, tourniquets, syringes, electrode pads, surgical masks, goggles, rubber aprons, erasers, catheters, injection ports, rubber tops of multidose vials, condoms, and dental dams are among items that are likely to contain latex. One of the major reasons to use nonpowdered gloves is that the dust produced by removing powdered gloves from a box or wrapper disperses powder into the air that conveys latex allergens. The particles may now be inhaled, contacting skin and mucous membranes and producing irritations and allergenic responses. They may also settle into upholstered furniture and carpet and become deposited on the duct work of ventilation units. This once again reinforces the fact that fabric surfaces that cannot be deep cleaned on a regular basis should not be used in clinical environments. It also serves to emphasize the need for frequent filter changes in duct work and on vacuum cleaners used in the area.

The problem of latex allergies is significant. All healthcare facilities are now required to have a plan for dealing with latex-sensitive patients or staff members. It is imperative that all screenings for living patients include determination of latex allergies. The use of HEPA filters may be beneficial in reducing the risks associated with this problem. In addition, all furnishings and equipment in the room should be latex-free.

Herpes

Herpes simplex viral infections of importance to the forensic nurse are herpetic whitlow and herpes labialis.

Herpetic whitlow is a painful infection of the finger accompanied by lymphangitis and regional adenopathy. It may result from exposure to HSV-1 or HSV-2. Oral or other lesions that are secreting may be involved in transmission; protective eyewear is indicated for any procedure in which splash or splatters could occur. Lost time from work for such occupational conditions may be up to seven weeks. Gloves, masks, and protective gowns may minimize some hazards, but micropunctures in gloves pose the greatest risks. Scrupulous and frequent hand washing is imperative.

Herpes labialis can be transmitted by contact for up to two hours after exposure; nurses with active lesions must wear masks to protect patients. Kaposi's sarcoma is associated with herpesvirus (e.g., peripheral blood, body cavities, central nervous system, gastrointestinal tract, liver, and bone marrow). Because there is obvious clustering within geographical regions and association with certain sexual practices, it is thought that a transmissible agent is present within the neoplasm itself. Forensic nurse death investigators (FNDI) and others who work with AIDS patients should be aware of this risk and don appropriate barrier precautions.

Respirators and Fit-Testing for Tuberculosis

Forensic nurse examiners should be fitted for N-95 respirators used for protection against tuberculosis. Healthcare facilities will provide appropriate protective masks and ensure proper fittings before use in accordance with Occupational Health and Safety Administration's (OSHA) and Centers for Disease Control (CDC) guidance.

Rare and Exotic Contagious Diseases

The forensic nurse examiner may encounter a number of rare, exotic, and life-threatening illnesses, especially during death investigation procedures. For example, Ebola and Marburg viruses induce hemorrhagic conditions that are often fatal. Individuals who die after experiencing signs and symptoms of such illnesses (fever, chills, myalgia, maculopapular rash, and eventually jaundice, and multisystem organ failure) should be managed with extreme caution during autopsy procedures and other forensic examinations because these diseases are thought to spread directly from body fluids and cell cultures.

Lassa fever is an acute viral illness that has been found largely in West Africa. The disease is spread by rodents. The majority of victims have no observable symptoms, but about one out of five persons develop multisystem crises. When caring for patients with Lassa fever, further transmission of the disease through person-to-person contact or nosocomial routes can be avoided by taking precautions against contact with patient secretions (together called VHF [viral hemorrhagic fever] isolation precautions or barrier nursing methods). Such precautions include wearing protective clothing, such as masks, gloves, gowns, and goggles; using infection control measures, such as complete equipment sterilization; and isolating infected patients from contact with unprotected persons until the disease has run its course (CDC, 2004).

Smallpox remains a threat in the world, primarily as a weapon of bioterrorism. Patients who have an acute generalized body rash with vesicles or pustules (appearing after a febrile episode) are suspected of having smallpox until it is ruled out. Both airborne and contact precautions must be observed when in contact with the suspected individual.

Monkeypox is a rare viral disease that is spread to humans from infected animals (monkeys or prairie dogs) by either a bite or direct contact with the animal's lesions or body fluids. Face-to-face contact with infected animals and exposure to their respiratory droplets, bedding, or body fluids are likely modes of transmission.

These rare, but serious infectious diseases are typically encountered by healthcare workers and others who perform humanitarian services in countries where they are endemic. However, in the case of monkeypox, exposure is primarily from exotic or wild animals maintained as pets. It is vital in all forensic cases that foreign travel histories and contact with unusual animals are known to those working with a body, body fluids, or laboratory specimens.

Consultants are available at the Centers for Disease Control at all times to serve as resources in the event that there is suspicion of these rare infectious diseases (see Resources at the end of this chapter).

Infestations

Lice

Lice are not generally thought of as a medical concern because most people have never had association with them. However, they can create problems within the emergency setting, crime scene, and forensic examination room. It is important that staff recognize these creatures as being lice and take precautions against their spread by informing peers and taking proper care in cleaning the environment where the patient has been.

Three species of lice may be encountered when examining a patient:

1. Crab louse (*Phthirus pubis*)
2. Head louse (*Pediculus humanus capitis*)
3. Body louse (*Pediculus humanus corporis*)

Pediculosis is the medical term used when there is lice present on any part of the body. All three species of lice suck blood and cannot exist away from their host for very long periods of time.

Crab Louse. This louse is also called the pubic louse, and to have them is popularly known as having "crabs." This creature gets its name from its appearance–it looks like a crab. Crab lice are very stationary in habit and stay attached at a point on the skin for days. The louse attaches its eggs on the coarse hair of the body. They particularly infest the pubic region of adults but may also infest armpits, eyelashes, beards, and mustaches. Crab lice are often transmitted by sexual contact and can be considered, in a sense, a venereal disease. The lice may also be transmitted by contacting clothing used by the infested person. Crab lice generally infest human adults and not prepubertal individuals. The bites of crab lice cause extreme itching and the human skin usually discolors with long infestation.

Head Louse. This type of louse is about 2 to 3 mm in length and occurs most often on the head. These lice are easily transmitted by physical contact. The louse attaches its eggs onto the surrounding hair.

Body Louse. This louse can be found anywhere on the body but tends to be common where clothing comes in contact with the body for continual periods of time, such as areas covered by underwear, around the waistline, and the armpits. This louse usually stays on clothing, where it lays its eggs. It tends to move to the skin only when feeding. These lice may be transmitted by physical contact or by contacting objects (usually clothing) used by the infested person.

All lice irritate the skin and cause extreme itching. Their saliva causes small red pimple formations after a bite. Scratching the area, which is tempting for the victim with infestation, can lead to infection. Severe infestation can lead to fatigue, irritability, depression, and a generalized body rash. Persons who are continually infested with lice can develop pigmented and hardened skin, a condition known as "vagabond's disease."

All lice are generally treated in the same fashion. Persons who have been infested should be instructed to steam clean, burn, or fumigate clothing. A lotion such as Kwell may be used to clean the body, and gamma-benzene hexachloride (lindane or Kwell) shampoo may be used on hair. The shampoo should be worked into lather and left on for four minutes before washing it off. It must be used with caution in infants and children due to the potential for central nervous system (CNS) toxicity via absorption. After the shampooing is complete, the hair should be combed with a fine-tooth comb to remove the lice and nits. A cream or lotion (gamma-benzene hexachloride) may be left on for 8 to 12 hours and then washed off, with a second treatment following in a week. Body lice may be managed only with a bath and clean clothes. Body lice tend to live in clothing and bed linens, so these must be thoroughly laundered and then steam pressed with a hot iron to kill remaining nits.

All clothing should be changed and washed in hot water unless it is being retained for forensic evidence. Housekeeping should be notified of the problem to ensure proper cleanup of the room. If lice, nits, scabies, or other infestations are noted on the body, samples of these may be preserved as forensic evidence because they may be valuable in linking the victim and perpetrator.

Scabies

Scabies is probably the most common infestation of the human body. The female mite burrows into the epidermis and deposits eggs over a period of a month or two. After hatching, larvae mature within two weeks and the cycle continues. Lesions cause intense itching on the genitalia, in the axillae, and over the wrists. Nipple lesions are common in adult females. They can be identified by skin scrapings treated with potassium hydroxide solution. Burrows may be highlighted by use of ink or another staining agent on the skin. Using an alcohol wipe to remove the dye, small dark threadlike burrows can be detected.

Scabies are not uncommon in animal handlers and in health-care personnel who do not use standard precautions when dealing with infestations. Treatment consists of spreading 1% gamma-benzene hexachloride cream over the entire skin surface and permitting it to remain for 8 to 12 hours. Shorter therapy duration should be used for infants and young children. Two applications, 24 hours apart, complete the therapy. Re-treatment to rid the skin of eggs may be required within a week. Clothing and bedding should be handled as for pediculosis.

Personal Protection for Hazardous Environments

Forensic nurses often work within the many perils that are associated with the scene to be investigated. Crime scenes, disasters, terrorism aftermaths, fires, and aircraft and other transportation or industrial accidents each pose unique challenges. It is imperative that the forensic nurse examiner be equipped and attired to cope with on-scene hazards.

Eye Protection

Appropriate eye protection, such as safety glasses and goggles, should be worn when handling biological, chemical, or radioactive materials. Face shields offer better protection to the face when there is potential for splashing or flying debris. Face shields must be worn in combination with safety glasses or goggles because face shields alone are not considered appropriate eye protection.

Contact lens users should wear safety glasses or goggles to protect the eyes. In the event of a chemical splash into the eye, it can be difficult to remove the contact lens to irrigate the eye. For those who wear prescription glasses, protective eyewear is available and should be worn over prescription glasses.

Foot Protection

Shoes that completely cover and protect the foot are essential. Protective footwear should be used at crime scenes when there is a danger of foot injuries or rolling objects piercing the sole and when feet are exposed to electrical hazards. The standard recognized by OSHA for protective footwear is the American National Standard for Personal Protection–Protective Footwear, ANSI Z41-1991. In some cases, nonpermeable shoe covers can provide barrier protection to shoes and prevent contamination outside the crime scene.

Head Protection

In certain crime scenes, such as bombings where structural damage can occur, protective helmets should be worn. The standard recognized by OSHA for protective helmets is ANSI's Requirement for Industrial Head Protection, Z89.1-1997.

Routes of Exposure

The *FBI Handbook on Forensic Services* (FBI, 1999) summarizes important information about routes of exposure. For most nurses, this section will cover material that is usually a mandatory requirement for yearly educational reviews, but this information can never be repeated enough. Much of the information is the same whether taking care of a patient or working a crime scene.

Inhalation

Airborne contaminants at a crime scene can be in the form of dust, aerosol, smoke, vapor, gas, or fumes. Depending on the contaminant, immediate respiratory irritation or destruction might ensue upon inhalation. Some airborne contaminants can enter the bloodstream via the lungs when inhaled. Once in the bloodstream, the contaminant can circulate throughout the body and cause chronic damage to liver, kidneys, CNS, heart, and blood-forming organs. Proper work practices along with adequate ventilation can minimize airborne contaminant inhalation. In extreme cases, respiratory protection is required.

Skin Contact

Skin contact is the frequent route of entry into the body of contaminants that can result in localized or systemic health effects. Localized effects can result in irritation or damage to the tissues at the point of contact. These effects can include irritation, redness, swelling, and burning. The severity of the injury will depend on the concentration of the substance and the duration of the contact. Systemic effects, such as dizziness, tremors, nausea, blurred vision, liver and kidney damage, shock, or collapse, can occur once the substances are absorbed through the skin and circulated throughout the body. Exposure can be prevented by the use of appropriate gloves, safety glasses, goggles, face shields, and protective clothing.

Ingestion

Ingestion is a less common route of exposure. Ingestion of a corrosive material can cause damage to the mouth, throat, and digestive tract. When swallowed, toxic chemicals can be absorbed by the body through the stomach and intestines. To prevent entry of chemicals or biological contaminants into the mouth, wash hands before eating, smoking, and applying cosmetics. Also, it is a good idea to not bring food, drinks, or cigarettes into areas where contamination can occur.

Injection

Needle sticks and mechanical injuries from contaminated glass, metal, or other sharp objects can inject contaminants directly into the bloodstream. Extreme caution should be exercised when handling objects with sharp or jagged edges. The use of wire-mesh gloves may be appropriate for some settings.

Light Source Safety

When using ultraviolet (UV) lights, lasers, and other light sources, the eyes must be protected from direct and indirect exposure. Prolonged exposure to the skin should also be avoided. Protective eyewear appropriate for the light source in use should be worn by all personnel in the vicinity of the light source.

Eyewear must have sufficient protective material and fit snugly to prevent light from entering at any angle and be clearly labeled with optical density and wavelength. Not all laser beams are visible, and irreversible eye damage can result from exposure to direct or indirect light from reflected beams.

Confined Space Safety

A confined space is an enclosed area large enough for personnel to enter and work. It has limited means for entry or exit and is not designed for continuous occupancy (for example, open pits, tank cars, and vats). Confined spaces can expose personnel to hazards including toxic gases, explosive or oxygen-deficient atmospheres, electrical dangers, or materials that can engulf personnel entering. Conditions in a confined space must be tested by experts with appropriate testing instruments and equipment. Do not enter these spaces until it is confirmed that it is safe to do so. Rescues in these settings are performed only by a member of a designated rescue team who has proper knowledge, training, skills, and equipment to perform a safe rescue.

In recent years there has been an increase in the number and types of hazardous materials that can pose threats for hospital personnel who are not adequately equipped to handle and care for the contaminated victim. Although the prehospital personnel (e.g., fire, HAZMAT [hazardous materials] and EMS [emergency medical services]) may have accomplished field decontamination procedures, victims still require special handling when they arrive at the emergency facility.

Specific federal regulations mandate personal protective clothing and equipment (PPE) to shield or isolate individuals from the chemical, physical, and biological hazards that may be encountered at a hazardous waste site or at an incident involving hazardous materials. OSHA standards outline training requirements (40 hours of initial training and at least three days of initial field experience) for employees at uncontrolled hazardous waste operations. All hazardous waste site operators must develop a safety and health program and provide for emergency responses. These standards are also designed to provide additional protection for those who respond to hazardous materials incidents, such as firefighters, police officers, and EMS personnel. OSHA's directive, as it applies to emergency medical personnel, states that "training shall be based on the duties and functions to be performed by each responder of an emergency response organization" (OSHA, 1992). This, of course, includes emergency department personnel who continue the care of a victim of a hazardous material exposure.

No combination of protective equipment and clothing is capable of protecting an individual against all hazards. There are specific types of protection which are recommended for protection when dealing with a known or unknown substance (Box 54-1). Personnel must receive in-depth training in regard to using any PPE (*FBI Handbook*, 1999).

Respiratory Protection

Two types of respirators are used for hazardous materials: (1) air-purifying respirators and (2) air-supplying respirators, which include self-contained breathing apparatus (SCBA) and supplied air respirators (SAR).

Air-Purifying Respirators

An air-purifying respirator (APR) depends on ambient air purified through a filtering element before inhalation. The three types of APRs utilized by emergency personnel are chemical cartridges or canisters, disposables, and powered-air units. One advantage of the APR system is that it permits the wearer considerable mobility. Since APRs only filter the air, the ambient concentration of oxygen must be sufficient (>19.5%) for the user. The most commonly used APR is the cartridge or canister unit, which purifies inspired air by a chemical reaction, filtration adsorption, or absorption. Disposable APRs are used for particulates, such as asbestos. Some may be used with other contaminants. These respirators often are half-masks that cover the face from nose to chin, but do not provide any eye protection. This type of APR depends on a filter to trap particulates. Filters may also be used in combination with cartridges and canisters to provide an individual with increased protection from particulates.

Air-Supplying Respirators

Air-supplying respirators (ASRs) are available in two basic designs: the self-contained breathing apparatus (SCBA), which has its own air supply, and the supplied-air respirator (SAR), which depends on an air supply from a distant source. The self-contained apparatus has a facemask connected to a source of compressed air for breathing, which is then exhaled into the atmosphere. There are also closed units that rely on a "rebreather" mask. The most popular SCBA is an open-circuit, positive-pressure unit in which air is supplied from a positive-pressure cylinder. In contrast with the negative-pressure unit, there is a higher air pressure maintained within the mask, which affords maximum protection against airborne contaminants, so that any leakage forces the contaminant

Box 54-1 Specific Precautionary Measures for Crime Scene Investigators

1. Wear the appropriate protective clothing when conducting crime scene searches.
2. Surgical masks or facemasks with appropriate filter cartridges should be worn when aerosol or airborne pathogens may be encountered. This caution may apply to dried blood particles as well.
3. Double latex gloves, surgical masks, and protective eye wear should be used when handling bodies, liquid blood, body fluids, dried blood particles, and evidence containing trace amounts of these materials.
4. Latex gloves, eye coverings, surgical masks, and a gown should be worn when attending an autopsy.
5. When processing the crime scene, constantly be alert for sharp and broken objects or surfaces.
6. Do not place hands in areas where one is unable to see when conducting a search. If this is necessary, wear specially designed search gloves, which can give added protection.
7. Under no circumstances should anyone at the scene be allowed to smoke, eat, or drink.
8. When liquid blood and body fluids are collected in bottles or glass vials, such containers must be prominently labeled "blood precautions" or "biohazard."
9. Clothing and objects stained with blood and body fluid must be dried and packaged in double paper bags and labeled properly. If evidence is collected from a suspected infected person or scene, the package should be labeled "caution—potential AIDS (hepatitis, etc.) case." However, be aware of confidentiality laws that mandate nondisclosure of that information and handle evidence accordingly.
10. If practical, use only disposable items at a crime scene where infectious blood is present. All nondisposable items must be decontaminated after each use.
11. Any reports, labels, or evidence tags splashed with blood should be destroyed with information duplicated on clean forms or labels.
12. After completing the search of a scene, investigators should clean their hands with diluted household bleach solution, soap, and water. Alternatively, when out in the field and away from water, some commercially available cleansing reagents may be used.
13. Any contaminated clothing or footwear should be properly disposed of.

out (with a negative-pressure type apparatus, contaminants may enter a poorly sealed facemask). SARs are connected to an air source outside the contaminated area. These are used only at hazardous waste sites where an individual may need to work for a long period of time around a potentially dangerous substance.

Best Practice *54-2*

Personnel must be fit-tested for use of all respirators. A fit-test is usually conducted on a yearly basis and is performed using a substance such as amyl acetate (banana oil) and irritating fumes to test the adequacy of the seal of the wearer's APR device.

Case Study 54-1 Henhouse Hanging

A forensic death investigator is called to investigate the hanging death of an elderly farmer whose body was found in an abandoned henhouse. His neighbors report that he has been extremely ill for many years with "lung disease" and that after his wife died a year or two ago, he "never went anywhere." Upon entering the henhouse, from the initial signs and smells, the investigator knows the man has been dead for several days. There are piles of trash, feathers, garbage, manure, and other debris in the henhouse, but no chickens are noted. The investigator will need to crawl under the roosting areas to reach the body. This will not be easy because old boards, fencing, and broken glass are scattered everywhere.

Personal protective attire must include an air-purifying respiratory facemask, a helmet, impermeable body suit, reinforced footwear, and gloves suitable for a hazardous waste environment.

Chemical Protective Clothing

The intent of chemical protective clothing (CPC) is to prevent the individual from coming into direct contact with a chemical contaminant. No CPC will provide protection against all substances, so emergency personnel must know the capabilities and limitations of the garments provided for their use. Furthermore, they must have received specific information on how to don and remove the various items such as suit, gloves, mask, shoe covers, and head gear to ensure that accidental contamination does not occur during these maneuvers.

The level of protection that is required to protect an individual against contact with known or anticipated toxic chemicals has been divided into four categories:

Level A: Highest level of respiratory, skin and eye protection is needed.

Level B: Highest level of respiratory protection is needed, but a lesser level of skin protection is required.

Level C: Air purifying is required.

Level D: Provides minimal protection against skin hazards and no protection against respiratory hazards. This level is not used for situations in which there is any risk to respiratory tract or skin.

The level of protection required is determined by the type of hazardous substance, its toxicity, and the concentration of the substance in the ambient air. Another factor involves the potential for exposure to this substance from the air, splashes of liquids, or other direct contact with materials that may occur during work. Emergency personnel may use CPC gear which is typical for level D protection and occasionally may use certain items associated with level C protection.

Forensic nurses are natural extenders of emergency teams at scenes of a fire. Their role in preserving evidence at the scene, especially on the bodies of victims and rescuers, is extremely valuable. However, many fire scenes are punctuated by the unknown. What caused the fire? If it was an incendiary device, is there potential for yet another explosion? Have toxic fumes been released? Are they merely bothersome and unpleasant, or noxious, posing threats to health and life? What are the possibilities for becoming burned or contaminated at the fire scene while sifting through the area for survivors or evidence? Could one be subject to heat stress during long hours of vigorous work in heavy personal protective clothing when the scene temperature can already be excessively high? Answers to these questions must be considered prior to engaging in forensic duties at a scene of a fire.

Burns

The fire scene invariably poses dangers to rescuers, forensic personnel, and others who work to recover bodies and other evidence associated with the event. Objects at the scene often reach incredibly high temperatures and when hidden among the ashes or other debris may remain "hot" for hours and even days. Heat-resistant personal protective garments and shoes, as well as heat-proof gloves, should always be worn. Metal tongs are recommended to retrieve small metallic items.

Explosions

Explosions can occur with or without an associated fire. After any type of explosion, there can be many hazards to personnel involved in either rescue and recovery, or in forensic investigation processes. The scenes are managed like fire and arson scenes, and concerns for personal safety are similar. Recurrent blasts from unexploded materials can be a potential risk, and caution should be exercised by everyone on the scene until the integrity of the site can be ensured. Among risks at scenes of explosions are building structural damage, secondary explosive devices, unconsumed explosive materials, failed utilities, and a wide array of hazardous materials (Lee, 2001).

Toxic Inhalations

In scenes involving fire or explosions, toxic inhalations may pose real dangers for on-scene personnel. There are many toxic by-products that are generated by burning common materials. Polyvinyl chloride, a common component of electrical insulation, wall coverings, car and airplane interiors, and even plastic bottles produces hydrochloric acid and carbon monoxide as by-products of combustion. Polyurethane, a typical foam used in mattresses, seat cushions, and carpets, produces carbon monoxide, toluene, 2 hydrocyanic acid, and 4-diisocyanate when it burns. Styrene, acrylics, and nylon, found in many household textiles, wood finishes, furniture, carpeting, clothes, and upholstery, also yield similar by-products. When fires are still smoldering or gases have been trapped within the confines of a building, these toxic materials that are released when items burn can create a series of symptoms that range from annoying to life-threatening. If workers at a fire or explosion scene experience dyspnea or other respiratory distress, lightheadedness, chest pain, nausea, rhinorrhea, conjunctivitis, or burning sensations of mucous membranes, they should immediately be removed from the team and transported promptly to a medical treatment facility.

Smoke Inhalation Injuries

Fire scenes are hazardous zones, especially immediately after the incident, but also for many hours and even days, as fires continue to smolder and yield harmful products of combustion. Inhalation injuries greatly affect the morbidity and mortality data related to fire scenes. Firefighters, fire scene examiners, and industrial workers exposed to products of combustion in closed spaces are at risk. The upper airway is a prime target for inhalation injury from toxic fumes, superheated gases, and irritating substances, both dry and moist. During the fire and in the immediate aftermath, facial burns, singed nasal hair, and carbonaceous deposits in the airway and sputum are hallmarks of inhalation injury, but the absence of these does not rule out the possibility of injury. The forensic nurse who is investigating a fire or arson scene, hours or days later, should be cognizant of stridor, hoarseness, difficulty speaking, and chest retractions that indicate irritation of the upper airways. Laryngospasm, although rare, may be present in highly sensitive personnel. The lower airway becomes involved when there are exposures to high concentrations of toxic fumes or irritating substances for a prolonged period of time. Tracheobronchitis, bronchospasm, bronchorrhea, and pulmonary edema can occur if irritation extends deep into the tracheobronchial structures. Bronchial blood flow will intensify, and edema in the airways and alveolar tissue may be aggravated. Other problems include surfactant dysfunction, increased lung water, decreased lung compliance, increased airway resistance, and increased pulmonary vascular resistance (Lanros & Barber, 1997).

If rescue or forensic investigators become confused, obtunded or unconscious at a scene, there is a high likelihood of carbon monoxide and hydrogen cyanide poisoning. All such workers must be able to promptly recognize the classic indices of these two life-threatening inhalation-related poisonings.

Carbon Monoxide

This toxic inhalation injury occurs when individuals breathe the products of incomplete carbon combustion. Examples of places where such fumes may be present are automobile exhaust and confined areas where gas-flame heating units and charcoal grills are used. Because carbon monoxide (CO) has a 200 times greater affinity for hemoglobin than oxygen, it will preferentially bind, thus limiting oxygen availability. Furthermore, recent studies indicate that CO may also bind to myoglobin and cytochrome oxidase, thus interfering with intracellular respiration (Ayres et al., 1995). CO is readily taken up by a fetus because the fetal hemoglobin has even greater affinity for CO than the child or adult, so pregnant patients and their unborn are at significant risk even in the presence of low levels of exposure. Pregnant forensic nurses should not investigate scenes in which there is a significant potential for carbon monoxide or other toxic gas accumulations.

Treatment must be based on presenting signs and symptoms and the presence of CO in the blood. CO poisoning cannot be evaluated properly with a pulse oximeter because oxyhemoglobin and carboxyhemoglobin have similar light absorption spectra. The documented pulse oximetry reading will be falsely elevated in CO poisoning (Wilkins & Dexter, 1993). Arterial blood gases are also unreliable since PO_2 is a measurement of the partial pressure of oxygen in millimeters of mercury, not of the oxygen saturation of hemoglobin (Ayres et al., 1995). Carboxyhemoglobin spectrophotometry is the standard measurement for CO poisoning. CO breath analyzers have also been shown to reliable (Ayres et al., 1995).

The clinical manifestations of CO poisoning are obscure until the blood level reaches 20% to 40%. Up to that point, only mild headache, exercise-induced angina (in susceptible individuals), and mild headache occur. However, at higher levels, these symptoms worsen, and vomiting, muscular weakness, visual disturbances, dizziness, and impaired judgment are noted. Tachypnea, tachycardia, seizures, syncope, and irregular breathing follow when levels reach 40% to 60%. Above 60%, shock, coma, apnea, and death occur. The classic "cherry-red skin" sign of CO poisoning is an unreliable determinant of this life-threatening condition.

Persons with indices of CO inhalation require oxygen administration at 100% flow rates. The half-life of carboxyhemoglobin is three to five hours in room air; in oxygen, it is 30 to 80 minutes. Moderate acidosis is not aggressively treated because hydrogen ions shift the hemoglobin-dissociation curve to the right, thus improving oxygen delivery to tissues. Hyperbaric therapy is often used in severe cases, but there are no controlled studies that confirm its superiority to regular modes of oxygen therapy. Considerations for its use include coma, cardiovascular involvement, pregnancy, and carboxyhemoglobin levels above 40% (Ayres et al., 1995).

Cyanide Poisoning

Cyanide is extensively used in industrial and agricultural applications and is liberated in fires by the burning of wool, silk, nylon, and polyurethanes. It occurs naturally in some plants and in fruit pits. Hydrogen cyanide gas has been used for suicide, judicial executions, and mass executions (e.g., Nazi extermination camps, Jonestown massacre). Because cyanide can be inhaled, injected, ingested, or absorbed through intact skin and mucous membranes, it is of great concern in chemical warfare and terrorist tactics. Some drugs (e.g., sodium nitroprusside) also contain cyanide that is liberated during metabolism. Cyanide binds to the ferric ion and interrupts electron transport so that pyruvate is no longer metabolized in the Krebs cycle. Metabolic acidosis follows.

The patient with cyanide poisoning experiences symptoms that are nonspecific and include anxiety, agitation, flushing, tachycardia, tachypnea, and dizziness followed soon by seizures, metabolic acidosis, coma, and death. The odor of bitter almonds is classically associated with cyanide poisoning, but only about 65% of all individuals can detect this using their own olfactory sense (Ayres et al., 1995).

Forensic personnel who may have signs or symptoms of cyanide poisoning should be promptly transported to the emergency department. Treatment includes ventilatory support with supplemental oxygen and prompt use of amyl nitrite, sodium nitrite, and sodium thiosulfate. Most emergency departments have "cyanide kits" for specific management of this poisoning.

Key Point *54-3*

It is imperative that all personnel wear protective clothes when dealing with suspected cyanide poisoning cases because skin, vomitus, and other body fluids can contain the agent.

Hydrogen Sulfide

Hydrogen sulfide is a cellular asphyxiant, too, and although carboxyhemoglobin from carbon monoxide inhalation and cyanide are classic examples, hydrogen sulfide can also produce rapid morbidity and death, depending upon the concentration and duration of exposure. Like cyanide, hydrogen sulfide produces cytotoxic anoxia by binding with ferric iron in cytochrome oxidase. It is a natural product, generated by putrefaction of sewage and animal waste products, and has a characteristic rotten-egg odor. A high concentration of hydrogen sulfide accumulating in a small closed space can be rapidly fatal.

Presenting signs and symptoms include several ocular phenomena including blepharospasm, pain, conjunctival injection, and blurred, iridescent vision. Confusion, dyspnea, stupor, cyanosis, coma, and respiratory arrest are seen in severe cases (Barber, 1996).

Both hydrogen sulfide and cyanide have the same mechanism of action, and both respond to almost the same treatment. The immediate administration of the amyl nitrite and sodium nitrite contained in the Lilly cyanide kit will rapidly reverse the profound metabolic acidosis of the cytotoxic anoxia caused by hydrogen sulfide. Sodium thiosulfate should not be administered, however. Beyond reversing the metabolic acidosis, careful monitoring and oxygen administration are indicated.

Heat-Related Hazards

Forensic personnel, especially scene investigators, are often responding to outdoor scenes or to buildings that are not temperature controlled. Occasionally, scenes involve walk-in refrigerated rooms, foundries, and other industrial sites in which extraordinary temperatures are routine. Extreme heat, cold, and altitude can impair or even disable the heartiest forensic nurse. In the intensity and excitement of the search for evidence, personnel must continually monitor their own safety and well-being to ensure that they do not become victims of environmental stressors.

Case Study 54-2 Operating Room Fire

Starting in a hospital operating room, a fire quickly spread to a storage area that contained tanks of compressed gases, including oxygen, helium, and nitrous oxide. The circulating nurse reported a flash and then an explosion, which immediately was followed by a fire. In addition to the patient and five members of the staff who were critically burned, other OR personnel incurred only minor burns while attempting to rescue the original victims. Although the fire was quickly contained when firefighters arrived, there were lingering odors, smoke, and fumes as well as considerable debris from linens, instrument trays, and medical supplies. All burned victims had been evacuated by the time the nurse arrived on the scene to launch a forensic investigation and to collect critical evidence.

Occupational hazards would include toxic exposures to hazardous fumes and gases, lack of oxygen consumed by helium, potential flash fires, and further explosions. Sharp injuries or other wounds are potential threats in an environment that is strewn with debris from the OR suite.

Personal protective attire for the investigator should include a helmet, an air-supplying respirator, a hazardous materials suit, wire-mesh gloves, and protective footwear. Forensic nurses would enter the scene for their survey and evidence collection *after* the area had been cleared for safe entry by the fire department and safety personnel.

Humans are homeothermic beings with a core temperature ranging from 97.5° F to 99.5° F. Thermal regulation is controlled in the hypothalamus, which receives information from the temperature of the circulating blood and from skin sensors that relay data about environmental temperature. When the hypothalamus is stimulated, the respiratory rate increases to enhance heat loss via expired air; cardiac output is increased to facilitate cutaneous and muscular blood flow, which helps dissipate heat; and sweat glands become active in their role of sustaining evaporative heat loss.

Normally, metabolic processes continuously produce heat, and it is dissipated to the outside environment, which is usually cooler. In certain instances, however, the body may gain heat. If there is increased metabolic production (600 to 900 kcal/hour with maximal work), poor heat dissipation, uptake of heat from a hot environment, or any combination of these three, the hypothalamus is stimulated. Initially, shivering is inhibited and sweating occurs (nearly 600 kcal of heat is lost as 1 L of sweat is evaporated). Vasodilation follows promptly, and the cardiac output increases in response. The enhanced blood flow to the skin surface assists in heat loss via radiation and convection. These regulatory mechanisms work together to continually balance the amount of heat produced and lost by the human body.

Acclimatization is the process that enables the body to cope with heat stress. Acclimatization benefits are usually only apparent, however, when the individual has had daily exposure to heat stress for three to six weeks. During this time the body gradually develops defenses against hyperthermia. Aerobic metabolism increases, thus ensuring that the body uses energy more efficiently and that heat production is lessened. The body also develops a new, lower point at which sweating begins, and even the rate of sweat production is increased. Fully acclimatized individuals nearly double their loss of heat by perspiring and therefore can dissipate heat more rapidly. The heart muscle responds by improving cardiac output and stroke volume. Cutaneous circulation improves, and again heat dissipation is augmented. Finally, increased secretion of aldosterone aids in sodium conservation by the kidneys and sweat glands. Of course, the additional sodium enhances extracellular fluid volumes, which play a part in accelerated cutaneous blood flow and heat dissipation, too. Nurses working in hot climates need to appreciate that environmental heat stress can cause a loss of 1 to 3 L of fluid per hour, each liter containing 20 to 50 mEq of sodium chloride. Individuals who are not acclimatized can fall victim to heat-related syndromes rather rapidly. Other predisposing factors include a high ambient temperature or humidity, obesity, wearing of heavy clothing, sweat gland dysfunction, potassium depletion, dehydration, and cardiovascular diseases.

Types of Heat-Related Illness

Although various authorities categorize heat-related illness in unique ways, the forensic nurse must be familiar primarily with four such problems: heat cramps, heat syncope, heat exhaustion, and heat stroke.

Heat Cramps

Heat cramps are a rather common disorder; the painful cramps, or contractions, of skeletal muscle are due to the sodium depletion that typically accompanies profuse sweating. Water and sodium replacement by the oral route is usually all that is required to curb the annoying problem of heat cramps. Popular thirst quenchers for sports enthusiasts, such as Gatorade, Sportade, and Body Punch, are appropriate for this minor heat-related problem, as both preventive and therapeutic measures.

Heat Syncope

Heat-related fainting episodes may occur through the interaction of several phenomena. Vasodilation and peripheral pooling of blood, volume deficit, and sluggish vasomotor tone may all contribute to this problem. Venous return does not support the required cardiac output, and syncope occurs. Treatment consists of water and sodium replacement, usually by the oral route, and avoidance of prolonged standing, which encourages venous pooling.

Heat Exhaustion

Heat exhaustion is a more serious heat-related problem that tends to occur when the core body temperature reaches 39° C to 40° C, or 103.5° F to 104° F. It may encompass heat cramps and heat syncope, as previously described, but is also characterized by altered mental status, gastrointestinal upsets (i.e., anorexia, nausea, vomiting), headache, dizziness, irritability, weakness, and marked volume depletion. Thirst, hypotension, tachycardia, and syncope may occur along with hyperventilation. Typically, at first, the victim sweats profusely, and body temperature is normal or mildly elevated. Treatment consists of oral water and sodium replacement and rest in a cool, quiet environment.

Heat Stroke

Heat stroke is the most serious of heat-related emergencies; this condition is associated with high morbidity and mortality rates. Essentially, heat stroke results from the failure of the hypothalamus to regulate body temperature. The usual heat loss mechanisms are simply overwhelmed. The core body temperature ranges from 40° C to 42° C, or 104° F to 107° F (42° C is the temperature level normally established for the onset of heat stroke). Temperature elevations above this lead to physiologic disaster and collapse. Enzymes denature, membranes liquefy, mitochondria do not function, protein coding is disrupted, and most essential physiologic processes cease normal functioning.

Signs and symptoms of heat stroke are evident in several body systems. Irrational behavior, confusion, and sudden changes in the level of consciousness often mark the onset of heat stroke. Seizures are common and may occur early or late in the course of this illness. When there are suggestions that heat stroke may be occurring, prompt transport to an emergency department is imperative. As in all other emergencies, airway and breathing should be supported as necessary. Sequelae of heat stroke include pulmonary edema, myocardial ischemia, infarction, and life-threatening dysrhythmias. Liver and renal failure, as well as widespread coagulopathy, are also common.

When victims of heat stroke reach emergency departments, an initial priority is body cooling. Sponge baths, cooling blankets, peritoneal dialysis, rectal lavage, cardiopulmonary bypass, gastric lavage, and administration of phenothiazines are useful techniques for lowering body temperature. Invasive procedures, such as peritoneal dialysis and cardiopulmonary bypass, however, are reserved for the most severe cases. Aspirin should not be used because it cannot correct the underlying problem and may aggravate associated coagulopathy. Alcohol sponges should not be used, either, because enough alcohol can be absorbed through a widely dilated periphery to induce deep coma from toxic blood levels of alcohol. Temperature should be reduced to 39° C as measured by rectal thermometer or thermistor probe. Once the temperature reaches the desired level, it must be monitored and maintained carefully because rebound hyperthermia can easily occur.

Heat-related illness, with its devastating effects, can be avoided or at least reduced in severity through simple preventive measures. These measures include becoming acclimatized; avoiding alcohol during exposure in hot, humid areas; wearing protective, light-colored clothes and hat; ingesting adequate amounts of balanced liquids to maintain fluid and electrolyte homeostasis; and pacing personal activities through awareness of heat stress.

Cold-Related Hazards

The human body loses heat in five ways: radiation, conduction, convection, evaporation, and respiration. Radiation loss occurs any time the body temperature exceeds that of the surrounding environment. Because the head and neck are especially vascular, and often unprotected, heat loss can occur readily from these areas.

Conduction heat loss occurs when there is a direct transfer of heat from the body to another object. When any body part comes into contact with a cooler object, heat is conducted to the external object until its temperature is equal to that of the body. Thereafter, the object becomes an insulating device, actually preventing further heat loss. Much body heat is lost this way in cold environments.

When working in cold climates, it is vital that forensic investigators dress appropriately for the cold, wearing mittens rather than gloves so that their fingers can benefit from the heat given off by adjacent digits. Cotton socks worn next to the skin should be supplemented by wool socks, and tight-fitting shoes or boots should be avoided because they tend to interfere with circulation. Wearing several layers of clothing is ideal; they trap air and form an insulating zone around body tissue. Hoods, hats, and scarves are always "in fashion" in cold weather. Alcohol should be avoided because it dilates peripheral circulation, thus encouraging heat loss. Food ingested should be high in calories to generate heat. Activity is desirable, too, because muscle work tends to produce heat and enhance the circulation. Of course, as with all cold-related problems, wet clothes and wind chill should be avoided.

Convection heat loss requires that heat be conducted to the air and then carried away by convection currents. Wind chill that combines the forces of lower temperature and the velocity of air currents can be a devastating form of heat loss from the human body. Charts are available that convert environmental temperature and wind velocity to a wind-chill index. Heat transfer in water is about 25 times faster than in air of the same temperature. It is obvious, then, that victims exposed to cold water in immersion accidents can succumb rapidly to hypothermia.

Evaporative heat loss occurs when wind sweeps across the skin and vaporizes the water of perspiration. This type of heat loss is an aggravating circumstance when an individual is wearing perspiration-soaked clothing and is exposed to a very cold environment.

The body also loses heat through the process of breathing. As cold air enters the respiratory tract, it is warmed by the body heat before exhalation. Prolonged breathing of cold air, therefore, contributes to a gradual loss of total body heat. In considering cold-related emergencies or hypothermic events, one must take these several factors into account; they usually occur in some combination to create a serious decline in body temperature. Injuries due to cold exposure may be local tissue injury only, or they may be generalized (i.e., a reduction of the body core temperature or hypothermia).

Local Tissue Injury

The pathophysiology of local, cold-related tissue injury occurs at the arteriole, capillary, and venule levels of the circulatory system. When the body is chilled, the arterioles constrict to conserve body heat. This is tolerated well for a brief period. After prolonged vasoconstriction and flow redirection, however, the microvasculature becomes occluded, and the capillary bed becomes inactive. Eventually, the associated cells become compromised as aerobic metabolism ceases. Furthermore, the shunted blood returning to the heart is chilled by the cold surrounding tissue, contributing to a gradual cooling of the core. The involved tissue is compromised in terms of its vital processes, and if the temperature is below freezing, ice crystals begin to form and expand extracellularly at the expense of adjacent tissue that may yet be functioning normally. Dehydration occurs promptly, and surrounding cells are adversely affected. Muscles, nerves, and blood vessels are initially insulted, followed later by the more resistant tissue, such as ligaments, tendons, and bones. It is important to note that critical tissue injury can occur in temperatures above the freezing point. Any prolonged exposure to cold that results in significant vasoconstriction and sluggish circulation can create injury to exposed areas of flesh.

Frostnip or Incipient Frostbite

Frostnip occurs in cold weather and primarily affects exposed areas of the body farthest from the trunk, such as the nose, ears, cheeks, chin, hands, and feet. Initially the nipped area blanches, and the victim experiences a burning, tingling sensation that eventually evolves to numbness. The condition comes on gradually, and very active persons may be oblivious to its early warning signs.

Frostnip, if not treated promptly, progresses to frostbite. In superficial frostbite, the skin and superficial tissue layers become solid from freezing, but the deeper tissues remain resilient. The skin has a waxy, white appearance and is numb. After rewarming, the area becomes mottled and purplish, but the numbness persists. Edema and burning and stinging sensations follow. The damaged tissue is often marked by blisters that dry up and become hard and black within 10 to 14 days. Resting the part encourages the early resolution of edema, but the throbbing and burning may last for weeks. Eventually, the skin peels away, and the underlying red, tender area retains its sensitivity to the cold and tends to perspire abnormally for an extended time.

Deep frostbite includes damage to the skin, the subcutaneous tissue, muscle, and blood vessels. The area is hard and cannot be depressed when touched; its color is pale or gray. Tremendous swelling that may last for weeks occurs after rewarming. Blisters form within three days, and a blue-violet or blue-gray discoloration persists. A sharp, throbbing pain is typical, and this may be present for several weeks. The blisters dry, turn black, and slough, leaving a new red layer of tender skin that is very sensitive to the cold and perspires and itches for up to six months. In rare instances in which rewarming has not been promptly executed, gangrene of the affected part may occur and amputation is ultimately required.

Treatment of Local Tissue Injury

Frostnip can be treated rather simply, merely by applying warmth to the affected part. If the feet or hands are involved, the socks or gloves, respectively, should be removed before rewarming. Never rub the affected parts because friction increases tissue damage. For actual frostbite, a warm water bath is useful for rewarming. The bath temperature should be 100° F to 110° F (37.8° C to 43.3° C) as measured by a thermometer, not an estimate. Feet, hands, and other affected body parts should be suspended in the bath and not permitted to touch the bottom or sides of the container. The part should be completely surrounded by bath water. Measure the temperature of the water periodically, and maintain it at the desired level. Of course, never add hot water without removing the body parts and stirring the water carefully afterward. Check the temperature with a bath thermometer before reimmersing the part. Remember that pain is not reliably perceived with cold injury. The affected part usually begins to thaw within 10 minutes, but up to an hour may be required for complete thawing. The victim does not experience pain at first, but as thawing nears completion, the area throbs, aches, and burns. Analgesics may be required. When rewarming is complete, the part should be patted (not rubbed) dry and covered lightly with dressings. Areas between fingers and toes should be packed with cotton or gauze to prevent tissue-to-tissue contact. Deep frostbite requires hospitalization.

Hypothermia

Hypothermia is a life-threatening condition occurring when the core body temperature is less than 95° F, or 35° C. Most adverse physiological problems do not manifest themselves, however, until the body reaches 90° F, or 32.2° C. This is the point at which shivering stops and muscles become rigid. When the core temperature falls below 78° F, or 25.5° C, death usually occurs. Forensic personnel must bear in mind that hypothermia protects the brain and vital physiological processes that would ordinarily fall victim to anoxia associated with circulatory arrest. If a hypothermic victim at a crime scene is cold and stiff, resuscitation may still be attempted; successful recoveries have been reported two and three hours after apparent clinical death. Some authorities have advocated that no hypothermic patient be declared dead until rewarming has taken place and resuscitation been attempted with the "warm" body. Hopefully, one will never have to make such a decision!

When the hypothermic victim is encountered, the ABCs of basic life support receive attention first. Peripheral pulses may not be palpable because of intense vasoconstriction. It should be recalled that pulse rate and respirations slow in relation to the degree of hypothermia, so the pulse may be only 40 to 50 beats per minute and the respiration rate can fall below 10 at core temperatures of 28° C to 30° C. If oxygen is available, it should be given to restore the PaO_2 to normal without inducing hyperventilation. A sudden lowering of $PaCO_2$ and changes in pH increase the likelihood of ventricular fibrillation. All essential care must be provided with as little manipulation of the patient as possible, for even routine handling can precipitate ventricular fibrillation. Conservative approaches are in order because airway maneuvers and chest compressions, for example, can induce an arrest state. Obviously, however, if such measures are required for resuscitation, they should be promptly executed by a technically competent member of the team to minimize iatrogenic injury. In the meantime, all wet clothing should be removed, and warm and dry linens are provided. Other care (intravenous lines, electrocardiographic monitoring, blood sampling, etc.) will be dependent upon the capabilities of available field medical personnel at the scene.

Active rewarming through both core and external approaches must be attempted as soon as the patient's basic life support has been assured. Rewarming must be judiciously managed to ensure that the core temperature increases along with the external temperature to avoid ventricular fibrillation complications. If the periphery is rewarmed rapidly, the demand for oxygen will be initially high and the hypothermic heart will be unable to keep pace with the high demands by merely increasing cardiac output. Myocardial hypoxia and acidosis can quickly compromise resuscitation in this instance. Recommendations for rewarming include a variety of traditional and novel measures. A thermal blanket or a radiant warming hood may be used initially to increase the body temperature on a gradual basis by 1 or 2 degrees hourly. The desired setting is 98° F to 100° F. Immersion baths of 104° F are also useful if vital processes are relatively stable and if the effects of vasodilation (i.e., reduction in central circulatory volume) will not compromise the patient. Core rewarming techniques are reserved for the hospital setting and may include warmed IV fluids, warm lavages (peritoneal, thoracic, rectal, mediastinal, etc.), dialysis, cardiopulmonary bypass, and respiratory therapy with warm, humidified air. Monitoring parameters should include laboratory values (arterial blood gases, electrolytes, blood sugar, blood urea nitrogen, hematocrit, clotting studies), intake and output, central venous pressure, neurological status, electrocardiogram, blood pressure, and of course, core temperature.

The objective of gradual rewarming must constantly be in front of the therapeutic team in order to prevent overly aggressive, rapid external rewarming that exceeds core rewarming, thus predisposing the patient to ventricular fibrillation and cardiac arrest. Restraint during rewarming must be every team member's responsibility because haste in this critical period can result in the death of a potentially salvageable patient.

Altitude Illness

Forensic scenarios may occur at any altitude and the forensic nurse may be exposed to altitude-related illness. Altitude-related illness becomes apparent when nonacclimatized persons are exposed to altitudes of 2000 m (7200 ft) or higher. At this level, physiological adaptation is required by several body systems, and this process usually takes up to two or three days to complete. In the meantime, because of the reduced partial pressure of oxygen, hypoxemia and alkalosis occur.

During the initial physiological stress at high altitudes in a nonacclimatized individual, the heart rate increases but the cardiac output remains unchanged. The net result, of course, is a decreased ability by the body's muscles to perform work (it is estimated that people have only about 75% efficiency at such altitudes). Respirations increase because of chemoreceptors in normal individuals, but such compensatory responses are not possible in patients with chronic obstructive pulmonary disease who have already maximized their adaptation; thus, they experience an even more severe oxygen deprivation. The red blood cell mass increases gradually to increase its oxygen-carrying power, and this phenomenon, coupled with increased breathing, facilitates satisfactory adjustment to the reduced partial pressure of oxygen. However, because of the fact that a respiratory alkalemia and a reduced stroke volume occur as well, illness may result before the body experiences the spontaneous bicarbonate diuresis that occurs 24 to 36 hours after altitude stress has been realized.

Signs and symptoms of altitude illness include lethargy, headache, nausea, and difficulty sleeping. Although insomnia can be annoying, sedatives should never be taken during altitude stress because they can induce catastrophic respiratory depression and life-threatening hypoxemia. Acetazolamide (Diamox) is useful, but it increases the excretion of bicarbonate by the kidneys and must be used with caution, for it can lead to systemic dehydration when other stressors, such as overexercise or heat, are present. Acute "mountain sickness" can produce serious problems for some individuals who fail to adapt. The onset of retinal hemorrhages, cerebral edema, or coma signal that the individual requires immediate emergency care at a lower altitude. Oxygen should be given as soon as it is available. When the victim reaches definitive medical care, electrolyte imbalances should be corrected.

High-Altitude Pulmonary Edema

High-altitude pulmonary edema (HAPE) is a serious altitude-related problem that presents in a manner similar to that of other cases of pulmonary edema. The signs and symptoms include increased respirations and shortness of breath; a cough producing pink, frothy sputum; lethargy; nausea and vomiting; cyanosis; and rales. A slight temperature elevation may be present that may confuse the presentation with that of a minor infection.

Emergency care should include oxygen administration and immediate evacuation to a low altitude where the individual can receive definitive care.

Lightning

After considering the foregoing environmental dangers, the forensic nurse may believe that things can't get worse in an outdoor setting; just then, lightning strikes! Lightning-related injuries can be devastating, capable of inducing unresponsiveness and cardiac arrest. When an individual is hit by lightning, cardiopulmonary resuscitation (CPR) should be started immediately, regardless of the time that has elapsed since the injury. Successful resuscitations have occurred when CPR has been delayed far longer than the four- to six-minute "brain death" period, perhaps because of the fact that when an electrical force passes through the body, all cell metabolism is halted. A longer period of time than usual is required for cell degradation to occur. The individual struck by lightning usually becomes unconscious or has an altered state of consciousness that ranges from being "stunned," with retrograde amnesia, to coma. Motor paralysis and hyporeflexia that correspond to spinal cord levels often accompany the accident. Paralysis of the respiratory center is thought to be the cause of death in many cases, perhaps closely linked to the phenomenon of ventricular fibrillation. For individuals who are somewhat responsive after a lightning strike, deafness and loss of speech are common. The cardiovascular system is compromised by massive vasomotor spasm that causes loss of peripheral pulses, loss of sensation and color in the extremities, and the sequelae of peripheral arterial thrombosis, which may require fasciotomy or even amputation at a later time. Other signs and symptoms related to lightning injury include hysteria and personality changes, deafness, cataracts, optic atrophy, retinal detachment, hyphema, vitreous hemorrhage, and other eye injuries.

In addition to the usual resuscitation efforts, careful attention should be paid to assessing for electrical burns that often accompany lightning injuries. The "featherlike" lightning printing may be the real key to recognizing the lightning injury in the comatose patient. This "printing" is a linear, spidery, arborescent, and erythematous skin discoloration that relates to the pathways of decreased skin resistance. In assessing victims of suspected lightning strikes, pay careful attention to obscure areas for exit wounds, such as the bottom of the feet and the anus.

Emergency care should encompass the following considerations: providing a patent airway (intubated if the patient is apneic) and ensuring that oxygen is administered at 4 to 6 L/minute; monitoring for ventricular fibrillation (one of the most common complications); and attaining an IV access route for drugs if resources are available at the scene. Later care at the hospital, of course, will include management of the electrical burn wound characteristically associated with lightning injuries and strict monitoring and support of renal function, which may be impaired by myoglobinuria that often occurs after lightning injuries.

Documentation of Occupational Health and Safety Issues

Nurses and others who work in forensic settings are aware of their responsibilities for notifying agencies and authorities under specific sets of circumstances. These personnel also must be aware of regulatory guidance, standards of practice, and mandatory reporting of occupational health and safety issues. In healthcare facilities, the occupational health nurse and the infection control practitioner will be able to provide advice and recommend courses of actions in the event of accidents or injuries. Prompt reporting and precise actions are in order to avoid unfortunate outcomes from occupational exposures to infectious diseases, toxins, and work-related injuries.

Summary

Forensic nurses work in many settings ranging from hospitals and homes to a variety of other locations with multiple physical, chemical, environmental, and biological hazards. Personal protection attire is vital for safety and survival in many of these scenarios. In addition to being in optimal physical condition, the forensic nurse examiner should be well versed and compliant in regard to infection control and occupational health standards of practices.

Blood-borne pathogens, physical injuries, and contagious diseases are among major perils for the forensic examiner. These perils may be associated with both living and deceased individuals. The work environment itself can also pose additional risks. Accident sites involving mass casualties such as fires, explosions, or acts of terrorism are steeped with conditions that could contribute to injury or illness of the forensic nurse examiner or investigator. Among these conditions are extremes of heat, cold, altitude, and weather that affect job performance and physiological equilibrium and even threaten survival.

Forensic nurses must understand the dangers posed by their work environments and educate themselves about the use and wear of recommended personal protective attire. Finally, the impact of long hours and difficult working conditions should be appreciated in regard to their negative effects on personal health status. Each nurse should be sure to contact appropriate resources for periodic immunizations, screenings, routine medical interventions, and emergency care needs.

Resources

Publications

AORN Recommended Practices Committee. (March 2002). Recommended practices for cleaning and caring for surgical instruments and powered equipment. *AORN J*, *75*(3), 627-641.

Bartley, J., & Bjerke, N. B. (2001). Infection control considerations in critical care unit design and construction: A systematic risk assessment. *Crit Care Nurs Q*, *24*(3), 43-58.

Froede, R. C. (Ed.). (1990). *Handbook of forensic pathology*. Northfield, IL: College of American Pathologists.

Garner, J. S. (1996). Guidelines for isolation precautions in hospitals (from USPHS, USDHHS, CDCP, Atlanta, GA). *Infect Control Hosp Epidemiol, 17*(1), 53-80.

Gruendemann, B. J. (2002). Taking cover: Single-use vs. reusable gowns and drapes. *Infect Control Today, 6*(3), 32-34.

HICPAC/SHEA/APIC/IDSA Hand Hygiene Task Force and the Healthcare Infection Control Practices Advisory Committee. (2002). *Guidelines for hand hygiene in healthcare settings.* Washington, DC: Centers for Disease Control and Prevention; www.cdc.gov.

Leighner, L. A. (1997). Don the barriers. *Crit Care Nurs Q, 24*(2), 30-38.

Mandell, G. L., Douglas, R. G., Bennett, J. E., et al. (1996). *Principles and practice of infectious diseases, antimicrobial therapy, 1996-1997.* New York: Churchill Livingstone.

Morbidity and Mortality Weekly Report (multiple issues). (1996-1997). Waltham, MA: Massachusetts Medical Society.

National Institute for Occupational Safety (NIOSH) HealthAlert. (2003). *Preventing allergic reactions to natural rubber latex in the workplace.* Washington, DC: U.S. Department of Health and Human Services; www.cdc.gov/niosh.

Pugliese, G. (1995). Increase in vancomycin-resistant enterococci. *Morbid Mortal Weekly Rep, 44*(17), 504-506.

Pyrek, K. M. (2002). Follow standard precautions when handling soiled linens. *Infect Control Today, 6*(3), 12-14.

Sussman, G., & Gold, M. (Eds.). (1998). *Guidelines for the Management of Latex Allergies and Safe Latex Use in Health Care Facilities.* Milwaukee, WI: American College of Allergy, Asthma and Immunology and the Canadian Healthcare Association.

Wenzel, R. A. (Ed.). (1997). *Prevention and control of nosocomial infections* (3rd ed.). Baltimore: Williams & Wilkins.

Organizations

American College of Allergy, Asthma and Immunology

85 West Algonquin Road, Suite 550, Arlington Heights, IL 60005; Tel: 847-427-1200; www.acaai.org

American Latex Allergy Association

3791 Sherman Road, Slinger, WI 53086; 888-972-5378 (toll-free)

Association for Professionals in Infection Control and Epidemiology, Inc.

1275 K Street NW, Suite 1000, Washington, DC 20005-4006; Tel: 202-789-1890

Centers for Disease Control and Prevention

1600 Clifton Road, Atlanta, GA 30333; Tel: 404-639-3311

National Post-Exposure Hotline

University of California, San Francisco, Tel: 888-448-4911

Occupational Safety and Health Administration (OSHA)

Department of Labor, 200 Constitution Avenue NW, Washington, DC 20210; Tel: 866-4-USA-DOL; www.osha.gov

References

Ayres, S. M., Grenvik, A., Holbrook, P. R., et al. (1995). *Textbook of critical care* (3rd ed.). Philadelphia: W.B. Saunders.

Barber, J. S. (1996). Life-threatening infection in the critically ill. Pathophysiology, antibiotics and clinical management (course syllabus). Lewisville, TX: Barbara Clark Mims Associates.

Bjerke, N. B. (2004). The evolution: Handwashing to hand hygiene guidance. *Crit Care Nurs Q, 27*(3), 295-307.

Centers for Disease Control (CDC). (2004). *Updates on infectious diseases.* Atlanta, GA: Author.

Federal Bureau of Investigation. (1999). *FBI handbook on forensic services.* Washington, DC: US Government Printing Office.

Henderson, D. K. (2001). Raising the bar: The need for standardizing the use of "standard precautions" as a primary intervention to prevent occupational exposures to bloodborne pathogens. *Infect Control Hosp Epidemiol, 22*(2), 70-72.

Lanros, N., & Barber, J. S. (1997). *Emergency nursing* (4th ed.). Stamford, CT: Appleton & Lange.

Larson, E., & APIC Guidelines Committee. (1995). APIC guidelines for handwashing and hand antisepsis in health care settings. *Am J Infect Control, 23,* 251-269.

Lee, H., Palmbach, T., & Miller, M. (2001). *Henry Lee's crime scene handbook.* San Diego: Academic Press.

O'Boyle, C. A., Henly, S. J., & Larson, E. (2001). Understanding adherence to hand hygiene recommendations: The theory of planned behavior. *Am J Infect Control, 29*(6), 352-360.

Occupational Safety and Health Adminstration. (1992). Standard 29 CFR 1910.120: *Hazardous waste operations and emergency response.* Washington, DC: US Department of Labor.

Wilkins, R. L., & Dexter, J. R. (1993). *Respiratory disease: Principles of patient care.* Philadelphia: F. A. Davis.

Chapter 55 Education and Credentialing for Forensic Nurses

Virginia A. Lynch, Cynthia Whittig Roach, and David W. Sadler

Forensic nursing education and credentialing is highly variable throughout the world. Scotland has been included here because it represents one of the earliest efforts in formal educational processes for forensic scientists, and important interdependencies of medicine and nursing are emphasized. Additional information on education can be found in Chapters 56 and 57.

Forensic Nursing Education in the US

VIRGINIA A. LYNCH AND CYNTHIA WHITTIG ROACH

A number of forces are acting in concert to exert enormous pressures on professional nursing to change. New trends in healthcare are also changing the face of services provided by nursing professionals. The arena in which nursing care has traditionally been played is expanding, as are the variables, which determine adjustment, coping, and resolution of problems associated with the medical diagnosis. Thus, the need for baccalaureate prepared and advance practice nurses capable of independent nursing activities is growing rapidly. In the face of these changes, programs producing professional nurses must also change. A necessary change in the character of the faculty must also be accomplished to ensure that each student is provided with skilled clinical role models in every major curriculum area, including a sincere and earnest desire to engage significantly in a helping profession to teach and educate students to share those values.

Best Practice *55-1*

Academic institutions will require that forensic nursing faculty be qualified by both education and practical experience in a forensic specialty in order to ensure that students are mentored by a skilled clinical role model in each major curriculum area.

The educational preparation of today's forensic nurse represents diverse pathways; formal curricula in undergraduate, graduate, and doctoral programs have only been introduced within the past two decades in the US.

In 1986, the University of Texas at Arlington opened a graduate level forensic nursing option for its master's degree candidates. Approximately 10 students completed the curricula over the next two years, but in 1990 the program was discontinued by the School of Nursing owing to lack of human and fiscal resources to support the offering. In 1994 Beth-El College in Colorado Springs offered forensic nursing courses at the undergraduate level, later advancing toward a degree option for advanced practice nurses. In 1996 Fitchburg State College (MA) opened a graduate program designed to prepare the clinical nurse specialist. Other formal offerings have occurred at Gonzaga State University, Xavier University, Quinnipiac University, Johns Hopkins University, and at least a dozen other schools throughout the US.

The barriers to introducing this specialty are largely attributed to the lack of understanding about the discipline itself. Many nurses cannot appreciate the relationships and close associations between the scientific methods of forensic science and the nursing process. Because nurse educators have traditionally lacked indoctrination in the forensic sciences, a shift of paradigm has been difficult. Furthermore, forensic nursing is a new discipline and therefore lacks nursing educators with doctoral preparation who can champion the specialty within faculty groups who determine the curricular structure of undergraduate and graduate study. At the dawn of this millennium, there are fewer than 10 forensic nurses with doctoral preparation who have aligned themselves with forensic nursing science. Although there is a larger pool of forensic nurses with a master's degree, they usually must work outside the specialty for their earning power, pursuing forensic nursing as a secondary field of interest because currently there are few paid positions for forensic clinical nurse specialists or forensic nurse practitioners. This, however, is changing in the clinical arena and in death investigation, government institutions, and law enforcement agencies. Although the catch-22 represented by this lack of qualified educators and thus a lack of programs to prepare forensic specialists in nursing is frustrating, it is commonly experienced with emerging scientific disciplines. In the meantime, a small, but highly motivated group of qualified educators in both nursing and in medicine are carrying the banner.

Challenges and Opportunities

The inevitability of change and the emphasis of greater diversity in nursing education has defined baccalaureate nursing as the standard by which the profession of nursing in the US is measured. The American Nurses' Association Congress of Nursing Practice has established entry level standards and certification requirements for various nursing specialties. Most require a minimum of a baccalaureate degree. Certain specialties, however, designate graduate preparation, advanced practice status, and minimal levels of experience. The Core Curriculum Committee of the International Association of Forensic Nurses is currently working to establish certification requirements for forensic nurses in several subspecialties.

The development of educational programs preparing forensic nurses for optimal clinical application of the standards and philosophies of forensic nursing science, role clarification, investigative case management, multidisciplinary team relationships, certification examination, and advance practice comprise the nuclei of preparation for forensic nursing practice. The forensic nurse examiner's (FNE) biomedical skills benefit hospital administration, trauma centers, centers for evaluation of mental health, forensic psychiatric evaluations, and medicolegal research to meet the clinical forensic standards defined by the Joint Commission on Accreditation of Healthcare Organizations (JCAHO) and legal statutes. These biomedical skills also contribute significantly to the scientific investigation of death for the forensic nurse death investigator (FNDI) who assists the forensic pathologist in the analysis of fatal injuries and medical deaths. The unlimited potential for the FNE in both the clinical arena and in death investigation is directly related to the specific body of knowledge and skills associated with the quality of existing forensic nursing education programs and those currently developing. Education founded on sound clinical evidence and research is essential to the future of forensic nursing. The rapid growth and development of forensic nursing practices has provided an impetus for universities and colleges to incorporate forensic nursing curricular options into their strategic plans in both developing and developed countries.

Educational Preparation

Subsequent to the first formal graduate program in forensic nursing at the University of Texas in Arlington, numerous programs have developed and continue to develop at universities, colleges, and technical schools as well as hospitals and educational offerings within professional associations across the US, Canada, Australia, UK, Africa, and India. These course offerings include electives, minors, certificate programs, master's degrees, and post-master's certificates in forensic nursing science for nurses and nursing students and nonnursing majors from other schools and colleges on campuses interested in the forensic health sciences.

Forensic nursing science may stand alone as a degree major, entailing all traditional nursing requirements with the forensic specialty as the focus of career options (similar to pediatrics, psychiatric, critical care, geriatrics, adult health, and other specialty areas), or it may be offered as a thread within the curriculum major, being linked to emergency/trauma nursing or other specializations as well as integrated within courses such as women's studies, healthcare ethics, victimology, or other specialty courses.

The most common model for today's forensic nurse is postlicensure education in a selected aspect of the specialty. For example, diploma nurses, as well as those with degrees (associate, baccalaureate, and master's), have obtained their forensic education by "piecing together" content from continuing education courses, workshops, professional meeting programs, and certificate offerings. Some have been fortunate enough to be able to obtain sufficient credentials for employment as a sexual assault nurse examiner, death investigator, or other forensic specialist. Most, however, still await the opportunity to enroll in degree-granting academic programs. In the meantime, in response to the outcry for forensic educational courses, distance learning programs have become popular as a method for accessing forensic nursing information, because few nurses are fortunate enough to live in proximity to the programs now offering formal academic curricula. Although the Internet and distance learning courses are effective tools for some content, they have limitations, of course. Many skills associated with forensic nursing require practical "real world" opportunities to collect physical and biological evidence and to interface with the human situations germane to the discipline. In addition, clinical experience with law enforcement, members of the judiciary system, and other forensic scientists is imperative for preparing the forensic nurse as a specialist. Well-designed simulations, supervised chat rooms, and written scenarios are indeed valuable learning tools, but they cannot fully provide what is gained from a well-qualified clinical mentor.

Undergraduate programs with required or elective forensic nursing courses are still a minority even today. New strategies for nursing education must be forthcoming in order to meet the needs for those individuals who want to pursue this nursing specialty.

Baccalaureate Programs

The foundation for strong clinical practice is the foundation for a specialty practice in forensic nursing. One cannot emphasize the value of this foundation enough in order to provide the basis for the specialization of the forensic nurse examiner. Thus, it is the basic knowledge gained from clinical nursing, nursing theory, anatomy and physiology, pharmacology, and psychosocial nursing that separates the nursing professional from the criminal justice professional at a *scene of crime* or in the investigation of abuse, neglect, sexual assault, or questioned deaths.

Key Point 55-1

> The nursing process is the design for the investigation of trauma, injury, illness, and death. Once a nurse has demonstrated a successful and confident acquisition of knowledge as a registered nurse and has completed specific studies in forensic nursing science, then he or she should be considered prepared to effectively fulfill the role of a forensic nurse.

Because basic requirements for a bachelor of science (BS) in nursing degree generally offer two nursing electives or nonnursing electives within the degree plan, these requirements can be filled with forensic nursing and forensic health science courses, which also may provide the required classes for a certificate in forensic nursing with the exception of a requisite clinical internship.

Master's Degree Programs

Advanced forensic nursing curricula pursue subjects not addressed in undergraduate programs, such as pathophysiology, research, epidemiology, consulting, curriculum design, and informatics. Beth-El College of Nursing and Health Sciences, University of Colorado at Colorado Springs, offers the most complete curricular options. Through advanced nursing education, clinical nurse specialists are prepared in forensic nursing, a certificate program, and degree transferable elective courses in forensic health science and nursing. Forensic photography, human rights, sexual assault, both theory and clinical, law and legal issues are among the special electives offered in addition to the required courses.

Doctoral Programs

As generally happens, the greater desire for knowledge promotes higher academic goals. To date, four accredited US universities offering doctorate level degrees in nursing have opted to extend these opportunities to students who are designing their own program and research in forensic nursing science. As principal research investigators these doctoral students have identified areas within forensic nursing science as instrumental in nursing education, practice, and research. The development of core and specialty competencies has been a significant initiative for affirming the need for this quality education, but it also requires programs to reevaluate their curricula and make the necessary adjustments (Sperhac and Clinton, 2005). The solution lies in a different model for educating advanced practice nurses: the practice doctorate. For forensic nurses who want a terminal professional degree representing the highest level of competency, the practice doctorate provides the benefits and challenges of a united effort to prepare the forensic nurse examiner for the challenges of tomorrow. Although several practice doctoral nursing programs exist and others are in the approval stage, the University of Tennessee College of Nursing is the only one to offer a doctor of nursing practice in forensic nursing.

Online Education

The availability of online educational programs in forensic nursing has proved to be of special interest to nurses who live in areas in which there are no appropriate educational opportunities in on-site classrooms. It is also a desirable option for military nurses, traveling nurses, and those with irregular schedules that are incompatible with standard university course requirements. Returning nurses who may not be comfortable with a young campus peer group, can do online study without regard for social considerations that often accompany other educational settings. Individuals who are self-motivated and self-directed thrive in online learning, and often success with these endeavors provides the courage and incentive to return to a formal academic setting or other educational opportunities. High-quality online programs offer legitimate academic credits or continuing education units that support some state's licensure requirements. A few online offerings grant certificates after completion of a basic curriculum of sequential modules covering the fundamentals of forensic nursing.

Preceptorships and Internships

Any innovative forensic nursing program must conclude with the opportunity to obtain practical experience. The internship or practicum generally requires a minimum of 120 contact hours under the supervision of a forensic nursing specialist, law enforcement officer, prosecutor, or other appropriate professional. There are also options for informal practicums in settings where nurses can design their own learning experiences. Forensic nurses often arrange such preceptorships with selected mentors who possess outstanding reputations for teaching and practice.

One example of an internship is titled "Introduction to Medicolegal Death Investigation: A Nursing Internship." Susan Chewning, Coroner, Charleston County, South Carolina, has served as the elected coroner since 1992 and directs a team of forensic nurse investigators as deputy coroners. Chewning has established a program that provides a hands-on opportunity to learn about death investigation. Nurses interested in advancing their knowledge base in the forensic field can apply to spend a one-week internship shadowing the coroner's all-nurse investigator staff, observing and participating in scene investigation and autopsy procedures, reviewing computer systems related to the National Crime Information Center (NCIC) and the Automated Fingerprint Identification System (AFIS), and attending lectures on forensic odontology and forensic anthropology, firearms and ballistics, blood spatter techniques, drugs, child death management, and other categories of deaths such as suicides, traffic accidents, and homicides. This innovative and pioneering program has given nurses the necessary experience to evaluate the knowledge gained in both formal and informal classes on death and crime scene investigation. Graduate nursing students may wish to apply for an internship at the Houston medical examiner's office where the investigative staff are exclusively degreed forensic nurse death investigators (FNDI). The experiences are essentially the same, but contrast between the coroner system and the medical examiner system is an excellent learning opportunity.

Certificate and Short Courses

Beth-El College of Nursing and Health Sciences, University of Colorado, Colorado Springs, was the first to offer a forensic certificate program. The course work requirements include four courses (12 semester hours) and a 120-contact-hour internship (two semester hours). This certificate program includes a one-semester course (17 weeks or equivalent) in the Investigation of Injury and Death. Other one-semester course requirements incorporate an Introduction to Forensic Nursing Science, Crime Lab and Crime Scene Investigation, and the Psychosocial and Legal Aspects of Forensic Health Care.

One important consideration that makes this program attractive for the students is flexible programming for the adult learner. For example, some programs are delivered in one-week blocks so that individuals can come from across the US or from other countries to complete a 40- to 46-hour minisemester, the equivalent of a 17-week semester. Three academic credits can be earned in one week. Dr. Mary Dudley, currently the Chief Medical Examiner, Wichita, Kansas, initiated the first courses at Beth-El College of Nursing and has continued to educate nurses through an extensive series of courses in death investigation and other forensic nursing subjects.

Continuing Education Offerings

There are several schools of nursing and organizations offering singular programs and forensic series in forensic nursing. In response to the lack of faculty support for establishing forensic nursing within the undergraduate or graduate programs as formal offerings, the University of Texas at Austin's School of Nursing offered a highly successful series of continuing education programs in forensic issues from 1992 to 1999. It was hoped that if the value of the offering could be demonstrated, and students were enthusiastic about participating, the faculty might be leveraged to support formal courses when fiscal and human resources permitted. Topics in the CEU series included introductory concepts, education and career opportunities, forensic photography, crime scene investigation, environmental issues in forensic science, sexual assault, child and elder abuse, domestic violence, correctional and forensic psychiatric issues, and the role of the forensic nurse in legal proceedings. Guest experts in the various subjects provided lectures, discussion sessions, and supervised clinical practice. However, in 1999, the Continuing Nursing Education Program division was closed, and forensic nursing educational opportunities were lost. In the meantime, the champions of forensic education have moved on, channeling their energies into other pursuits. In 1999, the School of Nursing at the University of New Mexico initiated a series of forensic programs to meet the needs of students clamoring for forensic education. Two types of students enrolled in the offerings, undergraduate for credit and graduate for CEUs only. Along with these two examples, there are several other resources for continuing education in forensic nursing, but what is sorely needed is a widespread proliferation of undergraduate exposure to the subject. Two approaches can be used effectively, namely, elective or required courses on certain forensic topics, or forensic principles or concepts woven throughout the curriculum. Examples of such threads include human abuse, forensic assessments and collection of evidence, documentation and reporting of crimes of abuse and negligence, social justice, jurisprudence, and prevention strategies for societal violence. The value of using curricular "threads" would be to effect a highly flexible way to ensure that students would be exposed to the core curriculum of forensic nursing. They could be introduced early in the curriculum and expanded as the student builds other components of a generic nursing education. There is not a singular clinical area to which the student is exposed that would be an inappropriate locus for testing forensic principles and concepts.

Best Practice *55-2*

Nursing education will incorporate key concepts and principles of forensic nursing throughout all courses in order to ensure that students are exposed to essential information about human abuse, forensic assessments and collection of evidence, documentation and reporting of crimes of abuse and negligence, social justice, jurisprudence, and prevention strategies for societal violence.

In recent years, undergraduate, graduate, and postgraduate programs in forensic nursing science have been developed and are continuing to develop across the US and abroad. These programs offer specific forensic curricula in the scientific investigation of injury and death, human abuse, forensic chemistry, crime scene/crime laboratory, forensic photography, toxicology, victimology, traumatology, sexual violence, human rights, and psychosocial and legal aspects of forensic science, among others. Highly specialized courses in this field are currently available through medical examiner/coroner systems and universities offering formal and informal coursework in forensic nursing education.

Other sources for medical forensic education include the Miami Dade County Medical Examiner Department at the Joseph E. Davis Forensic Institute, Miami, Florida, which provides a 40-contact-hour course entitled "The Investigation of Injury and Death: Through the Eyes of the Forensic Nurse." St. Louis University School of Medicine provides another resource in education and training in medicolegal death investigation for (lay) coroners, nonmedical investigators, police officers, and forensic nurses.

Scientific Meetings

In tribute to the American Academy of Forensic Sciences (AAFS), forensic nursing was first recognized as a scientific discipline at the 43rd annual meeting in 1991 (Anaheim, California). The International Association of Forensic Nurses (IAFN), patterned after the AAFS, was founded in 1992. In 1995 the American Nurses' Association (ANA) Congress of Nursing Practice bestowed formal recognition to forensic nursing as an official nursing specialty, and in 1997, the IAFN, in conjunction with the ANA, published the Scope and Standards of Forensic Nursing Practice. The American Board of Forensic Nursing, one component of the American College of Forensic Examiners, has developed a generalist certification, which will accept forensic nurses with or without degrees, as does the American Board of Medicolegal Death Investigators for lay-investigators. The goal of IAFN credentialing is to promote advanced practice in the clinical environs, sexual assault examination, forensic psychiatric nursing, correctional healthcare, and death investigation to meet the requirements of clinical nurse specialists, nurse practitioners, and doctoral prepared forensic nurse specialists in the decades ahead.

Issues in Forensic Education

Determining Resources

In academic settings, considerable negotiation and debate are required to permit the introduction of a new curricular offering. This process is often difficult since monies, faculty, and other resources must be realigned to permit new courses. Few institutions have the luxury of being able to add new courses or hire new faculty without some compromises or sacrifices in other curricula. In some instances, grant support and public funding have assisted schools of nursing in program launches.

Faculty Preparation and Credentials

In addition to offering unique curricula, other variables that contribute to a successful program include the quality and experience of the faculty, both full-time and part-time. Most forensic faculty members are experts in their areas, and most have extensive clinical experience as well as a strong theory base to support these programs. The arguments for greater diversity in nursing education and to include basic and advanced education in forensic nursing science are significant. This has been reflected in the need to draw larger numbers of scholars into the field of nursing. With the shortage of competent professionals in varied areas of nursing, forensic nursing poses only one of many new challenges. In addition to nursing scholars, resources from law enforcement, the legal system, and subspecialties within the forensic sciences must be readily available as resources to forensic nursing faculty. Although these additional individuals often are willing to participate as guest lecturers in educational programs with little or no remuneration, their credentials must undergo the scrutiny of the university system to attest to their qualifications.

Availability of Textbooks and Teaching Resources

Textbooks and other teaching resources for forensic nursing curricula have generally come from the legal sciences, forensic medicine, political and police sciences, and other associated disciplines. Although several new forensic nursing textbooks are in various stages of development and production, ephemeral materials, Internet information, journal articles, and books from associated forensic disciplines continue to be needed for amplification of classroom lectures. Because forensic nursing is a collegial discipline and requires a sound understanding of community and public services, other agencies that may cooperate in the program include police departments, crime laboratories, local courts, and various social services. Field trips to the hospital emergency department, pediatric clinics, and morgues are typically included.

Core Curricula Considerations

Advanced Practice and Clinical Specialization

Specialty practice is at the growing edge of the profession of nursing. According to the ANA, when nurse specialists are employed in clinical or community healthcare settings, descriptions of their positions and functions ought not to be standardized, for their nature and scope change as new knowledge develops. Graduate programs that prepare specialists in nursing practice are initiated, established, and conducted by universities and colleges, which have the primary social responsibilities for the education of scientists and professionals. Specific criteria are used by the ANA to decide if an area of specialization in nursing merits establishment of a program. There must be evidence of a previously unrecognized area that lies within or would be a reasonable expansion of nursing's scope of practice. Furthermore, there must be a sufficient need existing in society for the area that has been identified and evidence to believe that the field of nursing would be diminished or limited in its long-range aim if the recognized need were ignored.

ANA has asserted that the wide diversity in clinical experience that exists among nurses must be recognized and seen as a constructive response of nurses to social needs in a time of rapid, complex, and sophisticated changes in present-day healthcare systems. As the boundaries of nursing are expanding in response to changing social needs and demands, nursing's social responsibility must address the diagnosis and treatment of human responses to actual and potential health problems. In relevance to forensic nursing there are several consideration.

New degrees in forensic nursing broaden one of many choices of career opportunities in nursing for the future. A curriculum blending psychosocial and clinical nursing with biomedical education and the basic principles of law and human behavior utilized in the medicolegal field has brought a new perspective to nursing roles. Forensic nursing not only prepares the registered nurse to assist law enforcement officers investigating injury and death in systems of inquiry regarding health and justice, but provides a new role for psychosocial nursing in community mental health, for emergency nurses in death and dying, and for clinical nurses in general related to a more encompassing concept of holistic nursing when including the entirety of body, mind, spirit, *and* the law. The entirety of this principle of forensic nursing represents a long overdue concern for victims of crime and for those who are accused, convicted, or executed for crimes they did not commit, as well as the significant others left behind in the traumatic aftermath of human tragedy.

With the ever-increasing challenges to the profession of nursing faced in these demanding times, recent advances in the field of forensic nursing, and the shift toward community-based rather than institutional care, forensic nursing recognizes the importance of community mental health (CMH) in the reduction and prevention of violence. Instead of waiting for illness, CMH seeks to find people who are responding to losses of various kinds and assist them in working through grief states as a form of preventive psychiatry or preventive medicine. Intervention in grief must be seen and supported as a means toward adaptation and health.

The experienced, educated forensic registered nurse provides a uniquely qualified clinician capable of a valuable professional contribution on behalf of the victims, perpetrators, the deceased, the families, and the community. This emphasis is on the use of clinically oriented investigators combining their healthcare orientation with the field of trauma and death investigation while providing a support system to the living and the deceased's immediate and extended family members and the community as a whole.

Nurse educators are urged to include these relevant aspects of social and biological content to be included in the nurse's basic education in order to integrate pertinent ideas from these disciplines into the basic and advanced forensic curricula. Nurses must use their own powers of observation and their own intellect and must strive to develop independence in thought and practice.

The relationship of this new era of nursing practice affects both nursing education and nursing services through the facts, concepts, and principles upon which the education of forensic nurses and their services to families and communities are based. Society has a right to expect that the responsibility for nursing services will rest with persons possessing a substantial theoretical foundation for making judgments and assuming responsibility. Forensic nurses must continue to be probing the frontiers of knowledge in force.

Nursing's perspective evolves from the practical aim of the optimization of human environments for health. One area of major conceptualizations in nursing deals with human characteristics and natural processes, such as consciousness, abstraction, adaptation and healing, growth, change, self-determination, interconnectedness, development, aging, dying, reproducing, drive, satisfaction, assimilating, and relating.

Key Point 55-2

The discipline of forensic nursing is defined by social relevance and value orientations that must be continually reexamined in terms of societal need and scientific discoveries.

Further, some members of the profession must engage in inquiry that is not immediately applicable to current clinical practice, requiring researchers to employ a variety of approaches to forensic nursing's perspective. Its scope goes far beyond that required for current clinical practice. If the discipline were so narrowly defined, professional nursing could be limited to functioning in the realm of disaster relief rather than serving as a moving force in the promotion of world health.

Part of nursing's struggle in evolution stems from the slow emergence of recognition of its social relevance. Forensic nurses give service related to the quality of human life and death. This service is only recently being valued. Therefore, forensic nursing as a discipline is broader than nursing science or forensic science and its uniqueness stems from its perspective of life and death. What is needed is a new philosophy of nurse educators in curricula development and of nurse researchers in its inquiry and methodology. Forensic nursing is essentially a special type of caring. Science can be an effective tool of the humanist. If forensic scientist-nurses are to contribute to the development of nursing, however, there must be some values that forensic scientist-nurses and other nurses hold in common. It is hoped that one such value would be service to society in prevention and intervention of violence in the living and expressed in concern, and care regarding the dead.

Though it has long been accepted that nursing's contribution goes beyond effective assistance in the nursing care plan, knowledge of people and how they respond biologically, physically, and socially to stress is needed. The provisions of comprehensive nursing care, which are provided to individuals or groups under stress of a death-related nature, has as its primary purpose the relief of tension and discomfort with the end of restoring or maintaining internal and interpersonal equilibrium. This is the ultimate goal held by all forensic nurses.

Science can be defined as a branch of study concerned either with a connected body of demonstrated truths or with observed facts systematically classified and more or less colligated by being brought under new laws, which includes trustworthy methods for the discovery of new truths within its own domain (*Oxford Dictionary*, 2003). It is proposed that the body of knowledge called the science of forensic nursing consists of a synthesis, reorganization, and or extension of concepts drawn from the basic or other applied sciences that, in their reformulation, tend to become new concepts. It is further proposed that these new concepts will be concerned largely but not exclusively with the causation, character, and progress of the tensions growing out of stress and disturbing internal or interpersonal equilibrium to both. They will lead to the development of theories of forensic nursing intervention that will yield predictable and desired responses when implemented into nursing care. If there is a need for a specifically defined body of knowledge in nursing and if nursing scholars are going to contribute to that knowledge, then keeping pace is not an option but a requirement. Perspectives on forensic nursing theory, knowledge, and university education must reflect a theoretical area of social exchange associated with current and changing needs.

Since its inception, forensic nursing science as a health and justice profession has come a long way, but it still has much to achieve. This will entail countless challenges and risk, but the process should help create an entity of forensic nurse-scientists capable of developing knowledge that reflects sensitivity to the inherent problems in clinical and community death investigation. It is reasonable to expect that as this body of knowledge develops corresponding substance in clinical mandates, nursing will adapt forensic science concepts to nursing behaviors and role expectations in the clinical environs, using and evaluating this knowledge.

Preparation for Advanced Practice

The major thrust of any developing discipline needs to consider the issue of basic versus advanced nursing preparation and the differentiation of roles for forensic nurses in advanced practice, describing the roles they need to assume for graduate leadership to manage and supervise other forensic nurses.

- *Leadership and administration of forensic nursing and other health-related forensic services:* Especially during times of economic and human resource limitations, advanced skills and knowledge base are required for good decision making, allocation of resources, promotion of human rights, and patient advocacy (staff nurses are on the first line of intervention, but advanced practice nurses and those with doctorates have more power and influence in systems in which other practitioners and healthcare administrators have advanced degrees).
- *Advancing forensic nursing science in forensic healthcare applications:* These applications are particularly important in the area of promoting evidence-based practice, developing outcomes and sensitive nursing interventions, developing of nursing assessment instruments, and using those advanced assessment instruments to provide comprehensive healthcare, health promotion, and disease prevention among forensic clients and populations. This calls for site leadership in participation in clinical trials involving forensic populations, particularly in the areas concerning violence as a public health problem. The role of the forensic nurse is to define interpersonal violence as a healthcare issue and to be able to demonstrate through practice and research how providing care to victims can decrease healthcare costs in a time of limited healthcare resources.
- *Creation of a critical mass of forensic nurses prepared at the advanced practice level*: These nurses are needed to assume roles in specialized services and direct client care (collaborative and independent) in order to increase access to at-risk and vulnerable populations, serve as nursing faculty to basic and advanced practice students, conduct research, and serve as major professors for graduate students doing research with forensic populations or developing forensic concepts and roles. Growing numbers of doctoral students are involved with forensic nursing research and clinical applications that will impact future nursing practice.
- *Nurses must be prepared to develop policy and influence legislation related to nursing and healthcare of forensic populations:* These nurses need to interact with government agencies (CDC, OVC, etc.) that will provide funding in the future for the care of the forensic patient. As government and regulatory laws (HIPAA, EMTALA, etc.) continue to have a greater impact on forensic healthcare, the forensic nurse should have an understanding of how the law impacts healthcare. Graduate nurses are needed to help minimize the financial impact of new regulations on healthcare systems and patients.

Specialty Practice in Forensic Nursing

Nursing is the most optimistic of sciences, and all that nurses do is based on the assumption that human caring makes a difference in the health of individuals and societies. Nursing as a profession serves society's health and well-being, and confronts issues of humanism, ethics, legalities, and economics that shape public policy (Lindberg, Hunter, & Kruszewski, 1998). Nurses thus may view their role toward the care of victimized women as requiring consideration of health and human rights. The Universal Declaration of Human Rights of 1948 emphasized that "everyone has the right to life, liberty and security of person" and that ". . . no one shall be subjected to torture or to cruel, inhuman, or degrading treatment or punishment." As Gilligan (1982) asserted, "While an ethic of justice proceeds from the premise of equality–that everyone should be treated the same–an ethic of care rests on the premise of nonviolence–that no one should be hurt."

Because nurses are generally women, making up 96% to 98% of the entire nursing population, in most male-dominated areas of the world, they too must work against cultural norms and may find themselves in denial of their own victimization. Awareness and attention to individual victimization of oneself is a priority for nurses applying the tenets of forensic nursing science. Forensic nurses must first address their own victimizations prior to providing forensic care to others lest they become a part of secondary victimization that may decrease their ability to nurture and heal others.

Certification and Specialized Credentialing

The IAFN is currently developing a core curriculum for the specialty, utilizing an advanced practice and clinical specialization model. A preliminary report of the Core Curriculum Committee was delivered at IAFN's Scientific Assembly in Chicago in October 2004. Earlier, in 2001, certification was launched for adult and pediatric sexual assault nurse examiners. Development of specific standards and national certification in biomedical investigation for the forensic nurse death investigator is currently in progress through the IAFN. This certification will include professional standards in postmortem sexual assault examination for those who practice in this field.

Educational Program Development

Program development is a challenge whether it is for one class or ten classes. Many questions need to be answered before content development is initiated. These questions include: What are the primary objectives and goals for the program? Are there specific outcomes that the participants must obtain? How will one know that goals have been reached? What standards will be used in order to present the most comprehensive and accurate information? These are just a few of the questions to be answered in this chapter. Readers no doubt will add a few more of their own.

Establishing Objectives

Principles of curriculum and instruction always begin with identification of the objectives to be accomplished. Program objectives are broad and encompass in a general way all the content to be presented. Examples of program objectives commonly used are (1) to discuss the principles of injury and death investigation and (2) to describe the role of the forensic nurse in the clinical setting and emergency department. Individual class objectives are more specific and limited in scope; for example, (1) to differentiate specific caliber gunshot wounds and (2) to describe the procedure for collection of a victim's clothing. Verbs within the objectives also indicate the educational level or depth to which the content will be delivered. For instance, *discuss* is a relatively low level action verb to describe an objective and can be made more specific by changing to *analyze* or *synthesize*. Specific course content and evaluation methodologies must reflect the level of the objective as well. Attention to these details provides direction so that a program does not teach at one intellectual level and evaluate at another level. Thus, if more time is spent on the overall program objectives in the initial development, the objectives will become the blueprint or outline that the program content will then follow.

Considerations for content planning include the faculty, the students, and the institution. The best planned presentations are not appreciated if they are above the educational level of the students. Likewise, students attend conferences in order to learn new information, not to have the majority of the information a repeat of what they already know. Teaching and learning strategies must also be considered. Is the student to be a passive learner who sits in the chair taking copious notes? Or is the student actively involved with the speaker in discussion or specific classroom exercises? The environment in which the class is held, as well as the number of students, will also affect the strategies that can be implemented. These strategies are usually integrated within each speaker's lesson plan or content outline. Use of a variety of strategies is beneficial so that all students' learning styles can be addressed.

The mission and policies of the institution should be congruent with the program objectives. Imagine all the time and energy spent on a wonderful program that is canceled due to administration policy conflicts. Are there religious or cultural implications that might affect program implementation? These examples provide just a few considerations to guide the development of any program. Administrative support is crucial in the early planning stages.

Standards

It is also important that the educational program goals are based on accepted standards of practice. Standards that should be considered include the Scope and Standards of Forensic Nursing Practice (IAFN, 1997) and standards promoted by the Joint Commission on Accreditation of Healthcare Organizations (2004). Depending on program content, specific standards, such as those adopted by the sexual assault nurse examiners or the Emergency Nursing Standards, might also be useful. Use of an identified core curriculum that is endorsed by the specialty organization is also important and may save the program development committee many hours of work and frustration.

Practical Aspects

Practical considerations must address whether the program is for academic credit, continuing education credit, or both. In either case, usually administrative committees will have policies or procedures that apply. For instance, if the program offers academic credit (i.e. semester credit hours), the objectives, course description, content outline, evaluation methodologies, textbooks, total content hours, and faculty credentials may need to be approved by the institution's curriculum review committee. The program objectives should be congruent with the mission of the institution and the conceptual framework of the college in which the course is being offered. Review committees usually have structured time frames in which materials must be submitted prior to approval. This may delay program scheduling. Approval for continuing education hours may be done locally, within the state board of nursing or within a specialty organization. This, too, may place time constraints upon when the program may be offered for credit. A time line assists program planners to anticipate and control for a variety of administrative details, such as changes in dates, faculty, and location. An example of a time line is provided in Table 55-1.

Fiscal roles and responsibilities must also be carefully planned. Academic institutions generally have separate fees for in-state and out-of-state students; rules and regulations related to residency and in-state fees may also exist. Conflict may be averted by simultaneously offering a course for academic credit and continuing education credit. Commuter students then have an opportunity to pay similar fees without being penalized as out-of-state students. Faculty may not be locally available and an expense budget should be established to plan for travel, meals, lodging, and materials. If the program is not held at a hotel, there is the additional consideration of transportation, for the faculty and for the students. A primary administrative contact person is critical to handling questions that both the faculty and students will have.

Scheduling of courses can be a challenge on a college campus. Accelerated courses given over five to six days need a classroom nine hours per day; a classroom may not be available during the regular semester due to classroom shortages or scheduling difficulties. Individual institutions may not have a classroom available for extensive time periods either. Colleges may want to use the intersession period between semesters in order to facilitate classroom scheduling. One drawback can be that the college may also decrease services, meaning reduced cafeteria hours, bookstore hours, etc., which should be anticipated.

Lodging is also a concern for commuter students. Local hotel room rates may be subject to peak holiday periods and this may create additional expense for students. Commuter students need flexible scheduling that supports being able to obtain economical

Table 55-1 Program Planning Time Table for Forensic Nurses in the US

INITIAL PLANNING MEETING	FORMALIZE PLANS	IMPLEMENTATION PHASE I	IMPLEMENTATION PHASE II	PROGRAM DATE	EVALUATION PHASE
1. Establish program objectives and goals (draft). 2. Assess time frame needed for credit hours or continuing education hours applications. (Assign member to obtain necessary paperwork and instructions.) 3. Identify target audience. 4. Discuss marketing plan.	1. Obtain final approval of program objectives. 2. Complete and submit necessary approval forms for credit or continuing education contact hours. 3. Develop brochures, Web site, and advertising plan. 4. Plan marketing, distribution, and advertising. 5. Set target date for program. 6. Make initial contact with faculty.	1. Identify target date for return of approval credit 2. Reserve tentative dates with faculty. 3. Begin site planning and make tentative reservations. 4. Initial plans for materials, books, etc.	1. Final approval for credits or continuing education. Assign member to coordinate forms for credits, grades, etc. 2. Final date(s) confirmed for a. Location b. Faculty c. Brochure 3. Finalize plan for distribution of brochures, Web site, and advertising.	1. Establish program coordinator for day(s) of program (check room, equipment, etc). 2. Committee member available to handle administrative details for credits, continuing education, grades.	1. Review critiques and student comments. 2. Document changes for next program. 3. Celebrate!

airfare rates; a class that is offered Tuesday through Saturday allows students to avoid peak travel times. A map of the region and of the facility should be provided with registration information or confirmation.

Program development requires a multifaceted approach. Content experts and quality presentations based on current standards of practice are very important. Program administrators must plan in detail in order to predict and avoid potential problems before they occur. Every program needs someone with vision and expertise to guide the development and someone with management skills to direct the day-to-day details in order for the program to run smoothly.

Strategies for teaching and learning experiences will be briefly discussed. The reader is encouraged to consult the references at the end of this chapter to obtain additional information on this extensive topic. One question to be answered is: Is the student to be an active participant in learning or a passive learner? In the past, continuing education has received a negative reputation for sometimes requiring little more from students other than being warm bodies. Participants may or may not have been interested in the content presented, but attend only for the CEU certificate. Students who are accustomed to this passive approach may be shocked when they learn that the course being offered for academic credit requires that they take examinations, write papers, and earn a specific grade!

Specific approaches to teaching may also be of interest to the faculty and the program planners. Case study scenarios provide an opportunity for small group exercises and discussion. Policy and procedure development is an advanced level of learning and allows students to apply concepts to their clinical practice. Owing to the inherent nature of forensic material, faculty may find it useful for the student to maintain daily reflections or logs in which the instructor can provide feedback. Debriefing sessions at the end of each day may also allow students to ventilate fears, concerns, or generalized apprehension.

Another means for students to apply forensic content in a clinically focused manner can be with an internship. The clinical experience should have specific general objectives that can be customized into a specific area of interest for the student. Students may be interested in death and injury investigation and tailor their specific clinical objectives to this area. Other students may want to study violence in their own community. Students may also want to examine in depth the criminal justice system and how it responds to victims of violence as well as the perpetrators. Single or multiple preceptors in various agencies can provide effective learning experiences. The internship or clinical experience can provide a vehicle for adult learners to structure their learning experience in a way that is meaningful for them. Structure for the internship is necessary but should not limit the vast potential of experiences available. Most important is the need for the students to do their internship in their area of interest and within their own geographical region, if desired.

Evaluation and critique of each program is integral to the quality of subsequent programs. Students should have an opportunity to voice their opinions in a safe and nonjudgmental manner, both verbally and in writing. Faculty must receive critiques in a timely manner that allows for reflection and provides information on how they can make improvements for the future. Additional analyses should include the logistics of the course, the financial statistics, and the market demand for future courses or programs.

Forensic Nursing: Global Perspectives

Dr. Dora Maria Carbonu, an international nurse educator, has championed forensic nursing in Asian countries as a futuristic trend in health and justice ethics, stating that "nurses worldwide must be educated in the principles and techniques of forensic nursing science in order to provide appropriate forensic care that address legal issues." Programs have been established or are developing in countries outside the US, including Canada, Australia, England, Scotland, El Salvador, Singapore, Japan, Africa, India, Turkey, and Iran. The University of Bari, in Italy, recently held an International Conference on Forensic Nursing to lay groundwork for developing formal curricula there.

The Future of Forensic Nursing Education

Forensic nursing practice today differs significantly from that of 20 years ago. At that time, we were few in number and had no formal title, education was primarily on-the-job, and the diverse roles of nurses who provided forensic services were striving for credibility within the arena of the law. Physicians, prosecutors, police, and scientist were skeptical of those nurses who were seen as infringing on the role of forensic specialists. Physicians criticized nurses for their lack of educational preparation, viewing them as less academically qualified to pronounce death, perform sexual assault examinations, or recover trace and physical evidence at a homicide scene, much less to testify as an expert witness. Yet, the medicolegal communities had always relied on law enforcement personnel who were far less educated or qualified than nurses to perform the same services.

With the 1986 implementation of a master's degree preparing a clinical nurse specialist in forensic nursing, the medicolegal community began to take notice. Now, 20 years have passed and revision of the original and subsequent curricula is essential to keep pace, not only with medicine, law, and science, but also with nursing itself.

The American Nurses Association has urged RNs to achieve a bachelor's degree and nurses with master's degrees to achieve advanced practice status. The American Association of Colleges of Nursing (AACN) position paper has moved to support the practice doctorate as essential for all advanced practitioners to meet the changing needs and advances of the healthcare delivery system. Change is necessary to meet the long-term goals of forensic nursing science as advanced associates to forensic physicians. These advances continue to put legal issues in the forefront of nursing practice, such as licensure issues, independent practice without direct physician supervision, prescriptive authority, admitting privileges, and direct reimbursement for services. Can we afford not to be prepared?

Summary

Forensic nursing, a concept that emerged in professional nursing in the early 1990s, can be related to the four components of nursing as a profession: (1) education, (2) practice, (3) administration, and (4) research and theory. According to the IAFN forensic nursing represents nothing less than "the cutting edge issue in education, practice and research in healthcare in the 21st century." In this context forensic nursing calls for new educational programs to facilitate the *transmission* of new knowledge, direct patient care practices through the clinical *application* of new knowledge, manage administrative functions through the *use* of new knowledge, and foster research and theory through the *development* of new knowledge. These components must be articulated and coordinated toward the full attainment of forensic nursing as a professional practice discipline. McGraw's (1994) adaptation of Maslow's hierarchy of needs, paralleled with empowerment and its antecedent, Chally's (1992) tools for empowerment and Keen's (1988) assertion of power, can be used to conceptualize the world view of forensic nursing and the empowerment of vulnerable populations. The forensic nurse employs these concepts in discussions and decision making to facilitate the integration of victims into all aspects of society.

Empowerment is defined as the enabling of individuals and groups to participate in actions and decision making within a context that supports an equitable distribution of power and requires a commitment to connect between self and others. Antrobus (2001) states that empowerment is a process that enables victims to develop autonomy, self-control, and confidence as well as a collective influence over oppressive social conditions. Empowerment has great utility for nursing practice, education, administration, and research. The forensic nurse appreciates empowerment as a process that can be acquired through teaching and is characterized by caring, commitment, creativity, interaction, and recognition of humanity. The empowered forensic nurse demonstrates caring responses toward complex and sensitive issues related to victims (Lynch, 1993; Watson, 1990). Forensic nurse examiners assist in court-ordered evaluations of the mentally disordered offender, investigations of questioned deaths, and care of survivors of violent crimes and provide support to grieving family members as part of the forensic nursing process. Through empowerment and caring responses, clinical observation, and communication skills, the forensic nurse examiner can bring empathy, compassion, and credibility to the forensic investigation.

Case Study 55-1 Education of the Forensic Nurse in the US

In 1986 there were no options for nurses who considered the value of forensic science in nursing education. At this point nurses were learning about forensic nursing through independent lecture series and educational programs through police department and forensic science organizations.

One nurse, G.P., an emergency department specialist, expert photographer, and one who strongly fought for victim's rights among the patients she cared for, learned that the role she filled was conceptually identified as the role of the forensic nurse examiner. At once, she began to seek more information, opportunities, and education to increase her knowledge in this new field. She soon discovered that every door that could possibly lead to such preparation was closed to her, but she was determined to become a forensic nurse examiner. G.P. joined the forensic science organizations, registered for forensic lectures, and sought training in forensic and criminal justice conferences. She wanted a formal forensic nursing education program, but none was available where she lived. In frustration, she decided to enroll in a master's degree program in forensic science. Although this decision would limit her opportunities in nursing, she felt strongly that it would enhance her visibility and knowledge in the forensic sciences, which she would then apply to her nursing practice.

After succeeding in this degree program and becoming one of the first nurses to have a degree in forensic science, she learned that a new graduate program in forensic nursing had evolved on the East Coast and that they were searching for teachers for these courses. She applied but was told that an advanced degree in nursing was required to teach in a nursing college. Although she had more education in forensic science than any of the faculty, she was denied the opportunity to teach. She knew she wanted to teach and the only option was to enroll as a student in this new forensic nursing program. She did and subsequently obtained a master's degree in nursing.

G.P. is now a forensic nurse leader who is nationally recognized in teaching, consulting, publishing, and clinical practice.

Forensic Nursing Education in Scotland

DAVID W. SADLER

Clinical forensic medicine and forensic nursing have been struggling to achieve proper recognition as academic disciplines worldwide. Although there has been considerable resistance to the recognition of clinical forensic medicine as a specialty in the UK, the increasing need for clinical skills at the medicolegal interface continues to drive improvements in the clinical forensic training of doctors and nurses (Davis, 1994). Currently, the police call upon the services of a doctor for a wide variety of reasons. The commonest request is for provision of healthcare to those detained in police custody, with particular regard to the impact of illness, injury, and drug intoxication/withdrawal on their fitness to be detained or interviewed. Other common requests include assessment of a police officer's fitness to continue his or her duties; examination and collection of evidence from the victims and perpetrators of sexual offenses and other criminal assaults (both adults and children); assessment of intoxication (particularly in relation to road traffic offenses); management of acute psychiatric emergencies in the community; and attendance at the scene of sudden or unexpected deaths.

The History of the Police Surgeon

In the UK and Commonwealth countries, doctors employed by police forces (traditionally known as police surgeons) are now becoming increasingly known as forensic physicians, forensic medical examiners, or forensic medical officers. Most police surgeons are general practitioners working for the National Health Service who make their services available to the police on a part-time contractual basis upon payment of an annual retainer fee plus a fee per item of service.

The first official recognition of the appointment of a doctor to the police in the UK was in 1805 (Summers, 1988). A medical officer was paid £100 per annum to examine recruits and provide medical attention to the Mounted Bow Street Patrol, known as the Robin Redbreasts on account of their red waistcoats. The Association of Police Surgeons of Great Britain (APS) was founded in 1951 to protect the interests of doctors serving various police forces and to facilitate continuing education. Membership of the APS is only about a third of the total number of doctors undertaking police work (Davis, 1994). The clinical diploma in medical jurisprudence (DMJ clin.) of the Society of Apothecaries of London has been the principal postgraduate qualification in clinical forensic medicine since 1961 but has always been better supported by overseas doctors than by those in the UK (Davis, 1994). The society has recently introduced a mastership in medical jurisprudence (MMJ) for physicians wishing to progress beyond the basic diploma. Steps have also been taken to discuss concerns and formalise training in clinical forensic medicine, both in the UK and in Australia (Robinson, 1997; Wells & Cordner, 1998).

Clinical Forensic Nursing in the Police Environment

There is a growing tendency toward the development of a two-tier clinical forensic medicine service (Davis, 1994): (1) *specialists* have appropriate training, qualifications, and court experience to deal with serious forensic cases such as assault, child abuse, and sexual abuse, and (2) *generalists* deal with therapeutic cases requiring the assessment, observation, and treatment of detainees. Although forensic nursing is in its infancy outside the US, the use of forensically trained nurses, primarily in the therapeutic role, is attracting growing worldwide interest (Moon, Kelly, & Savage et al., 1995; Howitt, 1995). An Australian trial successfully utilised trained nurses as the primary medical contact in police custody situations to perform initial triage, basic medical assessment, and administration of appropriate treatments (Young, Wells, & Jackson, 1994). Forensic physicians provided medical consultation and support, as necessary. This service was widely commended by police, nurses, physicians, prison workers, and community groups alike and represented a cost-effective addition to the provision of quality forensic care in larger centres. Although this approach is untried in the UK, initial reaction to the secondment of forensic nurses from emergency departments to certain larger police stations in Central London has also been encouraging.

Key Point *55-3*

Forensic knowledge and skills acquired by a nurse while working in the police setting are valuable assets when they return to staffing positions in the hospital emergency department.

Clinical Forensic Practice in the Emergency Department

Nurses and doctors working in any department have a primary duty of care to the living patient that cannot be compromised (Smialek, 1983). However, patients and society are best served by staff who can also recognise, document, and preserve trace evidence on the assumption that it may later assume great medicolegal significance. In the emergency department, nurses are usually first to see the victims of trauma, to handle their clothing and property, and speak to witnesses. It follows that they may also be the first to suspect the possibility of criminal liability (Hoyt, 1996). The responsibilities associated with treating the victims of trauma reach beyond immediate emergency management and include accurate documentation of injuries, collection and preservation of trace evidence, maintenance of the legal chain of custody, and ensuring that evidentiary procedures are adequately documented and witnessed (Mittleman, Goldberg, & Waksman, 1983; Marsh, 1978). Clothing may harbour vital and invisible trace evidence, such as hairs, fibres, bloodstains, semen, gunshot residues, paint, glass, and soil. Careful removal and separate packaging of clothing and evidence is essential if it is to be preserved for useful scientific and legal evaluation. Even specimens of blood, urine, and stomach contents, collected as a matter of routine, may assume great importance to forensic toxicologists when poisoning is a possibility.

When death from accidental or deliberate trauma occurs in the emergency department, operating theatre or hospital ward, that location becomes the scene of a medicolegal inquiry. The responsibility for "preserving the scene," collecting evidence, and managing the immediate medicolegal issues lies with nursing and medical staff. Under these circumstances, careless disposal of property and clinical material is tantamount to destroying forensic evidence. Personnel must anticipate which deaths are likely to require medicolegal investigation and deal with the issues likely to arise.

Best Practice *55-3*

The forensic nurse must maintain a high index of suspicion about abuse because victims may be unwilling or unable to report the facts.

Detection of physical abuse, sexual abuse, child abuse, and elder abuse requires that health workers are able to recognise the associated injury patterns. Early recognition of stab wounds and gunshot wounds is of particular importance because both are commonly misinterpreted, with serious consequences for both the patient and the attending staff (Smock, 1994; Smialek, 1983).

In many parts of the US clinical forensic practice has passed into the capable hands of forensic nurse specialists (Lynch, 1995). The clinical forensic responsibilities mentioned earlier have been fully embraced by the nursing profession with the development of clinical forensic nursing as a specialty in its own right; other countries could learn from this role. Forensic nurse specialists are specifically trained to deal with cases of sexual assault (McMair & Finegan, 1996), child abuse, acute psychiatric emergencies, and death investigation. Expert witness testimony by forensic nurse specialists is now accepted (Lynch, 1995). In this way the forensic nurse in the US can provide true continuity of care "from trauma to trial."

Forensic Nursing Education

The undergraduate forensic training of nursing and medical students in the UK is inadequate. It is therefore not surprising that nurses and doctors who work with victims of trauma frequently find themselves in difficult situations in the witness box. Feedback previously sought from Scottish nurses indicated that they felt ill-equipped to deal with such important forensic problems as recognising injury patterns, collecting trace evidence, and appearing in court. In view of this, the Department of Forensic Medicine at Dundee introduced an annual three-day Forensic Medicine for Nurses course in 1995. It is commendable that clinical forensic medicine has been incorporated into the training curriculum of emergency physicians in some centres, most notably in Louisville, Kentucky (Smock, 1994). The provision of nursing and medical staff equipped with the knowledge base and technical skills necessary for proper forensic evaluation of living patients should be the rule, not the exception, and widespread adoption of this approach should be encouraged.

The University of Dundee Schools of Nursing, Medicine, and Dentistry have recently merged into a single academic faculty. The new nursing curriculum is implementing problem-based learning techniques with multiprofessional education, shared modules, and integration of nursing and medical students. February 2001 saw the introduction of an optional clinical forensic module as part of the bachelor of nursing degree program. This module comprises 36 contact hours, spread over six days, with self-directed learning and interactive, problem-solving assessment tasks. Content includes injuries, gunshot wounds, trace evidence, bloodstains, alcohol and drugs, suicide, rape, child abuse, death investigation, and court evidence. The module makes full use of Internet and multimedia technologies. Assessment is based on exploration and interpretation of clinical/forensic cases presented as a CD-ROM-based interactive "clickable" multimedia format. Although the module is designed primarily for nursing students, it is also open to other interested health professionals, including lawyers and police personnel. This shared approach has a positive effect on bringing doctors, nurses, and other professionals together, and this will also be of benefit to their patients (Casey & Smith, 1997). Better clinical forensic education will enable the caring professions to instinctively "think forensic" as well as "thinking clinical." The forensic needs of patients should not be overlooked out of ignorance but rather addressed out of knowledge and awareness, as part of the forensic nurse's duty to "do no harm" (Smock, 1994).

Summary

The need for forensic nursing education has been identified. Courses can be provided through academic institutions or continuing education formats. Information may also be provided on site or through distance education modalities. Specialization in forensic nursing is well established and imperative for the future of nursing. Educational programs need identified goals and objectives. The roles and responsibilities of the educational organization, the faculty, and the students cannot be overemphasized. The curriculum must be based on scientific fact and recognized standards of practice. Content must be applied to all the various roles of the forensic nurse. Teaching strategies should focus on active learning principles that provide students with applications to clinical practice. Continuous evaluation is an inherent quality improvement mechanism that can promote quality education. The establishment of a body of knowledge is important for the future of forensic nursing.

Resources

Organizations

American Nurses Credentialing Center

8515 Georgia Avenue, Suite 400, Silver Spring, MD 20910-3402; Tel: 800-284-2378

International Association of Forensic Nurses (IAFN)

East Holly Avenue, Box 56, Pitman, NJ 08071-0056; Tel: 856-256-2425; www.iafn.org

References

United States

Antrobus, P. (2001). Towards an empowerment framework. In S. Bisnath & D. Elson (Eds.), *Background paper for progress for the world's women.* New York: UNIFEM. Retrieved from: www.enterprise-impact.org.uk/pdf/Modedale.pdf.

Chally, P. (1992). Empowerment through teaching. *J Nurs Educ, 31*, 117-120.

Gilligan, C. (1982). *In a different voice: Psychological theory and women's development.* Cambridge, MA: Harvard University Press.

International Association of Forensic Nurses and the American Nurses' Association. (1997). Scope and standards of forensic nursing practice. Washington, DC: ANA Press.

Joint Commission on Accreditation of Healthcare Organizations (JCAHO). (2004). *Accreditation manual for hospitals.* Oakbrook, IL: Author.

Keen, P. (1988). *Manifestations of empowerment.* Unpublished paper.

Lindberg, J. C., Hunter, M. L., & Kruszewski A. Z. (1998). *Introduction to nursing: Concepts, issues and opportunities* (3rd ed.). Philadelphia: J. B. Lippincott.

Lynch, V. (1993). Forensic aspects of health care: New roles, new responsibilities. *J Psychosoc Nurs, 31*(11), 5-6.

McGraw, J. (1994). The road to empowerment. In Hein, E., Nicholson, & M. J., (Eds.). *Contemporary leadership behavior: Selected readings* (4th ed., pp. 227-230). Philadelphia: J.B. Lippincott.

Oxford dictionary of the English language (3rd ed.). (2003). London: Oxford.

Watson, J. (1990). The moral failure of the patriarchy. *Nursing Outlook, 28*(2), 62-66.

Scotland

Casey, N., & Smith, R. (1997). Bringing nurses and doctors closer together. *Br Med J, 314*, 617-618.

Davis, N. (1994). What now–what next? The future of clinical forensic medicine in the UK. *J Clin Forensic Med, 1*, 47-49.

Howitt, J. B. (1995). Clinical forensic medical services: London and Melbourne contrasted. *J Clin Forensic Med, 2*, 17-24.

Hoyt, C. A. (1996). Forensic nursing implications and the autopsy. *J Psychosoc Nurs Ment Health Serv, 34*(10), 24-31.

Lynch, V. (1995). Clinical forensic nursing: A new perspective in the management of crime victims from trauma to trial. *Crit Care Nurs Clin North Am, 7*(3), 489-507.

Marsh, T. O. (1978). A nurse's guide to sleuthing (or how to collect evidence, hospital style). *RN, 41*(8), 48-50.

Mittleman, R. E., Goldberg, H. S., & Waksman, D. M. (1983). Preserving evidence in the emergency department. *Am J Nurs, 83*, 1652-1656.

McNair, S. M., & Finegan, A. B. (1996). The role of a forensic clinical nurse specialist in a sexual assault treatment program. *J Clin Forensic Med, 3*, 29-30.

Moon, G., Kelly, K., Savage, S. P., et al. (1995). Developing Britain's police surgeon service. *Br Med J, 311*, 1587.

Robinson, S. (1997). Future of education in clinical forensic medicine: Summary of multidisciplinary forum. *J Clin Forens Med, 4*, 145-150.

Robertson, G. (1993). The role of the police surgeon. Royal Commission on Criminal Justice Research Study number 6. London: HMSO.

Smialek, J. E. (1983). Forensic medicine in the emergency department. *Emerg Med Clin North Am, 1*(3), 693-704.

Smock, W. S. (1994). Development of a clinical forensic medicine curriculum for emergency physicians in the USA. *J Clin Forensic Med, 1*, 27-30.

Summers, R. D. (1988). *The history of the police surgeon.* London: Association of Police Surgeons of Great Britain.

Wells, D., & Cordner, S. (1998). Postgraduate education in clinical forensic medicine: A graduate diploma. *J Clin Forensic Med, 5*, 187-190.

Young, S., Wells, D., & Jackson, G. (1994). A tiered healthcare system for persons in police custody: The use of a forensic nursing service. *J Clin Forensic Med, 1*, 21-25.

Chapter 56 Global Perspectives on Forensic Nursing

Virginia A. Lynch

These are extraordinary times for personnel in the health sciences, and both challenges and opportunities abound in every sector of healthcare delivery. A healthy world cannot be achieved merely within a vacuum of highly industrialized nations. Antiquated laws and social policies, restrictive family values, and inequalities affect access and delivery of healthcare in various countries. Forensic medical and forensic nursing personnel have been among the first to step forward and become involved in the global issues of healthcare.

Contemporary healthcare curricula are being restructured to respond to many challenges, including preparation for practice in a global environment. This requires that healthcare professionals gain broad understandings of the complex social and political factors inherent in world cultures. The dynamics of archaic cultural traditions and religious practices will continue to have an impact and pose threats to the most vulnerable subjects in each of these societies, namely, women, children, the elderly, the disabled, and those in extreme poverty.

Nursing and other healthcare professionals in the US and other highly developed countries need to be reminded that their countries receive the greatest number of immigrants and refugees who are survivors of war, torture, and victims of cultural practices that have maimed and crippled them, physically and emotionally. Some of these individuals will have lived in countries where doctors, nurses, and police may have participated in their imprisonment, mutilation, and evaluation of survivability related to the extent of punishment or torture. An awareness of cultural and traditional practices such as female genital mutilation, honor killings, bride burning, dowry deaths, child prostitution, and lack of education for women must be fostered within basic educational programs. Opportunities must be provided to assist nurses in understanding the diseases, psychological scarring, and other human conditions that emerge as a result of such practices. Perhaps most essential, nurses need to appreciate their role and responsibilities in taking action required to successfully cope with the sequelae of adverse social, cultural, and ethnic phenomena.

The following sections provide examples of the historical development and contemporary trends of forensic nursing in selected countries.

United Kingdom

LYNDA FILER

Police Surgeons and Forensic Medical Examiners

Since Victorian times, the medical care of people in custody in police stations in the UK has been undertaken by registered medical practitioners, who are general practitioners (family doctors) that combine their general medical practice with clinical forensic medicine (Summers, 1988). They held the "courtesy" title of *police surgeon,* which was a courtesy because, except for possibly the suturing of prisoners, very little surgery was performed in the police station and they were certainly not viewed as part of the ranks of the local police force. In recent years, to emphasize their independence from the police, these individuals have been designated as forensic medical examiners (FME) in many parts of the UK.

The duties of the FMEs are wide ranging and include determining the fitness of a prisoner for custody, providing care for prisoners in custody, examining the victims of assault, and obtaining samples of bodily fluids or tissues for forensic examination (McLay, 1990). In addition, FMEs have become involved in assessing "fitness for interview"–an exercise that can be very time-consuming. By the mid-1980s the workload of the then police surgeons in urban areas was rising considerably, in part due to the general increase in the use of illicit drugs (Wright & Pearl, 1995) and the introduction of the Police and Criminal Evidence Act 1984.

The Police and Criminal Evidence Act 1984 states that the custody officer must immediately call the police surgeon if a person brought to a police station and detained there exhibits the following:

- Appears to be suffering from physical illness or a mental disorder; or is injured;
- Fails to respond normally to a question or conversation (other than through drunkenness alone);
- Or otherwise appears to need medical attention. (Police and Criminal Evidence Act, 1984, revised Codes of Practice, 1995, p. 47)

Furthermore, it states, "If a detained person has in his possession or claims to need medication relating to a heart condition, diabetes, epilepsy or a condition of comparable potential seriousness, then the advice of the Police Surgeon must be obtained" (Police and Criminal Evidence Act, 1995, p. 48). In the notes for guidance concluding the Section on "Medical Treatment of Detained Persons," custody officers are told "the need to call a Police Surgeon need not apply to minor ailments or injuries that do not need medical attention" (Police and Criminal Evidence Act, 1995, p. 49). The way the act is worded, it does require the custody officer to use discretion as to whether an FME needs to be called; however, the officers usually err on the side of caution and call the FME.

On the purely practical aspects of management, the problems or difficulties associated with the monitoring of "patient's" level of consciousness, while in police custody, has been a source of concern to FMEs for decades. Representatives of the Association of Police Surgeons gave the House of Commons, Home Affairs Committee evidence on death investigations in police custody dating as far back as 1980.

Box 56-1 Nursing Role in Police Stations

Patients*	Professional monitoring
	Supervise the administration of medicine
	Reduction in level of apprehension
Police	Presence of immediate medical care
	Release from medical responsibilities, e.g., administration of drugs
	Release of manpower, e.g., chaperone for female prisoners
Physician	Nursing assistance with prisoners
	Nursing assistance to victims
	"Peace of mind"

*Patient is a generic term for anyone needing medical attention within the confines of a police station.

By 1988, consideration was starting to be given to the possibility of having suitably trained nurses in police stations. In 1989, it was acknowledged that although there was an increase in the standard of forensic medicine of the UK, there continued to be poor backup facilities in police stations (Filer & Filer, 1989). At the World Police Medical Officers Conference at Harrogate in 1993, (Filer & Filer, 1993) the potential advantages of skilled nurses in police stations were identified (Box 56-1).

The Audit Commission (1998) reviewed the provision of forensic medical services and found that 85% of the role of the FME was nonforensic and was actually therapeutic in nature. This nonforensic role included treatment of minor injuries and ailments, which could be carried out by nurses in the same manner that they are in other healthcare settings.

General Forensic Nursing

Until recent years, the concept of forensic nursing in the UK had generally been limited to that of the role of the forensic psychiatric nurse; the concept of general forensic nurses in England is new (Whyte, 1997). Although there had been advancements in forensic nursing in the US, Canada, and other parts of the world (Lynch, 1995; McNair & Finigan, 1996), the roles that had been identified differed from those envisioned in the English police station. Because FMEs are not resident in the police station, nurses may well find themselves involved in critical situations without the usual support provided in hospitals. FMEs are also not resident in the accident and emergency department, which leaves an interval between the time a forensic patient is admitted and intervention of forensic services. The FME does not provide emergency medical treatment, but rather provides documentation of injury and recovery of evidence, among other forensic services. Conversely, the presence of a clinical forensic nurse on duty 24-7 can provide immediate forensic services, decreasing the interval prior to forensic intervention, and further decreasing an unnecessary workload on the FME as it parallels the role of the custody nurse examiner.

In January 2000, a three-month pilot scheme was started, with nurses working in custody suites in the county of Kent, England. The custody nurses provided 24-hour cover and their duties involved assessment and treatment of minor injuries and monitoring the fitness of detainees, particularly those with drug- and alcohol-related problems. Most of the nurses employed for the pilot study came from nursing posts in accident and emergency departments, and they all undertook an induction course to assist with the adaptation to their forensic nursing role in the custody suite environment (Moore, 2001). An independent evaluation of the pilot custody nursing scheme was positive, and since then the use of custody nurses has been extended throughout Kent (Moore, 2001). The use of forensic nurse examiners in custody suites is now being explored in other parts of the UK. Two recent initiatives in forensic and nursing science have included the introduction of the sexual assault nurse examiner role in Manchester, and the use of custody nurses for certain death investigation duties within secured environments.

The police station is the only place in clinical medical practice outside the home where ill patients are "nursed" by laypersons, very often young inexperienced police officers. The use of forensic nurses in the police station setting can assist in improving the standard of care to the detained person and also ensure that the specialist skills of the FME are concentrated on the more forensic aspects of their role.

England and Wales

JANE E. RUTTY

The Coroner's Role

The majority of medical and nursing professions in the UK confuse the forensic nurse as being synonymous with forensic psychiatric nursing. However, the discipline of forensic nursing is a broad field that encompasses not only forensic psychiatric nursing, but also nurses working within the arena of death investigation, sexual assault, legal nurse consulting, correctional nursing, and clinical forensic nursing, among other forensic nursing roles (Lynch, 1997). Forensic psychiatric nursing has a long history within the UK and is recognized in its own right as a nursing profession.

The close association of the forensic nurse examiner in death investigation and the role of the coroner has become a significant faction within forensic pathology and clinical forensic medicine in many progressive countries, such as the US, Canada, Singapore, and South Africa. Sexual assault nurse examiners, legal nurse consultants, forensic nurse clinicians, and forensic nurse death investigators are only now emerging within England and Wales.

Historically, the coroner is one of the oldest judicial positions of the English legal system. Indeed, as long ago as Saxon times (fifth century) there is evidence of the existence of a coroner at least in name (McGee & Mason, 1990). It was not until soon after the Norman Conquest in 1066 that the power of the coroner was reinforced, as officials whose purpose it was to inquire into sudden unexpected deaths, with the primary duty of determining whether the deceased was English or Norman.

The establishment of the office, though, is commonly assigned to over 100 years later during King Richard's reign in the publication of the Articles of Eyre in 1194, an Eyre denoting a periodical circuit of justices. King Richard placed in office during this time some of his knights as "custos plactitorum coronae," which translates as "keeper of the pleas of the crown." This title across the centuries has transformed into "crowner" and finally to "coroner" (Dorries, 1999). The responsibilities of the original coroners included taking charge of the records and financial concerns of the crown, especially in accordance to the deaths of the monarch's subjects.

The coroner has survived a long and eventful history including the near extinction of the position in the seventeenth and eighteenth centuries. Nevertheless, the office has regained a position of importance in the English legal system in the last 100 years as the principal route for the investigation of sudden death (McGee & Mason, 1990).

Today, the coroner is a registered medical practitioner or a lawyer who has held a general qualification within Section 71 of the Courts and Legal Services Act 1990 for a minimum of five years (HMSO, 1988; 1990). The appointment is still made by the local authority to a geographical district known now as a jurisdiction. However, the coroner is an independent judicial officer, responsible only to the crown (Her Majesty Queen Elizabeth II) and cannot be dismissed by anyone other than the Lord Chancellor.

Currently, whenever a person dies, the law requires the death to be registered. In order for this to be effected there are two strict and rigid essential conditions that must be satisfied: a valid certificate supplying the cause of death must be completed and signed by a registered medical practitioner who attended the deceased during his last illness; and the cause of death must be shown to be entirely natural and prove satisfactory to the registrar of deaths in accordance with the Registration of Births and Deaths Regulations (1987). It is in all other cases that the death must be referred to the coroner.

The purpose of the coroner is still to investigate the causes of sudden or unexpected deaths (those that have to be reported to the coroner are listed in Box 56-2). If the death is violent or accidental, or there are suspicious circumstances, the police will also have to be informed (HMSO, 1988).

Generally, with regard to all deaths in England and Wales, approximately 33% demand the coroner to be informed. In a certain number of cases preliminary explorations with the deceased's general practitioner will indicate that the death was caused by natural causes and therefore no more additional investigations are needed. Despite this, with regard to the deaths informed to the coroner, approximately 75% will need further investigation by way of an autopsy examination.

The Autopsy

The autopsy, from the Greek word "autopsia," meaning "seeing with one's own eyes," is a medical examination of a body after death, with the basic purpose of determining, among other things, the ultimate cause of death (Petrakis, 1995). The relatives have no right to refuse an autopsy when requested by the coroner, but they do have a right to have a doctor of their own choice present, at their own expense (HMSO, 1984).

The autopsy is carried out following the coroner's consent and direction, by a fully registered medical practitioner (HMSO, 1988). When the circumstances surrounding the death are considered to be suspicious a Home Office–approved forensic pathologist is usually directed by the coroner following the request of the police to perform the autopsy. The autopsy examination will uncover a natural cause of death in the majority of cases; however, a coroner's inquest will be required by law for about 12% of cases which remain to be uncovered as an unnatural cause of death (Dorries, 1999). Additionally, an inquest can be conducted at the discretion of the coroner if the coroner considers it desirable to allay suspicion or public disquiet (Burton, Chambers, & Gill, 1985).

Coroner's Inquest

The coroner's inquest is an inquiry, not a trial; in other words, it is confined to discovering who the deceased person was and how, when, and where that person came to their death, together with information needed by the registrar of deaths, to enable the death to be registered (HMSO, 1996). Therefore, there are no parties, indictments, prosecutions, defenses, trials, legal aid, or award of costs, and no enforceable judgments or orders can be made.

Witnesses to the death are likely to be asked to provide a statement and may well be called to give evidence at the inquest, which is usually held in public. Witnesses are not obliged to answer questions if this may incriminate themselves (HMSO, 1984), as the motive of the inquest is not to ascertain any criminal liability against any named person, or any question of civil liability, as a trial would. On the contrary, the intent of the inquest is to purely establish the facts. Nevertheless, it ought to be realized that the facts exposed in the evidence could provide possible foundations for an action of civil damages.

The inquest may proceed without a jury unless the circumstances of the death indicate that there may be a continuing risk to the health and safety of the public (HMSO, 1988). In other cases, coroners have a discretion to hold jury inquests if they choose.

As well as defining the actual cause of death, there is a suggested range of verdicts that can be delivered at the end of a coroner's inquiry (HMSO, 1984). Decisions concerning the cause of death range from unlawful killing to death aggravated by lack of care (Montgomery, 1997). An open verdict would indicate that the means have not been found as to how the cause of death arose (Dorries, 1990).

In summary, it can be seen that the coroner's inquiry begins when a registered medical practitioner is unable to ascertain that the cause of a person's death was natural and so the case is consequently referred to the coroner. The inquiry is complete when the cause of death is known and the information for registration of death has been gathered and completed.

Box 56-2 Deaths That Must Be Reported to Her Majesty's Coroner

1. There is reasonable cause to suspect a person has died a violent or unnatural death.
2. There is reasonable cause to suspect a person has died a sudden death of which the cause is unknown.
3. The person has died in prison or in such place or under such circumstances as to require an inquest.

Causes of death that should be reported to the coroner include abortions; accidents and injuries; acute alcoholism; anesthetics and operations; crime or suspected crime; drugs; ill-treatment; industrial diseases; infant deaths if in any way obscure; pensioners for whom death might be connected with a pensionable disability; persons in legal custody; poisoning; septicemias if originating from an injury; and stillbirths if there is a possibility or suspicion that the child may have been born alive.

Data from Dimond, B. (1995). *Legal aspects of nursing* (2nd ed.) Upper Saddle River, NJ: Prentice Hall.

The Concealed Forensic Nurse

Green (1994) suggests that nursing staff in general is becoming increasingly more involved in legal processes with relevance to their observations, records, and recall of events. Internationally, nurses have embraced their role more extensively within aspects of the legal profession with the ultimate example of the ability of nurses to be coroners in the US. Sadly, within England and Wales the role of the nurse has been poorly addressed, with many nurses themselves not considering this as an area that they should be involved in. Additionally, except for the research by Rutty (2000), there are minimal peer-reviewed published articles within the nursing or medical literature to date that evaluates or reflects on nursing within this area of practice in England and Wales. Death investigation is an area of great upheaval in people's lives, yet it is one the nursing profession seems to have forgotten.

Over 20 years ago, the Department of Health and Social Security stated that no matter what changes occur regarding the nurse's professional role, the essence of the profession will always be about caring for people. In 1996, Henderson, too, referred to care when she said that nursing would never be seen as anything less than essential to the human race. The Royal College of Nursing (RCN) stated that nursing is based on a combination of professional knowledge and skills, with the desire to care for others. It is with these beliefs in mind and the foresight regarding the contributions that forensic nursing already makes to death investigation that this research was completed (Rutty, 2000). In fact, it can now be seen that the nursing profession in England and Wales has a great deal to offer the coroner's inquiry.

According to Home Office forensic pathologists and coroners in England and Wales, nurses of all specialties as part of their everyday work are contributing in some way to death investigation (Rutty, 2000). Such roles can be split into those that contribute indirectly to the coroner's inquiry to those that are more directly involved.

Indirect Contributions to the Coroner's Inquiry

Nurses contribute regularly to coroners' inquiries, but in the majority of cases will never be aware of their input (Rutty & Rutty, 2000). Such indirect nursing roles include record keeping and knowing nursing policy. Coroners and forensic pathologists, to aid in death investigations, commonly read records from all nursing specialties. These nursing records are perceived as being extremely valuable and depicted as being a way to gain a perspective of a situation that extends beyond the presented facts. Medical notes are affected by the nurses having a certain intimacy or closeness with their patients. Interestingly, though, computerized records are not favored, as there is a fear that a valuable nursing tool is being lost by the inability to record unusual events. Nurses, more than other professions, understand, empathize, and present patient views holistically. Nursing records are conceptually part of a large and sometimes complicated puzzle during a coroner's inquiry in England and Wales.

Key Point *56-1*

In England, the old saying in forensic pathology is, "If you want to know what should have happened, read the medical notes, but if you want to know what really happened, read the nursing records" (Rutty 1998).

The role of "knowing" is described as the importance of all nurses acquiring knowledge about the coroner's inquiry (RCN, 1992). Gaining such knowledge enables nurses to perform their role when required to a higher standard concerning death investigation, in turn promoting family care of the deceased patient. This may be having the knowledge to advise families about organ transplantation or by explaining why an autopsy is required or by providing information on death certification.

Nursing policies are designed to clarify what constitutes acceptable practice and guards against risk by incorporating suitable safeguards (Grimshaw, Freemantle, & Wallace et al., 1995). Developing and strengthening nursing policy from a forensic perspective is a role particularly important to coroners who come from a legal professional background (Rutty, 2000). Nursing policies provide the coroners with guidelines and directives that assist them in determining whether or not the acceptable standards of practice were followed in a given case. However, being able to clarify and justify nurse practice decisions through strong evidence aids not only the coroner but significantly assists the bereaved family in understanding the circumstances surrounding their loved one's death.

Direct Contributions to the Coroner's Inquiry

The potential for nurses to be directly involved in a coroner's inquiry is gaining recognition. As part of a multidisciplinary team in healthcare, the nurse need not attempt to deal with issues surrounding patient death by themselves. The nurse can, however, act after the death of a patient as a resource provider to relatives by sharing knowledge with them concerning the coronial process. For example, if the death is to be investigated by the coroner or even the police, the nurse can assist relatives by directing the family to other relevant professionals such as bereavement counselors and coroners' officers who can help them further. This role is performed after a patient has died, but before relatives have left the ward/unit in a hospital environment. The guidance provided to grieving family members and friends may prove invaluable in helping them to comply with unfamiliar procedures at a difficult time in their lives (Davis, 1994).

Best Practice *56-1*

Nurses should ensure that they care for the decedent's family and significant others at the time of death.

A parallel role for the nurse is that of communicator (Rutty, 2000). This role embraces initial communication between bereaved relatives and the multidisciplinary team. Without frequent and direct communication by nurses to all concerned, good multidisciplinary team interaction cannot always be guaranteed (Kyle, 1995).

Benner (1984) suggested that nurses are often educated to believe that they are most effective when doing something practical for a patient. Several nurses in her study, however, noted the essential importance and value of just being with a patient, otherwise known as *presencing*. Similar to this, coroners believe, too, that if an inquiry is held, the role of the nurse in *presencing* is perceived as becoming important (Rutty, 2000). *Presencing* is described as the presence of a nurse known to the relatives during the coroner's inquest in court. It is believed that *presencing* can have a tremendous calming effect on relatives at such a difficult time in their lives.

Davis (1994) has previously suggested that families involved in a coroner's inquiry may suddenly feel pushed aside or helpless, particularly if they were involved in care decisions while their loved one was alive. The caring relationship that nurses have established with relatives extends the role of patient advocacy throughout the coroner's inquiry.

A final role in which nurses are contributing directly to the coroner's inquiry in England and Wales relates to that of evidence giver, either in the form of written or verbal evidence. When nurses are required to give evidence regarding their witness to fact, first they write a statement, which in some hospital and community trusts are then formally submitted to their managers, who forward this on to the coroner. No more may be required from the nurse. However, in some cases, nurses will be needed to give evidence verbally in a coroner's inquest in the coroner's court, where they will answer questions related to the case. Many nurses, though, have minimal or no training or education in preparing written statements (Rutty & Rutty, 2000).

Similarly, the arts of verbal evidence giving and dealing with cross-examination of nurses in court are not highly valued by coroners and forensic pathologists, who often perceive nurses as confused and unprepared (Rutty, 2000). Despite these views, the nurse as evidence giver makes a major contribution to the coroner's inquiry; the contribution is one that is predicted to develop through experience and education and, more important, one that is required more than ever before.

The Future of Forensic Nursing

The coroners and forensic pathologists of England and Wales (Rutty, 2000) proffered and debated two future nursing roles in the area of death investigation. One role is "verifying (or certifying) the fact of death" as opposed to determining the cause of death, which by law remains purely within the domain of medical practitioners. Coroners are open-minded and ready to consider that this could be a role for nurses, but forensic pathologists are deeply divided. Some hospitals are now educating nurses in the verification of death relating it to the scope of professional practice (UKCC, 1992). This means some nurses can now perform last offices and transfer the deceased to the mortuary without a doctor needing to attend to confirm patient death. Nevertheless, the situations in which it would be appropriate or inappropriate for the nurse to verify death have not as yet been clearly defined.

The second future nursing role proffered is that of nurses as expert witnesses. Coroners and forensic pathologists on the whole embrace this concept positively. All grades of nurses may qualify as either an ordinary or professional witness, but qualifying as an expert witness when opinions are provided concerning nursing practice is considered a role relevant only to senior nurses and a role that would be accepted in the coroner's inquiry only occasionally at present. Despite its current infrequency, it is a role that will expand in the future as the roles of the advanced nurse practitioner, the nurse consultant, and nurse-led healthcare services in the UK continue to proliferate and advance in scope and practice (RCN, 2000).

The coroner's inquiry in England and Wales has existed for centuries. The coroner's aim remains the same: to discover who the deceased was and how, when, and where that person came to death. Henderson (1966) believed that part of the nurse's role is to assist patients to a peaceful death. Davis (1994) took this one step further by suggesting that the role of patient advocacy goes beyond death. Rutty (2000) has shown that nurses are contributing on a regular basis to the coroner's inquiry and death investigation. It is a role that needs recognition, exposure, acceptance, and development before it can be maximized to its best potential in enhancing family care. It is time for nursing in the UK to take the lead in building partnerships in clinical practice, education, and research, but it is imperative that the underlying intention of upholding and promoting patient advocacy and family care remains.

Canada

SHEILA EARLY

Forensic nursing in Canada has been identified as an emerging trend over the past 30 years. Canada has focused on the areas in which nursing interfaces with the law, primarily pertaining to the forensic aspects of psychiatry, emergency medicine, criminology, corrections, and death investigation. Four forensic nursing subspecialties are strongly represented in Canada: forensic psychiatric nursing, forensic correctional nursing, the medical examiner's investigator, and sexual assault nurse examiner. In the earliest stages of development, the role of the forensic nurse examiner in Canada has expanded to include this subspecialty of nurses who provide care for the sexual assaulted patient, both living and deceased. The moving forces in each of these fields have worked collaboratively to define and differentiate these roles in respect to each unique subspecialty of forensic nursing as a scientific discipline.

Death Investigation

In the office of the Chief Medical Examiner a forensic nurse investigator is one who applies nursing knowledge in the investigation of any medicolegal death. Medicolegal death includes expected and unexpected or violent deaths, wherever the cause of death is unclear or remotely suspicious.

The forensic nurse has become a valuable associate in the role of the medical examiner (ME) or coroner's investigator when biomedical deaths, catastrophic accidents, and criminal violence require a forensic review. In specific provinces the forensic nurse examiner may be appointed to the position of coroner. Any death that must be reported to a legal agency is categorized as a forensic case and is mandated by law to be investigated. In 1975, Dr. John Butt, Chief Medical Examiner, in Calgary, Alberta, was the first to recognize that the registered nurse represented a valuable resource to the field of death investigation, and he established a program whereby registered nurses functioned as medical examiner's investigators. At that time he cited nurses' biomedical education (with emphasis on their knowledge of medical terminology and pharmacology), psychosocial skills, the ability to empathize, and experience in public relations as necessary qualifications. These skills prepare nurses to effectively carry out the role of the forensic nures examiner (FNE): being present at the death scene, handling confidential material, and relaying sensitive information to family members. (Lynch, 1993a).

More than half of the medical examiner's caseload comprises natural deaths that require no high investigative profile involving law enforcement agencies, so the use of forensic nurse examiners (FNEs) in these cases allows police officers to devote more time to criminal investigations. Butt stressed the importance of teamwork between the criminal and biomedical investigative personnel, expressing concern that medically untrained officers often disregarded medical evidence, maintained poor sensitivity, and were noncommunicative with grieving families. Conversely, healthcare professionals recognized the importance of the integrity of criminal evidence, the suspect interview, and the investigation of leads (Lynch, 1993a).

Since that time, Canadian nurses function as ME investigators or coroner in several provinces and territories. In 1990, Kent Stewart, BSN, RN, became the chief coroner of the Yukon Territory, maintaining jurisdiction over 483,000 square miles and involving a vast group of native people. This required an incisive knowledge of cause of death, cultural traits, and social and religious perspectives among this population. Other provinces continue to evaluate this unique approach to legal inquires into the deaths of their citizens. One constraint that has prevented a greater application of nurse investigators has been certain stipulations in the law that require only physicians to serve as the officiator of death. However, those provinces are currently considering ways to reinterpret or change these statutes in order to incorporate nurses into their systems. When this role became recognized as a valuable resource to death investigation systems across Canada, the US began to take notice.

As a result of the Canadian experience, the forensic nurse investigative role became preferred in many death investigation systems in the US. The nurses' expertise in death investigation is being recognized in numerous archaic systems in which lay officiators of death have been outdated in today's concerned society (Lynch, 1993a). However, integrating the forensic nurse investigator in certain provinces has been difficult owing to different statutes defining the coroner system in some provinces. Resistance to change due to the lack of knowledge and recognition of this new concept is also a deterrent in incorporating the forensic nurse investigator in Canada. According to Vernon McCarty, "the application of nursing science to the law in death investigation is probably the least understood of societal and governmental processes, because it has not been a traditional role for nurses in the past" (McCarty, 1985).

Key Point *56-2*

In forensic nursing, the healthcare profession is represented in a holistic concept of human relationship to all health processes. Dying, as well as living, produces important needs in a society concerned with disease prevention and health maintenance (Lynch, 1993).

The achievement of Dr. Butt represents results of the long overdue quest for an improved method of death investigation. This pioneering project has helped to extend a vital resource to forensic pathologists beyond the borders of Canada and into other countries concerned with an accurate, scientific cause and manner of death.

Forensic Psychiatric Nursing

According to Kent-Wilkinson, forensic psychiatric nursing in Calgary began in 1976, with the opening of an eight-bed forensic unit at the Calgary Remand Center. In 1978, the forensic unit moved to the specially designed 20-bed unit on the eighth floor of the Calgary General Hospital. In 1980, the forensic unit was granted a Significant Achievement Award, by the American Psychiatric Association of Hospital and Community Psychiatry. It was recognized as unique, being the only one of its kind providing forensic psychiatric services in a general hospital setting.

In February 1993, the World Health Organization (WHO) designated the Calgary General Hospital's Department of Psychiatry a collaborating center for research and training in mental health. Only seven other such centers in mental health exist throughout the world. Under the directorship of Dr. Arboleda-Flo'rez, this department became the first center in the world in the area of forensic psychiatry to offer policy advice, education, and research to the World Health Organization.

Offenders from the justice system are most often sent to the unit for comprehensive psychiatric assessments to determine fitness to stand trial. Assessments include presentence, pretrial, and occasionally parole assessments. Offenders may also be sent from the justice system for treatment.

Forensic Correctional Nursing

Forensic correctional nursing is defined as the provision of bio-psycho-social nursing care to individuals who have been charged with or convicted of a crime. Since the mid-1960s, nurses have worked in corrections in Calgary, in adult and young offender centers, offering a full range of on-site healthcare services. Correctional nurses are primary practitioners and caregivers who coordinate the effort of all other healthcare professionals (physicians, dentists, psychiatrists, and psychologists). Correctional nurses provide a critical liaison with operations and administration of the facility.

Key Point *56-3*

The role of the correctional nurse is a dynamic combination of primary care, health promotion and education, physical and mental healthcare, and the delivery of emergency medical services to a forensic population in a forensic institution.

The Blair Report in 1974 brought with it many proposals for needed change to healthcare in Canadian prisons. It cited the deplorable state of healthcare conditions in Canadian penal institutions. In 1975, Shirley Hinds, RN, was hired by the Department of Corrections to provide nursing care and establish systems to improve the quality of healthcare. At first, Hinds was not allowed access behind security. At that time it was an all-male population and because Hinds was female, she was not allowed into the living units. Through perseverance and hard work, she was able to successfully cross the barriers. In 1984, Hinds chaired a committee to develop standards of practice for correctional nurses (Hinds, 1994).

Sexual Assault Care

The forensic nurse examiner (FNE) who specializes in the care of the sexually assaulted patient of any age or gender as a sexual assault nurse examiner (SANE) is performing one of the eight roles of the FNE recognized by the International Association of

Forensic Nurses (IAFN). The term sexual assault nurse examiner refers to the registered nurse who has advanced education in forensic examinations of sexual assault victims (Ledray, 1999). Because the categories of victim specifications and the circumstances of the assault often fall within the domain of child physical abuse, elderly abuse, gunshot wounds, knife wounds, or victim of homicide, enhanced forensic nursing skills are now recognized as crucial in the practice of the SANE. According to Lynch (2003) the FNE is cross-trained in a wide range of forensic interventions and reaches beyond the individual role of one subspecialty.

Canada consists of 10 provinces and three territories with a population of 32.5 million people. The mandate of healthcare is a provincial one with the costs of healthcare shared between the national and provincial/territorial governments. The Ministry of Health provides national direction for healthcare, and each provincial/territorial branch of the Ministry of Health is responsible for the management of healthcare within that locale.

SANE Programs in Canada

The SANE role in Canada is potentially the forensic nursing role with the greatest opportunity for expansion over the next decade. The first SANE program in Canada was implemented in April 1993 in Winnipeg, Manitoba, at the Health Sciences Center adult emergency department. The second Canadian SANE program followed in November 1993 in Surrey, British Columbia, at Surrey Memorial Hospital. Utilization of the SANE in a network of provincial sexual assault care and treatment centers began in Ontario in 1995 with 75 nurse examiners trained to work in 28 centers throughout the province. BC Women's Hospital sexual assault service (SAS) in Vancouver, British Columbia, added nurse examiners to its physician-based program in 1995. Victoria, British Columbia, developed a SANE program in 1996. In 1999, Edmonton, Alberta, initiated a two-year pilot project: Sexual Assault Response Team of Edmonton (SARTE) program as the first SANE program in that province. In the short time span of 11 years from 1993 to 2004, FNE programs have developed in five of Canada's 10 provinces.

Impetus for Forensic Nurse Examiners in Canada

Awareness of the SANE role in Canada was recognized in two provinces early in 1991 in Manitoba and in British Columbia in 1992. Information from programs in the US provided the basis for examining the possibilities of training nurses to care for patients who present for sexual assault examination. Physician-based programs were present in centers across Canada, but were mainly located in populous areas of each province. Patient care issues cited as being influential in developing SANE programs included long waits for patients to be examined, inexperienced or untrained nurses and physicians, insensitive reactions to victims/survivors by emergency staff, lack of support for patients and family, no follow-up patient care, difficulty in maintaining physician rosters to provide care, inadequate or incomplete forensic evidence collection, inconsistent chain of custody for evidence practices, and inconsistent case documentation. In Alberta, prior to the implementation of the sexual assault response team (SART), patients waited up to five hours.

The Sexual Assault Center of Edmonton (SACE) provided two nonmedical volunteers to wait with the patient. The role of the volunteer was to support the patient during the wait for the emergency department examination and to provide community resource information. The volunteer was often subpoenaed to court for testimony as to the emotional state of the patient, which is beyond the expertise of nonmedical volunteers and should remain strictly within the scope of nursing practice.

Ontario recognized that the role of the FNE was accomplished within the scope of nursing practice and that the utilization of healthcare professionals could be maximized through a SANE program. The success of these existing programs provided the impetus for the development of a provincial network of care centers. With the initiation and implementation of successful FNE programs in Winnipeg, Manitoba, and Surrey, British Columbia, in 1993, FNEs and SANEs became new titles in the vocabulary of nursing. Ontario developed its provincial SANE program in a quest to establish standardization in service provision of accessible, comprehensive, high-quality care for sexually assaulted patients and, more recently, domestic violence patients as well, thus advancing to a full FNE program. Established SANE programs assisted new programs to become reality.

In 1995, BC Women's Hospital SAS was designated the provincial resource for sexual assault care and received special funding to assist communities throughout the province in developing and implementing nurse examiner programs. The impetus for Alberta's program also originated from a need to provide timely care to patients who presented to emergency departments, with standardization of methods of collecting forensic evidence, taking of photographs, and providing treatment via medical protocols. Nova Scotia's only program was initiated after researching other programs in North America to address the identified need for care for the sexually assaulted patient within 72 hours, providing medical treatment, forensic evidence collection, expert testimony in courts of law, and appropriate referrals for patients. The Moncton, New Brunswick, nurse examiner program was initiated following a regional National Emergency Nurses' Affiliation conference in 2002 when two BC forensic nurse examiners, Janet Calnan and Sheila Early, presented a workshop on SANE programs. Early met with medical, nursing, law enforcement, victim services, and government officials to provide guidance in program development.

Developing and Maintaining SANE Programs

Developing and maintaining SANE programs has not been without difficulties, as witnessed by programs that have trained nurse examiners but have not been able to either become established or continue to maintain a service. The difficulties cited for the demise of programs include lack of resources for programs, inability to retain nurse examiners, lack of adequate salary, lack of support from other healthcare professionals, lack of sustained clinical experience (numbers of patients examined too low), sustained funding issues, and lack of clinical and administrative support for programs. Funding SANE programs is an ongoing problem. Hospitals often do not have the money in their budgets, and sexual assault care is not viewed as a fiscal healthcare priority. Smaller communities often want to start a SANE program but are unable to find enough interested nurses within a small community to maintain a 24-hour roster and to offer enough examinations for SANEs to obtain the necessary experience, skills, and confidence.

The funding structure for SANE programs in Canada is very individual, depending on the province and the community in which the program exists. Ontario, with its network of sexual assault care and treatment centers, is the most stable of the Canadian programs. The funding for Ontario's network comes from the provincial Ministry of Health, which also funds a provincial coordinator, who is based in Women's College Hospital (WCH), Toronto. Toronto provides provincial training for nurse examiners twice a year, and approximately 50 nurse examiners from centers across the province are trained at WCH in Toronto each year. The Manitoba Health Plan is billed for forensic examinations, and nurse examiners are also paid from this budget, which funds the Winnipeg, Manitoba, sexual assault program. In British Columbia each SANE program is independent and the funding structure is varied. The first SANE program in Surrey, BC, was initially funded as a pilot project through the Surrey Memorial Hospital Foundation. When the pilot project was completed, obtaining alternate funding was a monumental task. Programs also obtain funding by invoicing each police detachment for cases in which forensic evidence is collected and released to police for investigation. Alberta's SART funding is shared with Capital Health covering the nursing and administrative costs and local police departments paying the policing and court costs. The birth control center staff provides additional direct and indirect support, as does the administrative structure of the Capital Health region. British Columbia has a unique program from the provincial ministry of the attorney general's office for cases in which a sexual assault is not reported to police. Although each program identifies a different rate of cases unreported to police, the number of these unreported cases remains as high as 40% at any given time. Nova Scotia's SANE program was funded as a three-year pilot project (2001 to 2003) from the provincial Department of Health. The program is community-based out of the Avalon Sexual Assault Center, which is unique in the Canadian environment considering that the coordinator of the program reports to the Avalon Board of Directors and an advisory committee with key players from hospitals, police, justice system, local university, victim services, and community organizations

Standards of Practice

To date, Canadian standards of practice for SANE at a national level do not exist. Each program or network, such as Ontario, has developed standards of practice that are program-specific. The templates for the standards of practice, however, are often based on the IAFN SANE Standards of Practice developed by the SANE Council of IAFN in 1999. Each developing SANE program may research standards of practice, policies, and guidelines of existing Canadian and US programs and formulate their own standards to meet the needs of their community and program mandate. Training programs also are similarly developed with constant revision and updating as the programs progress along the spectrum of forensic nursing care. Each provincial professional body has standards of nursing practice for all registered nurses within the province, and the national Canadian Nurses' Association governs nursing practice nationally. In addition, the National Emergency Nurses Affiliation (NENA) has Standards of Emergency Nursing Practice. Because most SANE programs are based in the emergency department, the NENA standards are applicable to FNEs.

Response to Forensic Nurse Examiners

In Canada, the judicial response to testimony of FNEs thus far has been quite positive. "Police and crown attorneys like having nurse examiners involved in court because we take it more seriously, are available and don't *overtestify*. Since the FNE program started, more of us have been declared expert witnesses than ever before," remarked Sheila MacDonald, Ontario Network Provincial Coordinator. "Consistently forensic nurse examiners who testify in sexual assault cases are accepted as expert witnesses," said BC Women's Hospital Sexual Assault Service Coordinator, Lianne Ritch. The proven expertise of FNEs in the court system is a positive factor when the introduction of a FNE program is being considered in a community. Similar responses have been given by law enforcement, citing numerous benefits, including time saving, examination quality and consistency, and improved care for the victim, starting at the crime scene.

National Issues

FNEs who are SANEs are part of the larger field of forensic nursing, which has only recently begun to look beyond the present to future development in Canada. Significant national issues for FNE programs are centered on a number of different areas and foci including development of national standards of practice for the FNE, increased educational programming, and research. There are also initial plans to expand the use of the FNE into other areas such as domestic violence, child abuse, death investigation, and interpersonal violence across Canada.

Future of Forensic Nurse Examiners

From the inception of the first SANE program in 1993 to the present, with five out of 10 provinces having established SANE programs, the future of FNE programs in Canada is indeed bright. The ability of FNE programs to promote a coordinated sexual assault response team that ensures comprehensive optimal care, treatment, and support for the sexually assaulted patient has been established. The success of one program has led to the development of more programs, even to the extent of a provincial network in one province. Interest in the role of the SANE has also led to a general interest in forensic nursing in the student, basic, and postgraduate nursing programs. Increasingly, articles in nursing journals speak to forensic nursing issues and clinical application of the forensic nursing skills. Forensic nursing courses are appearing in college calendars and Internet education opportunities. Forensic issues are being introduced at all levels of nursing education but not on a consistent basis from province to province. There is much work to be done to move forensic nursing to a specialty status in Canada.

Currently, the process to become a specialty in nursing is to do so through the Canadian Nurses' Association. Forensic nursing must come together nationally in all its diverse forms to work toward the common goal of specialty nursing. For the last 10 years, nurses working in forensic nursing fields have belonged to one of many specialty groups, including emergency nursing, psychiatric nursing, critical care, and pediatrics, rather than selecting the common thread of forensic nursing and joining these differing roles. Ideally, membership in the International Association of Forensic Nurses has incorporated aspects of each specialty group and integrated those roles into the role of the FNE.

Australia

CHRISTINE VECCHI

The history of forensic services in Australia dates back to the earliest times when the British sent their criminals and mentally ill to this Pacific island, which served as a penal colony. It has been the tradition of all in Australia to approach each public service endeavor from the perspective of a rule of law and respect for human rights. The development of forensic nursing services in Australia is in its infancy and is now beginning to emerge as a specialty area within the profession of nursing. The expanding movement of forensic nursing and its deviation from the more traditional nursing roles within Australia has evolved through the influence of forensic nursing progress in other countries.

Forensic Psychiatric and Correctional Nursing

Australia's history of receiving transported British criminals has been instrumental in this country's developing forensic healthcare services. Mental health services in Australia began in 1805 after a member of the first fleet, Charles Bishop, was declared a "lunatic." In 1811, the first asylum in Australia was established in Castle Hill, New South Wales. Since these early times, trends in Australian mental health have mimicked those in the British system.

Forensic nursing services have developed in a similar fashion to that of the mental health services–ad hoc across the various states and territories. Therefore, there is little documented history of the true beginnings of forensic nursing in the current published literature. Today, forensic nursing in Australia primarily focuses on work with patients who are in some way connected to the criminal justice system, usually individuals who have been accused or convicted of a criminal offense. Mason (2002) believes that the term "forensic" is generally accepted within nursing literature to denote those who work with mentally disordered offenders in secure psychiatric services of some description.

Various state organizations throughout Australia provide support for forensic nurses involved in forensic mental health care. There is little national recognition, organization, or collaboration for the broader specialty of forensic nursing science. This situation is in extreme contrast to the North American and Canadian forensic nursing movement (Vecchi, 2003).

Forensicare

The Australian healthcare system began with the most basic circumstances of prison life for those who were incarcerated more than 300 years ago. However, today mental healthcare and prison forensic healthcare have risen to the forefront as a consummate example of contemporary health and justice service. One of Australia's prime exemplary systems is the Victorian Institute of Forensic Mental Health under the trade name of Forensicare. During 1999, Forensicare opened a purpose-built, 120-bed inpatient hospital in Fairfield, Melbourne, and has undertaken a major redevelopment of its community program.

Forensicare is an international center of excellence in understanding and treating mental disorders associated with criminal behavior. Its vision is to provide effective mental health services in a safe and secure environment to those who have both mental disorders and a history of criminal offending or who present a serious risk of such behavior.

The treatment and standard of care for individuals with mental disorders are equal to or greater than those provided to people suffering from other forms of illness and are delivered in accordance with international and national covenants relating to forensic mental health. Advances within Forensicare have provided support to the field of forensic nursing and aided its need to be recognized as a specialized area of nursing. Up until the last few years, forensic nurses have developed their expertise in relative isolation, with scarce and random communication between nurses working in other states. Often forensic colleagues have had little knowledge of other nurses who work in a similar forensic capacity, their existence, or what it was that forensic nursing entailed. In the last few years, Australian forensic nurses have begun to present at conferences, publish papers, and generally heighten the profile and role diversity of the Australian FNE. The IAFN provides a global network of professionalism to link the diverse roles of forensic nurses worldwide within a common boundary of forensic nursing practice.

Emerging Trends

Prison Healthcare

Several emerging trends have had an impact on Australian forensic nurses. Historically, the security and delivery of healthcare to prisoners have been a public function, administered and operationally managed by the seven individual states and territorial governments. However, in the last few years, Australia has seen the emergence of private prison operators as well as the employment of forensic nurses (FNs) in these privately operated facilities. This will no doubt have some bearing on the way FNs proceed and communicate in the future.

Advanced Practice and Collaboration

The development of the nurse practitioner role in Australia will no doubt be relevant to the advancement of the FN roles. Such role development is a mainstream movement that FNs can access, contribute to, and assist in its development.

There is no national profile or details of Australian FNs as a group. Owing to the vast landscape and the relatively small population, there is a greater potential for FNEs feeling and experiencing significant isolation. The Australian landscape is vast (approximately the same size as the US), with only a national population of 18 million (1 million less than the state of Texas in the US). The issue of isolation is compounded by the very small number of practicing FNs and the even smaller number of opportunities that are available to meet, network among colleagues, and attend educational seminars. In addition to this, most Australian FNs work behind great walls in state and territory prisons or in secure forensic psychiatric centers. Individual national and state or provincial chapters of the IAFN serve a unifying purpose to reduce isolation among these members.

Educational Needs

FNs require a working knowledge of the criminal justice system and how that system impacts the patient. How involved the nurse becomes with the criminal justice system is dependent on a number of factors, the least of which are the policy directives of those who manage the services and employ the FNE. Curriculum for FNs in Australia does not include information on expert testimony, the collection and preservation of crime evidence, or the other FN roles that are recognized in the US and Canada.

Most FNEs have learned about the criminal justice system "on the job" and generally refer any legal concerns the patient has to the police or the patient's solicitor. Therefore, the focus for Australian registered nurses is to provide generalized nursing care to the patient and to dissociate themselves from any judicial aspect of patient care. The nurse stays focused on nursing care and becomes concerned with the criminal aspects only if and when they impact on the patient's immediate healthcare status. This philosophy has no doubt been borne out of a desire to provide nonjudgmental care and not to become a voyeur of the patient's criminal affairs. Although this has been the approach historically taken by forensic nurses in Victoria toward the criminal aspect of the forensic patients care, times are changing. There is beginning to be some questioning of the effect and foundation of historical approach to forensic patient care, wondering whether this approach to care effectively acts as a defense against perceiving the forensic psychiatric patients in all their entirety and complexity.

Role in Legal Proceedings

The role of the Australian general forensic nurse is not as described by Coram (1993, p. 26), writing from Washington state, who reports that the "client of the physiologically oriented forensic nurse is the victim." There has been an historical decision to keep nurses out of the courtroom, in part to ensure they are not taken away from their routine duties where their services are always in desperate need.

The requirement of a nurse in court causes a disruption to service delivery as well as additional costs to employ another nurse to provide cover if one is available. Due to the current nursing shortages across the country, sufficient nursing staff has become a major concern for all healthcare institutions. Traditionally, most health-related court evidence is given by doctors. This has also limited the progression of the forensic nursing role.

In addition, there are no Australian forensic nursing services to assist victims of crime. This fact is sadly lamented by many nurses, for the result is a restriction of healthcare options for victims of crime. This area of role development is long overdue for FNEs.

There are many prison- and hospital-based forensic physicians who provide services to offenders/alleged offenders that do not require any forensic specific training. However, these doctors, in addition to their clinical caseloads, do not hesitate to take up their place in court.

Role development for FNEs who provide expert testimony in court has never fully developed. This is unlike the role of the forensic nurse in North America who gives expert testimony, and can be engaged to focus on the defendant's thinking and behavior prior to and during committing the crime (Coram, 1993). Similarly, involvement in evaluating the legal sanity and competence of the felony defendant is a forensic nursing role in other countries (Lynch, 1993a). Again, this is an area of role development long overdue for the Australian FNE. Forensic nurses in some other countries are greater in number, have become well organized, and have had the benefit of some driving and entrepreneurial personalities.

Australia can learn much from the international perspective of forensic nursing. The advances made in other countries must become learning opportunities for forensic nurses in this country. International communication is therefore vital to furthering the development of forensic nursing in Australia. Membership and participation in the IAFN is one way to promote such dialogue.

Advances in Nursing Education and Practice

Progress in forensic nursing education has taken on a new and exciting perspective. Flinders University in Adelaide, South Australia, has initiated the first graduate program in the field of clinical forensic nursing. Linda Saunders, JD, RN, has been the moving force in this emerging new field that will address the need for FNEs in the clinical environs to minister to the survivors of medicolegal cases. This program was established in 2000 along with the first world conference in the Southern Hemisphere to address the International Association of Forensic Nurses.

In Perth, Western Australia, forensic clinical nurse specialist, Christine Vecchi, MSN, BSc, RN, has addressed the roles of the SANE, forensic photographer, and clinical forensic nurse to the Dean of Nursing at Notre Dame University. This presentation stimulated an interest to design and develop a course of study in clinical forensic nursing principles. In August 2003, the first class of its type successfully began at a postgraduate level.

Expanded Practice Roles in Corrections

In Melbourne, Victoria, a pilot program was instigated to reduce the workload of forensic medical officers. The research design was to incorporate a forensic nursing service that provided a 12-hour night-time (7:00 p.m. to 7:00 a.m.) referral and primary care nursing service to police detainees. Before this pilot study, the responsibility for all the primary healthcare to this group was that of the forensic medical officer (FMO). With the advent of this service the forensic nurse became the health professional of first-line services, excluding emergency response.

Lynch (1993b) reports the model of the police surgeon service used in the UK served as the prototype for the pilot study. A proposed plan to implement and develop a nurse practitioner service to police detainees was presented at the Association of Police Surgeons in Harrogate, England, in 1993. For the police surgeons in the UK, an overwhelming demand for forensic services was the drive to promote and develop the forensic nurse role. In Melbourne, in 1991, FMOs (formerly known as police surgeons) found themselves in a similar situation to their UK colleagues. Lynch links the need for and the development of the Australian FNE pilot program to an overwhelming demand for specialized forensic services. Due to the limited number of trained forensic professionals, physicians required help. This situation was one of the antecedents to the development of the role of the forensic nursing service to police detainees in Victoria.

Following extensive evaluation during its pilot phase, a forensic nursing program was developed as an ongoing forensic nursing service and remains operational today. The forensic nursing service was found to reduce the nighttime call-out rate of the FMO by 73%. Of the detainees referred to the FNE (both of whom held psychiatric and general nursing registrations), 79% of their healthcare needs were managed by the nurse without referral to the FMO. Of the 21% referred to the FMO via a phone call from the nurse, 4% were seen by the FMO. Most of the remaining 17% were resolved by either a phone order for prescription medication or transferred to the local emergency department for further investigation.

In addition, this forensic nursing service reduced overnight delays in responding to health assessment referrals and was shown to improve the continuity of care between police- and prison-based health services (Young, Wells, & Jackson, 1994; Evans & McGilvray, 1996). Most important in this economic age, the program was cost effective. As a result of this success, the police were some of the keenest advocates and lobbied for the forensic nursing service to be extended from 12 to 24 hours (McGilvray & Evans, 1996). This type of demonstrable result for the advanced forensic nurse role provides evidence that research into the advancement of the various other areas of forensic nursing is a vital component for the future.

The Forensic Nurse Examiner's Role

With rare exception, the Australian forensic nurse does not have a role in the care or treatment for victims of crime. Internationally, forensic nursing roles include sexual assault nurse examiner (SANE), nurse coroner/death investigator, forensic psychiatric nurse, forensic correctional nurse specialist, legal nurse consultant, forensic geriatric nurse specialist, forensic photographer, and forensic clinical nurse specialist (Lynch, 1993b). This breadth of role definition provides the Australian forensic nurse with a vision for future development. Forensic nursing as a discrete discipline, however, was recognized with the first formal paper delivered on the subject by Virginia Lynch at the American Academy of Forensic Sciences (AAFS) annual meeting in New Orleans in 1986 (Lynch, 1986).

This type of national recognition for forensic nursing is required in Australia. It is imperative that Australian forensic nurses develop a higher profile. If there is to be role development, advancement, and future recognition as a specialty in nursing, there first needs to be increased awareness of forensic nursing's scope of practice throughout all health and justice professions.

New Career Opportunities

Forensic nurses will become more visible and gain recognition by participating in mainstream nursing movements. The emerging recognition, development, and promotion of the nurse practitioner role is one such movement across Australia. Forensic nurses frequently work in the capacity of nurse practitioners and have much to offer and much to gain by their participation in this trend to formalize the role of the nurse practitioner.

The eastern Australian state of New South Wales saw the birth of a nurse practitioner pilot project in 1992. Government funding was made available to establish and research the effectiveness of nurse practitioner services. "Evidence from the research conducted by each of the pilot projects and the Across-Project research supports that nurse practitioners are feasible, safe and effective in their roles and provide quality health services in the range of settings researched" (NSW Dept. of Health, 1996, p. ii). Since that time the prospect of formalizing the nurse practitioner role has progressed in other states. The role of the nurse practitioner is emerging in western Australia, both as an independent practitioner (in private practice) and one employed and paid by a service provider.

Challenges for the Future

Forensic nursing in Australia has developed independently in each state and territory in response to a myriad of factors. The vast expanse of land and the relatively small population of the country have compounded the isolation that occurs when nurses work "behind bars." Just keeping in touch with developments in forensic nursing across the country can be a daunting task. Australian forensic nursing is based almost entirely on the nursing care to the offender/alleged offender/released offender.

There is great potential for role development for FNEs in Australia. The well-organized and developed roles of forensic nurses, especially in the US, give rise to great expectations in this area. Coupled with specific education, Australian forensic nurses have the potential to expand their horizons. The developing role and recognition of the nurse practitioner can only enhance the potential for forensic nurse practitioners. It is to these ends that forensic nurses need to include themselves in mainstream movements to gain recognition for developed nursing roles.

South Africa

GLENDA WILDSCHUT

The discipline of forensic nursing is a new and emerging concept in the Republic of South Africa. Although some activities of the forensic nurse are carried out by a variety of other practitioners, the discrete functions of this forensic specialist are yet not clearly defined.

Recently, with the frequent courses developed and presented by Virginia Lynch, in South Africa the discipline has taken on a momentum of its own. The conceptual model of a clinical forensic specialist in nursing was first introduced by Lynch in 1995 at the Seventh International Congress on Caring for Survivors of Torture in Cape Town. To date, six training programs have been offered, two of which were presented by Lynch in Kimberley and were sponsored by the Office of the Attorney General in the Northern Cape Province of South Africa in 1998 and subsequently in 1999 (Lynch & Weaver, 1998). In 2001 Lynch taught two courses in Durban, South Africa. These programs were sponsored by the Provincial Minister of Health in Kwa Zulu Natal and the Independent Medico-Legal Unit (IMLU) in conjunction with the University of Natal and the Nelson Mandela School of Medicine. In that same year, Lynch and Dr. Tromp Els taught two courses in Pretoria and Paarl to law enforcement and legal professionals, including the South African police, magistrates, and attorneys. These courses were sponsored by the International Criminal Training and Assistance Program (ICTAP) in Washington, D.C.

Lynch's tenure coincided with South Africa's emergence from more than three decades of authoritarian rule, announcing a new era of democracy. Despite peaceful change at a political level, lasting peace cannot be achieved if the abuses of the past are not addressed. To that end, the South African Truth and Reconciliation Commission (TRC) was established to uncover as much as possible of the truth about past gross violations of human rights (Truth and Reconciliation Commission [TRC], 1998). This task was necessary for the promotion of national unity and reconciliation.

Best Practice *56-2*

In cases of human rights violations, a forum for truth-telling should be utilized as a method for helping victims to understand the past and integrate it into their total life experiences.

The aims and objectives of the TRC coincide with that of forensic nursing: to develop leadership in the healthcare response to violence. As part of the responsibility as commissioner on the TRC, this author was tasked to facilitate special hearings for children and youth who had suffered violations during the period 1960-1994 (TRC, 1998).

Truth as a Central Paradigm

As the truth recovery process in South Africa was not only a judicial mechanism but also an exercise of healing, the principles of forensic nursing assisted this author to develop a program of support for those who testified while the important task of exposing the horrors of the past were under way. According to Lynch (2002, 2004), "*Truth* is the central issue in resolution to questioned issues involving the physical, psychological and social health or ills of a human population; both past and future truths. *Truth*, as the central implicit assumption to all forensic investigations brings enlightenment to unknown, unanswered and questioned issues related to the origin of manifestations of pathological conditions impacting the person, environment, health and nursing."

The philosophy of forensic nursing practice is based on the discovery of truth, diagnosis, treatment, evaluation, rehabilitation, recovery, and prevention. Without *truth*, reconciliation and justice are denied. Forensic nursing theory incorporates the various human dimensions pertinent to all nursing theories of care, yet projects beyond the aspects of biopsychosocial, spiritual, and cultural beings to introduce and incorporate a dimension of law (Lynch, 2004).

Children Subjected to Violation of Human Rights

Holding special hearings for children and youths provided an opportunity to focus on the impact of apartheid in South Africa on them. Over the years, children and young people were the victims of and witnesses to the most appalling human rights violations in South Africa's history. The effect of the exposure to the ongoing violence may have had serious consequences on the development of these children. It was therefore considered imperative that the trauma inflicted on children and youth be heard and shared within the framework of the healing ethos of the Commission. The basic propositions within the theory of forensic nursing science include truth, presence, perceptivity, and regeneration (Lynch, 2004). The regeneration of victims of human violence is essential to the fulfillment of a meaningful future.

An important, yet lesser-known role of the forensic nurse is identifying victims of human rights abuse and investigating related violations of international law. This specialized role focuses on the loss of life and function as a result of violations related to, among others, political or religious domination based on mass interpersonal aggression. The forensic nurse in this domain is a new health and justice specialist blending biomedical knowledge with the basic principles of jurisprudence and human behavior. "*Truth* is the mantra of the forensic sciences and central to the field of all scientific investigation" (Lynch, 2004). In this way the forensic nurse is contributing to the dissemination of the rule of law (Lynch & Weaver, 1998). In 1995, South Africa ratified the United Nations Convention on the Rights of the Child (CRC), an important step toward securing South Africa's rightful place in the world community of nations (TRC, 1998). The CRC imposes important obligations and responsibilities on its signatories, including that of "honoring the voice" of children and youth by giving them an opportunity to express their feelings and relate their experiences as part of the national process of healing. It was in the spirit of honoring that treaty that the children's hearings were held. Children from across the country were given the chance to tell their stories as they experienced them.

Format of the Hearings

The special hearings on children and youth were more flexible than other hearings of the Commission in that they allowed the participants to reflect on or critically analyze the root causes of apartheid and its effects on children. Most parties providing testimony supplied written submissions ahead of the hearing and were asked to summarize their submissions orally and answer questions posed by the panel. The hearings also allowed for the participation of the children in ways other than testifying; these included finding creative ways to access and share the children's experience.

Case Study 56-1 Political Activism and Torture

Mrs. M. told the commission of her son, Siphiwe. He was a determined political activist in the Eastern Cape Province in South Africa. He was detained several times, subjected to severe torture, and faced constant police harassment. To protect his family from harassment, he was continually on the run, and when he did not return home, he lived in a dog kennel. In 1981, after his release from yet another arrest, his health deteriorated rapidly and he was diagnosed as having been poisoned with thalium. His body swelled, and his hair fell out. He could not urinate and was confined to a wheelchair. He fought to recover and began slowly regaining his health. Throughout his convalescence, Siphiwe continued with his political activities and filed a claim for damages against the police. In 1982, he left home for a checkup at the local provincial hospital. He never returned home. It was later revealed that the police had killed him.

Fig. 56-1 Child's drawing depicting trauma of violence.

In some of the regions, the children spent a day telling their stories in the presence of mental health practitioners and making drawings that reflected those experiences. These drawings were shared at the hearings the following day (Fig. 56-1).

Children in Police Custody

In large and often arbitrary police action, thousands of children, some as young as seven years old, were arrested and detained in terms of South Africa security legislation. Some times entire schools were arrested en masse. Torture often occurred while children were in detention. Types of abuse reported by the children included food and sleep deprivation, solitary confinement, beating, kicking, enforced physical exercise, being kept naked during interrogation, suspension from poles, and electric shock. Other forms of torture included verbal insults, banging a detainee's head against a wall or floor, use of tear gas in a confined space, enforced standing in an unnatural position, near suffocation, and cigarette burns. These forms of torture were compounded by the lack of intellectual stimulation, false accusations, threatened violence to the detainee and his or her family, misleading information, untrue statements about betrayal by friends, pressure to sign false documents, and interrogation at gun point. This information has been derived from testimonies of witnesses who appeared before the TRC at the special children's hearings held nationally in South Africa (TRC, 1998).

Witness Support Strategy

As part of the hearings for children and youth, attention was given to the fact that children would need special support as they testified in public about abuse perpetrated against them. Support for the witnesses at the hearings was an important part of the work of the mental health unit of the Commission. This type of intervention included the preparation and briefing of the witness before public hearings, the containment and advocacy of the witness during the hearings, and after the hearings, the debriefing and referral of those who testified to regionally appropriate service providers who had knowledge of local resources and who followed up accordingly.

Best Practice *56-3*

The forensic nurse specialist must ensure that the victims of violence are given professional support during their quest for justice.

The development of the witnesses' support strategy could best be described as the quest to bridge the gap between the need for and the provision of emotional support. Although constrained by the limitations of the legal act that controlled the activities of the Commission and overwhelmed by witnesses' understandably high expectations of direct and immediate service delivery, the Commission, on the whole, managed to navigate a path that went toward restoring human dignity and facilitating the delivery of support. Community debriefing also assumed the critical task of supplying longer-term support for the families and witnesses in need. As local service providers, community debriefers endeavored to ensure that the people received the sustained interest and support that they required, although they met with different levels of success. The ability to provide ongoing support to those in need of counseling was, ultimately, beyond the resources of the commission.

Impact of Violations against Children

Political and community violence characteristically expose children and youth to suffering long after the event. Although many are able to recover with the support of friends, family, and community, others may suffer lasting psychological damage. Young people may suffer from concomitant conditions similar to those of adults, including post-traumatic stress disorder, depression, substance abuse, and antisocial behavior. Straker (1994) and Dawes (1994) have reported significant depression, anxiety, and other post-traumatic symptoms at levels that impaired functions of daily living in South African youth (Pynoos, Kinzie, & Gordon, 1998).

Children who have been contiguously exposed to violence may experience a significant change in their beliefs and attitudes. Loss of trust may occur when children have been abused by people they previously considered as trusted adults. Fear, hatred, and bitterness may be the greater, therefore, after intra- or intercommunity violence where children not only know who the perpetrators are, but are forced to live in the same community as them, despite simmering rage and possibly continued fear (Machel, 1996).

The purpose of the TRC in South Africa in uncovering the abuses perpetrated against children and youth and the contribution forensic nursing has made toward understanding the consequences of trauma and how witnesses should be supported as they break the silence of their abuse have helped to initiate the recovery process.

Forensic Nursing in the New South Africa

Forensic nursing was first introduced in South Africa in 1997 in the Northern Cape Province under the direction of Dr. Tromp Els, chief forensic medical officer. Since that time, the hearings of the Truth and Reconciliation Commission have ended, and the national Minister of Health, Dr. Tsabalala-Msimang, has proposed a strategy to implement forensic nursing programs in each of the nine provinces. The Minister further recognized forensic nursing as a national priority program and as one step in the reduction and prevention of violence against women and children. In an address to the National Intersectoral Sexual Offences Forum held in Cape Town in 2000, Dr. Tsabalala-Msimang acknowledged this futuristic insight as she stated, "Dr. Tromp Els is hereby saluted for his pioneering work in the field of Forensic Nursing in South Africa."

Violence, as a primary method of conflict resolution, often becomes an automatic response in the aftermath of civil strife and war. It is not uncommon for social defense mechanisms to take two generations to recover and heal. In spite of the initial progress of the new South African government in addressing interpersonal and sexual violence, by 2001 gender-based discriminatory treatment of girls and women continued. In response, both the South African government and women's rights organizations are working to improve the state's response to domestic and sexual violence. The new South African constitution prohibits unfair discrimination against anyone directly or indirectly on the ground of gender, sex, or pregnancy, among others. International human rights law requires states to address persistent violations of human rights and take measures to prevent their occurrence. The Convention on the Elimination of All Forms of Discrimination against Women (CEDAW), ratified on December 15, 1995, requires the government to take action to eliminate violence against women as a form of discrimination that inhibits women's ability to enjoy rights and freedoms on a basis of equality with men.

The International Covenant on Civil and Political Rights (ICCPR), ratified by South Africa on December 10, 1998, requires the government to ensure the rights to life and security of the person of all individuals in its jurisdiction. Yet, violence against women in South African society generally is widely recognized to have reached the highest incidence in the world.

After an intensive study by Human Rights Watch, recommendations to the government of South Africa included abuse prevention, victim support, provision of medical assistance, appropriate treatment for HIV/AIDS, prevention of virginity testing, and investigation and documentation of abuse, among other pertinent issues. Interventions to these issues are defined within the Scope and Practice of Forensic Nursing by the International Association of Forensic Nurses (1997). Through the initial endeavors of Dr. Els, the education and training of forensic nurse examiners has been recognized as one important response to South Africa's obligations under international and national law methodology.

With the support of the Minister of Health, Minister of Justice, Minister of Police, and the National Attorney General, among other provincial officials, this recognition of forensic nursing has initiated a course of progress that has come "from virtually nothing and evolved into a moving force" that will help to heal the wounds of yesterday. What remains an important challenge for nurses globally is not only to deal with consequences of violations, but also to work toward creating environments and societies that value life and prevent the occurrence of human right abuses. In this regard forensic nursing, particularly in South Africa, has an important education and advocacy role.

Turkey

MIRA GÖKDOĞAN, SEVIL ATASOY, AND M. FATIH YAVUZ

Although the history of professional nursing has been well established for over a century, forensic nursing is a new phenomenon in Turkey. The few nurses working in the fields of legal medicine and the forensic sciences, until recently, did not have specialty postgraduate education. In addition, many nurses working in related sections of forensic medicine (emergency departments, traumatology, drug dependence, forensic psychiatry, etc.) also have no postgraduate education or knowledge of forensic sciences.

The Institute of Legal Medicine and Forensic Sciences (LEMFOS) of the Istanbul University teaches graduates of diverse disciplines the forensic aspects of their field. Trusting in the importance of forensic nursing, LEMFOS, as the only institution in the field of forensic sciences available to graduates of various disciplines, started also to enroll nurses in 1995 as a general education, training, and public service project. The focus of this program was to address the reduction and prevention of sexual assault, which is being reported at an alarming rate, traumatizing women, men, and children.

Sexual Assault Management

After a sexual assault, the scene that follows in the majority of hospitals is almost as traumatic as the assault itself. Forensic examinations for rape victims are conducted by physicians in the emergency department. Over the years, problems such as lack of experience and insensitivity to victims were associated with physicians, who were reluctant to conduct the examination. This reaction often occurs because no specific education in sexual assault evaluation is given to general practitioners. Victims wait several hours for an examination, and in some regions, they have to travel to another city to find a hospital where the examination can be accomplished.

After making a legal statement, the victims are sent to the Council of Forensic Medicine to have another examination by court order. These experiences only prolong the trauma associated with sexual violence for sexual assault victims.

LEMFOS introduced the Section of Sexual Assaults (SSA) in 1996 to ensure more timely and accurate collection of forensic evidence for use in prosecution of perpetrators. In the process, SSA developed unique, professional instructions on the physical examination and collection of evidence, information on pregnancy and cessation, sexually transmitted diseases, suggestions on providing support to the victim, and a variety of report forms.

SSA provides training on sexual assault examination protocol to health professionals to ensure these victims receive sensitive treatment and that evidence is properly and efficiently collected to ensure prosecution. SSA provides training materials, including an evidence collection kit and a video titled *Caring for the Sexual Assault Victim: Forensic Evidence Collection and Medical Examination Guidelines.*

Role Development

Currently, forensic nurses are trained as specialists who will apply their dual expertise in nursing and forensic sciences (Gorea & Jasuja, 2003). Previously, there have been no more than six nurses with master's level education from LEMFOS having general legal medicine, criminology, and natural sciences education. In the near future, with increasing numbers, forensic nurse examiners (FNEs) will play important roles in different areas of forensic sciences, especially in sexual assault investigation, forensic traumatology, and forensic psychiatry. With the participation of nurses, legal medicine and the forensic sciences will achieve great acceleration in this country (Lynch, 2003).

Furthermore, with the effort of LEMFOS, courses in forensic medicine were established within the College of Nursing at Istanbul University in the 1997-1998 academic year. Forensic nursing was added to the nursing curriculum in the 2002-2003 academic year. With continued support, these educational programs will continue in the future, establishing a foundation for the development of forensic nursing science and practice.

Although the role of a forensic specialist in nursing remains a new concept in Turkey, support is given from the forensic physicians and scientists, police, and attorneys. With the force of knowledge provided by effective postgraduate studies, seminars and courses, research, and articles, FNEs will designate their own place within the forensic sciences in Turkey.

In 1995, Mira Gökdoğan, the initial pioneer in forensic nursing, enrolled in the academic program at the Institute of Legal Medicine and Forensic Sciences at the Istanbul University. One important aspect of the LEMFOS program is to prepare students of science, medicine, and sociology in the legal aspects of healthcare. The program is also committed to the education of the professionals who are most frequently involved in the medicolegal management of forensic cases because these professions assist in the administration of justice through data collection and documentation of information that will help to complete complex forensic investigations. In an unprecedented movement, this program was developed and directed through the endeavors of the faculty of the Istanbul University and the Public Health Department, the Ministry of Justice, and the Ministry of the Interior.

As a result of Gökdoğan's interest in forensic nursing, she became the first nurse in Turkey to attend the sexual assault nurse examiner (SANE) program at Palomar Medical Center in San Diego, California, where she also participated in a clinical internship to gain experience in sexual assault evaluation.

Achieving Credentials

The future of forensic nursing education will require a great deal of clarification and direction as FNEs move toward qualification and credentials in this field. In a questionnaire regarding the field of work as a forensic nurse, nursing students and registered nurses were queried regarding such topics as the role of the sexual assault nurse examiner and the criminal, legal, and nursing behaviors in the care of victims of crime. The results indicated many were aware of the interface between the forensic sciences and sexual assault investigation, but were lacking in knowledge regarding other forensic nursing behaviors (Khodakarami, 2003).

For the past seven years, nurses who have been taught these concepts in practice while working with practitioners have also learned to care for the victims of sexual assault at the forensic medical examination center. Currently, there are two registered nurses studying in the University of Istanbul program who will have earned a doctoral degree in forensic sciences upon completion. With this degree these nurse educators will help spread forensic nursing throughout the country and help all nurses take advantage of this new opportunity in healthcare.

Modeling Forensic Practice

At the LEMFOS, a special room has been prepared to provide care for the victims of sexual assault. There the victim will be looked after in the immediate aftermath of an assault, regarding physical, sexual, psychological, and emotional needs. This special examination room will also be used in the education experiences of sexual assault nurse examiners, providing a harmony of theoretical and practical education.

Registered nurses throughout the country will take note of operating instructions to use the evidence collection kits to recover biological material such as hair, physical fluids, or tissue. Nurses will also learn to write reports and document patient statements. The evidence kits will be transferred to the central laboratories by officers of the government to maintain the chain of custody. Presently, there are two forensic laboratories, one located in Istanbul and one in Ankara. DNA analysis will be performed in these specially equipped forensic hemogenetic laboratories.

In Turkey, specific education programs in the field of forensic nursing will be developed and implemented in the near future. This will provide a major step forward to assist in the reduction and prevention of sexual violence. The unpublished component of statistics in sexual assault is suspected to be quite high, sustaining false beliefs and remaining myths. Therefore, fearful of being unable to prove their statements, victims often remain silent. In these cases, a FNE will be the best person to help the victim. A forensic nurse will have the time and the knowledge and will give the appropriate attention, not only to the victim but to the family as well.

Japan

NANAKO YONEYAMA

Historically in Japan, healthcare, law enforcement, and the public have not acknowledged interpersonal violence. Crimes against women have not been recognized as a violation of human rights. Therefore, it is not surprising that women seldom ask for help. Although some Asian countries have well-established domestic violence law, Japan has only now recognized violence against women as an interpersonal crime. In 2002, the Law for the Prevention of Spousal Violence and the Protection of Victims was established into legislation. Presently, with rare exception, there are few safe harbors for battered women. This is just the beginning of judicial protection.

In 1997, a program for battered women was established at a private clinic at the Institute of Family Function (IFF) in Tokyo (Yoneyama, 2000; Lynch, 2000). Because of the stigma related to domestic violence and the lack of legal recourse, few women sought protection. Unfortunately, because of the low number of individuals presenting for treatment the program was unable to continue. New interest was awakened with the Shelter-Net Conference in Tokyo in 2000, a national symposium on domestic violence and women's shelters. The attendance of a cadre of nurses indicated a greater interest and commitment to this vulnerable population.

In 1999, the 145th Diet addressed the challenges related to violence against women in contemporary Japanese society. A Committee of Issues consisting of 25 members related to the Men and Women Symbiosis Society in the House of Councilors, the Diet is responsible for evaluating existing laws and recommendations for revision to meet contemporary social needs. Nanako Yoneyama, associated with the International Association of Forensic Nurses, was among the witnesses called to testify before this committee regarding women's issue. Topics included identifying current problems, the previous failure to resolve these concerns, and how nursing is supporting this population. Other witnesses, all women, included a psychiatrist and a lawyer (Lynch, 2000).

Although public health services and public social welfare services in Japan are increasing in each of the areas concerned with social injustice and human abuse, nurses in Japan are hopeful for their country and believe that forensic nursing will offer considerable assistance to victims of violence. It is necessary to understand the characteristics of Japanese culture in order to provide solutions to contemporary social crime.

Understanding Characteristics of Japanese Society

Conditions contributing to societal conflict, gender bias, and domestic abuse include three main characteristic elements of the cultural background of Japan:

1. Codependency
2. Harassment or bullying by the majority
3. Social hierarchy derived from educational background

These are issues requiring a generation or more to effect societal changes. Presently, Japanese motivation is nearly the same as portrayed in the book by Ruth Benedict, *The Chrysanthemum and the Sword* (Benedict, 1989). What motivates the Japanese is not "what do I want to do?" but rather "how does society see me?" Especially in an enterprise organization, the values within the organization are set prior to individual philosophy or belief. A husband works like a robot for the organization, and his wife also becomes a robot who places her husband before herself. A wife, as an excellent robot, has no identity of her own and gives priority to other family members before herself. Thus, she gives little thought to her own values, and as a result, she loses sight of them. The "robot wife" allows her husband to need her while taking care of him. Though the husband takes some pride in supporting his wife, she manages him. Each of the couple needs the other for existence and depends on the other, without knowledge or consciousness, which is a typical case of codependency.

The child learns how to endure the relationships within the family or the community while trying not to assert himself or herself. Being the same as others or not being conspicuous in a group is given the top priority. A sense of superiority or consciousness carries with it the threat of being excluded. As with adults, the children's motivations are not "what do I want to do?" but "how do others see me?" When children are harassed, they endure it because they cannot depend on adults to help them. In fact, the harassment or bullying will be the harsher when it is reported to some adult. After learning that nobody can change anything, feelings of helplessness arise, and the person assumes a demeanor of silence and passiveness, or in the worst case, commits suicide.

The school is not in the least a safe place for children. When choosing an advanced school, others make their decision. Students will enter a university, not because they want to go there, but because its ranking matches their educational results. After graduation, they will not select their own career; instead, they allocate themselves to any company that matches their schooling.

Japan has long been and remains a society where educational background is respected. Most bureaucratic organizations noticeably cherish this tradition as national university graduates. The bureaucrats sustain the bureaucratic society, sending retired bureaucrats into the management boards of private companies under their supervision, which is called "amakudari," literally meaning "descending from heaven." Few bureaucrats give thought to their own benefit but rather consider the national benefit or welfare. Some need a society full of subjugation and codependency to sustain these customs, while others secretly envy and would follow their own path but are afraid of making themselves too conspicuous. Learning may often fall into the trap of learned helplessness or depression, as evidenced by a recent increase of suicide in the population of middle age males. Japan may well be called a society full of silent violence.

Substance Abuse

Substance abuse is another concern that has brought forensic nurses into the pioneering field of addictions nursing in Japan. Addiction was another critical social issue little understood by those in healthcare, with few options for treatment and rehabilitation. To help meet this challenge, Addiction mondai wo Kangaeru Kai (AKK), a nonprofit organization of citizens against addiction, was established in 1986 (Lynch, 2000). At that time, addictions were not recognized as psychosocial and mental health problems. In 1993, AKK successfully established a shelter for women whose batterers are addicted, as well as for other women who are victims of battering in their homes.

Domestic Violence Shelter Movement

Several years ago, a high official of Japanese government stated at an international conference that there was rarely domestic violence from a man to an intimate woman in Japan. Yet, the number of cases identified as battered women indicate that this is not the case. In a society in which domestic violence or violence against women is not realized as violence against human rights, it is understandable that women seldom ask for help. Most batterers are able to live an otherwise respectable social life. In 1997, there were 88 public women's shelters in Japan. Although the total number of private shelters remains over 40 today, there will be a greater number of resources in the near future. A public shelter, however, has many limitations that complicate services for women and their children, such as a two-week residency limit.

For more than 15 years, AKK has intervened with a wide range of addictions. Recovering addicts, their family members, physicians, psychiatrists, nurses, public health nurses, caseworkers, and social workers serve as volunteers in the spirit of community service. The principal activities of AKK are to create an environment for free discussion on overcoming addiction, telephone consultation, and self-help groups, such as Alcoholics Anonymous. Reflecting the battered women's voice that public (government-supported) shelters are not satisfactory, the mission of AKK is to provide emotional support, peace, and a safe environment for the battered woman's recovery. Recently, AKK shelter changed its name to Abused Women's Shelter (AWS).

In February 1997, the third anniversary of the opening of AKK Women's Shelter, seven other shelters joined in celebration of the event, coming together for the first time to network and to share knowledge. In March 1997, "Forum Yokohama" opened a problem-solving workshop for battered women that was attended by almost 80, including counselors from women's centers, a surgeon, a psychiatrist, nurses, staffs of women's shelters, journalists, police officers, and lawyers. These professionals affirmed the following:

- All people can have the common recognition of what constitutes domestic violence.
- Professionals may have a better understanding of battered women's mental process.
- Professionals must insist upon the arrangement of the legal system that covers violence against women.
- Professionals have to extend the network to support battered women.

This movement in Japan is similar to that in the late 1970s in the US. Only a limited number of nurses are interested in working with domestic violence victims, although some general nurses and public health nurses take responsibility in providing private care.

A pilot program on "Domestic Violence and the Victim's Support" was initiated at a private educational center in Tokyo. This program included a series of 12 lectures and was open to all interested persons, both professionals and the community. Although small in attendance, there was strong initial support for the program by those who participated.

Critical Incident Stress Intervention

Japanese mental health nursing is considered to be two decades behind that in the US. The need for mental healthcare for victims of catastrophic accidents or natural disasters is now being recognized. Events such as the Hanshin-Awaji earthquake, along with its victims and their families, traffic fatalities, or crimes against persons are now being recognized as the type of scenarios that require specific interventions for post-traumatic stress. In addition, in recently reported cases, some patients who had been given a diagnosis of schizophrenia or personality disorders are now known to have been exposed to various degrees of violence in their families. With an emphasis on progressive change, it has been recognized that there is a need to analyze present social conditions and to apply forensic psychiatric nursing processes as a component of interventions.

Educational Needs

Education for healthcare professionals is one immediate initiative for nurses and physicians alike in order to improve their knowledge and recognition of violence and abuse. For example, when a battered woman presents to the emergency department with injuries resulting from domestic violence, it is very important who copes with her problem and how it is managed. One surgeon said that battered women hate the nurses' way of treating them, so he took care of those patients without the assistance of a nurse. It is possible that both the physician and the nurse are misunderstanding the battered woman's mental state. In the past, the Japanese police usually did not cope with domestic violence because they thought, under civil law, they were not supposed to interfere with problems between husband and wife or intimate partner. Japanese police and the legal system were powerless to intervene with the perpetrator. Few lawyers have adequate knowledge to file suit for divorce or to try a criminal lawsuit for battered women.

Case Study 56-2 Psychological Abuse and Support Systems

A woman requested a consultation regarding her marital relationship and psychological abuse and was assured confidentiality by the nurse because the woman lived near the clinic. The woman stated that at times she thought she would become sick if she had to endure her husband's treatment any longer and that she had wanted to talk to someone for a long time but knew of no one who would listen. Although the nurse was unfamiliar with the term psychological abuse at that time, she immediately recognized the husband's behavior as unacceptable and unfair to the woman. By providing affirmation of her feelings, the woman requested to be able to continue the discussion at a later time. She was told that she was welcome to return any time she pleased.

Advances in Child Protection

Hospitals, public health centers, and child welfare bureaus are the organizations that are most frequently concerned in the cases of child abuse. Pediatricians, but also other doctors and nurses working in emergency services, must have adequate knowledge about child abuse. Today with the inception of the new Law for the Prevention of Spousal Violence and the Protection of Victims, the nurse has the responsibility to notify the police when the victim agrees to report. Nurses are also required to record the evidence of violent injuries in the medical chart. Follow-up intervention is subsequently required and is the responsibility of the nurse in cases of family violence.

Japan is now beginning to acknowledge the issues of child abuse. It has not been recognized generally because it was not identified by Japanese society as criminal behavior. Cases of child abuse traditionally have been concealed within the ancestral structure and remained largely unreported. Although the Child Abuse Prevention Law was passed in 1933 and the Child Welfare Act in 1947, Japanese parental authority is respected so highly that many suspected cases of abuse remain unreported. Unlike the American and European legal systems, under the Japanese legal system no penalty exists for specialists who fail to report child abuse. Recently, however, an increase in the number of reports made by public health nurses shows that healthcare professionals are attentive and concerned about child abuse. Concurrently, prevention efforts are increasing, primarily by nongovernmental organizations at a grassroots level. A more extensive child abuse law was established in June 2000.

Child Abuse and Public Health Nursing

In Japan, the Child Abuse Prevention Law was passed in 1933 and was included in the Children's Welfare Act in 1948. Yet, generally, the cases of child abuse were in the name of discipline. In other cases the minimum care was neglected, where children were provided with little food or cleanliness. However, these cases were considered ordinary and weren't recognized as abuse. In the statistics of child welfare in 1994, there were 2961 reports of child abuse from the Children's Welfare Bureau–and this is just the tip of the iceberg.

Best Practice *56-4*

Nurses and their colleagues should facilitate child protection and contribute to the improved laws surrounding violence against women.

In 1987, Osaka Prefecture, located in western Japan, initiated the investigation of abused children's care. The results of the investigation showed that there were increasing reports of child abuse each year: 40% of the reports were sent to Children's Welfare Bureau, 25% to Public Health Center, and 23% to hospitals and clinics. In 1988, the Conference for Coping with Child Abuse and the Committee for Establishing Measures against Child Abuse were implemented. The Conference for Coping with Child Abuse consisted of the supervising Osaka Prefecture's Health-Welfare Medical Officer, medical organizations, lawyers, and the court of family affairs, police, and Osaka Prefecture's officers in charge of welfare, health, and education. They examined the possibility of prevention of child abuse, early reporting, and support programs. A manual based on information gathered from this conference was developed and made available for every organization that was responsible for identifying child abuse.

In Tokyo, the Center of Child Abuse Prevention offered services such as telephone consultation for the community at large and case examination conferences for specialists. In this corporation, besides the citizens, many specialists who are public health nurses, general nurses, pediatricians, lawyers, mother-and-child counselors, child welfare officers, and case workers join as volunteers.

Through the expansion of these grassroots movements, the phrase "child abuse" has now started to be acknowledged in Japanese society. In the past, through the Children's Welfare Act, the parental authority was respected so highly that many cases of possible abuse were unreported.

Key Point *56-4*

Presently, it is a rare case in which the Child Welfare Bureau can stop the parental authority.

Under the Japanese law, unlike American or European law, specialists are not penalized for failing to report child abuse. This has resulted in a misinterpretation of crime rates as well as unsanctioned abuse of children. In Japan, the Public Health Center Act was recently revised into the Community Health Act, and the administration of mother and child health activities has been handed over from the prefecture to city, town, or village authorities. Hopefully, this will instill greater security for the child, and punishment will be implemented to those who abuse the children of Japan.

In spite of changing laws, there is not enough education or training for public health nurses who are responsible for distinguishing abuse. In metropolitan Tokyo, there are a few programs for mother-and-child community care. The public health nurse can often detect child abuse because in addition to seeing the parent and child in the public health center, the nurse also visits the home and provides supportive care. Recently a mother's self-help group has been started at a private psychiatric clinic in Tokyo.

Nursing Education Needs

Nursing education rarely addresses the issue of family-related violence as a public health disturbance in Japan. It has only recently initiated discussion on post-traumatic stress disorder, codependency, and child abuse by adults. However, nursing research on child abuse has made an appearance in the mental health/psychiatric nursing arena. Although no formal academic programs offer forensic nursing within the curricula, Kobe University was the first to initiate an interest in forensic nursing in 1997, when Virginia Lynch was invited to introduce this new field of studies. Owing to the interest stimulated by this first endeavor, Lynch was requested to provide an expanded program in 2004. Judging from the interest expressed by students and faculty alike, forensic nursing is expected to become a new academic program in the near future.

Currently, few pioneers are in the forefront of forensic nursing in Japan, but these nurses continue to promote and develop forensic nursing through their clinical practice and faculty appointments. Nurses involved in pioneering forensic nursing in Japan are primarily involved in psychiatric/mental health nursing, in which these skills are applied within the forensic patient population. Initial studies that interface with forensic nursing roles include such subjects as substance abuse and violence against women and children, areas that have not previously been included in Japanese nursing curricula. Today, lectures on communication, family therapy, addictions, interpersonal relationships, domestic violence, child abuse, and community health and education are being addressed and have stimulated interest in the field of forensic nursing. It was not until 1997 that mental-health and psychiatric nursing was included in the curriculum as a required subject, rather than an elective. This should significantly benefit the advancement of forensic nursing in Japan.

Forensic Nurse Examiners

The first sexual assault nurse examiner (SANE) program in Tokyo was established in June 2000 by the Women's Support and Education Center for Women's Safety and Health, a nonprofit and nongovernmental organization that offers basic and advanced training programs. By following this course of study, these nurses are able to testify as experts. There is at present no special license, but a certificate is awarded. In 2003, the Women's Support and Education Center presented a series of lectures and a workshop by Virginia Lynch. These lectures prepared nurses in the transition from a SANE program to that of a forensic nurse examiner (FNE) program as an expansion of forensic nursing services. This is seen as the pathway to the future of forensic nursing education and practice across Japan. This previously unavailable resource is recognized for the benefits and credibility it brings into the health and justice systems and will become an invaluable asset to the judiciary and the courts.

FNE and advocate services also contribute to the successful prosecution of offenders and the exoneration of those who have been falsely accused, as well as to the medicolegal management of forensic patients in clinical and community public health and safety. In the near future, these forensic specialists in nursing will reach beyond their limited role and become clinical forensic specialists, addressing all patients with medicolegal concerns. Although presently there are few forensic nurses in Japan, it is firmly believed those practicing today are committed to influencing nursing education, clinical practice, and forensic nursing services in the future.

New Role Perspectives Needed

In Japan, most nurses do not recognize that the role of forensic nursing should be included in their daily activities. On the contrary, nurses have little appreciation about their responsibilities for recognizing health problems and injuries that result from acts of violence or prolonged physical and emotional abuse. Because of the lack of education in traditional nursing programs, nurses are generally unaware of the interrelationship between public heath and interpersonal violence.

However, should suspicion of abuse be recognized, conventional accepted policies would imply that identifying crime victims and reporting to legal agencies are outside their responsibilities and that this role is too difficult. Nurses are especially naïve about their roles in areas in which the law is involved because forensic nursing is not traditionally included in the Japanese nursing education.

Southeast Asia

DORA MARIA CARBONU

Establishing forensic nursing in Asia is a challenge beyond any experience nursing faces as a profession. The most recent country to address the benefits of forensic nursing has been Brunei Darussalam, a tropical rainforest country located in the northwest region of the Island of Borneo, in the South China Sea. Brunei is an Islamic monarchy, with a history that dates to the fourteenth century. It has a population of 340,800 citizens, 51.0% are male; 49.0% are female; 29.9% are 14 years old or younger; 67.2% are 15 to 64 years old; and 2.9% are 65 years old and above. Two-thirds (67.0%) of the population is Malay by race and Muslim by religion; 11.0% are Chinese; 3.6% are of indigenous origins; and 18.8% are of other origins (Brunei Yearbook, 2003).

Nursing in Brunei Darussalam

Nursing education was launched in Brunei in 1946 under the Ministry of Health and Medical Services. This was conducted on an informal basis until 1951, when a hospital-based school of nursing was established in collaboration with the World Health Organization (WHO) and the United Nations Children's Emergency Fund (UNICEF). The goal was to provide formal training to assistant nurses, who would assist in the care of the sick and needy. A structured three-year nursing educational program was introduced in 1954 to train high school graduates for the position of certified trained nurses. This program was based on the recommendations of what is currently known as the Nursing and Midwifery Council (NMC).

In the 1960s, there were a number of Brunei national candidates receiving their education in the UK through the award of government scholarships. The graduates qualified as state registered nurses. A number of the graduates stayed on to acquire post-basic diplomas in midwifery or psychiatric nursing before returning home to Brunei. A midwifery training school was later established as a component program of the School of Nursing, with the goal to train midwives for the national needs of women and children. The Ministry of Health has been and continues to be the main "employer" of the nurses and midwives for the four district hospitals, health centers, and clinics in the country.

In 1985, His Majesty and Yang Di Pertuan of Brunei Darussalam, Sultan Hassanal Bolkiah, granted his consent for the establishment of the College of Nursing. University of Wales College of Medicine in Cardiff acts in an advisory capacity and ensures that the programs of the college attain their goal of achieving levels of competency as designed by the NMC. The linkage and affiliation continue today.

The College of Nursing, which is named after its patron, Her Royal Highness Pengiran Anak Puteri Rashida Sa'adatul Bolkiah (PAPRSB), had graduated 792 basic diploma candidates by 2002 (Carbonu & Abdul Rahim, 1998; Ninth Convocation Program, 2003). In 1998, the School of Nursing merged with the College of Nursing to become one institutional body for nursing educational programs in the country.

Forensic Agenda in Southeast Asia

Domestic violence is as common a problem in Asia as it is in other parts of the world, making the continent a fertile ground for a forensic nursing program that would address violence against women from a holistic health, social, and legal point of view (Carbonu, 2000; Carbonu & Soares, 1997)

In Brunei Darussalam, dialogue regarding forensic nursing has been initiated with leaders in nursing education and practice, and there have been efforts to enlist the cooperation of leading personnel of health, education, social services, the legal system, and law enforcement in the establishment of a forensic nursing program in the country. This endeavor has come as a result of the lecture series presented in November 1999 by Virginia Lynch. Her series of lectures on how nurses have become a primary resource to legal and government agencies, healthcare, and victim services has stimulated interest within the Brunei community. Conclusions and recommendations have been considered to critically address the issue of domestic violence–through the development of and enhancement of awareness among members of the society about the serious impact of this health issue and the establishment of a forensic health science multidisciplinary team for the prevention, management, control, reduction, and even eradication of domestic violence in the country (Carbonu, 2000).

Singapore

Singapore, an independent island country, is located in Southeast Asia, between Malaysia and Indonesia. It has a population of 4,608,595, the majority (75.5%) of whom are between 15 and 64 years old; 17.3% are 0 to 14 years old; and 7.2% are 65 years old or older. The population is predominantly Chinese (76.7%), 14% Malay, 7.9% Indian, and 1.4% for others (CIA).

Singapore was the first Asian country to employ forensic nurse examiners as investigators in the medical examiner system at the Singapore Institute of Legal Medicine and Forensic Sciences, and did so with great success. The Singapore Ministry of Health has arranged for five Singaporean nurses to participate in a forensic nursing certificate program and internship in forensic psychiatric nursing at the University of Colorado. Upon return to Singapore, internship in the scientific investigation of death is arranged at the medical examiner's office to continue the broad perspective of knowledge between the living and the dead.

Although Singapore was the first among Asian countries to send nurses to the US to study the expanded role of forensic nursing and to employ forensic nurses, the implementation of clinical forensic practice has been slow to develop (Lynch, 1999). On the other hand, even though the concept of a forensic nurse in clinical practice is new to this area of Asia, it appears to be progressing with an acceptance not found in other Asian countries. The need, nonetheless, is greater in these countries than in many other areas of the world, and with perseverance and support from government and nongovernment agencies, forensic nursing will no doubt become an important component of healthcare services in Asia and neighboring eastern countries.

Violence against Women

Domestic violence is seen not only in the disabilities of women who are victims, but also throughout the entire culture–the home, social circles, community, and workplace (Haji Abu Salam, 2000; Haji Badarudin, 2000; Salaam, 2003). Some international statistics suggest that the incidence of violence against women continues to yield higher figures, more particularly in developing countries, with the highest figures recorded in Asian countries: 25% in India; 35% in South Korea; 50% in Thailand; 59% in Japan; 60% in Papua New Guinea and People's Republic of North Korea; and as high as 80% in Pakistan.

Women of Brunei Darussalam experience various forms of domestic violence, including rape, incest, wife battery, concealment of birth by secret disposal of dead body, procuration of a minor, trafficking in women and children, prostitution of minors, and abuse of domestic helpers (Royal Brunei Police Force, 2000). These and other forms of domestic violence plague the female population of the country. Yet, measures to explore and address these problems are poor and inadequate.

Evidence suggests that healthcare professionals in the country do not have adequate training in managing cases of domestic violence. For example, a four-year-old victim of sexual molestation was brought to the accident and emergency department. The doctor sent back the girl with her mother to report the incident to the police first, before the doctor would attend to the child. In another example, the death of a female foreign worker, which was a strongly suspected case of homicide, was left for more than three hours without police involvement. After several phone calls and persuasions by a concerned expatriate nurse, the police finally arrived in the emergency department, and even then, they decided to have the body moved to the morgue, where they planned to conduct the forensic examination the next day! Several other cases of abuse are poorly handled and documented. Similarly, no counseling services are available to the victims of abuse.

In Pakistan, women have a uniquely defined identity as a Muslim, a Pakistani, and a woman. This identity dictates the way women live and is influenced by custom, religion, norms, mores, laws, rules, and regulations. Even though women make up 48% of the national population (Khan, 2000), their role is limited predominantly to childbearing and childrearing, and their contributions to society are considered trivial (Carbonu & Soares, 1997; Khan, 2000; Shahin, 2000). Consequently, women are vulnerable to victimization through inequity in activities of daily living, and many are victims of domestic violence, sexual assault, drug addictions, and suicide attempts. Women in Pakistan also fall prey to emotional trauma, which further leads to low self-esteem, low self-confidence, feelings of worthlessness and hopelessness, and fatalistic tendencies.

In recent years, the Aga Khan University School of Nursing in Pakistan was using the conceptual framework of Maslow's hierarchy of needs, paralleling empowerment and its antecedents. However, the contemporary definition of a forensic holistic hierarchy of needs is *body, mind, spirit,* and the *law* (Lynch, 1999); Maslow does not specifically examine these critical legal concerns. It is essential to consider the legal issues surrounding patient care if the body, mind, and spirit are to be successfully healed and the patient returned to a homeostatic preabuse status.

The prevention and identification of abuse and subsequent intervention are important areas of nursing involvement. Nurses are always the first professionals to interact with those affected by family violence. As members of the interdisciplinary team, nurses can play a significant role in addressing the issue of violence against women in Asia (International Council of Nursing, 2001; Lynch, 1999). However, there may be reluctance on the part of some nurses to intervene because of the perception that violence is a private, family matter rather than a social health problem. In addition, nurses may be uncertain about what to say or do when a person acknowledges that abuse has occurred (ICN, 2001).

New Awareness

Although the origins of women's issues are prehistoric and a global phenomenon, only within the last few decades has vivid testimony of the change in the expectations of Asian women been provided, highlighted by the World Health Organization's (WHO) Universal Declaration of Human Rights in 1948; Declaration of the United Nations International Decade for Women (1975-1985); and the emergence of women's and affirmative action movements. In more and more countries, attempts are being made to bring women's health issues and problems into the open, to help victims, and to expose the causes (Physicians for Human Rights, 2001; Salaam, 2003).

Women's issues tend to be more pronounced in developing countries, where they include extremely limited resources, lack of communication, vast distances with limited mobility and inability to access services, lack of education, individual and community poverty, and poor nutrition. These conditions lead to low standards of living, inadequate food intake, poor housing, poor health and hygiene, and poor medical care. These problems, in turn, result in maternal and infant morbidity and fatality, various health burdens, taboos on sexuality, risk of exposure to sexually transmitted diseases, sexual violence and exploitation, and in extreme cases, even death (Khan, 2000; Physicians for Human Rights, 2001; Salaam, 2003).

The Brunei Initiative

Brunei Darussalam embraced a bold initiative in 1987, when a special committee was set up by the government to address the issue of domestic violence, more specifically child abuse. In 1993, the Social Affairs Services Unit (SASU) was established within the Ministry of Culture, Youth and Sports. One specific goal of the unit is to work in collaboration with the National Committee in enhancing and promoting the effectiveness of the national protocol on child abuse. In addition, SASU would provide special services to the vulnerable, needy groups of the country, including the destitute, handicapped, pregnant teens, children, youth, and female adults who are victims of abuse of various forms (SASU, 2000). The government has instituted several measures as penalty for such offenses. These penalties range from two years of imprisonment for concealment of birth by secret disposal of dead body or a fine, or both, to 30 years of imprisonment with whippings, for rape, and for other forms of violence (Table 56-1).

Table 56-1 Range of Sentences for Forms of Abuse in Brunei Darussalam

SENTENCES	NATURE OF VIOLENCE
2 years, or a fine, or both	Concealment of birth by secret disposal of dead body
3 years	Causing hurt
5 years with whipping and $20,000 maximum fine	Outraging modesty
	Act for purposes of prostitution
	Trafficking in women and children
	Living on or trading in prostitution
2-7 years with whipping (up to 12 whippings maximum)	Carnal knowledge of a child under age 16
Up to 24 whippings maximum	Carnal knowledge of a youth 12 years of age or under by an adult of 24 years and over
7 years with whipping or a fine, or both	Causing hurt by dangerous weapons or other means
	Exposure of child under 12 years
10 years with a fine and whipping	Infanticide
	Causing grievous hurt
	Unnatural offenses
	Incest
15 years with whipping	Causing grievous hurt by dangerous weapons or other means
30 years with 12 whippings minimum	Rape
	Procuration of a minor
	Selling or let to hire a minor for prostitution
	Buying or obtaining a minor for prostitution
	Importing for purposes of prostitution

Data from Police Headquarters, Royal Brunei Police Force, Brunei Darussalam.

Limitations of Domestic Violence Initiatives

The problem of domestic violence is so pervasive and voluntary sector agencies, including senior policy and strategy developers, have the role to provide services to the public. Yet, these measures have not been successful because of several factors, including the ineffective and inadequate services available. There are limited educational programs that teach and prepare health professionals, legal, police, and social services staff, as well as other members of the multidisciplinary team, to provide adequate care, and to be understanding and sensitive to the needs of victimized patients. In spite of these limitations, the SASU in Brunei continues in its efforts to initiate a dialogue for a forensic science program in the country, and to work closely with the Domestic Violence Committee to improve the health and welfare of the women and children of Brunei.

Pakistan

In spite of increased urbanization and industrialization, as well as the revolution in modern communications, Pakistani women are still entrapped within the traditional and religious beliefs and values, and in their predominantly childbearing and childrearing roles, which are highly regarded as a woman's natural function. Women generally are deprived of equal participation in many social activities, including labor, economy, and politics (Khan, 2000; Salaam, 2003).

The Dowry System

The dowry system has many implications that result in various forms of violence being inflicted on women through family quarrels, wife battery, acid baths, permanent disability, and even murder (Rosen & Conly, 1996; Salaam, 2003; Akanda & Shamin, 1985). In marriage, a woman's in-laws consider the dowry system, a customary practice, as the symbol and measure of her status as a bride in the family. As a wife, her status is very low and she is regarded as property. Her ownership is transferred to the husband's family until her death, and she is one of the chattels to be "inherited" after the death of her husband (Ali, 1993; Khan, 2000; Salaam, 2003). A woman's own family would rather have her dead, and her body brought back home for burial, than have her return from an abusive marital home as a divorced individual.

Marriage and Childbirth

On average, the Pakistani woman has six children during her lifetime (Anderson, 1999; Gudeta, 1995; Shahin, 2000). This birth rate is considered to be the highest in the world. In Brunei, a woman has four children during her lifetime, on average.

In Pakistan, adolescents make up 22% to 25% of the national population. The average age at marriage for women is 22 and this age is increasing. A 1998 report indicated that 17% of adolescent girls aged between 15 and 19 were married, and over half of women 20 to 24 years old were married before 20 (Khan, 2000; Shahin, 2000). UNICEF defines a "child" as someone between the ages of 5 and 19, while UNFPA (United Nations Population Fund) terms "youth" as all those people between 15 and 24 years old and those below this age are categorized as "children." The government of Pakistan, on the other hand, defines "child" as 14 years old or younger (Khan, 2000). In the Punjab, the ideal age of marriage expressed by girls is between 20 and 25 (Khan 2000). In the rural area of Sindh, fertility is highest among women between 15 and 39, indicating an early marriage for girls. According to Kazmi (1992), in the urban area of Sindh Province, the highest fertility rate recorded is in the age group of 20 to 34, in which 75% of births take place. Rural girls are at a disadvantage compared to their urban counterparts when it comes to marrying early. Khan (2000) further reports that low female status and little decision-making power among younger women suggests that those who marry young may not be doing so out of their own choice and that preparation for married life is likely to be inadequate.

Gudeta (1994) and Akhtar (Khan, 2000) report that early marriage leads to childbearing before physical development is complete. Married adolescent girls are likely to find motherhood the sole focus of their lives, at the expense of development in other areas, such as formal education, training for employment, work experiences, and personal growth. These factors lead to depletion in maternal nutrition, increase in susceptibility to diseases, and complications during pregnancy, during delivery, and in the postpartum phase. These complications include increased risk of premature labor, miscarriage, and stillbirth (Zaidi, Wajid, & Rehan, 1996). According to PDHS (Pakistan Demographic and Health Survey) 1990-1991 data (Khan, 2000), 17% of women 20 to 24 years old have given birth by age 18. Maternal morbidity and mortality rates are very high. Rosen and Conly (1996) report that only a third of Pakistani women have access to a trained healthcare worker in pregnancy and childbirth. Tinker reports only 20% of women as receiving assistance from a trained healthcare provider during delivery. Rosen and Conly also note that 600 women die for every 100,000 live births. Tinker records maternal mortality ratio as 340 per 100,000 live births (Khan, 2000). Shaikh (2003) conducted a study to assess the magnitude and type of domestic violence inflicted on women by their husbands in Rawalpindi and Islamabad. The majority (97.0%) of the 216 women involved in the study reported enduring multiple types of violence, and 24.9% reported that violence in general increased during pregnancy.

Death of women in pregnancy and childbirth is rivaled by the violence inflicted on them by their male partners (Khan, 2000). A survey by Jafarey (2002) of 30 hospitals and private clinics across Pakistan, and covering 104,561 live births, found 703 maternal deaths. Adolescents figured prominently in deaths associated with childbearing; 10% of those whose ages were determined, were between 15 and 20 years old (Khan 2000). Patients who were not enrolled in regular antenatal care and suffering primarily from direct causes, such as hemorrhage, hypertensive diseases, eclampsia, and sepsis, accounted for most of the deaths (Lodhi & Yusaf, 1997; Kolachi, 1999; Khan, 2000).

Jafarey and Korejo (Khan, 2000) conducted a study of 150 pregnant or recently delivered women, who entered hospitals in Karachi "dead on arrival." The purpose of the study was to determine the causes of delay that resulted in the women arriving at the hospitals dead. Another study by Ashraf (Khan, 2000) also involved a similar group of women, who had arrived in Quetta Hospital already dead. Both studies found similar results. Reasons for delay included lack of available transport and finances, reluctance of the family to bring the woman to hospital, absence of husband from the house, and inadequate maternal services that failed to refer the patient to the tertiary care facility in time. The findings further showed that most of the causes of death were preventable had health services been accessed in time. The most disturbing finding was that all but five of the DOA women in the Karachi study lived only 5 to 10 kilometers away from a hospital.

A situational analysis of maternal health in Sindh Province was conducted from a 1997 Provincial database. The results showed very poor maternal health indicators. Out of 1,601,740 pregnancies, only 10.2% obtained prenatal care; pregnancy loss was 11.1%, and only 3.2% of maternal deliveries had supervision from trained healthcare workers (Kolachi, 1999). The risk of death increases with high parity and infant fatality is strongly linked with mother's age at first birth (Khan, 2000).

The Value of a Male Child

The woman's status increases with the birth of a male child, which makes it an imperative to produce sons (Joshi, 1999). As boys are more "desirable," however, they are given special care from infancy. As a result of lack of attention and nurturing, many girls are believed to die in childhood. The period of adolescence for Pakistani children marks an increase in a trend of gender differentials in nutrition levels, access to healthcare, education, and other social services. This further suggests a general attitude of negligence toward women.

Adultery as a Weapon

Female sexuality is tightly controlled, and this is expressed most severely in restrictions placed on unmarried girls (Khan, 2000). The charge of adultery has been used as a weapon against women. A member of the current wife's family purports the "accusation" as a convenient way for the husband who wants to marry a second time to get rid of his current wife. A father may use the accusation or threat of accusation to punish a "disobedient" daughter who does not follow the family's dictates. This is reflected in the practice of "honor killing," which is prevalent in certain sectors of society (LeGood, 1999). The charge of adultery may also be used as a ploy to get a woman out of the way if she is to inherit property (Ahmed, 1993). Other forms of domestic violence against women include physical abuse, throwing acids, burns, and sexual abuse, including incest, sexual exploitation, and pornography, with the most vulnerable age group being girls 10 to 18 years old (Niaz, 1994; Salaam, 2003).

The Civil and Legal Systems

Women generally are considered unaware of their legal, civil, and human rights, which leads to their exploitation. In Pakistan, legal controls, among them the 1979 Hudood Ordinances, and customary practices, such as *karo kari* (honour killings) in Sindh and Balochistan (Khan, 2000), make sex outside of marriage by a man or a woman punishable by death by a community on the suspicion that both man and woman have committed adultery. Those killed include adolescent girls, although the proportion of those deaths cannot be ascertained (Khan, 2000).

According to Khan (2000), unfortunately, the reality of young people's lives continues to expose the paucity of policies that affect them. Adolescent boys appear to be prime targets of sexual abuse, while discrimination in the laws will make an adolescent girl liable to adult prosecution for illegal sex if she has attained puberty. Adolescent girls, whether or not they are married, face the greatest social restrictions in accessing healthcare, which is likely to have serious implications for their gynecological well-being as well as for their ability to control their own fertility (Khan, 2000).

Only a fraction of violent abuses are recorded and dealt with by the police or the legal system. Certain anomalies are present within the legal systems that at times work against women. Husbands may inflict grievous injury on their wives for the "purpose of correcting her." An abused female victim who approaches the legal system for protection may rather become the target of further abuse.

Discriminatory laws that have enhanced the climate for tolerance of violence against women must be revisited and revised.

Outcome

Isolation may be the worst of women's suffering. Lack of respect, influence on decision making, opportunity to grow, control over one's life or circumstances, and time with family, as well as having too many births and feelings of powerlessness, are forms of abuse and part of the woman's struggles between self and society. Added to the Pakistani woman's plight is the practice of *purdah*, or seclusion, or segregation of the sexes. This strict norm has historical significance and represents an adoption of attitudes that are consistent with traditional beliefs and values (Joshi, 1999; Khan, 2000; Rosen & Conly, 1996). Purdah is enforced at the time of puberty and is not relaxed until the time of menopause; it permits less formal education for women and limits their activities outside the home. Purdah norms interfere with access of women to medical treatment, demands that husbands accompany their wives to the clinic, as well as demands for the presence of a lady doctor only to attend to the women if they are able to access health services. In this respect, women, especially adolescent girls, have minimal involvement within their respective communities, including limited access to education and employment opportunities (Khan, 2000; LeGood, 1999; Rosen & Conly, 1996).

This fear is a major factor in favor of marrying girls off young, as a means to ensure that control over their sexuality is not lost (Khan, 2000). Kazi and Sathar (Khan, 2000) found that Southern Punjabi communities were more restrictive of women's freedom of movement than the more developed villages of Central Punjab, most especially in women younger than 25 years old. This normative practice and bias captures the dilemma of being adolescent in Pakistani society, where a girl's biological development signals her "entry into a world in which her value is largely determined by her sexual and reproductive functions" (Niaz, 1994; Rosen & Conly, 1996; Khan, 2000).

Issues and problems of abuse are not unique to Pakistani women. Various authors have deliberated on the issues of women in different parts of the globe. In a comprehensive report on human rights developments, the Human Rights Watch looked at the issues of violence or abuse from a global point of view. Bilimoria (Khan, 2000) examined Muslim personal laws in India, with some emphasis on women's issues in that country. Joshi (1999) critically considered gender equity and the demographic implications for women, while Joshi (1999) revisited the contrasts in social development between Pakistan and India. Consistently, commonalities, comparisons, and contrasts could be drawn from these various researchers and analysts, in relation to the plight of the Pakistani woman, supporting the fact that Pakistani women are not alone; violence against women and its related implications and complications are universal and pertain to women of all races, colors, religions, cultures, social classes, and status.

Psychosocial Nursing

Forensic nurses provide psychological or psychosocial support to their patients through empathy and assertiveness and by sustaining the emotions, morale, culture, and spirituality of the individual. The philosophical approach to nursing is grounded in caring for the whole person, and nurses who care for victims of violence have the responsibility to protect the women's legal rights by proper collection of forensic evidence. With the nature of crimes against women in Asia, as well as the general status of women, there is a great need for psychosocial support that can be provided by the forensic nurse examiner at the time of intervention for trauma. Forensic psychiatric nurses also provide care for the suspects and perpetrators of crime who are awaiting trial or execution. In South Asia, a Singaporean forensic psychiatric nurse identifies components of his work as caring for the mental health of prisoners condemned to die by hanging as well as support for their mothers, wives, and children who come to say goodbye.

Forensic Psychiatry

The forensic nurse examiner must not only work therapeutically with the patient through assessment and treatment planning and implementation; he or she must understand and respect the goals of the correctional system to work most effectively with the person. In Pakistan, the need to ensure the link among these systems may be regarded as a demand, because failure to ensure such a link is believed to result in misinterpretation, mishandling, or omission of valuable forensic evidence. Evidence collection should never interfere with timely patient treatment (Lynch, 1995).

Nursing Education

The history of nursing education in Pakistan parallels the country's independence. In 1947, the nursing curriculum was adapted, leading to the granting of certificates in general nursing. The curriculum was revised and updated in 1973 by the Pakistan Nursing Council (PNC) for implementation by all schools of nursing in the country, and the graduates were issued a diploma in nursing education. The International Declaration (Alma Ata) of "Health for All by the Year 2000" led to further revisions of the basic nursing education with special emphasis on primary healthcare. The emphasis on community health nursing was influenced further as a result of various health issues, including population. During that same period, the provision and promotion of mental healthcare was endorsed as one of the eight components of community-based primary healthcare in Pakistan (Ahmed, Ahmed, & Khan, 1988).

The need to improve mental health services for the citizens in Pakistan was recognized with emphasis on the most vulnerable, underserved, and inappropriately served rural population (Mabbashar, 1988). The aim was to achieve the following:

- Include community participation in the development of mental health services to support the nongovernmental organizations
- Generate a spirit of self-help in the community
- Create awareness in the general public and mental health workers regarding the harmful effects of such factors as broken homes, juvenile delinquency, drug abuse, and the impaired performance of roles due to rapid social change (Mabbashar, 1988)

The demand for the specialized field of psychiatric or mental health nursing in Pakistan is great, yet its practice continues to remain in the medical mode with a high psychiatric morbidity rate in the country (Kazi, 1988; Mirza, 2002). Psychiatric or mental health nursing also forms a strategic part of the curriculum and is a specialization course, yet there is an acute shortage of such specialists in the country, and the few in practice are mostly hospital-based (Islam, 2002; Mirza, 2002; Qidwai, 2003). This suggests that the impact of psychiatric nursing in the protection and management of victimized individuals is limited. Ahmed and associates (1988) identified the need for the revision of a specialized training program for nurses and recommended the training of nursing auxiliary aids/mental nursing assistants and training and orientation in psychiatry for administrators, with the aim of changing attitudes toward mental health.

Although these recommendations were made almost two decades ago, evidence suggests that implementation and achievement have been insignificant (Mirza, 2002; Qidwai, 2003; Shahin, 2002). The World Health Organization launched "Mental Health: New Understanding, New Hope" on October 10, 2001, highlighting the burden of mental disorders as a major public health challenge in the twenty-first century and beyond. This drive by WHO further prompts the desperate need for educational and health authorities in Asian countries, including Pakistan, to consider making the undergraduate syllabus of psychiatric and behavioral sciences rigorous in the light of WHO report in an effort to curb the "chronic" mental health issues facing these countries (Anderson, 1999; Mirza, 2002; Qidwai, 2003).

The Role of Pakistan Nursing Council in Forensic Nursing Initiatives

As the professional licensing body responsible for the standards of education for nurses in Pakistan, the PNC may recommend the inclusion of forensic nursing education in the diploma nursing program. The concept may be introduced in the second year, when the students learn about such subjects as rape and trauma. This measure was taken from 1995 to 1997 with a very positive outcome among the three-year diploma students at The Aga Khan University School of Nursing (AKUSON) (Carbonu & Soares, 1997). There are countless areas of nursing in which a stronger background in forensic science would help the nurse better serve the patient, the victim, or in some cases, the criminal.

The Aga Khan University School of Nursing (AKUSON) has worked collaboratively with the PNC (the regulatory body), Pakistan Nursing Federation (the professional body), provincial nursing examination boards, other schools of nursing, and various health service institutions throughout the country to improve nursing education and professional standards in the country. The contributions of AKUSON toward nursing in Pakistan are tremendous and include the development of curricula for post-basic courses at a college of nursing under the World Bank Family Health Project; facilitation for the inclusion and development of community health nursing and mental health nursing subjects in the PNC diploma curriculum; as well as advocacy of changes in PNC regulations, so that married women, and those women between the ages of 35 and 40 would be eligible to enroll in the diploma program. There is no doubt that the AKUSON can be very instrumental in a forensic nursing initiative in Pakistan.

Continuity and Follow-Up Care

Continuity and follow-up care is essential, and victimized women should have the opportunity to discuss their individual needs with the forensic nurse examiner. The women should be provided with information about support groups that deal with victimization of women, such as safe homes, halfway houses, and religious institutions. In Pakistan, these include affirmative action groups such as Women's Action Forum (WAF), Women Against Rape (WAR), and the Sexual Harassment Group (Salaam, 2003; Shamim, 1993); reemphasis on education, training, and development of women through workshops and seminars to raise awareness and to control or prevent various forms of verbal, nonverbal, and physical abuse is important (Mirza, 2002; Qidwai, 2003; Shahin, 2000).

In Pakistan, this is a great challenge for the forensic nurse examiner. As Anderson (1999) observed, Pakistan is a country where women are generally suppressed and constrained by religious rules and have to follow these rigid rules and behaviors. However, in that same country, there are a good number of women who are working on advancing their education and are actively involved in the learning process. They are willing to talk about their problems, and their expectations in "this new Pakistan," at least among the upper class, are changing. Anderson (1999) noted further that female medical students, psychologists, social workers, nurses, and occupational therapists see a world in which they, as women, will have power to control their own lives.

Empowering Victimized Women: The Conceptual Process

The empowerment process encompasses the individual responsibility of the forensic nurse in the healthcare delivery system, the victimized women, and the broader institutional and societal responsibilities of governmental and nongovernmental organizations. These include considering religious values, marital issues, customs, and other values in enabling victimized women to assume responsibility for their own health and destiny (Darlington & Mulvaney, 2003). Maslow's (1954) hierarchy of needs, which is a motivational concept for human behavior that builds from the most basic physiological needs to safety and social needs, self-esteem, and the most sophisticated self-actualization needs, is a conceptual tool that can be utilized by the forensic nurse in the process of empowering the victimized women.

Empowerment of Victims of Violence through Caring

The concept of empowerment has become a common loosely used expression wherever women's issues are being discussed, particularly throughout the developing world. The Platform for Action and the Beijing Declaration frame the issue of women's equality as a human right and advocate the active facilitation of women's empowerment to ensure their full participation in every aspect of development.

Physiological Needs

The basic needs of the victimized woman are physiological, and are congruent with a clean, safe, comfortable environment in the home, the community, within society, and at work. The cleanliness of the environment conveys to the woman a message of respect and value. These needs include stable homes as opposed to separated or divorced families.

Safety Needs

Once physiological needs are met, the woman moves on to the next level: home, family, community, and workplace environmental safety and security. Emotionally hostile conditions provide barriers to the woman's sense of safety and security, particularly when she is a victim of violence from other hostile members of the family, community, or society (McGraw, 1994).

Social Needs

Social needs include a sense of belonging and commitment. Home, workplace, and societal environments that do not provide social support or encourage contribution of risk-taking by women render them powerless and helpless (Jezewski, 1994; Watson, 1994). This phenomenon is common in Pakistan and other developing countries, where women are not encouraged to take risks and are rendered powerless and helpless, particularly through the patriarchal societal system (Islam, 2002; Qidwai, 2003; Salaam, 2003; Shahin, 2000).

Esteem Needs

Women need recognition, trust, a positive image, and a sense of value. The Pakistani woman generally is not provided with messages of thanks and appreciation; therefore, she feels that her deeds are not good enough or are trivial.

Self-Actualization

According to McGraw (1994), empowerment can occur only when its antecedents are present. For the victimized woman, empowerment is possible only when her basic needs for safety and security are met and she knows that she belongs to a family, group, community, or society, and that she is rewarded and cared about.

Success of Empowerment

The success of empowerment further depends on five tools: support, information, resources, creativity, and positive self-concept (Chally, 1992).

Support for victimized women in personal and professional ways, such as a smile, positive feedback, and acknowledgment of frustrations and achievements, can enhance a feeling of accomplishment of important tasks by the women. Women's support for one another is important for empowerment. They bring their support systems to the learning environment, which in turn is a support for empowerment. As female nurses in Southeast Asia studied forensic nursing and conceived the potential for practicing as a forensic nurse examiner it was obvious by their body language, comments, and appearance that their confidence had been elevated.

Information

Information is considered the key to empowerment through teaching. As Sohail asserted in relation to women's fertility and childbearing in Pakistan, the solution lies in the education and empowerment of women and that if they can get a seventh grade education, they will take over control of family size (Anderson, 1999). The forensic nurse must be politically intelligent to be able to positively work with these women (Batliwala, 2003; Darlington & Mulvaney, 2003; Anderson, 1999).

Resources

The success of empowerment is further linked to resources available to the victimized women, who need these assets in learning situations. The forensic nurse examiner plays a significant role in having access to resources or advocating for resources (Batliwala, 2003; Qidwai, 2003; Tabassum & Baig, 2002). Because the role of the forensic nurse in areas of Southeast Asia has been recognized as that of expert in forensic services, the ability to relegate authority as a resource in acquiring and providing materials, information, technology, funding, and facilities is being asserted.

Creativity

The forensic nurse further assists victimized women to obtain resources for their cause through various means, including creativity, which evolves from the women's imagination and thoughts. Creativity is necessary for the advancement of the forensic nurse examiner and for the women, in achieving their goals and overcoming victimization (Anderson, 1999; Chally, 1992). The imagination served to assert their empowerment as they perceived the forensic nursing role: working with police, attorneys, judges, and forensic pathologists and serving as an expert witness in court. The status of nurses as forensic experts has not previously existed in Asia.

Positive Self-Concept

Positive self-concept is critical if victimized women are to become empowered to identify and achieve their goals. The victimized woman must believe that she is capable and worthy. Self-concept develops through a variety of experiences and relationships and is enhanced through a positive forensic nurse–victimized woman interaction. One aspect of the *presence* of the forensic nurse is to ensure that victims do not blame themselves for their victimization, but rather learn that the crime is always the fault of the perpetrator, which in Asia is commonly related to the entrenchment of a patriarchal society.

Power

At the core of the concept of empowerment is the idea of *power*. Power is a positive force that has an impact on the decisions that govern women's lifestyles personally, socially, and professionally.

Chally (1992) asserts a need to change from power over the woman to power to her. Keen (1988) conceptualizes empowerment as manifesting itself in many forms. *Power of inclusion* arises from coalition building with women's groups, support groups, self-help groups, nongovernmental organizations, and various societies (human resources). In *power of affirmation*, sharing positive messages (intellectual resources) allows for feelings of self-esteem and self-worth. The empowered Asian woman then realizes that the *possibilities* for achieving her goals are *endless* (Batliwala, 2003; Bisnath & Elson, 2001). Through the advent of forensic nursing in Asia, women have found a new source of support and empowerment from those who understand her pain and the law.

The Asian woman is victimized in various forms, and as long as she hides behind abuse and finds it shameful to discuss, the matter will never be open to cure. Batliwala (2003) and Bisnath and Elson (2001), among others, emphasize that every person has a power potential; however, only a few use it or know that it exists. This is true of the Asian woman, and her acknowledgment that she and other victimized women have power is the beginning of limitless possibilities.

Mental health nursing in Pakistan is very young. It currently is under the aegis of psychiatric nursing and slowly is becoming a recognized field of practice. Existing mental health services are limited, poorly promoted, and practiced within the medical model. The PNC has been striving to promote the concept of mental health (psychiatric) nursing and to inculcate in society the importance of this field of practice. The introduction of forensic nursing will, at this stage of PNC's efforts, have a tremendous impact on the promotion of positive attitudes toward mental health, including community mental health, and in raising awareness of the health needs and demands of society, which is plagued by various forms of abuse, violence, and victimization of women. Through support, understanding, team effort, determination, and the use of the tools of empowerment as vital resources, the forensic nurse examiner and Pakistani women can translate a shared vision into reality by the integration of victimized women into all aspects of society.

Southeast Asia has been the first in the Southern Hemisphere to introduce and implement forensic nursing in the area of death investigation. Since the 1960s, in Singapore, male nurses had been appointed by the Minister of Health to provide forensic services pertaining to the investigation and certification of "natural" death in residence. In 1984 these nurses began working with the forensic pathologist in the Department of Forensic Pathology. This position now requires duties that include knowledge of autopsy procedures, forensic pathology, and medicolegal investigation of death. Today, they are the designated death investigators in the Center for Forensic Medicine, Health Sciences Authority–the name of the department, too, underwent changes.

The Singapore Center for Forensic Medicine and Health Sciences Authority employs a full staff exclusively comprising forensic nurse examiners as scene investigators. This forensic nurse death investigator program was implemented by Professor Chao Tzee Cheng, one of the pioneers in forensic medicine in Asia. His futuristic insight has proved to be a catalyst for the forensic nursing movement in Asian countries. Although forensic psychiatric nursing has long existed, the need to move beyond and into the arena of clinical forensic nursing science is essential in order to keep pace with the rest of the rapidly progressing countries.

Summary

Those who have reached out to countries in need of a new resource to address violence and its associated trauma have discovered the similarities of interpersonal crime common to each society. Crimes against women, children, and the elderly are inherent. Other commonalties include homicide, sexual violence, alcohol abuse, and suicide. In any country, culture, or society, children are often those most violated by mistreatment, neglect, brutality, sexual abuse, forced labor, and consequences of war.

For forensic nurse examiners to understand the necessary approach to forensic assessment and management of medicolegal cases requires the incorporation of trans-cultural nursing perspectives, ethical and moral dimensions of human care, healthcare practices of diverse cultures, and a review of the law, meaning local, national, and international as well as an in-depth knowledge of the United Nations Declaration of Human Rights. A strong working knowledge of the law promotes interaction with local law enforcement agencies, helps to develop an accurate approach to forensic nursing interventions, and protects healthcare providers outside their own national boundaries.

Resources

Organizations

International Association of Forensic Nurses (IAFN)

East Holly Avenue, Box 56, Pitman, NJ 08071-0056; Tel: 856-256-2425; www.iafn.org

International Council of Nurses

3, Place Jean Marteau, 1201, Geneva, Switzerland, Tel: 41-22-908-01-00; www.icn.ch

References

United Kingdom, England, and Wales

Audit Commission. (1998). *The doctor's bill* (p. 16). London: Belmont Press.

Benner, P. (1984). *From novice to expert: Excellence and power in clinical nursing practice.* Palo Alto, CA: Addison-Wesley.

Burton, J., Chambers, D., & Gill, P. (1985). *Coroners' inquiries: A guide to law and practice.* Middlesex: Kluwer Law.

Davis, G. (1994). Your role in death investigations. *Am J Nurs, 94*(9), 39-41.

Dorries, C. (1990). *Coroner's courts: A guide to law and practice.* Chichester: John Wiley & Sons.

Filer, D. S., & Filer, L. R. (1989). *The role of the forensic nurse. Congress handbook.* Madras, India: Third Indo Pacific Congress on Legal Medicine and Forensic Sciences.

Filer, D. S., & Filer, L. R. (1993). Whither or whither not forensic nursing in the UK. Harrogate, UK: Third International Conference Clinical Forensic Medicine. Programme of Papers. 1993.

Green, L., & Ottoson, J. (1994). *Community health* (7th ed., pp. 383-413). St. Louis: Mosby.

Grimshaw, J., Freemantle, N., Wallace, S., et al. (1995). Developing clinically valid practice guidelines. *J Eval Clin Pract, 1*(1), 37-48.

Henderson, V. (1966). *Nature of nursing.* New York: Macmillan.

Her Majesty's Stationary Office (HMSO). (1988). *The coroner's act.* London: HMSO.

HMSO. (1984). *The coroner's rules.* London: HMSO.

HMSO. (1990). *The courts and legal services act.* London: HMSO.

HMSO. (1987). *The registration of births and death regulations.* London: HMSO.

HMSO. (1996). *What to do after a death in England and Wales: A guide to what you must do and the help you can get.* Oldham: HMSO.

Islamabad Ministry for Population Welfare and London School of Hygiene. (1994). *Issues and opportunities* (2nd ed). Philadelphia: Lippincott.

Kyle, M. (1995). Collaboration. In M. Snyder & M. P. Mirr (Eds.), *Advanced nursing practice: A guide to professional development.* New York: Springer.

Lynch, V. (1997). *Clinical forensic nursing: A new perspective in trauma and medico-legal investigation of death.* Divide, CO: Bearhawk Consulting Group.

Lynch, V. (1995). Clinical forensic nursing: A new perspective in the management of crime victims from trauma to trial. *Crit Care Nurs Clin North Am, 7*(3), 489-507.

McGee, D., & Mason, J. (1990). *The courts and the doctor.* Oxford: Oxford University Press.

McGraw, J. (1994). *The road to empowerment. Contemporary leadership behavior: Selected readings* (4th ed., pp. 227-230). Philadelphia: J. B. Lippincott.

McNair, S., & Finigan, A. The role of a forensic clinical nurse specialist in a sexual assault treatment program. *J Clin Forensic Med, 3*(1), 29-30.

McLay, W. D. (Ed.). (1990). *Clinical forensic medicine.* London: Panther Publishers for the Association of Police Surgeons.

Montgomery, J. (1997). *Health care law.* Oxford: Oxford University Press.

Moore, A. (2001). Knowing their station. *Nurs Standard, 16*(5), 18-19.

Petrakis, P. (1995). Autopsy. In S. Pickstock (Ed.), *Grolier multimedia encyclopaedia compact disc.* England: Future Publishing.

Police and Criminal Evidence Act, 1994. Revised Codes of Practice. (2001). London: HMSO.

Royal College of Nursing (RCN). (2000). *Guidance on nurse expert witnesses.* London: Author.

Royal College of Nursing (RCN). (1992). *Issues in nursing and health: Nursing, the nature and scope of professional practice.* London: RCN.

Rutty, J. (2000). Her Majesty's coroners and Home Office forensic pathologist's perception of the nurses' role in the coroner's inquiry. *Int J Nurs Studies, 37*, 351-359.

Rutty, J., & Rutty, G. (2000). Giving evidence: Why and how. *Nurs Times, 96*(32), 40-41.

Summers, R. D. (1988). *The history of the police surgeons.* London: The Association of Police Surgeons.

United Kingdom Central Council for Nursing, Midwifery and Health Visiting (UKCCN). (1992). *The scope of professional practice.* London: Author.

Whyte, L. (1997). Forensic nursing: A review of concepts and definitions. *Nurs Standard, 11*(23), 46-47.

Wright, J., & Pearl, L. (1995). Knowledge and experience of young people regarding drug misuse, 1969-94. *Br Med J, 310*(6971), 20-24.

Canada

Hinds, S. (1994, March 6). Personal communication to Arlene Kent-Wilkinson.

Ledray, L. (1999). *Sexual assault nurse examiner development and operational guide.* Washington, DC: US Department of Justice, Office of Justice Programs, Office for Victims of Crime, 7.

Lynch, V. (2003). *Forensic nursing science.* Course for British Columbia Institute of Technology (BCIT). Vancouver, BC, Canada.

Lynch, V. (1993a). Forensic aspects of health care: New roles, new responsibilities. *J Psychosoc Nurs, 31*(11), 5-6.

McCarty, V. (1985). *Washoe County Nevada handbook on death investigation.*

Australia

Coram, J. (1993). Forensic nurse specialists: Working with perpetrators and hostage negotiation teams. *J Psychosoc Nurs, 31*(11), 26-30.

Evans, A., & McGilvray, L. (1996). RNs trial a forensic nursing service. *Aust J Adv Nurs, 14*(2), 11-15.

Lynch, V. (Feb. 1986). *AAFS proceedings* (p. 59). Presented at annual meeting in New Orleans.

Lynch, V. (1993a). Forensic aspects of health care: New roles, new responsibilities. *J Psychosoc Nurs, 31*(11), 5-6.

Lynch, V. (1993b) Forensic nursing diversity in education and practice. *J Psychosoc Nurs, 31*(11), 7-14.

Mason, T. (2002). Forensic psychiatric nursing: A literature review and thematic analysis of role tensions. *J Psychiatric Mental Health Nurs, 9*(5), 511-520.

McGilvray, L. & Evans, A. (1996). *The sole practitioner in a police setting.* Paper presented at Australia's Third International Psychiatric Nursing Conference, Melbourne.

NSW Department of Health. (1996). Nurse Practitioner Project Stage 3: Final Report of the Steering Committee (NB 96 0027), NSW Department of Health, Australia. *Overview of Human Rights Developments.* Human Rights Watch: Kyrgyzstan. Retrieved from http://docsmgmt.hrw.org/kyrgyzstan-pubs.php.

Vecchi, C. (2003). Implementing a forensic educational package for registered nurses in three emergency departments in Western Australia. Unpublished doctoral thesis research proposal, Notre Dame University, Western Australia.

Young, S., Wells, D., & Jackson, G. (1994). A tiered healthcare system for persons in police custody–The use of a forensic nursing service. *J Clin Forensic Med, 1*, 21-5.

South Africa

Dawes, A. & Donald, D. (Eds.). (1994). Childhood and adversity: Psychological perspectives from South African research. Cape Town: David Philip.

Weaver, J., & Lynch, V. (1999). Forensic nursing: A unique contribution to international law. *J Nurs Law, 5*(4), 23-34.

Machel, G. (1996). UNICEF, The impact of armed conflict on children. Report of Gracia Machel, expert of the 5. Secretary-General of the United Nations, Selected Highlights, New York.

Pynoos, R. S., Kinzie, J. D., & Gordon, M. (1988). Children, adolescents, and families exposed to torture and related trauma. In E. Gerrity, T. M. Keane, et al. (Eds.), *The Mental Health Consequences of Torture.* New York: Kluwer Academic/Plenum.

Straker, G. (1994). Integrating African and Western healing practices in South Africa. *American Journal of Psychotherapy, 48*(3), 455-467.

Truth and Reconciliation Commission (TRC). (1998, Vol. 4). *A summary of reparation and rehabilitation policy, including proposals to be considered by the president.* Cape Town: Author.

Turkey

Gorea, R. K., & Jasuja, O. P. (2003, Nov. 16). Forensic nursing in India: Benefits to the society. Paper presented at the First Turkish and US Conference on Forensic Science. Istanbul, Turkey.

Lynch, V. (2003, Nov. 16). Evolution of a forensic nurse: Medicolegal solutions. Special Session address presented at the First Turkish and US Conference on Forensic Science, Istanbul, Turkey.

Nahid, K., Njai, H., Godarz, G., et al. (2003, Nov. 16). The relation between women and abuse and pregnancy outcome in Iranian pregnant women. Paper presented at the First Turkish and US Conference on Forensic Science, Istanbul, Turkey.

Japan

Benedict, R. (1989). *The chrysanthemum and the sword* (reprint ed.). Routledge and Kegan Paul, London: Mariner Books.

Lynch, V. (2000). Pioneering efforts in Japan. *On the Edge* (IAFN newsletter), *6*(3), 1-3.

Yoneyama, N. (May 27, 2000). Personal communication with Virginia A. Lynch.

Southeast Asia

Ahmed, N. (1993). The position of women with reference to the Pakistani criminal justice system. *Pakistan J Women's Studies: Alam-E-Niswan, 1,* 57-63.

Ahmed, S. H., Ahmed, Q. I., & Khan, J. R. (1988). *Psychiatry in Pakistan.* Karachi: Pakistan Psychiatric Society.

Akanda, L., & Shamim, I. (1985). Women and violence: A comparative study of rural and urban violence against women in Bangladesh. *J Women's Studies: Alam-E-Niswan, 1,* 21-26.

Ali, S. (1993). Are women also human? Women's rights in tribal areas: A case study of the provincially administrated tribal area of Pakistan. *Pakistan J Women's Studies: Alam-E-Niswan, 1,* 21-26.

Anderson, W. (1999). *Progress amid chaos: Team trains violence-worn Pakistanis.* University of Missouri School of Medicine. Retrieved from www.hsc.missouri.edu/~umicpt/pakistan99.shtml.

Batliwala, S. (2003). *Defining women's empowerment: A conceptual framework.* Retrieved from www.genderatwork.org/updir/Batliwala_empowerment_framework.htm.

Bisnath, S., & Elson, D. (2001). Women's empowerment revisited. *UNIFEM.* Retrieved from www.undp.org/unifem/progressww/empower.html.

Brunei yearbook: Key information on Brunei. (2003). Bandar Seri Begawan: Borneo Bulletin.

Carbonu, D. M., & Soares, J. M. (1997). Forensic nursing in Pakistan: Bridging the gap between victimized women and health care delivery systems. *J Psychosoc Nurs, 35*(6), 19-27.

Carbonu, D. M. (2000). Diploma in accident and emergency nursing: Curriculum document. Brunei Darussalam: College of Nursing.

Chally, P. (1992). Empowerment through teaching. *J Nurs Educ, 31,* 117-120.

Darlington, P. S. E., & Mulvaney, B. M. (2003). *Women, power, and ethnicity: Working toward reciprocal empowerment.* New York: Haworth Press.

Gudeta, T. (1994). Obstetric fistulae: The silent shame. *Populi, 21*(2), 6-11.

Haji Abu Salam, H. R. (2000). Women as victims of domestic violence in Brunei Darussalam: Implications for nursing in the accident and emergency nursing. A research proposal, Diploma in Accident and Emergency Nursing, College of Nursing, Brunei Darussalam.

Haji Badaruddin, S. (2000). The caring role of forensic nurses in the accident and emergency department toward the victims of family violence. A research proposal, Diploma in Accident and Emergency Nursing, College of Nursing, Brunei Darussalam.

International Council of Nurses (ICN). (2001). *Nurses, always there for you: United against violence.* Geneva, Switzerland: International Council of Nurses.

Islam, A. (2003). Health sector reforms in Pakistan: Future directions. *J Pakistan Med Assoc, 52*(4), 174-182. Retrieved from www.pakmedinet.com/view.php?id=2329.

Jafarey, S. (2002). Maternal mortality in Pakistan: Compilation of available data. *J Pakistan Med Assoc, 52*(12), 539-544. Retrieved from www.pakmedinet.com/view.php?id=3497.

Jezewski, M. (1994). *Culture brokering as a model for advocacy. Contemporary leadership behavior: Selected readings* (4th ed., pp. 3-15). Philadelphia: Lippincott.

Joshi, H. (June 21, 1999). Gender and development workshop: Gender equity and the "democratic dividend" (pp. 1-5). World Bank ABCDE Europe Meeting, Paris.

Kazi, H. A. G. (1988). Forensic psychiatry in Pakistan. *Psychiatry in Pakistan.* Karachi: Pakistan Psychiatric Society.

Kazmi, S. (1992). *Statistical profile: Women of Sindh.* Karachi, Pakistan: Association of Business, Professional and Agricultural Women, Panjwani Press.

Keen, P. (1988). *Manifestations of empowerment.* Unpublished manuscript.

Khan, A. (2000, June). Adolescents and reproductive health in Pakistan: A literature review. *Research Report No. 11, Final Report.* Islamabad, Pakistan: The Population Council. Retrieved from www.shirazi.org.uk/family.htm.

Kolachi, H. B. (1999). Maternal health in Sindh: Situational analysis 1997. *Mother and Child, 37*(1), 24-26. Retrieved from www.pakmedinet.com/view.php?id=1907.

LeGood, J. (1999, Jan. 18). The price of honor. *Time,* p. 4.

Lodhi, S. K., & Yusaf, A. W. (1997). Maternal mortality at Lady Wellingdon Hospital: A comparison of causes twenty years apart. *Ann King Edward Med Coll, 3*(4), 90-92. Retrieved from www.pakmedinet.com/view.php?id=1738.

Lynch, V. (1999, Sept.). Clinical forensic nursing: Approaching a new century. Address to the Brunei Ministry of Youth, Culture and Sports, Brunei Darussalam.

Lynch, V. (1995). Clinical forensic nursing: A new perspective in the management of crime victims from trauma to trial. *Crit Care Nurs Clin North Am, 7*(3), 489-507.

Mubbashar, M. (1998). Community mental health care program in Pakistan. In I. al Issa (Ed.) *Al-Junun* (pp. 187-203).

Maslow, A. (1954). *Motivation and personality.* New York: Harper & Row.

McGraw, J. *The road to empowerment. Contemporary leadership behavior: Selected readings* (4th ed., pp. 227-230). Philadelphia: Lippincott.

Mirza, I. (2002). Mental health services rooted in primary care: Why is this so relevant for Pakistan? *Ann King Edward Med Coll, 8*(3), 142-143. Retrieved from www.pakmedinet.com/view.php?id=3929.

Niaz, U. (1994). Sexual harassment at workplace. *Pakistan J Women's Studies: Alam-E-Niswan, 1*(2), 47-50.

Ninth Convocation. (2003). College of Nursing, Brunei Darussalam.

Physicians for Human Rights (PHR). (2001). Women's health and human rights in Afghanistan: A report by PHR: Win news: Women and violence (review). Retrieved from www.findarticles.com/cf_0/m2872/4_27/80089785/print.jhtml.

Qidwai, W. (2003). Accessibility and effectiveness of healthcare providers. *J Coll Physicians Surg* (Pakistan), *13*(3), 174-177. Retrieved from www.pakmedinet.com/view.php?id=3632.

Rosen, J., & Conly, S. (1996). *Pakistan's population program: The challenge ahead.* Washington, DC: Population Action International.

Royal Brunei Police Force. (2000). *Violence on women: 1994-1999.* Brunei Darussalam: Police Department.

Salaam, T. (2003). For struggle, solitarity and socialism in Nigeria: A brief analysis on the situation of women in Nigeria today. Retrieved from Democratic Socialist Movement, www.socialistnigeria.org/women/1-3-03.html.

Social Affairs Services Unit (SASU). (2000). Carbonu, D. M. Seminar on domestic violence: A forensic agenda for the new millennium–Resolutions and recommendations. Brunei Darussalam: Social Affairs Services Unit, Ministry of Culture, Youth and Sports.

Shahin, S. (2000). India vs. Pakistan–Contrasts in social development. The observer of business and politics. Retrieved from www.hvk.org/articles/0400/30.html.

Tabassum, F., & Baig, L. (2002). Child labor a reality: Results from a study of a squatter settlement of Karachi. *J Pakistan Med Assoc, 52*(11), 507-510. Retrieved from www.pakmedinet.com/view.php?id=3487.

Zaidi, K., Wajid, G., & Rehan, N. (1996). Utilization pattern of different health facilities for MCH services in the three areas of district Lahore. *Mother & Child, 34*(1), 11-14. Retrieved from www.pakmedinet.com/view.php?id=1840.

Chapter 57 Career Paths for the Forensic Nurse

Virginia A. Lynch

The career opportunities for healthcare personnel in this century are immense, especially for nurses. However, few practice arenas offer the potential rewards that parallel those of forensic nursing. Until the last few years, nursing education offered few options for students desiring to pursue the specialty. Now there are courses offered at both the graduate and undergraduate levels, and continuing education offerings, workshops, and short courses are available in certain locales. The central challenge for individuals who want to specialize in forensic nursing is identifying the various educational and experiential components required for achieving the knowledge and skills required for the chosen specialty. This chapter will discuss career choices within forensic nursing.

During the last two decades, public officials and their partners in the healthcare industry have been challenged to coalesce human resources to address the social issues and physical injuries that occur from acts of interpersonal violence. Schools of nursing and medicine are beginning to respond to pleas of law enforcement and the courts to provide both personnel and programs, but efforts must be accelerated in order to meet the growing needs for victim services, perpetrator care, and rehabilitation.

Forensic nursing, as a scientific discipline, evolved in response to this challenge and to identified needs in society. Because of the overwhelming number of victims, offenders, and associated forensic functions, the need for increased forensic services required new resources. Historically, physicians have been expected to provide the evaluation of forensic patients, both living and dead. Yet, forensic medicine in the clinical and pathology sectors has not been an academic requirement of physicians in the US, as opposed to the majority of other countries that incorporate clinical forensic medicine as a component of medical studies (American Academy of Forensic Sciences, 1991).

Factors such as the lack of preparation, a loss of confidence in treating forensic patients, loss of time in court, and financial considerations have limited the number of qualified physicians available for a timely, competent identification of victims, documentation of injury, and recovery of evidence. In countries where the clinical physician is a designated forensic medical officer, an identified system of legal and civil services specific to the forensic client is available.

This service varies in quality and quantity of forensic skills based on the opportunity and availability of education and training for physicians. The UK was first to recognize and establish a clinical forensic medical system and maintains an organized and highly skilled medicolegal body of forensic medical examiners under the direction of the Department of Forensic Medicine at Scotland Yard. Although most systems are not comparative to the UK, many provide similar structured systems but lack the sophistication or availability of clinical forensic examiners. Forensic pathology, however, in North America equals or surpasses the skills and requirements of other government systems of death investigation.

Nursing and the Forensic Patient

Nurses have always been expected to provide care regarding crime victims, patients in legal custody, traumatic accidents, and other liability-related injuries, as well as clinical and community deaths. Yet, no specialty role or explicit education existed to ensure that these legal responsibilities, along with traditional nursing interventions, were met with reasonable certainty. The complex legal needs of the patient were often in jeopardy owing to the emergency medical response team's and the nurse's or physician's ignorance of forensic issues. Investigating officers lacked status in the trauma room and generally depended on the nurse or physician to accurately document injury and to recover evidence. However, without specialized knowledge, neither objective was fulfilled.

The evolution of a forensic clinician in nursing has provided healthcare's direct response to violence. This new discipline was intrinsic to the role nurses would fill in the challenge to decrease the threat to public health and the financial impact on both individuals and society, as well as to help correct injustices. As nurses acknowledged their role in the health and justice movement, they recognized crime-related issues as legitimate elements for healthcare professionals to integrate into their individual practice models. They accepted the challenge to reach beyond immediate treatment concerns, into the often-shadowed areas of legal issues surrounding patient care.

Key Point 57-1

The concept of an integrated practice model in forensic nursing science has firmly established a skilled clinician, cross-trained in the principles and philosophies of nursing science, forensic science, and criminal justice.

Attributes and Characteristics of the Forensic Nurse

Forensic nursing has created an exciting new trend in nursing education and practice. Nurses involved in any nursing specialty have discovered that the application of forensic science to healthcare has granted new roles, new responsibilities, and new insight into the combination of nursing, public health, human behavior, and issues of law. Forensic nursing is applicable to any specialty practice in nursing, crossing all boundaries in the healthcare institution: public, private, clinical, and community. Forensic healthcare stimulates critical thinking and ways of knowing in the investigation of crime-related trauma in which previously nurses were admonished from participating. Forensic nurses must recognize that they are not criminal investigators, but rather clinical investigators assisting legal agencies with the direct mandate to identify crime-related injuries and to recover, preserve, and secure a system of transfer for forensic evidence to the appropriate legal agency.

Forensic nursing as a discipline has existed for more than a century, involving nurses who care for patients in secured environments, fulfilling the legal requirements of the court and care of patients in custody. It has expanded into the relatively new role of the clinical forensic nurse, an investigator of injury and death in the clinical patient as a specialty practice. Other roles have evolved from this base of nursing practice. Forensic nurses also practice their nursing skills in the scientific investigation of death, working at the crime scene, in clinics, in hospitals, and in the autopsy laboratory. Forensic nurses are direct service providers, administrators, educators, and consultants. Thus, the forensic nursing professional provides a resource previously unavailable to the patient, to the police, and to the courts involving social crimes that impact public health.

Forensic nursing does not shy away from the atrocities of human abuses such as child and elder maltreatment, sexual violence, crimes against women, homicide and murder, self-inflicted injury, and death as well as the psychopathology of the criminal offender (Lynch, 1997). Responding to the intensity necessary to deal with such social scourges, the forensic nurse requires an insightful evaluation of person, personality, and outcomes. One must consider the secondary trauma associated with the work of the forensic professional who comes in contact daily with the darker side of human nature.

Career Motivation

Nurses and others who have been victims of violence are frequently drawn into this field as a means of understanding what has happened to them in the past, to gain control over their victimization, or to help prevent interpersonal crimes from happening to someone else. Often, unresolved victimization issues long thought to have healed will resurface during the interview, investigation, or examination of the victim or offender of criminal violence. Knowing how to recognize one's own vulnerabilities and an awareness of interventions specific to one's personal needs is an essential requirement for the forensic nurse. It is difficult, if not impossible, to be a support system to the patient when the professional is experiencing a personal crisis. Burnout is a frequent symptom of nurses who commit too much of themselves, for too long, to the far-reaching ill effects of social inequity, morbidity, and mortality.

Criminal offenders may also become involved as public servants (police officers, firefighters, paramedics, nurses, physicians, etc.), especially if they have attained these skills prior to committing a crime or committed a crime while in the professional role. This is not a role for individuals who have not yet come to terms with their own criminality, received treatment and therapy, and paid restitution to society. However, healthcare professionals are often involved in legal issues related to drug abuse, neglect, or malpractice, as well as intimate violence in interpersonal relationships; thus, incisive background evaluations are imperative for the forensic nursing candidate. A discerning evaluation of rehabilitation and recommendation from authority or supervisory personnel should be considered for nurses who have overcome these issues.

In addition to being motivated by health and justice issues, many nurses now experience longer professional working lives and may desire a "second career" to refresh and renew their spirits after toiling for decades in a more traditional role within healthcare. These nurses are ideal candidates for forensic nursing because they bring with them the wealth of knowledge and skills they have accumulated while working with a wide array of patients.

Human and Professional Qualities

The arena of forensic nursing is unique in the wide range of forensic subspecialties involved in the care and treatment of forensic patients. The commonality of each individual role is the dedication and commitment of the professional to seek out answers to the questioned issues involved in each specific case. The intrigue and intellectual stimulation of their objective is related to determining "the truth." In order to succeed as a forensic nursing professional, the individual must be ethical, compassionate, empathic, assertive, and nonjudgmental.

The nurse's clinical education and experiential background offer a major strength in forensic investigation by providing analytical and observational skills, allowing these nurses to venture beyond their traditional roles. Vision, commitment, and endurance are strengths that support new and challenging roles for nurses and sustain their capacity for performance in this field. Collaboration and innovation are two significant qualifications of the forensic nurse that implement positive change in antiquated health and justice systems. Prevention is a major goal of the forensic nurse that parallels the major goals of traditional medicine and nursing. These qualities help to prevent needless human tragedy as well as advance progress in this field of specialization.

Forensic nurses base their investigations of trauma on assessment of the patient's injury, disease, or disorder; predicting danger in the home, community, or secured environment; securing of the patient's physiological safety; and planning to bring about change in the person's life. Forensic nursing relies on the concept of empowerment to bring about self-confidence and change in women and men, children and the elderly, and those who have been deprived of education, decision-making authority, and autonomy from generations of abuse. Behavioral scientists have long recognized the impact of abuse on each of these patient populations as the substructure that initiates the damaged personality, loss of identity, and initiation of anger that often, without intervention or a positive role model, results in the sociopathic personality devoid of conscience, the victim affect and attitude, as well as the repetitive behavior of the abuser. These definitions parallel the definitions of other specialty nurses.

Dr. Patricia Rowell, Senior Policy Fellow, ANA Congress of Nursing Practice, states: "There is no specialty in nursing that requires graduate education in order to identify a nurse with a specialty area of practice. The difference that distinguishes levels of recognition is between specialization vs. advanced practice nursing which does require master's preparation. It is within the purview of the governing body of the individual specialty to define the criteria for those who practice in that specialization and whose practice is recognized as an area of specialization apart from other nursing roles" (Lynch, 1996).

A registered nurse whose primary focus is on the investigation of trauma and the identification, collection, preservation, and documentation of evidence is practicing forensic nursing. Cases may include crime victims, liability-related injury, and psychological evaluations for use in a court of law. Patients may be living or deceased.

The forensic nurse must be committed to working with diversity; the economic, social, cultural, and emotional composition of each patient or subject will be unique. They will include victims of violence and their families and offenders of the law and their families.

When the forensic nurse clinician is authorized to provide a sexual assault examination, evaluation of a battered child near death, or the investigation of a questioned death and subsequent notification of next-of-kin, a forensic caring intervention reaches beyond a skilled technique of injury assessment and quality collection of biological evidence. This intervention must also incorporate concern for physical, mental, emotional, psychological, and sexual well-being. In order to be effective, however, the sociocultural, spiritual, and social justice components cannot be ignored. This is what, again, separates the forensic nurse from the police officer, the forensic physician, or scientist. This service answers a need of the community, which has historically been unmet in times of public and private trauma.

In addition to a strong sense of caring and concern, the forensic nurse must possess a sound ethical framework and be willing to "stand the ground" when interfacing with law enforcement, the judicial system, and other individuals and groups. They must be able to put aside emotions and biases and base their forensic examinations on science. Although they bring the component of human caring into the discipline, forensic nursing cannot survive on merely rhetoric or the intention to help the victims. It must be able to stand with other scientific disciplines and pursue the scientific method as the basis for establishing the truth (Barber, 2001).

Educational Approaches to Forensic Nursing

Core Competencies

The techniques, type of communication, and focus of the investigation or examination vary among law enforcement, health scientists, and the forensic nurse examiner (FNE). Consider the differences outlined in Table 57-1. The FNE relies on skilled communication, balanced with controlled sensitivity, to obtain both objective and subjective data.

Trauma is the central underlying issue involved in the majority of cases prosecuted as crimes against persons. Such cases involve physical assault, sexual assault, drug abuse, homicide, murder, accidental injury or death, injuries associated with worker's compensation, medical malpractice, environmental hazards, and myriad others. Yet trauma is the common thread that ties these cases together. Would it not make intuitive sense to have someone skilled in trauma to provide the clinical investigation of these crimes?

Table 57-1 Comparison of Background and Training for Forensic Fields

CRIMINAL INVESTIGATION	HEALTH SCIENCE INVESTIGATION	FORENSIC NURSE EXAMINER
Interrogative technique	Investigative technique	Skilled communication
Objective	Subjective	Balance of objective/subjective
Controlled distance	Sensitive	Controlled sensitivity

Courses offered to nurses through forensic nursing programs involving trauma and aspects of forensic pathology, clinical forensic practice, and victimization experience from the perspective of the victim, the offender, the family, and society bring a skilled clinician into touch with the forensic aspects of the patients they care for. A forensic psychiatrist's perspective regarding the behavior of the criminal mind, understanding statistical data on the rise and fall of crime rates, and crime scene investigation as well as equivocal death and the principles of death notification also provide a unique background for the nurse who will work with the police, medical examiner/coroner, and the judiciary.

With the emphasis on education in the professional world today, it has become imperative for those seeking employment to have attained a degree and, often, specialized training beyond that degree. Postgraduate education may be required in order to fulfill highly specialized positions in the forensic field. For example, a criminalist has a basic degree in chemistry, perhaps a master's degree in forensic science, and a doctorate in biology or a relevant physical science. Forensic pathologists must first become a medical doctor, then become board-certified in clinical and anatomical pathology before becoming eligible to receive a fellowship in forensic medicine. Only then can they sit for board certification in forensic medicine.

Forensic nursing parallels these specialties in forensic science and medicine because FNEs must be registered nurses with a specialization in forensic nursing or forensic health science. Advances in nursing science have continued to accelerate along with that of medicine and other sciences. This progress has demanded that nursing education keep pace with these sciences in order to remain credible in complex sciences and technology. In the past 20 years, requirements for nursing have focused on maintaining an ever-increasing level of knowledge on this progressive movement in education, practice, and research. Typically, nurses are expected to hold a bachelor's degree in order to practice forensic nursing. Although some nurses practicing in this field do not have degrees, they have many years of experience and became indoctrinated in forensic nursing before even specialty courses or degrees were offered in this field. These nurses are adequately qualified to practice within their specialty. However, if looking for a new career or for advances in a current career, one would do well to commit to a degree program in order to ensure a position or specialty role in the future. For example, in San Francisco, nurses who had been practicing as sexual assault nurse examiners for 15 to 20 years were told that they would be replaced by nurse practitioners. This was a great disappointment to these forensic nurses, as well as to the legal agencies that had worked with these well-trained, experienced professionals and had established a strong working relationship with this team. The nurse felt displaced and unappreciated, specifically when those replacing them had no forensic experience. The point is that management felt that to maintain progressive credibility in the professional world, it was easier to replace this team with advanced practice nurses than to require or provide higher education for the existing team members.

Certainly, forensic nursing must continue to work toward establishing entry level academic criteria, national certification, and standards of practice; these criteria will establish the credibility of forensic nursing. As nurses monitor advances in science and medicine, it will become essential for nursing education to keep pace by providing curricula for both generalists and specialists who will fill positions that will become available for forensic nurses in the future. As new employment opportunities evolve, peers in the forensic and nursing sciences will set the pace and expectations of the forensic nurse in the future. Nurses must ask themselves where they want to be 10 years from now. For those who expect to become leaders in forensic nursing, preparation must include advanced nursing education.

A lack of formal degrees, however, should not deter the basic forensic nurse or the forensic nursing generalist. There will always be a need for nurses educated on all levels of forensic practice to provide forensic nursing services. Remember however, as in other specialties, if education is minimal, so may be the level of opportunity. Those who are prepared to operate the increasingly intricate technologic equipment, who develop instructional design via digital distance delivery, who understand genetics and appreciate its impact on the health and justice systems, and who can relate the epidemiology of crime to nursing practice are the forensic nurses who will be the leaders in forthcoming decades.

Career Expanding Courses and Continuing Education

Although some nurses will want to become full-time forensic nursing specialists, others may choose to pursue forensic nursing as an area of special interest to combine with another nursing role. Emergency nurses often move into this specialty because it has so many applications within that particular setting. Trauma nurse specialists may choose to move into death investigation; in-patient nurses may develop an interest in elder abuse or domestic violence. Often nurses are motivated toward a career in forensic science as a result of a patient contact or clinical situation that compelled them to get more involved in specific interventions for violence. Because certificate courses may be more readily available than formal academic offerings, and more feasible for the working nurse, many individuals develop their forensic acumen one certificate course or workshop at a time. Nurses who are fortunate enough to have colleges or universities within their communities may enroll in part-time study in one or more courses, leading to a major or minor in forensic nursing. Forensic nurses who are well-motivated tend to be very creative in constructing a pathway to forensic practice.

Web-based learning opportunities abound now, so academic preparation can occur at the student's convenience, and many requirements may be met online from the comfort of one's own home. However, to achieve the clinical experience and practical knowledge from interfaces with the law enforcement and judicial components, a mentor must be secured.

Role of the Mentor

A mentor is essentially a coach. A mentor encourages, instructs, and keeps the student "on a steady course," moving toward the goal. Although most mentors will be seasoned practitioners within the discipline, others may bring a wealth of life and career experiences to the student, even though they may not be primarily engaged in forensic practice on a full-time basis. Professional associations such as the American Academy of Forensic Sciences (AAFS) provide matches of students with mentors in the various forensic disciplines.

Evaluating Educational Offerings

With forensic nursing being a relatively new discipline, there are entrepreneurs in the marketplace, seducing eager nurses into courses that may be marginal and into programs that lead virtually nowhere. Before investing in any program, ensure that it provides the type of credit or recognition that is expected. Check with other students who have completed the course. Has it led to further learning opportunities or to a job? If not, was the information gained in the course of practical value in the clinical arena?

Certificates versus Certification

It is not uncommon for nurses to be confused about certificates and certification. A certificate of course completion rarely can be directly linked to any certification in a discipline. Such certificates usually record facts about course completion and continuing education credit. One can accumulate dozens of certificates and not be certified in anything!

Most organizations, including the International Association of Forensic Nurses (IAFN), must demonstrate that its published core curriculum is consistent with the Scope and Standards of Practice, jointly endorsed by the American Nurses' Association (ANA). Certification for excellence in nursing practice is obtained by a combination of formal study and clinical experience. Most professional associations have identified the core competencies required for practice within a nursing specialty. This core consists of the body of knowledge, the technical competencies for practice, and the role behaviors inherent in the discipline. Certification does not only encompass a demonstration of proficiency through a formal testing program; most also require validation of a clinical acumen via a mentor, work supervisor, or other designee. In certain nursing specialties, there is a strict requirement for a specific number of hours of clinical practice with competency demonstrated through a presentation of case studies by the candidate for certification. The IAFN is currently exploring various approaches to forensic nursing certification, and have already launched their initial pilot test for sexual assault nurse examiner certification. Texas, New Jersey, Virginia, and California had previously been the only states offering certification for sexual assault nurse examiners. It is expected that certification opportunities will be expanded into the other areas of specialization, including clinical forensic nursing, death investigation, geriatrics, pediatrics, and others as the field demands. Although some states and localities have already sanctioned certification programs for some forensic nurse practice roles, national certification is highly desirable for nurses who often are geographically mobile in their career. National certification also "levels the playing field" in the courtroom and helps to ensure a consistent recognition of the forensic nurse credential.

Professional Identity

The Scope and Standards of Forensic Nursing Practice provide the authoritative statements that describe member responsibilities. The standards, written in measurable terms, define accountability to the public and articulate outcomes for which all forensic nurses are accountable.

Credentials for clinical specialization, advanced practice, and certification are based on specific criteria established by the ANA, state boards of nursing, and specialty organizations.

Credentialing is an important part of establishing the credibility of the forensic nurse. It is difficult to identify the skills, education, experience, training, and subspeciality of practice without recognized credentials. Forensic nurses have begun to develop their forensic résumés and establish respected credentials through academic programs and professional organizations. One of the earliest recognized titles was that of the sexual assault nurse examiner

(SANE), which became a readily identified title. This specifically pertains to the nurse specializing in the examination and evaluation of the sexual assault patient. Initially, this specialist was credentialed by the hospital or agency that had trained them and was recognized only by that authority.

In one state the SANE became an essential component of the state office of the attorney general and became certified by that state agency. This state service also allowed for credentialing as an expert in pediatric or adult sexual assault assessment. This type of certification involved only a few states; the remainder of SANEs were developing individual training programs and credentials without continuity of curricula requirements.

Today, the IAFN has developed the first national certification examination for sexual assault nurses based on the specific requirements approved by the Council of Sexual Assault Nurse Examiners. Future certification for other forensic nursing specialization will include those involved in death investigation, clinical forensic practice, forensic psychiatric nursing, and other specialties within the scope of forensic nursing as they develop. Some forensic nurses are certified by their specific nursing organizations, such as the Association of Legal Nurse Consultants, and the state bar credentials nurse attorneys where they practice.

Another respected credential among forensic nurses dedicated to the advancement of forensic science in nursing is FAAFS, indicating this individual has become an elected Fellow of the American Academy of Forensic Sciences. The Academy is among the oldest and most prestigious forensic organizations, was founded in 1948, and includes a wide range of forensic disciplines from countries worldwide. This organization was the first to recognize the forensic nurse as a unique specialty within the forensic sciences as early as 1991. The advancement to fellow is one earned by participation, attendance, and contribution to the organization and to forensic science. Qualifications for fellowship involve active involvement and action for approximately seven years.

DABFE is a credential indicating a diplomate status within the American Board of Forensic Examiners. DABFN is recognized as a diplomate of the American Board of Forensic Nursing. Both boards are part of the American College of Forensic Examiners. This relatively new (founded in 1992) organization has rapidly gained a rather large (over 15,000) following of forensic specialists in a variety of fields. The college hosts excellent annual conferences, and its size provides exceptional networking opportunities among a wide variety of occupations and skills. Diplomate status for these boards is awarded through credential review of education and experience, as well as three examinations in ethics, law, and the individual specialties. There are continuing education requirements for the retention of diplomate status.

In applying for employment positions that require indications of credibility in a specific field, one may wish to consider the requirements for nurses who will need to be qualified in a court of law. The term forensic implies, by the nature of the profession, that this individual is an expert in a specific field and will be called to court to testify at an advanced level of knowledge. Thus, it should be the standard by which forensic nurses in any subspecialty would evaluate skills and credentials as they move further into the forensic science arena. In other words, the qualifications of a nurse expert witness, whether a forensic nurse or a specialist in any field of nursing, is defined by the following criteria: credibility, education, experience, degrees, position held, specialty training, publications, and professional organization membership. Among these, one of the most readily accessible and motivating qualifications is membership in the official organization of the professional body of the specialty. Professional organizations provide opportunities for members to network and to become involved in initiatives for advancing the discipline. Most organizations also offer multiple options for continuing education through journals, newsletters, and scientific membership.

Although nurses new to a professional practice may not have achieved multiple degrees, attained years of experience, advanced to a management position, or published any literature in the field, they are generally eligible for membership in one of these professional associations. This may include an associate or student membership or as a trainee affiliate until the individual is qualified for full membership. Identification with a professional organization affords the forensic nurse the opportunity to interact with specialists of noted expertise in the field. This alone is motivating and encouraging.

Advancing Clinical Forensic Practice

Although the UK was the first to practice the concept of clinical forensic medicine, the initial reluctance to use nurses as an extension of the forensic medical examiner has delayed the advancement of forensic nursing in the UK as a viable resource in forensic services. However, with entry into the forensic science service in England, it is reasonable to expect that this system of forensic nursing services will eventually spread across the UK and to other neighboring countries (Pratley, 2001).

Emergency and Trauma Networks

One system initiated by Memorial Hermann Hospital, a major trauma center in Houston, Texas, has established a position entitled Director, Forensic Nursing Services, and has replaced the way crime victims, perpetrators, and liability-related cases are facilitated through the health and justice system. The incorporation of a clinical forensic nurse to coordinate these cases has provided a positive change and improvement. Recognizing the need and the opportunity, Russell Rooms, EMT-P, MSN, RN, proposed and filled this new role (Box 57-1).

The proposal for such positions can be initiated through the presentation of information to the appropriate department head that will address the needs and benefits of establishing a system of forensic nursing services. Information proving to be persuasive may include a cover letter outlining the intent of this service, a copy of the job description, and an attached copy of a published article that provides an overview of the role of the forensic nurse in the clinical setting. Box 57-2 presents an example of a cover letter.

Investigative Staff

Similar approaches may be used when the benefits of a forensic nurse would be of value to other institutions or agencies. Considering the many legal agencies mandated to investigate crimes against persons or those who provide victim or offender services, it is reasonable to expect that a forensic nurse could be integrated into the investigative staff. In order to balance the perspective of a team of medicolegal investigators, the nurse would contribute the forensic/medical component, while the rest of the team would supply the legal or law enforcement element. Agencies that have embraced this approach have encouraged like agencies to evaluate the return invested in the inclusion of an FNE. One such agency is the Coos County Office of the Chief Medical Examiner.

Box 57-1 Position Description: Forensic Nurse Examiner

REQUIREMENTS

Registered professional nurse, bachelor of science in nursing required, master's degree in nursing preferred.
Clinically proficient in trauma related issues.
Evidence of personality characteristics and skill consistent with positive leadership. Also exhibit excellent interpersonal and organizational skills.
Certificate in forensic nursing or equivalent thereof.

PART I. MAJOR FUNCTIONS OF POSITION

Responsible for:

1. Consulting with hospital personnel and individuals in the investigation of medicolegal-related trauma and questioned deaths in the emergency department, and other hospital departments.
2. Assisting with the notification of family members or significant others of death and providing immediate crisis intervention.
3. Informing law enforcement agencies and other appropriate authorities of circumstances surrounding trauma deaths that impact medicolegal actions.
4. Serving as a liaison between the hospital departments and the county attorney's office and law enforcement.
5. Maintaining current knowledge of case law, legal evidence collection procedures, and working knowledge of law enforcement and medical investigative responsibilities.
6. Participating in the educational programs of the hospital that have forensic implications.
7. Consulting with the emergency department and other hospital departments as requested.
8. Assisting the hospital with preparation for civil or criminal cases.
9. Developing and maintaining standards, policies, and procedures and activities/programs essential to the forensic application to traumatic injuries in nonfatal assaults, accidents, or self-inflicted wounds.
10. Applying knowledge and skills of biomedical/medicolegal investigation in the immediate nursing interventions and follow-up care of victims of violence.
11. Performing sexual assault examinations as an expert practitioner in forensic gynecology.

PART II. ORGANIZATIONAL RELATIONSHIPS

Reports to appropriate supervisor identified by institution.
Affiliates with:

1. Law enforcement agencies
2. Pathologist
3. Risk management officer
4. County attorney's office
5. Faculty of the local school of nursing
6. Social services staff

PART III. SPECIFIC RESPONSIBILITIES

1. Meets with the director of the emergency department, the pathologist, law enforcement agencies, and emergency department staff regarding current medicolegal cases of trauma and death in order to process information in a constructive manner.
2. Educates personnel in techniques of crisis intervention and grief counseling.
3. Serves as a preceptor for students and staff members seeking additional knowledge and skills related to medicolegal management of victims.
4. Maintains documentation and evidence files that would assist in subsequent investigation of medicolegal cases.
5. Reports medicolegal cases to law enforcement or other appropriate agencies.
6. Participates in staff orientation programs in order to convey critical information regarding medicolegal implications of care.
7. Provides ongoing staff education in medicolegal nursing content.
8. Manages training activities for the sexual assault nurse examiner program.
9. Coordinates the care of sexual assault victims from the emergency department entry through any judicial processes involved in the resolution/disposition of the case.

PART IV. IMPROVEMENT OF PATIENT CARE

Responsible for:

1. Identifying problems associated with the coordination of medicolegal activities and services.
2. Participating in problem-solving processes with agencies and services in order to improve or refine medicolegal management of victims of violence.
3. Reviewing and revising protocols associated with medicolegal aspects of care.
4. Maintaining current knowledge in forensic science and the emerging trends in clinical practice that impact the medicolegal management of victims of violence.
5. Assisting the hospital departments and personnel in upgrading the practices and care protocols.
6. Initiating and participating in research related to clinical forensic issues.
7. Monitoring and evaluating clinical forensic activities as an integral part of the quality improvement/risk management program.
8. Providing expert care for the victims of violence.

PART V. PROFESSIONAL AND COMMUNITY SERVICE ROLES

Responsible for:

1. Educating the community regarding the devastating effects of trauma.
2. Raising community awareness of trauma prevention through education and outreach endeavors.
3. Serving as a change agent through role-modeling and educational activities.
4. Interfacing with agencies/services that are associated with the prevention of trauma/violence and subsequent management within the community.

Kris Karcher, BSN, RN, has been employed there as the Chief Deputy Medical Examiner since 1998.

Karcher also works as a clinical FNE in the management of sexual assault cases. Her duties include serving as a member of the Child Advocacy Center Board, the Homicide Investigation Team, Child Fatality Review Committee, and CRASH Team (vehicular accident reconstruction and investigation team). Karcher is also regularly used as an expert witness in homicide, sexual assault, and domestic violence cases and serves as a member of the Oregon Attorney General's Sexual Assault Taskforce. According to Paul Burgett, Coos County District Attorney, when elaborating on the benefits of an FNE, "[Karcher] is an invaluable partner in the

Box 57-2 Sample Letter Accompanying Proposal for Forensic Nurse Examiner

To Whom It May Concern:

_____________ Hospital represents a name synonymous with excellence in trauma care. Patients presenting to the trauma center require attention to their immediate needs including physiologic, psychological, and forensic (medicolegal) issues. Currently, inattention to forensic needs of victims of interpersonal violence results in less than comprehensive care. Recent initiatives by governments and healthcare organizations worldwide have empowered healthcare providers and hospital administrators to embrace measures ensuring holistic care for victims of crime. Attention to lifesaving intervention alone no longer suffices without addressing the patient's legal, civil, and human rights.

Advances in social justice and contemporary trauma care require new roles and new responsibilities. Forensic nurses are uniquely skilled to address issues of interpersonal violence based on core nursing curricula, strengthened with additional education and training in the forensic arena. The American Nurses' Association Congress of Nursing Practice has recognized this role as a formal specialty in nursing and one of the four major areas for nursing development in the twenty-first century.

I propose that_____________ Hospital will benefit from the creation of such a position by ensuring JCAHO standards are addressed, providing a visionary model of comprehensive care for patients subjected to interpersonal violence. Enclosed is a job description for a forensic nurse examiner that is currently implemented in other clinical facilities. Initial objectives include policy development essential to facilitate the medicolegal management of forensic patients and the development of a multidisciplinary approach to the health and justice systems. This position will create opportunities for research and publication in the field of trauma care, forensic nursing, and interpersonal violence.

Funding represents a major challenge in the development of any new program or position. Yet forensic nursing services, as with any consultant position such as an ostomy or wound care nurse, are billable to the patient. Uniquely, the forensic nurse examiner can assist crime victims in accessing funds provided by local law enforcement agencies, the Crime Victims Compensation Fund, as well as private insurance. Benefits include liability protection to the healthcare institution when the patient's legal needs are met. Assisting law enforcement and the judicial system benefits the community in providing a safer place to live.

Please consider this proposal as a further commitment to comprehensive patient care and the advancement of humanity in our society. I am available to answer any questions at your convenience. You may contact me by cellular phone at_________ or digital pager at _________. I look forward to your reply.

Respectfully submitted,

_________________, RN

investigation of our most serious cases. She brings forensic-medical expertise and information to the crime scenes, emergency departments and the courtroom with equal facility and grace. Our forensic nurse examiner is a financial bargain for our local criminal justice system" (Burgett, 2002).

When addressing the criminal justice system's perspective of the FNE, Coos County law enforcement officer and state police laboratorist Jim Pex (2000) affirmed the role filled by Karcher with an endorsement (Box 57-3).

Box 57-3 Coos County Endorsement of Forensic Nurse Examiner

RE: Coos County Forensic Nurse Examiner

Prior to entering a law enforcement profession, I worked 10 years in the medical profession. I spent a lot of time in the emergency department and watched the interaction between law enforcement and the ED. I have worked 24 years in law enforcement and have many stories to tell about the LE/ER relationship. Within any group of people, you have different views on civil liberties, crimes and people in uniform. Compounding the issue is that hospitals get their advice from private attorneys who often have an anti-police attitude and discourage the hospitals from interaction with police. "If they want the evidence, they can get a search warrant." "You are not obligated to answer any questions." These are common responses that I have heard over the years. The unfortunate side is that the patient has to go back into the community after he or she has received treatment and needs to go back into a safe environment.

The advent of the forensic nurse has opened the door to a new era in criminal justice. We now have someone at the hospital that knows the laws and understands their role in the community. It begins with having an identified person for the patrol officer to contact. Someone to talk with about a person or their injuries. Someone who can document injuries or collect important sexual assault evidence. Just knowing how long semen may be detectable in the vaginal vault already exceeds the knowledge of a patrol officer. From here a decision can be made about how to collect important evidence that may lead to the apprehension of a dangerous person or the exoneration of an innocent person.

The value of the forensic nurse extends outside the medical facility. Attorneys need someone who can read medical reports and tell them what is there. The strength or weakness of the medical evidence is also important. From here, the diversity of expertise expands in many directions. Elder abuse, child abuse, mental health all need assistance from the forensic nurse. When a senior citizen has suspicious bedsores, a nurse from outside the care facility is the best qualified to determine if this constitutes abuse and to work with local law enforcement to get the problem resolved.

In our community, a forensic nurse is active in death determinations, crime scene response, domestic violence cases and training to law enforcement. Nursing is about service to others through medicine. Law enforcement is about service to others through protection. Forensic nursing is about service through building bridges between medicine and law enforcement for the long-term benefit of others within their community.

—Jim Pex

Law Enforcement

In other areas, police officers are incorporating forensic nursing into their armamentarium of equipment and methods to combat violence involving crimes against persons and society. Police officers have recognized the need to grasp a greater understanding of the medical aspects of medicolegal cases, as well as the psychosocial needs of the citizens they serve to protect. Nurses have as well recognized the need to grasp a greater understanding of the legal aspects of forensic cases and their responsibilities to law enforcement and the courts. With this combination of skills and authority, a new clinical role in law enforcement is emerging. Some officers have retired from their law enforcement duties before initiating their nursing education and forensic nursing practice, and some nurses have moved away from the clinical setting and into the community as a police officer. Yet, unique to both roles, nurses exist who simultaneously hold a nursing license and a law enforcement badge.

One such individual is police officer Jane Weiler, RN, MSN, forensic clinical nurse specialist, in Hastings, Nebraska. Weiler is also a critical care nursing specialist who provides both the legal and forensic/medical services to her community. She serves the Hastings Police Department in a distinct and separate role from her nursing duties at the Mary Lanning Memorial Hosptial. Weiler has qualified as a SANE, completed a certificate program in forensic nursing from Beth-El College of Nursing at the University of Colorado, Colorado Springs, and holds a certificate in forensic science from the University of Nebraska in Lincoln, Nebraska. She has designed and implemented her degree plan to obtain her Master's of Science Degree in Nursing with a specialization in forensic nursing. Weiler is a member of the IAFN, AAFS, and the American Board of Forensic Nursing. She also participates in law enforcement training programs and professional organizations. Weiler is an exemplary role model of the consummate forensic nurse.

Sergeant Dan Losada of the Hastings Police Department reflects on the professionalism and advantages of having a forensic nurse in the service of the community's law enforcement team (Box 57-4) (Losada, 2004). He emphasizes the unique value of an officer with an acumen that includes medical knowledge and forensic science.

These examples represent only a few of the unparalleled opportunities that nurses are gaining within and outside the immediate treatment environment. As the boundaries of nursing continue to expand into the evolving field of forensic nursing science, opportunities are unlimited. Although the initial perspective of the nurse who seeks employment in a forensic role is often one of discouragement and disappointment, opportunities are commonly equated with the extent of one's education and experience. When education is limited, so are opportunities. Roles held by forensic nurses in these early stages of development are most often roles carved out by the nurses themselves. It is difficult to establish a definitive list of potential roles, salaries, benefits, or career advances. However, it is inevitable that as forensic nursing grows in stature and credibility, so will the availability of opportunities within the forensic nursing field.

Box 57-4 Forensic Nurse's Value to Law Enforcement

Jane Weiler is a Reserve Officer with the Hastings Police Department serving since March 1996. While her primary duties are as a police officer her forensic nurse's training is quite helpful. When working as an officer she has encountered numerous incidents where her medical background has helped officers in determining the severity of injuries and the cause or mechanism of trauma. Jane is also able to compare the injury and the statement of the victim to the physical evidence and determine when the victim may not be telling the truth about an incident.

As a forensic nurse she has conducted numerous exams of individuals and has the ability to communicate her findings in a manner that is easily understood by other law enforcement personnel. Also, in one attempted homicide case she was able to accompany the victim into surgery and recover evidence reducing the chain of custody. Chief Larry Thoren considers Jane to be a valuable asset to the Hastings Police Department. Jane's accomplishments in the forensic nursing field have also reflected positively upon the Hastings Police Department.

—Dan Losada

Employment Opportunities

As the healthcare delivery systems and medical science grow in intricacy and sophistication, so does the need for nurses with specialized skills and knowledge. Forensic nursing is one of the emerging specialties that offer an array of interesting professional possibilities, each vastly different from the other in specific rewards and responsibilities, yet each expands the nurse's opportunities to exert a meaningful influence on the delivery of healthcare. Most nurses today have become aware of the evolution of forensic nursing and its role in the clinical settings. Hospitals, however, are slow to realize the benefits and rewards of providing forensic nursing services in most regions of the US.

Forensic nurses have proved to be beneficial in providing a new approach to policies, education programs, patient intervention, and administrative functions that improve patient care and outcome. They also provide unique functions as a direct service provider and agency consultant and can represent the healthcare institution as an expert witness in liability or criminal cases. However, one of the most positive benefits has been in public relations with the police and with families of crime victims.

Police have often experienced negative treatment from nurses and physicians when bringing a patient in custody into the emergency department for evaluation or when requesting numerous items, from evidence to medical records, from the healthcare providers on duty. This treatment has resulted in complicating an already difficult situation for the police and the prisoner/patient. Having a designated forensic nurse on duty at all times will facilitate the forensic services and patient treatment in a more acceptable manner for all personnel involved, further extending a positive image from the hospital to the community concerned with social crime and public safety.

Internationally, few countries have become aware of the role of the clinical forensic nurse. Yet others, such as Finland, have a country-wide network of municipal health centers where 70% to 80% of the healthcare personnel are nurses. Each center has a first aid clinic to provide emergency services, and physicians who work in these clinics also serve as police surgeons. Most forensic cases are brought into the clinic by police officers, and each clinic routinely provides forensically skilled nurses to assist the police surgeon. In cases involving wounds and other injuries or sexual assault, the nurse assists in the forensic examination as well as performing other forensic nursing functions. Although these nurses have not advanced to the level of forensic nurses in the US, they are expected to be skilled in forensic behaviors and participate in forensic interventions.

With a continuing awareness of the evolution of forensic nursing in the US, enlightened administrators and directors of hospitals and trauma centers in developing and developed countries are beginning to recognize that it is in their best interest to develop a system of forensic nursing services. The forensic nurse is available to assist the nonforensic physician and, when necessary, is qualified to provide the forensic examination and the collection of evidence.

In 1987, a paper entitled "The Role of the Forensic Nurse," was presented at the First Meeting of the World Police Medical

Officers encouraging the participation of nurses in the forensic medical services. Dr. David Filer, a police surgeon and his daughter, forensic nurse Linda Filer, RN, BSN, from the UK, stated that "whilst during the past decade, the standards of clinical forensic medicine have risen with increased training for new entrants and upgrading of facilities at police stations, there are still problems in its application. These relate to the examination of victims, the need for disassociation of examining physician with the police, and the lack of trained assistants when treating prisoners. The purpose of this paper is to demonstrate the advantage of the presence of a nurse, trained in addition to general nursing, in basic clinical forensic medicine" (Filer, 1987).

This proposal framed the beginning of a new approach to forensic nursing that was integrated into the Metropolitan Police Services in London in 2001, following a pilot program established in Kent in 2000 with funding sources provided by Scotland Yard (Pratley, 2001). This historical advancement in forensic services will eliminate the problem of police officers administering medication to inmates or assessing circumstances of injury and illness to determine if a physician should be called. This program has initiated new opportunities and challenges for nurses throughout the UK where police stations will eventually be staffed with forensic nursing personnel, providing a screening system for medical complaints and assuming other forensic functions as their responsibilities are increased.

Career Barriers

The initial phase of all new fields of practice limits employment opportunities. New paradigms in healthcare are expected to take 12 to 15 years to become accepted practices. As ever-changing medical and scientific advances continue to move forensic nursing forward, employment opportunities that have been limited in the recent past are becoming recognized as essential, expanded roles within the clinical arena. In spite of the growing number of nurses seeking forensic education, experience, and positions, the medical and legal worlds have been initially hesitant to consider the forensic nurse as a member of the alliance of forensic investigators involving healthcare and the law.

Traditionally, these roles have been defined as a clinical physician–only role, that of a forensic pathologist, or one that required a law enforcement background. Negative responses to an employment search may provide an incentive to the entrepreneurial nurse resulting in a creative forensic service offered to hospitals and other agencies by way of independent consulting through private practice.

Forensic services can be independently contracted to hospitals, community clinics, police departments, coroner/medical offices, jails, prisons, and long-term care facilities, as well as abuse screening to elementary schools, sexual assault assessments in college and university clinics; domestic violence shelters, human rights organizations, and any environment where issues of threats to public well-being interface with the law. As forensic nurses have continued defining new parameters in the medicolegal arena, greater opportunities are evolving.

In jurisdictions where nurses have not previously participated in forensic investigations, it is not uncommon for the first line of resistance to be from those who feel threatened by nurses invading a territory not previously open to nurses. Physicians, police and public prosecutors, magistrates, and traditional medical investigators are often unaware of the acceptance or the benefits identified by agencies that have experienced and valued the contributions of the forensic nurse. Once the nurse has been tried, tested, and proven to be a skilled forensic examiner, these same authorities are among the strongest advocates of the forensic nurse. Initially, prosecutors and judges questioned the veracity of a forensic nurse giving testimony in court: How could the nurse replace a physician on the witness stand? Would the jury believe a nurse? What would happen if the nurse were asked a question he or she couldn't answer?

These times seem to have passed. In an article published in the *Prosecutor*, the official publication of the National District Attorneys Association, this prestigious organization stated that "forensic nurses make formidable allies in court" (NDAA, 1997). Prosecutors find that nurses often make excellent expert witnesses when they have developed the communication skills essential to educate and persuade a jury. Nurses can be superb teachers. Because patient teaching is one of their most basic nursing skills, nurses are able to extend these teaching skills into the courtroom. And so, issues that have been obstacles to forensic nursing in the recent past are dissipating as forensic nurses gain the attention and respect of peers in all areas of the forensic sciences.

One of the most troublesome concerns, however, is when nursing itself becomes the major obstacle to the forensic nurse. When nursing administration does not understand the implications of crime-related injuries resulting in liability issues facing the hospital, or violations of law without a standardized, systematic approach to case management of forensic patients, the progress of forensic nursing is limited. It is the responsibility of nurse managers to persuade hospital administration of the needs and benefits of this liaison to the legal world. It is interesting to note, however, that once an agency becomes familiar with the skills and ability of the forensic clinician, it readily becomes dependent on these services and begins to request a greater number of forensic services and eventually to implement the forensic nursing role.

Combining Present Interests with Forensic Nursing

Because all areas of nursing and all departments of clinical care can involve forensic issues, forensic patients, and forensic responsibilities, it is not difficult to see ways to combine a current position or even outside interest into a forensically challenging adventure. In a sense, this is how new fields, new interventions, and concepts of forensic functions evolve. For example, consider that the forensic professional has an initial practice in a specific field; recognizing the need for a forensic specialization of that practice could result in unlimited career innovation. Consider the fields of forensic accounting, forensic rehabilitation, forensic sculpting, computer image enhancement, forensic social work, or speech analysis.

Even more innovative in the realm of forensic nursing is the role of a forensic nurse canine handler. Combining the skills of the forensic nurse with those of the forensic canine handler has been proposed as an exciting and fulfilling career opportunity. One innovative forensic nursing student identified the forensic search dog and the accelerant detection canine as an area of research for nurses involved in crime scene investigation. Linking this unique approach with an internship, the nurse is working with the K-9 unit in order to better understand the role of the investigator/handler and the canine in this working environment. After all, not only police personnel can be canine handlers. Nurses are taught to assess a situation, identify the problem, plan interventions and goals, implement

Box 57-5 Example of Internship Objectives

Objectives of the forensic nurse canine handler combine the nursing process and the role of the forensic canine investigator:

- Identify source of problem at the crime scene (arson or chemical explosion, tracking scent of a perpetrator or missing person)
- Plan strategy of best use of nurse/handler/canine skills
- Plan activation during the implementation phase
- Evaluation of effectiveness of plan, nurse handler, and the canine

their plan, and evaluate its effectiveness. Whether investigating an arson scene or tracking a scent, the forensic nurse canine handler would assess the situation through a systematic collection of data while relating the nursing process to the scientific investigation of injury and death (Box 57-5).

Forensic nurse canine handler is an example of but one of the many fascinating concepts that can evolve from combining personal or professional interests with the intrigue of forensic science and the pragmatic tools of combating crime.

International Perspectives on Educational Opportunities

In this era of globalization, nurses worldwide are seeking forensic nursing education. Yet, primary resources for formal forensic education in nursing are limited mainly to North America. Because of the cost involved for foreign students who wish to apply for a student visa in the US, most are unable to provide the financial statement required to cover tuition, books, housing, sustenance, transportation, and medical care during the period of tenure expected to achieve a degree emphasizing forensic nursing.

Scholarships available for education in the US are commonly restricted to US citizens only. Students from indigent countries must rely on gifts from relatives or agencies willing to fund their education. In most developing countries where war, civil and political unrest, famine, and the devaluation of currency are common, opportunities for sponsorship are rare.

Education in forensic nursing emanated from an extensive field of the broader forensic sciences, involving forensic medicine, police science, political science, sociology, criminology, and others depicted within the model of forensic nursing science. Therefore, as an integrated model of practice, forensic nursing education also incorporates integrated theoretical and scientific studies of other related forensic specialties. With the evolution of Internet digital distance learning, forensic studies in many fields are becoming available to nursing students worldwide.

With access to the Internet, availability to education is increasingly reaching even the poorest areas of the world. In India, free Internet access provided as part of a public research project placed computers in the walls of a courtyard in several of the most economically depressed areas. Without any instructions or directions available, the village children accessed and explored the innumerable avenues of educational experiences via digital formats and virtual classrooms. Thus, Internet learning programs are the future of forensic nursing education until it becomes an integrated component of basic nursing curriculum.

Currently, however, few distance-learning programs specific to forensic nursing education are available. Those that are online may provide sound introductory foundations to forensic nursing practice or may lead students to believe that after a single Internet distance program, they are qualified to provide sexual assault examinations or are qualified as a criminal profiler. Care must be taken to evaluate the educational program provider, their credentials, experience, and credibility. Frequently, students fail to realize that a certificate of completion of this course is only as good as the accreditation of the institution that provides it. Unethical and unscrupulous individuals offer courses known to appeal to nurses eager to gain forensic expertise and who often fail to recognize the lack of accreditation proffered by the provider.

Where clinical skills are required, the nurse hoping to attain FNE status must realize that hands-on instruction and evaluation of technique are requisites of the ethical provider. The forensic clinical instructor is a critical component of the forensic educational expertise.

The number of nursing and medical universities and colleges offering forensic nursing education programs internationally continues to escalate. Forensic education options available for nurses that offer advanced degrees as well as specialty courses include university and college programs in Australia, Canada, Africa, Scotland, and England. Outside the formal academic setting, one of the most sought-after programs provides a six-week, 240-contact-hour, didactic and clinical program provided by international forensic experts in nursing, medicine, and criminology from the US and Australia. This residency program has been provided for registered nurses from varied backgrounds in education and experience, as well as from a wide range of geographical locations in Zimbabwe and South Africa since 1997 (Els, 1997). This unique approach in preparing a forensic specialist in nursing has created a synergistic effect, extending this educational opportunity throughout the international forensic community. Ideally, this program will become a "train the trainer" approach, whereby each group of graduate FNEs will become the forensic educators of the future.

The forensic nurse, no less than the forensic pathologists, magistrates, or victim advocates, should be aware of the international laws and crimes against persons worldwide. Cultural and social crimes may be specific to a particular geographical location, or specific to individual religious groups, as well as to regional trends in crime and violence. Laws generally differ from one country to another as well as in individual jurisdictions within a country.

Because most victims of interpersonal crimes are admitted to hospitals and clinics in any country, the nursing personnel will find themselves caring for patients with legal implications. The law may or may not require reporting, collection of evidence, or security of medical records in criminal cases. Yet, the International Council of Nurses (ICN) addresses these ethical concepts for professional nurses worldwide. ICN policy statements address accepted standards of practice as well as the human rights of all patients.

Laws and categories of crimes most commonly committed in a specific area should be included in basic nursing education, along with guidelines to direct the nurse faced with a forensic dilemma. This would be defined as a situation in which the law requires reporting of a particular type of injury or an individual associated with a political group, yet culture, religion, or ethics indicate that this would compromise the life or freedom of an innocent person. For example, during the apartheid period of South Africa, many of the freedom fighters sought treatment in private clinics or homes where they knew they would not be reported to the South

African police. Because most developing countries are in a constant struggle for democracy and human rights, there remains a continuing struggle for nurses faced with these legal dilemmas. Most developing countries are faced with a lack of local forensic personnel, funding, resources, or facilities for training healthcare providers. The challenge must be addressed within the institutions of nursing education in order to clarify and define appropriate ethical and forensic behaviors.

Initiating a Forensic Career through Education

A beginning student or a returning student interested in developing a career in the forensic sciences will face challenges after completing one's education and looking for a position as a forensic nurse. However, taking a few steps now to prepare for this career can help overcome many obstacles. Careful planning can help one get that first position in forensic nursing and ensure it is the right position.

Develop a forensic résumé early in educational and experiential framework. This is essential when approaching an agency for work or prospective learning experiences. Often, individuals starting out think they have to have far more information and achievements before starting a résumé. Yet, with any forensic organization programs, training courses, or elective classes, the forensic nurse is beginning to develop important information for the curriculum vitae (CV). Be sure to save all certificates of completion or attendance to these programs or classes and encase them in clear protective sheets, placed in a ring binder along with the CV, to present to a potential employer or agent with the authority to provide permission to spend time in their agency. This collection of material and information can provide an impressive statement and show one's interest in the forensic sciences.

First, focus on the forensic courses offered in the local area. Explore those offered within the university system as electives or certificate programs. If currently enrolled in a university or college that does not offer forensic courses, seek permission to take a forensic course taught at another accredited institution, or approved as an independent study through a nonaccredited program and have the credit transferred. By designing objectives to address the nursing goals necessary for the elective course, one should be able to provide the necessary outcomes to satisfy the requirements. After determining the field of study of interest, expand to a wider selection of courses offered nationally and internationally.

Use every opportunity to attend any programs on campus associated with the multidisciplinary team involved in the forensic sciences. Get involved with student organizations related to other majors in this field; offer to participate in their programs or other aspects of their training. Learning about other fields will provide a broader field of reference and will provide contacts and opportunities that may come from outside the field of nursing.

Community Service and On-the-Job Immersion

Next, look beyond campus environs into the community resources available through local training programs at the police academy, fire department, or social services. Each of these agencies interrelate with others involved in victim services, public safety, or crime and violence, creating opportunities for further cross-training or employment options otherwise missed.

When requesting permission to participate in an agency's work area, remember that these are primarily legal agencies with highly classified information and where the security of evidence is at risk. First file an application for employment. This will allow access to the recommendations and requirements for the positions available within that agency while displaying a serious interest. Because these positions are commonly few and difficult to obtain, ask to leave the application on file for future reference.

Sergeant Dan Losada, Hastings police department, advises that many agencies have volunteer and reserve officer programs. Volunteer programs allow interested and qualified individuals to work within the organization. Reserve programs allow qualified individuals to become certified officers when working under certain conditions. Normally, reserves are required to carry and qualify with firearms. Anyone with strong feelings against handguns should not apply for reserve status (Losada, 2002).

Use this opportunity to also inquire if one is eligible to serve as a reserve investigator, officer, or agent. This is generally a volunteer position, with little or no salary, but is open to individuals interested in training or citizens interested in donating their time to the community. The term *reserve* is generally preferred in most legal agencies because it projects a more professional or confidential image than *volunteer.*

For example, many sheriff and police departments have reserve units, in both rural metropolitan areas. These are volunteer positions without salaries in most agencies. Reserve officers help to supplement the agency's investigative staff during medical emergencies or crisis situations. Requirements for reserve deputy sheriff candidates generally include the same training and background check as a full-time officer. Criteria for candidacy in a state peace officer training program in Texas include a 640-contact-hour academy course, an academic examination that must be passed with a score of at least 70%, and the option to retake the examination, if necessary, before repeating the entire program. To be accepted into the state program, one must be a high school graduate, have no felony convictions, and be of high moral character, among other requirements. It takes approximately eight months to complete this program and qualify for the examination.

Reserve deputies are scheduled to work a minimum number of hours per month, or they may replace regular officers as needed. They maintain the same authority as regular officers. Considering that the individual candidate assumes the total cost of training, the amount of time involved, and the hazardous duties of a peace officer, the volunteer reserve officers must be commended for service to their communities. Police departments also rely on reserve officers for services in times of dire need such as search and rescue for a lost child, help during natural disasters, or to replace off-duty officers.

Considering that the forensic nurse is a unique professional, cross-trained in nursing science, forensic science, and criminal justice, it may be that such a program in law enforcement training will provide that essential component of the equation not offered in traditional nursing education. One must never lose sight of one's major status, which is nursing (unless a sworn officer of the law), when on duty. The forensic nurse/police officer is one of the new creative occupational positions that is commonly referred to as a hyphenated professional, referring to the duality of the role. Not only is it useful to complete a specialized training in a different field, but this training may open the door to opportunities as a forensic nurse. Some agencies will not hire anyone without police training.

Reserve Officer versus Volunteer

Although law enforcement training is not a requirement for forensic nursing, forensic nurses have the opportunity to demonstrate a combination of skills developed through a multidisciplinary education, perhaps create an awareness of the value of a forensic nurse on the investigative team. If nurses are finding it difficult to obtain training and experience in the forensic or criminal justice field, regard the volunteer position and cost of training as one more educational investment in the future. Even Patricia Cornwell served as a reserve police officer in Richmond, Virginia, in order to gain the necessary experience to work in the medical examiner system where she initiated her famous career as the author of forensic science novels.

The Colorado Springs Police Crime Laboratory offers a volunteer position for citizens interested in donating time to their agency. This has proved to be an excellent placement for students in the forensic nursing internship program. Once they have completed the specified training and security check, time spent assisting professionals in their particular areas of expertise will provide an invaluable experience not offered through any other avenue. Some police agencies offer similar programs in their communities, such as the explorer program for youths, citizens on patrol, citizen police academy, or a police auxiliary.

One medical examiner system provided a reserve investigator position to select university students majoring in related areas, such as criminal justice or reserve officer training corps (ROTC). With the continuing recognition of forensic nurses as a viable resource to the forensic community, nurses have also been accepted as reserve investigators in some death investigation agencies.

If the agency does not have a reserve program, explain the benefits of having someone familiar with their system, policies, computers, and personnel, with the set of skills of a forensic nurse. Explain that a qualified individual will be available to train their personnel, at no cost to the agency, in specific areas like reviewing medical records, checking and confirming investigator reports related to medical information, and providing telephone replies and responses to individuals and families.

This approach allows an opportunity to become familiar with the office personnel, learn about specific system approaches, and be available during periods of crisis. It is an important benefit to have extra skilled personnel available when disasters strike. Nurses who have provided these skills on a volunteer basis have also demonstrated the value of having an individual with a nursing background on the staff.

Be innovative in exploring the options to get started, expect rejection, and be tenacious. Eventually, an opportunity will become available and may lead to other opportunities. Be active, participate, and become involved, and one will excel in forensic nursing.

Mentor Relationships

Mentoring is one of the initial avenues of any new member of an organization or in a designated professional field. Some organizations, such as the IAFN and the AAFS, have offered a mentorship service to new members. This affords the new member to feel attached to the organization as well as the opportunity to ask questions regarding advice, direction, guidelines, and opportunities available in the field. One of the basic principles of those who are true professionals is to pass down the knowledge and expertise of their years of study and experience to those who will follow and carry on the work they have established. The consummate professional is not threatened by the most recent individual to join the field; rather, they will entrust the future of their visions to the one who will extend their work.

The value mentoring holds for the next generation of forensic nurses is immense. Forensic specialists who serve as mentors not only pass on knowledge and skills; they impart confidence, providing inspiration and encouragement. Mentoring is a give and take process. Those eager to seek knowledge must identify goals and objectives in order to attain them; they must know what they have to offer and what they would like to gain. Mentors have a critical role to fill in assuring that the future of forensic nursing maintains an ongoing, quality educational experience for decades to come.

Continuing Education

Maintaining a current knowledge in the latest techniques and advances in forensic nursing is an essential component of a competent qualified practitioner as well as an expert witness in forensic nursing practice. Trends, technique, and law change rapidly in the scientific and nursing world. Individual responsibility remains a high priority of those that practice their nursing skills within the arena of the law. This includes researching literature to maintain awareness of changes and advancements in forensic nursing relating to education, training, certification, and clinical practice.

National Association Meetings

Attending the professional meetings of forensic organizations not only provides a wealth of educational offerings, but it also affords the practitioner the opportunity to network with peers and other colleagues. Research and scientific papers, workshops on vital topics, and stimulating presentations by leaders in the field will not only add to the professional acumen of the participant, but will revitalize enthusiasm for the forensic sciences. It is amazing how immersion with the discipline is a strong motivator for both students and the tenured members of the profession.

On-the-Job Training

In the past, many if not most forensic positions were considered on-the-job training. Because there were few formal education programs, especially at an entry level, those who wished to initiate a role in the forensic field had to seek their own training or be trained after hiring. This involved high-level positions as well as those that allowed laypersons to be trained on the job. Positions were initially recognized by the basic education, experience, and credentials, such as a medical doctor, engineer, psychiatrist, psychologist, nurse, and other professional presenting with a designated certification, and then that individual was provided with in-house specialty training in the forensic aspects of that field. As the professionalism of each specialty advanced, they began to define their own standards and criteria for quality expertise, developing formal education, board examinations, and credentials to state their qualifications. Forensic nurses are following this same avenue of attaining professional respect and recognition.

One example of a successful program involving clinical forensic nurse examiners was established by Dr. George Nichols in 1995. Nichols was the Chief Medical Examiner of the Commonwealth of Kentucky for over 20 years and recognized the benefits of a cadre of clinical forensic nurses to his investigative staff. Although most forensic nurses employed in a medical examiner system serve as death scene investigators, this new team of nurses would serve

Box 57-6 Example Advertisement for Louisville Clinical Forensic Nurse Investigators

NURSE SPECIALIST

Three positions, 20 hr in office/20 hr on-call status in rotation with physician staff, 1 in 3 weekends on-call. Utilize clinical nursing skills to examine human subjects who are victims of physical/sexual assault.

Take specimens, perform physical examinations, use photographic and infrared technology to provide documentation for Living Forensic Pathology Project. Provide assistance in statistical analysis of traumatic injuries sustained to live human subjects by way of criminal assault. Requires a bachelor's degree in nursing, Kentucky license, one year related nursing experience.

Additional experience may be substituted for up to two years of related education. Prefer experience as emergency nurse, sexual assault nurse examiner, or death scene investigator.

Send resume or apply in person by ________ on Mon., Wed., or Fri., 8 a.m.-3 p.m. to Personnel Services, University of Louisville, Louisville, KY 40292. Affirmative Action.

patients who presented to the clinical arena with crime- or liability-related injuries. These nurses would be selected based on their nursing education and experience as well as their interest in medicolegal evaluation of living patients with forensic injuries (Box 57-6).

This team of three nurse investigators received on-the-job training in investigative technique and evaluation of traumatic forensic injury within the system, as well as attending specialized courses outside the system, once they had been selected for employment. This was the first identified team to serve as a pilot program in clinical forensic nursing under the direction of a forensic pathologist. This program proved to be of great value to the police and the prosecutors as well as the university hospital system. It continues to be a model program that has influenced forensic services wherever healthcare interfaces with the law.

Other Pathways to Forensic Science and Nursing

As nurses begin to explore options and opportunities to become established in the forensic field, with law enforcement agencies, crime laboratories, medical examiner or coroner systems, prosecutor offices, and other agencies within the forensic services, they often turn to other academic programs outside the nursing field. It is commonly believed that it will benefit their stature in forensic nursing to have a degree in criminal justice, criminology, forensic science, or another associated field in order to attain a professional position. In terms of gaining employment, perhaps it may, for some agencies, require police training for any employee in a specific role. In terms of gaining stature as a forensic nurse, however, a basic or advanced degree in nursing is a prerequisite for becoming a leader in the evolution of forensic nursing.

Consider that the forensic nurse's major status is in nursing. This is the role of the forensic specialist in nursing, not a nursing specialist in forensic science or criminal justice. If one truly wishes to advance the notion of forensic nursing, it must be remembered that it is nursing education and experience that makes the FNE unique. This is what separates the forensic nurse from the police officer, from the lay death investigator or lay coroner, and from the criminalist or criminologist. Forensic nursing is the only discipline in the forensic sciences that brings with it the unique body of knowledge attained only through a nursing education and practice.

The special skills nurses contribute to the forensic sciences include, among others, communication, documentation, and observation skills; the ability to speak the medical language and understand and interpret nurse's notes, physician's progress notes, medical records, surgical interventions, pharmacology, natural disease processes, emotional trauma; and of great importance, to understand the parameters of trauma and victimology and to provide a scientific, yet empathic, approach to the evaluation of injury and death.

Trauma is the issue at hand, at the core of forensic nursing. Most often this trauma is physical, yet subtle trauma may be readily overlooked. Even more often and more readily overlooked is psychological trauma, including the covert psychological trauma of the silent victim of child abuse, domestic violence, or elder abuse that speaks volumes without words. It may also include the psychopathology of the accused that must be confirmed or ruled out in order to establish the ability of that client to stand trial. Psychopathology may also be an indicator of the initial or ongoing trauma to the psyche that has causative links to criminal behavior that research is trying to identify in order to establish preventive guidelines.

Although the behavioral sciences are continually exploring these avenues to trauma or traumatic events related to violent behavior, it is the forensic nurse who most frequently will come in contact with the victims of trauma, physical or psychological, in the earliest stages as these patients are admitted for evaluation or interview during major or minor episodes. The nurse is most commonly the first to see the patient, to identify trauma, to document information and to interview the parent or caretaker while obtaining health history. It is through these unique opportunities to be on the front line of defense that forensic nurses are contributing a special service to the forensic sciences. No other professional is in this initial position. These unique nursing skills are combined with the nurse's forensic expertise to incisively explore, examine, evaluate, and identify forensic issues requiring investigation and reporting to the appropriate legal agency.

In a science that stresses the careful collection and accurate documentation of evidence, it is interesting to note that the psychological impact of traumatic death and human violations on the survivors receive little attention in actual practice in the forensic sciences. The forensic nurses base their assessment on outcomes that evaluate each of these areas of trauma. This includes the patient, the family, the community, and without reservation, the forensic nurse's overall ability to provide the competence and efficacy required to achieve professional goals. When these areas of trauma affect the forensic nursing professional's well-being, stress management for secondary or vicarious trauma must be addressed.

Nursing and Jurisprudence

Medical jurisprudence has long set the standard for the answers to medicolegal questions that require answers in the courtroom pertaining to the interface between healthcare and the law. Questioned issues that require the expertise of medical knowledge have become one of the most respected, demanded and most readily understood issues of a case at trial. In the US, the juror system is the accepted rule of law, yet the average educational level of most jurors is between the fourth and 12th grades. It is difficult for a juror of this level to understand the advanced scientific information, DNA evidence, insanity defenses, or mechanical engineering data that may be essential to the prosecution or the defense's case. Yet, most people are familiar with the medical doctor of their community and associate medical testimony with the care, intervention, surgery, or prescriptions of their past experiences in some way. Therefore, the medical expert is often the most believable of those providing explanations to the questions presented.

Therefore, nursing jurisprudence is the complementary component of medical jurisprudence. Nurse attorneys and legal nurse consultants are in the unique position of being able to analyze medical records and interpret healthcare practices for jurors and others in the courtroom.

Nursing and Criminalistics

Criminalistics provides another potential opportunity for those interested in the analysis of trace and physical evidence as a career option. Those with a skill for chemistry and who have an analytical personality may enjoy working in crime laboratories where many answers are actually determined via sophisticated technology and analysis. Options range from serving as a citizen "volunteer" in the crime lab to gain experience for application to other career paths in which this information provides important knowledge, to obtaining more specialized training leading to the position of a forensic scientist or criminalist. With specific interest in DNA, these positions could lay the foundation for higher education and opportunities to receive training in this exciting new field. With the concept of genetic engineering and further legal issues surrounding human identification, DNA will continue to become even more important in the future.

Nursing and Mental Health

The combination of psychiatry and nursing has been one of the earliest forms of forensic nursing. For centuries, nurses have provided care and intervention for patients in legal custody who required psychiatric evaluations to determine the state of mind at the time a crime was committed or if the individual accused is mentally stable to stand trial, as well as the nursing management of the criminally insane. Psychiatric nurses with an interest in these patients and the controlled environments in which they must work are invaluable to the forensic psychiatric staff.

This role provides a perspective with the opposite viewpoint from those nurses who work primarily with victims. The forensic psychiatric nurse is responsible for the accused or the perpetrator of criminal acts. Kent-Wilkinson defines forensic psychiatric nursing as the provision of psychiatric mental health nursing care in the assessment and treatment of individuals who have been charged with criminal act(s) and who may have a mental disorder (Kent-Wilkinson, 1995).

Career Rewards

Evaluation of outcomes not only involves the reparation, recovery, or atonement for the victim, punishment for the offender, and exoneration for the innocent, but it must also include the personal and professional compensation for the forensic nurse. Through this avenue of compensation, the nurse is able to regenerate mental and physical energies that provide the courage, the incentive, and the desire to continue after having faced, and won or lost, the ongoing conflict with crime and violence. This compensation is the antidote to burnout, to job-related depression, and hopelessness when faced with the refuse of human behavior.

In consideration of the nurse investigator's psychological burden that may create a sense of guilt, a common trait among those who have not yet developed a system of "empathic distance," when the expected outcome is flawed, one must remember that although it is the nurse's role to help the patients make decisions, it is not the nurse's responsibility to solve their problems. Such circumstances include victims who make choices that can further endanger themselves and their family, or offender recidivism that returns the patient to the criminal justice system.

The nurse may experience a sense of failure, betrayal, or loss of self-esteem with the behavior of the patient in the same way that a clinical nurse may experience the death of a patient after intensive life-saving intervention. Yet, it is the compassion inherent in nursing that also gives us the ability to provide that intangible gift of caring, of presence in the face of great sorrow, to reach out and touch patients, to encourage them to cry without shame and to feel secure in closeness. What makes one vulnerable also makes one strong. The skillful FN makes victims feel secure and the accused feel confident. Families will feel the forensic nurse is involved, conscientious, and concerned about their loved one, about the welfare of the community, and about the outcome of the case.

Best Practice *57-1*

Forensic nurses should obtain specialized knowledge, skills, and credentials beyond basic nursing education in order to be perceived as a credible expert in a court of law.

Summary

Career opportunities in forensic nursing are limited only by the vision, dedication, and enthusiasm of its aspiring students, teachers, and mentors. Because this specialty is so new and essentially starting with a clean slate, it can determine its own destiny. Although framed within time-honored traditions of nursing, forensic nursing can break out of the mold and launch forward into territory formerly considered off-limits for nurses.

As society struggles with the fallout from interpersonal violence, a burgeoning population of incarcerated persons, acts of terrorism, and record levels of medicolegal liability claims, it is obvious that there is indeed ample justification for a cadre of forensic nurses. Even though the precise parameters for various subspecialty careers are not clearly defined, the nurse who desires to be among forensic resources in the future must not wait for all the answers that will eventually emerge. Nurses must possess a broad forensic education and essential core skills so that when career opportunities present themselves, forensic nurses can take their places among other professionals with confidence.

Resources

Organizations

American Academy of Forensic Sciences (AAFS)

410 North 21st Street, Colorado Springs, CO 80904, Tel: 719-636-1100; www.aafs.org

American Association of Legal Nurse Consultants (AALNC)

401 North Michigan Avenue, Chicago, IL 60611, Tel: 877-402-2562; www.aalnc.org

The American Association of Nurse Attorneys

PO Box 515, Columbus, Ohio 43216, Tel: 877-538-2262; www.taana.org

American College of Forensic Examiners International

2750 East Sunshine, Springfield, MO 65804, Tel: 800-423-9737; www.acfei.com

International Association of Forensic Nurses (IAFN)

East Holly Avenue, Box 56, Pitman, NJ 08071-0056; Tel: 856-256-2425; www.iafn.org

Sigma Theta Tau International, Honor Society of Nursing

550 West North Street, Indianapolis, IN 46202; Tel: 800-634-7575; www.nursingsociety.org

Publications

Journal of Clinical Forensic Medicine

Journal of the Association of Police Surgeons, subscription department, Harcourt Publishers, Ltd, Foots Cray High Street, Sidcup, Kent DA14 5HP, UK; www.harcourt-international.com/journals/jcfm/

On the Edge

IAFN newsletter, East Holly Avenue, Box 56, Pittman, NJ 08071-0056; www.forensicnurse.org

Forensic Nursing

Virgo Publishing, 3300 N. Central Avenue, Suite 2500, Phoenix, AZ 85012

Journal of Forensic Sciences

Published by the American Academy of Forensic Sciences, Michael A. Peat, PhD, Editor, 7151 West 135th Street, PMB 410, Overland Park, KS 66223

Journal of Emergency Nursing

Published by Mosby, a division of Elsevier Health Sciences, , Tel: 800-654-2452; www.mosby.com/jen

Forensic nursing and multidisciplinary care of the mentally disordered offender

David Robinson and Alyson Kettles (Eds.), Jessica Kingsley Publishers, London and Philadelphia, 2000.

References

American Academy of Forensic Sciences. (Feb. 16, 1991). Proceedings of the General Section, presented at Anaheim, CA.

Barber, J. (Aug. 27, 2001). Keynote address: Core Values in Forensic Nursing. Presented at Carl T. Hayden Veterans Administration Forensic Nursing Conference, Phoenix, AZ.

Burgett, P. (Feb. 20, 2002). Personal communication.

Els, J. F. *Report on forensic nursing in South Africa.* Unpublished manuscript.

Filer, D., & Filer, L. (1987). Role of forensic nurse. Abstract 33, Proceedings of the First Meeting of the World Police Medical Officers, Wichita, KA.

Kent-Wilkinson, A. (1995). Spouse abuse/homicide: A current issue in health risk management. *J Psychosoc Nurs Mental Health Serv*, 34, 10.

Losada, D. (Feb. 24, 2002). Personal communication.

Lynch, V. (1997). Clinical forensic nursing: New perspectives in the management of victims from trauma to trial. *Crit Care Clin North Am*, 7(3), 492.

Lynch, V. (1996). Dimensions of a forensic nurse. On the Edge, Fall (2), 3.

Nichols, G. (1995, September). Job description: Nurse specialist. Louisville Courier.

Pex, J. (Feb. 20, 2000). Personal communication.

Pratley, K. (Nov. 12, 2001). Personal communication from Director, Forensic Medicine, Scotland Yard, London.

National District Attorneys Association (NDAA). (1997). What is forensic nursing? *The Prosecutor*, Nov./Dec., 12-14.

THE FORENSIC NURSE

Carmen Henesy, RN, SANE, Forensic Nurse

At the dawn of a new millennium, there has evolved a need,
For a new group of nurse professionals, a pioneering breed,
On the cutting edge of nursing, to fight crime's vicious curse,
Health care responds to violence, in the role of forensic nurse.

The tasks are many and varied, each sharing a common thread,
A search for truth and justice as this specialty forges ahead.
Fighting interpersonal violence, making note of multiple clues,
Learning to hear the unspoken, recognizing the tiniest bruise.

A commingling of nursing science, forensic science and the law,
From this vast wealth of knowledge, the forensic nurse must draw,
From sociology, and psychology, criminology and fields diverse,
An arsenal of such education, arms the forensic nurse.

Easing the trauma of rape, responding to a criminal scene,
Compassionate notification of kin, judging nothing as routine,
Dealing with drug and alcohol abuse, calling for a hearse,
Providing care for inmates, these are roles of the forensic nurse.

Facilitating organ donation, expert witness testimony in court,
Investigating workplace injuries, writing a medicolegal report,
Assisting in forensic research, providing specialized quality care,
Educating and consulting with colleagues, making the public aware.

From birth to death, and far beyond, there is a difference made,
By nurses who have undertaken to embrace a new crusade,
In the fight against crime and violence, helping in its reverse,
Is the commitment and dedication of the forensic nurse.

Dedicated with love and respect to Virginia Lynch,
founding president of the International Association of Forensic Nurses,
and to all my colleagues in the International Association of Forensic Nurses

Courtesy of Carmen Henesy, October 1996.

Appendix A
The Forensic Nurse's Code of Ethics
Used by permission of the International Association of Forensic Nurses

The International Association of Forensic Nurses expects its members to adhere to the highest standards of ethics. Forensic nurses have professional obligations to colleagues, to science, and to the public, and especially to those members of the public who are demonstrably disadvantaged.

Accordingly, the International Association of Forensic Nurses expects its members and associate members to abide by its Code of Ethics as a condition of initial and continued membership.

Code of Ethics

Responsibility to the Public and the Environment

Forensic nurses have a professional responsibility to serve the public welfare, especially its most disadvantaged citizens, and to further the cause of science and justice. Forensic nurses should be actively concerned with the health and welfare of the community at large. Forensic nurses must understand and anticipate the environmental consequences of their work on the work of others in their communities. Forensic nurses must be prepared to stand up and oppose environmental pollution and other environmental degradation. Public comments on scientific matters should be made with care and precision, devoid of unsubstantiated claims, exaggeration, and/or premature statements.

Obligation to Science

Forensic nurses should seek to advance nursing and forensic science, understand the limits of their knowledge, and respect the truth. Forensic nurses should ensure that their scientific contributions, and those of their collaborators, are thorough, accurate, and unbiased in design, operationalization, and presentation.

Care of the Profession

Forensic nurses should remain current with developments in their field, share ideas and information, keep accurate and complete records, maintain integrity in all conduct and publications, and give due credit to the publications of others. Conflicts of interest and scientific misconduct, such as fabrication, falsification, slander, libel, and plagiarism, are incompatible with and a violation of this Code.

Dedication to Colleagues

Forensic nurses, as employers, should promote and protect the legitimate interest of their employees, perform work honestly and competently, fulfill obligations, and safeguard proprietary information. As employees and managers, forensic nurses should treat subordinates with respect for their professionalism and concern for their well-being, and provide them with safe, congenial working environment, fair compensation, and proper acknowledgments of their scientific contributions. Forensic nurses should regard the tutelage of students as a trust conferred by society for the promotion of the student's learning and professional development. Each student should be treated respectfully and without exploitation. Forensic nurses should treat associates with respect, regardless of the level of their formal education, and encourage them, learn with and from them, share ideas honestly, and give credit for their contributions.

Fidelity to Clients

Forensic nurses should serve clients faithfully and incorruptibly, respecting confidentiality, advising honestly, and charging fairly.

Appendix B

Nursing Diagnoses for Forensic Nursing Problems and Issues

(Partial List)

Cris Finn

Victim Management: Psychological and Emotional

- Fear related to perceived inability to control situation
- Ineffective individual or family coping skills
- Anxiety related to situational crisis
- Body image disturbance
- Potential for violence–self-directed or directed at others
- Disturbance in self-concept related to self-esteem, body image, and personal identity
- Social isolation related to situational depression
- Disturbance related to self-esteem
- Fear related to perceived retaliation or physical harm (fear of blame for activity, fear of punishment, fear of threats)
- Fear related to cognitive confusion
- Disturbance in sleep pattern related to manifestations of anxiety
- Anxiety related to prognosis and feelings of helplessness
- Anxiety related to discussion of intimate information, diagnosis, and concerns for partner and/or children
- Disturbance in self-concept related to loss of control
- Ineffective coping related to inability to manage situational crisis
- Anxiety related to pain, treatment methods, and lifestyle implications
- Alteration in thought process, perception
- Body image disturbance related to lifestyle changes necessitated by treatment
- Anxiety related to loss of self-control
- Altered thought process related to depression
- Potential disturbance in self-concept due to abuse from caregiver

Victim Management: Physical Injuries and Disabilities Associated with Violence

- Risk of infection due to interruption in integrity of skin barrier
- Knowledge deficit related to prevention of injury
- Knowledge deficit related to diagnosis and therapeutic procedures
- Potential for injury related to helplessness
- Pain related to tissue, nerve, or vessel disruption from penetrating, blunt, or extremity trauma
- Pain related to swelling and dislocation
- Potential for infection related to unsafe sexual exposure
- Alteration in comfort due to pain
- Risk of injury due to altered state of consciousness and neurological defects
- Ineffective breathing pattern related to altered ventilator mechanisms
- Ineffective airway clearance related to mechanical obstruction (asphyxia)
- Fluid volume deficit–actual or potential–related to blood loss
- Impaired physical mobility related to injury and pain
- Alteration in tissue perfusion related to hypovolemia (impaired blood supply) or vascular compromise from fractures
- Risk of altered body temperature due to loss of skin integrity and environmental heat losses
- Anxiety related to hemorrhage and uncertainty of treatment
- Knowledge deficit related to cause of bleeding
- Potential for activity intolerance related to weakness
- Potential for secondary infection
- Alteration in skin integrity due to animal or human bite
- Altered thought process related to cerebral hypoxia
- Potential for self-care deficit related to visual impairment
- Anxiety related to prognosis
- Potential for infection secondary to immunocompetence
- Ineffective bowel elimination due to inflammation, obstruction, or ileus
- Ineffective breathing pattern related to hyperventilation
- Alteration in thought processes due to delirium or coma
- Sensory-perceptual alteration–visual, auditory, kinesthetic
- Knowledge deficit related to discharge instructions
- Impaired or ineffective verbal communication
- Alteration in health maintenance
- Potential for injury related to hopelessness (elder)
- Anxiety related to discomfort, procedures, surgery, prognosis, loss of function, and alteration of body image
- Sensory-perceptual alteration regarding self and situation
- Disturbance in sleep pattern related to manifestations of anxiety

Appendix C
Body Diagrams
Courtesy of the Metropolitan Dade County Medical Examiner Department, Dade County, Florida

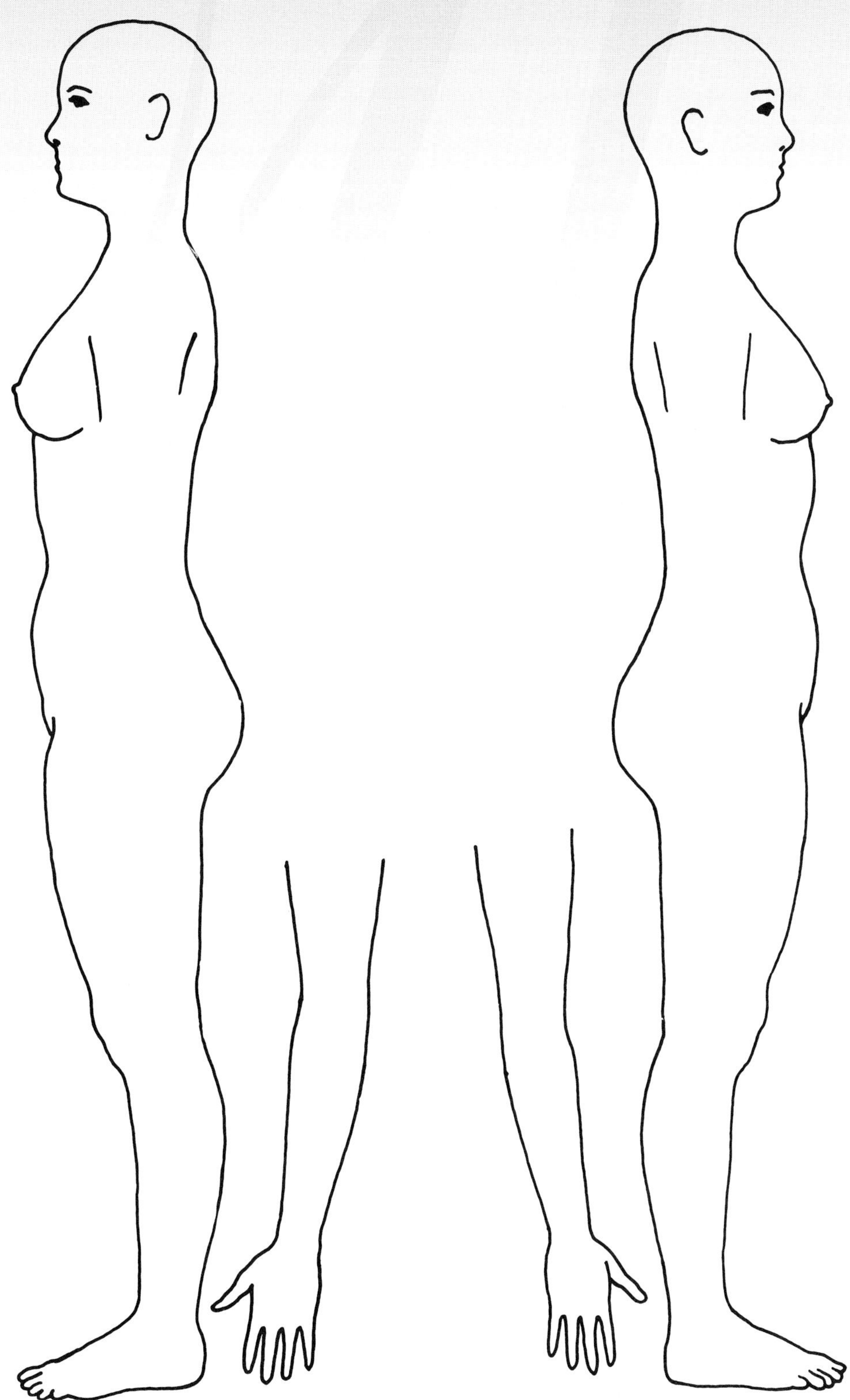

Fig. 1 Full body, female, lateral view

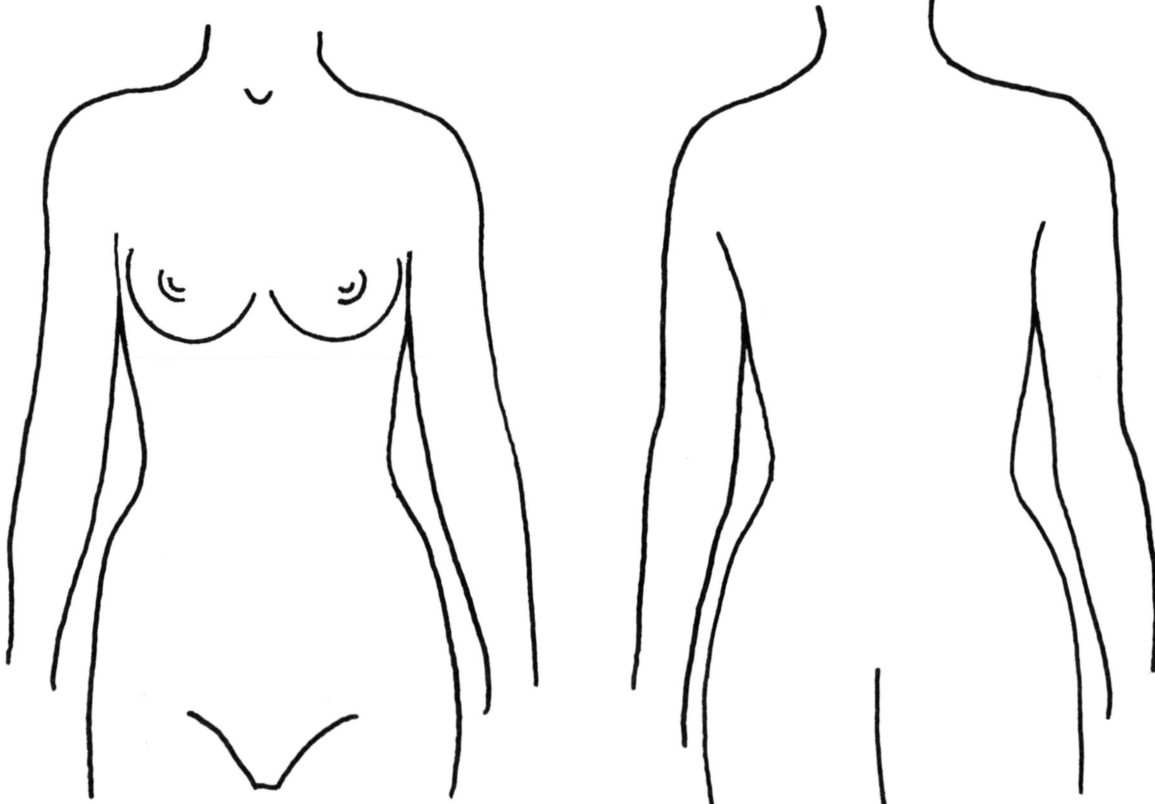

Fig. 2 Thoracic abdominal, female, anterior and posterior view

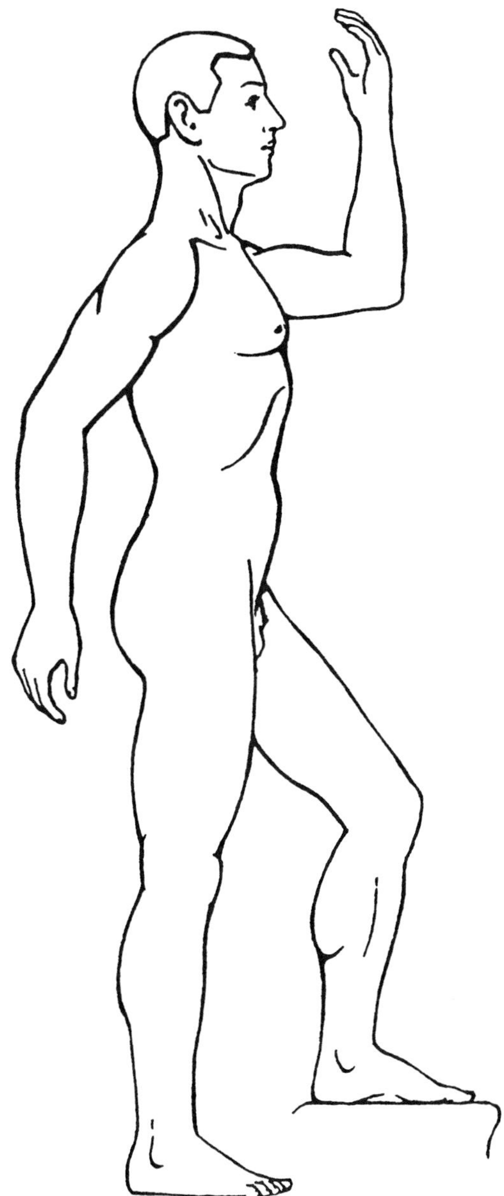

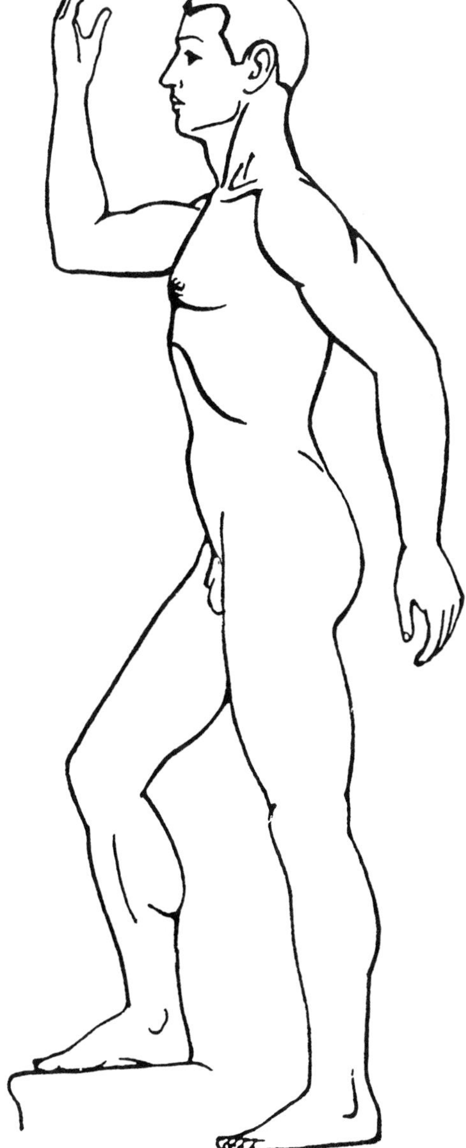

Fig. 3 Full body, male, lateral view

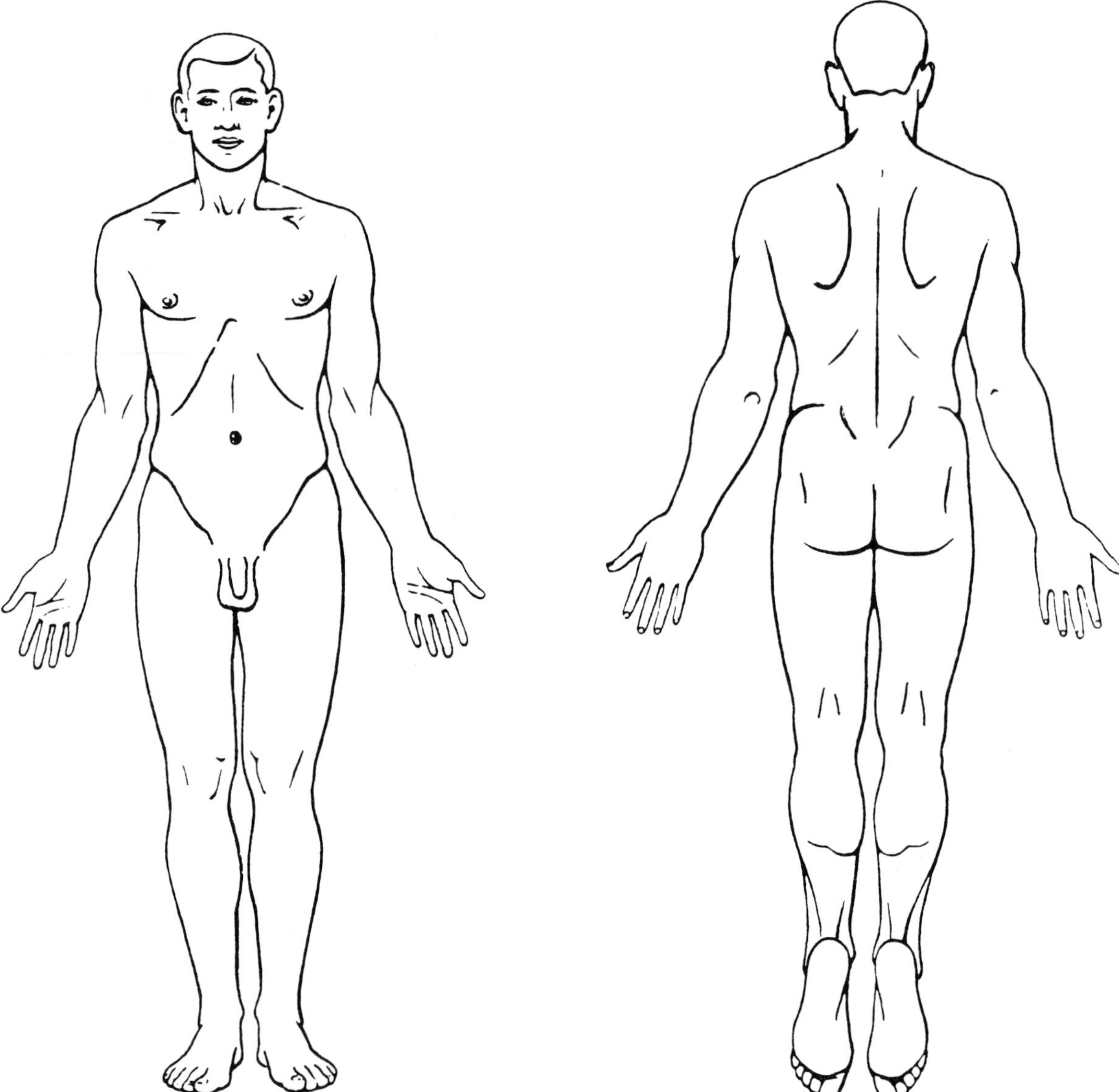

Fig. 4 Full body, male, anterior and posterior view

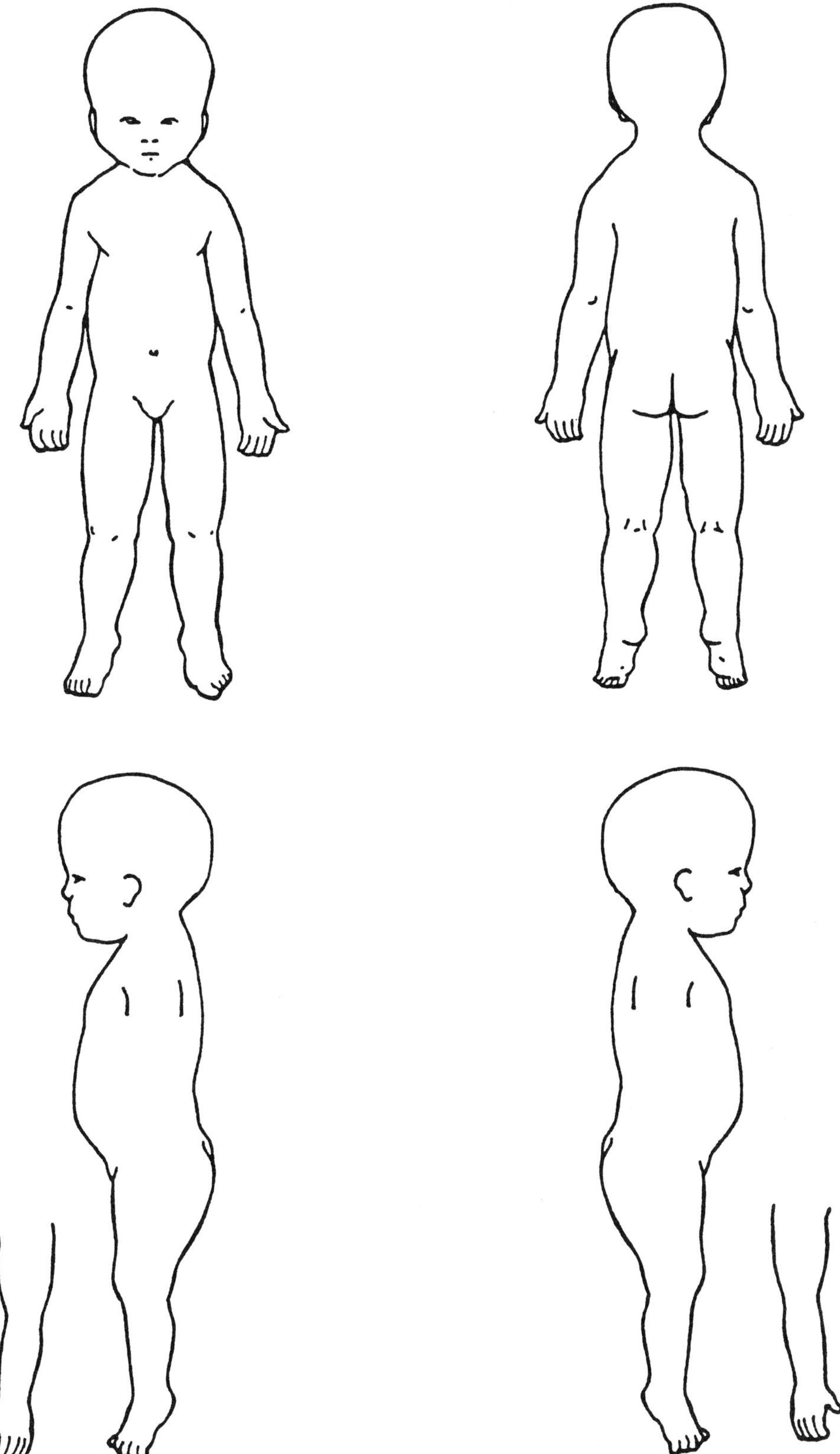

Fig. 5 Infant, ventral, dorsal, and left and right lateral view

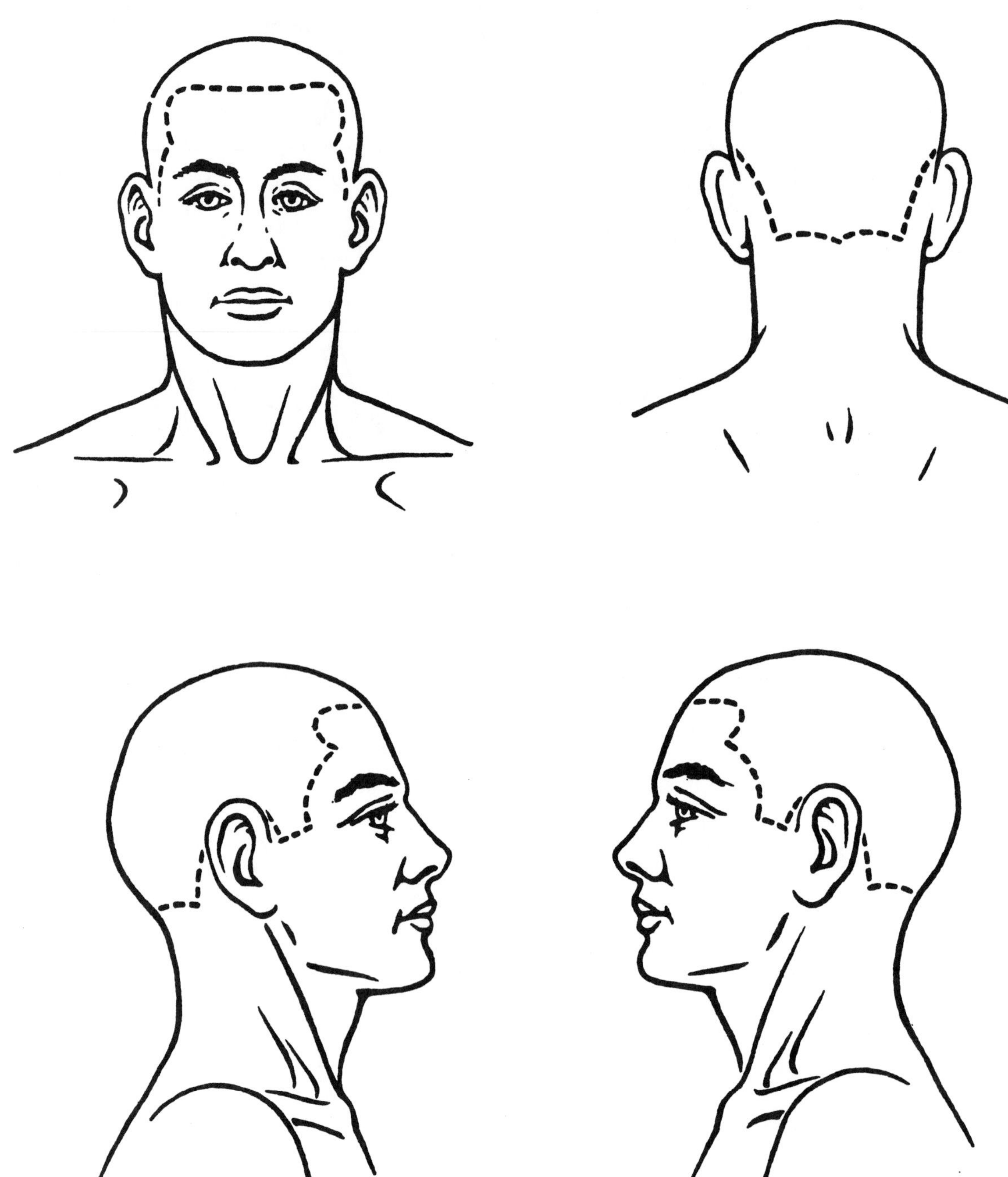

Fig. 6 Head and face diagrams

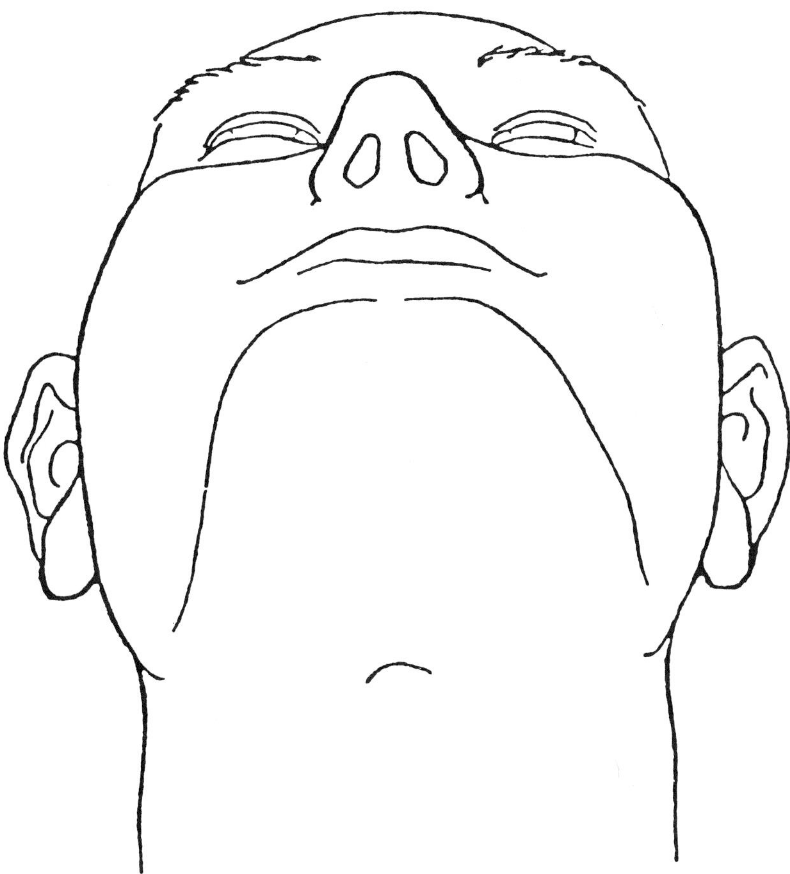

Fig. 7 Submental view

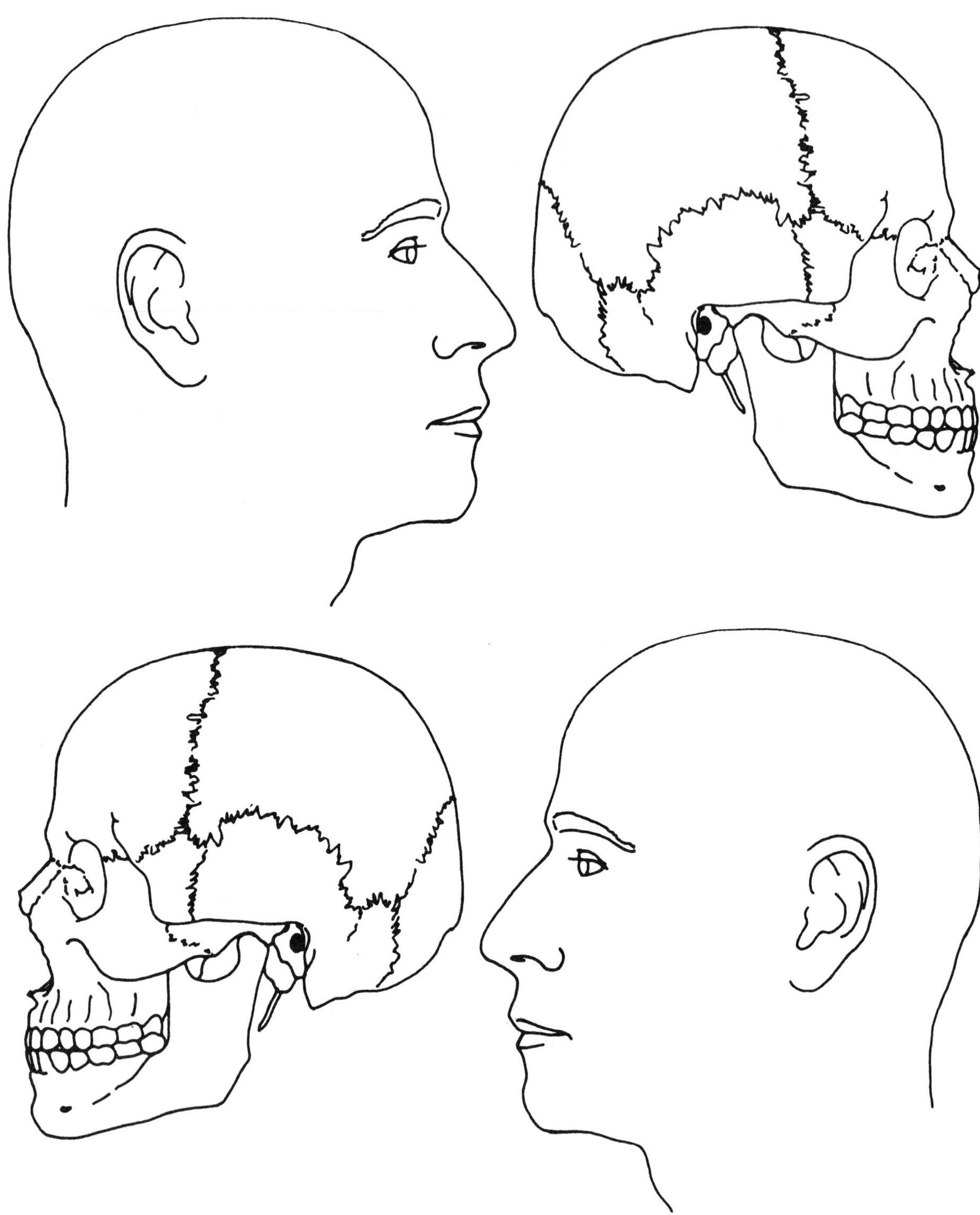

Fig. 8 Head and skull, lateral view

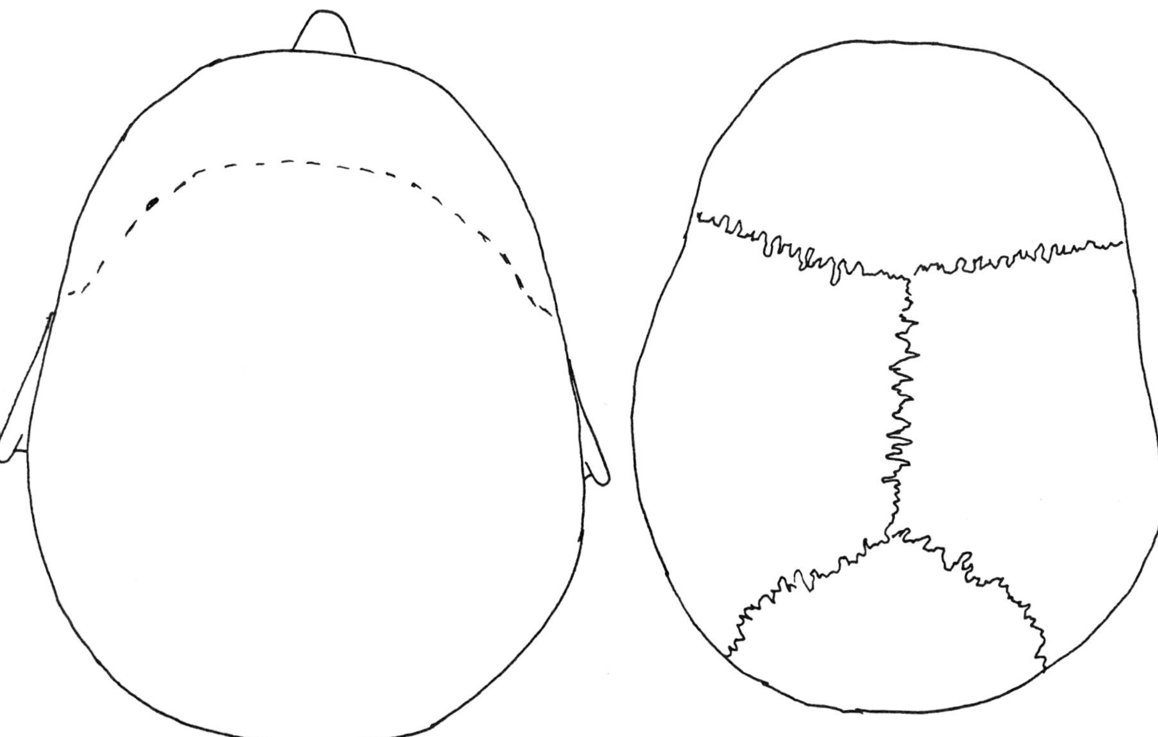

Top of head and skull

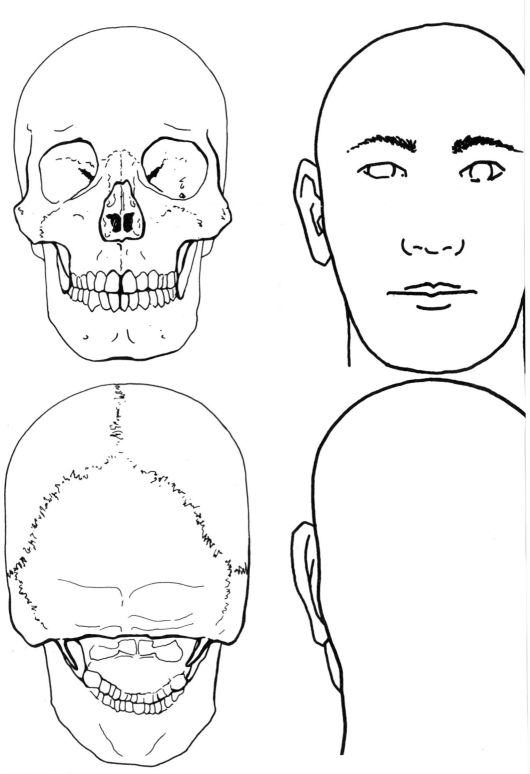

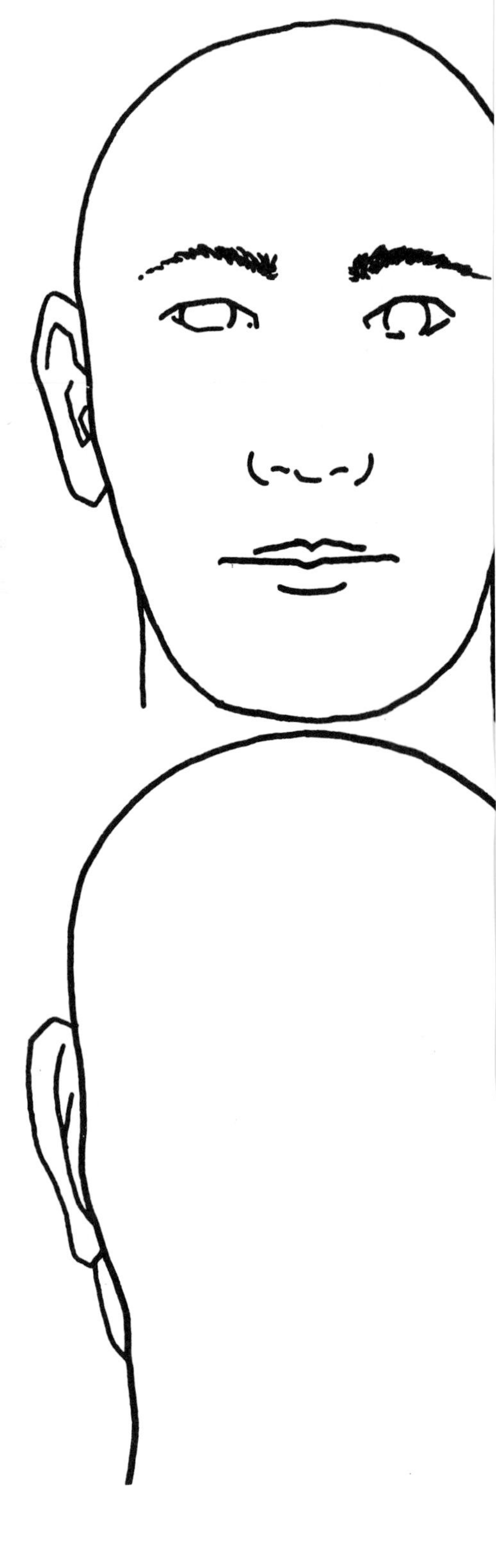

Fig. 9 Head and skull, anterior and posterior view

Fig.

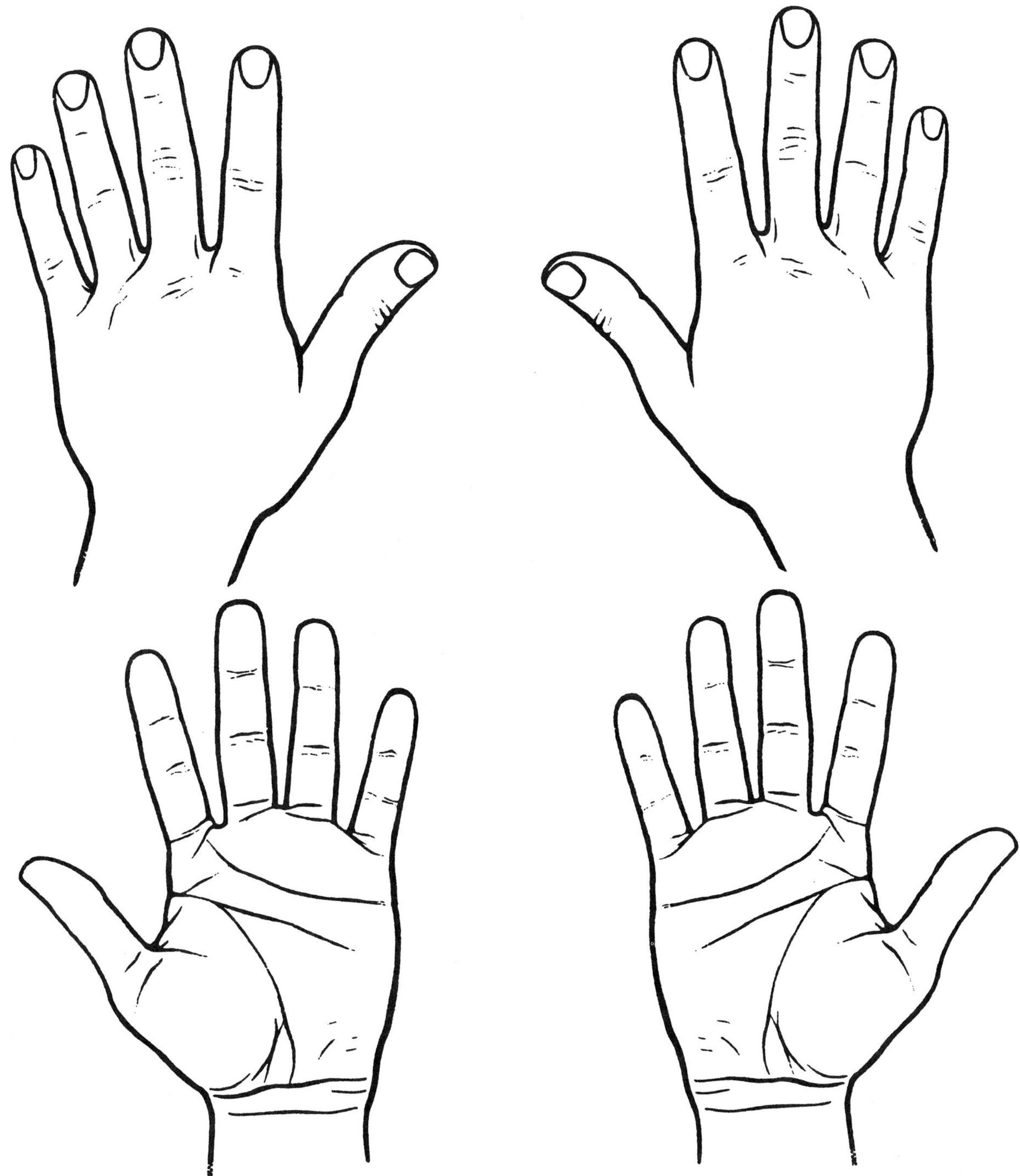

Fig. 11 Left and right hands

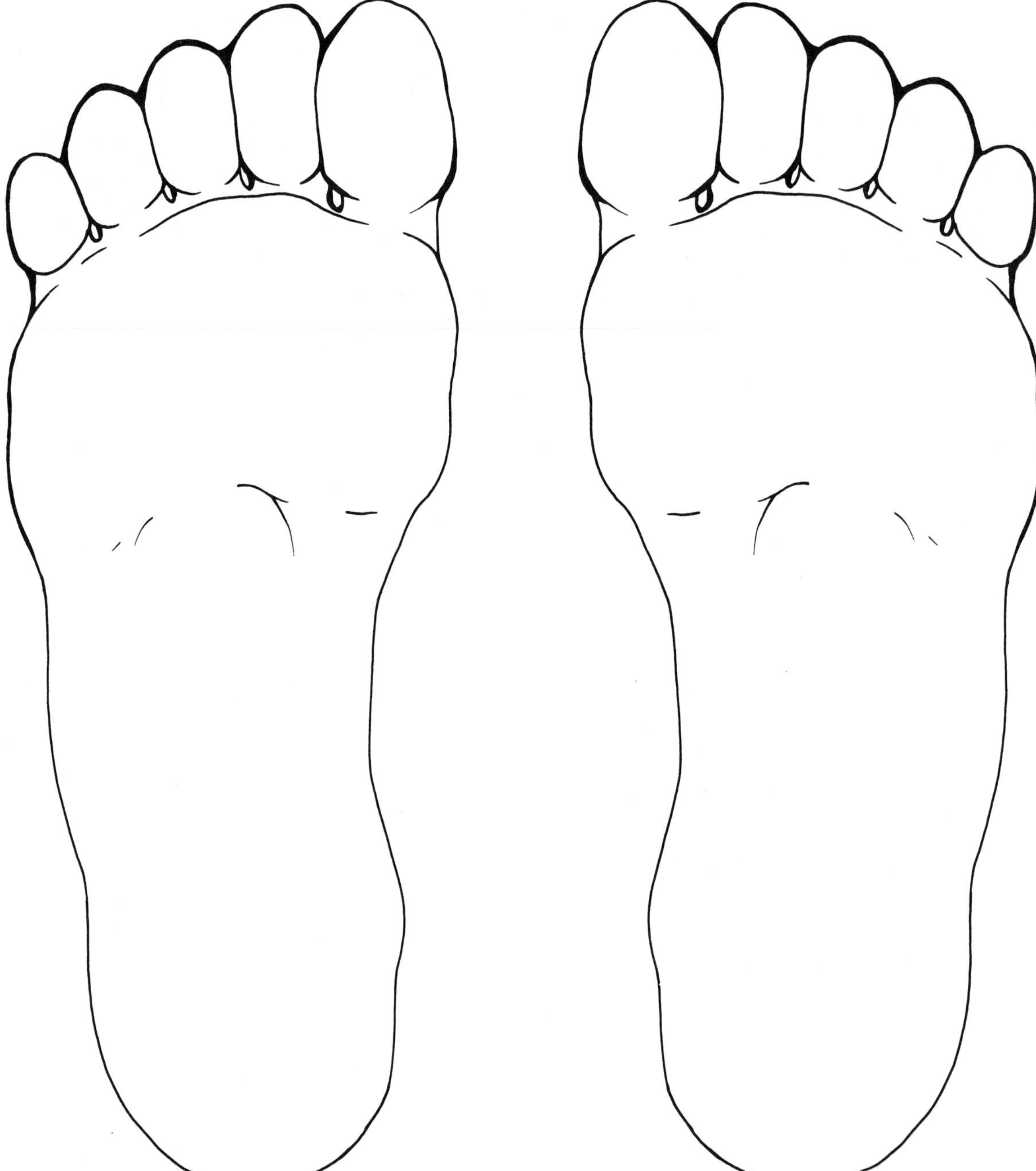

Fig. 12 Feet, left and right plantar surfaces

Appendix D
Forms for Evidence Collection in Sexual Assault
Courtesy of the California Governor's Office of Criminal Justice Planning

Every healthcare practitioner who conducts a medical examination of a sexual assault victim or suspect for evidence must use a form to record findings. The following pages are forms used by the state of California and are excellent sources for all forensic examiners.

Forms must be filled out as completely and accurately as possible. These forms are intended to help document the forensic evidence but are not the complete medical record.

Complete and detailed instructions are available for each of the three forms included in this appendix. For these instructions and more information about completing these forms, go to the California Governor's Office of Criminal Justice Planning Web site at www.ocjp.ca.gov or the forms Web site at www.oes.ca.gov/Operational/OESHome.nsf/CJPD_Documents?OpenForm. The University of California–Davis California Medical Training Center can be reached by telephone at 916-734-4141.

FORENSIC MEDICAL REPORT: ACUTE (<72 HOURS)
ADULT/ADOLESCENT SEXUAL ASSAULT EXAMINATION

STATE OF CALIFORNIA
OFFICE OF CRIMINAL JUSTICE PLANNING

OCJP 923

Confidential Document

Patient Identification

A. GENERAL INFORMATION (print or type) — Name of Medical Facility:

1. Name of patient — **Patient ID number**

2. Address | **City** | **County** | **State** | **Telephone (W) (H)**

3. Age	DOB	Gender M F	Ethnicity	Arrival Date	Arrival Time	Discharge Date	Discharge Time

B. REPORTING AND AUTHORIZATION — Jurisdiction (☐city ☐county ☐other):

1. Telephone report made to law enforcement agency
Name of Officer | **Agency** | **ID Number** | **Telephone**

Reported by: **Name** | **Date** | **Time**

2. Responding Officer | **Agency** | **ID Number** | **Telephone**

3. I request a forensic medical examination for suspected sexual assault at public expense.

Law enforcement officer | **ID number** | **Agency**

Telephone | **Date** | **Time** | **Case Number**

Telephone Authorization
Agency:
Authorizing party:
ID number:
Date/time:

C. PATIENT INFORMATION

- I understand that hospitals and health care professionals are required by Penal Code Sections 11160-11161 to report to law enforcement authorities cases in which medical care is sought when injuries have been inflicted upon any person in violation of any state penal law. The report must state the name of the injured person, current whereabouts, and the type and extent of injuries. ________ (Initial)
- I have been informed that victims of crime are eligible to submit crime victim compensation claims to the State Victims of Crime (VOC) Restitution Fund for out-of-pocket medical expenses, psychological counseling, loss of wages, and job retraining and rehabilitation. ________ (Initial)

D. PATIENT CONSENT

Minors: Family Code Section 6927 permits minors (12 to 17 years of age) to consent to medical examination, treatment, and evidence collection for sexual assault without parental consent. See instructions for parental notification requirements for minors.

- I understand that a forensic medical examination for evidence of sexual assault at public expense can, with my consent, be conducted by a health care professional to discover and preserve evidence of the assault. If conducted, the report of the examination and any evidence obtained will be released to law enforcement authorities. I understand that the examination may include the collection of reference specimens at the time of the examination or at a later date. I understand that I may withdraw consent at any time for any portion of the examination. ________ (Initial)
- I understand that collection of evidence may include photographing injuries and that these photographs may include the genital area. ________ (Initial)
- I hereby consent to a forensic medical examination for evidence of sexual assault. ________ (Initial)
- I understand that data without patient identity may be collected from this report for health and forensic purposes and provided to health authorities and other qualified persons with a valid educational or scientific interest for demographic and/or epidemiological studies. ________ (Initial)

Signature ________________________________ ☐ Patient ☐ Parent ☐ Guardian

DISTRIBUTION OF OCJP 923

☐ Original - Law Enforcement ☐ Copy within evidence kit - Crime Lab ☐ Copy - Child Protective Services (if patient is a minor) ☐ Copy - Medical Facility Records

E. PATIENT HISTORY

1. Name of person providing history:	Relationship to patient:	Date	Time

2. Pertinent medical history:

- Last menstrual period
- Any recent (60 days) anal-genital injuries, surgeries, diagnostic procedures, or medical treatment that may affect the interpretation of current physical findings? ☐ No ☐ Yes
  If yes, describe:
- Any other pertinent medical condition(s) that may affect the interpretation of current physical findings? ☐ No ☐ Yes
  If yes, describe:
- Any pre-existing physical injuries? ☐ No ☐ Yes
  If yes, describe:

3. Pertinent pre- and post-assault related history:

	No	Yes	Unsure
• Other intercourse within past 5 days?	☐	☐	
If yes,			
anal (within past 5 days)? When ______	☐	☐	
vaginal (within past 5 days)? When ______	☐	☐	
oral (within past 24 hours)? When ______	☐	☐	
If yes, did ejaculation occur?	☐	☐	☐
If yes, where? ______________			
If yes, was a condom used?	☐	☐	☐
• Any voluntary alcohol use within 12 hours prior to assault?	☐	☐*	
• Any voluntary drug use within 96 hours prior to assault ?	☐	☐*	
• Any voluntary drug or alcohol use between the time of the assault and the forensic exam?	☐	☐*	

* If yes, collection of toxicology samples is recommended according to local policy. ☐ Blood ☐ Urine

4. Post-assault hygiene/activity: ☐ **Not applicable if over 72 hours**

	No	Yes
Urinated	☐	☐
Defecated	☐	☐
Genital or body wipes	☐	☐
If yes, describe: ______________		
Douched	☐	☐
If yes, with what ______________		
Removed/inserted tampon ☐ diaphragm ☐	☐	☐
Oral gargle/rinse	☐	☐
Bath/shower/wash	☐	☐
Brushed teeth	☐	☐
Ate or drank	☐	☐
Changed clothing	☐	☐
If yes, describe: ______________		

5. Assault-related history:

	No	Yes
Loss of memory? If yes, describe:	☐	☐ *
Lapse of consciousness? If yes, describe:	☐	☐ *

*If yes, collection of toxicology samples is recommended according to local policy. ☐Blood ☐Urine

	No	Yes
Vomited? If yes, describe:	☐	☐
Non-genital injury, pain and/or bleeding? If yes, describe:	☐	☐
Anal-genital injury, pain, and/or bleeding? If yes, describe:	☐	☐

Patient Identification

F. ASSAULT HISTORY

1. Date of assault(s):	Time of assault(s):

2. Pertinent physical surroundings of assault(s):

3. Alleged assailant(s) name(s)	Age	Gender	Ethnicity	Relationship to patient: Known	Relationship to patient: Unknown
#1.		M F			
#2.		M F			
#3.		M F			
#4.		M F			

4. Methods employed by assailant(s):

	No	Yes	If yes, describe:
Weapons	☐	☐	
Threatened?	☐	☐	
Injuries inflicted?	☐	☐	
Type(s) of weapons?	☐	☐	
Physical blows	☐	☐	
Grabbing/holding/pinching	☐	☐	
Physical restraints	☐	☐	
Choking/strangulation	☐	☐	
Burns (thermal and/or chemical)	☐	☐	
Threat(s) of harm	☐	☐	
Target(s) of threat(s)	☐	☐	
Other methods	☐	☐	

Involuntary ingestion of alcohol/drugs ☐No ☐Yes ☐ Unsure

If yes, ☐ Alcohol ☐ Drugs

If yes, ☐ Forced ☐ Coerced ☐ Suspected

If yes, toxicology samples collected: ☐ Blood ☐ Urine ☐None

5. Injuries inflicted upon the assailant(s) during assault? ☐No ☐Yes
If yes, describe injuries, possible locations on the body, and how they were inflicted.

G. ACTS DESCRIBED BY PATIENT

- **Any penetration of the genital or anal opening, however slight, constitutes the act.**
- **Oral copulation requires only contact**
- **If more than one assailant, identify by number.**

Patient Identification

1. Penetration of vagina by:

	No	Yes	Attempted	Unsure
Penis	☐	☐	☐	☐
Finger	☐	☐	☐	☐
Object	☐	☐	☐	☐

If yes, describe the object:

Describe:

2. Penetration of anus by:

	No	Yes	Attempted	Unsure
Penis	☐	☐	☐	☐
Finger	☐	☐	☐	☐
Object	☐	☐	☐	☐

If yes, describe the object:

Describe:

3. Oral copulation of genitals:

	No	Yes	Attempted	Unsure
Of patient by assailant	☐	☐	☐	☐
Of assailant by patient	☐	☐	☐	☐

Describe:

4. Oral copulation of anus:

	No	Yes	Attempted	Unsure
Of patient by assailant	☐	☐	☐	☐
Of assailant by patient	☐	☐	☐	☐

Describe:

5. Non-genital act(s):	No	Yes	Attempted	Unsure
Licking	☐	☐	☐	☐
Kissing	☐	☐	☐	☐
Suction injury	☐	☐	☐	☐
Biting	☐	☐	☐	☐

Describe:

6. Other act(s):	No	Yes	Attempted	Unsure
	☐	☐	☐	☐

Describe:

7. Did ejaculation occur?	No	Yes	Unsure
	☐	☐	☐

If yes, note location(s):
- ☐ Mouth
- ☐ Vagina
- ☐ Anus/Rectum
- ☐ Body surface
- ☐ On clothing
- ☐ On bedding
- ☐ Other

Describe:

8. Contraceptive or lubricant products:

	No	Yes	Unsure
Foam used?	☐	☐	☐
Jelly used?	☐	☐	☐
Lubricant used?	☐	☐	☐
Condom used?	☐	☐	☐

Describe Type/Brand, if known:

H. GENERAL PHYSICAL EXAMINATION

Record all findings using diagrams, legend, and a consecutive numbering system.

1. Blood Pressure	Pulse	Resp	Temp	2. Exam Started		Exam Completed	
				Date	Time	Date	Time

3. Describe general physical appearance	4. Describe general demeanor

Patient Identification

5. Describe condition of clothing upon arrival.

6. Collect outer and underclothing if indicated. ☐ Not indicated

7. Conduct a physical examination. ☐ Findings ☐ No Findings

8. Collect dried and moist secretions, stains, and foreign materials from the body. Scan the entire body with a Wood's Lamp.
☐ Findings ☐ No Findings

9. Collect fingernail scrapings or cuttings according to local policy.

Diagram A

Diagram B

LEGEND: Types of Findings

AB	Abrasion	DF	Deformity	FB	Foreign Body	MS	Moist Secretion	PE	Petechiae	TB	Toluidine Blue ⊕
BI	Bite	DS	Dry Secretion	IN	Induration	OF	Other Foreign Materials (describe)	PS	Potential Saliva	TE	Tenderness
BU	Burn	EC	Ecchymosis (bruise)	IW	Incised Wound			SHX	Sample Per History	V/S	Vegetation/Soil
CS	Control Swab	ER	Erythema (redness)	LA	Laceration	OI	Other Injury (describe)	SI	Suction Injury	WL	Wood's Lamp ⊕
DE	Debris	F/H	Fiber/Hair					SW	Swelling		

Locator #	Type	Description	Locator #	Type	Description

RECORD ALL CLOTHING AND SPECIMENS COLLECTED ON PAGE 8

I. HEAD, NECK, AND ORAL EXAMINATION

Record all findings using diagrams, legend, and a consecutive numbering system.

1. **Examine the face, head, hair, scalp, and neck for injury and foreign materials** ☐ Findings ☐ No Findings
2. **Collect dried and moist secretions, stains, and foreign materials from the face, head, hair, scalp, and neck.** ☐ Findings ☐ No Findings
3. **Examine the oral cavity for injury and foreign materials (if indicated by assault history). Collect foreign materials.** **Exam done:** ☐ Not applicable ☐ Yes ☐ Findings ☐ No Findings
4. **Collect 2 swabs from the oral cavity up to 12 hours post assault and prepare one dry mount slide from one of the swabs.**
5. **Collect head hair reference samples according to local policy.**

Patient Identification

Diagram C

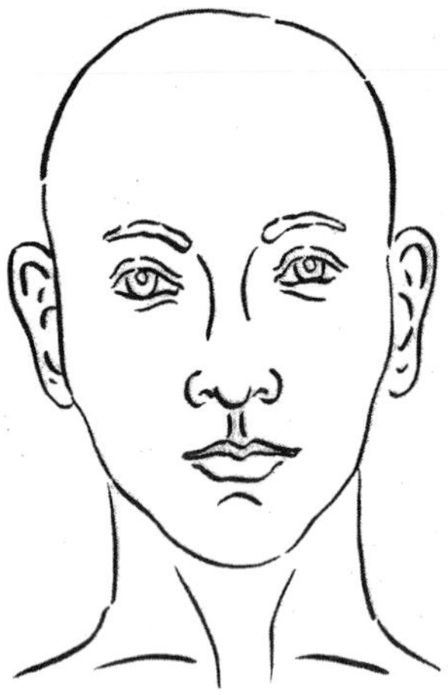

Diagram D

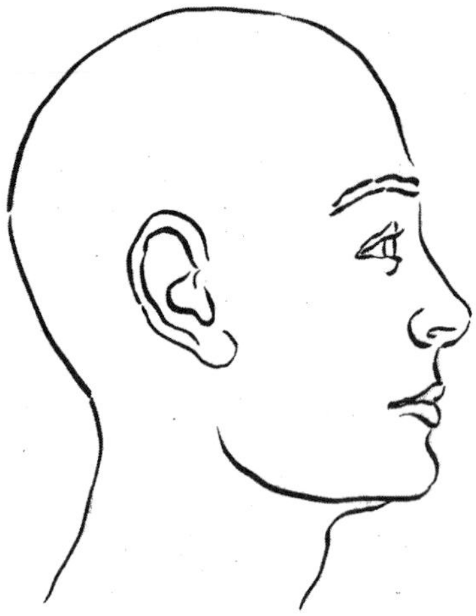

Diagram E

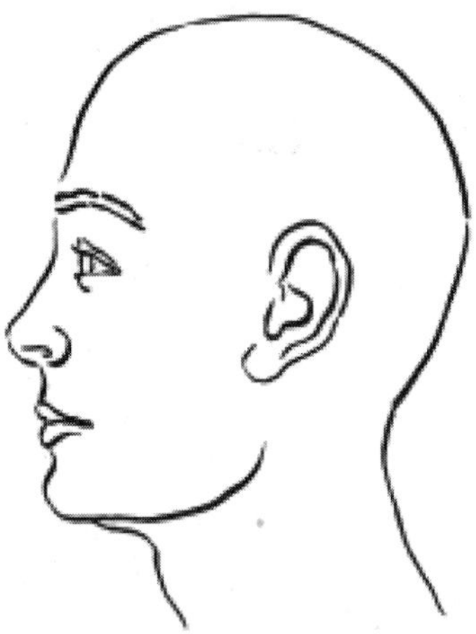

Diagram F

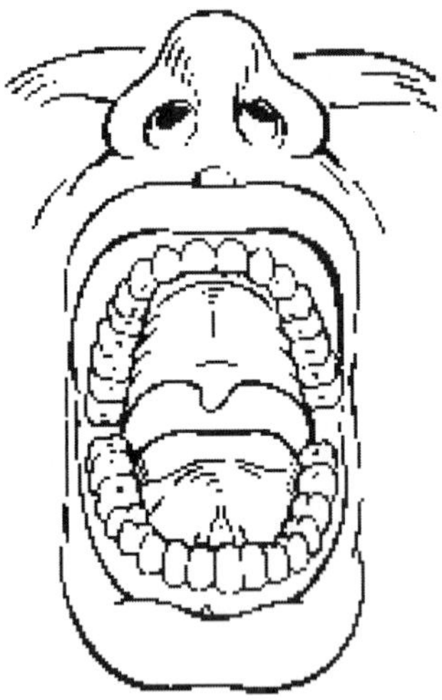

LEGEND: Types of Findings

AB Abrasion	**DF** Deformity	**FB** Foreign Body	**MS** Moist Secretion	**PE** Petechiae	**TB** Toluidine Blue ⊕
BI Bite	**DS** Dry Secretion	**IN** Induration	**OF** Other Foreign Materials (describe)	**PS** Potential Saliva	**TE** Tenderness
BU Burn	**EC** Ecchymosis (bruise)	**IW** Incised Wound		**SHX** Sample Per History	**V/S** Vegetation/Soil
CS Control Swab	**ER** Erythema (redness)	**LA** Laceration	**OI** Other Injury (describe)	**SI** Suction Injury	**WL** Wood's Lamp ⊕
DE Debris	**F/H** Fiber/Hair			**SW** Swelling	

Locator #	Type	Description	Locator #	Type	Description

RECORD ALL SPECIMENS COLLECTED ON PAGE 8

J. GENITAL EXAMINATION - FEMALES

Record all findings using diagrams, legend, and a consecutive numbering system.

1. **Examine the inner thighs, external genitalia, and perineal area. Check the box(es) if there are assault related findings:**
   ☐ No Findings

   ☐ Inner thighs ☐ Periurethral tissue/urethral meatus
   ☐ Perineum ☐ Perihymenal tissue (vestibule)
   ☐ Labia majora ☐ Hymen
   ☐ Labia minora ☐ Fossa navicularis
   ☐ Clitoris/surrounding area ☐ Posterior fourchette

2. **Collect dried and moist secretions, stains, and foreign materials. Scan the area with a Wood's Lamp.** ☐ Findings ☐ No Findings
3. **Collect pubic hair combing or brushing.**
4. **Collect pubic hair reference samples according to local policy.**
5. **Examine the vagina and cervix. Check the box(es) if there are assault related findings.**
   ☐ No Findings ☐ Vagina ☐ Cervix
6. **Collect 4 swabs from the vaginal pool. Prepare one wet mount slide and one dry mount slide.**
7. **Collect 2 cervical swabs (if over 48 hours post assault).**
8. **Examine the buttocks, anus, and rectum (if indicated by history).**
   Exam done: ☐ **Yes** ☐ **Not applicable**
   Check the box(es) if there are assault related findings:
   ☐ No Findings

   ☐ Buttocks ☐ Anal verge/folds/rugae
   ☐ Perianal skin ☐ Rectum
9. **Collect dried and moist secretions, stains, and foreign materials.**
   ☐ Findings ☐ No Findings
10. **Collect 2 anal and/or rectal swabs and prepare one dry mount slide.**
11. **Conduct an anoscopic exam if rectal injury is suspected or if there is any sign of rectal bleeding.**
    Rectal bleeding ☐ No ☐ Yes
    If yes, describe:____________________
12. **Exam position used:**
    ☐ Supine ☐ Other Describe:

LEGEND: Types of Findings

AB	Abrasion	**EC**	Ecchymosis (bruise)	**MS**	Moist Secretion	**SI**	Suction Injury
BI	Bite	**ER**	Erythema (redness)	**OF**	Other Foreign Materials (describe)	**SW**	Swelling
BU	Burn	**F/H**	Fiber/Hair			**TB**	ToluidineBlue⊕
CS	Control Swab	**FB**	Foreign Body	**OI**	Other Injury (describe)	**TE**	Tenderness
DE	Debris	**IN**	Induration	**PE**	Petechiae	**V/S**	Vegetation/Soil
DF	Deformity	**IW**	Incised Wound	**PS**	Potential Saliva	**WL**	Wood's Lamp⊕
DS	Dry Secretion	**LA**	Laceration	**SHX**	Sample Per History		

Locator #	Type	Description

Patient Identification

Diagram G

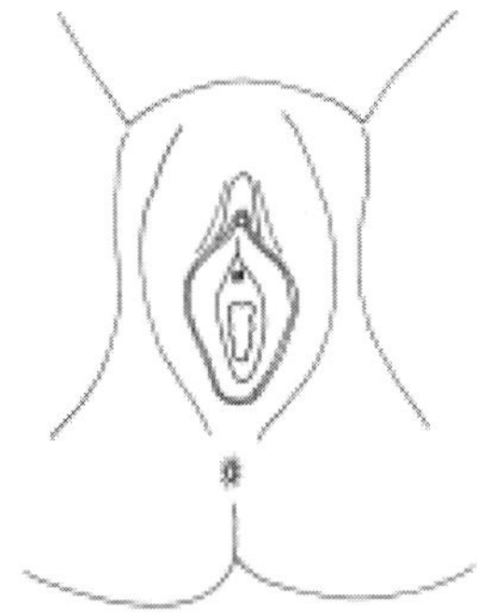

Diagram H

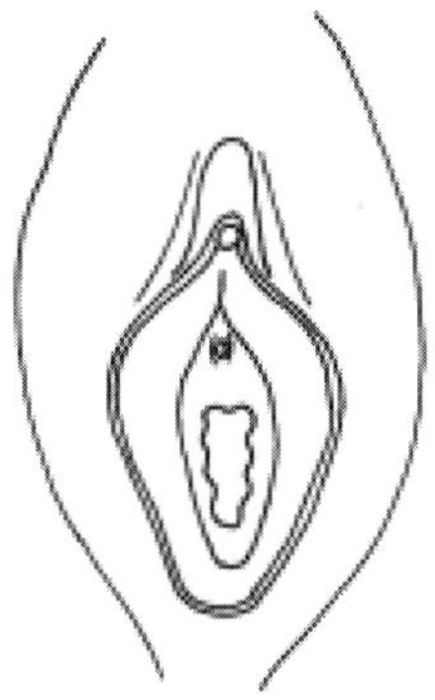

Diagram I

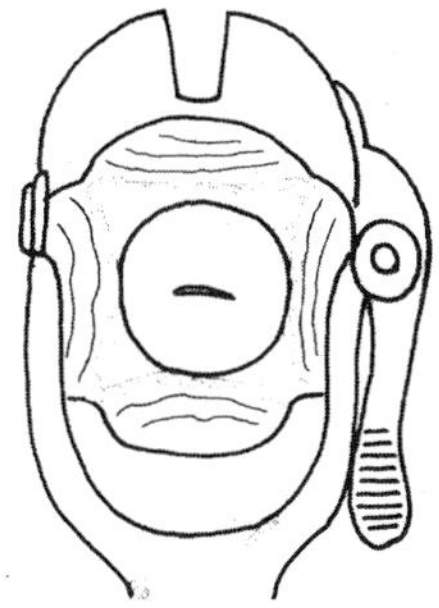

Diagram J

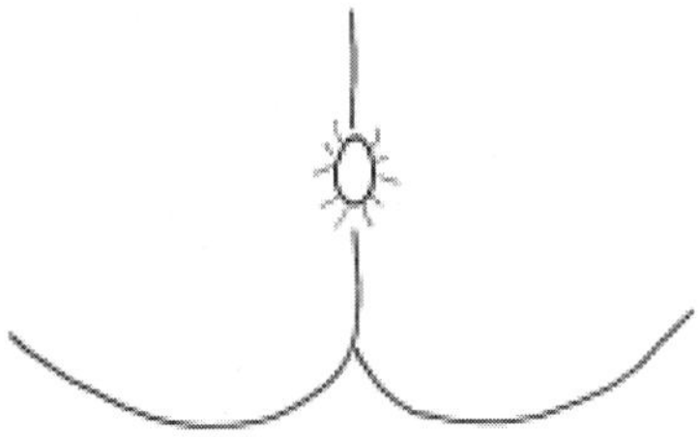

RECORD ALL SPECIMENS COLLECTED ON PAGE 8

K. GENITAL EXAMINATION – MALES

Record all findings using diagrams, legend, and a consecutive numbering system.

1. **Examine the inner thighs, external genitalia, and perineal area. Check the box(es) if there are assault related findings:**
   ☐ No Findings

   ☐ Inner thighs ☐ Glans penis ☐ Scrotum
   ☐ Perineum ☐ Penile shaft ☐ Testes
   ☐ Foreskin ☐ Urethral meatus
2. **Circumcised:** ☐ No ☐ Yes
3. **Collect dried and moist secretions, stains, and foreign materials. Scan the area with a Wood's Lamp.** ☐ Findings ☐ No Findings
4. **Collect pubic hair combing or brushing.**
5. **Collect pubic hair reference samples according to local policy.**
6. **Collect 2 penile swabs, if indicated by assault history.** ☐ N/A
7. **Collect 2 scrotal swabs, if indicated by assault history.** ☐ N/A
8. **Examine the buttocks, anus, and rectum (if indicated by history)**
   Exam done: ☐ **Yes** ☐ **Not applicable**
   Check the box(es) if there are assault related findings:
   ☐ No Findings

   ☐ Buttocks ☐ Anal verge/folds/rugae
   ☐ Perianal skin ☐ Rectum
9. **Collect dried and moist secretions, stains, and foreign materials.**
   ☐ Findings ☐ No Findings
10. **Collect 2 anal and/or rectal swabs and prepare one dry mount slide.**
11. **Conduct an anoscopic exam if rectal injury is suspected or if there is any sign of rectal bleeding.**
    Rectal bleeding: ☐ No ☐ Yes
    If yes, describe: ______________________
12. **Exam position used:**
    ☐ Supine ☐ Other Describe:

LEGEND: Types of Findings

AB	Abrasion	**EC**	Ecchymosis (bruise)	**MS**	Moist Secretion	**SI**	Suction Injury
BI	Bite	**ER**	Erythema (redness)	**OF**	Other Foreign Materials (describe)	**SW**	Swelling
BU	Burn	**F/H**	Fiber/Hair			**TB**	ToluidineBlue⊕
CS	Control Swab	**FB**	Foreign Body	**OI**	Other Injury (describe)	**TE**	Tenderness
DE	Debris	**IN**	Induration	**PE**	Petechiae	**V/S**	Vegetation/Soil
DF	Deformity	**IW**	Incised Wound	**PS**	Potential Saliva	**WL**	Wood's Lamp⊕
DS	Dry Secretion	**LA**	Laceration	**SHX**	Sample Per History		

Locator #	Type	Description

Patient Identification

Diagram K

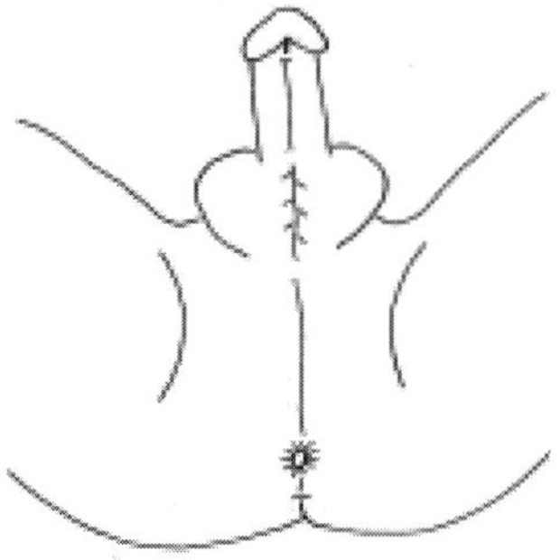

Diagram L

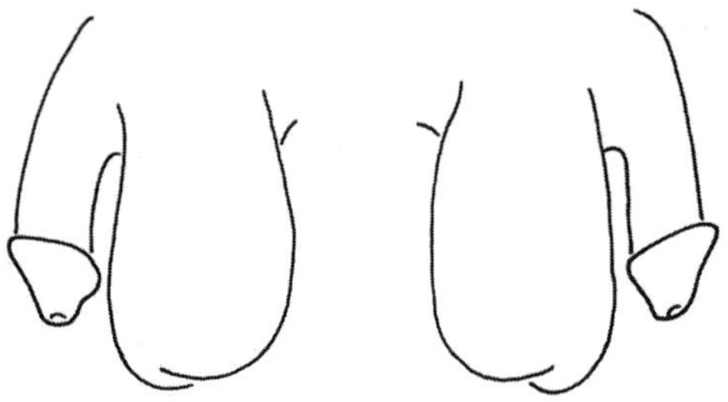

Diagram M

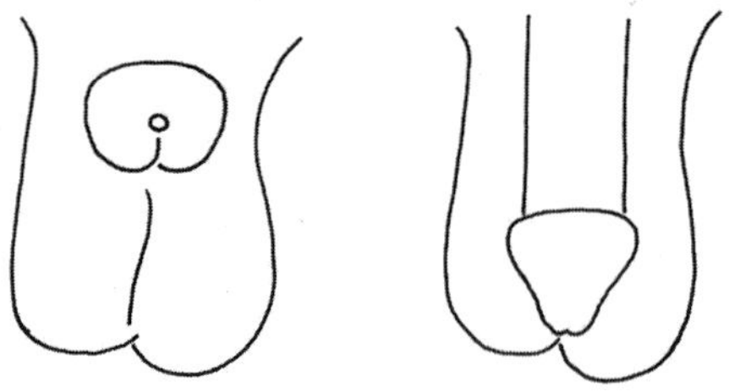

Diagram N

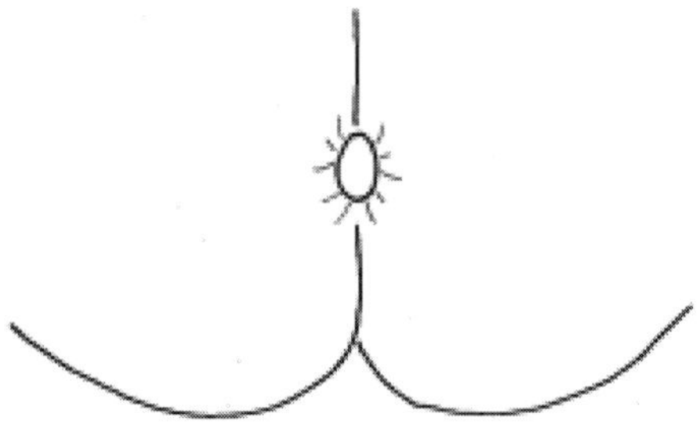

RECORD ALL SPECIMENS COLLECTED ON PAGE 8

L. EVIDENCE COLLECTED AND SUBMITTED TO CRIME LAB

1. Clothing placed in evidence kit | **Other clothing placed in bags**

Clothing placed in evidence kit	Other clothing placed in bags

2. Foreign materials collected

	No	Yes	Collected by:
Swabs/suspected blood	☐	☐	
Dried secretions	☐	☐	
Fiber/loose hairs	☐	☐	
Vegetation	☐	☐	
Soil/debris	☐	☐	
Swabs/suspected semen	☐	☐	
Swabs/suspected saliva	☐	☐	
Swabs/Wood's Lamp⊕ area(s)	☐	☐	
Control swabs	☐	☐	
Fingernail scrapings/cuttings	☐	☐	
Matted hair cuttings	☐	☐	
Pubic hair combings/brushings	☐	☐	
Intravaginal foreign body	☐	☐	
If yes, describe:			
Other types	☐	☐	
If yes, describe:			

3. Oral/genital/anal/rectal samples

	# Swabs	# Slides	Time collected	Collected by:
Oral				
Vaginal				
Cervical				
Anal				
Rectal				
Penile				
Scrotal				

Aspirate/washings (optional) ☐ No ☐ Yes

4. Vaginal wet mount slide

	No	Yes	Time	Examiner:
Slide prepared				
Motile sperm observed				
Non-motile sperm observed				

M. TOXICOLOGY SAMPLES

	No	Yes	Time	Collected by:
Blood alcohol/toxicology (gray top tube)				
Urine toxicology				

N. REFERENCE SAMPLES

	No	Yes	Collected by:
Blood (lavender top tube)			
Blood (yellow top tube)			
Blood Card (optional)			
Buccal swabs (optional)			
Saliva swabs			
Head hair			
Pubic hair			

O. PHOTO DOCUMENTATION METHODS

	No	Yes	Colposcope/ 35mm	Macrolens/ 35mm	Colposcope/ Videocamera	Other Optics
Body	☐	☐	☐	☐	☐	☐ ________
Genitals	☐	☐	☐	☐	☐	☐ ________

Photographed by:

Patient Identification

P. RECORD EXAM METHODS

	No	Yes		No	Yes
Direct visualization only	☐	☐	Toluidine Blue Dye	☐	☐
Colposcopy	☐	☐	Anoscopic exam	☐	☐
Other magnifier	☐	☐	Anal speculum exam	☐	☐
Other	☐	☐			

If yes, describe: ______

Q. RECORD EXAM FINDINGS

☐ **Physical Findings** ☐ **No Physical Findings**

R. RECORD ASSESSMENT OF FINDINGS

☐ Exam consistent with history
☐ Exam inconsistent with history

S. SUMMARIZE FINDINGS

T. PRINT NAMES OF PERSONNEL INVOLVED

	Telephone:
History taken by:	
Exam performed by:	
Specimens labeled and sealed by:	
Assisted by: ☐ N/A	
Signature of examiner	License No.

U. EVIDENCE DISTRIBUTION

U. EVIDENCE DISTRIBUTION	GIVEN TO:
Clothing (item(s) not placed in evidence kit)	
Evidence Kit	
Reference blood samples	
Toxicology samples	

V. SIGNATURE OF OFFICER RECEIVING EVIDENCE

Signature: ______

Print name and ID #: ______

Agency: ______

Date: Phone:

FORENSIC MEDICAL REPORT: ACUTE (<72 HOURS)
CHILD/ADOLESCENT SEXUAL ABUSE EXAMINATION
STATE OF CALIFORNIA
OFFICE OF CRIMINAL JUSTICE PLANNING

OCJP 930

Confidential Document | **Patient Identification**

A. GENERAL INFORMATION (print or type) | **Name of Medical Facility:**

1. Name of patient | Patient ID number

2. Address | City | County | State | Telephone

3. Age	DOB	Gender M F	Ethnicity	Arrival Date	Arrival Time	Discharge Date	Discharge Time

4. Name of : ☐ Mother ☐ Stepmother ☐ Guardian | Address | City | County | State | Telephone W: H:

5. Name of : ☐ Father ☐ Stepfather ☐ Guardian | Address | City | County | State | Telephone W: H:

6. Name(s) of Siblings	Gender	Age	DOB	Name(s) of Siblings	Gender	Age	DOB
	M F				M F		
	M F				M F		

B. REPORTING AND AUTHORIZATION | **Jurisdiction (☐city ☐county ☐other):**

	Name	Agency	ID number	Telephone
1. Telephone report made to Law Enforcement ☐ and/or Child Protective Services ☐				
2. Responding Personnel (to medical facility) Law Enforcement ☐ and/or Child Protective Services ☐				
3. Assigned Investigator (if known) Law Enforcement ☐ and/or Child Protective Services ☐				

4. Authorization for evidential exam requested by law enforcement or child protective services agency

I request a forensic medical examination for suspected sexual abuse at public expense.

☐ **Law enforcement officer** | **ID number** | ☐ **Child Protective Services**

Telephone | **Date** | **Time** | **Case number**

Telephone Authorization
Agency:
Authorizing party:
ID number:
Date/time:

C. CONSENT FOR EXAMINATION BY PATIENT/PARENT/GUARDIAN Note: Parental consent is not required for a suspected child sexual abuse examination if the child is in protective custody. Family Code Section 6927 permits minors (12 to 17 years of age) to consent to medical examination, treatment, and evidence collection for sexual assault without parental consent. See instructions regarding parental notification requirements for minors.

- I hereby consent to a forensic medical examination for evidence of sexual abuse. I understand that collection of evidence may include photographing injuries and that these photographs may include the anal-genital area (private parts). I further understand that medical providers are required to notify child protective authorities of known or suspected child abuse; and, if child abuse is found or suspected, this form and any evidence obtained will be released to a child protective agency.
- I have been informed that victims of crime are eligible to submit crime victim compensation claims to the State Victims of Crime (VOC) Restitution Fund for out-of-pocket medical expenses, psychological counseling, loss of wages, and job retraining/rehabilitation.
- I understand that data without patient identity may be collected from this report for health and forensic purposes and provided to health authorities and other qualified persons with a valid educational or scientific interest for demographic and/or epidemiological studies.

Signature ______________________ ☐ Patient ☐ Parent ☐ Guardian

DISTRIBUTION OF OCJP 930

☐ Original – Law Enforcement ☐ Copy – Child Protective Services ☐ Copy within evidence kit – Crime Lab ☐ Copy – Medical Facility Records

D. PATIENT HISTORY

1. Record time or time frame of the incident(s)	Date(s)	Time or time frame
☐ Less than 72 hours		
☐ Multiple incidents over time		

2. **Pertinent physical surroundings of abuse/assault:**

3. Record patient's name for:	4. Alleged perpetrator(s) name(s)	Age	Gender	Patient Identification Ethnicity	Relationship to Patient Known	 Unknown
Female genitalia						
Male genitalia	#1.		M F			
Breasts	#2.		M F			
Anus	#3.		M F			

E. ACTS DESCRIBED BY HISTORIAN

Name of historian	Relationship to patient	History obtained by:	Telephone	Agency	☐ Not applicable

	No	Yes	Attempted	Unsure	N/A	Describe pain and/or bleeding and additional pertinent history:
Genital/vaginal contact/penetration by:						
Penis	☐	☐	☐	☐	☐	______
Finger	☐	☐	☐	☐	☐	
Object (Describe)	☐	☐	☐	☐	☐	______
Associated pain?	☐	☐		☐	☐	
Associated bleeding?	☐	☐		☐	☐	______
Anal contact/penetration by:						
Penis	☐	☐	☐	☐	☐	______
Finger	☐	☐	☐	☐	☐	
Object (Describe)	☐	☐	☐	☐	☐	______
Associated pain?	☐	☐		☐	☐	
Associated bleeding?	☐	☐		☐	☐	______
Oral copulation of genitals:						
Of patient by assailant	☐	☐	☐	☐	☐	______
Of assailant by patient	☐	☐	☐	☐	☐	
Oral copulation of anus:						______
Of patient by assailant	☐	☐	☐	☐	☐	
Of assailant by patient	☐	☐	☐	☐	☐	______
Anal/genital fondling:						
Of patient by assailant	☐	☐	☐	☐	☐	______
Of assailant by patient	☐	☐	☐	☐	☐	
Non-genital act(s)?	☐	☐				______
If yes: ☐ Fondling ☐ Licking ☐ Kissing ☐ Suction Injury ☐ Biting						
Other acts? (Describe)	☐	☐	☐	☐	☐	______
Did ejaculation occur?	☐	☐		☐	☐	
If yes, note location(s):						______
☐ Mouth ☐ Vagina ☐ Body surface ☐ On bedding						
☐ Anus/Rectum ☐ On clothing ☐ Other						______

			N/A	
Contraceptive or lubricant products?	☐ No	☐ Yes	☐	
If yes, note type/brand: ☐ Foam ☐ Jelly ☐ Lubricant ☐ Condom				______
Were force or threats used?	☐ No	☐ Yes ☐ Force ☐ Threats	☐	
Were weapons used?	☐ No	☐ Yes	☐	______
If yes, describe: ______				
Were pictures/videotapes taken ☐ or shown ☐?	☐ No	☐ Yes		______
If yes, note type(s):	☐ Pictures	☐ Videotapes		
Were drugs ☐ or alcohol ☐ used?	☐ No	☐ Yes*	☐	______
Loss of memory?	☐ No	☐ Yes*	☐	
Lapse of consciousness?	☐ No	☐ Yes*	☐	______
Vomited after act(s)?	☐ No	☐ Yes	☐	
Behavioral changes in patient?	☐ No	☐ Yes	☐	______

***Collection of toxicology samples is recommended according to local policy.**

F. ACTS DESCRIBED BY PATIENT

1. Acts disclosed by patient to:
☐ Medical Examiner
☐ Social Worker
☐ Law Enforcement Officer
☐ Multi-disciplinary Interview Team
☐ Other:

	No	Yes	Attempted	Unsure	N/A
Genital/vaginal contact/penetration by:					
Penis	☐	☐	☐	☐	☐
Finger	☐	☐	☐	☐	☐
Object (Describe below)	☐	☐	☐	☐	☐
Associated pain?	☐	☐		☐	☐
Associated bleeding?	☐	☐		☐	☐
Anal contact/penetration by:					
Penis	☐	☐	☐	☐	☐
Finger	☐	☐	☐	☐	☐
Object (Describe below)	☐	☐	☐	☐	☐
Associated pain?	☐	☐		☐	☐
Associated bleeding?	☐	☐		☐	☐
Oral copulation of genitals:					
Of patient by assailant	☐	☐	☐	☐	☐
Of assailant by patient	☐	☐	☐	☐	☐
Oral copulation of anus:					
Of patient by assailant	☐	☐	☐	☐	☐
Of assailant by patient	☐	☐	☐	☐	☐
Anal/genital fondling:					
Of patient by assailant	☐	☐	☐	☐	☐
Of assailant by patient	☐	☐	☐	☐	☐
Non-genital act(s)?	☐	☐			☐

If yes: ☐ Fondling ☐ Licking ☐ Kissing ☐ Suction injury ☐ Biting

	No	Yes	Attempted	Unsure	N/A
Other acts? (Describe below)	☐	☐	☐	☐	☐
Did ejaculation occur?	☐	☐		☐	☐

If yes, note location(s):
☐ Mouth ☐ Vagina ☐ Body surface ☐ On bedding
☐ Anus/Rectum ☐ On clothing ☐ Other

Contraceptive or lubricant products? ☐ No ☐ Yes ☐
If yes, note type/brand: ☐ Foam ☐ Jelly ☐ Lubricant ☐ Condom

Were force or threats used? ☐ No ☐ Yes ☐ Force ☐ Threats
Were weapons used? ☐ No ☐ Yes ☐
If yes, describe: ____________

Were pictures/videotapes ☐ taken or ☐ shown? ☐ No ☐ Yes ☐
If yes, note type(s): ☐ Pictures ☐ Videotapes

Were drugs ☐ or alcohol ☐ used? ☐ No ☐ Yes* ☐
Loss of memory? ☐ No ☐ Yes* ☐
Lapse of consciousness? ☐ No ☐ Yes* ☐
Vomited after act(s)? ☐ No ☐ Yes ☐
Behavioral changes? ☐ No ☐ Yes ☐

***Collection of toxicology samples is recommended according to local policy.**

2. Describe pain and/or bleeding (using patient's exact words) and additional pertinent history from above.

____
____
____
____
____
____

Patient Identification

G. MEDICAL HISTORY (to be completed by medical personnel)

1. Name of person providing history	Relationship to patient	Date	Time

	No	Yes
2. Any recent (60 days) anal-genital injuries, surgeries, diagnostic procedures, or medical treatment that may affect the interpretation of physical findings?	☐	☐
3. Any other pertinent medical conditions that may affect the interpretation of physical findings?	☐	☐
4. Any pre-existing physical injuries?	☐	☐
5. Any previous history of physical abuse and/or neglect?	☐	☐
6. Any previous history of sexual abuse?	☐	☐
7. Other intercourse? (For adolescents only)	☐	☐
If yes,		
anal (within past 5 days)? When ______	☐	☐
vaginal (within past 5 days)? When ______	☐	☐
oral (within past 24 hours)? When ______	☐	☐
If yes, did ejaculation occur?	☐	☐
If yes, where? ____________		
If yes, was a condom used?	☐	☐
8. Menstrual periods? If yes, age of menarche: ______	☐	☐
Last menstrual period: ______	☐	☐

9. Other symptoms disclosed	by patient: No	by patient: Yes	by historian: No	by historian: Yes	by historian: Unk
Abdominal/pelvic pain	☐	☐	☐	☐	☐
Pain on urination	☐	☐	☐	☐	☐
Genital discomfort or pain	☐	☐	☐	☐	☐
Genital itching	☐	☐	☐	☐	☐
Genital discharge	☐	☐	☐	☐	☐
Genital bleeding	☐	☐	☐	☐	☐
Rectal discomfort or pain	☐	☐	☐	☐	☐
Rectal itching	☐	☐	☐	☐	☐
Rectal bleeding	☐	☐	☐	☐	☐
Constipation	☐	☐	☐	☐	☐
Other ______	☐	☐	☐	☐	☐

If yes, describe onset, duration, and intensity:

10. Post-assault hygiene activity
☐ Not applicable if over 72 hours

	by patient: No	by patient: Yes	by historian: No	by historian: Yes	by historian: Unk
Urinated	☐	☐	☐	☐	☐
Defecated	☐	☐	☐	☐	☐
Genital or body wipes	☐	☐	☐	☐	☐
If yes, describe: ______	☐	☐	☐	☐	☐
Douched					
If yes, with what? ______					
Removed/inserted ☐ tampon ☐ diaphragm	☐	☐	☐	☐	☐
Oral gargle/rinse	☐	☐	☐	☐	☐
Bath/shower/wash	☐	☐	☐	☐	☐
Brushed teeth	☐	☐	☐	☐	☐
Ate or drank	☐	☐	☐	☐	☐
Changed clothing	☐	☐	☐	☐	☐

If yes, describe:

H. GENERAL PHYSICAL EXAMINATION

Record all findings using diagrams, legend, and a consecutive numbering system.

1. BP	Pulse	Resp	Temp	Height	Weight	2. Exam Started		Exam Completed	
						Date	Time	Date	Time

3. Female Tanner Stage – Breast 1☐ 2☐ 3☐ 4☐ 5☐
4. Describe general physical appearance.
5. Describe general demeanor and relevant statements made during exam.
6. Describe condition of clothing upon arrival.
7. Collect outer and underclothing if indicated. ☐ Not indicated

Patient Identification

8. Conduct a physical examination. ☐ Findings ☐ No Findings
   General exam within normal limits: ☐ Yes ☐ No ☐ If no, describe:
9. Collect dried and moist secretions, stains, and foreign materials from the body. Scan the entire body with a Wood's Lamp.
   ☐ Findings ☐ No Findings
10. Collect fingernail scrapings or cuttings according to local policy.

Diagram A

Diagram B

LEGEND: Types of Findings

AB	Abrasion	CS	Control Swab	DS	Dry Secretion	HC	Hymenal Cleft	OI	Other Injury (describe)	PE	Petechiae	SW	Swelling
AHT	Absent Hymenal Tissue	CV	Congenital Variation	EC	Ecchymosis (bruise)	IN	Induration			PGW	Possible Genital Wart	TB	Toluidine Blue⊕
				ER	Erythema (redness)	IW	Incised Wound	OSC	Other Skin Condition	PS	Potential Saliva	TE	Tenderness
AL	Anal Laxity	DE	Debris	FB	Foreign Body	LA	Laceration	OT	Other	SH	Submucosal Hemorrhage	V/S	Vegetation/Soil
BI	Bite	DF	Deformity	F/H	Fiber/Hair	MS	Moist Secretion	PW	Perianal Wart	SHX	Sample Per History	VL	Vesicular Lesion
BU	Burn	DI	Discharge	GT	Granulation Tissue	OF	Other Foreign Materials (describe)			SI	Suction Injury	WL	Wood's Lamp⊕

Locator #	Type	Description	Locator #	Type	Description

RECORD ALL CLOTHING AND SPECIMENS COLLECTED ON PAGE 8

I. HEAD, NECK, AND ORAL EXAMINATION

Record all findings using diagrams, legend, and a consecutive numbering system.

1. **Examine the face, head, hair, scalp, and neck for injury and foreign materials.**
   ☐ Findings ☐ No Findings
2. **Exam method:**
   ☐ Direct visualization ☐ Colposcope ☐ Other magnification
3. **Collect dried and moist secretions, stains, and foreign materials from the face, head, hair, scalp, and neck.**
   ☐ Findings ☐ No Findings
4. **Examine the oral cavity for injury and foreign materials. Collect foreign materials.**
   ☐ Findings ☐ No Findings
5. **Collect 2 swabs from the oral cavity up to 12 hours post assault and prepare one dry mount slide from one of the swabs.**
6. **Collect head hair reference samples according to local policy.**

Patient Identification

Diagram C

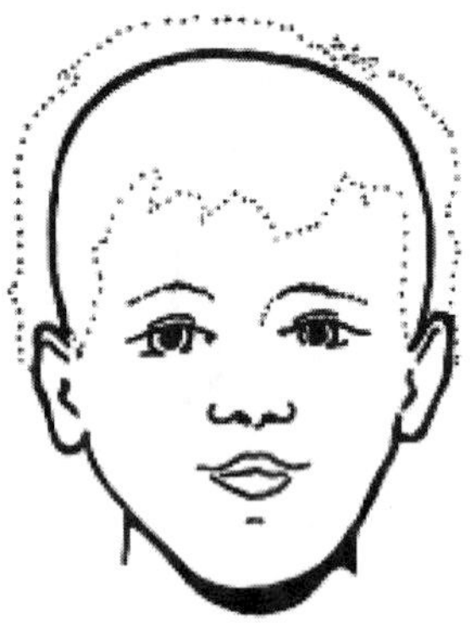

Diagram D

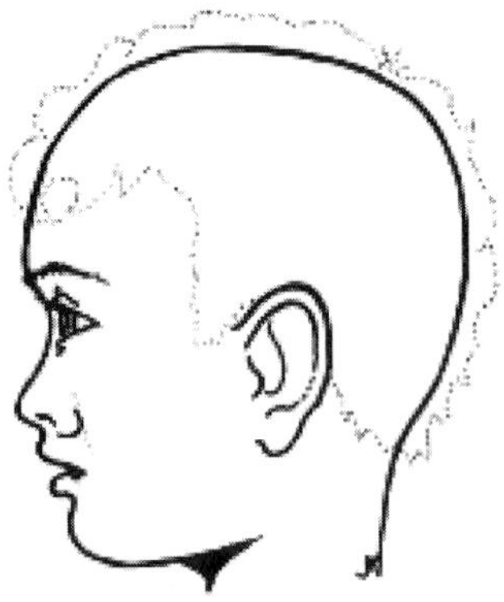

Diagram E

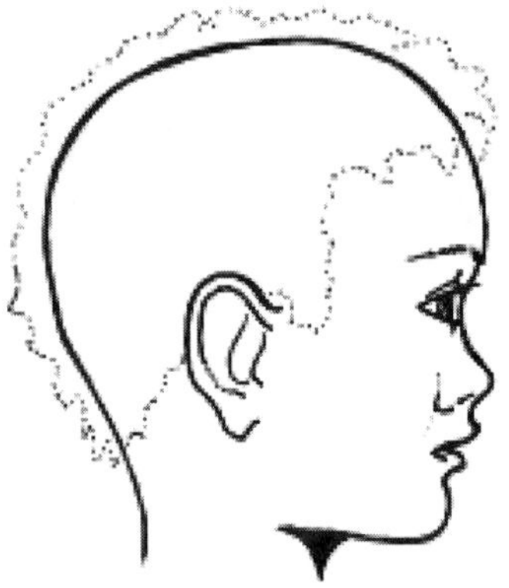

Diagram F

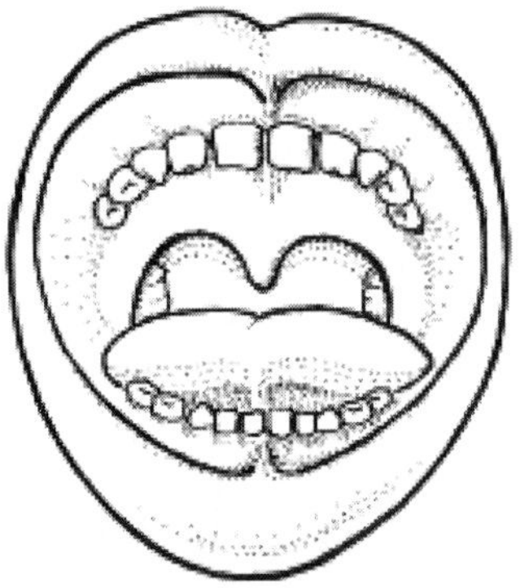

LEGEND: Types of Findings

AB Abrasion	**CS** Control Swab	**DS** Dry Secretion	**HC** Hymenal Cleft	**OI** Other Injury (describe)	**PE** Petechiae	**SW** Swelling
AHT Absent Hymenal Tissue	**CV** Congenital Variation	**EC** Ecchymosis (bruise)	**IN** Induration		**PGW** Possible Genital Wart	**TB** Toluidine Blue⊕
AL Anal Laxity	**DE** Debris	**ER** Erythema (redness)	**IW** Incised Wound	**OSC** Other Skin Condition	**PS** Potential Saliva	**TE** Tenderness
BI Bite	**DF** Deformity	**FB** Foreign Body	**LA** Laceration	**OT** Other	**SH** Submucosal Hemorrhage	**V/S** Vegetation/Soil
BU Burn	**DI** Discharge	**F/H** Fiber/Hair	**MS** Moist Secretion	**PW** Perianal Wart	**SHX** Sample Per History	**VL** Vesicular Lesion
		GT Granulation Tissue	**OF** Other Foreign Materials (describe)		**SI** Suction Injury	**WL** Wood's Lamp⊕

Locator #	Type	Description	Locator #	Type	Description

RECORD ALL CLOTHING AND SPECIMENS COLLECTED ON PAGE 8

J. GENITAL EXAMINATION - FEMALES

Record all findings using diagrams, legend, and a consecutive numbering system.

1. **Examine the inner thighs, external genitalia, and perineal area.**
2. **Exam method:** ☐ Direct visualization ☐ Colposcope ☐ Other magnification

Exam positions/methods:

	Separation	Traction	Knee Chest
Supine	☐	☐	☐
Prone	☐	☐	☐

☐ Saline/Water ☐ Moistened swab ☐ Toluidine Blue Dye
☐ Catheter ☐ Other:

3. **Genital Tanner Stage** 1☐ 2☐ 3☐ 4☐ 5☐
4. **Examine the genital structures. Check the ABN box(es) if there are abuse/assault related findings and describe.**

	WNL	ABN	Describe:
Inner thighs	☐	☐	______
Inguinal adenopathy	☐	☐	______
Labia majora	☐	☐	______
Labia minora	☐	☐	______
Clitoral hood	☐	☐	______
Perineum	☐	☐	______
Periurethral tissue/urethral meatus	☐	☐	______
Perihymenal tissue (vestibule)	☐	☐	______
Hymen ☐ Supine ☐ Prone	☐	☐	______
Record morphology:			
☐ Annular			______
☐ Crescentic			______
☐ Imperforate			______
☐ Septate			______
Fossa navicularis	☐	☐	______
Posterior fourchette	☐	☐	______
Vagina (pubertal adolescents)	☐	☐	______
Cervix (pubertal adolescents)	☐	☐	______

Discharge ☐ No ☐ Yes
If yes, describe: ______

No Findings ☐

5. **Collect dried and moist secretions, stains, and foreign materials. Scan the area with a Wood's Lamp.** ☐ Findings ☐ No Findings
6. **Collect swabs and prepare slides.**
   - ☐ **Prepubertal female**
     - ☐ **Collect at least 2 vulvar and 2 vestibular swabs.**
   - ☐ **Pubertal female**
     - ☐ **Collect 4 swabs from the vaginal pool.**
     - ☐ **Prepare one wet mount and one dry mount slide.**
     - ☐ **Collect 2 cervical swabs (if over 48 hours post assault).**
7. **Collect pubic hair combing or brushing.** ☐ Not applicable
8. **Collect pubic hair reference samples according to local policy.** ☐ Not applicable

LEGEND: Types of Findings

AB	Abrasion	DF	Deformity	LA	Laceration	SH	Submucosal Hemorrhage
AHT	Absent Hymenal Tissue	DI	Discharge	MS	Moist Secretion	SHX	Sample Per History
AL	Anal Laxity	DS	Dry Secretion	OF	Other Foreign Materials (describe)	SI	Suction Injury
BI	Bite	EC	Ecchymosis (bruise)	OI	Other Injury (describe)	SW	Swelling
BU	Burn	ER	Erythema (redness)	OSC	Other Skin Condition	TB	Toluidine Blue⊕
CS	Control Swab	FB	Foreign Body	OT	Other	TE	Tenderness
CV	Congenital Variation	F/H	Fiber/hair	PW	Perianal Wart	V/S	Vegetation/Soil
DE	Debris	GT	Granulation Tissue	PE	Petechiae	VL	Vesicular Lesion
		HC	Hymenal Cleft	PGW	Possible Genital Wart	WL	Wood's Lamp⊕
		IN	Induration	PS	Potential Saliva		
		IW	Incised Wound				

Locator #	Type	Description

Patient Identification

Diagram the position that best illustrates your findings.

Diagram G Genitalia - Supine

Diagram H Genitalia - Knee-Chest

RECORD ALL CLOTHING AND SPECIMENS COLLECTED ON PAGE 8

K. GENITAL EXAMINATION – MALES

Record all findings using diagrams, legend, and a consecutive numbering system.

1. **Examine the inner thighs, external genitalia, and perineal area.**
2. **Exam method:** ☐ Direct visualization ☐ Colposcope ☐ Other magnification
   Exam positions/methods:
   ☐ Supine ☐ Prone ☐ Moistened swab
   ☐ Toluidine Blue Dye ☐ Other:__________
3. **Genital Tanner Stage** 1☐ 2☐ 3☐ 4☐ 5☐
4. **Circumcised:** ☐ No ☐ Yes
5. **Check the ABN box(es) if there are abuse/assault related findings and describe.**

	WNL	ABN	Describe:
Inner thighs	☐	☐	________
Inguinal adenopathy	☐	☐	________
Perineum	☐	☐	________
Foreskin	☐	☐	________
Glans Penis	☐	☐	________
Penile shaft	☐	☐	________
Urethral meatus	☐	☐	________
Scrotum	☐	☐	________
Testes	☐	☐	________

Discharge ☐ No ☐ Yes If yes, describe: ________
No Findings ☐

6. **Collect dried and moist secretions, stains, and foreign materials. Scan the area with a Wood's Lamp.** ☐ Findings ☐ No Findings
7. **Collect pubic hair combing or brushing.** ☐ Not applicable
8. **Collect pubic hair reference samples according to local policy.** ☐ Not applicable
9. **Collect 2 penile swabs, if indicated by assault history.** ☐ Not applicable
10. **Collect 2 scrotal swabs, if indicated by assault history.** ☐ Not applicable

L. FEMALE/MALE ANAL AND RECTAL EXAMINATION

1. **Examine the buttocks, perianal skin, and anal folds for injury, foreign materials, and other findings.**
2. **Record exam positions, methods, observations:**
   ☐ Direct visualization ☐ Colposcope ☐ Other magnification

Exam positions	Observation	Observation with traction
Supine	☐	☐
Supine knee chest	☐	☐
Prone knee chest	☐	☐
Lateral recumbent	☐	☐

Exam methods: ☐ Moistened swab ☐ Toluidine blue dye ☐ Anoscopy ☐ Other:______

3. **Check the ABN box(es) if there are abuse/assault related findings and describe any abnormal or unusual findings.**

☐ No Findings	WNL	ABN	Describe:
Buttocks	☐	☐	________
Perianal skin	☐	☐	________
Anal verge/folds/rugae	☐	☐	________
Rectum	☐	☐	________

Anal dilation ☐ No ☐ Yes If yes: ☐ Immediate ☐ Delayed
Stool present in rectal ampulla ☐ No ☐ Yes ☐ Undetermined

4. Collect dried and moist secretions, stains, and foreign materials.
   ☐ Findings ☐ No Findings
5. **Collect 2 anal and/or rectal swabs and prepare one dry mount slide.**
6. **Rectal bleeding:** ☐ No ☐ Yes If yes, describe:

LEGEND: Types of Findings

AB	Abrasion	**DF**	Deformity	**LA**	Laceration	**SH**	Submcosal Hemorhage
AHT	Absent Hymenal Tissue	**DI**	Discharge	**MS**	Moist Secretion	**SHX**	Sample Per History
AL	Anal Laxity	**DS**	Dry Secretion	**OF**	Other Foreign Materials (describe)	**SI**	Suction Injury
BI	Bite	**EC**	Ecchymosis (bruise)	**OI**	Other Injury (describe)	**SW**	Swelling
BU	Burn	**ER**	Erythema (redness)	**OSC**	Other Skin Condition	**TB**	Toluidine Blue⊕
CS	Control Swab	**FB**	Foreign Body	**OT**	Other	**TE**	Tenderness
CV	Congenital Variation	**F/H**	Fiber/hair	**PW**	Perianal Wart	**V/S**	Vegetation/Soil
DE	Debris	**GT**	Granulation Tissue	**PE**	Petechiae	**VL**	Vesicular Lesion
		HC	Hymenal Cleft	**PGW**	Possible Genital Wart	**WL**	Wood's Lamp⊕
		IN	Induration	**PS**	Potential Saliva		
		IW	Incised Wound				

Locator #	Type	Description

Patient Identification

Diagram I - Penis

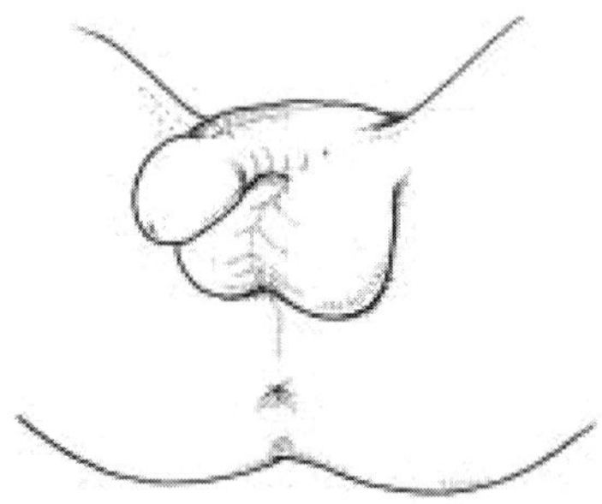

Diagram J - Penis

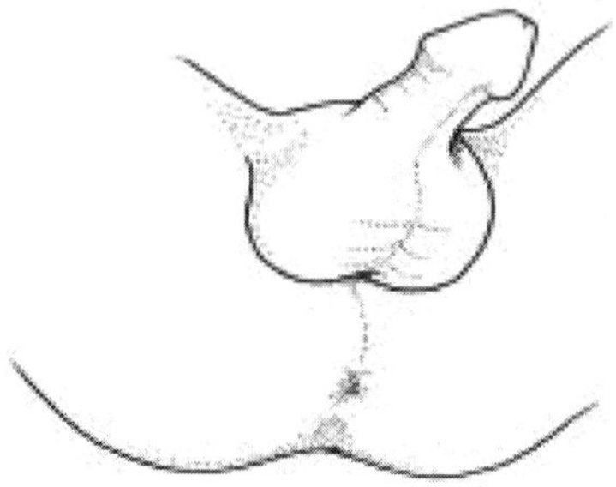

Diagram K - Anus Supine

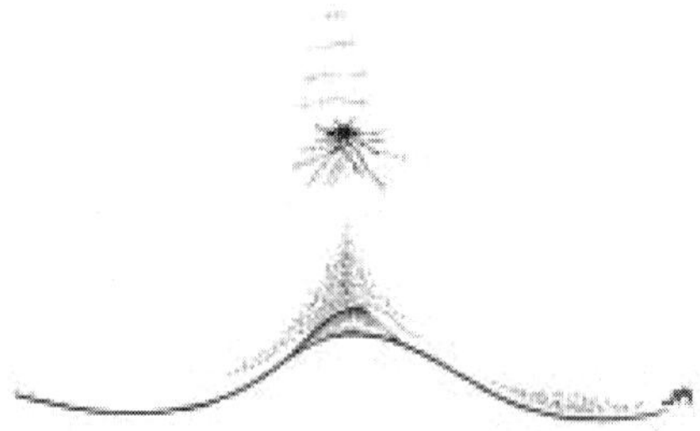

Diagram L - Anus Prone

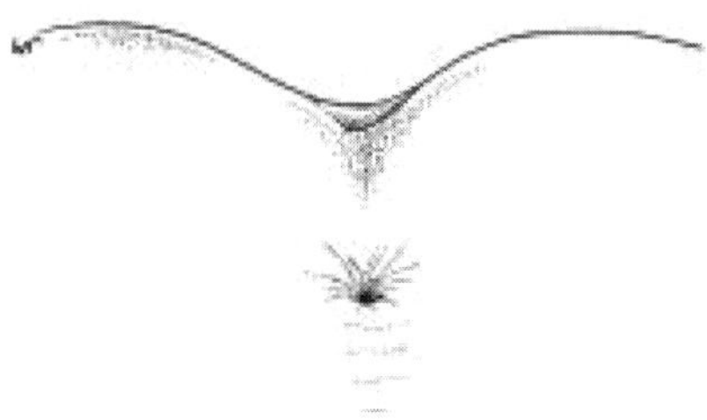

RECORD ALL CLOTHING AND SPECIMENS COLLECTED ON PAGE 8

M. EVIDENCE COLLECTED AND SUBMITTED TO CRIME LAB

1. Clothing placed in evidence kit	Other clothing placed in bags

Patient Identification

2. Foreign materials collected

	No	Yes	Collected by:
Swabs/suspected blood	☐	☐	
Dried secretions	☐	☐	
Fiber/loose hairs	☐	☐	
Vegetation	☐	☐	
Soil/debris	☐	☐	
Swabs/suspected semen	☐	☐	
Swabs/suspected saliva	☐	☐	
Swabs/Wood's Lamp⊕ area(s)	☐	☐	
Control swabs	☐	☐	
Fingernail scrapings/cuttings	☐	☐	
Matted hair cuttings	☐	☐	
Pubic hair combings/brushings	☐	☐	
Intravaginal foreign body Describe:	☐	☐	
Other types If yes, describe:	☐	☐	

3. Oral/genital/anal/rectal samples

	# Swabs	# Slides	Time collected	Collected by:
Oral				
Vulvar		■		
Vestibular		■		
Vaginal				
Cervical		■		
Anal				
Rectal				
Penile		■		
Scrotal		■		
Aspirate/washings (optional) ☐ No ☐ Yes				

4. Vaginal wet mount slide

	No	Yes	Time	Examiner:
Slide prepared				
Motile sperm observed				
Non-motile sperm observed				

N. TOXICOLOGY SAMPLES

	No	Yes	Time	Collected by:
Blood alcohol/toxicology (gray top tube)				
Urine toxicology				

O. REFERENCE SAMPLES

	No	Yes	Collected by:
Blood (lavender top tube)			
Blood (yellow top tube)			
Blood Card (optional)			
Buccal swabs (optional)			
Saliva swabs			
Head hair			
Pubic Hair			

P. PHOTO DOCUMENTATION METHODS

	No	Yes	Colposcope/ 35mm	Macrolens/ 35mm	Colposcope/ Videocamera	Other Optics
Body	☐	☐	☐	☐	☐	☐ ______
Genitals	☐	☐	☐	☐	☐	☐ ______

Photographed by:

Q. FINDINGS AND INTERPRETATION

1. **Anal-Genital Findings**
   - ☐ Normal anal-genital exam
   - ☐ Abnormal anal-genital exam
   - ☐ Indeterminate anal-genital exam
2. **Assessment of Anal-Genital Findings**
   - ☐ Consistent with history
   - ☐ Inconsistent with history
   - ☐ Limited/Insufficient history
3. **Interpretation of Anal-Genital Findings**
   - ☐ Normal exam: can neither confirm nor negate sexual abuse
   - ☐ Non specific: may be caused by sexual abuse or other mechanisms
   - ☐ Sexual abuse is highly suspected
   - ☐ Definite evidence of sexual abuse and/or sexual contact
4. ☐ **Need further consultation/investigation**
5. ☐ **Lab results or photo review pending (may alter assessment)**
6. **Additional comments regarding findings, interpretations, and recommendations:**

R. MEDICAL LAB TESTS PERFORMED

STD Cultures	GC	Chlamydia	Other	Describe:	Collected by:
Oral	☐	☐	☐		
Vestibular	☐	☐	☐		
Vaginal	☐	☐	☐		
Cervical	☐	☐	☐		
Rectal	☐	☐	☐		
Penile	☐	☐	☐		
Wet mount	☐	☐	☐		
Serology	Syphilis ☐	HIV ☐	Hepatitis ☐		
Pregnancy test	Blood ☐	Urine ☐			
Other test(s)					

S. PRINT NAMES OF PERSONNEL INVOLVED

	Telephone
History taken by:	
Exam performed by:	
Specimens labeled and sealed by:	
Assisted by: N/A	
Signature of examiner	License No.

T. EVIDENCE DISTRIBUTION

	GIVEN TO:
Clothing (item(s) not placed in evidence kit)	
Evidence Kit	
Reference blood samples	
Toxicology samples	

U. SIGNATURE OF OFFICER RECEIVING EVIDENCE

Signature: ______

Print name and ID#: ______

Agency: ______

Date: Telephone:

FORENSIC MEDICAL REPORT:
SEXUAL ASSAULT SUSPECT EXAMINATION
STATE OF CALIFORNIA
OFFICE OF CRIMINAL JUSTICE PLANNING

OCJP 950

Confidential Document | **Patient Identification**

A. GENERAL INFORMATION (print or type) **Name of Medical Facility:**

1. Name of patient				Patient ID number			
2. Address			City	County		State	Telephone (W) (H)
3. Age	DOB	Gender M F	Ethnicity	Arrival Date	Arrival Time	Dishcarge Date	Discharge Time

B. AUTHORIZATION Jurisdiction (☐ city ☐ county ☐ other):

1. Name of Law Enforcement Officer	Agency	ID Number	Telephone

2. **I request a forensic medical examination for suspected sexual assault at public expense.**

Law enforcement officer signature	Date	Time	Case number

C. MEDICAL HISTORY

1. **Any recent (60 days) anal-genital injuries, surgeries, diagnostic procedures, or medical treatment that may affect the interpretation of current physical findings?** ☐ **No** ☐ **Yes**
   If yes, describe: ____________
2. **Any other pertinent medical condition(s) that may affect the interpretation of current physical findings?** ☐ **No** ☐ **Yes**
   If yes, describe: ____________
3. **Any pre-existing physical injuries?** ☐ **No** ☐ **Yes**
   If yes, describe: ____________

D. RECENT HYGIENE INFORMATION ☐ Not applicable if over 72 hours

	No	Yes		No	Yes
Urinated	☐	☐	Bath/shower/wash	☐	☐
Defecated	☐	☐	Brushed teeth	☐	☐
Genital or body wipes	☐	☐	Ate or drank	☐	☐
If yes, describe: ____________			Changed clothing	☐	☐
Oral gargle/rinse	☐	☐	If yes, describe: ____________		

E. GENERAL PHYSICAL EXAMINATION

1. Blood Pressure	Pulse	Respiration	Temperature	2. Exam Started		Exam Completed	
				Date	Time	Date	Time
3. Height	Weight	Hair color	Eye color	☐ Right-handed ☐ Left-handed			

4. **Describe general physical appearance**

5. **Describe general demeanor**

6. **Describe condition of clothing upon arrival.**

7. **Collect outer and under clothing, if indicated.** ☐ **Not indicated**

DISTRIBUTION OF OCJP 950

☐ Original - Law Enforcement ☐ Copy within evidence kit - Crime Lab ☐ Copy - Medical Facility Records

E. GENERAL PHYSICAL EXAMINATION

Record all findings using diagrams, legend, and a consecutive numbering system

8. **Conduct a physical examination. Record scars, tattoos, skin lesions, and distinguishing physical features.** ☐ Findings ☐ No Findings
9. **Collect dried and moist secretions, stains, and foreign materials from the body. Scan the entire body with a Wood's Lamp.** ☐ Findings ☐ No Findings
10. **Collect fingernail scrapings or cuttings according to local policy.**
11. **Collect chest hair reference samples according to local policy.**

Patient Identification

Diagram A

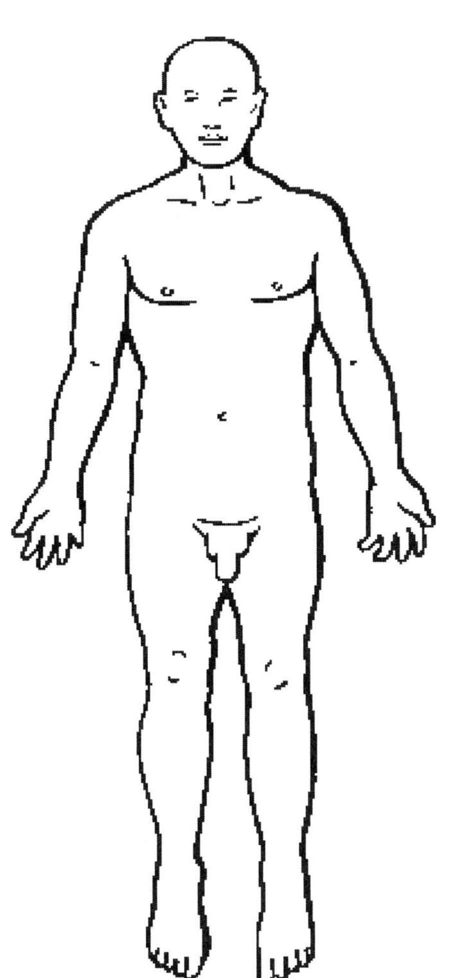

Diagram B

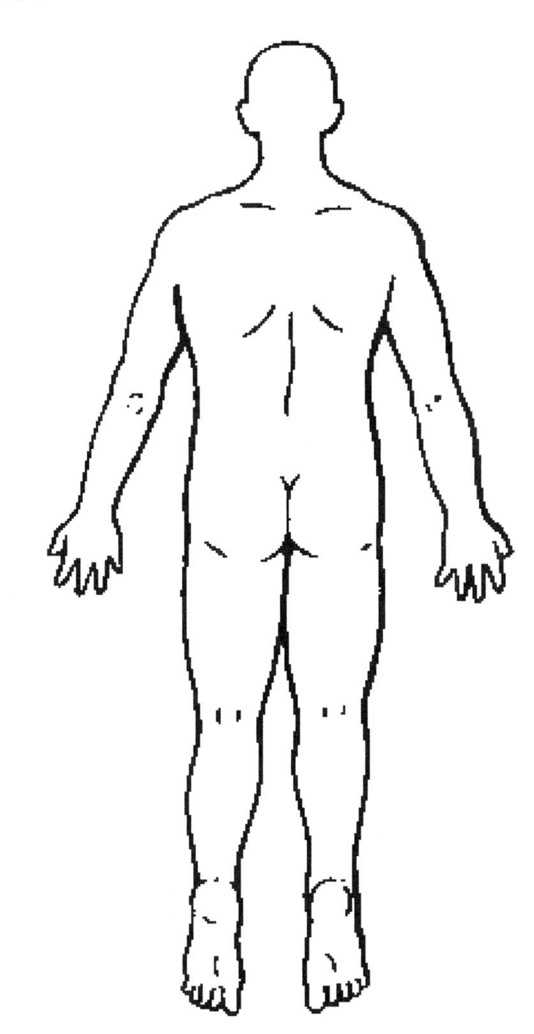

LEGEND: Types of Findings

AB	Abrasion	**DE**	Debris	**F/H**	Fiber/hair	**OF**	Other Foreign Materials (describe)	**SC**	Scars	**TA**	Tattoos
BI	Bite	**DF**	Deformity	**IN**	Induration			**SHX**	Sample Per History	**TB**	Toluidine Blue⊕
BP	Body Piercing	**DS**	Dry Secretion	**IW**	Incised Wound	**OI**	Other Injury (describe)			**TE**	Tenderness
BU	Burn	**EC**	Ecchymosis (bruise)	**LA**	Laceration	**PE**	Petechiae	**SI**	Suction Injury	**V/S**	Vegetation/Soil
CS	Control Swab	**ER**	Erythema (redness)	**MS**	Moist Secretion	**PS**	Potential Saliva	**SW**	Swelling	**WL**	Wood's Lamp⊕

Locator #	Type	Description	Locator #	Type	Description

RECORD ALL CLOTHING AND SPECIMENS COLLECTED ON PAGE 5

F. HEAD, NECK, AND ORAL EXAMINATION

Record all findings using diagrams, legend, and a consecutive numbering system.

1. **Examine the face, head, hair, scalp, and neck for injury and foreign materials.**
   ☐ Findings ☐ No Findings
2. **Collect dried and moist secretions, stains, and foreign materials from face, head, hair, scalp, and neck.**
   ☐ Findings ☐ No Findings
3. **Examine the oral cavity for injury and foreign materials (if indicated by assault history). Collect foreign materials.**
   Exam done: ☐ Not applicable ☐ Yes ☐ Findings ☐ No Findings
4. **Collect 2 swabs from the oral cavity up to 12 hours post assault and prepare one dry mount slide from one of the swabs.**
5. **Collect head and facial hair reference samples according to local policy.**

Patient Identification

Diagram C

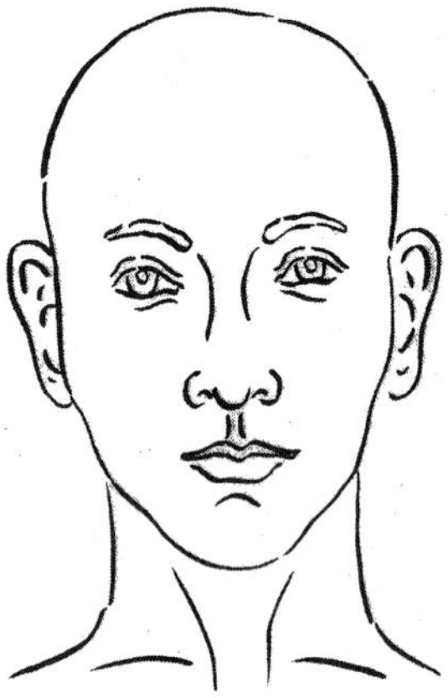

Diagram D

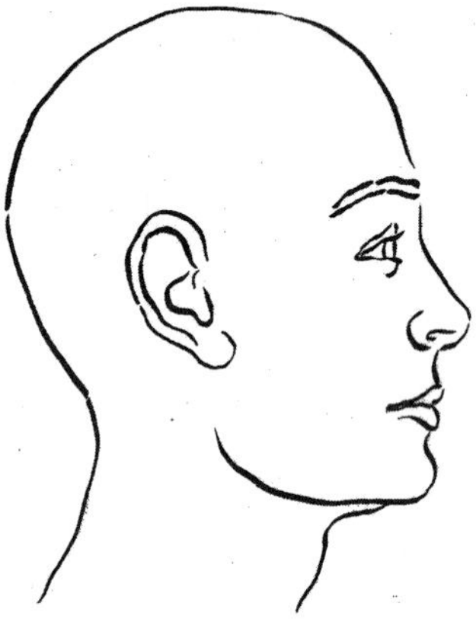

Diagram E

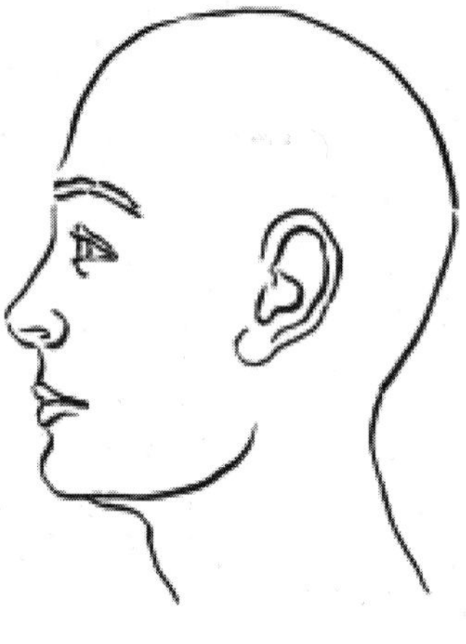

Diagram F

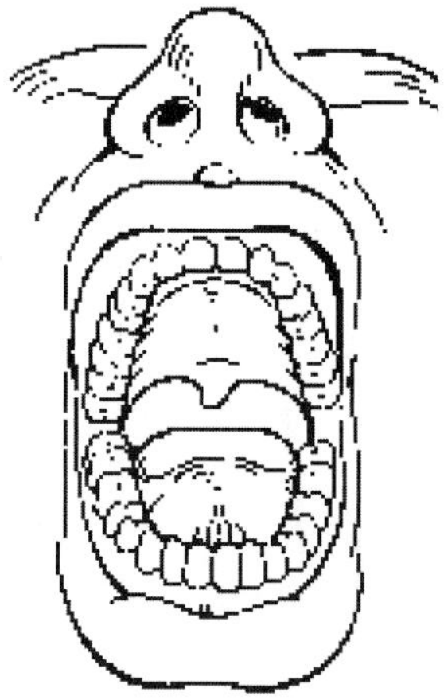

LEGEND: Types of Findings

AB	Abrasion	**DE**	Debris	**F/H**	Fiber/hair	**OF**	Other Foreign Materials (describe)	**SC**	Scars	**TA**	Tattoos
BI	Bite	**DF**	Deformity	**IN**	Induration			**SHX**	Sample Per History	**TB**	Toluidine Blue⊕
BP	Body Piercing	**DS**	Dry Secretion	**IW**	Incised Wound	**OI**	Other Injury (describe)			**TE**	Tenderness
BU	Burn	**EC**	Ecchymosis (bruise)	**LA**	Laceration	**PE**	Petechiae	**SI**	Suction Injury	**V/S**	Vegetation/Soil
CS	Control Swab	**ER**	Erythema (redness)	**MS**	Moist Secretion	**PS**	Potential Saliva	**SW**	Swelling	**WL**	Wood's Lamp⊕

Locator #	Type	Description	Locator #	Type	Description

RECORD ALL CLOTHING AND SPECIMENS COLLECTED ON PAGE 5

G. GENITAL EXAMINATION

Record all findings using diagrams, legend, and a consecutive numbering system.

1. **Examine the inner thighs, external genitalia, and perineal area. Check the box(es) if there are assault related findings:**
   ☐ No Findings
   ☐ Inner thighs ☐ Glans penis ☐ Scrotum
   ☐ Perineum ☐ Penile shaft ☐ Testes
   ☐ Foreskin ☐ Urethral meatus
2. **Circumcised** ☐ **No** ☐ **Yes**
3. **Collect dried and moist secretions, stains, and foreign materials. Scan the area with a Wood's Lamp.** ☐ Findings ☐ No Findings
4. **Collect pubic hair combing or brushing.**
5. **Collect pubic hair reference samples according to local policy.**
6. **Collect 2 penile swabs, if indicated by assault history.** ☐ **N/A**
7. **Collect 2 scrotal swabs, if indicated by assault history.** ☐ **N/A**
8. **Record other findings per history.** ☐ **No** ☐ **Yes**
   If yes, describe:

Patient Identification

Diagram G

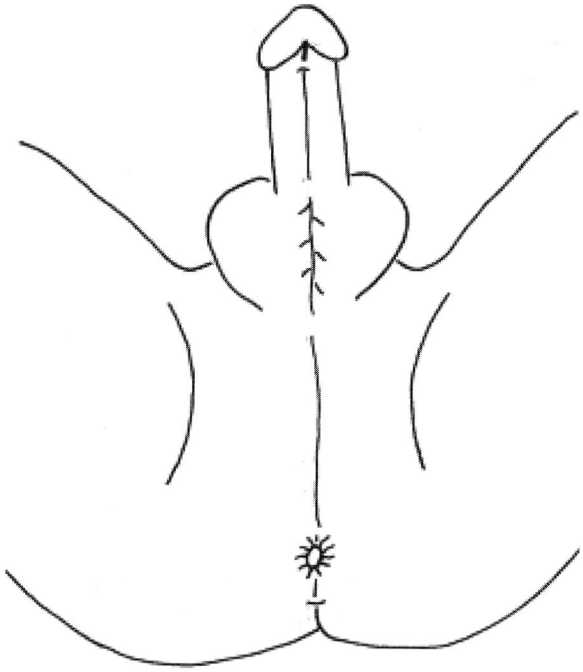

Diagram H

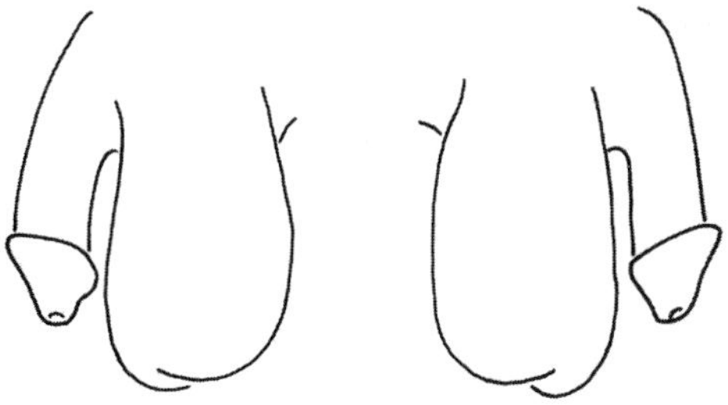

Diagram I

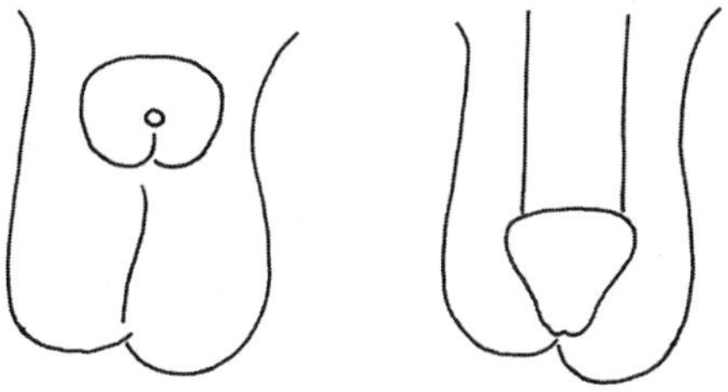

Diagram J

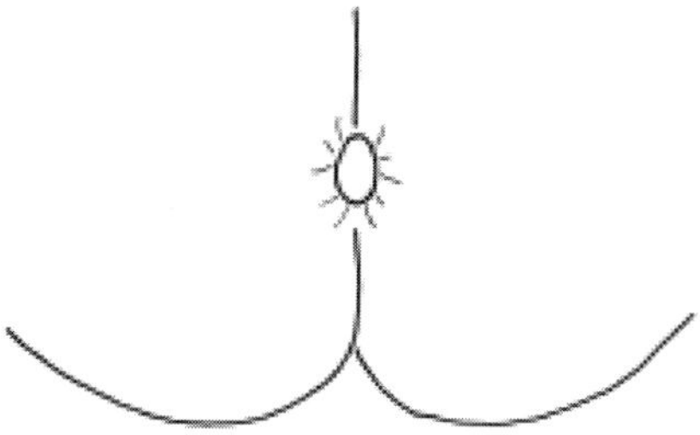

LEGEND: Types of Findings

AB	Abrasion	**ER**	Erythema (redness)	**PE**	Petechiae	**V/S**	Vegetation/Soil
BI	Bite	**F/H**	Fiber/hair	**PS**	Potential Saliva	**WL**	Wood's Lamp⊕
BP	Body Piercing	**IN**	Induration	**SC**	Scars		
BU	Burn	**IW**	Incised Wound	**SHX**	Sample Per History		
CS	Control Swab	**LA**	Laceration	**SI**	Suction Injury		
DE	Debris	**MS**	Moist Secretion	**SW**	Swelling		
DF	Deformity	**OF**	Other Foreign Materials(describe)	**TA**	Tattoos		
DS	Dry Secretion			**TB**	Toluidine Blue⊕		
EC	Ecchymosis (bruise)	**OI**	Other Injury (describe)	**TE**	Tenderness		

Locator #	Type	Description

RECORD ALL CLOTHING AND SPECIMENS COLLECTED ON PAGE 5

H. EVIDENCE COLLECTED AND SUBMITTED TO CRIME LAB

1. Clothing placed in evidence kit / Other clothing placed in bags

Clothing placed in evidence kit	Other clothing placed in bags

2. Foreign materials collected

	No	Yes	Collected by:
Swabs/suspected blood	☐	☐	
Dried Secretions	☐	☐	
Fiber/loose hairs	☐	☐	
Vegetation	☐	☐	
Soil/debris	☐	☐	
Swabs/suspected semen	☐	☐	
Swabs/suspected saliva	☐	☐	
Swabs/Wood's Lamp⊕ area(s)	☐	☐	
Control swabs	☐	☐	
Fingernail scrapings/cuttings	☐	☐	
Matted hair cuttings	☐	☐	
Pubic hair combings/brushings	☐	☐	
Other types	☐	☐	

If yes, describe: ____________

3. Oral/genital samples

	# Swabs	# Slides	Time collected	Collected by:
Oral				
Penile		■		
Scrotal		■		

I. TOXICOLOGY SAMPLES

	No	Yes	Time	Collected by:
Blood alcohol/toxicology (gray top tube)				
Urine toxicology				

J. REFERENCE SAMPLES

	No	Yes	Collected by:
Blood (lavender top tube)			
Blood (yellow top tube)			
Blood Card (optional)			
Buccal swabs (optional)			
Saliva swabs			
Chest hair			
Facial hair			
Pubic hair			
Head hair			

K. PHOTO DOCUMENTATION METHODS

	No	Yes	Colposcope/35mm	Macrolens/35mm	Colposcope/ Videocamera	Other optics
Body	☐	☐	☐	☐	☐	☐ ________
Genitals	☐	☐	☐	☐	☐	☐ ________

Photographed by:

Patient Identification

L. RECORD EXAM METHODS

	No	Yes
Direct visualization only	☐	☐
Colposcopy	☐	☐
Other magnifier	☐	☐
Other	☐	☐

If yes, describe:

____

M. RECORD EXAM FINDINGS

☐ **Physical Findings** ☐ **No Physical Findings**

N. SUMMARIZE FINDINGS

____

O. PRINT NAMES OF PERSONNEL INVOLVED

History taken by:	Telephone
Exam performed by:	
Specimens labeled and sealed by:	
Assisted by: ☐ N/A	
Signature of examiner:	License No.

P. EVIDENCE DISTRIBUTION	GIVEN TO:
Clothing (item(s) not placed in evidence kit)	
Evidence kit	
Reference blood samples	
Toxicology samples	

Q. SIGNATURE OF OFFICER RECEIVING EVIDENCE

Signature: ____________

Print name and ID#: ____________

Agency: ____________

Date: ____________ Phone: ____________

Appendix E

Procedure for Sexual Assault Examination for Male Victims

Sheila D. Early

General Guidelines

- Male patients presenting for sexual assault medical forensic examination are more likely to have suffered physical trauma and genital injuries than female patients.
- Male patients are at greater risk of secondary traumatization by caregivers due to the lack of experience and expertise of the examiner in situations of male assault.
- Male patients are more likely to show symptoms of behavioral disorders than female patients on first presentation.

Process

A signed consent for care is needed prior to commencing the sexual assault medical forensic examination and forensic evidence collection protocol. The patient's options for care and the procedure for examination need to be thoroughly explained and discussed.

The examiner will:

- Obtain an accurate medical and event history
- Provide a medical forensic examination
- Collect forensic evidence according to facility protocols and local forensic lab procedures
- Document the medical and forensic findings
- Initiate and maintain chain of custody for forensic evidence
- Provide or arrange for treatment of physical injuries, sexually transmitted infection prophylaxis, and referrals for aftercare resources
- Provide a legal report of medical forensic examination
- Testify in court as a neutral, objective witness

Procedure

1. Explain all procedures and the forensic evidence collection process to the patient.
2. Obtain a history of the event from the patient and law enforcement officer if present:
   - Date and time of the event
   - Location of the event–geographic area as well as physical location, e.g. house, park, car (may correlate history with findings)
   - Nature of injuries and any use of weapons, force, threats, or restraints (may correlate with physical findings)
   - Nature of events:
     - oral-penile
     - penile-rectal
     - digital-rectal
   - Penetrations or attempted penetrations
   - Condom usage
   - Ejaculation occurrence
   - History of foreign object(s); include site and object
   - Loss of consciousness and, if occurred, for how long
   - Ingestion of drugs, medications, or alcohol before or after presenting event
3. Obtain a history of postevent behaviors including bathing, showering, urinating, defecating, changing clothes, eating or drinking, brushing teeth, gargling, chewing gum. These activities may result in loss of forensic evidence.
4. Obtain a pertinent personal history including last consensual coitus, whether oral-penile, penile-anal, or penile-vaginal as appropriate (within 72 hours is an accepted guideline). Include date and time if possible.

Personal History

- Medical problems or conditions, e.g. diabetes; cardiac, renal, hepatic conditions; history of thrombus or pulmonary embolism; blood disorders; carcinomas; surgical procedures on genital organs
- Pertinent anal/rectal history, e.g. hemorrhoids, surgery, fistulas, fissures, carcinoma, bleeding
- Medications, including antiepileptic medication, antidepressant and antipsychotic medication, and nonprescription medication (especially antihistamines and antacids); this information is needed for possible drug interactions with medications to be administered
- Allergies to drugs
- Tetanus/diphtheria and Hepatitis B immunization status
- HIV status if known by patient

Body Evidence

- Use powder-free gloves for all specimen collections.
- With the patient standing on two sheets of paper, have him remove all items of clothing separately and place each article in a *separate paper bag.* As clothing is removed, examiner labels each bag and lists contents on appropriate program or agency documentation.
- Retain top sheet of paper, bundle, and place in a paper bag. Label with patient's personal data and forensic evidence label, and initial it. Discard bottom sheet of paper.
- Document any stains, tears, cuts, or foreign material that may be present on clothing.
- Inspect for any area of staining on patient's body. Use alternate light source or ultraviolet light to identify area of stains. Remove sample with a swab moistened with *sterile water.* Document location swab is taken from on appropriate documentation forms. Repeat for every area of staining.
- Inspect entire body for T.E.A.R.S.:
  T = tears or tenderness
  E = ecchymosis (bruises are different from ecchymosis and are documented as Bruises)
  A = abrasions
  R = redness
  S = swelling or signs of physical injury
  Document each finding on appropriate body diagrams.
- Query bite marks are swabbed for DNA in the following manner:

- With a sterile swab moistened with sterile water, swab the entire inside and edges of the query bite mark.
- With a second sterile swab, remove all moisture from the inside and edges of the query bite mark left by previous swabbing. Both swabs can usually be submitted as one sample with the location from which swabs were taken clearly identified.
- Each query bite mark area needs to be swabbed and identified separately.

- Check for broken fingernails on patient's hands. Fingernails should be clipped with either scissors or clippers and collected from each hand separately.
- Debris under patient's fingernails can be collected by using a sterile nail pick or by using a sterile swab moistened with sterile water to swab under the fingernails, using a separate swab for each hand.

Oral Examination

- Inspect mouth, tongue, buccal surfaces, uvula, hard and soft palate, and upper and lower lips for signs of trauma. If patient wears orthodontic appliances inspect for intactness of appliances.
- Semen may be collected in the areas where gums meet the teeth if oral penetration and ejaculation has occurred. Collect oral swab from these areas.
- Obtain medical specimen swabs for gonorrhea if oral penetration has occurred.

Anal/Rectal Examination

- Inspect for T.E.A.R.S., blood, signs of semen, lubricant, or any other foreign substance. Spread buttocks with thumb and index finger. Lacerations or other injuries may occur at 6 and 12 o'clock positions.
- Patient may be examined in chest-knee position (sigmoid position) or left lateral position.
- If there is a history of penetration with foreign objects or any concern regarding rectal trauma, examiner or physician will examine anal/rectal area using anoscope.
- Obtain anal swab from anal sphincter.
- Obtain rectal swab. In chest-knee position it will take approximately 2-3 minutes for anal sphincter to dilate.
- Collect medical specimen swab for gonorrhea if rectal penetration has occurred.

Medical Laboratory Examinations

Collect medical samples according to facility procedures.

Securing the Evidence

- When the examiner is collecting evidence for the police, he or she must collect and identify each specimen separately, noting the date and in some cases the time, and initialing the labels. Each item is identified by patient data and forensic evidence label.
- When evidence collection has commenced, evidence must never leave the sight of the examiner until it is either transferred to law enforcement or secured as per facility protocols. This maintains a chain of evidence, and the examiner may have to testify in court proceedings that this chain was never broken.
- Forensic evidence is collected and given to the law enforcement officer for all cases when patient has reported to law enforcement. Documentation is completed as per facility protocols.
- The receiving officer's name and badge number and the case file number are documented.

Baseline Status and Prophylaxis

The patient should be offered protection or prevention for tetanus/diphtheria, Hepatitis B, sexually transmitted infections (including gonorrhea, chlamydia, and others depending on local protocols), and HIV postexposure prophylaxis as per facility protocols.

Appendix F
Operative Assessment of Organ Donors
Documentation for the Medical Examiner

Teresa J. Shafer

Operative Note: Organ Donors
(to be completed by Recovery Surgeon)

Surgeon Name: ____________________ ***Donor Name:*** ____________________

Date: ____________________ ***Time:*** ____________________

Crossclamp: ____________________ ***LG Coordinator:*** ____________________

Incision location: ____

Time closed: ____________________ *Surgeon's signature:* ____________________

KIDNEYS

Size: ☐ **normal** ☐ **abnormal**
If abnormal, describe:

Texture: ☐ **normal** ☐ **abnormal**
If abnormal, describe:

Surface Abnormalities: ☐ **yes** ☐ **no**
If yes, describe:

Lacerations: ☐ **yes** ☐ **no**
If yes, describe:

Hematoma: ☐ **yes** ☐ **no**
If yes, describe:

Ecchymosis: ☐ **yes** ☐ **no**
If yes, describe:

Anatomy:

Arteries:	**number:**	______		
	plaque:	☐ **yes**	☐ **no**	
Veins:	**number:**	______		
Ureter	**number:**	______		
	length:	______		

Masses: ☐ yes ☐ no
If yes, describe:

LIVER

Size: ☐ normal ☐ abnormal
If abnormal, describe:

Texture: ☐ normal ☐ abnormal
If abnormal, describe:

Lacerations: ☐ yes ☐ no
If yes, describe:

Ecchymosis: ☐ yes ☐ no
If yes, describe:

Anatomy ☐ normal ☐ abnormal
If abnormal, describe:

Masses: ☐ yes ☐ no
If yes, describe:

Gallbladder: ☐ distended
☐ not distended
☐ present ☐ absent

HEART

Size: ☐ normal ☐ abnormal
If abnormal, describe:

Surface Abnormalities: ☐ yes ☐ no
If yes, describe:

Contusion: ☐ yes ☐ no
If yes, describe:

Mediastinal Hematoma: ☐ yes ☐ no
If yes, describe:

Ecchymosis: ☐ yes ☐ no
If yes, describe:

Pericardial Effusion: ☐ yes ☐ no
If yes, describe:

Valves:	**pulmonary**	☐	**normal**	☐	**abnormal**
	aortic	☐	**normal**	☐	**abnormal**
	mitral	☐	**normal**	☐	**abnormal**
	tricuspid	☐	**normal**	☐	**abnormal**

If abnormal, describe:

Evidence of Coronary Artery Disease: ☐ **yes** ☐ **no**
If yes, describe:

Masses: ☐ **yes** ☐ **no**
If yes, describe:

<u>LUNGS</u>
Size: ☐ **normal** ☐ **abnormal**
If abnormal, describe:

Texture: ☐ **normal** ☐ **abnormal**
If abnormal, describe:

Lacerations: ☐ **no** ☐ **yes**
If yes, describe:

Ecchymosis: ☐ **no** ☐ **no**
If yes, describe:

Masses: ☐ **yes** ☐ **no**
If yes, describe:

Contusion: ☐ **yes** ☐ **no**
If yes, describe:

Hematoma: ☐ **yes** ☐ **no**
If yes, describe:

Pleural Effusion: ☐ **yes** ☐ **no**
If yes, describe:

Evidence of : **Pneumonia** ☐ **yes** ☐ **no**
If yes, describe distribution:

Fractured ribs ☐ **yes** ☐ **no**
If yes, describe:

Pulmonary emboli: ☐ **yes** ☐ **no**
If yes, describe:

Pneumothorax: ☐ yes ☐ no

Emphysema: ☐ yes ☐ no

PANCREAS

Size: ☐ normal ☐ abnormal
If abnormal, describe:

Texture: ☐ normal ☐ abnormal
If abnormal, describe:

Lacerations: ☐ yes ☐ no
If yes, describe:

Ecchymosis: ☐ yes ☐ no
If yes, describe:

Anatomy: ☐ normal ☐ abnormal
Describe if abnormal:

Masses: ☐ yes ☐ no
If yes, describe:

Calcification: ☐ yes ☐ no
If yes, describe:

SMALL BOWEL

Surface Abnormalities: ☐ yes ☐ no
If yes, describe:

Lacerations: ☐ yes ☐ no
If yes, describe:

Hematoma: ☐ yes ☐ no
If yes, describe:

Ecchymosis: ☐ yes ☐ no
If yes, describe:

SPLEEN

Surface Abnormalities: ☐ yes ☐ no
If yes, describe:

Lacerations: ☐ yes ☐ no
If yes, describe:

Hematoma: ☐ yes ☐ no
If yes, describe:

PROSTATE:

Size: ☐ normal ☐ abnormal
If abnormal, describe:

Masses: ☐ yes ☐ no
If yes, describe:

Surface Abnormalities: ☐ yes ☐ no
If yes, describe:

The Istanbul Protocol

International Guidelines for the Investigation and Documentation of Torture

The effective investigation and documentation of torture is the most important tool in exposing the problem of torture and in bringing those responsible to account.

The Manual on the Effective Investigation and Documentation of Torture and Other Cruel, Inhuman or Degrading Treatment or Punishment (the Istanbul Protocol) is the first set of international guidelines for the investigation and documentation of torture. The Protocol provides comprehensive, practical guidelines for the assessment of persons who allege torture and ill treatment, for investigating cases of alleged torture, and for reporting the findings to the relevant authorities.

Leading International Guidelines & Standards

Initiated and co-ordinated by Physicians for Human Rights USA (PHR USA) and the Human Rights Foundation of Turkey (HRFT), the Istanbul Protocol represents the work of more than 75 experts in law, health, and human rights, representing 40 organisations from 15 countries, including the IRCT.

The Istanbul Protocol was submitted to the UN High Commissioner for Human Rights (UNHCHR) in 1999, and the Istanbul Principles have subsequently received support in resolutions of the UN Human Rights Commission and General Assembly. In international forums and in dialogue with national governments, the IRCT has called for the full and effective implementation of the Protocol and Principles, encouraging Governments to establish effective procedures reflecting the Istanbul Protocol for all Government officials who undertake forensic investigations.

Medical and legal experts directly benefit from the Istanbul Protocol's detailed procedures and practical content for conducting investigations into allegations of torture. The IRCT provided training on the Istanbul Protocol in 2001, as part of a technical co-operation programme between the Office of the UNHCHR and the Government of Mexico. A significant outcome was the development of a 'short-form' torture detection procedure, used to rapidly identify those cases where torture or ill treatment may have occurred and where the full investigation procedure as described in the Protocol should be applied.

The short-form procedure is particularly useful in facilitating screening in restrictive circumstances; e.g. during prison visits by teams of independent observers with a very limited time to assess several hundred detainees. The short-form procedure enables an initial screening to be undertaken of all detainees, with a view to identifying those who may have been subjected to torture or other cruel treatment. This information can then form the basis for a subsequent in-depth examination of that detainee in accordance with the format recommended in the Protocol. This format is sensitive to the need to maintain confidentiality in order to protect detainees from possible further abuse by prison authorities, and is designed to minimise the risk of victim re-traumatisation.

Towards Global Implementation

In spite of its international standing, awareness of the Istanbul Protocol is still limited. In many cases, medical and legal university curricula do not provide instruction on the examination or treatment of torture victims or on the consequences of torture. As a result, many health and legal professionals have little or no training in the investigation and documentation of torture, which requires specific technical skills and knowledge to be conducted effectively.

In response, the IRCT in partnership with the World Medical Association, the HRFT, and PHR USA and with the support of the European Commission, is undertaking the 'Istanbul Protocol Implementation Project', initially targeting five countries between March 2003 and March 2005. The overall objective of the project is to develop a framework for the universal implementation of the Istanbul Protocol, thereby making an important and sustainable contribution to the prevention of torture and an end to the vicious cycle of impunity.

At the start of the project, the five countries were selected, and subsequently preparatory missions were carried out in Morocco, Georgia, Uganda, Mexico and Sri Lanka. Great progress in the development of the training material was made, and legal and medical training committees were established which are now developing the generic training materials. An interactive CD-ROM has been developed for the training, containing pictures of torture methods and the physical signs of torture. In the training, participants will be asked to describe and discuss the allegation of torture and the signs, and to come up with a conclusion.

Local adaptation will take place in collaboration with the partners identified at the preparatory missions. In the autumn of 2004, the five training seminars will ultimately increase the capacity in the five countries for investigating and documenting torture, and this should lead to a marked increase in the number of torture cases reported. This will then enable the provision of authoritative documentation on the prevalence of torture on which national authorities will be increasingly pressured to take action: to acknowledge the problem of torture, to commit towards its prevention, and to punish the perpetrators. This will further enable torture victims to seek justice and to obtain reparation, including the right to rehabilitation.

The Istanbul Protocol:
Manual on the Effective Investigation and Documentation of Torture and Other Cruel, Inhuman or Degrading Treatment or Punishment is part of the UN Professional Training Series, No. 8. Arabic, Chinese, English, French, Spanish and Russian versions are available in pdf. format on the UNHCHR website: www.unhchr.ch/html/menu6/2/training.htm.

International Rehabilitation Council for Torture Victims, IRCT • Borgergade 13 • P.O. Box 9049 • 1022 Copenhagen K • Denmark
Phone: +45 33 76 06 00 • Fax: + 45 33 76 05 00 • E-mail: irct@irct.org • http://www.irct.org

Appendix H
ABFO Ruler

Courtesy of Lightning Powder Company, Inc.

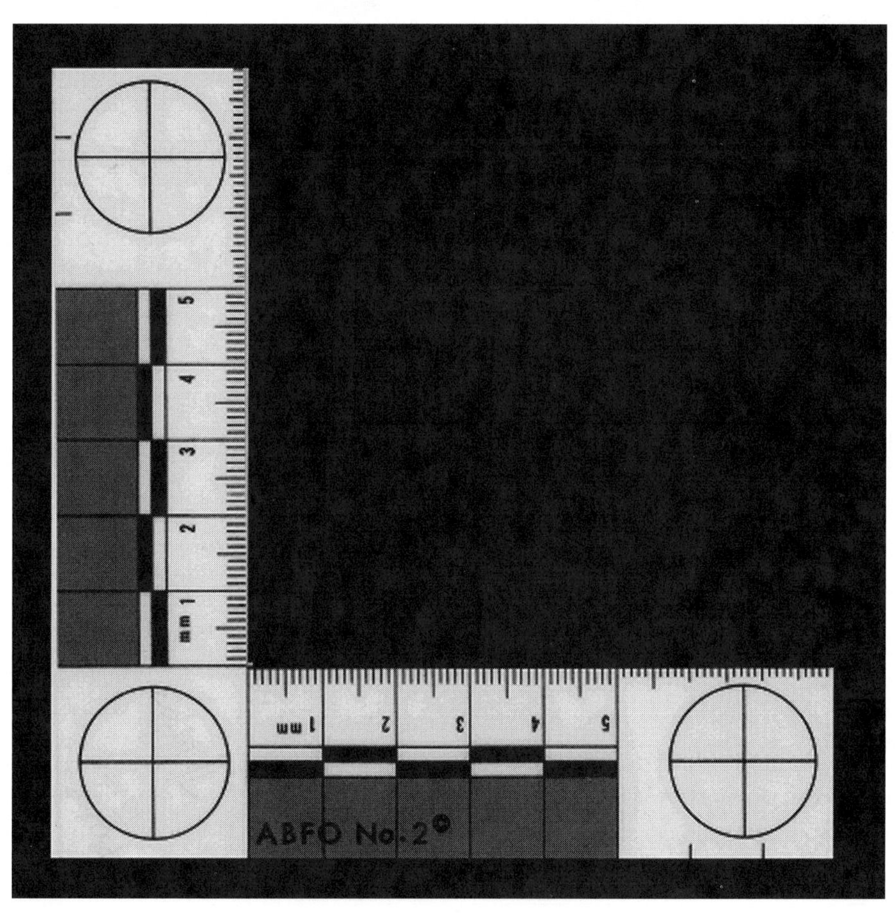

Glossary

A

Abrasion

Removal of the outermost layer of skin by a compressive and/or sliding force over a rough surface or object. Abrasions result when the skin contacts a rough object or surface with sufficient force to rub away part of the surface. This type of injury includes what are commonly referred to as scratches and grazes.

Acclimatization

The process that enables the body to cope with environmental stressors such as heat or cold through gradual changes permitting physiological adaptations that are compatible with routine functioning.

Accumulative stress

A mixture of life's stresses merged together.

Acute stress response

Onset of physical, emotional, or cognitive stress symptoms occurring at the scene of the event or within 24 hours of the event.

Air-purifying respirator (APR)

A face mask device that filters ambient air before inhalation; does not supply additional oxygen.

Air-supplying respirator (ASR)

A device consisting of a face mask for supplying air for breathing that is dependent on either self-contained or distant supply of compressed air.

Algor mortis

The cooling of the body after death.

Allograft

Tissue transplantation from one individual to another, usually after death

American Academy of Forensic Sciences (AAFS)

Professional society dedicated to the application of science to the law. Membership includes physicians, criminalists, toxicologists, attorneys, dentists, physical anthropologists, document examiners, engineers, psychiatrists, educators, and others who practice and perform research in the many diverse fields relating to forensic science. The organization is committed to the promotion of education and the elevation of accuracy, precision, and specificity in the forensic sciences.

Anthropopathy

The ascription of human emotions to nonhuman subjects.

Aperture

An adjustable opening in the lens that controls the beam of light that enters a camera and reaches the film or digital sensor. The aperture is known by several other names, including lens opening, iris, diaphragm, f-number, or f-stop.

Artificial lighting

Illumination produced by a source other than natural (which includes daylight, moonlight, starlight, and light aurora).

Autoerotic

An activity in which a potentially injurious agent is used to heighten sexual arousal.

Autoerotic fatalities

Deaths that occur as the result of or in association with masturbation or other self-stimulating activity.

Autopsy

Examination of a dead body for the purpose of determining the identification of the body and the medical cause and manner of death, and/or determining the nature and extent of any pathological process(es) that may be present.

Available light (ambient light)

Light that can be used at a scene without the photographer bringing in any other source.

Avulsed bite

A bite so severe in force that the bitten tissue has been completely separated from the victim.

B

Back dirt

Excess soil deposit near the perimeter of the grave.

Bag slap type injuries

Injuries incurred during the final stage of air bag deployment when the bag is at the peak of its excursion. When the canvas bag slaps the occupant's face, injuries to the eye and epithelium are commonly observed.

Battering

A term encompassing the range of behaviors that hurt, intimidate, coerce, isolate, control, or humiliate another, most commonly an intimate partner, most frequently a woman

Beneficence

The principle that requires researchers to ensure that participants in research achieve benefits, while at minimal risk.

Bereavement

To be deprived of something valuable, such as in suffering from the loss of a loved one in death.

Binocular microscopy

Use of a device with two eye pieces capable of magnification permitting visualization of otherwise occult or indistinguishable features of tissue or small objects; use of a microscope.

Biological evidence

Evidence derived from such sources as blood and bloodstains; semen and seminal stains; tissues and organs; bones and teeth; hairs and nails; and saliva, urine, and other biological fluids.

Biomechanics

The application of mechanical laws to living structures; the science that assists in understanding the mechanism of injury and the tolerance of the human body.

Blunt force trauma

Injury incurred by the crushing impact of, or when a moving body strikes a blunt object. The principal categories are abrasions, contusions, lacerations, and fractures.

Bondage

The use of physical restraining materials or devices that have sexual significance for the user.

Bore

The interior of a gun barrel forward of the chamber.

Bracketing

Taking a series of photographs with more and less light than the a light meter or in-camera meter is indicating; in other words, take one photograph at the meter reading; then one or more exposures that are underexposed and then overexposed with the intent of assuring that one is optimally or near-optimally exposed.

Brain death

A medically and legally valid declaration of death based on complete and irreversible cessation of brain and brainstem functions.

Breach of duty

An individual's failure to perform an agreed-on act or legal duty owed to another individual. The level of conduct falls below the standard of care required in a particular situation.

Bullet wipe (wipe-off)

The discolored area on the immediate periphery of a bullet hole caused by bullet lubricant, lead, soot, bore debris, or possibly by jacket material.

C

Caliber

When referring to firearms this measurement is the approximate diameter of the circle formed by the tops of the lands of a rifled barrel. When used in association with ammunition, this is a numerical term (use without the decimal point) included in a cartridge name to indicate the nominal bullet diameter.

Cartridge

A single unit of ammunition consisting of the case, primer, and propellant, with one or more projectiles; also applies to a shotshell.

Catapult type injuries

Injuries seen when occupants make contact with the airbag during midstage of its deployment. Injuries are consistent with the head and neck having been driven rapidly upward and rearward. Severe cervical spine hyperextension occurs with energy sufficient to rupture blood vessels and ligaments and to fracture cervical vertebrae.

Causation

A given outcome that is either the direct result of a nurse's negligent action or more probably attributable to the nurse's actions than to any other cause.

Cause of death

The entity that initiated the sequence of events that ended in death, such as a cancer or multiple injuries from a vehicle incident.

Centering

A shift in consciousness that provides the individual access to inner peace and tranquility and a shield from the violent energy patterns of the patient or victim. Centering provides the individual an opportunity to heal oneself and restore balance while moving beyond physical and emotional pain.

Centerfire

Any cartridge that has its primer central to the axis in the head of the case.

Certification

Formal recognition by an agency or professional organization that an individual has attained an advanced level of knowledge and skill.

Chain of custody

Written documentation signifying the link formed between each person who handles a piece of evidence.

Chamber

The rear part of the barrel bore that has been formed to accept a specific cartridge; revolver cylinders are multichambered.

Chemical agents

Poisons that incapacitate, injure, or kill through their toxic effects on the skin, eyes, lungs, blood, nerves, and other organs.

Chemical asphyxia

Lack of oxygen reaching the bloodstream that results from chemicals that prevent inhaled oxygen from reaching cells.

Child pornography

Any visual or print medium depicting sexually explicit conduct involving a child. More simply stated, child pornography is photographs or films of children being sexually molested.

Child sexual abuse

An expression of violence through the use of power and control in a sexual context where there is an age difference or caretaking responsibility between perpetrator and victim.

Choking

Blockage of an internal airway due to aspiration.

Circumstantial evidence

Physical evidence or statements that establish circumstances from which one can infer other facts.

Clinical forensic medicine

The medical specialty that applies the principles and practice of clinical medicine to the elucidation of questions in judicial proceedings for the protection of the individual's legal rights prior to death.

Clinical forensic nurse

A nurse who has the responsibility to evaluate and perform the root cause analyses of adverse patient events within a clinical setting, who has the ability to recognize forensic implications in any given patient care situation and set in motion the appropriate chain of events.

Clinical forensic nursing

The application of clinical nursing to trauma survivors or liability related injuries and to those whose death is pronounced within the clinical environs involving the identification of unrecognized, unidentified injuries and the proper processing of forensic evidence. The forensic nurse clinician further practices in secured environments with institutionalized patients in legal custody related to court-ordered evaluations, examinations, treatments, and rehabilitation issues or routine trauma intervention, which must be forensically documented.

Clitoridectomy

Removal of the clitoris and parts of the labia minora

Club drugs

Synthetic designer drugs or illegally diverted and trafficked therapeutic drugs popularized at nightclubs and parties with the false perception that they do not produce serious, harmful effects.

Close-up and macro lenses

Convenient and necessary for detailed images, these lenses allow the photographer to focus a few inches or centimeters away from the subject. Close-up photography can mean anything from one quarter life-size (1:4 or .2×) to 5× enlargement, depending on the equipment and the available attachments.

CODIS (Combined DNA Index System)

Federal Bureau of Investigation (FBI) program designed to type and catalog biological evidence for DNA typing permitting scientists to identify or eliminate suspects in forensic settings where biological evidence has been recovered; the national DNA data bank system, which allows states to compare their no-suspect profiles to a national DNA repository and solve additional crimes.

Colposcope

An instrument that provides illumination and magnification for the examination of the lower anogenital area of both adults and children. It is a stereoscopic or binocular microscope, similar to a dissecting microscope, with variable features including magnification from 5x through 30x; up to a 150-watt halogen ring-light source for bright illumination; a 300mm objective lens; and 35-mm photographic capabilities.

Colposcopy

Examination of the vagina and cervix by use of an instrument with a magnifying lens system.

Confirmatory analysis

A gas chromatography–mass spectrometry (GC-MS) test used to precisely identify and quantify drugs within the body.

Conjoint team approach

Being implemented by contemporary agencies, this approach to crime scene investigation involves both law enforcement investigators and forensic nurse examiners, specifically in sexual assault, homicide, child abuse, elder abuse, and domestic violence cases.

Consulting witness

A witness who provides knowledge and information upon which an expert may base his or her opinion, but who does not actually testify during the trial.

Contusions or bruises

Injuries that result from leakage of blood from vessels into soft tissues after sufficient force has been applied to distort soft tissue and to tear vessels.

Convicted Offender Index

CODIS data bank consisting of DNA typing of individuals convicted of felony sex crimes and other crimes, depending upon state legislation.

Coroner

An elected official who performs a legal role of death investigator within a given jurisdiction; but who does not necessarily possess medical or death investigation credentials.

Coroner's inquest

The investigation into a suspicious death by an elected or appointed officiator of death which includes a jury of lay persons to determine if the manner of death was suicide, homicide, accidental, or natural.

Correctional care nursing

Integration of the principles of nursing, forensic science, psychiatric health, primary care, and public health knowledge during the care of prisoners and parolees; the title used in England to identify this forensic caregiver is custody nursing; one subspecialty of forensic nursing.

Corpus delicti

A legal term refering to the body of the crime or offense, not the physical body of the decedent.

Criminalist

One who provides analysis of trace and physical evidence in a crime laboratory; this term is not to be confused with criminologist.

Criminal law

Deals with conduct that is offensive or harmful to society as a whole. Legal action is brought against the offender by the state, city, or an administrative body.

Criminologist

One who studies criminal behavior generally at the societal level through the use of large data sets or occasionally at the individual psychosociological level in attempts to explain deviant acts. Criminologists make recommendations concerning crime prevention and control and, although usually considered a part of the discipline of sociology, may be housed within the disciplines of political science, law, or medicine. This term is not to be confused with criminalist.

Crisis management plan

A document that outlines levels of authority and defined roles or responsibilities for identification, management, and resource application related to a crisis.

Critical incident stress

Symptoms that are precipitated by a specific event and might last two to six weeks.

Critical incident stress debriefing (CISD)

A CISD is a structured group process that uses a psychological and educational format with the aim of reducing the impact of the event.

Critical incident stress management (CISM)

The all-inclusive list of services offered by certified teams.

Cryopreservation

A tissue storage and preservation method using extremely cold temperatures.

Curriculum vitae (CV) or résumé

An organized summary of employment and educational history. It should include the nurse's legal name and contact information along with details regarding academic achievements, organizational affiliations, professional presentations, publications, and relevant work experiences.

Customary international law

The minimum standards of human behavior, also known as universal norms, consistently practiced by the majority of civilized nations because of a sense of legal obligation or custom.

Cut

A tissue wound resulting from a sharp object, under pressure, coming into contact with the skin.

Cyclic redundancy checking (CRC)

One of the newest technologies being used to safeguard digital photography as legal evidence. Originally used as a method for tracking errors in data that had been transmitted on a communication link, it is now being used successfully to establish authenticity and ensure integrity of digital images.

D

Damages

A sustained loss such as physical and emotional injury, monetary loss (lost personal property, lost earnings, relevant medical expenses, need to hire others to perform individual's customary duties), pain and suffering, or loss of consortium resulting from the unlawful conduct of another.

Daubert Test

A rule of evidence established with the Daubert and Kumho case (*Kumho Tire Company v. Patrick Carmichael*, 1999), which determined that expert opinions must be based on reliable methodology or analysis and not subjective belief or unsupported speculation.

Death

A permanent cessation of all vital functions: the end of life.

Defendant

The individual, individuals, corporation, governmental agency, or federal or state government against which a lawsuit is filed. In a civil case, the allegations against a defendant may include causes of action for personal injury, loss of money, or an invasion of a protected right. A person who is sued and against whom claims are made and relief or recovery is sought in an action or suit.

Defense wound

A characteristic injury, either blunt or sharp, incurred an attempt to ward off the blows (blunt) or thrusts (sharp) of a weapon by an assailant.

Delusional behavior

Term indicating the presence of a mental disorder (psychosis).

Deponent

The individual witness who answers questions during a deposition.

Deposition

The testimony of a witness taken outside of court where the witness is subject to both direct and cross-examination; usually reduced to writing and taken under oath; a type of pretrial discovery method whereby a party or witness statement concerning the case is taken under oath with all parties and their attorneys present.

Delayed stress response

Onset of stress symptoms occurring 48 hours to several months after an incident. In extreme cases, it may occur up to one to two years later.

Delta V

Sudden change in velocity, which measures the severity of forces in a vehicle crash or impact. Note that this term includes the change in forward velocity plus that of rebound.

Depth of field

A measurement of the zones in front of and beyond the subject of a photograph that are in acceptably sharp focus.

Digital photography

Electronically capturing an image through the use of a filmless camera. Other than the absence of film, the physical features of the digital camera are relatively similar to a film camera.

Direct evidence

An eyewitness account of what happened; statements from witnesses who possess firsthand knowledge of the event in question.

Disaster

Any major human-created or natural event of such severity and magnitude to warrant disaster responses

Disturbance

A physical disruption associated with burial processes.

Diversionary wound

An injury inflicted in the course of an attack in order to promote a response, which will facilitate the exposure of a previously guarded, less exposed, or more vital area of the body.

Domestic stalking

Stalking that occurs when a former boyfriend, girlfriend, family member, or other household member threatens or harasses another member of the household. This definition includes common-law relationships as well as longterm acquaintance relationships.

Double grid search

A linear scene search that involves doubling back on the original search pattern at 90-degree angles to provide multiple coverage of the same area from different points of view. This search pattern is useful when visual or physical obstructions make observations difficult. The double grid search pattern is most useful in small outdoor areas.

Dowry

A gift of money or valuable possessions to the groom's family by the bride's family at the time of marriage, a common practice in many Asian countries.

Drug-facilitated sexual assault

The use of chemical agents such as drugs and alcohol to assist in or procure sexual contact by impairing the victim.

Duty

What a reasonably prudent person would do in the same or similar situation.

E

Elder abuse

Abuse of the elderly by a caretaker, either a relative, friend, or individual upon whom the elderly person is dependent, which is manifested in several ways including physical or sexual abuse, financial abuse or exploitation, neglect, and emotional or psychological abuse.

Empowerment

Instilled confidence and self-worth or authority in an individual, which gives that person the ability to raise his or her level of social functioning within a group.

Epidemiology

Study of the distribution and determinants of health-related states and events in populations with the primary goal of providing critical information for control of health problems.

Erotomania-related stalking

Stalking motivated by an offender-target relationship that is based on the stalker's fixation. This fantasy is commonly expressed in such forms as fusion (the stalker blends his personality into his target's) or erotomania (a fantasy-based idealized romantic love or spiritual union of a person [rather than sexual attraction]). The stalker can also be motivated by religious fantasies or voices directing him to target a particular individual.

Evidence

Data presented to a court or jury to prove or disprove a claim; any item or information that may be submitted and accepted by a competent tribunal for the purpose of determining the truth of any matter it is investigating; may be physical or informational by a witness, records, documents, or exhibits.

Evidence recovery kits

Supply kit containing sufficient qualities of suitable containers (test tubes, bottles, plastic and paper bags, boxes, rubber gloves, rubber bands, tweezers, print and impression recovery materials, and syringes) to recover a variety of substances.

Excited delirium syndrome

A condition manifested by irrational, delusional, and violent behavior in which catecholamine-mediated physiological responses result in sudden death.

Exemplar

A fractional specimen, representative of the whole.

Expert witness

One who is qualified by the court, based on education, experience, employment, publications, or research to render an opinion on certain facts where the knowledge is beyond that of a judge or jury; one who has special knowledge of the subject about which he or she is to testify.

F

Fact witness

A witness testifying to actual events or occurrences observed.

Factitious disorder by proxy

The intentional production or feigning of symptoms in another person who is under the individual's care.

Failure to thrive (FTT)

A diagnostic term used to describe a lack of growth according to expected norms for age and gender (Frank and Drotar, 1994).

Far-field

Factors that are outside a range of influence on burial systems.

Female circumcision (FC)

Surgical removal of the labia minora.

Female genital mutilation (FGM)

One of several procedures designed to alter the sexual responses of women by altering their anatomical structures:

Type I: May include removal of the prepuce or hood of the clitoris and partial or total removal of the clitoris.

Type II: May be known as excision and includes removal of clitoris and labia minora. The vagina is typically not covered but copious scar tissue and adhesions may obliterate the vaginal introitus over time.

Type III: Also known as infibulation or pharaonic circumcision, it includes removal of the clitoris, labia minora, and part of the labia majora.

Type IV: An unclassified grouping of all other mutilations of the female genital area such as pricking, piercing, cutting, and scraping of vaginal tissue, incisions to the clitoris and vagina, and burning, scarring, or cauterizing of tissue.

Financial abuse or exploitation

The misuse of another individual's funds or assets without his or her knowledge or consent, for perpetrator's benefit.

First responders

Skilled personnel who respond to medical emergencies outside a hospital setting; includes emergency medical technicians (EMTs), paramedics, and members of rescue squads and search-and-rescue teams

Fluorescent photography

A technique that is often used to bring out bodily fluid stains on clothing, bedding, or other material. *Fluorescent* refers to luminescence caused by the absorption of radiation at one wavelength followed nearly immediately by reradiation usually at a different wavelength, which ceases almost at once when the incident radiation stops. Various light sources and filters are used.

Focal length

The distance measured from the optical center of a lens to the film plane; it determines the reproduction ratio and thus the field that you see through the lens

Forensic

Pertaining to courts of justice, it commonly refers to the application of science to the resolution of legal issues, for example, forensic pathology, forensic chemistry, forensic medicine, forensic botany, or forensic engineering.

Forensic anthropology

The analysis and identification of human remains for criminal and legal investigation.

Forensic archaeologist

Application of archaeological recovery techniques to death scene exhumations.

Forensic botanist

One who utilizes training in taxonomy, morphology, plant anatomy, and plant ecology to identify plant evidence for the purpose of placing a suspect at the crime scene or determining the time of death.

Forensic cases

Any case that potentially involves criminal or civil liability or other legal implications.

Forensic clinical nurse specialist

An individual specifically educated at the graduate level (master of science in nursing) in a clinical nurse specialist program in forensic nursing at a regionally accredited institution of higher learning offering such a degree.

Forensic entomologist

One who analyzes insects and other invertebrates in determining manner of death, movement of a cadaver from one site to another, and length of the postmortem interval.

Forensic Index

CODIS data bank consisting of DNA typing of individuals derived from lawfully collected specimens obtained during the course of a criminal investigation; contains DNA records from cases without a suspect.

Forensic medicine

Application of medical knowledge and skills to questions of law and/or patient treatment involving court related issues.

Forensic nurse (FN)

A registered nurse qualified by education and experience in the evaluation and investigation of trauma, injury, or death involving individuals in need of medicolegal intervention and court-ordered evaluations.

Forensic nurse death investigator (FNDI)

A licensed nurse who carries out the duties of a death investigator in accordance with the performance standards and procedures established under the medical examiner or coroner's system of death investigation and the jurisdictional standards of practice; one subspecialty of forensic nursing.

Forensic nurse examiner (FNE)

The forensic nurse who provides a medicolegal examination, whether physical, psychological, or sexual, for the documentation and recovery of trace and physical evidence, whether the patient is living or dead. Those who review and investigate or examine medical records and other documents of record and those who examine a crime seen may also be referred to as FNEs. Forensic nurses who fill other roles would be referred to as consultants, educators, scientists, attorneys, or related terms associated with their field of expertise. This term parallels the forensic medical examiner (FME) of a multitude of countries who provide forensic services.

Forensic nurse practitioner

A master's prepared registered nurse specifically skilled in a nurse practitioner program with a specialty focus on forensic nursing as an advanced practice at a regionally accredited institute of higher learning offering such a program.

Forensic nursing

The application of nursing to the law; the forensic aspects of healthcare combined with the bio/psycho/social/spiritual education of the registered nurse in the scientific investigation and treatment of trauma or death of victims and perpetrators of violence, criminal activity, and traumatic accidents. The forensic nurse provides direct services to individuals; consultation services to nursing, medical, and law-related agencies; and expert court testimony in areas dealing with questioned death investigative processes, adequacy of services delivered, and specialized diagnoses of specific conditions as related to nursing.

Forensic nursing science

A body of diverse and collective scientific knowledge, drawn from the application of the forensic sciences to the nursing process in public or legal proceedings; the forensic aspects of healthcare involving the physiological, psychological, and behavioral sciences relevant to the scientific investigation of trauma and death or related medicolegal issues.

Forensic odontology

The branch of dentistry that deals with the collection, evaluation, and proper handling of dental evidence to provide assistance to law enforcement and civil and criminal judicial proceedings; applying knowledge of development, structure, and function of the teeth to the identification or age of individuals.

Forensic pathologist

Pathologists who are specially trained to recognize, interpret, and document features of injury and disease in the human body.

Forensic pathology

One subspecialty of forensic medicine involving the scientific investigation of death charged with the responsibility of determining the cause and manner of questioned deaths.

Forensic physical anthropologist

A discipline that identifies and interprets remains such as skeletal or body elements.

Forensic processing center

A collection area organized to process a large number of bodies and body parts to aid in victim identification.

Forensic role behaviors

Enactment of differentiated performance or action relevant to a specific position providing an in-depth clinical focus in the investigation of trauma, death, or related medicolegal issues.

Forensic science

The application of science to the just resolution of legal issues.

Forensic toxicologist

Applying the science of the nature of poisons, their effects, and detection to legal cases.

Forensic toxicology

Investigation of drugs and poisons practiced within a legal domain for the purpose of upholding the law.

Forensicare

The trademarked name of a forensic facility that provides care to forensic patients in custody.

Fouling

A dustlike residue of burned gunpowder (soot) that is deposited when the muzzle of a weapon is within a few inches of the target; also refers to the residual deposits remaining in the bore of the firearm after firing.

Fracture

Discontinuity, break, or rupture of bone caused by blunt trauma; can be direct or indirect.

Fraud

Falsely representing a fact or concealment of information that should have been disclosed.

Frye Rule

A term derived from the case of *United States v. Frye*, 293 F. 1013 (1923). It established in the rules of evidence that results of scientific tests or procedures are admissible as evidence only when the tests or procedures have gained general acceptance in the particular field to which they belong.

G

Genocide

Any of the several acts committed with intent to destroy, in whole or in part, a national, ethnic, racial, or religious group

Good faith

Honest belief, without malice or design to defraud or seek an unconscionable advantage.

Graze

A wide area of abrasion.

Grid search

Involves searching in linear patterns and is suited to small outdoor crime scenes that do not involve obstructions (such as underbrush) that may pose physical and/or visual obstructions.

H

Health

A state of complete physical, mental, and social well-being and not merely absence of disease or infirmity.

Hearsay rule

A statement other than one made by the declarant while testifying at the trial or hearing, offered in evidence to prove the truth of the matter asserted (Uniform Rules of Evidence, Rule 801). This means that a witness is not permitted to provide testimony about something that someone else has told her or him.

Hematoma

A localized mass of blood that is relatively or completely confined within an organ, tissue, space, or potential space, and which is usually or partly clotted.

High-altitude pulmonary edema

A form of respiratory compromise that occurs in vulnerable individuals who are not acclimated, but quickly immersed in altitudes exceeding 2000 meters.

Holistic forensic nursing care

Nursing care for the body, mind, spirit, and legal aspects of total patient care.

Human bite

The prototypical human bite is generally ovoid or circular and consists of two opposing U-shaped patterns separated at their bases by open space. Frequently there is a central area of ecchymosis or contusion between the opposing arches.

Hysteresis

The variable effects of a given drug based on the elapsed time since it entered the body.

I

Immunoassay

An antibody-based test that provides presumptive screening data based on competitive binding reactions between antidrug antibodies and either labeled or unlabeled drug.

Incision

A soft-tissue wound created by a sharp object or instrument; characterized by a defect that is longer than it is deep and has clean-cut edges.

Independent medical examination (IME)

An evaluation of the plaintiff or claimant conducted at the request of the defendant's insurance company and performed by an individual (e.g., physician, dentist, psychologist, therapist) not involved in the care of the plaintiff.

Infibulation

(1) See Type III FGM (above); (2) the passing of needles or pins through the body, most often through the scrotum, penis, or nipples, but sometimes through an earlobe or the nose.

Informed consent

Permission given for a procedure after full disclosure of all aspects of the procedure, including risks, benefits, complications, and consequences.

International Association of Forensic Nurses (IAFN)

A professional organization of registered nurses working in the medicolegal nursing arena whose purpose is to develop, promote, and disseminate information about the science of forensic nursing.

International law

The body of rules and principles governing, controlling, or affecting the dealings of nations with each other as based on the customs and usages of civilized nations, treaties, statutes, and judicial decisions of international tribunals.

Internship

A course of supervised learning experiences outside the classroom, designed to achieve specific learning objectives over a predetermined period of time.

Investigative profiler

A forensic specialist who develops profiles of perpetrators based on evidence, situation reconstruction, and hypothetical constructs using experience and data collected from multiple cases.

Ionizing radiation

Any radiation, as either particles or electromagnetic energy, that has sufficient energy to produce ions in matter.

J

JCAHO standards

Regulatory guidance derived from the Joint Commission on Accreditation of Healthcare Organizations; specifically, guidelines for identification and management of victims of abuse and neglect.

JPEG format

Abbreviated from the Joint Photographic Experts Group, who created a standard for compressing digital images made available in 1991. Digital files (images) are compressed to a fraction of their original size by a lossy compression method; quality is lowered, but images can be uploaded at a faster rate.

Justice

Principle based on society's need to protect people's dignity and rights; the administration of law; act of determining rights and assigning reward or punishment within the judicial system.

K

Knowing

Ways of knowing that range from the empirical to the intuitive, which define the nurse's ability to accept and understand situations that affect patients' behavior.

L

Laceration

A defect in soft tissues resulting from blunt forces (tear, rip, crush, overstretch, bend, or shear).

Legal nurse consultant (LNC)

A registered nurse who uses clinical knowledge and expertise in any context where law and medicine overlap; one subspecialty of forensic nursing.

Legal sanity

A person's ability to know right from wrong with reference to the act charged; the capacity to know the nature and quality of the act charged, and the capacity to form the intent to commit the crime.

LEMFOS

Title of the Turkish Institute of Legal Medicine and Forensic Sciences in Istanbul, Turkey.

Lividity

Discoloration of tissue due to settling or hypostasis of the blood after death. Blood remains in the vessels.

Living forensic patients

A patient base distinct from deceased individuals who are subject to forensic investigations: survivors of rape, drug and alcohol addiction, domestic violence (including spousal, child, and elder abuse), nonfatal assaults, automobile and pedestrian accidents, suicide attempts, work-related injuries, disputed paternity, incest, medical malpractice, police and corrections custody abuse, drug and food tampering, the incarcerated and institutionalized mentally ill offender.

Living forensics

A recently contrived term referring to clinical forensic practice; that component of the forensic sciences addressing the application of science to the just resolution of legal issues in cases involving living persons, as opposed to forensic pathology, which focuses on the deceased; clinical forensic practice that focuses on the civil and criminal investigation of traumatic injury or patient treatment with legal-related issues. It encompasses both victims and perpetrators who survive.

Livor mortis

Early postmortem change caused by the pooling of blood in the dependent extremities; discoloration of dependent tissue surfaces due to the settling or hypostasis of blood post-death; the bluish-red discoloration of the dependent portion of the external surface of the body resulting from postmortem stasis of blood.

Locard's Principle

A tenet that states that when a person or object comes in contact with another person or object, there exists a possibility that an exchange of materials (a cross-transfer of evidence) will take place.

Lossless compression method

A data compression technique in which no data is lost. For most types of data, lossless compression techniques can reduce the space needed by approximately 50%; method used when compressing data and programs.

Lossy compression method

A method used to gain more compression of data or programs; the final image is not the pixel-by-pixel equivalent of the original. A method of storage used for graphics, audio, and video.

Lyophilization

A tissue storage and preservation method using a freeze-drying technique.

M

Malpractice

Misconduct or the improper discharge of duty by a professional that results in harm to another person; failure to meet the standard of care expected of a reasonably prudent person in a similar situation.

Manner of death

The fashion of circumstances in which the cause of death arose, and whether it was natural, accidental, homicidal, suicidal, or undetermined.

Mass graves

Locations where three or more victims of extrajudicial, summary, or arbitrary executions are buried.

Medical examiner

A forensic pathologist who is appointed or hired to determine the cause and manner of death, and who possesses medical knowledge and skills associated with a medical degree and license to practice.

Medicolegal or legal medicine

Areas of common interest to medicine and law, where medical knowledge is applied to the administration of justice.

Mental defect

Developmental disability or some physiologic condition affecting cognition, such as head injury, meningitis, brain tumor, or dementia.

Mentor

A senior professional who provides information, advice, and emotional support to a junior member or protégé; the mentor has advanced job-related knowledge and experience and may possess some power in an organization based on his or her ability to help others succeed.

Mentoring

A two-party relationship designed to assist a junior member in a work environment or other organization to achieve upward mobility in her or his career.

Mitochondrial DNA typing

An important new forensic tool involving PCR amplification followed by direct sequencing of the DNA. The mitochondrial genome contains 16,569 bp of circular DNA. Mitochondrial DNA exists outside the nucleus and is present in multiple copies per cell.

Munchausen syndrome by proxy (MSBP)

A highly documented variant of factitious disorder in which a parent or other caretaker fabricates or induces illness in a dependent, especially a child.

N

National DNA Index System (NDIS)

The single, central repository of DNA records submitted by all participating states to the Federal Bureau of Investigation (FBI).

Near-field

Factors that interfere with burial systems.

Necropsy

The evisceration and dissection of the dead; an examination of the dead; looking at the dead.

Necropsy pathology

The study of disease derived from studies of the dead.

NecroSearch

A project method used to search for clandestine graves using various technologies and disciplines pertinent to forensic science.

Neglect

The failure to fulfill a caretaking obligation to provide goods or services; typically involves acts of omission rather than commission and may or may not be intentional.

Negligence

Failure to exercise the appropriate degree of care that a prudent person would exercise under the same or similar circumstances; conduct that falls below the standard established by law for the protection of others against unreasonable risk of harm.

Newton's First Law of Motion

States that a body that is at rest tends to remain at rest, while a body that is in motion tends to remain in motion, unless it is acted upon by an unbalanced external force. This describes inertia.

Newton's Second Law of Motion

States that the acceleration of any body is directly proportional to the force acting on the body, while it is inversely proportional to the mass or weight of the body.

Newton's Third Law of Motion

States that for every force exerted on a body by another body, there is an equal but opposite force reacting on the first body by the second.

Nondelusional behavior

While reflecting a gross disturbance in a particular relationship, this term does not necessarily indicate a detachment from reality.

Nuisance stalker

One who targets an individual and interacts with that target through hang-up, obscene, or harassing telephone calls, unsigned letters, and other anonymous communications or continuous physical appearances at the target's residence, place of employment, shopping mall, or school campus. The stalker is often unknown to the target.

Nurse entrepreneur

A nurse who establishes and maintains a successful business and also makes quality nursing care and nursing services available to the public.

O

Older American Act (OAA)

An act providing grants to support state elder abuse prevention activities provided by state units on aging (SUA).

Ombudsman, forensic

A practitioner prepared in the discipline of nursing, gerontology, or social work who has jurisdiction to investigate complaints relative to poor resident care or violations of a patient's rights.

Orientation shots

Initial photographs that include the person's face and the wound or wounds prior to taking close-up photos of individual injuries; also refers to the initial photographs of the geographical location when forensic nurse examiners find themselves outside the clinical area, in a patient's home, or at a crime scene.

P

Pavulon

A nondepolarizing neuromuscular blocking agent used primarily for inducing a temporary paralysis of the muscles of respiration to facilitate endotracheal intubation.

Perceived importance

The product or effect of insight, intuition, or knowledge (through education and experience) regarding the value or significance applied to a personal judgment or evaluation of medicolegal behaviors in the treatment of forensic patients.

Performed frequency

Actions taken in accordance with the requirements of medical, legal, and forensic standards involving the number of times a specified event occurs in current nursing practice working with forensic patients.

Pharmacokinetics

The science of drug absorption, distribution, metabolism, and excretion used to determine the efficacy of drug action and the intensity and duration of effects within the body.

Pharmacological effects

The result of the drug's interactions with selected receptor sites within the body.

Physical abuse

The infliction of nonaccidental physical harm or injury through the use of excessive and inappropriate physical force. It may take the form of hitting, slapping, pushing, pinching, punching, burning, or sexual abuse.

Physical barriers

Barriers (e.g., crime scene/police line tape installed waist high where practical, guarded by uniformed official security personnel) used to secure the scene until the scene has been examined and cleared for release to the appropriate owner or tenant.

Physical evidence

Any matter, material, or condition that may be used to determine facts in a given situation.

Physical violence

Behavior that inflicts harm and includes threats and attempts to harm another individual; often found in cases of sexual violence and partners' violence

PLISSIT model

A theoretical framework for healthcare professionals to deal with sensitive issues including sexual assault and sexual abuse. This model provides specific guidelines designed to decrease inadequate feelings regarding asking questions.

Plaintiff

The individual or party initiating a civil lawsuit seeking damages.

Point and shoot (P&S) cameras

A camera system in which the viewfinder is placed near the lens so that the photographer's view and the camera's view are similar but not exactly the same. The difference between what you see through the viewfinder and what the lens sees and captures on film or digital sensor is referred to as parallax.

Police surgeon

A physician (generally a family doctor, but may be a specialist) hired by a police department to examine and treat detained persons and/or those in custody; a forensic medical examiner (FME).

Polymerase chain reaction

DNA typing method whereby small segments of DNA are amplified (duplicated); has been called molecular photocopying.

Population file

CODIS data bank of DNA types and allele frequency data from anonymous persons intended to represent major population groups found in the United States. These databases are used to estimate statistical frequencies of DNA profiles.

Postexercise peril

A time interval after exercise when an individual is subject to fatal cardiac arrhythmia.

Postmortem interval

The amount of time between death and the finding or initial examination of the remains.

Postmortem toxicology

Investigation of drugs and poisons in circumstances of death.

Post-traumatic rape syndrome

A syndrome characterized by physical, emotional, cognitive, behavioral, and interpersonal traumas experienced by victims who have been raped.

Post-traumatic stress disorder (PTSD)

A disorder recognized and defined by the American Psychiatric Association as a diagnosis in the *Diagnostic and Statistical Manual III*. Development of characteristic symptoms following a psychologically distressing event that is outside the range of usual human experience due to the victim's experiencing intense fear, terror, horror, and helplessness at the time of the crisis.

Postvention

Appropriate and helpful acts after the tragedy that can render immediate and on-the-scene crisis intervention.

Practicum

An internship or other clinical experience under the supervision of a specialist.

Preceptorship

A student-teacher relationship structured to achieve specific learning objectives for a portion or complete course of study in a discipline.

Presencing

The "being there" of a nurse, which reaches beyond the physical presence and develops an environment of caring, healing, and security.

Pressure pallor

A pale area of the body surface in which vessels are flattened by pressure and cannot develop. The discoloration is due to the settling of blood associated with postmortem lividity.

Primary prevention

Preventing the health problem from occurring through avoidance of risks to health or by preventing disease by prophylaxis (e.g. abstinence of tobacco use, vaccinating children). Also called pure prevention.

Primer

The ignition component of a cartridge.

Probate

Judicial proceedings to determine the validity of a purported last will.

Protective factors for suicide

Factors that make it less likely that an individual will engage in suicidal behavior; protective factors may encompass biological, psychological, or social factors in the individual, family, or environment.

Psychiatric forensic nurses

Professional registered nurses who assess perpetrators on issues of mental status, competency, legal sanity, and dangerousness; one subspecialty of forensic nursing.

Psychological abuse

Behaviors that are cruel, degrading, terrorizing, isolating, rejecting, demeaning, humiliating; intimidating verbal abuse.

Psychological personality profiling

A technique based on the rationale that behavior reflects personality and by examining behavior the investigator may be able to determine what type of person is most likely to have committed a crime by focusing on certain behavioral and personality characteristics; does not identify the perpetrator.

Punch-out wounds

Wounds incurred during the initial phase of air bag deployment. They include atlanto-occipital dislocations, cervical spine fractures, and brain stem resection; cardiac, hepatic, and splenic lacerations; diffuse axonal injuries; subdural and epidural hematomas; and decapitation.

Purdah

Seclusion of women from public observation; a restriction placed on married women who are kept within their homes, separated from society, particularly from male friends or relatives; practiced among Muslims or Hindus in India.

Q

Quality assurance

Planned internal process for the systematic monitoring, assessment, and improvement of the quality of a product (e.g., patient care).

R

Rape

An act of violence; nonconsensual sexual aggression involving the penetration of a body orifice; nonconsensual penile-vaginal or anal penetration.

Rape trauma syndrome (RTS)

A two-stage syndrome of response to a sexual assault; a specific type of PTSD pertaining solely to consequences of trauma related to sexual assault or childhood sexual abuse; not gender specific; also called post-rape trauma syndrome.

Raw

A type of digital image file that, unlike TIFF or JPEG, is not an acronym. It is "raw" in the sense of being unprocessed. The main advantage is that the image that originally came off the sensor can be processed later with special software.

Real evidence

A physical, tangible object that may prove or disprove a statement in question; such evidence may be direct or circumstantial

Reflective UV photodocumentation

A technique that produces an image that is otherwise not seen nor photographed by conventional techniques; records the reflection and absorption of long-wave UV light by the subject matter, excluding exposure of the film from all other visible light.

Reinfibulation

Resuturing the introitus to regain the perceived benefits of infibulation.

Relatives of Missing Persons Index

CODIS data bank of DNA typing from missing persons and their close relatives; used to identify individuals or body parts and relate them to a known group.

Remand center

A detention center for individuals in police custody who are awaiting trial. Many individuals in custody are also being examined physically and mentally to establish their capability to stand trial.

Rigor mortis

A postmortem change that presents as muscle rigidity; the stiffening of the body after death that is produced by chemical reactions within the muscle.

Rimfire

A flange-headed cartridge containing the priming mixture inside the rim cavity (compare to *centerfire*).

Risk factors for suicide

Those factors that make it more likely that individuals will engage in suicidal behavior; may encompass biological, psychological, or social factors in the individual, family, or environment.

Root cause analysis (RCA)

A process for identifying the basic or contributing causal factors that underlie variations in performance associated with adverse events or close calls.

S

Safety planning

Realistic planning for discharge and safety of the patient who will return home.

SANE-A

Credentials used by sexual assault nurse examiners who have passed the International Association of Forensic Nurses' national certification examination for adults and adolescents.

Scene documentation supplies and equipment

Items such as clipboards, paper, pencils and pens, measuring devices (small inch/metric rulers for photographic documentation and 100-foot tape measures for scene measurement), flags and other markers for outdoor scene identification, photographic equipment (35-mm camera, photoflash capability, and film), and adequate portable lighting.

Scene security supplies and equipment

Items such as physical barriers (saw horses, crime scene barrier tape) and rain protection devices (large plastic containers, waterproof tarpaulins) in the event footprints or tire tracks must be protected from inclement weather.

Scratch

A superficial abrasion that is long and narrow.

Secondary prevention

Involves prompt detection and successful management or treatment of the health condition to avoid actual damage to the person's health; early detection and treatment to prevent further damage to a body part or system.

Self-harm

A direct, deliberate, and often repetitive destruction or alteration of one's own body tissue without conscious suicidal intent; other terms include self-mutilation, self-injury, auto-aggression, and parasuicide.

Self-neglect

The neglect of personal well-being and home environment.

Sentinel event

An unexpected occurrence involving death or serious physical or psychological injury, or the risk thereof.

Sex ring crime

A term describing sexual victimization in which there are one or more adult offenders and several children who are aware of each other's participation.

Sexual assault

Sexually explicit conduct used as an expression of interpersonal violence against another individual; nonconsenting sexual acts achieved through the use of power and control.

Sexual assault nurse examiner (SANE)

A registered nurse (RN) who has advanced education in forensic examination of sexual assault victims.

Sexual assault response team (SART)

The group of professionals who work together to facilitate the survivor's recovery and the investigation and prosecution of the assailant by providing information, support, and crisis intervention, gathering evidence, and facilitating the movement of the sexual assault survivor through the legal system. SART members also work together or individually to improve the response to victims within their own disciplines and to educate the community they serve.

Sexual homicide

A death resulting from one person killing another in the context of power, control, sexuality, and aggressive brutality.

Sexually explicit conduct

Describes sexual intercourse, bestiality, masturbation, sadomasochistic abuse, and lewd exhibition of the genitals or pubic area.

Shaken baby syndrome

Intracranial injuries that are produced by acceleration-deceleration forces associated with vigorous shaking; may or may not involve blunt trauma to the head; also called shaken impact syndrome or whiplash shaken baby syndrome.

Short tandem repeats (STRs)

Method of DNA typing whereby multiple short tandem repeats (STRs) in a single reaction are studied by several fluorescent detection methods. Different STR types exhibit variation in the number of repeated core elements they contain and have tremendous discriminating power.

Shutter speed

The time that the shutter is actually open, which can vary from 1/8000 of a second or less, to slower, timed exposures of 30 seconds or more.

Single lens reflex camera (SLR)

A camera system that allows the photographer to look through the viewfinder to see exactly what will be reproduced on the film. It has a "what-you-see-is-what-you-get" viewing system. This is accomplished through an arrangement of internal mirrors similar to those on a submarine's periscope.

Smothering

Asphyxia due to obstruction of external airways.

Solo child sex rings

Sex ring crime characterized by the involvement of multiple children in sexual activities with one adult, usually male, who recruits the victims into his illicit behavior by legitimate means.

Spiral search

A crime search technique that begins from the "center" of the crime scene (where the principal item of evidence is, such as a dead body, where a reported assault reportedly took place, or where the majority of the physical evidence is located) and extends to the periphery (outside limits) of the scene.

Spree murder

Killings occurring at two or more locations and with no emotional cooling-off time between them.

Stab

A soft-tissue injury resulting from a relatively pointed and/or sharp object forced inward by a thrustlike force or by the forces created when an individual falls onto something with enough force for the object to pass through the tissue creating impalement. A stab wound is usually, but not always, deeper than it is long.

Standard of care

An authoritative statement of behavior expected of a reasonably prudent person developed by the profession so that the quality of the individual's practice, service, or education can be judged; a degree of care, expertise, and judgment exercised by a reasonable and prudent nurse under the same or similar circumstances.

Stewardship

Responsibility of overseeing or caretaking.

Stippling (tattooing)

Small abrasions and minute hemorrhages created when particles of unburnt or partially burnt gunpowder strike the skin. Such wounds are commonly consistent with a range of fire of about 24 to 30 inches but can be as great as 4 feet. The term may be interchanged with tattooing at times to simplify the evidence documentation; however, a distinction between the two is clarified as: tattooing is the indriving of gunpowder particles when a weapon was relatively near, and stippling is when a weapon was sufficiently far away that particles could no longer be driven into the skin.

Strangulation

Asphyxia due to hanging, ligature, or manual strangulation (throttling) that obstructs the main airways and/or blood vessels supplying the brain, impairing delivery of oxygen.

Stress

The nonspecific physiologic or psychological response of the body to any prolonged demand made upon it.

Strip search

(1) Involves searching the scene in long lines, most useful when the scene is long and narrow, as may be seen in roadway or roadside scenes; (2) the examination of an individual in custody involving the removal and examination of all clothing as well as the body for the identification and seizure of contraband.

Subpoena

An official notification or court order to appear in court for the purposes of participating in legal proceedings, usually to provide testimony or to provide specific evidence associated with a trial; also the act of delivering this notification.

Sudden traumatic death

Death that is usually violent in nature or the result of interpersonal violence or crime. This type of death is painful for the survivors (the family members and friends who are experiencing the associated loss).

Suffocation

Hypoxia or anoxia caused by the obstruction of the upper airways.

Suicide attempt

A suicidal act with a nonfatal outcome. Other terms that are sometimes used interchangeably include attempted suicide, act of deliberate self-harm, and parasuicide. Many researchers and clinicians avoid the term *attempted suicide* as it has negative connotations suggesting that such act is a failed (unsuccessful) suicide, although it may be the case.

Suicidology

The scientific study of suicide and suicide prevention.

Sunna

Removal of female prepuce.

Survivors by extension

The families and friends left behind in the wake of catastrophic death.

Suspiciousness factor

An intuitive sense of heightened alertness based on knowledge and experience that compels a nurse to action in response to a given circumstance or series of events.

Symbolic interaction

A sociological theory essentially contending that social reality is made up of shared verbal and nonverbal symbols that interacting individuals understand in more or less the same way through their interaction with significant others.

Syndicated child sex ring

A well-structured organization that involves the recruitment of children, the production of pornography, the delivery of sexual services, and the establishment of an extensive network of customers.

T

Tanner staging

A system of grouping periods of sexual development based on anatomical changes.

Taphonomy

The study of decomposition and dispersion of human remains after death.

Tardieu spots

Ecchymotic spots found in the dependent extremities secondary to vascular congestion and/or hypoxia.

Telephoto lense

A lense greater than the standard focal length for a particular size of camera. These lenses behave in much the same way as a telescope.

Tertiary prevention

Seeks to limit the impairment, increase the quality of life, and prolong life, for example, by providing emergency care for victims of automobile collisions or rehabilitative services to help maximize activity and independence after a stroke or heart attack.

Thanatology

The study of death.

Thermal imaging

Technique of using infrared cameras that generate an image based on objects that emit infrared radiation depending on temperature and characteristics of their surfaces.

Three-dimensional bite

A bite having all the components of the two-dimensional bite plus depth of penetration.

TIFF format

Tagged image format file; a lossless compression method where data is compressed but not lost. Describes and stores image data that comes from scanners and paint- and photo-retouching programs in order to be imported into desktop publishing programs.

Toluidine blue dye (TBD)

An aqueous blue dye used as a nuclear stain, which adheres to abraded skin and microlacerations; used to mark denuded tissue.

Tort

An act that occurs as a result of a careless or deliberate act producing harm or loss to another person or their property; unintentional violation of another person's rights.

Transcultural nursing theory

A theory that reflects the global relationship between cultural diversity, interpersonal intervention, and social issues for the individual, family, community, nurse, and environment in a culturally competent and appropriate care unique to that specific patient population.

Transitional child sex ring

Sex ring crime involving multiple offenders as well as multiple victims; the offenders are known to each other and collect and share victims.

Traumagram

Diagram used to annotate locations and types of injury on surfaces, anatomical parts, or within the human body cavities.

Treaty

A formal written agreement between two or more countries' governments intended to be legally binding in an international forum or at least be enforced via national law enforcement mechanisms.

Two-dimensional bite

A bite having width and breadth but no penetration of the epidermis.

U

Unidentifed Persons Index

CODIS data bank of DNA typing of individuals with uncertain identities.

V

Victim

Legal terminology that describes a person against whom a crime has been committed.

Victims' Index

CODIS data bank of DNA typing from victims, living or dead, from whom DNA may have been carried away by perpetrators.

Violence

The intentional use of physical force or power, threatened or actual, against oneself, another person, or a group or community, that results in or has a high likelihood of resulting in injury, death, psychological harm, maldevelopment, or deprivation.

Violence Against Women Act of 1994

An act of the U.S. Congress expressing the need for research addressing interpersonal violence. This is the first national act that addresses restructuring the philosophy, assessment, and prosecution of perpetrators while providing some privacy to the victim's lives.

VNTRs

The most common type of genetic variation studied in forensic DNA analysis whereby length differences produced by variable number of tandem repeats (VNTRs) are studied.

Vulnerable subjects

Populations whose participation in research brings elevated risks due to life circumstances. These include children, prisoners, pregnant women, mentally disabled persons, and economically or educationally disadvantaged persons.

W

Wheel search

Advanced as a supplementary search in outdoor areas; however, it is not particularly effective due to the ever-increasing space between search lines.

Wide-angle lense

A lense that is less than the standard size, allowing a wider than normal field of view.

Witness

Generally, a person who describes under oath (testifies) what she has seen, heard or otherwise observed, or, one who testifies to specific knowledge on issues relevant to the case.

Worker's compensation

Federal and state insurance programs enacted to provide benefits for employees injured while engaged in the performance of their duties.

Workplace violence

A wide range of behaviors occurring at a place of employment, including verbal abuse or threats, sexual and physical assault, hostage situations, homicide, kidnapping, armed robbery, arson, theft, vandalism, and bomb threats, that threaten or undermine the safety and security of coworkers in the environment.

Worksite analysis

A study of conditions within or surrounding an employment environment designed to determine whether conditions are conducive or contributory to acts of violence that would endanger employees and others in the workplace.

Z

Zone search

Used generally for indoor crime scenes; usually, specific zones are identified within a crime scene and then individually searched.

Zoom lense

A lense that has variable focal lengths and can be used to adjust the framing of an image (whereas perspective is controlled by the position of the lens and the camera).

Photo Credits

Illustrations borrowed from other sources are credited in the appropriate figure legend, except in the color insert. The authors would like to thank the following people for their illustrations:

Patrick E. Besant-Matthews for color plates 1-11, 13-18, 37-54, 65-66, 70, 79-81, 84-96
Virginia Lynch for color plates 12, 19-30, 69, 82-83
Dr. Michael J. Doberson for color plates 31-36
Dr. M. G. F. Gilliland for color plates 55-60
William S. Smock for color plates 61-64, 67
Kathy Bell for color plate 68
Judith Cook for color plates 71-72
Teresa M. Roe for color plates 73-78

Index

B

G

N

O

Scope and Standards of Forensic Nursing Practice

Used with permission of the International Association of Forensic Nurses

Standards of Care

Standard I. Assessment
The forensic nurse shall provide an accurate assessment, based upon data collected, of the physical and/or psychological issues of the client as related to forensic nursing and/or forensic pathology.

Standard II. Diagnosis
The forensic nurse shall analyze the assessment data to determine a diagnosis pertaining to forensic issues in nursing.

Standard III. Outcome Identification
The forensic nurse will identify expected individual outcomes based on the forensic diagnoses of the client.

Standard IV. Planning
The forensic nurse develops a comprehensive plan of action for the forensic client appropriate to forensic interventions to attain expected outcomes.

Standard V. Implementation
The forensic nurse implements a plan of action based on forensic issues derived from assessment data, nursing diagnoses, and medical diagnoses, when applicable, and scientific knowledge.

Standard VI. Evaluation
The forensic nurse evaluates and modifies the plan of action to achieve expected outcomes.

Standards of Professional Performance

Standard I. Quality of Care
The forensic nurse systematically evaluates the quality and effectiveness of forensic nursing practice.

Standard II. Performance Appraisal
The forensic nurse evaluates his/her own forensic nursing practice in relation to professional practice standards and relevant statutes and regulations.

Standard III. Education
The forensic nurse acquires and maintains current knowledge in forensic nursing practice.

Standard IV. Collegiality
The forensic nurse contributes to the professional development of peers, colleagues and others.

Standard V. Ethics
The forensic nurse's decisions and actions are determined in an ethical manner.

Standard VI. Collaboration
The forensic nurse collaborates with the forensic client, family members, significant others and multidisciplinary team members.

Standard VII. Research
The forensic nurse recognizes, values and utilizes research as a method for further forensic nursing practice.

Standard VIII. Resource Utilization
The forensic nurse considers factors related to safety, effectiveness, and cost in planning and delivering forensic services.

To obtain the complete Scope and Standards of Forensic Nursing Practice, please contact the International Association of Forensic Nurses at 856-256-2425.